Nancy Welling
CRNA

Evidence-Based Practice
of Anesthesiology

Evidence-Based Practice of Anesthesiology

Second Edition

Lee A. Fleisher, MD

Robert Dunning Dripps Professor and Chair
Department of Anesthesiology
Professor of Medicine
University of Pennsylvania School of Medicine
Philadelphia, Pennsylvania

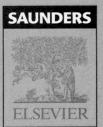
SAUNDERS

ELSEVIER

SAUNDERS
ELSEVIER

1600 John F. Kennedy Blvd.
Ste 1800
Philadelphia, PA 19103-2899

EVIDENCE-BASED PRACTICE OF ANESTHESIOLOGY, 2ND EDITION

ISBN: 978-1-4160-5996-7

Library of Congress Cataloging-in-Publication Data
Evidence-based practice of anesthesiology / [edited by] Lee A. Fleisher.
-- 2nd ed.
        p. ; cm.
Includes bibliographical references.
ISBN 978-1-4160-5996-7
1. Anesthesiology. 2. Evidence-based medicine. I. Fleisher, Lee A.
[DNLM: 1. Anesthesia. 2. Evidence-Based Medicine. WO 200 E928 2009]
RD81. E86 2009
617.9'6--de22

2008043224

Acquisitions Editor: Natasha Andjelkovic
Developmental Editor: Isabel Trudeau
Project Manager: Bryan Hayward
Design Direction: Karen O'Keefe Owens

Printed in the United States of America

Last digit is the print number: 9 8 7 6 5 4 3 2 1

Dedication

This book is dedicated to my children, Matthew and Jessica, for their unconditional love and support, as well as their constant desire to understand the justification of their parents' decisions (asking for the evidence). In addition, the book is dedicated to the residents of the University of Pennsylvania Department of Anesthesiology and Critical Care, who also constantly seek justification in the form of evidence for the faculty's and my decisions on how best to care for our patients.

Contributors

Sherif Afifi, MD, FCCM, FCCP
Associate Professor of Anesthesiology & Surgery
Chief, Division of Critical Care
Director of Critical Care Fellowship
Feinberg School of Medicine
Northwestern University
Chicago, Illinois

Seth Akst, MD, MBA
Assistant Professor
Department of Anesthesiology and Critical Care Medicine
George Washington University Medical Center
Washington, DC

James F. Arens, MD
Chair, Committee of Practice Parameters
American Society of Anesthesiology
Park Ridge, Illinois

Valerie A. Arkoosh, MD
Professor of Clinical Anesthesiology
University of Pennsylvania School of Medicine
Philadelphia, Pennsylvania

Barbara Armas, MD
Clinical Assistant Professor of Medicine
Robert Wood Johnson University Hospital
New Brunswick, New Jersey

Michael A. Ashburn, MD, MPH
Professor of Anesthesiology and Critical Care
  Medicine
University of Pennsylvania School of Medicine
Director of Pain Medicine and Palliative Care
Penn Pain Medicine Center
Tuttleman Center at Penn Medicine at Rittenhouse
Philadelphia, Pennsylvania

John G.T. Augoustides, MD, FASE
Assistant Professor
Department of Anesthesiology and Critical Care
University of Pennsylvania School of Medicine
Philadelphia, Pennsylvania

Michael Aziz, MD
Assistant Professor
Department of Anesthesiology and Peri-Operative
  Medicine
Oregon Health and Science University
Portland, Oregon

Daniel Bainbridge, MD, FRCPC
Assistant Professor and TEE Director
Division of Cardiac Anaesthesia
Department of Anaesthesia and Perioperative Medicine
London Health Sciences Centre
University of Western Ontario
London, Ontario, Canada

Jane C. Ballantyne, MD, FRCA
Associate Professor of Anesthesiology
Chief, Division of Pain Medicine
Department of Anesthesia and Critical Care
Massachusetts General Hospital
Harvard University
Boston, Massachusetts

Sheila R. Barnett, MD
Associate Professor of Anesthesiology
Harvard Medical School
Department of Anesthesiology and Critical Care
Beth Israel Deaconess Hospital Medical Center
Boston, Massachusetts

Joshua A. Beckman, MD, MS
Director, Cardiovascular Medicine Fellowship
Brigham and Women's Hospital
Assistant Professor of Medicine
Harvard Medical School
Boston, Massachusetts

Yaakov Beilin, MD
Associate Professor of Anesthesiology, and Obstetrics,
  Gynecology and Reproductive Sciences
Vice-Chair for Quality
Co-Director of Obstetric Anesthesia
Department of Anesthesiology
The Mount Sinai School of Medicine
New York, New York

Elliott Bennett-Guerrero, MD
Associate Professor
Department of Anesthesiology
Duke University Medical Center
Durham, North Carolina

Sanjay M. Bhananker, MBBS, MD, DA, FRCA
Assistant Professor
Department of Anesthesiology
University of Washington School of Medicine
Harborview Medical Center
Seattle, Washington

T. Andrew Bowdle, MD, PhD
Professor of Anesthesiology and Pharmaceutics
Chief of the Division of Cardiothoracic Anesthesiology
Department of Anesthesiology
University of Washington
Seattle, Washington

Lynn M. Broadman, MD
Clinical Professor of Anesthesiology
University of Pittsburgh Medical School
Children's Hospital of Pittsburgh
Pittsburgh, Pennsylvania

Daniel R. Brown, MD, PhD
Assistant Professor of Anesthesiology
Department of Anesthesiology
Mayo Clinic College of Medicine
Rochester, Minnesota

Robert H. Brown, MD, MPH
Professor
Department of Anesthesiology, Physiology and Radiology
Johns Hopkins University School of Medicine
Baltimore, Maryland

Robert A. Caplan, MD
Department of Anesthesiology
Virginia Mason Medical Center
Seattle, Washington

Jeffrey L. Carson, MD
Richard C. Reynolds Professor of Medicine
Chief, Division of General Internal Medicine
University of Medicine and Dentistry of New Jersey
   Robert Wood Johnson Medical School
New Brunswick, New Jersey

Maurizio Cereda, MD
Assistant Professor
Department of Anesthesiology and Critical Care
University of Pennsylvania School of Medicine
Philadelphia, Pennsylvania

Mark A. Chaney, MD
Associate Professor
Director of Cardiac Anesthesia
Department of Anesthesia and Critical Care
University of Chicago
Chicago, Illinois

Davy Cheng, MD, MSc, FRCPC, FCAHS
Professor and Chair
Department of Anaesthesia and Perioperative Medicine
London Health Sciences Centre and St. Joseph's
   Health Care
University of Western Ontario
London, Ontario, Canada

Grace L. Chien, MD
Associate Professor
Department of Anesthesiology
Oregon Health and Sciences University
Chief of Anesthesiology Service
Veterans Affairs Medical Center
Portland, Oregon

Vinod Chinnappa, MBBS, MD, FCARCSI
Clinical Fellow
Department of Anesthesia
University of Toronto
Toronto Western Hospital
University Health Network
Toronto, Ontario, Canada

Frances Chung, FRCPC
Professor
Department of Anesthesia
University of Toronto
Toronto Western Hospital
University Health Network
Toronto, Ontario, Canada

Neal H. Cohen, MD, MPH, MS
Vice Dean for Academic Affairs
Professor of Anesthesia and Perioperative Care
University of California, San Francisco
   School of Medicine
San Francisco, California

Nancy Collop, MD
Associate Professor of Medicine
Division of Pulmonary and Critical
   Care Medicine
Director, The Johns Hopkins Sleep Disorders Center
Baltimore, Maryland

Richard T. Connis, PhD
Chief Methodologist
Committee on Standards and Practice Parameters
American Society of Anesthesiologists
Park Ridge, Illinois

Douglas B. Coursin, MD
Professor of Anesthesiology and Medicine
University of Wisconsin School of Medicine and
   Public Health
Madison, Wisconsin

Stefan G. De Hert, MD, PhD
Professor of Anesthesiology
University of Antwerp
Vice-Chairman
Department of Anesthesiology
University Hospital Antwerp
Edegem, Belgium

Clifford S. Deutschman, MD, MS, FCCM
Professor of Anesthesiology and Critical Care
  and Surgery
Director, Stavropoulos Sepsis Research Program
University of Pennsylvania School of Medicine
Philadelphia, Pennsylvania

Karen B. Domino, MD, MPH
Professor
Department of Anesthesiology
University of Washington School of Medicine
University of Washington Medical Center
Seattle, Washington

Richard P. Dutton, MD, MBA
Associate Professor of Anesthesiology
Chief, Trauma Anesthesiology
University of Maryland Medical Center,
Baltimore, Maryland

R. Blaine Easley, MD
Assistant Professor
Department of Anesthesiology and Critical
  Care Medicine
Johns Hopkins Medical Center
Baltimore, Maryland

David M. Eckmann, PhD, MD
Horatio C. Wood Professor of Anesthesiology
  and Critical Care
Associate Professor of Bioengineering
University of Pennsylvania
Philadelphia, Pennsylvania

Nabil Elkassabany, MD
Clinical Assistant Professor
Department of Anesthesiology and Critical Care
University of Pennsylvania School of Medicine
Philadelphia, Pennsylvania

John E. Ellis, MD
Adjunct Professor
Department of Anesthesiology and Critical Care
University of Pennsylvania School of Medicine
Philadelphia, Pennsylvania

Kristin Engelhard, MD, PhD
Department of Anesthesiology
Johannes Gutenburg University
Mainz, Germany

Lucinda L. Everett, MD
Associate Professor
Harvard Medical School
Chief, Pediatric Anesthesia
Massachusetts General Hospital
Boston, Massachusetts

James Y. Findlay, MBChB, FRCA
Assistant Professor of Anesthesiology
Consultant, Anesthesiology and Critical Care Medicine
Department of Anesthesiology
Mayo Clinic
Rochester, Minnesota

Michael G. Fitzsimons, MD, FCCP
Instructor in Anesthesia
Fellowship Director, Adult Cardiothoracic Anesthesiology
Division of Cardiac Anesthesia
Department of Anesthesia and Critical Care
Harvard Medical School
Massachusetts General Hospital
Boston, Massachusetts

Lee A. Fleisher, MD, FACC, FAHA
Robert Dunning Dripps Professor and Chair
Department of Anesthesiology and Critical Care
Professor of Medicine
University of Pennsylvania School of Medicine,
Philadelphia, Pennsylvania

Nicole Forster, MD
Department of Anesthesiology
Johannes Gutenburg University
Mainz, Germany

Stephen E. Fremes, MD
Head, Division of Cardiac Surgery
Sunnybrook and Women's College Health Sciences Centre
Toronto, Ontario, Canada

Alan Gaffney, MBBCh
Registrar in Anaesthetics
University of Dublin
Dublin, Ireland

Tong J. Gan, MBBS, FRCA, FFARCSI
Professor
Department of Anesthesiology
Duke University Medical Center
Durham, North Carolina

Santiago Garcia, MD
Chief Cardiology Fellow
Division of Cardiovascular Medicine
University of Minnesota
Minneapolis, Minnesota

Adrian W. Gelb, MBChB
Professor
Department of Anesthesiology and Perioperative Care
University of California, San Francisco
San Francisco, California

Ralph Gertler, MD
Staff Anesthesiologist
Institute of Anesthesiology and Intensive Care
German Heart Centre of the State of Bavaria and the
    Technical University Munich
München, Germany

Satyajeet Ghatge, MD
Consultant Anesthetist
University Hospital of North Staffordshire
Stoke on Trent, United Kingdom

Barbara S. Gold, MD
Associate Professor
Department of Anesthesiology
University of Minnesota Medical School
Minneapolis, Minnesota

Allan Gottschalk, MD, PhD
Associate Professor
Department of Anesthesiology and Critical Care Medicine
Johns Hopkins Medical Institutions
Baltimore, Maryland

Anil Gupta, MD, FRCA, PhD
Associate Professor
Department of Anesthesiology and Intensive Care
University Hospital
Örebro, Sweden

Veena Guru, MD
Research Fellow
Department of Surgery
University of Pittsburgh Medical School
Pittsburgh, Pennsylvania

Ashraf S. Habib, MBBCh, MSc, FRCA
Associate Professor
Department of Anesthesiology
Duke University Medical Center
Durham, North Carolina

Carin A. Hagberg, MD
Professor
Department of Anesthesiology
Director of Neuroanesthesia and Advanced Airway
    Management
The University of Texas Medical School at Houston
Houston, Texas

Izumi Harukuni, MD
Assistant Professor
Department of Anesthesiology and Perioperative Medicine
Oregon Health and Science University
Portland, Oregon

Laurence M. Hausman, MD
Clinical Assistant Professor of
    Anesthesiology
Mount Sinai School of Medicine
New York, New York

Diane E. Head, MD
Assistant Professor
Department of Anesthesiology
University of Wisconsin School of Medicine and
    Public Health
Madison, Wisconsin

Robert S. Holzman, MD, FAAP
Associate Professor
Department of Anesthesia
Harvard Medical School
Boston Children's Hospital
Boston, Massachusetts

McCallum R. Hoyt, MD, MBA
Assistant Professor
Department of Anesthesia
Harvard Medical School
Brigham and Women's Hospital
Boston, Massachusetts

William E. Hurford, MD
Professor and Chair
Department of Anesthesiology
University of Cincinnati Academic
    Health Center
Cincinnati, Ohio

Aaron Joffe, DO
Department of Anesthesiology
University of Wisconsin School of Medicine
    and Public Health
Madison, Wisconsin

Edmund H. Jooste, MBChB
Assistant Professor
Department of Anesthesiology
University of Pittsburgh Medical School
Children's Hospital of Pittsburgh
Pittsburgh, Pennsylvania

Girish P. Joshi, MBBS, MD, FFARCSI
Professor of Anesthesiology and
    Pain Management
Director of Perioperative Medicine and
    Ambulatory Anesthesia
University of Texas Southwestern Medical Center
Dallas, Texas

Andrea Kurz, MD
Vice Chair
Department of Outcomes Research
Cleveland Clinic Foundation
Professor of Anesthesiology
Cleveland Clinic Lerner College of Medicine
Case Western Reserve University
Cleveland, Ohio

Martin J. London, MD
Professor of Clinical Anesthesia
University of California, San Francisco
Veterans Affairs Medical Center
San Francisco, California

Lynette Mark, MD
Associate Professor
Department of Anesthesiology & Critical Care Medicine
    and Department of Otolaryngology/Head and
    Neck Surgery
Johns Hopkins University
Baltimore, Maryland

Lynne G. Maxwell, MD
Associate Director, Division of General Anesthesia
Department of Anesthesiology and Critical
    Care Medicine
Children's Hospital of Philadelphia
Philadelphia, Pennsylvania

Edward O. McFalls, MD, PhD
Professor of Medicine
Division of Cardiology
Veterans Affairs Medical Center
Minneapolis, Minnesota

Michael L. McGarvey, MD
Department of Neurology
Hospital of the University of Pennsylvania
University of Pennsylvania Medical Center
Philadelphia, Pennsylvania

Kathryn E. McGoldrick, MD
Professor and Chair
Department of Anesthesiology
New York Medical College
Director of Anesthesiology
Westchester Medical Center
Valhalla, New York

Christopher T. McKee, DO
Attending Physician
Department of Anesthesiology
Nationwide Children's Hospital
Columbus, Ohio

R. Yan McRae, MD
Staff Anesthesiologist
Portland Veterans Affairs Medical Center
Assistant Professor
Department of Anesthesiology and Perioperative Medicine
Oregon Health and Science University
Portland, Oregon

Steven R. Messé, MD
Assistant Professor
Department of Neurology
University of Pennsylvania School of Medicine
Philadelphia, Pennsylvania

Amy L. Miller, MD, PhD
Fellow, Cardiovascular Medicine
Brigham and Women's Hospital
Instructor in Medicine
Harvard Medical School
Boston, Massachusetts

Marek Mirski, MD, PhD
Vice-Chair
Department of Anesthesiology and Critical
    Care Medicine
Director
Neuroscience Critical Care Units
Chief
Division of Neuroanesthesiology
Co-Director
Johns Hopkins Comprehensive Stroke Center
Associate Professor of Anesthesiology and
    Critical Care Medicine, Neurology, and Neurosurgery
Johns Hopkins Medical Institutions
Baltimore, Maryland

Vivek Moitra, MD
Assistant Professor
Department of Anesthesiology
Columbia University College of Physicians and Surgeons
New York, New York

Terri G. Monk, MD, MS
Professor
Department of Anesthesiology
Duke University Health System
Durham Veterans Affairs Medical Center
Durham, North Carolina

Michael F. Mulroy, MD
Clinical Associate Professor of Anesthesiology
University of Washington School of Medicine
Department of Anesthesiology
Virginia Mason Medical Center
Seattle, Washington

Glenn S. Murphy, MD

Associate Professor
Department of Anesthesiology
Northwestern University
Feinberg School of Medicine
Chicago, Illinois
Director of Cardiac Anesthesia
Evanston Northwestern Healthcare
Evanston, Illinois

Bradly J. Narr, MD

Associate Professor
Department of Anesthesiology
Mayo Clinic College of Medicine
Rochester, Minnesota

Patrick Neligan, MA, MB, FCARCSI

Clinical Senior Lecturer in Anaesthesia and
   Intensive Care
University College Hospital
Galway, Ireland

David G. Nickinovich, PhD

American Society of Anesthesiologists
Park Ridge, Illinois

Gregory A. Nuttall, MD

Professor
Department of Anesthesiology
Mayo Clinic College of Medicine
Rochester, Minnesota

E. Andrew Ochroch, MD

Assistant Professor
Department of Anesthesiology and Critical Care
University of Pennsylvania School of Medicine
Philadelphia, Pennsylvania

Catherine M.N. O'Malley, MBBS, FCARCSI

Department of Anaesthesia
St. James's Hospital
Dublin, Ireland

Alexander Papangelou, MD

Instructor
Department of Anesthesiology and Critical
   Care Medicine
Senior Fellow, Neurosciences Critical Care Unit
Johns Hopkins Medical Institutions
Baltimore, Maryland

Anthony N. Passannante, MD

Professor of Anesthesiology
Vice Chair for Clinical Operations
Department of Anesthesiology
University of North Carolina at Chapel Hill
Chapel Hill, North Carolina

L. Reuven Pasternak, MD, MPH, MBA

Chief Executive Officer
Inova Fairfax Hospital
Executive Vice President for Academic Affairs
Inova Health System
Falls Church, Virginia

Donald H. Penning, MD, MS, FRCP

Professor of Clinical Anesthesiology
Director, Obstetric Anesthesia
University of Miami Miller School of Medicine
Jackson Memorial Hospital
Miami, Florida

Beverly K. Philip, MD

Professor of Anesthesia
Harvard Medical School
Founding Director, Day Surgery Unit
Brigham and Women's Hospital
Boston, Massachusetts

Hugh Playford, MBBS, FANZCA, FFICANZCA

Assistant Professor of Anesthesia
Director of Cardiac Intensive Care Unit
Westmead Hospital
New South Wales, Australia

Catherine C. Price, PhD

Assistant Professor
Departments of Clinical and Health Psychology
   and Anesthesiology
University of Florida
Gainesville, Florida

George Pyrgos, MD

Professor
Department of Anesthesiology and Critical
   Care Medicine, Department of Medicine, and
   Department of Radiology
Johns Hopkins Medical Institutions
Baltimore, Maryland

Jeffrey M. Richman, MD

Assistant Professor
Department of Anesthesiology and Critical Care
   Medicine
Johns Hopkins University
Baltimore, Maryland

Hynek Riha, MD, DEAA

Clinical Assistant Profesor
Department of Anesthesiology and Intensive
   Care Medicine
Institute for Clinical and Experimental Medicine
Department of Cardiovascular and Transplantation
   Anesthesiology and Intensive Care Medicine
Postgraduate Medical School
Prague, Czech Republic

Stephen T. Robinson, MD
Associate Professor of Anesthesiology and Perioperative
    Medicine
Oregon Health and Sciences University
Portland, Oregon

Anthony M. Roche, MBChB, FRCA, MMed
Department of Anesthesiology
Duke University Medical Center
Durham, North Carolina

Peter Rock, MD, MBA
Martin Helrich Professor and Chair
Department of Anesthesiology
University of Maryland School of Medicine
Baltimore, Maryland

Stanley Rosenbaum, MA, MD
Professor of Anesthesiology
Internal Medicine and Surgery
Director, Section of Perioperative and Adult Anesthesia
Vice-Chair for Academic Affairs
Department of Anesthesiology
Yale University School of Medicine
New Haven, Connecticut

Meg A. Rosenblatt, MD
Associate Professor of Anesthesiology
Mount Sinai School of Medicine
New York University
New York, New York

Marc A. Rozner, PhD, MD
Professor of Anesthesiology and Perioperative Medicine
Professor of Cardiology
The University of Texas MD Anderson Cancer Center
Adjunct Assistant Professor of Integrative Biology and
    Pharmacology
University of Texas Health Science Center at Houston
Houston, Texas

Charles Marc Samama, MD, PhD, FCCP
Professor and Chair
Department of Anaesthesiology and Intensive Care
Hotel Dieu University Hospital
Paris, France

Rolf A. Schlichter, MD
Assistant Professor of Clinical Anesthesiology
University of Pennsylvania School of Medicine
Philadelphia, Pennsylvania

B. Scott Segal, MD
Vice-Chairman, Residency Education
Department of Anesthesiology, Perioperative and
    Pain Medicine
Brigham and Women's Hospital
Boston, Massachusetts

Douglas C. Shook, MD
Program Director, Cardiothoracic Anesthesia Fellowship
Department of Anesthesiology, Perioperative and
    Pain Medicine
Brigham and Women's Hospital
Harvard Medical School
Boston, Massachusetts

Ashish C. Sinha, MD, PhD
Assistant Professor of Anesthesiology and
    Critical Care
Assistant Professor of Otorhinolaryngology and
    Head and Neck Surgery
University of Pennsylvania School of Medicine
Philadelphia, Pennsylvania

Robert N. Sladen, MBChB, MRCP(UK), FRCP(C), FCCM
Professor and Vice-Chair
Department of Anesthesiology
College of Physicians and Surgeons of Columbia University
New York, New York

Clinton S. Steffey, MD
Department of Anesthesiology
State University of New York
Downstate Medical Center
Brooklyn, New York

Tracey L. Stierer, MD
Associate Professor and Medical Director, Johns Hopkins
    Outpatient Surgical Services
Department of Anesthesiology and Critical Care
    Medicine
Johns Hopkins University
Baltimore, Maryland

Wyndam Strodtbeck, MD
Department of Anesthesiology
Virginia Mason Medical Center
Seattle, Washington

Rebecca S. Twersky, MD, MPH
Professor and Vice Chair for Research
Department of Anesthesiology
Static University of New York Downstate
    Medical Center
Medical Director
Ambulatory Surgery Unit
Long Island College Hospital
Brooklyn, New York

Michael K. Urban, MD, PhD
Attending Anesthesiologist
Hospital for Special Surgery
Clinical Associate Professor of Anesthesiology
Weil Medical College of Cornell University
New York, New York

Jeffery S. Vender, MD

Professor and Associate Chair
Department of Anesthesiology
Northwestern University's Feinberg School of
    Medicine
Evanston, Illinois

Charles B. Watson, MD, FCCM

Chair, Department of Anesthesia
Deputy Surgeon-in-Chief
Bridgeport Hospital
Yale-New Haven Health System
Bridgeport, Connecticut

James F. Weller, MD

Staff Anesthesiologist
Bethesda North Hospital
Cincinnati, Ohio

David Wlody, MD

Interim Chief Medical Officer and Vice President for
    Medical Affairs
Medical Director of Perioperative Services
Chairman, Department of Anesthesiology
Long Island College Hospital
Professor of Clinical Anesthesiology
Vice Chair for Clinical Affairs and Director
Obstetric Anesthesia
State University of New York Downstate
    Medical Center
Brooklyn, New York

Christopher L. Wu, MD

Associate Professor
Department of Anesthesiology and Critical Care Medicine
Johns Hopkins University
Baltimore, Maryland

Foreword to the First Edition

This book is just what I want to read, and it appears just when I want to read it. When I look at the outline of questions and topics that Dr. Fleisher chose to present, it is obvious that those are the very questions I want answered; at least one of those questions seems to nag at me every day. Rather than just presenting the reader with a problem and laying out the evidence, then leaving the reader in a dilemma of having to make the choice, the authors state the actions they would take and explain why. This in no way restricts the readers, however; it just gives them an idea of what the experts in the field would do in a given situation. It is clear that Dr. Fleisher selected the authors carefully to have a balanced presentation by the experts in their fields. He did an outstanding job of editing this book (I am, of course, biased because he is my coeditor on *Essence of Anesthesia Practice*, and I know the great work he did on that book).

An example of why I think this is such an outstanding work is the chapter "Should a Child with Respiratory Tract Infection Undergo Elective Surgery?" Drs. Easley and Maxwell not only introduce the problem but also give the evidence that proceeding immediately with surgery increases risk. They present the evidence that delaying surgery may decrease risk, and, rather than leave the reader in the lurch, conclude that they would delay surgery for 2 to 4 weeks in patients with upper respiratory infection and symptoms and for 4 to 6 weeks in those with acute lower respiratory infection. They state clearly that this is their opinion and that the existing evidence is not conclusive enough to be definitive. They then offer the references if one wants to pursue the question in greater detail.

This book is a great educational tool for the private practitioner who wants to know what the experts in the field would do in a given situation. It is also a great book for the resident and faculty member who can learn how to handle a wide range of important issues, such as how to handle perioperative hypothermia, whether the choice of muscle relaxant affects outcome, what to do to prevent peripheral nerve injuries, or whether patients with obstructive sleep apnea should be admitted to the ICU.

I intend to buy two copies of this book—one to keep at home and use to prepare for the next day, and one to keep at work. I plan on relying heavily on this book for teaching in the operating room. I think it is a superb addition to our educational armamentarium and hope you enjoy it as much as I did.

Michael F. Roizen, MD

Preface

It has been 5 years since the publication of the first edition of *Evidence-Based Practice of Anesthesiology*. I am indeed fortunate to collaborate with my publisher at Elsevier, Natasha Andjelkovic, who, when I initially proposed this idea to Elsevier, had the foresight to recognize that this approach to the practice of medicine had become critical with respect to clinical care and education. I was extremely pleased that many practitioners, especially residents, found useful the approach taken to critical questions in the first edition. In editing the second edition, I maintained the approach and format of the earlier edition and updated important topics with ongoing controversy and added many new topics for which there is increasing evidence on how best to practice. It is my hope that the field of anesthesiology and perioperative medicine will continue to grow with increasing high-quality investigations, particularly randomized trials, to expand our evidence base and help practitioners provide the highest quality of care.

I am indebted to several people who were critical in the publication of the second edition of *Evidence-Based Practice of Anesthesiology*. I would like to particularly acknowledge my executive assistant, Eileen O'Shaughnessy, who kept the authors and myself on track and assisted with the editing of many chapters. In addition to my publisher, I would also like to thank Marla Sussman, our developmental editor. I hope this book will provide the answers to many of your daily anesthesia questions.

Lee A. Fleisher, MD

Contents

INTRODUCTION

1 Evidence-Based Practice Parameters—The American Society of Anesthesiologists Approach

David G. Nickinovich, PhD; Richard T. Connis, PhD; Robert A. Caplan, MD; and James F. Arens, MD

The American Society of Anesthesiologists (ASA) continues to improve and refine its evidence-based approach to the development of practice parameters. The intention of ASA practice parameters is to enhance and promote the safety of anesthetic practice and provide guidance or direction for the diagnosis, management, and treatment of clinical problems. Specifically, ASA evidence-based practice parameters consist of a "broad body of documents developed on the basis of a systematic and standardized approach to the collection, assessment, analysis and reporting of: (1) scientific literature, (2) expert opinion, (3) surveys of ASA members, (4) feasibility data and (5) open forum commentary."[1] Evidence-based practice parameters may take the form of standards, guidelines, or advisories.

Before 1991, ASA practice parameters were consensus-based documents, consisting primarily of practice standards. These practice standards focused on simple aspects of patient care and applied to virtually all relevant anesthetic situations, as reflected in the ASA *Standards for Basic Anesthetic Monitoring*.[2] The dissemination of these standards soon positioned the ASA and the Anesthesia Patient Safety Foundation of the ASA at the forefront of medical practice by demonstrating the benefits of a proactive approach to patient safety.

However, many aspects of clinical practice could not be adequately covered by the relatively limited and prescriptive recommendations of practice standards. When broader and more flexible clinical recommendations were needed, the ASA developed and published practice guidelines. Initially, practice guidelines were developed on the basis of evidence generated by the same methodology used in the development of practice standards at the time, namely the consensus of experts.

Recognizing that a more extensive and elaborate methodology was needed to evaluate the increasing breadth and complexity of issues addressed by practice guidelines, the ASA Committee on Standards and Practice Parameters (Committee) determined that the systematic evaluation of scientific evidence was necessary in addition to expert opinion. Consequently, in 1991, the ASA adopted an evidence-based model for the evaluation of scientific literature similar to that in use by the Agency for Health Care Policy and Research (now the Agency for Healthcare Research and Quality [AHRQ]). Combining a systematic synthesis of the literature with expert opinion, ASA published the first two evidence-based practice guidelines in 1993.[3,4] In developing these guidelines and recognizing the unique properties of the anesthesia literature and the practice of anesthesiology, the Committee realized that further changes in the methodology used were needed. Over the next few years, a multidimensional approach to guideline development evolved that contained four critical components: (1) a rigorous review and evaluation of all available published scientific evidence, (2) meta-analytic assessment of controlled clinical studies, (3) statistical assessment of expert and practitioner opinion obtained by formally developed surveys, and (4) informal evaluation of opinions obtained from invited and public commentary.

ORGANIZATIONAL CONTEXT

The ASA evidence-based practice parameter process typically begins with the Committee identifying an issue or clinical problem and appointing a task force of 8 to 12 anesthesiologists who are recognized experts on the issue or clinical problem and who therefore are able to advise the Committee on the need for a practice parameter. Task force members are carefully chosen to provide a balance between private practice and academia, and to ensure representation across major geographic areas of the United States. Non-anesthesiologists may also be appointed to a task force when the Committee has determined that such an appointment is appropriate (e.g., the appointment of a radiologist to the magnetic resonance imaging [MRI] task force).

If the task force determines that an evidence-based practice parameter is needed, it begins the process of defining goals and objectives within the mandate of the

Committee. In addition, it identifies approximately 75 to 150 peer-review consultants to serve as an external source of opinion, practical knowledge, and expertise. Consultants typically are recognized experts in the subject matter and, similar to task force members, represent a balance of practice settings and geographic locations. On occasion, individuals from non-anesthesia medical specialties or organizations are selected as consultants.

To begin development of an evidence-based practice parameter, a conceptual survey of the task force is conducted to identify target conditions, patient or clinical presentations, providers, interventions, practice settings, and other characteristics that help define or clarify the parameter. Members of the task force then collectively develop a list of evidence linkages based on their responses to this conceptual survey. These evidence linkages represent statements of explicit relationships between particular aspects of anesthetic or clinical care and desired outcomes. The linkages form the foundation on which evidence is collected and organized, thereby providing the structure within which recommendations and advice are formulated. When possible and appropriate, evidence linkages are designed to describe comparative relationships between interventions and outcomes. For example, the linkage statement "spinal opioids versus parenteral opioids improve maternal analgesia for labor" identifies a specific intervention (spinal opioids), a comparison intervention (parenteral opioids), and a specific clinical outcome (maternal analgesia) thought to be affected by the intervention. Once all of the evidence linkages for the parameter are specified, the task force then begins the process of collecting evidence.

SOURCES OF EVIDENCE FOR PRACTICE PARAMETERS

The ASA evidence-based process begins with the assumption that there is a sufficient body of scientific literature to produce evidence-based guidelines and clinical recommendations. Table 1-1 shows sources of information collected by a task force. The accumulated evidence will determine whether the document is either a guideline or an advisory. Three major sources of evidence are considered: (1) descriptive summary data from the literature (e.g., means, ranges, sensitivity/specificity), (2) consensus-based information obtained from formal surveys, and (3) when sufficient numbers of randomized controlled studies are available, meta-analytic findings.

The Literature Search

The initial literature search includes a computerized search of the National Library of Medicine and other large reference sources when applicable, and usually yields 2000 to 5000 citations for each practice parameter. Manual searches are also conducted, with supplemental references supplied by members of the task force and consultants.

In the selection of published studies, three conditions must be met. First, the study must address one or more of the evidence linkages being considered. Second, the study must report an anesthetic or clinical outcome or set of findings that can be tallied or quantified, thereby eliminating

Table 1-1	Sources of Evidence for Practice Parameters
Source of Evidence	**Type of Evidence**
Randomized controlled trials	Comparative statistics
Nonrandomized prospective studies	Comparative statistics
Controlled observational studies	Correlation/regression
Retrospective comparative studies	Comparative statistics
Uncontrolled observational studies	Correlation/regression/ descriptive statistics
Case reports	No statistical data
Consultants	Survey findings/expert opinion
ASA members	Survey findings/opinion
Invited sources	Expert opinion
Open forum commentary	Public opinion
Internet commentary	Public opinion

reports that contain only opinion (e.g., editorials, news reports). Third, the study must be an original investigation or report. Thus, review articles, books or book chapters, and manuscripts that report findings from previous publications are not used as a source of evidence. After the initial electronic review, letters, editorials, commentaries, and other literature with no original data are also removed from consideration. Typically, 1000 to 2500 articles remain that are suitable for library retrieval and further review.

Evaluating and Summarizing the Literature

The literature review focuses on evaluating studies that directly address an evidence linkage. When a study reports an outcome relevant to a given practice parameter, the findings related to that outcome are initially classified as directional evidence. *Directional evidence* refers to a designation of the extent to which beneficial or harmful clinical outcomes were found to be associated with a particular intervention. Each reported outcome is numerically classified as 1 (beneficial), −1 (harmful), or 0 (neutral). These values are then averaged across all studies to obtain an aggregate directional assessment of support or refutation. Although this aggregated directional assessment is not intended to provide a statistical finding, it nonetheless does provide a useful general indication of the positioning of a particular intervention on a continuum of clinical benefit and harm. Moreover, a directional finding may suggest that a one-tailed relationship exists between a clinical intervention and an outcome of interest, and it may justify proceeding with a statistical evaluation using meta-analysis when sufficient numbers of controlled studies are available.

All relevant articles, regardless of study design, are considered and evaluated during the development of an ASA evidence-based practice parameter. Although randomized prospectively controlled trials usually provide the strongest evidence, findings from studies using other research designs also provide critical information. For example, a nonrandomized comparative study may provide evidence for the differential benefits or risks of selected interventions. Observational studies may report frequency or incidence data that can indicate the scope of a problem, event, or condition or may report correlational findings suggesting associations among clinical interventions and outcomes. In addition, case reports may describe adverse events that are not normally reported in controlled studies and that can be the source of important cautionary notations within a recommendation or advisory. Case reports may also be the first indication that a new drug or technique is associated with previously unrecognized benefit or unwanted side effects.

One of the strengths of the ASA protocol for developing evidence-based practice parameters is that the primary search and evaluation of the literature is jointly conducted by the methodologists and clinicians who serve as members of the task force. Consequently, the research design and statistical aspects, as well as the clinical and practical significance of a study, are appropriately and thoroughly evaluated. In evaluating this protocol, formal reliability testing among task force members and methodologists is conducted. Interobserver agreement for research design, type of analysis, linkage assignment, and study inclusion is calculated using both two-rater agreement pairs (Kappa) and multirater chance-corrected agreement (Sav) values.[5,6] These values are reported in the final published document.

Evaluating and Summarizing Consensus Opinion

Literature-based scientific evidence is a crucial component of the process of evidence-based practice parameter development, but the literature is *never* the sole source of evidence in the development of evidence-based practice parameters. The task force always supplements scientific findings with the practical knowledge and opinions of expert consultants. The consultants participate in formal surveys regarding conceptualization, application, and feasibility issues, and they also review and comment on the initial draft report of the task force. Opinion surveys of the ASA membership are also conducted to obtain additional consensus-based information used in the final development of an evidence-based practice parameter. The evidence obtained from surveys of consultants and ASA members represents a valuable and quantifiable source of evidence, critical to formulation of effective and useful practice parameters.

In addition to survey information and commentary obtained from consultants and practitioners, the task force continually attempts to maximize the amount of consensus-based information available by obtaining opinions from a broader range of sources. These sources include comments made by readers of a Web posting of a draft of the practice parameter (www.asahq.org) and comments from attendees of one or more public forums scheduled during major national meetings. After collection and analysis of all scientific and consensus-based information, the draft document is further revised and additional commentary or opinion is solicited from invited sources, such as the ASA board of directors and presidents of ASA component societies.

Meta-Analysis

When sufficient numbers of controlled studies are found addressing a particular evidence linkage, formal meta-analysis for each specific outcome is conducted. For studies containing continuous data, either general variance-based methods or combined probability tests are used. When studies report dichotomous outcomes, an odds-ratio procedure is applied. In summarizing findings, an acceptable significance level typically is set at $p < 0.01$ (one-tailed) and effect size estimates are determined.

Reported findings in the anesthesia literature often use common outcome measures, thereby enhancing the likelihood that aggregated (i.e., pooled) studies will be homogeneous. Because homogeneity is generally expected, a fixed-effects meta-analytic model is used for the initial analysis. If the pooled studies for an evidence linkage are subsequently found to be heterogeneous, a random-effects analysis is performed, and possible reasons for the heterogeneous findings are explored. These heterogeneous findings are reported and discussed as part of the literature summary for an evidence linkage.

Whenever possible, more than one test is used so that a more complete statistical profile of the evidence linkage can be evaluated. For example, when a set of studies allows for more than one meta-analysis (e.g., using both continuous and dichotomous findings), separate meta-analyses are conducted and there must be agreement between the separate findings for the results of the analysis to be considered conclusive. Additionally, these analyses should be in agreement with the directional evaluation of the literature and with consensus opinion before an unequivocal supportive recommendation is offered. If disagreements occur, they are fully reported in the summary of evidence and usually acknowledged in caveats or notations following the recommendation for the evidence linkage.

GUIDELINE OR ADVISORY DETERMINATION

For an evidence-based practice parameter to be considered a guideline, all three sources of evidence (directional evidence from the literature, supporting agreement from the consultants and ASA members, and meta-analytic support) must be present. If, given the nature of the topic, sufficient controlled studies are not available, an evidence-based practice advisory is formulated to assist practitioners in clinical decision making and matters of patient safety.

The evidence-based practice advisory is a recent innovation developed by the Committee and authorized by the ASA in 1998 in response to the increasing need for expansion of the evidence-based process to areas where randomized controlled trials are sparse or nonexistent. This innovation allowed the ASA tremendous flexibility in applying the evidence-based process to a broader scope of topics.

The evidence-based protocol for a practice advisory is identical to that used in the creation of evidence-based practice guidelines. A systematic literature search and evaluation of the literature are formally conducted. Formal survey information is obtained from consultants and a sample of the ASA membership, as well as informal input from public posting of draft copies of an advisory on the ASA website, open forum presentations, and other invited and public sources.

The available evidence is then synthesized, and a practice advisory document is prepared. The intent is to produce a report that summarizes the current state of the literature, characterizes the current spectrum of clinical opinion, and provides interpretive commentary from the task force.

THE FINAL PRODUCT

A typical practice guideline or advisory requires approximately 2 years for completion at a cost of $200,000 to $300,000. Periodic updates occur 7 to 10 years after publication, unless circumstances require an earlier update. These documents are published in *Anesthesiology* and are available on the journal's website (www.anesthesiology. org), as well as on the ASA website (www.asahq.org). Supporting material is also available on the journal's website or can be requested from the ASA.

Since adopting the evidence-based model in 1991, the ASA has developed and approved 13 evidence-based practice guidelines, 6 guideline updates, and 6 evidence-based practice advisories. Currently, no evidence-based practice standards are planned.

ASA evidence-based practice guidelines and advisories are presented in a format that emphasizes the clinical use of the recommendations/advice for the practitioner. Anesthesiologists and other anesthesia care providers are generally interested in easily accessible, specific recommendations/advice about how to provide optimal care to their patients. Detailed rationales or descriptions of techniques, exhaustive critiques of the literature, or elaborate cost-benefit analyses are usually of secondary concern. The ASA has elected to provide documents that are brief and succinct, with supportive information available in summary form within the guideline or advisory, in an appendix, at the ASA website, or by request.

The general structure of ASA practice guidelines and advisories consists of an introductory section, a guidelines/advisory section, and supporting information (e.g., tables, figures, or appendices). The introductory section contains the ASA definition of practice guidelines or advisories, followed by a discussion of the focus, application, and methodology used in the guideline/advisory development process. The guidelines or advisories section is serially divided into subsections, each based on a separate evidence linkage. Each evidence linkage subsection is, in turn, divided into two parts: an evidence summary and recommendations or advice.

The *evidence summary* subsection contains a description of the literature, generally including statements concerning the availability of literature, the strength of evidence obtained from the literature, and details about particular aspects of the literature necessary for a clear interpretation as it pertains to the evidence linkage. Consultant and membership survey findings are also summarized, in addition to discussion of other opinion-based information when warranted.

Because it is assumed that the intended readers of the document are knowledgeable regarding the topic, the *recommendations or advisories* subsections are brief and to the point, with explanations added only if required for clarification. Cautionary notations may accompany a recommendation or advisory when deemed necessary by the task force. Extensive literature critiques are not presented in the main text of the document, but details of the literature evaluation, as well as opinion-based data, are included in appendices or are available on request.

The ASA evidence-based practice parameters are distributed worldwide and have been well received within both the anesthesia community and allied medical professions.

SUMMARY

Evidence-based practice parameters are important decision-making tools for practitioners, and they are particularly helpful in providing guidance in areas of difficult or complex practice. They can be instrumental in identifying areas of practice that have not yet been clearly defined. These documents also serve to improve research in anesthesiology by (1) identifying areas in need of additional study, (2) providing direction for the development of more efficacious interventions, and (3) emphasizing the importance of robust outcome-based research methods. By recognizing the value of merging broad-based empirical evidence with opinion and consensus, the ASA has taken a leadership role in improving specific areas of clinical practice, patient care, and safety.

The ASA is committed to the development of practice guidelines and practice advisories by using an evidence-based process that examines testable relationships between specific clinical interventions and desired outcomes (Table 1-2). This process recognizes that evidence is highly variable in quality and may come from many sources, including scientific studies, case reports, expert opinion, and practitioner opinion. By providing a consistent and transparent framework for collecting evidence and by considering its strengths as well as weaknesses, the ASA evidence-based process results in practice parameters that clinicians regard as scientifically valid and clinically applicable.

Physicians have voiced concern that guidelines and advisories will be treated as *de facto* standards, thereby increasing liability and creating unnecessary restraints on clinical practice. The ASA emphasizes the nonbinding nature of practice guidelines, in particular by defining them as "recommendations that may be adopted, modified, or rejected according to clinical needs and constraints." Because the process of evidence-based guideline and advisory development places a strong emphasis on consensus formation and communication throughout the practicing community, guidelines and advisories will continue to be relied on by anesthesiologists and other practitioners in their ongoing efforts to maintain a high quality of patient care and safety.

Table 1-2	**Strengths of the ASA Evidence-Based Process**

Specific outcome data related to a specific intervention are collected and evaluated.

A broad literature search from a wide variety of published articles.

Systematic evaluation of evidence from qualitatively different sources.

Randomized controlled studies used in meta-analyses to evaluate causal relationships.

Nonrandomized controlled studies to provide supplemental information.

Descriptive/incidence literature to provide an indication of the scope of a problem.

Case reports to describe adverse events not normally found in controlled studies.

Opinion-based evidence to evaluate clinical and practical benefits.

Evidence from the literature is directionally summarized to clarify and formalize evidence linkages and to reduce bias inherent in selective reviews.

Reliance on randomized clinical trials to demonstrate causal relationships and reduce bias inherent in nonrandomized studies or case reports.

General use of identical outcome measures rather than pooling different measures.

Consensus information obtained from both formal (e.g., surveys) and informal (e.g., open forums, Internet commentary) sources.

One-to-one correspondence between evidence linkages and recommendations.

Brevity in reporting evidence.

Simple summary statements of literature findings for each evidence linkage, thereby avoiding exhaustive literature reviews or critiques.

Specific clinical recommendations without lengthy discussion or detailed rationale.

Scientific documentation is provided in appendices or is available separately.

Bibliographic information is available separately.

Periodic updating to reflect new medications, technologies, or techniques.

REFERENCES

1. American Society of Anesthesiologists: Policy statement on practice parameters. In *ASA Standards, Guidelines and Statements, American Society of Anesthesiologists*, October, 2007: http://www.asahq.org/publicationsAndServices/standards/01.pdf.
2. American Society of Anesthesiologists: Standards for basic anesthetic monitoring. In *ASA Standards, Guidelines and Statements, American Society of Anesthesiologists Publication*, 5-6, October 1999.
3. American Society of Anesthesiologists: Practice guidelines for pulmonary artery catheterization. *Anesthesiology* 1993;78:380-394.
4. American Society of Anesthesiologists: Practice guidelines for management of the difficult airway. *Anesthesiology* 1993;78:597-602.
5. Sackett GP: *Observing behavior volume II: Data collection and analysis methods.* Baltimore, University Park Press, 1978, pp. 90-93.
6. O'Connell DL, Dobson AJ: General observer agreement measures on individual subjects and groups of subjects. *Biometrics* 1984;40:973-983.

SECTION II

PREOPERATIVE PREPARATION

2 Does Routine Testing Affect Outcome?

L. Reuven Pasternak, MD, MPH, MBA

Preoperative testing for patients undergoing elective surgical procedures is an issue that has received considerable attention during the past decade. This attention is not surprising because preoperative testing affects virtually all of the more than 30 million surgical procedures performed each year and is associated with costs that run well into the billions of dollars. Preoperative testing has become the focus of numerous studies and has also served as the cause for developing guidelines. The two most important of these are the American College of Cardiology/American Heart Association (ACC/AHA) recommendations[1] for cardiac patients undergoing noncardiac surgery and the more general advisory developed by the American Society of Anesthesiologists (ASA).[2]

The issue of routine testing as a method of screening for disease processes precedes the debate over this practice in anesthesiology. In the 1960s it was accepted as common knowledge in some of the most forward-thinking health systems that routine screening for various disease processes independent of the presence of symptoms or identification of risk factors would reveal potentially serious medical issues in their "preclinical" phase and thus allow for earlier intervention and reduced morbidity and mortality rates. These initiatives were undertaken without the benefit of any definitive outcomes research and were rapidly accepted as dogma. Conventional medical education imparted to medical students and residents (and patients) the concept that more testing was consistent with better medical care and may serve as a substitute for the history and physical examination as an indicator of distress.

The factors associated with this development are associated with the unique climate of that time. Those factors included a sense of almost infinite opportunity for expansion of health care resources and a failure to appreciate how increasingly complex health technology applied on a mass scale could rapidly deplete health care resources. The lack of appreciation of true risk-benefit analysis and evidence-based research was also a major contributor to this mindset. The sense that tests carried risk beyond cost was not appreciated, and the failure to link outcomes to interventions was consistent in almost all areas of medicine. At present, three factors have converged to reverse this trend. The first two are the new economic imperatives that make clear that resources are limited, and the drive for standardization and guideline development within and between specialties to ensure better communication and improved patient care. The ability to affect these two depends on the third development—the emergence of evidence-based outcomes studies as the accepted scientific foundation for recommendations, ranging from protocols to guidelines and advisories.[3-6] Note that this chapter will not address the issue of cardiac testing for noncardiac surgery.

EVIDENCE

Although quick to be accepted on faith, the cascade of evidence against routine testing is still met with grudging acceptance among professional and lay staff. The central tenet of the evidence-based approach is the value of any intervention, even an innocuous test of inherently low morbidity and cost, based on the extent that it can be demonstrated to have a beneficial effect as measured by defined outcomes. These can be either clinical (e.g., morbidity and mortality) or administrative (e.g., enhanced efficiency or patient satisfaction). In the absence of such evidence, the intervention should not be undertaken. Where the intervention has been standard practice for decades, as has been the case with preoperative testing, this change can be profound and unsettling but nonetheless scientifically appropriate.

Olsen and colleagues[7] were among the first to address this issue in the general medical arena in their study of multiphasic screening based on a 1972 study of adults in 574 families. Within the general category of chemistry tests that are routinely performed preoperatively, the rate of abnormalities was 1% to 3%, with the exception of serum glucose at 8%. Within these groups, fewer than 15% required any therapy. This study was the harbinger of others that started to reverse the trend to large batteries of tests for routine health screening.

When focusing more closely on the area of tests associated with preparation for surgery, the evidence is more profound for the lack of an association in outcomes. When the ASA did a literature review on this subject, the nature of the evidence by strict evidence-based criteria was deemed to be insufficient to provide recommendations for specific tests but did confirm the lack of associated benefit with routine testing. Kaplan and colleagues[8] addressed the issue of the utility of laboratory tests in a retrospective survey of 2000 patients who had undergone elective surgical procedures. Of the 2236 tests performed in this group (Table 2-1), 65.6% were done without indication. Of the 96 abnormalities encountered, only 10 were in

Table 2-1 Preoperative Screening Battery Tests

Test	Normal	Not Indicated (NI)	Abnormal (AB)	NI + AB	NI + AB and Significant
Prothrombin time (PT)	201	154	2	0	0
Partial thromboplastin time (PTT)	199	154	1	0	0
Platelet count	407	366	3	2	1
Complete blood count (CBC)	61	293	22	2	0
White blood cell count with differential	390	324	2	1	0
Chemistry 6 panel	514	176	41	1	1
Glucose	464	361	25	4	2
TOTAL	2236	1828	96	10	4

Adapted from Kaplan EB et al: *JAMA* 1985;253:3576.

the group without indication, and of these, only 4 were deemed to be clinically significant. In all cases, the surgery was performed without known morbidity. Kitz and colleagues[9] demonstrated how the lack of definitive criteria can cause considerable variance without altered outcome in virtually identical patient populations. Reporting on a naturally occurring experiment, patients undergoing arthroscopy and laparoscopy were assessed on test ordering. Performed before mandated outpatient management of these procedures, the two groups were inpatients and outpatients, with the decision on status determined by surgeon and patient preference without difference in clinical status. The ordering done by surgeons was substantially higher in all categories than by the anesthesia staff without difference in outcomes in the two groups (Table 2-2). Narr and colleagues[10] in reviewing the testing routinely done on 3782 healthy (ASA Class 1) patients, found that only 160 (4%) had abnormalities, of which 30 could have been predicted. None of the abnormalities were of a clinically significant nature, and all patients proceeded safely to surgery. On this basis, the Mayo Clinic in 1991 anticipated the more general trend and deferred all testing on healthy, asymptomatic patients for elective surgical procedures. In his study of 4058 standardized tests performed by protocol in ambulatory patients, Wyatt and colleagues[11] determined that only 1% were of sufficient importance to mandate delay or cancellation of surgery. Though not as precise as the studies of Kaplan and colleagues[8] and Kitz and colleagues,[9] the appearance of this item in the surgical literature brought this concept to the attention of the surgical community.

Within the context of specific tests the evidence is similarly lacking for an association for testing without indication and improvements in outcome. For example, Charpak and colleagues,[12] reporting on the utility of routine chest x-rays, found that of 1101 x-rays ordered on 3866 patients, only 51 (5%) had an impact on the surgical plan and anesthetic management and also that these could have been predicted on the basis of the patient's medical condition and anticipated surgery. Similarly, Rucker and colleagues,[13] in their review of 905 surgical admissions receiving chest x-rays, found that 368 had no risk factors and, of these, only 1 had a positive finding that did not affect surgery. Of the remaining 504 with risk factors, 114 (22%) had abnormalities, none of which were new or which changed planned surgical or anesthetic management. Similar findings have been found for urinalysis[14] and renal function studies.[15]

Dzankic and colleagues,[16] in their study of geriatric patients, documented the importance of medical and surgical risk as opposed to routine testing. In a retrospective review of 544 patients ages 70 and older undergoing elective procedures, the authors found a 6.8% prevalence of abnormal values, with the highest being for creatinine (12%), hemoglobin (10%), and glucose (7%), which is consistent with routine physiologic changes for this age-group. When a multivariate regression analysis was done to determine risk factors associated with adverse outcome, only ASA status greater than II and risk of surgery (per AHA/ACC classification) were found to be factors that in themselves had any predictive value in determining outcome. Age did not constitute a specific risk factor or

Table 2-2 Preoperative Screening Battery Tests

Test	ARTHROSCOPY		LEVEL 1 LAPAROSCOPY		LEVEL 2 LAPAROSCOPY	
	Outpatient (%)	Inpatient (%)	Outpatient (%)	Inpatient (%)	Outpatient (%)	Inpatient (%)
X-ray	12	30	24	58	0	79
ECG	11	30	12	50	2	83
Chemistry panel	3	92	0	75	2	86

Adapted from Kitz DS et al: *Anesthesiology* 1988;69:383.

Table 2-3	Effectiveness of a Preoperative Evaluation Center (PEC)		
Test	Surgical Service	PEC	% Reduction
Number of patients	3576	4313	—
Complete blood count	3417	3395*	17.7
Platelet count	3207	2620*	32.3
PT/PTT	2703	578*	82.3
Urinalysis	2489	309*	89.7
General survey panel	2199	811*	69.4
Electrolytes	1775	739*	65.5
Renal panel	1402	1022*	39.5
Electrocardiograms	2202	1362*	48.7
Chest x-rays	2510	1026*	66.1
TOTAL preoperative tests	21,904	11,862*	45.8
Tests per patient	6.13	2.75*	55.1

*$p < 0.001$.
Adapted from Fischer SP: *Anesthesiology* 1996;85:196.

indication for tests. This finding was consistent with that of the ASA Task Force, which could find no evidence that age alone was a risk factor that justified electrocardiograms (ECGs), chest x-rays, or other studies.

The preponderance of evidence thus has demonstrated that routine performance of tests is not indicated. This has been brought forward into the guideline development process[1,2] and in some official proceedings from outside of the United States as well.[17] Indeed, a study by Schein and colleagues[18] of cataract patients found no utility for any testing regardless of baseline health status when associated with outcomes from this minimally invasive procedure.

Having established that routine screening is of little merit, there is emerging evidence that appropriate screening systems are useful in eliminating this excess. Fischer,[19] in a study of patients undergoing elective surgical procedures, compared consultations, tests, and cancellations in a prestudy group that had tests and consultations ordered by surgical staff, while the posttest group had tests and consultations ordered by anesthesia staff based on the presence of specific clinical conditions in an anesthesia-managed preoperative assessment clinic. The group going through the preoperative screening system had a 55.14% reduction testing (Table 2-3) and associated reductions in cancellation were from 1.96% to 0.21%. This reduction was also matched with a 59.3% reduction in associated costs ($188.91 versus $76.82). Pollard and colleagues[20] demonstrated a similar reduction in cancellations and testing in a Veterans Administration hospital.

CONTROVERSIES

The movement toward less testing has created an environment that has opened the issue as to whether preoperative assessments are of any value. Clinicians and administrative staff look at studies such as Schein and colleagues'[18] and come to a conclusion not intended by these authors: that the assessment by the anesthesiologist has no inherent value with regard to safety or enhanced outcome. Roizen,[21] in his editorial response to these perceptions, notes that the real issue is substituting physician judgment for laboratory testing within the preoperative process, an assertion echoed in the ASA advisory on this subect.[2] The issue is not whether administration of anesthesia provides a risk to the patient, but whether that risk is modified by tests.

AREAS OF UNCERTAINTY

The issue of testing based on individual clinical symptoms may be subject to some revision based on emerging technologies. The first is the increasing bundling of tests. For example, it had been common in the past that each component of the routine chemistry panel was individually run and billed, making it necessary to order tests in a discriminating fashion. There is an increasing ability to perform large batteries of tests in a manner that is economically efficient. In fact, it is now more expensive to break apart these panels than to simply run the full series. Thus, any need to perform venipuncture for tests may in fact be a simple test-or-no-test decision with virtually all available values returned from this single decision point. If this is the case, the process for deciding on tests actually becomes a simple one that can be made by lower-level staff who can identify any one of several "triggers" to mandate this action.

The larger issue relates to what will be the emerging field of genomics in preoperative assessment. Based principally in cardiology research, genetic markers for patients with a predisposition to events such as perioperative arrhythmias have been identified, and the technology is being developed for rapid screening of individuals. As this new field expands, there will again be the pressure to screen and to perhaps let enthusiasm get ahead of evidence-based science in adopting these new technologies.

GUIDELINES/AUTHOR'S RECOMMENDATIONS

The recommended guidelines are consistent with those of the ASA in its Practice Advisory.[2] Testing should only be done for specific clinical conditions based on the patient's individual history, nature of surgery, and presenting symptoms. Age alone is not an indication for any of the tests; specific conditions that may be associated with the aging process would have to be identified. Thus, healthy patients of any age undergoing elective surgical procedures without coexisting medical condition should not require any testing unless the nature of the surgery might result in major physiologic stress or change for which baseline studies are indicated. Further testing is only as per the specific medical condition of the patient based on an appropriate review of the patient's history and examination before the day of surgery.

REFERENCES

1. American College of Cardiology/American Heart Association Task Force on Practice Guidelines: ACC/AHA guideline update for perioperative cardiovascular evaluation for noncardiac surgery—executive summary. *Anesth Analg* 2002;94:1052-1064.
2. American Society of Anesthesiologists Task Force on Preanesthesia Evaluation: Practice Advisory for Preanesthesia Evaluation. *Anesthesiology* 2002;96(2):485-496.
3. Eisenberg JM: Ten lessons for evidence-based technology assessment. *JAMA* 1999;282(19):1865-1872.
4. Evidence-Based Medicine Working Group: Evidence-based medicine. *JAMA* 1992;268(17):2420-2425.
5. Leape LL, Berwick DM, Bates DW: What practices will most improve safety? Evidence-based medicine meets patient safety. *JAMA* 2002;288(4):501-507.
6. Shojania KG, Duncan BW, McDonald KM, Wachter RM: Safe but sound: Patient safety meets evidence-based medicine. *JAMA* 2002;288(4):508-513.
7. Olsen DM, Kane RL, Proctor PH: A controlled trial of multiphasic screening. *N Engl J Med* 1976;294(17):925-930.
8. Kaplan EB, Sheiner LB, Boeckmann AJ, Roizen MF, Beal SL, Cohen SN, et al: The usefulness of preoperative laboratory screening. *JAMA* 2002;253(24):3576-3581.
9. Kitz DS, Susarz-Ladden C, Lecky JH: Hospital resources used for inpatient and ambulatory surgery. *Anesthesiology* 1988;69(3):383-386.
10. Narr BJ, Hansen TR, Warner MA: Preoperative laboratory screening in healthy Mayo patients: Cost-effective elimination of tests and unchanged outcomes. *Mayo Clin Proc* 1991;66:155-159.
11. Wyatt WJ, Reed DN, Apelgran KN: Pitfalls in the role of standardized preadmission laboratory screening for ambulatory surgery. *Am Surg* 1989;55:343-346.
12. Charpak Y, Blery C, Chastang C, Szatan M, Fourgeaux B: Prospective assessment of a protocol for selective ordering of preoperative chest x-rays. *Can J Anaesth* 1988;35(3):259-264.
13. Rucker L, Frye E, Staten MA: Usefulness of screening chest roentgenograms in preoperative patients. *JAMA* 1983;250(3):3209-3211.
14. Lawrence VA, Gafni A, Gross M: The unproven utility of the preoperative urinalysis: Economic evaluation. *J Clin Epidemiol* 1989;42(12):1185-1192.
15. Novis BK, Roizen MF, Aronson S, Thisted RA: Association of preoperative risk factors with postoperative acute renal failure. *Anesth Analg* 1991;78:143-149.
16. Dzankic S, Pastor D, Gonzalez C, Leung JM: The prevalence and predictive value of abnormal laboratory tests in elderly surgical patients. *Anesth Analg* 2001;93:301-308.
17. Munro J, Booth A, Nicholl J: Routine preoperative testing: A systematic review of the evidence. *Health Technol Assessment* 1997;1(12):1-63.
18. Schein OD, Katz J, Bass EB, Telsch JM, Lubomski LH, Feldman MA, et al: The value of routine preoperative medical testing before cataract surgery. *N Engl J Med* 2000;342(3):168-175.
19. Fischer SP: Development and effectiveness of an anesthesia preoperative evaluation clinic in a teaching hospital. *Anesthesiology* 1996;85(1):196-206.
20. Pollard JB, Zboray AL, Mazze RI: Economic benefits attributed to opening a preoperative evaluation clinic for outpatients. *Anesth Analg* 1996;83:407-410.
21. Roizen MF: More preoperative assessment by physicians and less by laboratory tests. *N Engl J Med* 2000;342(3):204-205.

3 Is a Preoperative Screening Clinic Cost-Effective?

Sheila R. Barnett, MD

Each year, between 11 and 30 million dollars are spent on preoperative testing, including laboratory tests and consultations.[1,2] Currently, 80% of all surgeries are outpatient or same-day admissions, and this has resulted in the development of preoperative assessment pathways to accommodate the outpatient surgical setting.

When evaluating the need or value of a preoperative testing clinic, it is important to understand the wide range of factors involved in the preoperative process—many beyond the anesthesiologist's usual realm of practice. Once a patient is scheduled for surgery there are several steps that occur; although the particular sequence of steps for an individual patient will depend on the individual health care institution, some requirements are common to all systems. For instance, the patient will need a hospital identification number to be booked in the operating room (OR) scheduling system and insurance and demographic information verified. The patient's prior medical record will need to be obtained for the holding area or preoperative assessment clinic. If testing has been done, the results will need to be collated in the chart for the day of surgery, and, in addition, the surgical history and physical, consent forms, anesthesiology paperwork, and nursing assessment forms must be in the patient's chart before entering the OR. Additionally, the finished chart should contain all the paperwork needed for the perioperative period—order sheets, requisition forms, prescriptions, and so on.

Ideally, a cost-effective preoperative screening clinic would fulfill these duties efficiently, reducing duplication of work in other areas of the hospital, and contribute positively to OR efficiency.

OPTIONS

The preoperative screening clinic is one example of a preoperative assessment alternative; others include the telephonic interview, Internet health screen, primary care physician evaluation, and mail-in health quiz. Frequently, a visit to a preoperative clinic is combined with another tool such as the health survey, and these results are used to identify patients requiring laboratory testing or a consultation with the anesthesiologist. Since the mid-1990s, preoperative testing clinics have gained in popularity. A survey of anesthesiology programs found the presence of a preoperative testing clinic in 88% of university and 70% of community hospitals in 1998.[3] Similar results were obtained following a survey in Ontario, Canada: 63% of 260 hospitals had preoperative clinics.[4]

EVIDENCE

The Preoperative Process

The evidence supporting the implementation of preoperative testing clinics is largely derived from retrospective studies, and there are no randomized controlled trials addressing the cost of having versus not having a clinic.[5,6] Despite this, historical data suggest that the introduction of a system for preoperative testing is associated with increased patient satisfaction,[7] as well as reductions in unnecessary laboratory testing and outside consultations.[8-10] More recent data also support a reduction in day-of-surgery cancellations and OR delays and reaffirm the cost savings gained through reductions in unnecessary laboratory testing.[11-13] From these studies, it is apparent that local factors such as OR volume and type, patient mix, and even geographic considerations[14] will weigh in heavily on the decision to have or use a preoperative clinic. Evidence in areas of benefit that have been attributed to preoperative clinics will be considered individually (Table 3-1).

The most recent American College of Cardiology/American Heart Association (ACC/AHA) perioperative guidelines[14] provide recommendations for the preoperative workup in patients with significant cardiac risk factors undergoing noncardiac surgery. In this group of individuals, additional preoperative workup and testing can be beneficial. In general, patients with known coronary disease should receive a careful cardiac baseline assessment; this includes a review of current testing results and new tests as warranted by the history and physical. When older than 50 years of age, even asymptomatic patients may require careful cardiac evaluation if there are associated cardiac risk factors. The advantage of the preoperative testing clinic is the ability of the anesthesiologists to oversee the appropriate testing and consultations.

Laboratory Testing

Inappropriate laboratory testing is costly. Large-scale preoperative laboratory testing in healthy individuals leads

Table 3-1   **Cost Savings**

Author, Year	Study Type	Reduction in Laboratory Testing	Reduction in Consultations	Reduction in Same-Day Cancellations	$ Saved per Patient
Fischer, 1996[8]	Retrospective	55.1%	Yes	116 (87.9%)	112.09
Pollard, 1996[25]	Retrospective			5 (19.4%)	
Starsnic, 1997[18]	Retrospective	28.63%			20.89
Vogt, 1997[2]	Retrospective	72.5%			15.75
Finegan, 2005[17]	Prospective double cohort	Yes			29.00
Tsen, 2002[10]	Retrospective		Yes		
Ferschel, 2005[13]	Retrospective			Yes: 50%	
Cantlay, 2006[24]	Retrospective			Yes	
Hariharan, 2006[11]	Prospective			Yes: 52%	
Correll, 2006[12]	Retrospective			Improved recognition of medical problems	

to an increase in false-positive results and inappropriate workups.[5,9,15,16] Several studies in healthy patients have demonstrated that screening laboratory testing rarely provides new information that would not otherwise have been obtained from a thorough history and physical examination.[1,9,16] When compared with outside referral physicians, anesthesiologists order fewer preoperative laboratory tests,[17-19] and this may be associated with financial benefit. Starsnic and colleagues[18] examined testing patterns in two groups of patients. Each group had approximately 1500 patients; laboratory tests were ordered by either their surgeon (group S) or by an anesthesiologist seeing them in the preoperative clinic (group A), although in group A surgeons were still allowed to order additional tests if required. Except for concurrence on the complete blood count, anesthesiologists consistently ordered fewer tests compared with surgeons, resulting in a 28.6% reduction in testing and an estimated cost savings of $20.89 per patient. In a similar study, Vogt and Henson[2] found that 72% of tests ordered by surgeons were "not indicated" according to anesthesiologists, and the net cost of unindicated preoperative tests was $15.75 per patient. Fischer[8] compared a 6-month period before and after the introduction of a clinic directed by anesthesiologists and observed a 59.3% reduction in laboratory testing, or $112.09 per patient. Power and Thackray[19] report a 38% reduction in preoperative laboratory testing, leading to an estimated saving of $25.44 per patient in 201 elective ear, nose, and throat (ENT) patients following the introduction of testing guidelines that included a review by an anesthesiologist. More recently, Finegan and colleagues[17] performed a prospective double-cohort study. In group 1, testing followed usual practice according to preestablished surgery-specific clinical pathway guidelines. In contrast, testing for group 2 was instituted only through the anesthesiologist attending's or resident's recommendation. Group 1 included 507 patients with a mean preoperative laboratory cost of $124 compared with only $95 for the 431 patients in group 2 ($p < 0.05$). When a subgroup

analysis was performed, the average cost of residents' ordering was $110, similar to group 1, whereas attending physicians' cost averaged $74, approximately $36 less than residents ($p < 0.05$). Although group 2 had slightly more complications, these were not related to the preoperative tests. This study supports a reduction in unnecessary laboratory testing when directed by anesthesiologists and demonstrates that education and experience may also contribute to laboratory savings.

Despite these positive results, reductions in laboratory testing cannot all be attributed to preoperative clinics because laboratory testing can be reduced even without a preoperative clinic visit. In one of the few randomized controlled trials (RCTs) available on preoperative testing, Schein and colleagues[1] looked at preoperative testing patterns in cataract surgery patients. They randomized 18,189 patients scheduled for cataract surgery into two groups; all patients had a history and physical by a health care provider. The "testing" group received additional routine laboratory tests and an ECG. In comparison, the "no-testing" group only had tests ordered if indicated by the history and physical examination. They found no difference in outcome of patients with or without testing, and both groups had a similar rate of 31 adverse events per 1000 surgeries.

Thus, despite the dearth of RCTs, the current evidence supports anesthesiology-directed preoperative laboratory testing. This practice can result in substantial cost saving and benefit to the patient.[20,21] The positive evidence does not mean that a preoperative testing clinic is always cost-effective because it may be possible to influence testing patterns in the absence of a clinic visit. Savings in preoperative laboratory screening may be achieved by improved education of other physicians and the development of clinical pathways by anesthesiologists for surgical patients.[22]

Consultations

Cardiology consultations are a frequent source of frustration in preoperative testing and often do not result in significant alterations in management, but instead may lead to delays, additional cost, and inconvenience to the patient and hospital. Fischer[8] found that the introduction of the preoperative clinic led to a significant reduction in the number of cardiology, pulmonary, and medical consultations. Following the introduction of stringent guidelines for consultation, Tsen and colleagues[10] reduced the rate of cardiology consultations in patients undergoing noncardiac surgery from 1.46% (914 patients) to only 0.49% (279 patients) ($p < 0.0001$), despite an increase in patient acuity over the 6-year study period. They also found that, following the introduction of an ECG educational program, they were able to reduce consultations for ECG from 43.6% to 28.5% ($p < 0.0001$).

These groups were able to demonstrate that through use of preoperative testing clinics they were able to reduce consultations and cancellations and delays in surgical bookings.[8,10] In addition, their data support the development of guidelines for preoperative assessment and education for those involved in preoperative assessment.[23,24]

Defining the "role of the consultant" is important in the preoperative setting. Unfortunately, many consultations are vague and do not lead to substantial requirements for additional testing or provide new recommendations for perioperative care. All consultations should provide a careful assessment of risk, and the success of a consultation is improved when the question is specific. An additional role of the consultant should be to advise on future health and additional postoperative strategies to reduce the patient's future risk, if possible.[14]

Same-Day Cancellations

One major purported benefit of the preoperative screening clinic is a reduction in cancellations on the day of surgery. There are several reports from individual institutions describing reduction of OR cancellations following the introduction of a preoperative testing clinic, although no randomized trials on preadmission testing screening clinics have been conducted. Correll and colleagues[12] collected data on more than 5000 patients seen in their preoperative clinic over a 14-month period. In that time, 680 medical issues were identified that required further investigation before surgery; 115 of these issues were new medical problems. New problems had a greater possibility of delay (10.7%) or cancellation (6.8%) compared with existing problems (0.76% and 1.8%). In a similar study, Ferschl and colleagues[13] compared preoperative testing status between patients assigned to same-day surgery and general ORs. Over a 6-month period, 6524 patient charts were reviewed. They found that 8.4% (98 of 1164) of same-day surgery patients were cancelled if seen in clinic versus 16.5% (366 of 2252) of those not seen in clinic ($p < 0.001$). This was even more dramatic for the general OR patients; they found a cancellation rate of 5.3% for those using clinic (87 of 1631) compared with 13.0% (192 of 1477) in those not using preoperative clinic. In addition, the preoperative clinic patients were more likely to go to the OR earlier or on time compared with those in the non-preoperative clinic group. These data support the findings reported by Fischer,[8] who was able to demonstrate an 87.9% reduction in OR cancellations from 1.96% (132 of 6722) to 0.21%

(16 of 7485) after the formation of the preoperative clinic. Earlier studies have also supported reductions in both cancellations and length of stay following the introduction of a preoperative testing clinic. However, these data were collected at the same time that institutions were changing from an inpatient to an ambulatory surgery model, so the impact of the clinic per se is questionable.[25-27]

Operating room efficiency can be affected by many factors. Inadequate preoperative preparation can result in OR delays, and same-day cancellations potentially leave costly gaps in the OR schedule.[21] Fischer[8] found that 90% of cancellations occurred just before the patient entered the OR. Fischer[8] evaluated all cancellations over a 2-year period and found that, on average, a cancellation resulted in 97 minutes of OR downtime; this was in addition to the usual 30 minutes of turnover time between cases. However, frequent causes of cancellation, such as alterations in the surgeon's schedule, patient's preference, and OR scheduling limitations (i.e., cases running overtime, emergency add-ons), will not be influenced by a preoperative screening clinic.[21] It is conceivable that the preoperative screening clinic could provide a "bank" of available patients for call-up at short notice in the event of a gap in the OR schedule, but there are no data documenting the success of this approach.

Preoperative Clinic Structure

The implementation of educational programs and the development of clear guidelines and protocols can result in improved efficiency in the clinic, as well as improved communication and patient satisfaction. The staffing models of preoperative clinics may be diverse, and clinics staffed by anesthesiology attendings, residents, dedicated nurse practitioners, and nurses have been described.[7,10,28,29] The structure of a preoperative clinic may present significant opportunities for cost savings. Cantlay and colleagues[24] described improved outcomes after introducing a clinic with consultant anesthesiologists to evaluate complex vascular patients. Varughese and colleagues[28] reported significant financial benefit with the creation of a nurse practitioner–assisted preoperative evaluation clinic. At this hospital, they substituted nurse practitioners for two anesthesiology attending staff in the preoperative clinic; one attending remained assigned to the clinic for consultations. The nurse practitioners received training in preoperative assessment. Following the introduction of the nurse practitioners into the clinic, the incidence of complications, preoperative patient time, and patient satisfaction were monitored at three intervals during a 1-year period. There was no change in patient satisfaction, complication rates, or time spent in preoperative clinic. Following the substitution of the nurse practitioners in the clinic, the group was able to provide two more anesthesiologists to the OR. The increase in anesthesiologist availability resulted in significant increases in margin for the hospital and the group—by increasing billable hours for the physicians and through the addition of two new ORs, leading to increased case numbers. Clearly, the opportunity at this institution was unique; however, it provides an example of redistribution of resources resulting in a more effective preoperative clinic.

The Patient

It is possible that the savings of the outpatient preoperative clinic may in fact represent cost shifted to the patient. For instance, a visit to the preoperative screening clinic may require additional time off work for the patient or the caregiver. Similarly, geographic constraints in rural areas of the country can make the preoperative clinic visit a scheduling challenge.[21-23] Seidel and colleagues[15] examined geographic barriers to visiting the preoperative clinic and found that for patients having surgery at an urban tertiary care center, the likelihood of attending preoperative clinic visits was diminished if the patient lived farther away from the hospital.

Unexpected Area of Benefit

One value of the preoperative clinic that is underappreciated is the opportunity for compliance with various regulations. Since the institution of the Patient Self-Determination Act in 1991, all health care facilities receiving Medicare and Medicaid funding need to recognize advance directives such as a living will and durable power of attorney. Most often, this involves providing patients with a written information sheet and inquiring if they have completed the forms. The preoperative clinic visit provides an unusual opportunity for discussion, at a time when families are frequently already involved and the patient is not yet hospitalized. Grimaldo and colleagues[30] randomized elderly patients attending preoperative evaluation clinic into "standard" and "intervention" groups. The "intervention" group attended a session addressing the importance of discussing end-of-life issues and preferences with their families. They found that 87% of patients in the intervention group discussed discussions with proxies versus 66% in the control group ($p = 0.001$). This is an unexpected benefit of the preoperative clinic. To assess the impact on cost, it would be useful to compare the preoperative screening clinic cost with the cost of compliance in a nonclinic setting in terms of hospital personnel, time, and space. Additionally, in any instance in which the preoperative screening clinic may improve compliance with hospital or government regulations, the cost of the clinic may be considered a wise investment if the risk of noncompliance is substantial and carries significant consequences.

AREAS OF UNCERTAINTY

Preoperative assessment should not be viewed as synonymous with a preoperative screening clinic, and although there appear to be demonstrable benefits of a preoperative screening clinic, there are few data directly comparing the clinic model with other approaches to preoperative assessment. Shearer and colleagues[22] describe a model of preadmission testing using general practitioners in Canada. In this model, the anesthesiology department provides a workshop to "accredit" general practitioners in preoperative assessment. Patients requiring a preoperative assessment are triaged to be seen in a preoperative screening clinic by anesthesiology, to go directly to surgery, or to be seen by an accredited general practitioner for preoperative assessment. They found a low rate of cancellations

(less than 1% of elective surgery), which was not different between the groups using this system. This type of model for preoperative assessment provides an alternative to the preoperative screening clinic but reemphasizes the need for patients to undergo a preoperative evaluation of some type.

AUTHOR'S RECOMMENDATIONS

An organized approach to the preoperative assessment is clearly beneficial to the patients, physicians, and institutions, and the preoperative screening clinic is a key component. There is good evidence that anesthesiology-directed laboratory testing results in a reduction in tests and costs, and a preoperative screening clinic can result in a reduction in operating room cancellations. The ultimate organization of the preoperative assessment at a given institution will depend heavily on factors such as the hospital size, patient mix and volume, types of surgery performed, referral bases, and geographic challenges of the area. Key points include the following:

- At a minimum, preoperative laboratory testing guidelines should be directed by anesthesiology.
- When possible, standards and guidelines for preoperative testing and consultation should be produced by anesthesiology.
- A preoperative screening clinic should be established for patients undergoing invasive surgery, and complex patients who may require further evaluation or interventions before surgery.
- An anesthesiologist should be available for consultation during the preoperative visit.
- If the establishment of a preoperative screening clinic is not feasible, the anesthesiologists should be involved in creating alternative preoperative pathways or protocols (e.g., telephone screens, medical chart reviews, and so on).
- Alternative preoperative pathways, for example, primary care visits or telephone interviews, should be established for patients who cannot visit the clinic and should be coordinated by the clinic.
- A system should be in place to monitor cancellations and delays attributed to the preoperative assessment.

REFERENCES

1. Schein OD et al: The value of routine preoperative medical testing before cataract surgery. *N Engl J Med* 2000;342:168-175.
2. Vogt AW, Henson LC: Unindicated preoperative testing: ASA physical status and financial implications. *J Clin Anesth* 1997;9:437-441.
3. Tsen LC, Segal S, Pothier M, Bader AM: Survey of residency training in preoperative evaluation. *Anesthesiology* 2000;93:1134-1137.
4. Bond D: Preanesthestic assessment clinics in Ontario. *Can J Anesth* 1999;46(4):382-387.
5. Matthews D, Klewicka M, Kopman A, Neuman G: Patterns and costs of preoperative testing: Preop clinic vs. outside testing. ASA 2001 meeting abstract.
6. Roizen M: Preoperative patient evaluation. *Can J Anesth* 1989;36:513-519.
7. Hepner DL, Bader AM, Hurwitz S, Gustafson M, Tsen LC: Patient satisfaction with a preoperative assessment in a preoperative assessment testing clinic. *Anesth Analg* 2004;98:1099-1105.
8. Fischer SP: Development and effectiveness of an anesthesia preoperative evaluation clinic in a teaching hospital. *Anesthesiology* 1996;85:196-206.

9. Roizen MF: The compelling rationale for less preoperative testing. *Can J Anesth* 1998;35:214-218.

10. Tsen LC, Segal S, Pothier M, Hartley LH, Bader AM: The effect of alterations in a preoperative assessment clinic on reducing the number and improving the yield of cardiology consultations. *Anesth Analg* 2002;95:1563-1568.

11. Harihan S, Chen D, Merritt-Charles L: Evaluation of the utilization of the preanesthesia clinics in a university teaching hospital. *BMC Health Services Research* 2006;6:59.

12. Correll DJ, Bader AM, Hull MW, Hsu C, Tsen LC, Hepner DL: Value of preoperative clinic visits in identifying issues with potential impact on operating room efficiency. *Anesthesiology* 2006;105:1254-1259.

13. Ferschl MB, Tung A, Sweitzer BJ, Huo D, Glick DB: Preoperative clinic visits reduce operating room cancellations and delays. *Anesthesiology* 2005;103:855-859.

14. Fleisher LA, Beckman JA, Brown LA, Calkins H, Chaikof E, et al: ACC/AHA 2007 guidelines on perioperative cardiovascular evaluation and care for non cardiac surgery (task force). *Circulation* 2007;116:e418-e499.

15. Seidel JE, Beck CA, Pocobelli G, Lemaire JB, Bugar JB, Quain H, Ghali WA: Location of residence associated with the likelihood of patient visit to the preoperative assessment clinic. *BMC Health Services Research* 2006;6:13.

16. Narr BJ: Outcomes of patients with no laboratory assessment before anesthesia and a surgical procedure. *Mayo Clinic Proc* 1997;72:505-509.

17. Finegan BA, Rashiq S, McAllister FA, O'Connor P: Selective ordering of preoperative investigations by anesthesiologists reduces the number and cost of tests. *Can J Anesth* 2005;52 (6):575-580.

18. Starsnic MA, Guarnieri DM, Norris MC: Efficacy and financial benefit of an anesthesiologist-directed university preadmission evaluation center. *J Clin Anesthesiol* 1997;9:299-305.

19. Power LM, Thackray NM: Reduction of preoperative investigations with the introduction of an anesthetist led preoperative assessment clinic. *Anaesth Intensive Care* 1999;27:481-488.

20. Boothe P, Finnegan BA: Changing the admission process for elective surgery: An economic analysis. *Can J Anaesth* 1995;42:391-394.

21. Holt NF, Silverman DG, Prasad R, Dziura J, Ruskin KJ: Preanesthesia clinics, information management, and operating room delays: Results of a survey of practicing anesthesiologists. *Anesth Analg* 2007;104:615-618.

22. Shearer W, Monagel J, Michaels M: A model of community based, preadmission management for elective surgical patients. *Can J Anesth* 1997;44(12):1311-1314.

23. Cheung A, Finegan BA, Torok-Both C, Donnelly Warner N, Lujic J: A patient information booklet about anesthesiology improves preoperative patient education. *Can J Anesth* 2007;54:355-360.

24. Cantlay KL, Baker S, Parry A, Danjoux G: The impact of a consultant anesthetist led pre-operative assessment clinic on patients undergoing major vascular surgery. *Anaesthesia* 2006;61:234-239.

25. Pollard JB, Zboray AL, Mazze RI: Economic benefits attributed to opening a preoperative evaluation clinic for outpatients. *Anesth Analg* 1996;83:407-410.

26. Pollard JB, Garnerin PH, Dalman RL: Use of outpatient preoperative evaluation to decrease length of stay for vascular surgery. *Anesth Analg* 1997;85:1307-1311.

27. Pollard JB, Olson L: Early outpatient preoperative anesthesia assessment: Does it help to reduce operating room cancellations? *Anesth Analg* 1999;89:502-505.

28. Varughese AM, Byczkowski TL, Wittkugel EP, Kotagal U, Kurth CD: Impact of a nurse practitioner assisted preoperative assessment program on quality. *Pediatr Anesth* 2006;16:723-733.

29. Kirkwood BJ, Pesudovos K, Coster DJ: The efficacy of a nurse led preoperative cataract assessment ad postoperative care clinic. *MJA* 2006;184:278-281.

30. Grimaldo DA, Wiener-Kronish JP, Jurson T, Shaughnessy TE, Curtis JR, Liu L: A randomized, controlled trial of advance planning discussions during preoperative evaluation. *Anesthesiology* 2001;95:43-50.

4 Who Should Have a Preoperative 12-Lead Electrocardiogram?

Barbara S. Gold, MD

INTRODUCTION

The utility of the preoperative electrocardiogram (ECG) has been under scrutiny for over two decades because of the volume of patients affected, as well as the associated medical and financial implications. During this period of time, the indications for the preoperative ECG have been refined as our understanding of the relationship between preoperative testing, patient selection, and the surgical procedure have evolved. In the United States, approximately 40 million surgical procedures are performed annually and roughly half of those patients are older than age 45.[1] Using conservative criteria, many of those patients would be considered for a preoperative ECG, yet there is no absolute consensus on who should actually have a preoperative ECG. Rather, there are general guidelines from several medical societies based on decades of clinical studies and observations. The aim of this chapter is to summarize the data that form the foundation for widely accepted recommendations and then to highlight relevant guidelines.

OPTIONS

As a diagnostic tool for assessing perioperative cardiovascular risk, the 12-lead ECG is limited. Because of the inherent limitations of the test's sensitivity and specificity, its usefulness depends on the population tested: populations with a higher prevalence or likelihood of cardiovascular disease are more likely to have abnormal ECGs. Our challenge is to determine which patients need a preoperative ECG because of the potential to affect their perioperative course. Among the ECG abnormalities that can significantly alter perioperative care are arrhythmias, heart block, ST-segment abnormalities consistent with ischemia, left ventricular hypertrophy (LVH), low voltage consistent with cardiomyopathy, previous myocardial infarction, Wolff-Parkinson-White syndrome, prolonged QT interval, or peaked T-waves. Many, but not all, of these abnormalities can be detected on standard ECG monitoring in the operating room before induction of anesthesia, albeit with potential impact on operating room scheduling.

Although the 12-lead ECG may detect significant abnormalities, its usefulness as a screening tool is quite limited. For example, the resting ECG is normal in approximately half of patients with chronic stable angina.[2] Conversely, even in healthy persons it has poor predictive value for heart disease. In a meta-analysis of long-term survival of patients who had a resting ECG, Sox and colleagues[3] concluded that there were insufficient data to support using the ECG as a screen for coronary artery disease (CAD) in asymptomatic persons or those without the following risk factors: diabetes, hypertension, hypercholesterolemia, or history of tobacco use. These findings are echoed in subsequent studies of surgical patients. However, when abnormalities suggestive of CAD appear, they are associated with a higher risk of coronary events and death.[4]

In summary, even though the resting 12-lead ECG is an imperfect tool, it has tremendous potential to detect disease that will affect perioperative care in selected patients. The potential of the preoperative ECG can be exploited if it is obtained in populations with a relatively high likelihood of cardiac disease.

EVIDENCE

Evidence to support the indications for the preoperative ECG is imperfect because study designs are variable and investigators examine different endpoints. Some studies ask how a preoperative ECG can prevent morbidity and mortality; others look for the incidence of abnormal ECGs; some ask whether a preoperative ECG resulted in an anesthetic intervention; still others look at abnormal ECGs resulting in case cancellation. Many studies are based on the premise that if a preoperative test were truly useful, it would have changed management. Therefore if, from chart review, management was not changed, the test was of questionable value. Most studies are retrospective or examine cohorts prospectively, without an intervention. Significantly, it is impossible to tell from any of the studies if the reading on the preoperative ECG subtly affected the anesthetic plan and hence the cardiovascular outcome. In addition, populations studied are vastly different in the risk profile and type of surgical procedures. Nevertheless, general principles emerge. We will examine the evidence to support obtaining a preoperative ECG in the following patient populations: asymptomatic patients, patients with cardiovascular risk factors, those of advanced age, and patients having "major" versus less invasive surgery.

Asymptomatic Patients

Circumstantial data have accumulated over the years refuting the utility of the preoperative ECG in asymptomatic patients undergoing elective, nonvascular procedures. Perez and colleagues[5] retrospectively studied 3131 ASA 1 and 2 patients of whom 2406 had an ECG (criteria not specified). Of those ECGs, 5.6% were unexpectedly abnormal and management was apparently altered in only 0.5% of patients. In a retrospective study of 2570 patients having elective cholecystectomy, Turnbull and Buck[6] found 101 abnormal ECGs, without any apparent impact on management. Goldberger and O'Konski,[7] in their review of the utility of "routine" preoperative ECG, found no evidence to support the "baseline" ECG in asymptomatic patients. However, the value of obtaining a baseline ECG in selected patients without evidence of cardiac disease was left to question. These relatively small observational studies should be interpreted with caution because the operative procedures were low to intermediate risk, and the findings on the preoperative ECG may have subtly influenced management, including the decision to proceed with surgery.

Epidemiologic data regarding incidence and prognosis of unrecognized myocardial infarction are the basis for the recommendation to obtain ECGs in asymptomatic patients.[8] The Framingham Study, begun in 1948, followed patients for 30 years with cardiovascular examination, including ECGs, every 2 years. Of all infarctions, 25% were detected only by new ECG findings and almost half of those new infarctions were "silent." These unrecognized infarctions were just as likely to cause serious cardiovascular sequelae as recognized infarctions. The incidence of both recognized and unrecognized infarctions increased dramatically after age 45 in men and 55 in women.

Risk Factors

Although patients are asymptomatic, they may have several cardiovascular (CV) risk factors, such as ischemic heart disease, diabetes, congestive heart failure, cerebral vascular disease, and renal insufficiency. Several studies, most of them within the past two decades, have correlated preoperative ECG abnormalities and CV risk factors. (Bear in mind that there is variance in the number and type of risk factors evaluated in most studies.) Tait and colleagues[9] retrospectively evaluated the efficacy of the routine preoperative ECG in 1000 ASA class 1 and 2 patients, including men older than age 40 years and women older than 50 years, or any patient with a history of CV risk factors or disease. About half of patients with CV risk factors had an abnormal ECG compared with 26% of patients without risk factors. However, in this small sample size, there was no difference in the prevalence of adverse perioperative CV events between groups. In another study examining CV risk factors and preoperative ECG abnormalities, of 354 patients who were to have a "routine" preoperative ECG, the ECG was abnormal in 62% of patients with known cardiac disease and 44% of patients with CV risk factors. Notably, only 7% of patients over 50 years old without cardiac disease or risk factors had ECG abnormalities.[10]

The presence of CV risk factors not only increases the likelihood of preoperative ECG abnormalities but also of adverse outcomes. Hollenberg and colleagues[11] used continuous 12-lead ECG monitoring preoperatively, intraoperatively, and postoperatively to identify predictors of postoperative myocardial ischemia. In this study of 474 men with or at risk for CAD, five major risk predictors were identified: left ventricular hypertrophy (LVH) by ECG, history of hypertension, diabetes mellitus, definite history of CAD, and use of digoxin. The risk of postoperative myocardial ischemia increased with the number of risk factors. For example, 22% of patients with none of those predictors had postoperative myocardial ischemia, increasing steadily to 77% with four predictors. To underscore the importance of the preoperative history and physical examination, of these five reported predictors, four are easily discernible by history and only one (LVH) by preoperative ECG.

Noordzij and colleagues[12] examined the value of the preoperative ECG in a large sample size (greater than 23,000 patients) to predict cardiovascular death. Not surprisingly, patients with abnormal ECG findings had a higher incidence of cardiovascular death (OR 4.5, CI 3.3 to 6.0). However, the invasiveness of the procedure was critical. Among patients undergoing low- or intermediate-risk surgery, the absolute difference in the incidence of cardiovascular death was only 0.5%.[12]

More recently, van Klei and colleagues[13] investigated records from almost 3000 noncardiac surgery patients. These investigators found that the preoperative ECG did not add value in the prediction of postoperative myocardial infarction when compared with clinical risk factors such as high-risk surgery, history of ischemic heart disease, history of congestive heart failure, renal failure, cerebrovascular accident, or insulin-dependent diabetes.[13]

In conclusion, if the goal is to detect ECG abnormalities preoperatively with the belief that this knowledge will positively affect perioperative management, it makes sense to obtain a preoperative ECG on persons at risk for heart disease. Potentially high-risk patients include those with known cardiac disease, diabetes, vascular disease, valvular disease, low functional capacity, and arrhythmias.

Age and the Preoperative Electrocardiogram

What age is considered advanced enough to warrant a preoperative ECG?

In a synthesis of four studies, Goldberger and O'Konski[7] reported that ECG abnormalities increase exponentially with age ($r = 0.99$). From these pooled data of men and women, 10% of patients aged 35 years are predicted to have an abnormal ECG, increasing to 25% by age 57 years. In a study of ambulatory surgery patients, all of whom had preoperative ECGs if they were older than 40 years, the odds of an abnormal ECG were significantly greater in the group aged 60 and older.[14] The strong relation between age and ECG abnormalities is hardly surprising given the substantial evidence correlating advancing age with cardiac disease, especially CAD.[4,8,12,15-17] The landmark study by Diamond and Forrester[15] analyzed autopsy data from 23,996 persons to determine the prevalence of CAD (Table 4-1).

Table 4-1	Autopsy Data Used to Determine the Prevalence of CAD	
Age (Years)	**Men (%)**	**Women (%)**
40–49	5	1.5
50–59	10	3
60–69	12	8

Adapted from Diamond GA, Forrester JS: Analysis of probability as an aid in the clinical diagnosis of coronary artery disease. *N Engl J Med* 1979;300: 1350-1358.

In spite of a documented correlation between CAD and age, published recommendations vary; consequently, there is tremendous latitude. The American College of Cardiology/American Heart Association (ACC/AHA) "Guidelines for Electrocardiography"[18] note that ECG abnormalities increase exponentially with age and their consensus is that patients older than 40 years with no apparent heart disease have a preoperative ECG. Roizen[19] has pooled data on age and ECG abnormalities and has stratified by age-groups. Based on at least 16 studies, and pooling both genders, the incidence of abnormalities on screening ECG exceeds 10% at 40 years of age and is approximately 25% by 60 years of age. Based on these data, screening ECGs were also recommended on men older than age 40 years and women older than age 50 years, for all moderately to highly invasive procedures. However, recent guidelines from ACC/AHA are silent on the need for a preoperative ECG based on age alone. As will be discussed, the predisposing risk factors and operative procedures are key elements in the decision to obtain a preoperative ECG.

Surgical Procedure

Several studies have demonstrated that cardiovascular risk correlates with the complexity of the surgery.[12,20-23] For example, in one study of 1487 elderly males, those having vascular surgery were more than three times as likely to have a postoperative myocardial infarction (PMI) as patients having nonvascular surgery.[21] Another study of 7306 patients found that "major surgery" (i.e., laparotomy, thyroidectomy, internal fixation of major fractures) increased the odds of a cardiopulmonary complication by fourfold to sixfold.[20] Consequently, recommendations for obtaining a preoperative ECG need to consider the type of procedure in addition to patient age, history, and risk factors. This is reflected in recommendations by both the AHA/ACC and the American Society of Anesthesiologists (ASA).

GUIDELINES

Because the decision to order preoperative ECGs affects a large population at considerable cost and potential benefit, there has been no shortage of recommendations from numerous medical societies on this issue. Following is a summary of two relevant recommendations from leading medical societies. Bear in mind that these guidelines are typically updated every 5 years.

ASA Practice Advisory for Preanesthesia Evaluation

The ASA published the "Practice Advisory for Preanesthesia Evaluation" in 2002,[24] which does not recommend a minimum age for obtaining a preoperative ECG. Specifically, the advisory states that age alone may not be an indication for testing. Important clinical characteristics to consider when deciding to order a preoperative ECG include cardiocirculatory disease, respiratory disease, type or invasiveness of surgery, and risk factors identified in the course of a preanesthesia evaluation.

ACC/AHA Guidelines

The American College of Cardiology and the American Heart Association first published guidelines for perioperative cardiovascular evaluation in 1996, updated them in 2002,[25] and most recently in 2007.[26] The 2007 guidelines emphasize (1) the level of evidence to support a recommendation, (2) how the test will change clinical management, and (3) the invasiveness of the procedure. Notably, the guidelines are silent on age and preoperative ECG testing.

Familiarity with the text is highly recommended to put guidelines into context. Recommendations are based on risk/benefit ratio in which Class I indicates that benefit greatly outweighs risk; Class IIa indicates that benefit is greater than risk, but additional focused studies are needed ("It is reasonable to perform procedure"); Class IIb indicates that benefits are equal to or greater than risks ("Procedure may be considered"); and Class III indicates that risks are greater than benefits and procedure is not indicated. Each of these risk/benefit classes is then paired with the amount of evidence that supports the conclusion, in which level A is the highest level of evidence (3 to 5 population strata evaluated) and C is the lowest. With respect to the preoperative ECG, the ACC/AHA recommendations, based on levels of evidence, are summarized as follows:

Class I

(Benefits greatly outweigh risks; ECG should be performed preoperatively)

- Patients undergoing vascular surgical procedures with at least one clinical risk factor
- Patients with known coronary, peripheral or cerebrovascular disease undergoing an intermediate-risk surgical procedure (e.g., head and neck surgery)

Class IIa

(Reasonable to consider)

- Patients without clinical risk factors undergoing vascular procedures

Class IIb

(May be reasonable to consider)

- Patients with at least one clinical risk factor undergoing intermediate-risk surgery

Class III

(Not indicated)

- Asymptomatic patients undergoing low-risk operative procedures

Bear in mind that each of these recommendations is qualified by the available evidence to support the recommendation and that "the ultimate judgment regarding care of a particular patient must be made by the healthcare provider and patient in light of all the circumstances."[26]

AUTHOR'S RECOMMENDATIONS

The author's recommendations are based on available evidence and synthesis of opinions and data; they are not clinical guidelines, nor do they represent consensus opinion. In general, the preoperative ECG should be considered in patients in whom there is a reasonably high likelihood of cardiac dysfunction, in which the test has the potential, in the judgment of the anesthesiologist, of affecting perioperative management. The patient's history, physical examination, and proposed surgical procedure are essential elements in this assessment.

A preoperative ECG should be considered in the following groups of patients:

- Asymptomatic patients or those with cardiovascular risk factors undergoing vascular surgery.
- Patients with one or more cardiovascular risk factor undergoing intermediate-risk procedures (e.g., orthopedic procedures, head and neck surgery, prostate surgery)
- Patients with known coronary, peripheral vascular, or cerebral vascular disease having an intermediate-risk procedure
- Patients with low (or unknown) functional capacity undergoing an intermediate-risk procedure
- Any patient in whom the results of the preoperative ECG will affect clinical management

REFERENCES

1. Owings MF, Kozak LJ: Ambulatory and inpatient procedures in the United States, 1996. National Center for Health Statistics. *Vital Health Statistics* 1998;13(139).
2. Zipes et al: *Braunwald's heart disease*, ed 7. Philadelphia, WB Saunders, 2005, Chapter 50, p 1277.
3. Sox HC, Garber AM, et al: The resting electrocardiogram as a screening test. *Ann Intern Med* 1989;111:489-502.
4. Tervahauta M, Pekkanen J: Resting electrocardiographic abnormalities as predictors of coronary events and total mortality among elderly men. *Am J Med* 1996;100:641-645.
5. Perez A, Planell J, et al: Value of routine preoperative tests: A multicentre study in four general hospitals. *Br J Anaesth* 1995;74:250-256.
6. Turnbull JM, Buck C: The value of preoperative screening investigations in otherwise healthy individuals. *Arch Intern Med* 1987;147:1101-1105.
7. Goldberger AL, O'Konski M: Utility of the routine electrocardiogram before surgery and on general hospital admission. *Ann Intern Med* 1986;105:552-557.
8. Kannel WB, Abbott RD: Incidence and prognosis of unrecognized myocardial infarction: An update on the Framingham study. *N Engl J Med* 1984;311:1144-1147.
9. Tait AR, Parr HG, et al: Evaluation of the efficacy of routine preoperative electrocardiograms. *J Cardiothorac Vasc Anesth* 1997;11(6):752-755.
10. Callaghan LC, Edwards ND, et al: Utilization of the pre-operative ECG. *Anaesthesia* 1995;50:488-490.
11. Hollenberg M, Mangano DT, et al: Predictors of postoperative myocardial ischemia in patients undergoing noncardiac surgery. *JAMA* 1992;268:205-209.
12. Noordzij PG, Boersma E, et al: Prognostic value of routine preoperative electrocardiography in patients undergoing noncardiac surgery. *Am J Cardiol* 2006;97:1103-1106.
13. van Klei WA et al: The value of routine preoperative electrocardiography in predicting myocardial infarction after noncardiac surgery. *Ann Surg* 2007;246:165-170.
14. Gold BS, Young ML, et al: The utility of preoperative electrocardiograms in the ambulatory surgical patient. *Arch Intern Med* 1992;152(2):301-305.
15. Diamond GA, Forrester JS: Analysis of probability as an aid in the clinical diagnosis of coronary artery disease. *N Engl J Med* 1979;300:1350-1358.
16. Kreger BE, Cupples LA, et al: The electrocardiogram in prediction of sudden death: Framingham study experience. *Am Heart J* 1987;113:377-382.
17. Nadelmann J, Frishman WH, et al: Prevalence, incidence and prognosis of recognized and unrecognized myocardial infarction in persons aged 75 years or older: The Bronx aging study. *Am J Cardiol* 1990;66(5):533-537.
18. Guidelines for electrocardiography. A report of the American College of Cardiology/American Heart Association Task Force on Assessment of Diagnostic and Therapeutic Cardiovascular Procedures (ACC/AHA). *JACC* 1992;19:473-481.
19. Roizen MF: Preoperative evaluation. In Miller RD, editor: *Anesthesia*, ed 6. Philadelphia, Churchill Livingstone, 2005, pp 951-954.
20. Pedersen T, Eliasen K, et al: A prospective study of risk factors and cardiopulmonary complications associated with anaesthesia and surgery: Risk indicators of cardiopulmonary morbidity. *Acta Anaesthesiol Scand* 1990;34:144-155.
21. Ashton CM, Petersen MS, et al: The incidence of perioperative myocardial infarction in men undergoing noncardiac surgery. *Ann Intern Med* 1993;118:504-510.
22. Kumar R, McKinney P, et al: Adverse cardiac events after surgery. *J Gen Intern Med* 2001;16:507-518.
23. Muir AD, Reeder MK, et al: Preoperative silent myocardial ischaemia: Incidence and predictors in a general surgical population. *Br J Anaesth* 1991;676:373-377.
24. Practice advisory for preanesthesia evaluation. *Anesthesiology* 2002;96:485-496.
25. Eagle KA, Berger PB, et al: ACC/AHA guideline update for perioperative cardiovascular evaluation for noncardiac surgery. *Circulation* 2002;105:1257-1267.
26. Fleisher LA: ACC/AHA 2007 guidelines on perioperative cardiovascular evaluation and care for noncardiac surgery: Executive summary. *Circulation* 2007;116:1971-1996.

5 Should Preoperative Hemoglobin Always Be Obtained?

Bradly J. Narr, MD, and Daniel R. Brown, MD, PhD

INTRODUCTION

Laboratory testing is part of perioperative patient evaluation. One of the most common tests performed is determination of venous hemoglobin concentration. The rationale for all preoperative testing has been based more on tradition than formal evidence.[1] However, testing guided by an anesthesiologist has been found to improve efficiency.[2]

To justify a "routine" test, the results of such a test should detect unsuspected abnormalities that can be modified, help identify conditions that may alter the risk of surgery, or serve as baseline results that will influence perioperative interventions.

A role of the anesthesia provider is to ensure that vital organs receive enough oxygen to meet metabolic demands throughout the entire procedure. The determinants of oxygen transport include pulmonary gas exchange, hemoglobin-oxygen affinity, total hemoglobin concentration, and cardiac output. As with all of the organ systems in the body, there is significant reserve capacity in the oxygen transport system of the normal individual. The system is regulated in such a way that an alteration in one component (decreased hemoglobin) results in changes in other components (increased cardiac output, increased red cell 2,3, biphosphoglycerate) to maintain oxygen delivery and homeostasis. Of the components of this system, the hemoglobin concentration has the greatest ability to be manipulated to augment oxygen transport. This understanding has always made anesthesiologists very interested in the preoperative hemoglobin concentration.

Preoperative hemoglobin levels predict the need for intraoperative blood transfusion.[3-5] Low hemoglobin levels are associated with increased perioperative morbidity in surgical patients,[6] longer recovery from procedures that involve blood loss,[7] and a higher likelihood of postoperative infection.[8] To decrease perioperative morbidity and optimally assist patients in understanding the risks and benefits of many procedures, the preoperative hemoglobin is useful.

THERAPIES

The hemoglobin concentration can be altered by blood transfusion or bone marrow stimulation, most commonly with recombinant erythropoietin. Red blood cell transfusion has attendant risks, including infection (viral and bacterial), immune modulation, and, in some circumstances, intravascular volume overload. Recombinant erythropoietin can be used before elective surgery with significant blood loss and has been shown in randomized prospective trials to result in higher postoperative hemoglobin levels and to decrease homologous transfusion.[9,10] However, recent studies in critically ill patients have shown that erythropoietin does not reduce overall red cell transfusion and this treatment is associated with an increased incidence of thrombotic events.[11]

EVIDENCE

No randomized prospective studies involving patients with anticipated blood loss have defined a specific minimum hemoglobin concentration as a risk factor for anesthesia and surgery. Modern anesthetic practice evolved to require hemoglobin of 10 g/dL before anesthesia and surgery from anecdotal case series and cohort studies. Older studies have implied that severe levels of preoperative anemia may be a factor for perioperative morbidity and mortality risk.[12-14] These studies were performed when anesthetic mortality risks were significantly higher than expected with modern practice. With the advent of dialysis in the 1960s, renal failure patients who were severely anemic were found to tolerate anesthesia and surgery well.[15] This was added to evidence that patients who refused blood transfusion tolerated normovolemic anemia, surgery, and anesthesia well and caused a reassessment of the "10 g/dL" rule.

The prevalence of preoperative hemoglobin concentration abnormalities has been studied in many different surgical populations. The incidence of abnormalities varies with how the abnormality is defined and the population studied. Table 5-1 summarizes several studies. Prospective studies have shown that screening baseline hemoglobin for surgeries that do not involve significant blood loss predicts no adverse outcome or specific perioperative risk.[16-18] A prospective consecutive case study in 395 hip fracture patients older than age 65 showed that patients with anemia on admission to the hospital have a lower functional status, longer hospital stays, and a higher mortality rate at 6 and 12 months after the fracture.[19] As noted previously, retrospective studies from the 1970s showed that mortality rates increased as hemoglobin levels decreased.[14] This has recently been

Year	Study Type	Surgical Population	N	% Abnormal	Outcomes
2007[20]	Retrospective cohort	Noncardiac surgery	310,311	Anemia: 42.8 Polycythemia: 0.2	30-day mortality rate and cardiac events increased with positive or negative deviations from normal hemoglobin levels; 1.6% increase in 30-day mortality rate with every percentage point increase or decrease in hematocrit level from normal range
2001[17]	Consecutive cohort	Noncardiac surgery	544	10	No prediction for cardiovascular, pulmonary, renal, hepatic, neurologic, surgical difficulty, reoperation, or death
2000[18]	Randomized prospective	Cataract	19,557	5.9	No difference in intraoperative or postoperative cardiovascular, cerebrovascular, pulmonary, or metabolic events
1989[33]	Retrospective	Hip replacement	86	4	Baseline useful for transfusion decisions; no effect on hospital course
1988[34]	Consecutive cohort	Ambulatory surgery	212	9	No cancellations, complications, or admissions to hospital
1987[35]	Prospective	Major and minor surgery with suspected hemoglobin abnormality	2138	32	Useful 22% of the time to transfuse red blood cells (RBCs) after minor perioperative blood loss in anemic patient or moderate perioperative blood loss not followed by RBC transfusion in patient with normal hemoglobin

Table 5-1 Hemoglobin Abnormalities

corroborated in a very large retrospective cohort study of elderly patients having noncardiac surgery looking at the adverse effects of preoperative anemia or polycythemia in more than 300,000 patients older than age 65 years.[20] In this study, 30-day mortality rate and adverse cardiac events increased monotonically with hemoglobin levels below 39% or in excess of 51%. Prospective data from the National Surgical Quality Improvement Program included more than 6000 noncardiac surgical patients; 39% of patients in this study had a preoperative hematocrit of less than 36%.[8] During the perioperative period the subgroup that had preoperative anemia required five times more blood than nonanemic patients. This study also documented that transfusion of more than 4 units of blood increased the risk of death.

Evidence That Preoperative Hemoglobin Predicts Transfusion Risk

The best evidence documenting the utility of preoperative hemoglobin regards perioperative transfusion. Approximately two thirds of all transfusions occur in the perioperative period, with a majority of these being given by anesthesia providers during the procedure.[15] Despite efforts to base all interventions on evidence, the decision to treat anemia in the surgical setting is difficult.[3]

Consideration of the physiologic consequences of anemia combined with the specific procedure and proceduralist help determine the transfusion threshold. It is important to remember that Hebert and colleagues'[21] study on transfusion and outcomes in critically ill patients excluded actively bleeding patients, and thus the applicability of this and similar studies advocating lower transfusion thresholds in operative patients is not clear. Although the indications for transfusion are debatable,

several studies suggest that the preoperative hemoglobin concentration predicts transfusion practice in cases associated with major blood loss.[8,22-26] Consequently, determination of preoperative hemoglobin concentration in cases associated with major blood loss helps determine perioperative transfusion risk and is needed to estimate the blood loss required before blood transfusion may be indicated.

AREAS OF UNCERTAINTY

The advent of recombinant erythropoietin has allowed for a means to endogenously increase preoperative hemoglobin, and advocates of this therapy suggest routine preoperative hemoglobin determination for every patient undergoing surgery associated with major blood loss.[24] Faris and colleagues[24] modeled data from two randomized double-blind placebo-controlled studies of 276 orthopedic patients assessing erythropoietin therapy to increase perioperative hemoglobin in patients having major orthopedic procedures. Patients treated with erythropoietin with hemoglobin greater than 10 to less than or equal to 13 g/dL had a significantly reduced transfusion risk compared with placebo patients. In patients with a hemoglobin greater than 13 g/dL, no significant benefit was observed. No data were reported in patients with hemoglobin less than 10 g/dL. A study in orthopedic patients undergoing elective joint arthroplasty showed that preoperative administration of erythropoietin significantly increased preoperative hemoglobin concentration and decreased blood transfusions compared with matched controls.[9] In addition, this practice has been determined to be as effective and safe as autologous preoperative blood donation.[10]

Despite these studies, several areas of uncertainty have limited widespread adoption of this practice. The preoperative hemoglobin concentration that warrants erythropoietin therapy, the dose and duration of therapy, and the cost and risk/benefit ratio between erythropoietin and conventional transfusion therapy are unknown. The risk of thrombosis may also increase with this therapy.[11]

Human studies have documented that rapid induction of isovolemic anemia is not associated with severe morbidity in the short term in healthy people. Studies have looked at rapid reductions in hemoglobin from normal to approximately 5 g/dL. Asymptomatic electrocardiographic changes of the ST segments suggesting myocardial ischemia occurred in 3 of 55 individuals.[27] Using the same model, formal psychometrics were performed at baseline and after isovolemic anemia at hemoglobins of 7, 6, and 5 g/dL. Immediate and delayed memory were degraded at the lowest hemoglobin levels, and reaction times were altered at hemoglobin levels less than 6 g/dL.[28] High levels of oxygen reversed these deficits,[29] but a nitrous oxide, fentanyl, and isoflurane anesthetic has been shown to significantly decrease the cardiac output response associated with acute normovolemic anemia.[30] Intraoperative anemia has also been a risk factor for ischemic optic neuropathy in adult cardiac surgery patients.[31] These studies show the uncertainty in the short- and long-term effects of isovolemic anemia. It is likely that specific procedures and patient-specific factors will determine minimum acceptable hemoglobin concentrations. Further studies are required to gain insight into this problem.

GUIDELINES AND AUTHORS' RECOMMENDATIONS

- Randomized prospective studies in patients having elective surgery without significant blood loss do not show that a preoperative hemoglobin predicts any adverse outcome.
- No routine laboratory tests are necessary for preanesthetic evaluation[32]; however, anesthesiologists should order tests when results may influence risks and management of anesthesia and surgery.[33-36] (Invasiveness of the procedure, liver disease, extremes of age or hematologic disorders should be considered as indications for preoperative hemoglobin levels.)
- Baseline hemoglobin level is a predictor of blood transfusion in those procedures involving significant blood loss.
- Although moderate isovolemic anemia is well tolerated in patients with cardiorespiratory reserve, there are limits to the degree of anemia that is tolerated without symptoms or sequelae. A baseline hemoglobin determination may be of use to guide therapy when employing hemodilution techniques.
- Patients with significant cardiac and or pulmonary disease will have a limited tolerance for perioperative anemia. The decision for perioperative transfusion should be based on preoperative hemoglobin concentration, anticipated blood loss, and cardiorespiratory status.
- Further studies are needed to determine the role of erythropoietin administration before elective procedures associated with significant blood loss and the minimum acceptable hemoglobin concentration for a given patient undergoing a given procedure.

REFERENCES

1. Bryson GL: Has preoperative testing become a habit? *Can J Anaesth* 2005;52:557-561.
2. Finegan BA, Rashiq S, McAlister FA, O'Connor P: Selective ordering of preoperative investigations by anesthesiologists reduces the number and cost of tests. *Can J Anaesth* 2005;52:575-580.
3. Gombotz H, Rehak PH, Shander A, Hofmann A: Blood use in elective surgery: The Austrian benchmark study. *Transfusion* 2007;47:1468-1480.
4. Guerin S, Collins C, Kapoor H, et al: Blood transfusion requirement prediction in patients undergoing primary total hip and knee arthroplasty. *Transfus Med* 2007;17:37-43.
5. Karkouti K, O'Farrell R, Yau TM, Beattie WS: Prediction of massive blood transfusion in cardiac surgery. *Can J Anaesth* 2006;53:781-794.
6. Kuriyan M, Carson JL: Anemia and clinical outcomes. *Anesthesiol Clin North Am* 2005;23:315-325, vii.
7. Carson JL, Terrin ML, Jay M: Anemia and postoperative rehabilitation. *Can J Anaesth* 2003;50:S60-S64.
8. Dunne JR, Malone D, Tracy JK, et al: Perioperative anemia: An independent risk factor for infection, mortality, and resource utilization in surgery. *J Surg Res* 2002;102:237-244.
9. Rauh MA, Bayers-Thering M, LaButti RS, Krackow KA: Preoperative administration of epoetin alfa to total joint arthroplasty patients. *Orthopedics* 2002;25:317-320.
10. Deutsch A, Spaulding J, Marcus RE: Preoperative epoetin alfa vs autologous blood donation in primary total knee arthroplasty. *J Arthroplasty* 2006;21:628-635.
11. Corwin HL, Gettinger A, Fabian TC, et al: Efficacy and safety of epoetin alfa in critically ill patients. *N Engl J Med* 2007;357:965-976.
12. Carson JL, Poses RM, Spence RK, Bonavita G: Severity of anaemia and operative mortality and morbidity. *Lancet* 1988;1:727-729.
13. Adams RC, Lundy JS: Anesthesia in cases of poor surgical risk. Some suggestions for decreasing the risk. *Surg Gynecol Obstet* 1942;74:1011-1019.
14. Lunn JN, Elwood PC: Anaemia and surgery. *BMJ* 1970;3:71-73.
15. Consensus conference. Perioperative red blood cell transfusion. *JAMA* 1988;260:2700-2703.
16. Olson RP, Stone A, Lubarsky D: The prevalence and significance of low preoperative hemoglobin in ASA 1 or 2 outpatient surgery candidates. *Anesth Analg* 2005;101:1337-1340.
17. Dzankic S, Pastor D, Gonzalez C, Leung JM: The prevalence and predictive value of abnormal preoperative laboratory tests in elderly surgical patients. *Anesth Analg* 2001;93:301-308, 2nd contents page.
18. Schein OD, Katz J, Bass EB, et al: The value of routine preoperative medical testing before cataract surgery. Study of Medical Testing for Cataract Surgery. *N Engl J Med* 2000;342:168-175.
19. Gruson KI, Aharonoff GB, Egol KA, et al: The relationship between admission hemoglobin level and outcome after hip fracture. *J Orthop Trauma* 2002;16:39-44.
20. Wu WC, Schifftner TL, Henderson WG, et al: Preoperative hematocrit levels and postoperative outcomes in older patients undergoing noncardiac surgery. *JAMA* 2007;297:2481-2488.
21. Hebert PC, Wells G, Blajchman MA, et al: A multicenter, randomized, controlled clinical trial of transfusion requirements in critical care. Transfusion Requirements in Critical Care Investigators, Canadian Critical Care Trials Group. *N Engl J Med* 1999;340:409-417.
22. Carson JL, Duff A, Berlin JA, et al: Perioperative blood transfusion and postoperative mortality. *JAMA* 1998;279:199-205.
23. van Klei WA, Moons KG, Leyssius AT, et al: A reduction in type and screen: Preoperative prediction of RBC transfusions in surgery procedures with intermediate transfusion risks. *Br J Anaesth* 2001;87:250-257.
24. Faris PM, Spence RK, Larholt KM, et al: The predictive power of baseline hemoglobin for transfusion risk in surgery patients. *Orthopedics* 1999;22:s135-s140.
25. Nuttall GA, Santrach PJ, Oliver WC Jr, et al: The predictors of red cell transfusions in total hip arthroplasties. *Transfusion* 1996;36:144-149.

26. Nuttall GA, Horlocker TT, Santrach PJ, et al: Predictors of blood transfusions in spinal instrumentation and fusion surgery. *Spine* 2000;25:596-601.
27. Leung JM, Weiskopf RB, Feiner J, et al: Electrocardiographic ST-segment changes during acute, severe isovolemic hemodilution in humans. *Anesthesiology* 2000;93:1004-1010.
28. Weiskopf RB, Kramer JH, Viele M, et al: Acute severe isovolemic anemia impairs cognitive function and memory in humans. *Anesthesiology* 2000;92:1646-1652.
29. Weiskopf RB, Feiner J, Hopf HW, et al: Oxygen reverses deficits of cognitive function and memory and increased heart rate induced by acute severe isovolemic anemia. *Anesthesiology* 2002;96: 871-877.
30. Ickx BE, Rigolet M, Van Der Linden PJ: Cardiovascular and metabolic response to acute normovolemic anemia. Effects of anesthesia. *Anesthesiology* 2000;93:1011-1016.
31. Nuttall GA, Garrity JA, Dearani JA, et al: Risk factors for ischemic optic neuropathy after cardiopulmonary bypass: A matched case/control study. *Anesth Analg* 2001;93:1410-1416.
32. Practice advisory for preanesthesia evaluation: A report by the American Society of Anesthesiologists Task Force on Preanesthesia Evaluation. Anesthesiology 2002;96:485-496.
33. Sanders DP, McKinney FW, Harris WH: Clinical evaluation and cost effectiveness of preoperative laboratory assessment on patients undergoing total hip arthroplasty. *Orthopedics* 1989; 12:1449-1453.
34. Johnson H Jr, Knee-Ioli S, Butler TA, et al: Are routine preoperative laboratory screening tests necessary to evaluate ambulatory surgical patients? *Surgery* 1988;104:639-645.
35. Charpak Y, Blery C, Chastang C, et al: Usefulness of selectively ordered preoperative tests. *Med Care* 1988;26:95-104.
36. American Society of Anesthesiologists: Standards, guidelines and statements. Statement on routine perioperative and diagnostic screening, October 14, 1987, and last amended on October 13, 1993. Website: www.asahq.org/publicationsServices.htm#phys.

6 Is Routine Preoperative Pregnancy Testing Necessary?

Clinton S. Steffey, MD, and Rebecca S. Twersky, MD, MPH

Surgery on a pregnant woman raises several concerns. These include the effect of surgery and anesthesia on the developing fetus and the potential to trigger preterm labor. The hazards to the fetus could come from teratogenic effects of drugs administered during the perioperative period or, in a more advanced pregnancy, alterations in uteroplacental blood flow and from maternal hypoxia or acidosis.[1] It is reported that up to 15% of known pregnancies miscarry before 20 weeks and up to 50% of unrecognized pregnancies miscarry during the first trimester.[2] Because the period of organogenesis is during the first trimester, elective surgery is usually postponed to avoid potential teratogenicity and intrauterine fetal death. Although it is unclear which factors account for it, increased risk of spontaneous abortion is observed in women undergoing general anesthesia during the first or second trimester of pregnancy.[1-5] Premature labor is more likely in the third trimester. Some studies have also suggested the presence of a strong association between central nervous system (CNS) defects and first-trimester anesthesia exposure.[6,7]

Consequently, the issue of ruling out pregnancy before surgery is a crucial one. Unfortunately, medical history alone is often unreliable in ruling out pregnancy, especially in the adolescent female population.[8] It is in this very population in which obtaining a routine pregnancy test may present an ethical and a legal problem. The patient may refuse to have the test done and may, in some states, have the legal right to keep that information private from parents.[9] On the other hand, the adult population of female patients of childbearing age may very well have the same or even a higher risk of unknown pregnancy before a surgical procedure.[10,11] Routinely testing those patients for pregnancy may present a trust issue with women who believe that their history excludes that possibility. Moreover, when calculating the cost incurred if pregnancy screening is done routinely before each surgery, this becomes an even more controversial issue.[12,13]

OPTIONS

Should preoperative pregnancy testing be performed on all female patients of childbearing age or just in selected populations? Whether these selected populations should include only those whose history is suggestive of pregnancy, or whose history is unclear, is still unresolved.

The general practice of anesthesiologists differs according to the institutions in which they work, as well as by their personal judgments and convictions. Instituting policies for preoperative pregnancy testing should be based on the patient's best interests in correspondence with state law and ethical responsibility.[11]

The American Society of Anesthesiologists (ASA) Committee on Ethics has stated that patients should be offered but not required to undergo pregnancy testing unless there is a compelling medical reason to know the patient is pregnant.[14]

The ASA Practice Advisory for Preanesthesia Evaluation was amended by the ASA House of Delegates on October 15, 2003, to reflect this. "The Task Force recognizes that patients may present for anesthesia with an early undetected pregnancy. The Task Force believes that the literature is inadequate to inform patients or physicians on whether anesthesia causes harmful effects on early pregnancy. Pregnancy testing may be offered to female patients of childbearing age and for whom the results would alter the patient's management."[15] The most common policies on preoperative pregnancy testing were outlined in a recent *ASA Newsletter*.[16] One approach is to test every female patient of childbearing potential whether or not she consents. The justification for this is that consent to surgery and anesthesia is also consent to a pregnancy test. An alternative policy is one that allows patients to refuse testing after anesthetic and surgical risks to a possible pregnancy have been explained. However, after refusal the patient is asked to waive all legal rights relating to undetected pregnancy. In some anesthesiology departments the patient is informed and consulted but may be tested whether or not she consents.[16]

In a survey distributed to members of the Society of Obstetric Anesthesia and Perinatology (SOAP), almost one third of 169 respondents required preoperative pregnancy testing for all childbearing-age female patients through mandatory departmental policy. Sixty-six percent (66%) of surveyed anesthesiologists, however, required testing only when history indicated possible pregnancy.[17] When surveyed, members of the ASA were asked whether pregnancy testing should be done routinely for all patients versus selected populations; 17% believed it was a necessary routine test, whereas 78% chose the latter.[15] The finding of a positive result has a very important impact on clinical management because it will lead to either delays or cancellations of surgery.[8,10,11,18,19]

EVIDENCE

Several studies have been conducted to examine the reliability of obtaining medical history preoperatively in indicating the possibility of pregnancy (Table 6-1). These studies included patients from different age-groups. One study by Malviya and colleagues,[20] in the adolescent population, showed that none of the patients who underwent testing were found to have a positive urine pregnancy test. Data from the study indicated that most of the patients denied the possibility of pregnancy, whereas very few were not sure. The authors concluded that a detailed history should be obtained in all postmenarchal patients, and unless indicated by that history, pregnancy testing would not be required. It is noteworthy that 17 patients in that study refused testing.

Several other studies, on the other hand, demonstrated that the medical history was often inconclusive and occasionally misleading. This was true for both adults and adolescents. Two studies, by Azzam and colleagues[18] and Pierre and colleagues,[8] demonstrated positive pregnancy test results in adolescent patients undergoing surgery. Incidence rates were 1.2% and 0.49%, respectively. The medical history in the Pierre study did not always correlate with test results.

Three additional studies included patients from all age-groups.[10,11,19] Manley and colleagues,[19] using either serum or urinary human chorionic gonadotropin (hCG), tested 2056 females undergoing ambulatory surgery. There was an incidence of 0.3% of unrecognized pregnancies. Wheeler and Cote[11] tested 261 patients ages 10 to 34 years, all of whom denied the possibility of pregnancy. Three patients (1.3%) had positive tests. Two of them were adults. Interestingly, the authors in the studies by both Azzam and colleagues[18] and Wheeler and Cote[11] point out that although positive results were documented

Table 6-1 Detecting the Incidence of Pregnancy during Preoperative Evaluation Using History and Laboratory Testing

Study	Design	Duration	No. of Cases	Patient Population	Age in Years	Type of Test	Time of Test	No. of Positive Results	Correlation with History
Manley and colleagues[19]	Prospective	36 mo	2056	All females of childbearing potential	*	Urine or serum β-hCG	Within 6 days of surgery	Total 7 (0.3%)	No[†]
Gazvani and colleagues[22]	Prospective	23 mo	125	Females undergoing laparoscopic sterilizations	*	Urine β-hCG	*	Total 6 (5%)	*
Azzam and colleagues[18]	Retrospective	24 mo	412	Adolescents	10.5-20	Urine β-hCG		Total 5 (1.2%) <14 old-0 (0%) ≥15 old-5 (2.4%)	*
Twersky and Singleton[10]	Prospective	*	315	All females of childbearing age	*	Serum β-hCG	*	Total 7 (2.2%) <23 old-0	No[†]
Malviya and colleagues[20]	Prospective	26 mo	525	Adolescents	10-17	Urine β-hCG	Day of surgery	1 (questionable result, deemed negative)	Yes[‡]
Pierre and colleagues[8]	Prospective	21 mo	801	Adolescents	12-21	Urine β-hCG	*	Total 6 (0.49%)	No[†]
Wheeler and Cote[11]	Prospective	15 mo	235	Adolescents and adults	10-34	*	*	Total 3 (1.3%) <15 old-0 (0%) ≥15 old-3 (2.3%)	No[†]
Hennrikus and colleagues[21]	Retrospective	36 mo	532	Adolescents	12-19	Urine β-hCG	Day of surgery	Total 5 (0.9%)	*
Kahn and colleagues[13]	Retrospective	12 mo	2588	All females of childbearing potential	*	Urine β-hCG	Day of surgery	Total 8 (0.3%)	No[†]

*Was not specified in the study.
[†]History indicated the possibility of pregnancy in all patients who tested positive.
[‡]History did not indicate possibility of pregnancy in all patients who tested positive.

in teenagers, no positive result was detected in patients younger than 15 years of age. In a study on adolescents, Hennrikus and colleagues[21] tested 532 females between ages 12 and 19. They found five patients to have positive urine hCG results, with the youngest being 13 years of age.

Evidence was most compelling in the adult population in the study done by Twersky and Singleton,[10] which examined 315 consecutive females of childbearing potential undergoing elective surgery. Seven patients (2.2%) tested positive for serum beta–human chorionic gonadotropin (β-hCG). None of them were teenagers. The highest percentage of positive pregnancy tests was found among patients undergoing laparoscopic sterilization. A study done in the United Kingdom including 125 patients undergoing laparoscopic sterilization detected 6 positive pregnancy tests (5%).[22] The authors did not specify if the history of these patients indicated the possibility of being pregnant.[23]

AREAS OF UNCERTAINTY

Cost

When doing a routine test, it is always important to consider if the findings obtained from that test provide an advantage over those not tested. Would a higher cost be incurred if those results were unknown? In a retrospective study, Kahn and colleagues[13] found the average cost per urine pregnancy test to be $5.03 and the cost per true positive result to be $3,273. Following these results, they speculated that the costs of preoperative pregnancy testing were validated by removing the potential risk to the mother and fetus along with a potential decrease in litigation. Based on the "numbers needed to treat" approach, Kettler[12] calculated the cost of detecting one pregnancy when using routine preoperative testing. The cost was $1,050 in the adolescent population and $7,750 in the adult population. Evaluation of cost needs to be weighed against the cost of spontaneous abortion, radiation exposure, or possible congenital abnormalities following an anesthetic and surgical procedure conducted in a patient with an unknown pregnancy.

Which Test to Be Done

Whether to do a urine pregnancy test versus a serum pregnancy test has also been a matter of inconsistency.[24] The studies mentioned earlier used them interchangeably (see Table 6-1). In general, it is believed that a urine pregnancy test, which is quicker and readily available, is a reliable one. It decreases the time required to obtain the result, in turn decreasing operating room delays.[25]

How Sensitive

Several urine hCG kits report a sensitivity of 99.4% and a specificity of 99.5%.[21,24] The significance of a positive pregnancy test is evaluated by the positive predictive value of the test processed. Based on the data and incidence of pregnancy detected from one preoperative evaluation study,[19] Lewis and Cooper[26] demonstrated that pregnancy testing had a low positive predictive value. This means that there will be patients with positive pregnancy tests who are not actually pregnant and will have their surgery delayed, secondary to the false-positive test result. A false-positive result could be due to ectopic production by neoplasms or from trophoblastic disease.[21] A false-negative result could occur if the sample was taken during the first 10 days after conception, or if the urine sample was too dilute (e.g., not a first morning specimen). However, given the low prevalence of actual pregnancy in the surgical population, positive predictive values vary and would be higher in other studies that resulted in higher incidence rates. Larger studies with bigger patient samples and unified testing methods are needed to resolve this issue.

When to Test

Levels of hCG are elevated 10 days after conception and remain elevated throughout gestation. In many cases, pregnancy testing takes place within 7 days before surgery. However, the concentration of β-hCG in early pregnancy doubles every 1.4 to 2 days.[21,26] Therefore there is a concern that an undetectable level at 7 days before surgery may become detectable on the day of surgery.[27,28] Thus it seems that testing on the day of surgery may identify more pregnant patients than when doing it earlier. It should be noted, however, that testing on the day of surgery opens up the chance for cancellation of surgery and hence complicates the surgical schedule, at a cost to the organization of a case that cannot be substituted.

GUIDELINES

The ASA, in its statement on routine preoperative laboratory testing, did not see any one test to be a requirement for all patients. Rather, testing guidelines should be tailored by each individual anesthesia department and according to its influence on selected populations.[29] In 2002, a task force was appointed by the ASA to review available literature, obtain expert and public opinion, and create the consensus-based "Practice Advisory for Preanesthesia Evaluation."[15]

The task force agreed that preoperative tests should not be ordered routinely. Rather, preoperative tests should be done or required on a selective basis for purposes of guiding and optimizing perioperative management. The indications for testing should be documented and based on medical and physical examination. The task force, however, recognized that a history and examination might be insufficient for identification of early pregnancy. In its 2003 amendment, in keeping with the ethical guidelines of anesthesia practice, it recommended that all female patients of childbearing potential should be offered pregnancy testing, rather than required to undergo testing, in light of the equivocal evidence-based linkages between pregnancy testing and anesthesia outcome. It gives individual physicians and hospitals the opportunity to set their own policies and practices relating to preoperative pregnancy testing. Though legitimate or illegitimate consequences can ensue (*Ballard v. Anderson*, 4 Cal. 3d 873, 1971; *Truman v. Thomas*, 27 Cal. 3d 285, 1980; *Rechenbach v. Haftkowycz*, 654 Ohio 2d 374, 1995), medicolegal concerns alone should not be the driving force to guide policies.

Some hospitals respect the patient's right of refusal after a thorough explanation of anesthetic risks during pregnancy, but require the patient to sign a waiver releasing the physicians and hospital from potential litigation over an unknown pregnancy.[16] Additionally, policies should address who shall discuss the results with the patient and

who is allowed to be notified of the results (partner, family, insurance company, employer, etc.).[14] Individual institutions should develop guidelines centered on the content and reliability of the patient's medical history, balanced by the physician's judgment.

AUTHORS' RECOMMENDATIONS

Medical tests are performed based on the contribution they offer to patient care and safety (Table 6-2). In this case we must ask ourselves the following question: How important is it to know if a patient is pregnant or not before performing surgery?

Even though the prevalence of pregnancy is expected to be low in patients undergoing surgery, the discovery of the fewest number of cases is extremely significant. As important as this would be to protect the patient and fetus, it is also important to protect the physician from unwarranted litigation. The argument has been, is this cost-effective? If we factor in the cost generated by abortions, miscarriages, and even malpractice lawsuits secondary to a suspected anesthetic teratogenic effect, one may conclude that pregnancy testing is indeed cost-effective. There have been concerns regarding the methods of informing patients before obtaining a pregnancy test. Some studies informed all patients, whereas others did not because the test was mandatory.

- We believe that even if the test is made to be mandatory, this should not preclude from obtaining a well-documented informed consent. Patients still have the right to refuse testing, at which point the physician also has the right to refuse to render services after explaining the rationale behind the test and the safety issues involved.
- Mandatory testing offers the advantage of avoiding the conflicts that physicians are presented with when some adolescent patients are asked about the test or their sexual history. The same applies to parents or adult patients, who may be offended by a detailed sexual history. As for young patients who are at the onset of their menses, there is no evidence that testing is helpful. Several studies have shown that patients under age 13 test negative. However, we prefer to have those patients tested if they consent because there are occasions where they may not disclose all of their history, or that history may be inaccurate.
- A policy must be in place addressing which physicians should be involved in informing the patient of the results and who may be informed of the results.
- In terms of what test to perform, serum testing is very sensitive and may be sufficient when done within a week of the surgical date. However, if a urine pregnancy test is used, it is preferably done on the day of surgery in order for it to identify the greatest number of pregnant patients.

In conclusion, based on current evidence, pregnancy testing is a cost-effective method and should be offered to all verbally consenting females of childbearing potential. This does not substitute for an appropriate pregnancy history and physical examination.

This will remain a controversial issue, and larger studies are needed. They should include a larger number of patients from all age-groups and use a unified method of testing, as well as a well-documented informed consent.

Table 6-2   Recommendations for Preoperative Pregnancy Testing

Population Type	Recommendations
Menstruating females under 13 years of age	No pregnancy test unless history is either indicative of sexual activity or is inconclusive.
Patients of childbearing age (over 13 years of age until 1 year after last reported menses)	Preoperative pregnancy test should be offered to all patients regardless of history, except in patients with a history of hysterectomy or bilateral salpingo-oophorectomy.
Testing on the day of surgery	Urine pregnancy test is sufficient.
Testing within 1 week of surgery	Serum pregnancy test is preferable.
All patients	Well-documented informed consent must be obtained from patients or their guardians.
All patients	A thorough and detailed history should be obtained from all patients.

REFERENCES

1. Kuzkowski KM: Nonobstetric surgery during pregnancy: What are the risks of anesthesia? *Obstet Gynecol Surv* 2004;59:52-56.
2. Wilcox AJ, Weinberg CR, O'Connor JF, Baird DD, Schlatterer JP, Canfield RE, et al: Incidence of early loss of pregnancy. *N Engl J Med* 1988;319:189-194.
3. Duncan PG, Pope WDB, Cohen MM, Greer N: The safety of anesthesia and surgery during pregnancy. *Anesthesiology* 1986;64:790-794.
4. Brodsky JB, Cohen EN, Brown BW Jr, Wu ML, Whitcher C: Surgery during pregnancy and fetal outcome. *Am J Obstet Gynecol* 1980;138:1165-1167.
5. Mazze RI, Kallen B: Reproductive outcome after anesthesia and operation during pregnancy: A registry study of 5405 cases. *Am J Obstet Gynecol* 1989;161:1178-1185.
6. Sylvester GC, Khoury MJ, Lu X, Erickson JD: First trimester anesthesia exposure and the risk of central nervous system defects: A population-based care-control study. *Am J Public Health* 1994;84:1757-1760.
7. Kallen B, Mazze RI: Neural tube defects and first trimester operations. *Teratology* 1990;41:717-720.
8. Pierre N, Moy LK, Redd S, Emans SJ, Laufer MR: Evaluation of a pregnancy-testing protocol in adolescents undergoing surgery. *J Pediatr Adolesc Gynecol* 1998;11(3):139-141.
9. Duncan PG, Pope WD: Medical ethics and legal standards. *Anesth Analg* 1996;82(1):1-3.

10. Twersky RS, Singleton G: Preoperative pregnancy testing: Justice and testing for all. *Anesth Analg* 1996;83(2):438-439.

11. Wheeler M, Cote CJ: Preoperative pregnancy testing in a tertiary care children's hospital: A medico-legal conundrum. *J Clin Anesth* 1999;11(1):56-63.

12. Kettler RE: The cost of preoperative pregnancy testing. *Anesth Analg* 1996;83(2):439-440.

13. Kahn RL, Stanton MA, Tong-Ngork S, Liguori GA, Edmonds CR, Levine DS: One-year experience with day-of-surgery pregnancy testing before elective orthopedic procedures. *Anesth Analg* 2008;106(4):1127-1131.

14. Palmer S, Jackson S: What's new in ethics, hot issues in legally sensitive times. *American Society of Anesthesiologists Newsletter* 2003; 67(10); www.asahq.org/Newsletters/2003/10_03/whatsNew10_03html.

15. American Society of Anesthesiologists Task Force on Preanesthesia Evaluation: Practice advisory for preanesthesia evaluation: A report by the American Society of Anesthesiologists Task Force on Preanesthesia Evaluation. *Anesthesiology* 2002;96(2):485-496; amended on page 492 by the ASA House of Delegates on October 15, 2003.

16. Bierstein K: Preoperative pregnancy testing: Mandatory or elective? *American Society of Anesthesiologists Newsletter* 2006;70(7):37.

17. Kempen PM: Preoperative pregnancy testing: A survey of current practice. *J Clin Anesth* 1997;9(7):546-550.

18. Azzam FJ, Padda GS, DeBoard JW, Krock JL, Kolterman SM: Preoperative pregnancy testing in adolescents. *Anesth Analg* 1996;82:4-7.

19. Manley S, de Kelaita G, Joseph NJ, Salem R, Heyman HJ: Preoperative pregnancy testing in ambulatory surgery. *Anesthesiology* 1995;83:690-693.

20. Malviya S, D'Errico C, Reynolds P, Huntington J, Voepel-Lewis T, Pandit UA: Should pregnancy testing be routine in adolescent patients prior to surgery? *Anesth Analg* 1996;83(4):854-858.

21. Hennrikus WL, Shaw BA, Gerardi JA: Prevalence of positive preoperative pregnancy testing in teenagers scheduled for orthopedic surgery. *J Pediatr Orthop* 2001;21(5):677-679.

22. Gazvani MR, Hawe J, Farquharson RG: Value of preoperative pregnancy test in risk management. *Lancet* 1996;347(9010):1271.

23. Wagman H: Value of preoperative pregnancy test in risk management. *Lancet* 1996;347(9016):1695-1696.

24. Twersky RS, Kotob F: Pregnancy testing. In Roizen MF, Fleisher LA, editors: *Essence of anesthesia practice*, ed 2. Philadelphia, WB Saunders, 2002, p 625.

25. O'Connor RE, Bibro CM, Pegg PJ, Bouzoukis JK: The comparative sensitivity and specificity of serum and urine HCG determinations in the ED. *Am J Emerg Med* 1993;11(4):434-436.

26. Lewis I, Cooper J: Preoperative pregnancy testing in ambulatory surgery. *Anesthesiology* 1996;84(5):1259-1260; discussion 1261.

27. Rosenberg MK: Preoperative pregnancy testing in ambulatory surgery. *Anesthesiology* 1996;84(5):1260; discussion 1261.

28. Zeig NJ, Herschman Z: Preoperative pregnancy testing in ambulatory surgery. *Anesthesiology* 1996;84(5):1260-1261.

29. American Society of Anesthesiologists: Statement on routine preoperative laboratory and diagnostic screening (approved by House of Delegates on October 14, 1987, and last amended on October 13, 1993).

7 What Are the Risk Factors for Perioperative Stroke?

Alexander Papangelou, MD, and Marek Mirski, MD, PhD

BACKGROUND

Perioperative stroke is a potentially devastating complication of surgery whose incidence varies widely with surgical procedure. A perioperative stroke can occur intraoperatively or in the postoperative period; however, this window of risk is not standardized, as studies have used intervals of 3 to 30 days.

A recent review on this topic illustrated the representative incidences based on surgical procedure.[1] These categories included general surgery (0.08% to 0.7%),[2] peripheral vascular surgery (0.8% to 3.0%),[3] resection of head and neck tumors (4.8%),[4] carotid endarterectomy in symptomatic patients (5.5% to 6.1%),[5] isolated coronary artery bypass graft (CABG) surgery (1.4% to 3.8%),[6,7] combined CABG with valve surgery (7.4%),[6,7] isolated valve surgery (4.8% to 8.8%),[6] double- or triple-valve surgery (9.7%),[6] and aortic repair (8.7%).[7] Beating-heart CABG has a lower incidence of stroke than does CABG on bypass (1.9% versus 3.8%, respectively).[6]

This variability in perioperative stroke incidence reflects the underlying surgical anatomy, risk of vascular compromise and injury, and the patient's overall preoperative health status. As such, there are likely no simple solutions for this complex perioperative complication. The problem has been approached by different specialties with a variety of preventive measures, including intense intraoperative monitoring, novel approaches to the surgical procedure, and development of predictive models. Regardless, the incidence of perioperative stroke has remained a concern.

The implication from the aforementioned reviews is that to achieve an appreciable reduction in the incidence of stroke, it will require universal as well as selective improvements by each surgical subspecialty. A fair appraisal of perioperative stroke thus requires that we present data for general surgery, carotid surgery, and cardiac surgery separately.

PATHOPHYSIOLOGY

Proposed mechanisms for perioperative ischemic stroke include thrombotic, embolic, lacunar, hematologic (hypercoaguable state), and hypoperfusion.[8] Evidence from studies of cardiac surgery supports that perioperative hemorrhagic stroke has a very low incidence. For example,

Likosky and colleagues[9] looked at 388 patients who suffered stroke after isolated CABG surgery. This study used the Northern New England Cardiovascular Disease Study Group classification system, and imaging was performed in the form of computed tomography (CT) or magnetic resonance imaging (MRI). The study revealed that 62.1% of strokes were embolic, 3.1% lacunar, 1.0% thrombotic, 8.8% due to hypoperfusion, 1.0% hemorrhagic, 10.1% multiple etiologies, and 13.9% unclassified. About 45% of strokes were detected within the first postoperative day, with a slow decrement of detection over time (about 20% additional by postoperative day 2, about 12% additional by postoperative day 3, and less than 5% beyond postoperative day 10).[9]

The source of emboli (cardiac or artery-to-artery) during any surgery could include arrhythmias such as atrial fibrillation, aortic arch atherosclerosis, perioperative myocardial infarction, and manipulations of the heart and carotid arteries.[10] The release of particulate matter from the cardiopulmonary-bypass pump must also not be forgotten. A rare source may also be paradoxic emboli from a patent foramen ovale or fat emboli during orthopedic procedures.[10] In a study of 2630 CABG patients,[11] 2.0% had postoperative strokes. The event occurred after a mean of 3.7 days. In 19 of 52 patients (36.5%), atrial fibrillation preceded the stroke, with a mean of 2.5 episodes of atrial fibrillation before the event.

Tissue injury from surgery results in a prothrombotic state, which lasts up to 14 to 21 days postoperatively. This is supported by decreased levels of tissue plasminogen activator and increased plasminogen activator inhibitor type 1 activity, fibrinogen-degradation products, thrombin-antithrombin complex, thrombus precursor protein, and D-dimer.[12-14] Other factors such as the use of general anesthesia, inadequate resuscitation leading to postoperative dehydration, and bed rest may all aggravate a hypercoaguable state.[8] Often, antiplatelet and anticoagulant agents are held in the perioperative period as well. This may exacerbate a hypercoaguable state and further increase the risk of perioperative stroke.[15,16] This practice has slowly changed, and it is being found that these agents are likely safe in the large majority of surgeries.[17]

Gottesman and colleagues[18] presented a different view of stroke in cardiac surgery. They studied 98 patients who had MRI after a clinical stroke. The group identified watershed infarcts in 68% of the diffusion-weighted imaging (DWI) sequences of MRI versus 37% of brain CTs.

In fact, 48% of DWI MRIs demonstrated bilateral watershed infarcts versus 22% of CTs. Bilateral watershed infarct patients were more likely to have undergone an aortic procedure than a simple or second CABG. These patients trended toward longer bypass times (nearly significant; $p = 0.055$). Univariate and multivariate logistic regression revealed that patients with a drop in mean arterial pressure (MAP) of at least 10 mm Hg from their preoperative baseline were greater than four times more likely to develop bilateral watershed infarcts than those with a small or no decrement in blood pressure. Importantly, absolute intraoperative blood pressure was almost identical in the bilateral watershed infarct group versus other infarct patterns. This author mentions the possibility that watershed infarcts may be due to a mechanistic interplay of hypoperfusion and embolization, citing a paper by Caplan and Hennerici.[19] The theory is that a state of reduced perfusion (due to reduced MAP or due to arterial narrowing, i.e., carotid) may impede washout of microemboli showered during cardiac surgery, and these particulates have a predilection to settle in watershed areas.

In keeping with this theory, a randomized study of 248 elective CABG patients by Gold and colleagues[20] revealed that patients maintained at a higher MAP (80 to 100 mm Hg) during bypass had a lower incidence of stroke. This study has been criticized for lack of power to draw any widely applicable conclusions. On the contrary, van Wermeskerken and colleagues[21] looked at outcomes from 2862 patients undergoing CABG. After controlling for bypass time and preoperative stroke risk index, patients with a lower pressure during bypass (MAP less than 50 mm Hg) had a decreased incidence of stroke and coma.

In general, hypoperfusion is believed to be an uncommon cause of perioperative stroke. The term *hypoperfusion* can imply global hypoperfusion (i.e., resulting in bilateral watershed infarctions) or relative hypoperfusion through a preexisting stenosis (i.e., unilateral watershed infarction due to carotid stenosis). The study by van Wermeskerken and colleagues[21] supports a limited role of hypoperfusion. In addition, Whitney and colleagues[22] concluded that hypoperfusion ischemia is rare during carotid endarterectomy (CEA), even when the contralateral carotid is occluded. Naylor and colleagues[23] reviewed the literature to assess the role of carotid stenosis as a perioperative stroke risk factor for CABG. Ninety-one percent of screened CABG patients had insignificant disease and had a less than 2% risk of stroke. The risk increased to 3% for asymptomatic unilateral stenosis of 50% to 99%, 5% in bilateral 50% to 99% stenosis, and 7% to 11% in those with an occluded carotid. As a consequence of such data, the current practice is to perform CEA before CABG or even intraoperatively immediately before CABG.

Studies looking specifically at the mechanisms of stroke in the general surgery patient are rare, and in general are not contemporary studies. Hart and Hindman[24] performed a retrospective review of 24,500 general surgery patients. Forty-two percent of strokes were believed to be embolic, with atrial fibrillation present in 33% of patients at the time of the events. Interestingly, most perioperative strokes in the general surgery population occur well into the postoperative period, on average on the seventh day.[2,24-28] A case-control study again reiterated the paucity of intraoperative stroke, with evidence of only 10 of 61 strokes occurring intraoperatively.[29] Of these studies, Parikh and Cohen[25] found the highest incidence (53%) of stroke within 24 hours following surgery.

Again, taken as a whole, these observations highlight the fact that the mechanisms of perioperative stroke should be reviewed in each surgical population separately.

EVIDENCE

There is no meta-analysis specifically assessing the risk factors for perioperative stroke in the general surgery population. The best evidence is in the form of prospective observational studies, but given that an extensive literature search identified only one such study, several retrospective and case-control investigations were included for review. A retrospective analysis of noncarotid vascular surgery patients was also included in Table 7-1.

The existing meta-analyses in cardiac surgery compared conventional CABG and off-pump CABG in terms of global outcomes. Table 7-2 only addresses stroke. The 2003 analysis included nonrandomized trials, but it was believed that the inclusion of these data did not bias the results.[30]

The existing data on perioperative stroke in cardiac surgery is limited to multiple prospectively collected, retrospectively analyzed observational studies. There is also one case-control design and multiple retrospective studies in the literature. The data are summarized in Table 7-3, and a small study with similar surgical breakdown as the article by Bucerius and colleagues[6] has been included for comparison. Also included at the end of the table are two recent larger prospective studies on thoracic aortic surgery, as these studies likely best fit in the cardiac surgery category.

There are several meta-analyses exploring different aspects of perioperative stroke in carotid surgery. These are applicable to this chapter only in a broad sense, but are interesting nonetheless. Only the most recent meta-analyses on this topic are included in Table 7-4.

Because these meta-analyses did not address the main theme of this section (risk factors for perioperative stroke), Table 7-5 includes the major multicenter randomized clinical trials for carotid endarterectomy.

INTERPRETATION OF DATA

The data presented are vast, but unfortunately the quality of many studies is suboptimal, especially in the general surgery group. Most studies of perioperative stroke in general surgery are older, and often without rigorous statistical analysis. Several risk factors are commonly seen in this subset: prior history of stroke, heart disease, hypertension, diabetes, peripheral vascular disease (PVD), and atrial fibrillation. The most powerful predictor is probably prior history of stroke.[29]

In the cardiac literature, the concept of increased surgical risk in women is prevalent and unique. In addition,

Table 7-1	Perioperative Stroke Studies in the General Surgery Population				
Study, Year	Number of Subjects	Study Design	Stroke Incidence	Significant Risk Factors	
1988[26]	2,463	PO	0.2%	Previous cerebrovascular disease Heart disease Peripheral vascular disease (eightfold increased risk) Hypertension (threefold-fourfold increased risk)	
1993[25]	24,641	R	0.08%	Hypertension Smoking Previous neurologic symptoms Abnormal rhythm on ECG	
1982[24]	24,500	R	0.07%	Atrial fibrillation Cardiac disease	
1990[62]	173 (patients with prior stroke)	R	2.9%	Use of preoperative heparin sodium (usually as a substitute for warfarin) General anesthesia (as opposed to regional)[63] Hypotension in recovery room[63]	
2004[64]	2,251 (abdominal aortic aneurysmectomy) 2,616 (aorto-bifemoral bypass) 6,866 (lower extremity bypass) 7,442 (major lower extremity amputation)	R	0.4%-0.6%	Preoperative ventilation (OR 11) Previous stroke or TIA (OR 4.2) Postoperative MI (OR 3.3) Need to return to operating room (OR 2.2)	
1998[29]	61 cases (general surgery) 122 random controls (matched for age, sex, procedure, and year of procedure)	CC	N/A	Previous cerebrovascular disease (AOR_1 12.57; AOR_2 14.70)* COPD (AOR_1 7.51; AOR_2 10.04) PVD (AOR_1 5.35) Higher MAP on admission (AOR_2 1.05) Blood urea at time of stroke (AOR_2 1.04) Postoperative MI (4 cases vs. 0 control) Diffuse intravascular coagulation (4 cases vs. 0 control)	
2000[65]	1,455 cases (surgery) 1,455 controls (age and gender matched)	CC	N/A	Perioperative period after general anesthesia extending for 30 days postoperatively (OR adjusted for known independent stroke risk factor = 3.9 for all surgeries and 2.9 for general surgery)	
2005[66]†	172,592	PO	0.03%	Most cases in ASA 3 patients 26% of stroke cases had prior history of stroke	

*Adjusted odds ratio 1 (AOR_1) is from the univariate analysis. AOR_2 is from the multivariate analysis. Noted values are only those that reached statistical significance.
†Requested copy of study from author. Unable to obtain. Data entered from abstract only.
AOR, adjusted odds ratio; *ASA*, anesthesia preoperative assessment score (1-5); *CC*, case control; *COPD*, chronic obstructive pulmonary disease; *MI*, myocardial infarction; *OR*, odds ratio; *PO*, prospective observational; *PVD*, peripheral vascular disease; *R*, retrospective; *TIA*, transient ischemic attack.

older age, a diseased proximal aorta, PVD, history of stroke, poor cardiac function, chronic renal insufficiency (CRI), hypertension, diabetes, atrial fibrillation, urgent surgery, and prolonged bypass time are prevalent risk factors in multivariate analyses. The most powerful predictors are likely prior stroke, surgery on the aorta, aortic disease burden, and perhaps female gender.[31,32] The two studies on aortic surgery again reveal female sex and surgery on the proximal aorta as substantial risk factors.[33,34]

Review of the carotid literature reveals that increased disease burden on the surgical side and contralateral occlusion (which will lessen collateral flow) are substantial factors. Prior stroke or transient ischemic attack (TIA; on the surgical side), hypertension (especially diastolic greater than 90), diabetes, and left carotid surgery are also

significant risk factors. Finally, it appears that women do not benefit from carotid surgery as much as men; this has been a constant significant finding or trend across nearly all studies.

In a retrospective review of 6038 patients after CEA in Ontario, the perioperative 30-day death or nonfatal stroke rate was 6.0%.[35] This study specifically aimed to identify predictors of stroke and reviewed substantially more surgical cases than any of the previously cited randomized controlled trials. In this study, a history of TIA or stroke (odds ratio [OR] 1.75), atrial fibrillation (OR 1.89), contralateral carotid occlusion (OR 1.72), congestive heart failure (OR 1.80), and diabetes (OR 1.28) were found to be independent predictors of a perioperative event.

Table 7-2	Meta-analyses of Conventional CABG and Off-Pump CABG: Outcome Analysis				
Study, Year	**Number of Trials**	**Number of Subjects (Intervention/No Intervention)**	**Intervention (30-day Stroke Percent)**	**Control (30-day Stroke Percent)**	**Outcomes (OR with Confidence Interval)**
2005[36]	37 (21 trials included data on stroke)	2859 (off-pump CABG vs. conventional CABG)	0.4	1.0	0.68 (0.33-1.40)
2003[30]	53 (38 trials included data on stroke)	34,126	Not noted	Not noted	0.55 (0.43-0.69)

Table 7-3	Perioperative Stroke Risk Factor Studies in the Cardiac Surgery Population			
Study, Year	**Number of Subjects**	**Study Design**	**Stroke Incidence**	**Significant Risk Factors (Multivariate Analysis Unless Otherwise Noted)**
2007[67]	5085	PO	2.6%	Female gender (OR 1.7), age > 60 (OR 1.2 per 5 yr interval), aortic surgery (OR 3.9), previous stroke (OR 2.1), critical preoperative state (OR 2.5), poor ventricular function (OR 2.0), diabetes (OR 1.7), peripheral vascular disease (OR 1.8), unstable angina (OR 1.7), pulmonary hypertension (OR 1.8)
2003[31]	2972 (1900 men, 1072 women)	PO	2.8% women, 0.95% men ($p < 0.001$)	Women: history of stroke (OR 44.5); ascending aortic atherosclerosis (OR 2.1); low cardiac output (OR 6.7); diabetes (OR 2.2) Men: history of stroke (OR 305.8)
2003[68]	4567	PO	2.5%	Cerebrovascular disease (OR 2.66); PVD (OR 2.33); number of periods of aortic cross clamping (OR 1.31 for each period); LV dysfunction (OR 1.82); increased age (OR 1.28 for each 10 years); nonelective surgery (OR 1.83, $p = 0.08$)
2007[69]	720	PO	3.9% in men; 1.3% in women ($p = 0.066$)	Prior cerebral infarction (OR 1.987 per grade); atherosclerosis of ascending aorta (OR 1.990 per grade)
2001[70]	6682	PO	1.5%	Age > 70 (OR 5.4); LVEF $< 40\%$ (OR 4.1); history of stroke/TIA (OR 3.0); normothermic CPB (OR 2.2); diabetes (OR 1.9); PVD (OR 1.9)
2000[71]	1987 CABG only 84 CABG and CEA	PO	1.7% CABG; 4.7% combo	Age: 76 vs. 71.9 yr (OR 1.09); hypertension (OR 2.67); extensively calcified aorta (OR 2.82); prolonged bypass time (OR 1.01, CI 1.00-1.02)
1996[72]	189	P	4.76% by 1 wk postoperatively	Univariate analysis on aortic atheromatous grade by TEE: advancing aortic atheroma grade was a predictor of stroke ($p = 0.00001$)
1992[73]	130	?P	3.85%	Protruding aortic arch atheroma (OR 5.8, CI 1.2-27.9)
2006[54]	810	PO	stroke and TIA 1.85%	Redo cardiac surgery (OR 7.45); unstable cardiac status (OR 4.74); history of cerebrovascular disease (OR 4.14); PVD (OR 3.55); preoperative use of statins (OR 0.24, CI 0.07-0.78)
2003[74]	11,825	P	1.5%	Prediction model incorporated known preoperative RF: age, DM, urgent surgery, EF $< 40\%$; creatinine ≥ 2.0; additional intraoperative and postoperative RF: CPB 90-113 min (OR 1.59); CPB ≥ 114 min (OR 2.36); atrial fibrillation (OR 1.82); prolonged ionotrope use (OR 2.59)

(Continued)

Table 7-3   Perioperative Stroke Risk Factor Studies in the Cardiac Surgery Population—Cont'd

Study, Year	Number of Subjects	Study Design	Stroke Incidence	Significant Risk Factors (Multivariate Analysis Unless Otherwise Noted)
2002[75]	2711	PO	2.7%	Past stroke (OR 2.11); hypertension (OR 1.97); age 65-75 (OR 2.39); age ≥75 (OR 5.02)
1999[76]	4518	PO	2.0% stroke; 0.7% TIA	Known cerebral vascular disease (OR 2.5); renal failure (OR 1.6); MI (OR 1.5); DM (OR 1.5); age >70 (OR 1.5); also associated with postoperative low EF and atrial fibrillation
2000[77]	472	P	3.4%	Severity of extracranial carotid artery stenosis (OR 6.59)
2003[6]	16,184 total: Group 1—8917 CABG only; Group 2—1842 beating-heart CABG; Group 3—1830 AV surgery; Group 4—708 MV surgery; Group 5—381 multiple-valve surgery; Group 6—2506 CABG + valve surgery	PO	4.6% overall; 3.8% in 1; 1.9% in 2; 4.8% in 3; 8.8% in 4; 9.7% in 5; 7.4% in 6	History of CVD (OR 3.55); PVD (OR 1.39); DM (OR 1.31); hypertension (OR 1.27); urgent operation (OR 1.47); preoperative infection (OR 2.39); prior cardiac surgery (OR 1.33); CPB time > 2 hr (OR 1.42); intraoperative hemofiltration (OR 1.25); high transfusion requirement (OR 6.04); beating-heart CABG (OR 0.53, CI 0.37-0.77)
2002[78]	4077 (45 stroke = cases; 4032 "no stroke" = controls)	P, CC	1.1%	Increasing age (OR 1.06 per yr); unstable angina (OR 2.69); preoperative creatinine >150 mol/L (OR 2.64); previous STROKE (OR 2.26); preexisting PVD (OR 2.99); salvage operation (OR 16.1)
1999[32]	2972	PO	1.6% (0.6% early and 1.0% delayed)	Early stroke (immediately after surgery): history of stroke (OR 11.6); ascending aortic atherosclerosis (OR 2.0); duration of cardiopulmonary bypass (OR 1.1); female sex (OR 6.9) Delayed stroke: history of stroke (OR 27.6); DM (OR 2.8); female sex (OR 2.4); ascending aortic atherosclerosis (1.4); combined end points of atrial fibrillation and low CO (OR 1.7)
2005[79]	4380	PO	1.2%	History of stroke (OR 6.3); DM (OR 3.5); older age (OR 1.1); temperature of CPB was insignificant
2000[41]	19,224	P	1.4%	Calcified aorta (OR 3.013); prior stroke (OR 1.909); increasing age—null of 60 (OR 1.522 per 10 yr); preexisting carotid artery disease (OR 1.590); duration of CPB (OR 1.27 per 60 min); renal failure (OR 2.032); PVD (OR 1.62); cigarette smoking in past year (OR 1.621); diabetes (OR 1.373)
2001[80]	16,528	PO	2.0%	CRI (OR 2.8); recent MI (OR 2.5); previous stroke (OR 1.9); carotid artery disease (OR 1.9) hypertension (OR 1.6); diabetes (OR 1.4); age >75 yr (OR 1.4); preoperative moderate/severe LV dysfunction (OR 1.3); postoperative low cardiac output syndrome (OR 2.1); postoperative atrial fibrillation (OR 1.7)
2005[81]	783 total: Group 1—582 CABG only; Group 2—101 single VR; Group 3—70 combined CABG+VR; Group 4—30 multi VR	R	Stroke and TIA 1.7% in 1; 3.6% in 2; 3.3% in 3; 6.7% in 4	Previous neurologic event (OR 6.8); age >70 (OR 4.5); preoperative anemia (OR 4.2); aortic atheroma (OR 3.7); duration of myocardial ischemia (OR 2.8); number of bypasses (OR 2.3); LV-EF <0.35 (OR 2.2); insulin-dependent diabetes (OR 1.5)
2007[33]	171 serial TEVAR cases	PO	5.8%	Prior stroke (OR 9.4); involvement of the proximal descending thoracic aorta (OR 5.5); CT demonstrating severe atheromatous disease of aortic arch (OR 14.8)
2007[34]	606 stent/graft cases	PO	3.1% stroke; 2.5% paraplegia	Stroke: duration of the intervention (OR 6.4); female sex (OR 3.3) Paraplegia: left subclavian artery covering without revascularization (OR 3.9); renal failure (OR 3.6); concomitant open abdominal aorta surgery (OR 5.5); three or more stent grafts used (OR 3.5)

CC, case control; *CI,* cardiac index; *CPB,* cardiopulmonary bypass; *CRI,* chronic renal insufficiency; *EF,* ejection fraction; *LV,* left ventricular; *MI,* myocardial infarction; *OR,* odds ratio; *PO,* prospective observational; *PVD,* peripheral vascular disease; *R,* retrospective; *TIA,* transient ischemic attack.

Table 7-4 Summary of Meta-analysis on Carotid Surgery and Stroke

Study, Year	Number of Trials	Number of Subjects (Intervention/No Intervention)	Intervention	Control	Outcomes
1999[82]	23 publications from 3 randomized studies (NASCET, ECST, VACSP)	6078 (3777/2301)	Surgery	Medical treatment	Stenosis 70%-99% (absolute RR 6.7%, NNT 15, to prevent stroke or death) Stenosis 50%-69% (absolute RR 4.7%, NNT 21) Stenosis <49% (absolute risk increase 2.2, NNH 45)
2004[83]	7 randomized; 41 nonrandomized	554 in randomized; 25,622 in nonrandomized	Local anesthesia for CEA	General anesthesia for CEA	Meta-analysis of nonrandomized studies showed significant reduction in risk of stroke (31 studies), but this was not shown in analysis of randomized studies Conclusion: insufficient evidence
2004[84]	7 randomized	1281 operations	Carotid patch angioplasty during CEA	Primary closure	Patch angioplasty associated with reduced risk of stroke of any kind ($p = 0.004$), ipsilateral stroke ($p = 0.001$), *perioperative stroke or death* ($p = 0.007$), long-term stroke or death ($p = 0.004$), perioperative arterial occlusion ($p = 0.0001$), long-term decreased recurrent stenosis ($p < 0.0001$)
2005[85]	62 (16 studies evaluated perioperative stroke and gender differences)	9131 female; 17,559 male	Female	Male	Female gender (OR 1.28; CI 1.12-1.46) Also evaluated risk of nonfatal perioperative stroke based on age: age $\geq$75 (OR 1.01, CI 0.8-1.3); age $\geq$80 (OR 0.95)
2005[37]	3 (asymptomatic carotid stenosis)	5223	CEA	Medical	Perioperative stroke or death rate: 2.9% Perioperative stroke or death or subsequent ipsilateral stroke: benefit for CEA (RR 0.71, CI 0.55-0.90)

CEA, carotid endarterectomy; *CI*, confidence interval; *NNH*, number needed to harm; *NNT*, number needed to treat; *OR*, odds ratio; *PVD*, peripheral vascular disease; *RR*, risk reduction; *TIA*, transient ischemic attack.

Table 7-5 Summary of Randomized Controlled Trials of Carotid Endarterectomy

Study, Year	Number of Subjects (Intervention/No Intervention)	Study Design	Intervention	Control (No Intervention)	Outcomes
1998[38] NASCET	1108 intervention; 1118 no intervention	RCT of symptomatic carotid stenosis (50%-69%)	CEA	Medical management	Perioperative stroke risk: 6.16% Univariate analysis: contralateral carotid occlusion (RR 2.3); left-sided carotid disease (RR 2.3); daily dose of less than 650 mg ASA (RR 2.3); absence of history of MI or angina (RR 2.2); lesion on imaging ipsilateral to operative artery (RR 2.0); DM (RR 2.0); diastolic BP >90 mm Hg (RR 2.0)
1998[86] ECST	1811 intervention; 1213 no intervention	RCT of all symptomatic carotid stenosis	CEA	Medical management (as long as possible)	Perioperative stroke risk: 6.8% Cox proportional-hazards model of major stroke or death within 5 postoperative days: female sex (hazards ratio: 2.39); age in years at randomization (HR 0.959 per year); occluded symptomatic carotid (HR 12.77)

(Continued)

Table 7-5	Summary of Randomized Controlled Trials of Carotid Endarterectomy—Cont'd				
Study, Year	Number of Subjects (Intervention/No Intervention)	Study Design	Intervention	Control (No Intervention)	Outcomes
1999[39] ACE	1395 "intervention"; 1409 "no intervention"	DBRCT of all patients scheduled for CEA	Low-dose ASA (81 or 325 mg)	High-dose ASA (650 or 1300 mg)	Perioperative any stroke/death (30 days): 4.7% in low dose and 6.1% in high dose (RR 1.29, CI 0.94-1.76) Univariate analysis for perioperative stroke/death: contralateral carotid occlusion (RR 2.3); history of DM (RR 1.9); taking ≥650 mg ASA (RR 1.8); endarterectomy of the left carotid (RR 1.6); ipsilateral TIA or stroke in prior 6 months (RR 1.4); history of contralateral stroke (RR 1.47); insulin therapy (RR 1.78)
2004[87] ACST	1560 intervention; 1560 no intervention	RCT of asymptomatic carotid stenosis ≥60%	Immediate CEA	Medical management	Perioperative stroke (30 days): 2.79% Perioperative stroke RF not assessed Conclusion: in those <75 years of age with asymptomatic stenosis of 70% or more, CEA cut 5-year stroke risk from 12% to 6%
1991[88] ECST	Mild stenosis (0%-29%): 219 intervention, 155 no intervention Severe stenosis (70%-99%): 455 intervention, 323 no intervention	RCT of symptomatic carotid stenosis	CEA	No CEA	Perioperative stroke/death (30 days): 3.7% severe stenosis, 2.3% mild stenosis Adverse 30-day outcome predicted by high blood pressure (SBP >160 mm Hg); rapid surgery (less than 1 hour)
1995[89] ACAS	825 intervention; 834 no intervention	RCT of asymptomatic carotid stenosis ≥60%	CEA	Medical management	Perioperative stroke/death (30 days after randomization): 2.3% Trend toward better outcome in men, but not statistically significant ($p = 0.1$) NNT 19 (to prevent one stroke in 5 years)
1991[90] NASCET	328 intervention; 331 no intervention	RCT of severe (70%-99%) symptomatic (TIA or nondisabling stroke within past 120 days) carotid stenosis	CEA	Medical management	Perioperative stroke (30 days): 5.5% Absolute risk reduction for intervention group for 2 years: 17% Medical management group*: • 0-5 RF—17% risk stroke in 2 years • 6 RF—23% risk stroke in 2 years • ≥7 RF—39% risk stroke in 2 years

*Selected RF = age >70, male sex, SBP >160, DBP >90, recency (<31 days), recent event was stroke not TIA, degree of stenosis (>80%), presence of ulceration on angiogram, history of smoking, hypertension, MI, CHF, DM, intermittent claudication, elevated lipids.

ASA, aspirin; *BP*, blood pressure; *CEA*, carotid endarterectomy; *CHF*, congestive heart failure; *CI*, confidence interval; *DB*, double-blind; *DM*, diabetes mellitus; *NNH*, number to harm; *NNT*, number to treat; *OR*, odds ratio; *P*, placebo controlled; *PVD*, peripheral vascular disease; *RCT*, randomized controlled trial; *RF*, risk factor; *RR*, risk reduction; *TIA*, transient ischemic attack.

AREAS OF UNCERTAINTY

In the cardiac literature, the most common question is whether off-pump CABG reduces perioperative stroke. This was assessed by two meta-analyses. It appears that off-pump CABG has a trend toward, if not being significantly superior to, conventional CABG in preventing perioperative stroke (OR [confidence interval, CI] 0.68 [0.33 to 1.40] and 0.55 [0.43 to 0.69]).[30,36] It is also likely that a "no touch" technique substantially reduces stroke risk in those with a heavily diseased aorta. In addition to technique, additional controversies revolve around intraoperative technologies to help prevent stroke (i.e., transesophageal echocardiography (TEE), epiaortic ultrasound, intraaortic filtration devices).

In the carotid literature, many of the controversies are addressed in the meta-analyses. One question is whether the use of local anesthesia instead of general anesthesia will reduce stroke risk. The conclusion is that we need more prospective studies to come to a verdict, although there is a suggestion that local anesthesia may be superior.[37] The NASCET trial showed that a daily dose of aspirin of less than 650 milligrams was associated with a higher relative risk of stroke.[38] The ASA and Carotid Endarterectomy (ACE) study[39] seemed to clear up that controversy, showing the opposite result, that conventional low-dose treatment was safer. This leads to current practice and guidelines to use 81 or 325 milligrams of aspirin.[40] Much of the current research in CEA is identifying the patient population who will benefit the most from surgery.

SUMMARY

Stroke is a devastating event, the incidence of which is augmented in the perioperative period. The most obvious consequence of perioperative stroke is worsened outcomes, particularly in terms of hospital mortality risk. A representative number for hospital mortality rate after CABG is about 24.8%,[41] and about 33% for thoracic endovascular aortic repair (TEVAR).[33] In another large database of 35,733 patients, the 1-year survival following stroke in the CABG population was 83%.[42] Additionally, intensive care unit (ICU) stay and hospital stay were increased, as well as health dollars spent.

One positive view of this phenomenon of perioperative cerebral ischemia is that, as an aggregate, surgery patients have a 0.08% to 0.7% base chance of having a perioperative stroke.[1] The risk of this event is altered by the presence or absence of risk factors (as noted in Table 7-1). This basic risk of stroke likely overlaps into all surgical procedures, including CABG and CEA. The success of the many predictive scales for postoperative stroke relies on accurately incorporating these risk factors. The augmented risk in CABG and CEA is likely from technical aspects of the surgery itself (accounting for the immediate postoperative ischemic events), as well as the more tumultuous postoperative course (electrolyte abnormalities, dehydration, arrhythmias, infections, redo procedures, etc.).

In the cardiac literature, it appears that continued improvement in stroke rates is very much feasible based on proper use of alternative techniques and multiple available technologies. As discussed earlier, off-pump CABG likely has a lower stroke risk as compared with conventional CABG.[36,30] One study revealed a promising off-pump CABG perioperative stroke/TIA rate of 0.14%,[43] an exceptionally low risk rate.

Another major issue is how to deal with clot burden in the ascending aorta and arch. A study by Mackensen and colleagues[44] demonstrated that cerebral emboli, as detected by intraoperative transcranial Doppler, were significantly associated with atheroma in the ascending aorta and arch but not the descending aorta. These emboli may be responsible for intraoperative stroke, but also other cerebral injury that may lead to postoperative delirium or long-term cognitive dysfunction. Logically, the use of novel available technologies may reduce these outcomes. In Europe, the use of intraaortic filtration appeared to improve postoperative neurologic outcome.[45,46] In one study, 402 patients were nonvoluntarily assigned intraaortic filtration.[45] The predicted number of strokes was estimated with the use of the Stroke Risk Index. Six neurologic events occurred, whereas the Stroke Risk Index predicted 13.7.

Both epiaortic ultrasound and TEE have been used to assess clot burden of the ascending aorta and aortic arch. In cases where aortic atheroma is severe (greater than 5 mm), altering technique ("no touch," off pump) may be paramount in importance. In one study, using both TEE and epiaortic ultrasound resulted in 0 strokes in the high-risk group (22 patients).[47] In cases of moderate disease (3 to 5 mm), careful choice of aortic cannulation site and minimal cross-clamping (single clamp) seemed to

have improved outcomes.[47,48] In addition to the studies already discussed, there is evidence that a "no touch" technique, in the right setting, may improve overall outcome, aside from overt stroke. In a review of 640 off-pump CABG cases,[49] 84 had their surgeries modified with a "no touch" technique. In the "no touch" group, the postoperative delirium rate improved (8% versus 15%, $p = 0.12$), and there was a lower incidence of stroke (0% versus 1%), although numbers were too small to reach statistical significance.

The improvements in carotid surgery will likely revolve, in part, around optimal patient selection, timing, and intervention approach. Currently, it is thought that severe (70% to 99%) symptomatic carotid stenosis benefits the most (5-year absolute risk reduction of 16%); followed by moderate (50% to 69%) symptomatic stenosis (5-year absolute risk reduction of 4.6%); and, finally, asymptomatic carotid stenosis of 60% to 99% (small benefit).[40] Also, current practice is to perform CEA within 6 weeks of a nondisabling carotid-related ischemic stroke. A prospective multicenter observational study directly assessed this question.[50] In this study, the perioperative stroke and death rate was 6.7%, comparable with ECST and NASCET. Interestingly, higher ASA grades of III and IV, as well as decreasing age, were predictive of higher perioperative risk, especially if surgery was done in the first 3 weeks. The perioperative risk was 14.6% in the first 3 weeks versus 4.8% beyond the first 3 weeks.

In the early part of this decade, carotid artery stenting (CAS) was used freely in all patient groups without the support of much evidence. Current investigations, however, are now considering the optimal use of CAS. A recent meta-analysis of seven trials (1480 randomized to CEA, 1492 to carotid angioplasty with or without stenting) significantly favored CEA over CAS with regard to death or any stroke at 30 days, risk of death, any stroke or myocardial infarction at 30 days, ipsilateral stroke at 30 days, any stroke at 30 days, death or stroke at 6 months, and the risk of procedural failure.[51] CAS, however, may be suitable in patients with concomitant coronary disease awaiting revascularization,[52] and in those patients with contralateral carotid occlusion.[53]

Finally, one must mention the possibility of identifying, using, or developing novel neuroprotective drugs. There is evidence that preoperative use of statins may be protective for cardiac surgery.[54] In addition, one study showed that perioperative beta-blockade during cardiac surgery may reduce the risk of neurologic injury.[54a] Several anesthetic agents, such as thiopental and isoflurane, may also provide some level of neuroprotection.[55]

For now, we must rely on identifying those patients at highest risk for a perioperative stroke. A commonly used scale for cardiac surgery is the Multicenter Study of Perioperative Ischemia (McSPI) Stroke Risk Index (SRI).[56] This scale is not quite ideal, however, as was shown by a recent study attempting to validate the SRI.[57] Other scales have been developed and are available for review. A different scale may be ideal for each surgical specialty. It is our hope that the contents of this chapter may help guide management of all patients at risk for stroke in the perioperative period.

AUTHORS' RECOMMENDATIONS

1. Precise history, especially with regard to history of stroke/TIA.
2. Optimal medical management for stroke risk factors. Consider initiation of statin therapy before CABG.[54]
3. Continuation of antiplatelet and anticoagulation whenever feasible.
4. Preoperative echocardiogram: to help risk stratify those patients with atrial fibrillation (heart failure and atrial fibrillation in combination increase risk of stroke).
5. Consider use of local anesthesia instead of general anesthesia when feasible.
6. Intraoperatively: maintain mean arterial pressure as near as possible to preoperative baseline, especially in patients at highest risk for stroke.
7. Intraoperatively: maintain glycemic control as per American Diabetes Association guidelines (as close as possible to 110, but less than 180). Some studies support this goal in cardiac surgery, but evidence remains controversial.[58-61]
8. CABG patients: screening carotid ultrasound with prior CEA if necessary.
9. CABG patients: intraoperative use of TEE and/or epiaortic ultrasound to optimize aortic cannulation and clamping (versus use of "no touch" technique).
10. CABG patients: consider perioperative use of beta-blockade.[51]
11. Postoperative CABG: monitor for atrial fibrillation with telemetry for at least 3 days; consider anticoagulation for 30 days after return of sinus rhythm.
12. Postoperative CABG: maintain electrolytes and intravascular volume.
13. Postoperative CABG and CEA: initiate antiplatelet therapy because this can reduce risk of perioperative stroke without increasing bleeding risk.[42,43]
14. Avoid and promptly treat postoperative (or preoperative) infections.
15. Prompt neurologic consultation once a potential deficit is identified. Depending on surgical procedure, options such as intravenous tissue plasminogen activator (IV tPA), intra-arterial tPA, mechanical thrombectomy, and clot retrieval may be considered.

REFERENCES

1. Selim M: Perioperative stroke. *N Engl J Med* 2007;356:706-713.
2. Kam PC, Calcroft RM: Peri-operative stroke in general surgical patients. *Anaesthesia* 1997;52:879-883.
3. Gutierrez IZ, Barone DL, Makula PA, Currier C: The risk of perioperative stroke in patients with asymptomatic carotid bruits undergoing peripheral vascular surgery. *Am Surg* 1987; 53:487-489.
4. Nosan DK, Gomez CR, Maves MD: Perioperative stroke in patients undergoing head and neck surgery. *Ann Otol Rhinol Laryngol* 1993;102:717-723.
5. Bond R, Rerkasem K, Shearman CP, Rothwell PM: Time trends in the published risks of stroke and death due to endarterectomy for symptomatic carotid stenosis. *Cerebrovasc Dis* 2004;18: 37-46.
6. Bucerius J, Gummert JF, Borger MA, et al: Stroke after cardiac surgery: A risk factor analysis of 16,184 consecutive adult patients. *Ann Thorac Surg* 2003;75:472-478.
7. McKhann GM, Grega MA, Borowicz LM Jr, Baumgartner WA, Selnes OA: Stroke and encephalopathy after cardiac surgery: An update. *Stroke* 2006;37:562-571.
8. Menon U, Kenner M, Kelley RE: Perioperative stroke. *Expert Rev Neurotherapeutics* 2007;7:1-9.
9. Likosky, DS, Marrin CA, Caplan LR, et al: Determination of etiologic mechanisms of strokes secondary to coronary artery bypass graft surgery. *Stroke* 2003;34:2830-2834.
10. Blacker DJ, Flemming KD, Link MJ, et al: The preoperative cerebrovascular consultation: Common cerebrovascular questions before general or cardiac surgery. *Mayo Clin Proc* 2004;79: 223-229.
11. Lahtinen J, Biancari F, Salmela E, et al: Postoperative atrial fibrillation is a major cause of stroke after on-pump coronary bypass surgery. *Ann Thorac Surg* 2004;77:1241-1244.
12. Dixon B, Santamaria J, Campbell D: Coagulation activation and organ dysfunction following cardiac surgery. *Chest* 2005;128:229-236.
13. Paramo JA, Rifon J, Llorens R, Casares J, Paloma MJ, Rocha E: Intra- and postoperative fibrinolysis in patients undergoing cardiopulmonary bypass surgery. *Haemostasis* 1991;21:58-64.
14. Hinterhuber G, Bohler K, Kittler H, Quehenberger P: Extended monitoring of hemostatic activation after varicose vein surgery under general anesthesia. *Dermatol Surg* 2006;32:632-639.
15. Maulaz AB, Bezerra DC, Michel P, et al: Effect of discontinuing aspirin therapy on the risk of brain ischemic stroke. *Arch Neurol* 2005;62:1217-1220.
16. Genewein U, Haeberli A, Straub PW, et al: Rebound after cessation of oral anticoagulant therapy: The biochemical evidence. *Br J Haematol* 1996;92:479-485.
17. Larson BJ, Zumberg MS, Kitchens CS: A feasibility study of continuing dose-reduced warfarin for invasive procedures in patients with high thromboembolic risk. *Chest* 2005;127:922-927.
18. Gottesman RF, Sherman PM, Grega MA, et al: Watershed strokes after cardiac surgery. *Stroke* 2006;37:2306-2311.
19. Caplan LR, Hennerici M: Impaired clearance of emboli (washout) is an important link between hypoperfusion, embolism, and ischemic stroke. *Arch Neurol* 1998;55:1475-1482.
20. Gold JP, Charlson ME, Williams-Russo P, et al: Improvements of outcomes after coronary artery bypass: A randomized trial comparing intraoperative high versus low mean arterial pressure. *J Thorac Cardiovasc Surg* 1995;110:1302-1311.
21. van Wermeskerken GK, Lardenoye JW, Hill SE, et al: Intraoperative physiologic variables and outcome in cardiac surgery: Part II. Neurologic outcome. *Ann Thorac Surg* 2000;69:1077-1083.
22. Whitney GE, Brophy CM, Kahn EM, et al: Inadequate cerebral perfusion is an unlikely cause of perioperative stroke. *Ann Vasc Surg* 2004;11:109-114.
23. Naylor AR, Mehta Z, Rothwell PM, Bell PR: Carotid artery disease and stroke during coronary artery bypass: A critical review of the literature. *Eur J Vasc Endovasc Surg* 2002;23:283-294.
24. Hart R, Hindman B: Mechanisms of perioperative cerebral infarction. *Stroke* 1982;13:766-772.
25. Parikh S, Cohen JR: Perioperative stroke after general surgical procedures. *New York State Journal of Medicine* 1993;93:162-165.
26. Larsen SF, Zaric D, Boysen G: Postoperative cerebrovascular accidents in general surgery. *Acta Anaesthesiol Scand* 1988;32: 698-701.
27. Carney WI, Stewart BS, Depinto DJ, et al: Carotid bruit as a risk factor in aortoiliac reconstruction. *Surgery* 1977;81:567-570.
28. Treiman RL, Foran RF, Cohen JL, et al: Carotid bruit: A follow up report on its significance in patients undergoing an abdominal aortic operation. *Arch Surg* 1973;106:803-805.
29. Limburg M, Wijdicks EFM, Li H: Ischemic stroke after surgical procedures: Clinical features, neuroimaging, and risk factors. *Neurology* 1998;50:895-901.
30. Reston JT, Tregear SJ, Turkelson CM: Meta-analysis of short-term and mid-term outcomes following off-pump coronary bypass grafting. *Ann Thorac Surg* 2003;76:1510-1515.
31. Hogue CW Jr, De Wet CJ, Schechtman KB, et al: The importance of prior stroke for the adjusted risk of neurologic injury after cardiac surgery for women and men. *Anesthesiology* 2003;98: 823-829.
32. Hogue CW Jr, Murphy SF, Schechtman KB, et al: Risk factors for early or delayed stroke after cardiac surgery. *Circulation* 1999;100:642-647.
33. Gutsche JT, Cheung AT, McGarvey ML, et al: Risk factors for perioperative stroke after thoracic endovascular aortic repair. *Ann Thorac Surg* 2007;84:1195-1200.

34. Buth J, Harris PL, Hobo R, et al: Neurologic complications associated with endovascular repair of thoracic aortic pathology: Incidence and risk factors. A study from the European Collaborators on Stent/Graft Techniques for Aortic Aneurysm Repair (EUROSTAR) Registry. *J Vasc Surg* 2007;46:1103-1111.

35. Tu JV, Wang H, Bowyer B, et al: Risk factors for death or stroke after carotid endarterectomy: Observations from the Ontario Carotid Endarterectomy Registry. *Stroke* 2003;34:2568-2573.

36. Cheng DC, Bainbridge D, Martin JE, et al: Does off-pump coronary artery bypass reduce mortality, morbidity, and resource utilization when compared with conventional coronary artery bypass? A meta-analysis of randomized trials. *Anesthesiology* 2005;102:188-203.

37. Chambers BR, Donnan GA: Carotid endarterectomy for asymptomatic carotid stenosis. *Cochrane Database Syst Rev* 2005;4:CD001923.

38. Barnett HJ, Taylor DW, Eliasziw M, et al: Benefit of carotid endarterectomy in patients with symptomatic moderate or severe stenosis. North American Symptomatic Carotid Endarterectomy Trial Collaborators. *N Engl J Med* 1998;339:1415-1425.

39. Taylor DW, Barnett HJ, Haynes RB, et al: Low-dose and high-dose acetylsalicylic acid for patients undergoing carotid endarterectomy: A randomized controlled trial. ASA and Carotid Endarterectomy (ACE) Trial Collaborators. *Lancet* 1999;353:2179-2184.

40. Chaturvedi S, Bruno A, Feasby T, et al: Carotid endarterectomy—an evidence-based review: Report of the Therapeutics and Technology Assessment Subcommittee of the American Academy of Neurology. *Neurology* 2005;65:794-801.

41. John R, Choudhri AF, Weinberg AD, et al: Multicenter review of preoperative risk factors for stroke after coronary artery bypass grafting. *Ann Thorac Surg* 2000;69:30-35.

42. Dacey LJ, Likosky DS, Leavitt BJ, et al: Perioperative stroke and long-term survival after coronary bypass graft surgery. *Ann Thorac Surg* 2005;79:532-536.

43. Trehan N, Mishra M, Sharma OP, et al: Further reduction in stroke after off-pump coronary artery bypass grafting: a 10-year experience. *Ann Thorac Surg* 2001;72:S1026-S1032.

44. Mackensen GB, Ti LK, Phillips-Bute BG, et al: Cerebral embolization during cardiac surgery: impact of aortic atheroma burden. *Br J Anaesth* 2003;91:656-661.

45. Schmitz C, Blackstone EH, International Council of Emboli Management (ICEM) Study Group. International Council of Emboli Management (ICEM) Study Group results: Risk adjusted outcomes in intraaortic filtration. *Eur J Cardiothorac Surg* 2001;20:986-991.

46. Wimmer-Greinecker G, International Council of Emboli Management (ICEM) Study Group: Reduction of neurologic complications by intra-aortic filtration in patients undergoing combined intracardiac and CABG procedures. *Eur J Cardiothorac Surg* 2003;23:159-164.

47. Gaspar M, Laufer G, Bonatti J, et al: Epiaortic ultrasound and intraoperative transesophageal echocardiography for the thoracic aorta atherosclerosis assessment in patient undergoing CABG. Surgical technique modification to avoid cerebral stroke. *Chirurgia (Bucur)* 2002;97:529-535.

48. Hangler HB, Nagele G, Danzmayr M, et al: Modification of surgical technique for ascending aortic atherosclerosis: Impact on stroke reduction in coronary artery bypass grafting. *J Thorac Cardiovasc Surg* 2003;126:391-400.

49. Leacche M, Carrier M, Bouchard D, et al: Improving neurologic outcome in off-pump surgery: The "no touch" technique. *Heart Surg Forum* 2003;6:169-175.

50. Eckstein HH, Ringleb P, Dörfler A, et al: The Carotid Surgery for Ischemic Stroke trial: A prospective observational study on carotid endarterectomy in the early period after ischemic stroke. *J Vasc Surg* 2002;36:997-1004.

51. Luebke T, Aleksic M, Brunkwall J: Meta-analysis of randomized trials comparing carotid endarterectomy and endovascular treatment. *Eur J Vasc Endovasc Surg* 2007;34:470-479.

52. Yadav JS, Wholey MH, Kuntz RE, et al: Protected carotid-artery stenting versus endarterectomy in high-risk patients. *N Engl J Med* 2004;351:1493-1501.

53. Kastrup A, Groschel K: Carotid endarterectomy versus carotid stenting: An updated review of randomized trials and subgroup analyses. *Acta Chir Belg* 2007;107:119-128.

54. Aboyans V, Labrousse L, Lacroix P, et al: Predictive factors of stroke in patients undergoing coronary bypass grafting: Statins are protective. *Eur J Cardiothorac Surg* 2006;30:300-304.

54a. Amory DW, Grigore A, Amory JK, et al: Neuroprotection is associated with beta-adrenergic receptor antagonists during cardiac surgery: Evidence from 2575 patients. *J Cardiothorac Vasc Anesth* 2002;16:270-277.

55. Turner BK, Wakim JH, Secrest J, et al: Neuroprotective effects of thiopental, propofol, and etomidate. *AANA J* 2005;73:297-302.

56. Newman MF, Wolman R, Kanchuger M, et al: Multicenter preoperative stroke risk index for patients undergoing coronary artery bypass graft surgery. Multicenter Study of Perioperative Ischemia (McSPI) Research Group. *Circulation* 1996;94:II74-80.

57. Elahi M, Battula N, Swanevelder J: The use of the stroke risk index to predict neurological complications following coronary revascularization on cardiopulmonary bypass. *Anaesthesia* 2005;60:654-659.

58. Doenst T, Wijeysundera D, Karkouti K, et al: Hyperglycemia during cardiopulmonary bypass is an independent risk factor for mortality in patients undergoing cardiac surgery. *J Thorac Cardiovasc Surg* 2005;130:1144-1150.

59. Gandhi GY, Nuttall GA, Abel MD, et al: Intraoperative hyperglycemia and perioperative outcomes in cardiac surgery patients. *Mayo Clin Proc* 2005;80(7):862-866.

60. Latham R, Lancaster AD, Covington JF, et al: The association of diabetes and glucose control with surgical-site infections among cardiothoracic surgery patients. *Infect Control Hosp Epidemiol* 2001;22:607-612.

61. Ouattara A, Lecomte P, Le Manach Y, et al: Poor intraoperative blood glucose control is associated with a worsened hospital outcome after cardiac surgery in diabetic patients. *Anesthesiology* 2005;103:687-694.

62. Landercasper J, Merz BJ, Cogbill TH, et al: Perioperative stroke risk in 173 consecutive patients with a past history of stroke. *Arch Surg* 1990;125:986-989.

63. Kim J, Gelb AW: Predicting perioperative stroke. *J Neurosurg Anesthesiol* 1995;7:211-215.

64. Axelrod DA, Stanley JC, Upchurch GR, et al: Risk for stroke after elective noncarotid vascular surgery. *J Vasc Surg* 2004;39:67-72.

65. Wong GY, Warner DO, Schroeder DR, et al: Risk of surgery and anesthesia for ischemic stroke. *Anesthesiology* 2000;92:425-432.

66. Lekprasert V, Akavipat P, Sirinan C, et al: Perioperative stroke and coma in Thai Anesthesia Incidents Study (THAI Study). *J Med Assoc Thai* 2005;88:S113-S117.

67. Anyanwu AC, Filsoufi F, Salzberg SP, et al: Epidemiology of stroke after cardiac surgery in the current era. *J Thorac Cardiovasc Surg* 2007;134:1121-1127.

68. Antunes PE, de Oliveira JF, Antunes MJ: Predictors of cerebrovascular events in patients subjected to isolated coronary surgery. The importance of aortic cross-clamping. *Eur J Cardiothorac Surg* 2003;23:328-333.

69. Goto T, Baba T, Ito A, et al: Gender differences in stroke risk among the elderly after coronary artery surgery. *Anesth Analg* 2007;104:1016-1022.

70. Borger MA, Ivanov J, Weisel RD, et al: Stroke during coronary bypass surgery: Principal role of cerebral macroemboli. *Eur J Cardiothorac Surg* 2001;19:627-632.

71. Bilfinger TV, Reda H, Giron F, et al: Coronary and carotid operations under prospective standardized conditions: Incidence and outcome. *Ann Thorac Surg* 2000;69:1792-1798.

72. Hartman GS, Yao FS, Bruefach M 3rd, et al: Severity of atheromatous disease diagnosed by transesophageal echocardiography predicts stroke and other outcomes associated with coronary artery surgery: A prospective study. *Anesth Analg* 1996;83:701-708.

73. Katz ES, Tunick PA, Rusinek H, et al: Protruding aortic atheromas predict stroke in elderly patients undergoing cardiopulmonary bypass: Experience with intraoperative transesophageal echocardiography. *J Am Coll Cardiol* 1992;20:70-77.

74. Likosky DS, Leavitt BJ, Marrin CA, et al: Intra- and postoperative predictors of stroke after coronary artery bypass grafting. *Ann Thorac Surg* 2003;76:428-434.

75. McKhann GM, Grega MA, Borowicz LM Jr, et al: Encephalopathy and stroke after coronary bypass grafting: Incidence, consequences, and prediction. *Arch Neurol* 2002;59:1422-1428.

76. Engelman DT, Cohn LH, Rizzo RJ: Incidence and predictors of TIAs and strokes following coronary artery bypass grafting: Report and collective review. *Heart Surg Forum* 1999;2:242-245.
77. Hirotani T, Kameda T, Kumamoto T, et al: Stroke after coronary artery bypass grafting in patients with cerebrovascular disease. *Ann Thorac Surg* 2000;70:1571-1576.
78. Ascione R, Reeves BC, Chamberlain MH, et al: Predictors of stroke in the modern era of coronary artery bypass grafting: A case control study. *Ann Thorac Surg* 2002;74:474-480.
79. Baker RA, Hallsworth LJ, Knight JL: Stroke after coronary artery bypass grafting. *Ann Thorac Surg* 2005;80:1746-1750.
80. Stamou SC, Hill PC, Dangas G, et al: Stroke after coronary artery bypass: Incidence, predictors and clinical outcome. *Stroke* 2001;32:1508-1513.
81. Boeken U, Litmathe J, Feindt P, et al: Neurological complications after cardiac surgery: Risk factors and correlation to the surgical procedure. *Thorac Cardiovasc Surg* 2005;53:33-36.
82. Cina CS, Clase CM, Haynes BR: Refining the indications for carotid endarterectomy in patients with symptomatic carotid stenosis: A systematic review. *J Vasc Surg* 1999;30:606-617.
83. Rerkasem K, Bond R, Rothwell PM: Local versus general anesthesia for carotid endarterectomy. *Cochrane Database Syst Rev* 2004;2: CD000126.
84. Bond R, Rerkasem K, Naylor AR, et al: Systematic review of randomized controlled trials of patch angioplasty versus primary closure and different types of patch materials during carotid endarterectomy. *J Vasc Surg* 2004;40:1126-1135.
85. Bond R, Rerkasem K, Cuffe R, et al: A systematic review of the associations between age and sex and the operative risks of carotid endarterectomy. *Cerebrovasc Dis* 2005;20:69-77.
86. European Carotid Surgery Trialists' Collaborative Group. Randomized trial of endarterectomy for recently symptomatic carotid stenosis: Final results of the MRC European Carotid Surgery Trial (ECST). *Lancet* 1998;351:1379-1387.
87. Halliday A, Mansfield A, Marro J, et al: Asymptomatic Carotid Surgery Trial (ACST) Collaborative Group: Prevention of disabling and fatal strokes by successful carotid endarterectomy in patients without recent neurological symptoms: Randomised controlled trial. *Lancet* 2004;363:1491-1502.
88. European Carotid Surgery Trialists' Collaborative Group: MRC European Carotid Surgery Trial: Interim results for symptomatic patients with severe (70-99%) or with mild (0-29%) carotid stenosis. *Lancet* 1991;337:1235-1243.
89. Executive Committee for the Asymptomatic Carotid Atherosclerosis Study: Endarterectomy for asymptomatic carotid artery stenosis. *JAMA* 1995;273:1421-1428.
90. North American Symptomatic Carotid Endarterectomy Trial Collaborators: Beneficial effect of carotid endarterectomy in symptomatic patients with high-grade carotid stenosis. *N Engl J Med* 1991;325:445-453.

8 Should We Delay Surgery in the Patient with Recent Cocaine Use?

Nabil Elkassabany, MD

INTRODUCTION

Prevalence and Epidemiology

Cocaine abuse and addiction continue to be a problem that plagues our nation. Data from the Drug Abuse Warning Network (DAWN) showed that "cocaine-related emergency department visits increased 33% between 1995 and 2002. Currently 5 million Americans are regular users of cocaine, 6000 use the drug for the first time each day, and more than 30 million have tried cocaine at least once".[1] Based on these data, the practicing anesthesiologist will likely come across the cocaine-abusing patient regardless of the setting of his or her practice.

The classic profile of patients reported to experience cocaine-related myocardial ischemia is typically a young, nonwhite, male cigarette smoker with no other significant risk factors for atherosclerosis.[2] However, this profile no longer holds true as the problem becomes more severe and is not confined to a particular race or gender. Cocaine abuse in parturients has been the focus of attention lately, with a reported incidence between 11.8% and 20%.[3]

Pharmacokinetics and Mechanism of Action

Cocaine produces prolonged adrenergic stimulation by blocking the presynaptic uptake of sympathomimetic neurotransmitters, including norepinephrine, serotonin, and dopamine. The euphoric effect of cocaine, the cocaine high, results from prolongation of dopamine activity in the limbic system and the cerebral cortex. It can be taken orally, intravenously, or intranasally. Smoking the free base (street name for the alkalinized form of cocaine) results in very effective transmucosal absorption and high plasma concentration of cocaine. It is metabolized by plasma and liver cholinesterase to water-soluble metabolites (primarily benzylecgonine and ecgonine methyl ester [EME]), "which are excreted in urine. The serum half-life of cocaine is 45 to 90 minutes; only 1% of the parent drug can be recovered in the urine after it is ingested.[4] Thus cocaine can be detected in blood or urine only several hours after its use. However, its metabolites can be detected in urine for up to 72 hours after ingestion, providing a useful indicator for recent use. Hair analysis can detect use of cocaine in the preceding weeks or months.[5] Table 8-1 summarizes the pharmacokinetics of cocaine with different routes of administration.

ANESTHETIC IMPLICATIONS OF COCAINE ABUSE

Acute effects of cocaine toxicity of interest to the anesthesiologist can be summarized as follows:

- Cardiovascular effects
- Pulmonary effects
- Central nervous system (CNS) effects
- Delayed gastric emptying
- Drug-drug interactions (DDIs)

Cardiovascular Effects

Cardiovascular effects of cocaine are largely due to the sympathetic stimulation resulting from inhibition of the peripheral uptake of norepinephrine and other sympathomimetic neurotransmitters. Central sympathetic stimulation has been suggested as an alternative mechanism to explain the exaggerated sympathetic response.[6,7] The resulting hypertension, tachycardia, and coronary artery vasospasm are responsible for the myocardial ischemia seen with cocaine toxicity. In addition, there is evidence that cocaine activates platelets, increases platelet aggregation, and promotes thrombus formation.[8] Knowledge of the mechanism of myocardial ischemia in patients with cocaine abuse is a key for effective treatment. Classically, beta-blockers are avoided because their use may lead to unopposed alpha-mediated coronary vasoconstriction.[9,10] This concept has been recently challenged, and there is some evidence to support the use of beta-blockers in cocaine-related myocardial ischemia.[11] Alpha-blockers and nitroglycerin have been used effectively for symptomatic treatment.[12] Esmolol is used for treatment of cocaine-induced myocardial ischemia because of its short duration of action and the ability to titrate the dose to a target heart rate.[13] Labetalol offers some advantage in that regard because of its combined alpha- and beta-receptor blocking effect.[14]

A major concern in the anesthetic management of the cocaine-abusing patient is the occurrence of cardiac arrhythmias. These include ventricular tachycardia, frequent premature ventricular contractions, or torsades de

Table 8-1	Pharmacokinetics of Cocaine According to the Route of Administration			
Route of Administration	**Onset of Action**	**Peak Effect**	**Duration of Action**	
Inhalation (smoking)	3-5 seconds	1-3 minutes	5-15 minutes	
Intravenous	10-60 seconds	3-5 minutes	20-60 minutes	
Intranasal/ intramucosal	1-5 minutes	15-20 minutes	60-90 minutes	
Gastrointestinal	Up to 20 minutes	Up to 90 minutes	Up to 180 minutes	

pointes. Myocardial ischemia has been suggested as the underlying mechanism for these arrhythmias; however, cocaine-induced sodium and potassium channel blockade is currently thought to be more important. This cation channel blockade results in QRS and QTc prolongation, which is considered to be the primary mechanism for induction of these cocaine-induced arrythmias.[15]

Aortic dissection[16] and ruptured aortic aneurysm[17,18] have been reported with acute abuse. Peripheral vasoconstriction may mask the picture of hypovolemia in the setting of acute cocaine toxicity.

Chronic use of cocaine can cause left ventricular hypertrophy, systolic dysfunction, and dilated cardiomyopathy.[19] Repetitive cocaine administration is associated with the development of early and progressive tolerance to systemic, left ventricular, and coronary vascular effects of cocaine. The mechanism of tolerance involves neither impaired myocardial nor coronary vascular responsiveness to adrenergic stimulation but rather attenuated catecholamine responses to repetitive cocaine administration.

Pulmonary Effects

Approximately 25% of individuals who smoke crack cocaine develop nonspecific respiratory complaints.[20] Within 1 to 48 hours, the smoking of cocaine may produce a combination of diffuse alveolar infiltrates, eosinophilia, and fever that has been termed *crack lung*.[21,22] Long-term cocaine exposure can produce diffuse alveolar damage, diffuse alveolar hemorrhage, noncardiogenic pulmonary edema, and pulmonary infarction.[23]

Central Nervous System

Stimulation in acute toxicity can lead to euphoria, hyperthermia,[24] and seizures.[25,26] Cocaine-induced psychomotor agitation can cause hyperthermia when peripheral vasoconstriction prevents the body from dissipating the heat being generated from persistent agitation. The resulting fever has to be differentiated from other causes of hyperthermia in the setting of general anesthesia. Cocaine is associated with both focal neurologic deficits and coma. Possible etiologies include vasoconstriction (i.e., transient ischemic attack or ischemic stroke) and intracerebral hemorrhage.[27,28] Minimum alveolar concentration (MAC) of halothane and other inhalational agents is increased

with the chronic use of cocaine.[29,30] Cocaine was found to delay gastric emptying via a central mechanism.[31] This effect becomes more relevant in the setting of trauma and obstetrics. Cocaine-amphetamine-regulated transcript (CART) is a chemical that acts in the CNS to inhibit gastric acid secretion via brain corticotropin-releasing factor system.

Drug-Drug Interactions

Even though cocaine is a known inhibitor of the enzyme cytochrome P450 2D6,[32] pharmacokinetic drug-drug interactions (DDIs) are generally unlikely to be clinically relevant. However, pharmacodynamic DDIs are a meaningful consideration to take into account in the perioperative period. Cocaine's potent sympathomimetic effects may act synergistically with other drugs (stimulants, anticholinergic agents, noradrenergic reuptake inhibitors) to produce an array of undesirable side effects (blurred vision, constipation, tachycardia, urinary retention, arrhythmias, etc.). Synergistic pressor effects can produce vascular compromise that can precipitate cardiac ischemia or cerebrovascular accidents. Ketamine may exacerbate the sympathomimetic effect of cocaine.[33] Halothane and xanthine derivatives sensitize the myocardium to the arrhythmogenic effect of epinephrine and should be avoided as well.[34] Cocaine has been reported to alter the metabolism of succinylcholine because they both compete for metabolism by plasma cholinesterases.[35] However, Birnbach[36] found that succinylcholine can be used safely in standard doses. Cigarette smoking was found to enhance cocaine-induced coronary artery vasospasm in the atherosclerotic segments when compared with the vasoconstriction produced by cocaine alone.[37] This effect was not evident in normal coronary arteries.

THE CONTROVERSY

Whenever it comes to taking care of cocaine-abusing patients, the questions that the anesthesiologist has to answer are, How safe is it to anesthetize patients with acute cocaine abuse? If the decision was made to delay the case as a result of a positive toxicology screening test or self-reported use, how much time should lapse before it would be "safe" to proceed? Particularly debatable is the case of elective surgery in a patient who tests positive for cocaine but does not show any signs of acute toxicity. Many anesthesia practitioners would prefer to delay such patients until the patient tests negative for cocaine or has not been using cocaine for 72 hours. This decision is more difficult nowadays because of the increased costs and wastage of resources associated with routine cancellations of these cases. The literature provides evidence to support both the safety of the anesthetic and the increased morbidity with the acute use of cocaine.

EVIDENCE

Perioperative Risk of General Anesthesia with Acute Cocaine Toxicity

The risk of acute myocardial infarction (MI) is increased by a factor of 24 in the 60 minutes after the use of cocaine in persons who otherwise are relatively low risk for myocardial ischemia.[38] A meta-analysis, done in 1992, reported a total of 92 cases of cocaine-related MI.[39] Two thirds of patients had their MI within 3 hours of the use of cocaine (with a range of 1 minute to 4 days). Data from the third National Health and Nutrition Examination Survey (NHANES III) found that 1 of every 20 persons ages 18 to 45 years reported regular use of cocaine.[40] This survey demonstrated that the regular use of cocaine was associated with an increased likelihood of nonfatal MI. One of every four nonfatal MIs in young patients was attributable to the frequent use of cocaine in this survey. There was no increased risk of nonfatal stroke in this population associated with frequent or infrequent use of cocaine. The focus of research in this area is to determine risk factors for developing MI in cocaine-abusing patients. A recent study suggested that age, preexisting coronary artery disease (CAD), hyperlipidemia, and smoking are associated with the diagnosis of MI among patients hospitalized with cocaine-associated chest pain.[41] Cocaine-induced myocardial ischemia can occur whether or not there was preexisting CAD. However, it has been shown that coronary artery vasospasm tends to be more severe in the diseased segments of the coronary vessels when compared with the normal coronary arteries in response to intranasal cocaine in a dose of 2 mg/kg of body weight.[42]

Most of the cases of cocaine-related myocardial ischemia are reported in the emergency medicine and internal medicine literature after recreational use of cocaine. There are seven case reports of cocaine-induced myocardial ischemia in the setting of the use of cocaine for topical anesthesia for ear, nose, and throat (ENT) procedures.[43-49] Some of these cases were done with the patient under general anesthesia. Two more cases of myocardial ischemia were reported under general anesthesia after recreational use of cocaine.[50-51] Other cardiac events reported under general anesthesia with acute use of cocaine include prolonged QT interval,[52] ventricular fibrillation,[53] and acute pulmonary edema.[54,55] One case report described a patient coming to the operating room (OR) after a motor vehicle accident with a white foreign body in the back of the oropharynx that proved to be crack cocaine.[56] This case goes on to report wide swings of blood pressure, patient agitation, and hypotension resistant to treatment with ephedrine.

One of the few studies that demonstrated the interaction between cocaine and general anesthesia was the study by Boylan and colleagues.[57] They found that increasing depth of anesthesia with isoflurane from 0.75 MAC to 1.5 MAC in their swine model was not associated with reversal of, or decrease in, the hemodynamic responses to cocaine infusion.[57] The observed responses were increase in systemic vascular resistance, ventricular arrhythmias, diastolic hypertension, and reversal of the endocardial/epicardial blood flow.

The half-life of cocaine ranges from 60 to 90 minutes. A reasonable assumption would be that most of the cocaine-related cardiac events in the perioperative period will happen at a time when the level of the metabolites, not the parent drug, is high in the circulation. The question now is, "How active are the metabolites of cocaine and can they affect the coronary vessels to the same extent as cocaine itself?" Brogan and colleagues[58] randomized 18 patients undergoing coronary artery catheterization for evaluation of chest pain to receive either intranasal cocaine or normal saline. They estimated the diameter of the coronary arteries and measured different hemodynamic variables at 30, 60, and 90 minutes. They found that coronary vasospasm happened twice, once at 30 minutes and the second at 90 minutes. The initial coronary artery vasospasm correlated with peak level of cocaine in the blood. The recurrent vasospasm occurred at 90 minutes when cocaine was hardly detected in the blood. The level of the main metabolites of cocaine (benzoylecgonine and EME) was at its peak at this point. Although this study was able to document a temporal relation between the recurrent coronary vasospasm and the peak level of the cocaine metabolites, it did not prove that these metabolites were the cause of the vasoconstriction. Such a proof will come only from assessment of the coronary vasoreactivity after direct administration of each metabolite.

Recent studies have suggested that various metabolites of cocaine may exert a substantial influence on a variety of tissues, including the heart, brain, and arterial smooth muscle. In rats, norcocaine, another pharmacologically active metabolite of cocaine, was found to be equipotent to cocaine in inhibiting norepinephrine uptake and in causing tachycardia, convulsions, and death.[59] In feline cerebral arteries in vitro, benzoylecogonine is a more potent vasoconstrictor than cocaine.[60]

Safety of General Anesthesia in Cocaine-Abusing Patients

The interaction between cocaine and general anesthesia is not well studied. Most of the information is derived from clinical case reports or animal studies. The few studies that looked into this interaction demonstrated that general anesthesia is probably safe in cocaine-abusing patients, especially in the absence of clinical signs of toxicity.

Barash and colleagues[61] studied 18 patients undergoing coronary artery surgery to examine whether cocaine in a clinically used dose exerts sympathomimetic effects during general anesthesia. Eleven patients received cocaine hydrochloride as a 10% solution (1.5 mg/kg) applied topically to the nasal mucosa. The other group received a placebo treatment. There were no important differences in cardiovascular function between groups. The rise in plasma cocaine concentration bore no relationship to any changes in cardiovascular function. Administration of topical cocaine did not exert any clinically significant sympathomimetic effect and appeared to be well tolerated in anesthetized patients with coronary artery disease. The results of this study should be interpreted cautiously as the doses used for recreational use may well exceed the doses used during this study.

A more recent study by Hill and colleagues[62] demonstrated that individuals undergoing elective surgery requiring general anesthesia who test urine positive for cocaine but are clinically nontoxic are at no greater risk than drug-free patients of the same ASA physical status. This study involved 40 ASA physical status I and II patients between 18 and 55 years of age. The authors of this study caution that these results may not be applicable to the cocaine-abusing patient with a QT interval of 500 ms or more on the preoperative electrocardiogram or to those patients whose vital signs indicate acute cocaine toxicity.

Another study looked into maternal morbidity in cocaine-abusing parturients undergoing cesarean section with general or regional anesthesia.[63] Cocaine-abusing parturients were at higher risk for peripartum events such as hypertension, hypotension, and wheezing episodes. However, when the analysis was done in a multivariate model, cocaine abuse was not an independent risk factor for these events. There was no increase in the rates of maternal morbidity or death in the cocaine-abusing group. The cocaine-abusing patients will often be seen in the OR with a complex medical history. It would be difficult to predict how our anesthetic is going to interact with cocaine in the presence of the multiple comorbidities based on the results of these two studies alone.

Regional Anesthesia and Cocaine-Abusing Patients

Any advantage of regional anesthesia over general anesthesia is controversial. The argument in favor of regional anesthesia, when possible, includes having an awake patient who will be able to communicate chest pain as a sign for myocardial ischemia. If regional anesthesia is selected, potential complications include combative behavior, altered pain perception, cocaine-induced thrombocytopenia, and ephedrine-resistant hypotension. Abnormal endorphin levels and changes in the mu and kappa receptors in the spinal cord may be responsible for pain sensation despite adequate sensory level with regional anesthesia.[64] The duration of action of spinal narcotics (sufentanil) in labor is shorter in cocaine-abusing parturients relative to controls.[65] Many theories have been proposed to explain cocaine-induced thrombocytopenia. These include bone marrow suppression, platelet activation, and autoimmune response with induction of platelet-specific antibodies. Gershon and colleagues[66] challenged this concept. They concluded that obtaining a routine platelet count before epidural or spinal analgesia in cocaine-abusing parturients is not necessary.

AUTHOR'S RECOMMENDATIONS

1. The decision-making process involving anesthetic care of cocaine-abusing patients should be individualized. History and associated comorbidities have to be considered when deciding whether or not to proceed with elective cases in the setting of recent cocaine abuse either by self-reporting or urine testing.
2. The level of invasive monitoring for each patient should be made on a case-by-case basis.
3. Routinely testing for cocaine is not necessary if the patient is not showing any signs of clinical toxicity.
4. Typically, we will not delay an elective case if the patient self-reported recent cocaine use, as long as the patient is clinically nontoxic and does not have an extensive cardiac history.
5. The issue of the interaction between cocaine and general anesthesia remains controversial. Until we have conclusive clinical trials to address this subject, the decision will remain to be individualized according to the setting of practice of each anesthesiologist and his or her level of comfort dealing with these cases.

REFERENCES

1. Department of Health and Human Services, Substance Abuse and Mental Health Service Administration: *National household survey on drug abuse main findings.* Rockville, MD, 2000.
2. Booth BM, Weber JE, Walton MA, Cunningham RM, Massey L, Thrush CR, Maio RF: Characteristics of cocaine users presenting to an emergency department chest pain observation unit. *Acad Emerg Med* 2005;12(4):329-337.
3. Kuczkowski KM: The cocaine abusing parturient: A review of anesthetic considerations. *Can J Anaesth* 2004;51(2):145-154.
4. Jones RT: Pharmacokinetics of cocaine: Considerations when assessing cocaine use by urinalysis. *National Institute of Drug Abuse Research Monograph* 1997;175:221-234.
5. Dupont RL, Baumgartner WA: Drug testing by urine and hair analysis: Complementary features and scientific issues. *Forensic Sci Int* 1995;70(1-3):63-76.
6. Vongpatanasin W, Mansour Y, Chavoshan B, Arbique D, Victor RG: Cocaine stimulates the human cardiovascular system via a central mechanism of action. *Circulation* 1999;100(5):497-502.
7. Tuncel M, Wang Z, Arbique D, Fadel PJ, Victor RG, Vongpatanasin W: Mechanism of the blood pressure-raising effect of cocaine in humans. *Circulation* 2002;105(9):1054-1059.
8. Egred M, Davis GK: Cocaine and the heart. *Postgrad Med J* 2005;81(959):568-571.
9. Lange RA, Cigarroa RG, Flores ED, McBride W, Kim AS, Wells PJ, et al: Potentiation of cocaine-induced coronary vasoconstriction by beta-adrenergic blockade. *Ann Intern Med* 1990;112(12):897-903.
10. Hollander JE: The management of cocaine-associated myocardial ischemia. *N Engl J Med* 1995;333(19):1267-1272.
11. Dattilo PB, Hailpern SM, Fearon K, Sohal D, Nordin C: Beta-blockers are associated with reduced risk of myocardial infarction after cocaine use. *Ann Emerg Med* 2007, June 19 (epub ahead of print).
12. Hollander JE, Hoffman RS, Gennis P, Fairweather P, DiSano MJ, Schumb DA, et al: Nitroglycerin in the treatment of cocaine associated chest pain—clinical safety and efficacy. *J Toxicol Clin Toxicol* 1994;32(3):243-256.
13. Cheng D: Perioperative care of the cocaine-abusing patient. *Can J Anaesth* 1994;41(10):883-887.
14. Boehrer JD, Moliterno DJ, Willard JE, Hillis LD, Lange RA: Influence of labetalol on cocaine-induced coronary vasoconstriction in humans. *Am J Med* 1993;94(6):608-610.
15. Lange RA, Hillis LD: Cardiovascular complications of cocaine use. *N Engl J Med* 2001;345(5):351-358.
16. Palmiere C, Burkhardt S, Staub C, Hallenbarter M, Paolo Pizzolato G, Dettmeyer R, La Harpe R: Thoracic aortic dissection associated with cocaine abuse. *Forensic Sci Int* 2004;141(2-3):137-142.
17. Rashid J, Eisenberg MJ, Topol EJ: Cocaine-induced aortic dissection. *Am Heart J* 1996;132(6):1301-1304.
18. Daniel JC, Huynh TT, Zhou W, Kougias P, El Sayed HF, Huh J, et al: Acute aortic dissection associated with use of cocaine. *J Vasc Surg* 2007;46(3):427-433.
19. Shannon RP, Lozano P, Cai Q, Manders WT, Shen Y: Mechanism of the systemic, left ventricular, and coronary vascular tolerance to a binge of cocaine in conscious dogs. *Circulation* 1996;94(3):534-541.
20. Heffner JE, Harley RA, Schabel SI: Pulmonary reactions from illicit substance abuse. *Clin Chest Med* 1990;11:151.
21. Forrester JM, Steele AW, Waldron JA, Parsons PE: Crack lung: An acute pulmonary syndrome with a spectrum of clinical and histopathologic findings. *Am Rev Respir Dis* 1990;142:462.
22. McCormick M, Nelson T: Cocaine-induced fatal acute eosinophilic pneumonia: A case report. *WMJ* 2007;106:92.
23. Baldwin GC, Choi R, Roth MD, Shay AH, Kleerup EC, Simmons MS, Tashkin DP: Evidence of chronic damage to the pulmonary microcirculation in habitual users of alkaloidal ("crack") cocaine. *Chest* 2002;121(4):1231-1238.
24. Marzuk PM, Tardiff K, Leon AC, Hirsch CS, Portera L, Iqbal MI, et al: Ambient temperature and mortality from unintentional cocaine overdose. *JAMA* 1998;279(22):1795-1800.
25. Koppel BS, Samkoff L, Daras M: Relation of cocaine use to seizures and epilepsy. *Epilepsia* 1996;37(9):875-878.

26. Brody SL, Slovis CM, Wrenn KD: Cocaine-related medical problems: Consecutive series of 233 patients. *Am J Med* 1990;88(4):325-331.
27. Daras M, Tuchman AJ, Marks S: Central nervous system infarction related to cocaine abuse. *Stroke* 1991;22(10):1320-1325.
28. Levine SR, Brust JC, Futrell N, et al: Cerebrovascular complications of the use of the "crack" form of alkaloidal cocaine. *N Engl J Med* 1990;323(11):699-704.
29. Bernards CM, Kern C, Cullen BF: Chronic cocaine administration reversibly increases isoflurane minimum alveolar concentration in sheep. *Anesthesiology* 1996;85(1):91-95.
30. Stoelting R, Creasser C, Martz R: Effect of cocaine administration on halothane MAC in dogs. *Anesth Analg* 1975;54:422-424.
31. Hurd YL, Svensson P, Pontén M: The role of dopamine, dynorphin, and CART systems in the ventral striatum and amygdala in cocaine abuse. *Ann N Y Acad Sci* 1999;877:499-506.
32. Tyndale RF, Sunahara R, Inaba T, Kalow W, Gonzalez FJ, Niznik HB: Neuronal cytochrome P450IID1 (debrisoquine/sparteine-type): Potent inhibition of activity by (-)-cocaine and nucleotide sequence identity to human hepatic P450 gene CYP2D6. *Mol Pharmacol* 1991;40(1):63-68.
33. Murphy JL: Hypertension and pulmonary edema associated with ketamine administration in a patient with a history of substance abuse. *Can J Anesth* 1993;40:160-164.
34. Hernandez M, Birnbach DJ, Van Zundert AJ: Anesthetic management of the illicit-substance-using patients. *Curr Opin Anaesthesiol* 2005;18:315-324.
35. Jatlow P, Barash PG, Van Dyke C, et al: Cocaine and succinylcholine sensitivity: A new caution. *Anesth Analg* 1979;58:235-238.
36. Birnbach DJ: Anesthesia and maternal substance abuse. In *Obstetric anesthesia*, ed 2. Philadelphia, Lippincott Williams & Wilkins, 1999, pp 491-499.
37. Moliterno DJ, Willard JE, Lange RA, Negus BH, Boehrer JD, Glamann DB, et al: Coronary-artery vasoconstriction induced by cocaine, cigarette smoking, or both. *N Engl J Med* 1994;330(7):454-459.
38. Mittleman MA, Mintzer D, Maclure M, Tofler GH, Sherwood JB, Muller JE: Triggering of myocardial infarction by cocaine. *Circulation* 1999;99(21):2737-2741.
39. Hollander JE, Hoffman RS: Cocaine-induced myocardial infarction: An analysis and review of the literature. *J Emerg Med* 1992;10(2):169-177.
40. Qureshi AI, Suri MF, Guterman LR, Hopkins LN: Cocaine use and the likelihood of nonfatal myocardial infarction and stroke: Data from the Third National Health and Nutrition Examination Survey. *Circulation* 2001;103(4):502-506.
41. Bansal D, Eigenbrodt M, Gupta E, Mehta JL: Traditional risk factors and acute myocardial infarction in patients hospitalized with cocaine-associated chest pain. *Clin Cardiol* 2007;30(6):290-294.
42. Flores ED, Lange RA, Cigarroa RG, Hillis LD: Effect of cocaine on coronary artery dimensions in atherosclerotic coronary artery disease: Enhanced vasoconstriction at sites of significant stenoses. *J Am Coll Cardiol* 1990;16(1):74-79.
43. Laffey JG, Neligan P, Ormonde G: Prolonged perioperative myocardial ischemia in a young male: Due to topical intranasal cocaine? *J Clin Anesth* 1999;11:419-424.
44. Minor RL Jr, Scott BD, Brown DD, et al: Cocaine-induced myocardial infarction in patients with normal coronary arteries. *Ann Intern Med* 1991;115:797-806.
45. Chiu YC, Brecht K, DasGupta DS, et al: Myocardial infarction with topical cocaine anesthesia for nasal surgery. *Arch Otolaryngol Head Neck Surg* 1986;112:988-990.
46. Ashchi M, Wiedemann HP, James KB: Cardiac complication from use of cocaine and phenylephrine in nasal septoplasty. *Arch Otolaryngol Head Neck Surg* 1995;121:681-684.
47. Littlewood SC, Tabb HD: Myocardial ischemia with epinephrine and cocaine during septoplasty. *J La State Med Soc* 1987;139:15-18.
48. Young D, Glauber JJ: Electrocardiographic changes resulting from acute cocaine intoxication. *Am Heart J* 1946;34:272-279.
49. Makaryus JN, Makaryus AN, Johnson M: Acute myocardial infarction following the use of intranasal anesthetic cocaine. *South Med J* 2006;99(7):759-761.
50. Liu SS, Forrester RM, Murphy GS, Chen K, Glassenberg R: Anaesthetic management of a parturient with myocardial infarction related to cocaine use. *Can J Anaesth* 1992;39(8):858-861.
51. Livingston JC, Mabie BC, Ramanathan J: Crack cocaine, myocardial infarction, and troponin I levels at the time of cesarean delivery. *Anesth Analg* 2000;91(4):913-915.
52. Kuczkowski KM: Crack cocaine-induced long QT interval syndrome in a parturient with recreational cocaine use. *Ann Fr Anesth Reanim* 2005;24(6):697-698.
53. Vagts DA, Boklage C, Galli C: Intraoperative ventricular fibrillation in a patient with chronic cocaine abuse—a case report. *Anaesthesiol Reanim* 2004;29(1):19-24.
54. Kuczkowski KM: Crack cocaine as a cause of acute postoperative pulmonary edema in a pregnant drug addict. *Ann Fr Anesth Reanim* 2005;24(4):437-438.
55. Singh PP, Dimich I, Shamsi A: Intraoperative pulmonary oedema in a young cocaine smoker. *Can J Anaesth* 1994;41(10):961-964.
56. Bernards CM, Teijeiro A: Illicit cocaine ingestion during anesthesia. *Anesthesiology* 1996;84(1):218-220.
57. Boylan JF, Cheng DC, Sandler AN, Carmichael FJ, Koren G, Feindel C, Boylen P: Cocaine toxicity and isoflurane anesthesia: Hemodynamic, myocardial metabolic, and regional blood flow effects in swine. *J Cardiothorac Vasc Anesth* 1996;10(6):772-777.
58. Brogan WC, Lange RA, Glamann B, Hillis D: Recurrent coronary vasospasm caused by intranansal cocaine, possible role of metabolites. *Ann Intern Med* 1992;116:556-561.
59. Hawks RL, Kopin IJ, Colburn RW, Thoa NB: Norcocaine: A pharmacologically active metabolite of cocaine found in the brain. *Life and Science* 1974;15:2189-2195.
60. Misra AL, Nayak PK, Bloch R: Estimation and disposition of benzoylecogonine and pharmacological activity of some cocaine metabolites. *J Pharm Pharmacol* 1975;27:784-786.
61. Barash PG, Kopriva CJ, Langou R, VanDyke C, Jatlow P, Stahl A, Byck R: Is cocaine a sympathetic stimulant during general anesthesia? *JAMA* 1980;243(14):1437-1439.
62. Hill GE, Ogunnaike BO, Johnson ER: General anaesthesia for the cocaine abusing patient. Is it safe? *Br J Anaesth* 2006;97(5):654-657 (epub 2006, Aug 16).
63. Kain ZN, Mayes LC, Ferris CA, Pakes J, Schottenfeld R: Cocaine-abusing parturients undergoing cesarean section. A cohort study. *Anesthesiology* 1996;85(5):1028-1035.
64. Kreek MJ: Cocaine, dopamine and the endogenous opioid system. *J Addict Dis* 1996;15(4):73-96.
65. Ross VH, Moore CH, Pan PH, et al: Reduced duration of intrathecal sufentanil analgesia in laboring cocaine users. *Anesth Analg* 2003;97:1504-1508.
66. Gershon RY, Fisher AJ, Graves WL: The cocaine-abusing parturient is not an increased risk for thrombocytopenia. *Anesth Analg* 1996;82:865-866.

9 Should All Antihypertensive Agents Be Continued before Surgery?

John G.T. Augoustides, MD, FASE

INTRODUCTION

Hypertension affects approximately 50 million individuals in the United States and approximately 1 billion individuals worldwide.[1] It is anticipated that this prevalence will further increase as the population ages. The relationship between sustained elevation in blood pressure and cardiovascular risk is continuous and independent of additional risk factors. The most recent classification of adult blood pressure in the seventh report of the Joint National Committee recognized this important relationship by introducing the classification of prehypertension to signal a patient cohort at increased future cardiovascular risk who would benefit from early intervention (Table 9-1).[1] This updated approach also classified hypertension as either stage 1 or stage 2, depending on systolic or diastolic pressure elevations (see Table 9-1). Furthermore, there are multiple oral antihypertensive medications that are used alone or in combination for pharmacologic control of hypertension (Tables 9-2 and 9-3). The cumulative evidence from multiple clinical trials demonstrates that successful ambulatory management of hypertension significantly reduces cardiovascular mortality and morbidity rates. From all of these considerations, it follows that hypertensive patients managed on various medication regimens will commonly undergo surgical procedures and hence compose a common and important part of daily anesthetic practice.

OPTIONS

Hypertensive patients undergoing surgery may or may not require adjustment of their antihypertensive regimen to optimize their perioperative management. The decision to continue or discontinue antihypertensive medication before surgery depends on a risk/benefit analysis (Table 9-4). The possible perioperative risks associated with the continuation or discontinuation of ambulatory antihypertensive medication may be divided as follows:

1. The risk of inadequate control of hypertension with possible increased perioperative cardiovascular risk, if a particular agent is discontinued before surgery

2. The risk of a clinically important withdrawal syndrome or increased perioperative cardiovascular risk if a particular agent is discontinued before surgery

3. The risk of an adverse perioperative cardiovascular event such as hypotension, if a particular agent is continued until surgery

EVIDENCE

What Is the Perioperative Risk of Hypertension?

In the absence of concomitant cardiovascular disease or hypertensive end-organ damage (e.g., left ventricular hypertrophy, renal dysfunction), stage 1 hypertension (systolic blood pressure less than 160 mm Hg or diastolic blood pressure less than 100 mm Hg) does not increase perioperative risk in noncardiac surgery. In a study of 4315 adults older than 50 years of age undergoing elective major noncardiac surgery, hypertension was not an independent predictor of postoperative cardiac complications.[2] A meta-analysis of over 30 observational studies found no clinically significant association between hypertension and perioperative complications.[3]

However, the perioperative risk associated with hypertension appears to be significant in cardiac surgery, carotid procedures, and pheochromocytoma resection. In 2417 patients undergoing coronary artery bypass grafting with cardiopulmonary bypass, baseline preoperative systolic hypertension (defined as a systolic blood pressure greater than 140 mm Hg) was associated with a highly significant 40% increase in adverse perioperative outcomes, including mortality, stroke, left ventricular dysfunction, and renal failure.[4] In a review of 80 adults undergoing off-pump coronary surgery, hypertension independently predicted hospital mortality ($p = 0.0185$) and hospital readmission ($p = 0.045$).[5] With respect to carotid procedures, perioperative hypertension was a significant risk factor for neurologic deficit not only in carotid endarterectomy but also in carotid stenting.[6-8] Furthermore, in 128 adults undergoing carotid endarterectomy, hypertension was a significant predictor of perioperative

Table 9-1 Classification and Suggested Management of Blood Pressure in Adults					
Blood Pressure Classification	**Systolic Blood Pressure**		**Diastolic Blood Pressure**	**Lifestyle Modification**	**Drug Therapy**
Normal	<120 mm Hg	and	<80 mm Hg	Encourage	None
Prehypertension	120-139 mm Hg	or	80-89 mm Hg	Yes	None
Stage 1 hypertension	140-159 mm Hg	or	90-99 mm Hg	Yes	Yes
Stage 2 hypertension	≥160 mm Hg	or	≥100 mm Hg	Yes	Yes

Adapted from Chobanian AV, Bakris GL, Black HR, et al: The seventh report of the Joint National Committee on prevention, detection, evaluation and treatment of high blood pressure. *JAMA* 2003;289:2560-2572.

myocardial ischemia ($p < 0.05$).[9] With respect to pheochromocytoma, progressive reduction in perioperative mortality rate from 3.9% to 0% has been attributed to contemporary perioperative control of hypertension.[10-12]

The presence of left ventricular hypertrophy (LVH) adds significant additional perioperative cardiovascular risk in noncardiac surgery. In the absence of aortic

Table 9-2 Oral Antihypertensive Agents	
Antihypertensive Drug Class	**Clinical Examples**
Thiazide diuretics	Chlorothiazide; indapamide; metolazone
Loop diuretics	Bumetanide; furosemide
Potassium-sparing diuretics	Amiloride; triamterene
Aldosterone-receptor blockers	Spironolactone; eplerenone
Beta-blockers	Atenolol; bisoprolol; metoprolol; nadolol; propanolol; timolol
Beta-blockers with intrinsic sympathomimetic activity	Acebutolol; penbutolol; pindolol
Combined alpha- and beta-blockers	Carvedilol; labetalol
Angiotensin-converting enzyme (ACE) inhibitors	Benzapril; captopril; enalapril; fosinopril; quinapril; ramipril; trandolapril
Angiotensin receptor blockers	Candesartan; eprosartan; irbesartan; losartan; valsartan
Calcium channel blockers (non-dihydropyridines)	Diltiazem; verapramil
Calcium channel blockers (dihydropyridines)	Amlodipine; felodipine; nicardipine; nifedipine; nisoldipine
Alpha-blockers	Phenoxybenzamine; doxazosin; prazosin; terazosin
Centrally acting agents	Clonidine; methyldopa; reserpine
Direct vasodilators	Hydralazine; minoxidil

Adapted from Chobanian AV, Bakris GL, Black HR, et al: The seventh report of the Joint National Committee on prevention, detection, evaluation and treatment of high blood pressure. *JAMA* 2003;289:2560-2572.

Table 9-3 Classes of Combination Drugs for Hypertension
• Angiotensin-converting enzyme inhibitors and calcium channel blockers
• Angiotensin-converting enzyme inhibitors and diuretics
• Angiotensin receptor blockers and diuretics
• Beta-blockers and diuretics
• Centrally acting anithypertensives and diuretic
• Diuretic and diuretic

Table 9-4 Considerations for Deciding on Continuing or Discontinuing Antihypertensive Medications before Surgery
• Is discontinuation of the antihypertensive agent associated with a clinically significant withdrawal syndrome?
• Is discontinuation of the antihypertensive agent associated with improved perioperative hemodynamics?
• Is discontinuation of the antihypertensive agent associated with increased perioperative cardiovascular risk?

outflow obstruction or hypertrophic cardiomyopathy, LVH typically is a result of systemic hypertension. In a prospective observational study of 405 patients undergoing major vascular surgery, LVH on preoperative electrocardiogram significantly predicted myocardial infarction and/or cardiac death (odds ratio [OR] 4.2; $p = 0.001$).[13] In a study of 474 men with coronary artery disease undergoing major noncardiac surgery, LVH significantly predicted perioperative myocardial ischemia.[14]

In the presence of severe baseline hypertension (systolic blood pressure greater than 180 mm Hg or diastolic blood pressure greater than 110 mm Hg), the relationship to perioperative cardiovascular risk is less clear. A recent meta-analysis demonstrated that these patients may be at more risk but that there was no evidence that delaying surgery reduces this risk.[3] Despite the lack of evidence, expert opinion recommends that when possible, surgery be delayed for medical control of baseline severe hyperetension.[1,15,16]

Furthermore, "white coat hypertension" (acute blood pressure elevation on the day of surgery due to anxiety) also confers no additional perioperative cardiovascular risk. This entity was the subject of a randomized controlled trial of 989 surgical patients with well-controlled baseline hypertension with diastolic blood pressures greater than 110 mm Hg on the day of surgery, despite anxiolysis with midazolam.[17] Study patients were then randomly assigned to surgery after intranasal nifedipine or delayed surgery with further medical control of hypertension. No outcome difference was detected between groups. However, an important qualifier is that all patients in this study had no previous myocardial infarction, unstable angina pectoris, renal failure, pregnancy-induced hypertension, LVH, prior coronary revascularization, aortic stenosis, preoperative arrhythmias, conduction defects, or stroke.

In summary, perioperative cardiovascular risk due to baseline hypertension alone is significant in the setting of left ventricular hypertrophy, carotid procedures, cardiac surgery, pheochromocytoma resection, and possibly when persistently severe. Thus, for surgical patients without these qualifiers, there is minimal additional cardiovascular risk due to worsening hypertension from discontinuing their antihypertensive medications before surgery. Therefore, for most hypertensive patients, perioperative decisions about their antihypertensive regimen are not based on the intrinsic risk due to hypertension, but rather on the considerations that follow.

Which Agents Decrease Risk If Continued Perioperatively?

Beta-Blockers

Perioperative beta-blockade has been extensively reviewed in a recent focused guideline by the American Council of Cardiology (ACC) and the American Heart Association (AHA).[18] This guideline recommends that hypertensive patients on beta-blockers should continue to receive beta-blockade perioperatively (Class I recommendation, that is, this recommendation should be followed because the benefit far outweighs the risk). The evidence for this recommendation was ranked as level C, that is, the evidence is limited to expert opinion and case reports, mainly about beta-blocker withdrawal.

The beta-blocker withdrawal syndrome was first recognized with propranolol, the first widely available beta-blocker introduced into clinical practice in the 1970s. In a case series, perioperative withdrawal of propranolol was associated with significant myocardial ischemia.[19] A recent prospective observational cohort study of 2588 adult outpatients found that the risk of myocardial infarction was further significantly increased by withdrawal of cardioselective beta-blockade.[20] Because it is already clear that perioperative beta-blockade withdrawal is dangerous, this question is unlikely to be further studied in a prospective trial.

Perioperative beta-blockade in certain at-risk populations is associated with significant reduction in cardiovascular risk. The role of beta-blockade in perioperative cardiovascular protection in patients with and without hypertension is covered in the recent AHA/ACC guidelines.[18,21]

Given their cardiovascular risk of withdrawal and their perioperative cardiovascular benefit, existing beta-blockade in hypertensive surgical patients should be continued up to the day of surgery, and throughout the perioperative period. This is the current recommendation from the American College of Physicians (ACP), as outlined in their physicians' information and education resource (www.acponline.org, accessed February 24, 2008).

Alpha-2 Agonists (Clonidine)

Clonidine is a centrally acting alpha agonist. It is available in oral, transdermal, and parenteral formulations. It is an alpha agonist with an alpha-2 to alpha-1 selectivity ratio of 39:1. Recent high-quality evidence has demonstrated its significant perioperative cardiovascular benefit. In a recent meta-analysis of 23 trials (total $N = 3395$), perioperative alpha-2 agonists reduced mortality rate (relative risk 0.76, 95% CI 0.63 to 0.91) and myocardial infarction (relative risk 0.66, 95% CI 0.46 to 0.94).[22] A recent randomized trial ($N = 190$) showed that perioperative clonidine significantly reduced myocardial ischemia (from 31% to 14%; $p = 0.01$) and long-term mortality rate (relative risk 0.43; 95% CI = 0.21 to 0.89).[23] The recent AHA/ACC perioperative care guideline has recommended alpha-2 agonists for control of hypertension in surgical patients with known or probable coronary artery disease (Class IIb recommendation, that is, benefit outweighs risk; level of evidence B, that is, evidence from trials that have evaluated limited populations).[21] The perioperative cardiovascular benefit of alpha-2 agonists is reviewed more comprehensively in Chapter 35 of this textbook.

Perioperative discontinuation of alpha-2 agonists such as clonidine is, however, dangerous in hypertensive patients chronically exposed to this drug class. Perioperative clonidine withdrawal is associated with severe delirium, hypertension, and myocardial ischemia.[24,25] In a clinical review, expert opinion has recommended careful supervision of perioperative clonidine therapy to avoid the deleterious effects of its cessation.[26] Given the risks of withdrawal and the potential cardiovascular benefit, existing therapy with alpha-2 agonists such as clonidine in hypertensive surgical patients should be continued up to the day of surgery and throughout the perioperative period. This is the current ACP recommendation, as outlined in their physicians' information and education resource (www.acponline.org, accessed February 24, 2008).

Calcium Channel Blockers

Calcium channel blockers, including the dihydropyridines, are widely used for the pharmacologic management of hypertension.[1,27,28] There are no described withdrawal syndromes related to perioperative discontinuation of calcium channel blockade. Furthermore, a recent meta-analysis (11 studies: total $N = 1007$) has demonstrated that perioperative calcium channel blockade, especially diltiazem, significantly reduced myocardial ischemia (relative risk 0.49; 95% CI 0.30 to 0.80), supraventricular tachycardia (relative risk 0.52; 95% CI 0.37 to 0.72), and mortality and major morbidity rates (relative risk 0.35; 95% CI 0.15 to 0.86).[28] Therefore, since there is net perioperative outcome benefit, it follows that existing calcium channel blockade in hypertensive surgical patients should be continued throughout the perioperative period. This is the current ACP recommendation, as outlined in their physicians' information and education resource (www.acponline.org, accessed February 24, 2008).

Alpha-Blockers

Alpha-blockers are a mainstay of preoperative preparation of patients with pheochromocytoma and are credited with improved perioperative survival in resection of this tumor.[10-12,29] Preoperative alpha-blockade, including with the long-acting phenoxybenzamine, is titrated to control hypertension by peripheral catecholamine blockade. Frequently, beta-blockade is added subsequently for control of tachycardia and arrhythmia in the setting of epinephrine-secreting tumors. It is recommended to continue the antihypertensive regimen up to and including the day of surgical resection to minimize preoperative catecholamine-related adverse events. This is the current ACP recommendation, as outlined in their physicians' information and education resource (www.acponline.org, accessed February 24, 2008).

Regardless of the preoperative antihypertensive regimen, alpha-blockade and/or beta-blockade will persist after tumor resection, depending on the half-life of the agents chosen. Consequently, severe intraoperative hypotension may ensue after tumor removal due to significantly reduced catecholamine secretion, as well as residual alpha- and beta-blockade. This severe hypotension may require aggressive volume resuscitation and support of systemic vascular resistance with vasopressin adminstration.[30] Because this intraoperative hypotension is readily managed, it is not an indication to recommend discontinuation of preoperative alpha-blockade on the morning of surgery for resection of pheochromocytoma. The resulting net perioperative benefit is the rationale for the ACP recommendation to continue aggressive catecholamine blockade up to the morning of surgery.

Which Agents May Increase Risk If Continued Perioperatively?

Angiotensin System Inhibitors

Pharmacologic blockade of the angiotensin system may be associated with significant intraoperative hypotension, whether due to angiotensin-converting enzyme (ACE) inhibitors or angiotensin receptor blockers. This hypotensive risk may be significantly reduced by preoperative discontinuation of these agents. In a randomized trial of 51 vascular surgical patients, discontinuation of ACE inhibitors 12 to 24 hours before anesthetic induction significantly protected against hypotension ($p < 0.05$).[31] In a prospective case-controlled clinical trial of 72 vascular surgical patients, preoperative angiotensin receptor blockade significantly increased hypotension ($p < 0.05$) and vasopressor requirement ($p < 0.001$).[32] A retrospective study of 267 hypertensive patients on both types of angiotensin inhibition demonstrated that discontinuation of the angiotensin blockade at least 10 hours before surgery was significantly associated with a reduced risk of intraoperative hypotension.[33] Furthermore, recent randomized trials have demonstrated that this intraoperative hypotension due to angiotensin inhibition may be treated effectively with ephedrine, norepinephrine, and/or vasopressin analogues such as terlipressin.[34,35] Therefore, based on this cumulative evidence, the ACP recommendation is that angiotensin blockade in hypertensive surgical patients be discontinued on the morning of surgery, as outlined in their physicians' information and education resource (www.acponline.org, accessed February 24, 2008).

Diuretics

Hypokalemia is common in hypertensive patients on chronic diuretic therapy. In a randomized trial of 233 hypertensive adults managed with chronic diuretic therapy, the prevalence of hypokalemia (defined as serum potassium less than 3.5 mEq/L) was 25%.[36] Perioperative hypokalemia, especially in cardiac surgery, is associated with an increased risk of arrhythmia. In a prospective multicenter trial of 2402 cardiac surgical patients, a serum potassium less than 3.5 mEq/L significantly predicted serious arrhythmia (relative risk 2.2; 95% CI 1.2 to 4.0), intraoperative arrhythmia (relative risk 2.0; 95% CI 1.0 to 3.6), and postoperative atrial flutter/fibrillation (relative risk 1.7; 95% CI 1.0 to 2.7).[37] Therefore, since chronic diuretic therapy for hypertension perioperatively may aggravate hypokalemia and risk of arrhythmia, it is reasonable to discontinue this therapy perioperatively, including the day of surgery. This is the current ACP recommendation, as outlined in their physicians' information and education resource (www.acponline.org, accessed February 24, 2008).

AREAS OF UNCERTAINTY

The first area of uncertainty is whether intraoperative hypotension associated with chronic ambulatory angiotensin blockade can be improved with modification of the induction technique. In the referenced prospective trials, the anesthetic induction technique (propofol and narcotic) was highly vagotonic, confounding the observed hypotension with the hypotensive effects due to bradycardia.[31,32,38] Perhaps vagolysis with preinduction glycopyrrolate would ameliorate hypotension associated with propofol induction in the setting of angiotensin blockade.[38,39] A recent trial documented a significant reduction in hypotension associated with etomidate induction in this setting.[40] Furthermore, it remains to be determined how variations in angiotensin genotype affect the perioperative hypotensive response associated with angiotensin blockade.[41]

The second area of uncertainty is about the perioperative effects of the following antihypertensives: direct-acting vasodilators such as hydralazine and centrally acting vasodilators such as reserpine and methyldopa.[42] These antihypertensive drugs are less commonly used, and consequently there is a paucity of published evidence about their perioperative applications. There are no clear indications to stop or continue these agents on the morning of surgery.

Table 9-5 Recommended Preoperative Management of Antihypertensive Medications

Antihypertensive Drug Class	Recommendation for Morning of Surgery	Sequelae with Discontinuation of Perioperative Therapy	Sequelae with Continuation of Perioperative Therapy
Beta-blockers	Continue	Withdrawal syndrome	Cardiovascular risk reduction
Clonidine	Continue	Withdrawal syndrome	Cardiovascular risk reduction
Calcium channel blockers	Continue	None described	Cardiovascular risk reduction
Alpha-blockers in association with pheochromocytoma	Continue	Severe preoperative and intraoperative systemic hypertension	Systemic hypotension, especially after tumor excision (readily treatable)
Angiotensin blockers (ACEI or ARB)	Discontinue	Significant reduction in risk of intraoperative hypotension	Significant risk of intraoperative hypotension
Diuretics	Discontinue	None described	Possible aggravation of hypokalemia with adverse outcome

ACEI, angiotensin-converting enzyme inhibitors; *ARB,* angiotensin receptor blockers.

In the author's opinion, it is reasonable to stop or continue these agents before surgery, depending on clinical circumstances.

In conclusion, recent evidence suggests that elevations in pulse pressure rather than systolic and/or diastolic hypertension may better predict perioperative risk such as renal injury.[43] Further perioperative studies are required to delineate the total risk associated with pulse pressure hypertension and the optimal interventions to ameliorate this adverse outcome.

GUIDELINES

The current guidelines for perioperative management of antihypertensive therapy are available from the American College of Physicians, as outlined in their physicians' information and education resource (www.acponline.org, accessed February 24, 2008). Furthermore, the AHA/ACC guidelines referenced in this chapter complement the perioperative approaches outlined in the ACP guideline.[18,21] Last, the overall guidelines for hypertension management (both inpatient and outpatient) are specified in the latest report from the Joint National Committee on prevention, detection, evaluation, and treatment of high blood pressure.[1]

AUTHOR'S RECOMMENDATIONS

The final recommendations are summarized by agent class in Table 9-5. This chapter is in full agreement with all of the current guidelines, including those from the ACP and the AHA/ACC. Perioperative management of ambulatory antihypertensives must account for the particular antihypertensive agents, the overall risk/benefit profile, and current guidelines, and then adjust the anesthetic plan accordingly.

REFERENCES

1. Chobanian AV, Bakris GL, Black HR, et al: The seventh report of the Joint National Committee on prevention, detection, evaluation and treatment of high blood pressure. *JAMA* 2003;289:2560-2572.
2. Lee TH, Marcantonio ER, Mangione CM, Thomas EJ, Polanczyk CA, Cook EF, et al: Derivation and prospective validation of a simple index for prediction of cardiac risk of major noncardiac surgery. *Circulation* 1999;1043-1049.
3. Howell SJ, Sear JW, Foex P: Hypertension, hypertensive heart disease and perioperative risk. *Br J Anaesth* 2004;92:570-583.
4. Aronson S, Boisvert D, Lapp W: Isolated systolic hypertension is associated with adverse outcomes from coronary artery bypass grafting surgery. *Anesth Analg* 2002;94:1079-1084.
5. Celkan MA, Uslunsoy H, Daglar B, Kazaz H, Kocoglu H: Readmission and mortality in patients undergoing off-pump coronary artery bypass surgery with fast-track recovery protocol. *Heart Vessels* 2005;20:251-255.
6. Asiddao CB, Donegan JH, Whitesell RC, Kalbfleisch JH: Factors associated with perioperative complications during carotid endarterectomy. *Anesth Analg* 1982;61:631-637.
7. Hans SS, Glover JL: The relationship of cardiac and neurological complications of blood pressure changes following carotid endarterectomy. *Am Surg* 1995;61:356-359.
8. Abou-Chebl A, Yadav JS, Reginelli JP, Bajzer C, Bhatt D, Krieger DW: Intracranial hemorrhage and hyperperfusion syndrome following carotid artery stenting: Risk factors, prevention and treatment. *J Am Coll Cardiol* 2004;43:1596-1601.
9. Kawahito S, Kitahata H, Tanaka K, Nozaki J, Oshita S: Risk factors for perioperative myocardial ischemia in carotid artery endarterectomy. *J Cardiothorac Vasc Anesth* 2004;18:288-292.
10. Desmonts JM, le Houelleur J, Remond P, Duvaldestin P: Anaesthetic management of patients with phaeochromocytoma. A review of 102 cases. *Br J Anaesth* 1977;49:991-998.
11. Kinney MA, Warner ME, van Heerden JA, Horlocker TT, Young WF Jr, Schroeder DR, et al: Perianesthetic risks and outcomes of pheochromocytoma and paraganglioma resection. *Anesth Analg* 2000;1118-1123.
12. Gifford RW Jr, Manger WM, Bravo EL: Pheochromocytoma. *Endocrinol Metab Clin North Am* 1994;23:387-404.
13. Landesberg G, Einav S, Christopherson R, Beattie C, Berlatzky Y, Rosenfeld B, et al: Perioperative ischemia and cardiac complications in major vascular surgery: Importance of the preoperative twelve-lead electrocardiogram. *J Vasc Surg* 1997;26:570-578.
14. Hollenberg M, Mangano DT, Browner WS, London MJ, Tubau JF, Tateo IM: Predictors of postoperative myocardial ischemia in patients undergoing noncardiac surgery. The Study of Perioperative Ischemia Research Group. *JAMA* 1992;268:205-209.
15. Casadei B, Abuzeid H: Is there a strong rationale for deferring elective surgery in patients with poorly controlled hypertension? *J Hypertens* 2005;23:19-22.
16. Fleisher LA: Preoperative evaluation of the patient with hypertension. *JAMA* 2002;287:2043-2046.
17. Weksler N, Klein M, Szendro G, Rozentsveig V, Schily M, Brill S, et al: The dilemma of immediate preoperative hypertension: To treat and operate or to postpone surgery? *J Clin Anesth* 2003;15:179-183.

18. Fleisher LA, Beckman JA, Brown KA, Calkins H, Chaikof E, Fleischmann KE, et al: ACC/AHA 2006 guideline update on perioperative cardiovascular evaluation for noncardiac surgery: Focused update on perioperative beta-blocker therapy. A report of the American College of Cardiology/American Heart Association task force on practice guidelines (writing committee to update the 2002 guidelines on perioperative cardiovascular evaluation for noncardiac surgery). *Anesth Analg* 2007;104:15-26.

19. Goldman L: Noncardiac surgery in patients receiving propranolol. Case reports and recommended approach. *Arch Intern Med* 1981;141:193-196.

20. Teichert M, Smet PA, Hofman A, Witteman JC, Stricker BH: Discontinuation of beta-blockers and the risk of myocardial infarction in the elderly. *Drug Saf* 2007;30:541-549.

21. Fleisher LA, Beckman JA, Brown KA, Calkins H, Chaikof E, et al: ACC/AHA 2007 guidelines on perioperative cardiovascular evaluation and care for noncardiac surgery. Executive summary: A report of the American College of Cardiology/American Heart Association task force on practice guidelines (writing committee to revise the 2002 guidelines on perioperative cardiovascular evaluation for noncardiac surgery): Developed in collaboration with the American Society of Echocardiography, American Society of Nuclear Cardiology, Heart Rhythm Society, Society of Cardiovascular Anesthesiologists, Society for Cardiovascular Angiography and Interventions, Society for Vascular Medicine and Biology, and Society for Vascular Surgery. *Circulation* 2007; 16:1971-1996.

22. Wijeysundera DN, Naik JS, Beattie WS: Alpha-2 adrenergic agonists to prevent perioperative cardiovascular complications. *Am J Med* 2003;114:742-752.

23. Wallace AW, Galindez D, Salahieh A, Layug EL, Lazo EA, Haratonik KA, et al: Effect of clonidine on cardiovascular morbidity and mortality after noncardiac surgery. *Anesthesiology* 2004; 101:284-293.

24. Brenner WI, Lieberman AN: Acute clonidine withdrawal syndrome following open heart operation. *Ann Thorac Surg* 1977; 24:80-82.

25. Simic J, Kishineff S, Goldberg R, Gifford W: Acute myocardial infarction as a complication of clonidine withdrawal. *J Emerg Med* 2003;25:399-402.

26. Feinberg LE: Perioperative care of patients with cardiac disease. *Postgrad Med* 1980;67:227-235.

27. Poelaert J, Roosens C: Perioperative use of dihydropyridine calcium channel blockers. *Acta Anaesthesiol Scand* 2000;44:528-535.

28. Wijeysundera DN, Beattie WS: Calcium channel blockers for reducing cardiac morbidity after noncardiac surgery: A meta-analysis. *Anesth Analg* 2003;97:834-841.

29. Pacak K: Preoperative management of the pheochromocytoma patient. *J Clin Endocrinol Metab* 2007;92:4069-4079.

30. Augoustides JG, Abrams M, Berkowitz D, Fraker D: Vasopressin for hemodynamic rescue in catecholamine-resistant vasoplegic shock after resection of massive pheochromoctyoma. *Anesthesiology* 2004;101:1022-1024.

31. Coriat P, Richer C, Douraki T, Gomez C, Hendricks K, Giudicelli JF, et al: Influence of chronic angiotensin-converting enzyme inhibition on anesthetic induction. *Anesthesiology* 1994;81:299-307.

32. Brabant SM, Bertrand M, Eyraud D, Darmon PL, Coriat P: The hemodynamic effects of anesthetic induction in vascular surgical patients chronically treated with angiotensin II receptor antagonists. *Anesth Analg* 1999;89:1388-1392.

33. Comfere T, Sprung J, Kumar MM, Draper M, Wilson DP, Williams BA, et al: Angiotensin system inhibitors in a general surgical population. *Anesth Analg* 2005;100:636-644.

34. Meersschaert K, Brun L, Gourdin M, Mouren S, Bertrand M, Riou B, et al: Terlipressin-ephedrine versus ephedrine to treat hypotension at the induction of anesthesia in patients chronically treated with angiotensin converting-enzyme inhibitors: A prospective randomized, double-blinded, crossover study. *Anesth Analg* 2002;94:835-840.

35. Boccara G, Ouattara A, Godet G, Dufresne E, Bertrand M, Riou B, et al: Terlipressin versus norepinephrine to correct arterial hypotension after general anesthesia in patients chronically treated with renin-angiotensin system inhibitors. *Anesth Analg* 2003; 98:1338-1344.

36. Siegel D, Hulley SB, Black DM, Cheitlin MD, Sebastian A, Seeley DG, et al: Diuretics, serum and intracellular electrolyte levels, and ventricular arrhythmias in hypertensive men. *JAMA* 1992; 267:1083-1089.

37. Wahr JA, Parks R, Boisvert D, Comunale M, Fabian J, Ramsay J, et al: Preoperative serum potassium levels and perioperative outcomes in cardiac surgery patients. Multicenter Study of Perioperative Ischemia Research Group. *JAMA* 1999;281:2203-2210.

38. Prys-Roberts C: Withdrawal of antihypertensive therapy. *Anesth Analg* 2001;93:767-768.

39. Skues M, Richards MJ, Jarvis AP, Prys-Roberts C: Preinduction atropine or glycopyrrolate hemodynamic changes associated with induction and maintenance of anesthesia with propofol and alfentanil. *Anesth Analg* 1989;69:386-390.

40. Malinowska-Zaprzalka M, Wojewodzka M, Dryi D, Brabowska SZ, Chabielska E: Hemodynamic effect of propofol in enalipril-treated hypertensive patients during induction of general anesthesia. *Pharmacol Rep* 2005;57:675-678.

41. Woodiwiss AJ, Nkeh B, Samani NJ, Badenhorst D, Maseko M, Tiago AD, et al: Functional variants of the angiotensinogen gene determine antihypertensive responses to angiotensin-converting enzyme inhibitors in subjects of African origin. *J Hypertens* 24: 1057-1064, 2006.

42. Sica DA: Centrally acting antihypertensive agents: An update. *J Clin Hypertens (Greenwich)* 2007;9:399-405.

43. Aronson S, Fontes ML, Miao Y, Mangano DT, for the Investigators of the Multicenter Study of Perioperative Ischemia Research Group and the Ischemia Research and Education Foundation: Risk index for perioperative renal dysfunction/failure: Critical dependence on pulse pressure hypertension. *Circulation* 2007; 115:733-742.

10 Is There an Optimal Timing for Smoking Cessation?

James Y. Findlay, MBChB, FRCA

INTRODUCTION

Cigarette smoking is the single most important avoidable cause of death in the United States. The long-term effects of cigarette smoking in causing cardiac disease, vascular disease, pulmonary disease, and a variety of cancers has been recognized for many years now.[1-4] The benefits of smoking cessation in reducing future risks of these diseases compared to those who continue to smoke are also well documented.[5] Despite this body of knowledge and its wide dissemination, approximately 25% of the adult population continues to smoke.[6] Thus the anesthesiologist is faced with providing preoperative advice and perioperative care to many current smokers. The questions that then arise are whether the smoker is at increased risk for perioperative complications and whether cessation of smoking in the short term before surgery influences these risks.

There are short-term effects of inhaling cigarette smoke that could cause intraoperative complications. Nicotine causes dose-related increases in heart rate and both systolic and diastolic blood pressure,[7] is a peripheral vasoconstrictor, and increases coronary artery resistance in diseased vessels.[8] Carbon monoxide (CO) inhaled in cigarette smoke combines with hemoglobin to form carboxyhemoglobin (COHb), and levels of COHb in smokers' blood are reported from 5% up to a peak of 20% depending on smoking practice.[9] Smokers under anesthesia have been demonstrated to have higher CO concentrations than nonsmokers.[10] The high affinity of CO for hemoglobin interferes with the oxygen-carrying capacity of Hb, as well as moving the oxygen dissociation curve to the left,[11] thus decreasing overall oxygen content and oxygen availability to tissues.

The long-term effects of smoking on the cardiovascular and respiratory systems could also be anticipated to cause perioperative problems. Cigarette smoking is a leading cause of atherosclerotic disease and a major risk factor for coronary artery disease.[12] It is also the leading cause of chronic obstructive pulmonary disease.[13] In addition, of particular relevance to anesthesia, smokers have a significantly greater upper airway sensitivity than nonsmokers.[14]

EVIDENCE

Relationship between Smoking and Perioperative Complications

This section will provide an overview of the literature linking smoking with perioperative complications. These studies are almost exclusively observational in nature. The literature pertaining to smoking cessation in the perioperative period is addressed in the subsequent section. Smoking is an important contributor to perioperative morbidity: Moller and colleagues[15] reviewed the postoperative complications and smoking histories of patients undergoing arthroplasty and found that smokers had significantly more cardiopulmonary and wound-related complications and more intensive care unit (ICU) admissions than nonsmokers; after multivariate analysis smoking was the single most important risk factor.

Pulmonary Complications

An increased incidence of postoperative pulmonary complications in smokers has been recognized since 1944 when Morton[16] reported that in a prospective series of 1257 patients undergoing abdominal surgeries, the incidence of pulmonary complications was approximately 60% in smokers versus 10% in nonsmokers. In the subsequent years the finding of increased pulmonary complications in smokers has been replicated in numerous studies, although the reported rates are lower. Smokers have an increased rate of all pulmonary complications,[17,18] an increased rate of infective pulmonary complications,[19,20] a higher rate of ICU admission after surgery,[21] and a higher rate of prolonged mechanical ventilation.[22] The mechanism behind these increased complication rates is suggested by the multivariate analysis carried out by Mitchell and colleagues[23] on 40 patients undergoing nonthoracic procedures. They found that although smokers had a higher rate of pulmonary complications, smoking per se was not an independent predictor of these complications, but that sputum production was.[23] A similar finding was reported by Dillworth and colleagues,[19] who found that the risk of postoperative chest infection in a prospective study of 127 patients undergoing abdominal surgery was markedly higher at 83% if a smoker had evidence of chronic bronchitis compared to 21% in its absence. Nonsmokers had a 7% rate of chest infection.

Airway Complications

Schwilk and colleagues[24] reviewed the occurrence of perioperative airway and respiratory events (reintubation, laryngospasm, bronchospasm, hypoventilation) in 26,961 anesthetics. They found an incidence of 5.5% in smokers compared to 3.1% in nonsmokers. Interestingly, the risk for all such events was higher in smokers less than 35 years of age and particularly in such patients with chronic bronchitis. Smoking was also identified as an independent predictor of bronchospasm in an analysis of a randomized trial of anesthetic agents involving 17,201 patients.[25]

Cardiovascular Complications

Choudhri and colleagues,[26] in an analysis of a database of 19,224 patients who underwent coronary artery bypass graft (CABG) surgery, identified smoking as an independent predictor of stroke. Smoking was also identified as an independent predictor of operative mortality in patients undergoing internal mammary artery grafting.[27] In patients undergoing abdominal aortic surgery smoking was found to be an independent predictor of postoperative complications, the most common being a deterioration in renal function.[28] In a prospective investigation of the short-term effects of smoking, Woehlck and colleagues[29] reported that patients under age 65 with no history of ischemic heart disease undergoing noncardiac, nonvascular surgery who smoked shortly before surgery had a higher rate of ST-segment depression than those who did not; however, postoperative outcomes were not reported.

Surgical Complications

Smoking has been identified as a significant risk factor for a number of postoperative surgical complications. In orthopedic surgery postoperative smoking has been identified as increasing the nonunion rate after spinal fusion[30] and after ankle arthrodesis,[31] increasing the need for reoperation, as well as the infection rate after amputation,[32] and increasing resource consumption after joint replacement, despite the smokers being younger and with less identified comorbidities than the nonsmokers.[33] Anastomotic leaks after colorectal surgery are more common in smokers than nonsmokers,[34] and smokers have more complications after plastic surgery to the extent that it has been suggested that plastic surgeons refuse to operate on those who fail to abstain.[35]

Smoking Cessation and Perioperative Complications

There are three published randomized controlled trials of smoking cessation in the preoperative period. Six pertinent observational studies are also discussed.

Observational Studies

In 1984 Warner and colleagues[36] reported a retrospective analysis of 500 randomly selected patients who had undergone CABG in 1 year. A history of smoking was noted for 456 patients. The rates of perioperative respiratory complications (chest infection, sputum retention, bronchospasm, pleural effusion, pneumothorax, and segmental pulmonary collapse) were reported in relation to the reported period of smoking cessation before surgery. Those who continued to smoke up to the time of surgery had a complication rate of 48%, whereas nonsmokers had a rate of 11%. Smokers who reported stopping 8 weeks or more before surgery had a complication rate of approximately 17%, not statistically different from that of nonsmokers. Those who stopped smoking for less than 8 weeks

before surgery had complication rates not statistically different from those who continued to smoke. When analyzed in 2-week blocks, the rate of complications rose slightly for those who stopped up to 4 weeks before surgery before falling toward that of nonsmokers.

A prospective study followed 200 consecutive patients undergoing CABG of whom 150 were current smokers or ex-smokers.[37] The same respiratory complications as in the previous study were sought and linked to the reported time of smoking cessation before surgery. The findings were similar to the previous study: respiratory complications occurred in 33% of continuing smokers and 11% of nonsmokers. Of those who had ceased smoking, complications occurred in 57% of those who stopped 8 weeks or less before surgery but only in 15% of those who stopped for more than 8 weeks. Those who had stopped smoking for more than 6 months had a complication rate of 11%, similar to that of those who had never smoked.

Brooks-Brunn[38] reported on the development of a predictive model for postoperative pulmonary complications following abdominal surgery using a prospective sample of 400 patients. Previously reported risk factors for postoperative pulmonary complications were collected, including length of smoking cessation before surgery. A history of smoking in the 8 weeks before surgery was one of six risk factors in the final model; this factor had an adjusted odds ratio (OR) of 2.3.

A further prospective series reported postoperative pulmonary complications in 410 patients undergoing noncardiac surgery.[39] This group again reported that current smokers had a higher complication rate (OR 5.5) than nonsmokers or past smokers (OR 2.9). A multivariate logistic analysis was performed to control for other known risk factors; this analysis resulted in a model including current smoking (OR 4.2).

Nakagawa and colleagues[40] reported similar findings in a retrospective study of 288 patients undergoing thoracic surgery, again focusing on pulmonary complications. The incidence of complications was 24% in nonsmokers, 43% in current smokers (here including those who smoked within 2 weeks of surgery), 54% in those who stopped smoking between 2 and 4 weeks preoperatively, and 35% in those who stopped more than 4 weeks before surgery. These differences persisted with the same ranking when the results were corrected for possible confounding factors. Four-week moving averages of the effect of smoking cessation were calculated; these showed that the rate of complications in smokers who stopped before surgery reached approximate equivalence with that of nonsmokers at an abstinence period around 8 weeks.

The influence of smoking cessation on wound complications was investigated by Kuri and colleagues[41] in a retrospective study of 188 patients who underwent reconstructive head and neck surgery. They divided patients into five groups based on preoperative smoking history—smokers (smoked within 7 days of surgery), late quitters (abstinence 8 to 21 days presurgery), intermediate quitters (abstinence 22 to 42 days presurgery), early quitters (abstinence 43 days or longer), and nonsmokers. Impaired wound healing was assessed by the need for subsequent surgical intervention. Impaired wound healing was significantly less frequent in the intermediate quitters (55%), early quitters (59%), and nonsmokers (47%) than in the smokers (85%). After multivariate analysis to control for other factors known to influence wound healing, intermediate and early quitters and nonsmokers continued to have a significantly lower risk of impaired healing than smokers. Late quitters had a lower incidence of impaired wound healing (68%) than smokers and a lower risk on multivariate analysis, but these changes were not statistically significant. The authors' conclusion was that 3 weeks of abstinence is required to reduce wound complications, but a moving average of impaired wound healing incidence they present suggests that this begins declining with 1 week of abstinence.

Taken together these studies indicate that the timing of smoking cessation in relation to surgery is of importance to the risk of complications. For pulmonary complications those patients who cease smoking before surgery can reduce their risk for pulmonary complications close to that of nonsmokers, but only if the period of abstinence is approximately 8 weeks or more. Also, the risk of complications appears not to fall from the time of cessation, but after 4 weeks of cessation, the risk during the first 4 weeks appears to increase, although in no individual study was this increase statistically significant. This effect is reported for all types of surgery addressed. For wound complications it seems that a shorter period of abstinence is required. All of the studies can be criticized for being observational in nature and also for relying on patient-reported information. In none of the studies is it clear if any advice to cease smoking was given to the patients involved, or whether the changes in smoking behavior observed reflected the patients' own assessment of the appropriate course of action, potentially resulting in a self-selected patient group. The clinician is then left asking whether general advice to stop smoking before surgery would be effective and would result in fewer complications.

Randomized Studies

Three randomized controlled trials have addressed these issues. In an experimental study, Sorensen and colleagues[42] compared wound healing in never-smokers and smokers randomized to either continued smoking or abstinence (with nicotine patch or placebo). Sacral wounds were made at 1, 4, 8, and 12 weeks after randomization. Continued smokers had greater rates of infection than abstinent smokers (and never-smokers) in wounds made 4 or more weeks after randomization. The use of a nicotine patch did not affect outcome.

Two randomized clinical trial have addressed the effectiveness of preoperative smoking intervention on postoperative outcomes. Moller and colleagues[43] performed a multicenter study in Denmark randomizing 120 smokers scheduled for elective hip or knee arthroplasty 6 to 8 weeks preoperatively to either a standard care group or to a smoking intervention group. Those in the smoking intervention group were offered weekly meetings with a nurse where they were strongly encouraged to stop smoking. Nicotine replacement was provided along with

smoking cessation education. Postoperative complications assessed included wound related (hematoma, infection), respiratory insufficiency (requiring ventilatory support in the intensive care unit), and cardiovascular insufficiency (myocardial infarction or congestive heart failure). Results were analyzed on an intention-to-treat basis. Thirty-six of the intervention group stopped smoking, and 14 reduced consumption. In the control group, only 4 patients stopped smoking. Postoperative complications were significantly less frequent in the intervention group (18% versus 52%), with the largest effect for wound-related complications. Cardiovascular complications were also more common in the control group (10% versus 0%), but this was not statistically significant. In a comparison of those who reduced their consumption versus those who stopped smoking, the reduction in complications was significant only for those who stopped; those who reduced consumption had the same complication rate as those who continued smoking.

In a similar study, also conducted in Denmark, Sorensen and Jorgensen[44] investigated the influence of a preoperative smoking intervention in patients undergoing colorectal surgery. Sixty patients were randomized to 2 to 3 weeks of either continued smoking or a smoking intervention program similar to that described previously. The intervention was successful in decreasing preoperative smoking (89% in the intervention group either quit or decreased consumption versus 13% in the control group). However, no difference in any postoperative complications was found.

These studies provide a strong indication that smoking intervention in the preoperative period is effective in reducing tobacco consumption, although a caveat is that in both studies approximately 25% of patients who were invited to participate refused, which may influence the generalizability of the findings.

The striking reduction in wound-related complications in the Moller study[43] and the tantalizing nonsignificant decrease in cardiovascular complications are noteworthy, although the lack of difference in pulmonary complications may seem surprising given the previous findings in observational studies. This may be related to study power; to definition, as mechanical ventilation was the only pulmonary complication collected; or to the selection of orthopedic surgeries in which pulmonary complications may be less frequent than in the surgeries reported in previous observational studies. The lack of effect of smoking cessation reported by Sorensen and Jorgensen[44] merits comment. It seems to support the concept that more than 3 weeks of abstinence is required to see decreased complications; however, the numbers are quite modest and patient details (such as comorbidities) scant, so this issue is not conclusively resolved.

Whether patients undergoing surgery in less than 3 weeks should be advised to quit may seem controversial given the current data on perioperative pulmonary complications; however, it should be noted that no long-term consequences have been identified, whereas the long-term consequences of continued smoking are well established. Given the chance of a "teachable moment" to advise smoking cessation, the physician should take it.

AREAS OF UNCERTAINTY

A number of issues require elucidation before definitive answers to the questions surrounding perioperative smoking cessation can be given.

- Does smoking in the immediate preoperative hours lead to a demonstrable effect on clinically relevant outcomes?
- Can the results reported by Moller and colleagues[43] be replicated in abdominal and thoracic surgeries?
- What is the minimum time period required for a formal smoking intervention program to reduce postoperative complications?
- Is the increase in postoperative pulmonary complications with cessation within 4 weeks of surgery seen in observational studies real? If so, can appropriate interventions reduce this?

GUIDELINES

The Veterans' Health Administration in the United States has an evidence-based guideline advising the cessation of smoking for 8 weeks before surgery in patients with chronic obstructive pulmonary disease (COPD) or asthma,[45] based on the studies by Warner and colleagues.[36,37] The Australian and New Zealand College of Anaesthetists statement on perioperative smoking concludes that preoperative cessation for at least 6 to 8 weeks is to be encouraged and smoking should not be permitted 12 hours before surgery.[46] A cursory Internet search reveals that many institutions have similar recommendations and many patient advice sites carry the same information. With reference to wound infection, the Centers for Disease Control and Prevention has recommended smoking cessation for at least 30 days preoperatively.[47]

SUMMARY

Smoking is the most important avoidable cause of disease in the United States. Smokers have a higher rate of perioperative complications than nonsmokers. Preoperative cessation of smoking reduces postoperative complications; the longer the time from cessation to surgery, the closer the complication rate becomes to that of never-smokers. Formalized preoperative smoking cessation programs are successful. When presented with a current smoker, physicians should recommend quitting.

MAIN POINTS

- Smokers have a higher postoperative complication rate than nonsmokers.
- Preoperative smoking cessation decreases the postoperative complication rate.
- The longer the preoperative cessation, the better.
- Formal preoperative smoking cessation programs are successful.

AUTHOR'S RECOMMENDATIONS

In an ideal world, all smokers would be identified 8 weeks or more before surgery and would give up entirely at that time. But, for our flawed reality, I suggest the following:

- All smokers scheduled for surgery are strongly encouraged to quit. Formal support to quit smoking, including nicotine therapy, should be made available.
- No smoking on the day of surgery for anyone.
- All smokers who undergo surgery should be advised to quit permanently.

REFERENCES

1. US Department of Health and Human Services: *Smoking and health. A report of the advisory committee to the Surgeon General of the Public Health Service.* Washington, DC, US Government Printing Office, 1964.
2. US Department of Health and Human Services: *The health consequences of smoking: Cardiovascular disease. A report of the Surgeon General.* Washington, DC, US Government Printing Office, 1983.
3. US Department of Health and Human Services: *The health consequences of smoking: Chronic obstructive lung disease.* Washington, DC, US Government Printing Office, 1984.
4. US Department of Health and Human Services: *The health consequences of smoking: Cancer. A report of the Surgeon General.* Washington, DC, US Government Printing Office, 1982.
5. US Department of Health and Human Services: *The health benefits of smoking cessation. A report of the Surgeon General.* Washington, DC, US Government Printing Office, 1990.
6. US Department of Health and Human Services: *Reducing tobacco use: A report of the Surgeon General.* Washington, DC, 2000.
7. Roth G, Shick R: The cardiovascular effects of smoking with special reference to hypertension. *Ann N Y Acad Sci* 1970;90:309-316.
8. Klein L, Ambrose J, Pichard A, Holt J, Gorlin R, Teichholz L: Acute coronary hemodynamic response to cigarette smoking in patients with coronary artery disease. *J Am Coll Cardiol* 1984;3:879-886.
9. Stewart R: The effect of carbon monoxide on humans. *J Occup Med* 1976;18:304-309.
10. Tang C, Fan S, Chan C: Smoking status and body size increase carbon monoxide concentrations in the breathing circuit during low flow anesthesia. *Anesth Analg* 2000;92:542-547.
11. Pearce A, Jones R: Smoking and anesthesia: Preoperative abstinence and perioperative morbidity. *Anesthesiology* 1984;61:576-584.
12. McBride P: The health consequences of smoking: Cardiovascular disease. *Med Clin North Am* 1991;76:333-353.
13. Sherman C: The health consequences of cigarette smoking: Pulmonary diseases. *Med Clin North Am* 1991;76:355-375.
14. Erskine R, Murphy P, Langton J: Sensitivity of upper airway reflexes in cigarette smokers: Effect of abstinence. *Br J Anaesth* 1994;73:298-302.
15. Moller A, Pedersen T, Munksgaard A: Effect of smoking on early complications after elective orthopaedic surgery. *J Bone Joint Surg [Br]* 2003;85-B:178-181.
16. Morton H: Tobacco smoking and pulmonary complications after operation. *Lancet* 1944;1:368-370.
17. Lawrence V, Dhanda R, Hilsenbeck S, Page C: Risk of pulmonary complications after elective abdominal surgery. *Chest* 1996;110:744-750.
18. Kocabas A, Kara K, Ozgur G, Sonmez H, Burgut R: Value of preoperative spirometry to predict postoperative pulmonary complications. *Respir Med* 1996;90:25-33.
19. Dillworth J, White R: Postoperative chest infection after upper abdominal surgery: An important problem for smokers. *Respir Med* 1992;86:205-210.

20. Garibaldi R, Britt M, Coleman M, Reading J, Pace N: Risk factors for postoperative pneumonia. *Am J Med* 1981;70:677-680.
21. Moller A, Maaloe R, Pedersen T: Postoperative intensive care admittance: The role of tobacco smoking. *Acta Anaesthesiol Scand* 2001;45:345-348.
22. Jayr C, Matthay M, Goldstone J, Gold W, Wiener-Kronish JP: Preoperative and intraoperative factors associated with prolonged mechanical ventilation. *Chest* 1993;103:1231-1236.
23. Mitchell CK, Smoger SH, Pfiefer MP, Vogel RL, Pandit MK, Donnelly PJ, et al: Multivariate analysis of factors associated with postoperative pulmonary complications following general elective surgery. *Arch Surg* 1998;133:194-198.
24. Schwilk B, Bothner U, Schraag S, Georgieff M: Perioperative respiratory events in smokers and non-smokers undergoing general anesthesia. *Acta Anesthesiol Scand* 1997;41:348-355.
25. Forrest JB, Rehder K, Cahalan MK, Goldsmith CH: Multicenter study of general anesthesia. III. Predictors of severe perioperative adverse outcomes. *Anesthesiology* 1992;76:3-15.
26. Choudhri J, Weinberg A, Ting W, Rose E, Smith C, Oz M: Multicenter review of perioperative risk factors for stroke after coronary artery bypass grafting. *Ann Thorac Surg* 2000;69:30-35.
27. He GW, Acuff TE, Ryan WH, Mack MJ: Risk factors for operative mortality in elderly patients undergoing internal mammary artery grafting. *Ann Thorac Surg* 1994;57:1460-1461.
28. Martin L, Atnip R, Holmes P, Lynch J, Thiele B: Prediction of postoperative complications after elective aortic surgery using stepwise logistic regression analysis. *Am Surg* 1994;60:163-168.
29. Woehlck H, Connolly L, Cinquegrani M, Dunning M, Hoffmann R: Acute smoking increases ST depression in humans during general anesthesia. *Anesth Analg* 1999;89:856.
30. Glassman S, Anagnost S, Parker A, Burke D, Johnson J, Dimar J: The effect of cigarette smoking and smoking cessation on spinal fusion. *Spine* 2000;25:2608-2615.
31. Cobb T, Gabrielsen T, Campbell D, Wallrichs S, Ilstrup D: Cigarette smoking and nonunion after ankle arthrodesis. *Foot Ankle Int* 1994;15:64-67.
32. Lind J, Kramhoft M, Bodtker S: The influence of smoking on complications after primary amputations of the lower extremity. *Clin Orthop Relat Res* 1991;267:211-217.
33. Lavernia C, Sierra R, Gomez-Marin O: Smoking and joint replacement: Resource consumption and short term outcome. *Clin Orthop Relat Res* 1999;367:172-180.
34. Sorensen L, Jorgensen T, Kirkeby L, Skovdal B, Vennits B, Wille-Jorgensen P: Smoking and alcohol abuse are major risk factors for anastomotic leakage in colorectal surgery. *Br J Surg* 1999;86:927-931.
35. Krueger J, Rohrich R: Clearing the smoke: The scientific rationale for tobacco abstention with plastic surgery. *Plast Reconstr Surg* 2001;108:1074-1077.
36. Warner M, Diverite M, Tinker J: Preoperative cessation of smoking and pulmonary complications in coronary artery bypass patients. *Anesthesiology* 1984;60:380-383.
37. Warner M, Offord K, Warner M, Lennon R, Conover M, Jansson-Schumacher U: Role of preoperative cessation of smoking and other factors in postoperative pulmonary complications: A blinded study of coronary artery bypass patients. *Mayo Clin Proc* 1989;64:609-616.
38. Brooks-Brunn J: Predictors of postoperative pulmonary complications following abdominal surgery. *Chest* 1997;111:564-571.
39. Bluman L, Mosca L, Newman N, Simon D: Preoperative smoking habits and postoperative pulmonary complications. *Chest* 1998;113:883-889.
40. Nakagawa M, Tanaka H, Tsukuma H, Kishi Y: Relationship between the duration of the preoperative smoke free period and the incidence of postoperative pulmonary complications after pulmonary surgery. *Chest* 2001;120:705-710.
41. Kuri M, Nakagawa M, Tanaka H, Hasuo S, Kishi Y: Determination of the duration of preoperative smoking cessation to improve wound healing after head and neck surgery. *Anesthesiology* 2005;102:883-884.
42. Sorensen L, Karlsmark T, Gottrup F: Abstinence from smoking reduces incisional wound infection: A randomized controlled trial. *Ann Surg* 2003;238:1-5.
43. Moller AM, Villebro N, Pedersen T, Tonnesen H: Effect of preoperative smoking intervention on postoperative complications: A randomised controlled trial. *Lancet* 2002;359:114-117.
44. Sorensen L, Jorgensen T: Short-term pre-operative smoking cessation intervention does not affect postoperative complications in colorectal surgery: A randomized clinical trial. *Colorectal Disease* 2002;5:347-352.
45. Management of chronic obstructive pulmonary disease. Washington, DC: VA/DoD Clinical Practice Guideline Working Group, Veterans Health Administration, Department of Veterans Affairs and Health Affairs, Department of Defense, August 1999 (Update 2007). Office of Quality and Performance publication 10Q-CP6/COPD-07.
46. Australian and New Zealand College of Anaesthetists: Statement on smoking as related to the perioperative period—2007. http://www.anzca.edu.au/resources/professional-documents/professional-standards/pdfs/PSR.pdf, accessed October 8, 2008.
47. Mangram AJ, Horan TC, Pearson ML, Silver LC, Jarvis WR: Guideline for prevention of surgical site infection. *Am J Infect Control* 1999;27:97-134.

11 Should Patients with Asthma Be Given Preoperative Medications Including Steroids?

George Pyrgos, MD, and Robert H. Brown, MD, MPH

INTRODUCTION

Asthma is a syndrome characterized by reversible airflow limitation that affects 5% to 9% of the population in the United States. The diagnosis of asthma is based on clinical evidence of recurrent symptoms such as wheezing, chest tightness, cough, and shortness of breath, and with airway hyperresponsiveness to various chemical, pharmacologic, or physical stimuli, such as endotracheal intubation. The diagnosis can be challenging because the clinical picture may be diverse and the possible pathophysiologic mechanisms are numerous. Patients with asthma are believed to be at increased risk for perioperative pulmonary complications, which may lead to increased morbidity. Perioperative pulmonary complications occur as frequently as cardiac complications and can lead to a prolonged hospital stay. Early studies reported overall rates of postoperative complications of 24% in patients with asthma compared with 14% in controls.[1-3] As with all anesthesia-related complications, the risks of pulmonary complications have decreased over time.

The goal of preparing a patient with asthma for anesthesia and surgery is to maximize the patient's pulmonary function. The physician must consider the maintenance or addition of antibronchospastic drugs such as sympathomimetic agents, leukotriene antagonists, and steroids. However, the role and benefit of preoperative medications to limit perioperative pulmonary complications in the asthmatic patient have not been determined.

PHARMACOLOGIC THERAPIES

The medications used in the management of asthma include sympathomimetic agents, leukotriene antagonists, steroids, and, most recently, anti–immunoglobulin E (anti-IgE) therapy. Other agents less commonly used include mucolytic agents, mast cell stabilizers, and parasympatholytic agents. There are no specific data with regard to these agents and their role in decreasing the incidence of perioperative pulmonary complications in the patient with asthma.

Sympathomimetic Compounds

There are no specific data that examine the use of perioperative treatment with beta-adrenergic agonists to reduce the incidence of pulmonary complications in the patient with asthma. It is common for patients with a history of asthma or patients who have evidence of wheezing preoperatively to receive beta-adrenergic therapy. Short-acting beta-adrenergic agents are routinely used in asthma exacerbations for quick relief of symptoms. Long-acting beta-adrenergic agents are used concomitantly with anti-inflammatory agents and have been shown in combination with low- to medium-dose inhaled steroids to improve lung function and reduce symptoms.[4] Beta-adrenergic agents cause smooth muscle relaxation by activation of adenylate cyclase and an increase in cyclic adenosine monophosphate (cAMP), which produce functional antagonism of bronchoconstriction.[4] Long-acting beta-adrenergic agents also help reduce nocturnal symptoms. Generally, patients should continue these agents at current dosages before surgery.

Leukotriene Modifiers

Leukotriene modifiers are considered an alternative to low-dose inhaled corticosteroids in patients with mild persistent asthma. Zafirlukast and montelukast are leukotriene receptor antagonists that selectively compete with LTD4 and LTE4 receptors. Zileuton is a 5-lipoxygenase inhibitor. Several studies have shown that these agents improve lung function while diminishing symptoms and the need for short-acting beta-adrenergic agents.[4] Most of the studies to date have been conducted in mild-to-moderate asthmatics with modest improvements noted. Zafirlukast has been demonstrated to attenuate the late response to allergen- and postallergen-induced bronchial hyperresponsiveness.[5] These classes of drugs are considered long-term control medications and have not been used for acute exacerbations.

Anticholinergics

Anticholinergic agents such as ipratropium bromide are used for relief of acute bronchospasm. These agents cause bronchodilation through competitive inhibition of muscarinic cholinergic receptors and reduce vagal tone to the airways. They may block reflex bronchoconstriction to irritants or to reflux esophagitis and may decrease mucus gland secretion. They are not effective against exercise-induced bronchospasm and are the treatment of choice for bronchospasm due to beta-blocker medication.

Corticosteroids

Corticosteroids are commonly used in the management of asthma. However, the significance and the role of corticosteroids in terms of reducing the incidence of perioperative pulmonary complications in the patient with asthma remain to be determined. Inhaled corticosteroids are the mainstay of treatment for persistent asthma. These drugs block the late reaction to allergens, reduce airway hyperresponsiveness, and inhibit cytokine production, adhesion protein activation, and inflammatory cell migration and activation. They also reverse beta-2-receptor downregulation and inhibit microvascular leakage.[4,6] Systemic corticosteroids are used for prompt control of moderate-to-severe exacerbations to prevent progression, reverse inflammation, speed recovery, and reduce rate of relapse. At high doses, inhaled corticosteroids may have systemic effects. Long-term systemic effects of corticosteroids are associated with adrenal axis and growth suppression, osteoporosis, dermal thinning, diabetes, hypertension, Cushing's syndrome, and impaired immune function.[4]

Anti-IgE Immunotherapy

The latest treatment for severe asthma is anti-IgE immunotherapy. Omalizumab is a recombinant humanized IgG monoclonal anti-IgE antibody that binds to IgE, a key molecule in the pathophysiology of allergic asthma.[7] Omalizumab binds to free IgE, effectively removing it from circulation, thus downregulating many of the inflammatory pathways involved in the pathogenesis of asthma. Although the role of omalizumab as a general treatment for asthma has not been effectively defined, it is generally reserved for patients with moderate persistent to severe asthma.[7] Although there are no data regarding omalizumab and surgery, patients on this drug should be considered to have moderate to severe disease and will likely need a more comprehensive evaluation.

EVIDENCE

Preoperative Assessment of the Patient with Asthma

Preoperative assessment of the patient with asthma should include a preoperative history with a focus on the patient's pulmonary status to determine the level of respiratory dysfunction and to assess the effectiveness of current therapy. Laboratory evaluation may include spirometry to assess the presence of airflow obstruction, the degree of obstruction, and reversibility with bronchodilators. Arterial blood gas measurement is helpful only if subsequent respiratory dysfunction occurs, and is usually normal at baseline. Oximetry may provide information with regard to desaturation with exertion. Measurement of inflammatory markers, such as exhaled nitric oxide, is used for the evaluation of asthma, but their measurement and interpretation require expertise and have not yet been well defined.[8] These markers are affected by steroids and other drugs, making their routine use as a preoperative test impractical. Routine chest x-rays are useful in ruling out comorbidities, such as infections, in the patient with asthma. In patients with mild intermittent disease there is no significant benefit to obtaining pulmonary function tests, arterial blood gases, oximetry, or chest x-ray. However, patients with moderate to severe symptoms or who are taking multiple medications for their asthma may require these evaluations to adequately assess their pulmonary risk.

Assessment of patients' asthma is important to establish the severity of their disease and how well their asthma is controlled. Recent guidelines define asthma severity in a step-wise fashion depending not only on spirometric measures but also the amount of treatment required to control symptoms. Asthma can be divided into four categories: (1) mild intermittent disease, those patients who typically use short-acting bronchodilators on an as-needed basis; (2) mild persistent disease, those patients who require a daily controller medication such as low-dose inhaled corticosteroid (ICS), leukotriene modifier, cromolyn, nedocromil, or theophylline; (3) moderate persistent disease, those patients who require a low- or medium-dose ICS with a long-acting bronchodilator; and (4) those patients with severe persistent disease who have established daily symptoms and typically are on multiple medications such as high-dose ICSs, oral steroids, bronchodilators, or biologic agents such as omalizumab (anti-IgE).[4] Categorization by disease severity should help to both stratify patients for risk of pulmonary complications and alert the anesthesiologist to the use of preoperative therapy to decrease potential bronchoconstriction and to plan perioperative care to decrease acute exacerbations.

Incidence of Pulmonary Complications in Patients with Asthma

No randomized clinical trials have examined the baseline prevalence of pulmonary complications in asthmatics stratified by severity of disease. Most of the studies were case series and retrospective in nature. Early studies reported overall rates of postoperative complications of 24% in patients with asthma.[1,3] More recent studies have reported rates of perioperative pulmonary complications for asthmatic patients of 1% to 2%.[9,10]

A retrospective study from the Mayo Clinic reviewed a database of 706 patients with asthma who underwent surgery and received either general anesthesia or regional anesthesia. The authors found an incidence of bronchospasm and laryngospasm of 1.7%, with respiratory failure occurring in one patient.[10] There were no reported episodes of pneumonia, pneumothorax, or death. The characteristics that were associated with complications included the recent use of asthma drugs, recent asthma exacerbation, and recent therapy in a medical facility for asthma. Complications were more prevalent in patients who were older at the time of diagnosis and at surgery. This study differed from earlier reports of increased complications of bronchospasm and barotrauma in patients with asthma, which reported an up to 24% complication rate.[1,3] Although the Mayo Clinic study had defined criteria for the diagnosis of asthma, the severity of the asthmatic symptoms of the subjects was not noted. The lower complication rate in these patients compared with the earlier studies may have been related to the strict definition used for asthma, thus excluding patients with chronic obstructive pulmonary disease (COPD). In addition, the trend toward safer anesthesia over the decades may account for the lower incidence of complications in the Mayo Clinic study. In addition, the database included all patients ever diagnosed with asthma rather than including only patients with active disease.[10,11] Whether preoperative medications were used was not noted, which may also affect the incidence of complications.

Risk Stratification of Asthmatics for Pulmonary Complications

There are no studies that provide baseline information with regard to the incidence of perioperative pulmonary complications stratified by severity of asthma symptoms. Although the Mayo Clinic study indicated a low incidence of perioperative pulmonary complications in patients with asthma,[10,11] it was not clear if this low incidence holds true for patients with symptomatic or severe disease, those who would most likely benefit from preoperative treatment. Moreover, of the four patients in the Mayo Clinic study who had respiratory symptoms at the time of surgery, two had complications.[10,11] Thus, the incidence of pulmonary complications in asthmatic patients by level of disease severity is important to assess the effectiveness of preoperative medications on potential pulmonary complications. Furthermore, if specific high-risk characteristics of patients with asthma can be identified, these may be treatable and thus potentially reduce perioperative pulmonary complications.

Use of Perioperative Medications for Asthma

It is common practice to continue currently prescribed medications for asthmatic patients up to the time of surgery. Furthermore, it is generally accepted practice to prophylactically administer a short-acting beta-adrenergic agonist to most asthmatic patients immediately before surgery and to administer systemic corticosteroids to severely asthmatic patients for a few days before surgery. However, it is important in general to establish outcome measures for the use of these various preoperative medications, and specifically for corticosteroids, for the patient with asthma because the use of these prophylactic treatment strategies has not been adequately supported by scientific evidence.

One study by Kabalin and colleagues[12] examined perioperative complications in asthmatic patients who were treated with corticosteroids. Patients were treated with systemic corticosteroids, prednisone 1 mg/kg 3 to 7 days preoperatively, along with hydrocortisone 100 mg intravenously (IV) every 8 hours perioperatively. The doses of steroids were similar for both mild and moderate asthmatics, with increased doses given to more severe asthmatics. Eighty-six of the 89 patients had no postoperative wheezing. Of the three patients who developed postoperative wheezing, two of them were treated with steroids preoperatively and the third patient was not a known asthmatic and did not receive any preoperative asthma treatment. This study found an incidence of postoperative pulmonary complications, as defined mainly by mild wheezing, of 4.5%. Two patients developed wound infections; however, there were no statistically significant differences between the incidence of infection among the patients with asthma versus the historical incidence of

wound infection for all surgical procedures. None of the outcome measures studied, including postoperative bronchospasm or pneumonia, were predicted by such variables as age, sex, severity of illness, smoking status, type of surgery, or pretreatment.

Another study performed at the same institution by Pien and colleagues[13] examined the prevalence of pulmonary complications following preoperative and perioperative treatment with steroids in 68 patients with asthma who underwent 92 surgical procedures. In the 92 procedures, a pretreatment regimen of 100 mg of hydrocortisone was given every 8 hours beginning the night before surgery. In 41 of the 92 procedures, prednisone was administered. The overall postoperative incidence of pulmonary complications with pretreatment with steroids was 9.7%. There were no deaths, wound infections, or evidence of adrenal insufficiency in the group. Conclusions for these studies are limited because of the lack of information about the patients' baseline pulmonary status, concurrent medications (specifically steroid use), and the use of historical controls.

Although both studies suggested a reduction in the incidence of pulmonary complications in the asthmatic patient treated preoperatively with corticosteroids, these studies used historical controls, which had a high incidence of complications,[2,3] and which may not be valid[9,10] because of the secular trend in the overall decrease in complication rates for anesthesia and surgery over time.

A more recent study by Su and colleagues[14] at Northwestern University found an overall low incidence of complications in 172 asthmatic patients who had 249 procedures treated with preoperative systemic steroids in 240 of the procedures. It was noted that 13 patients (5.2%) developed postoperative bronchospasm. In addition, 9 patients (3.6%) developed postoperative infections, 4 (1.6%) of which were wound infections. Although drawing conclusions from this study has limitations because of the retrospective cohort design employed,[14] it should be noted that even when asthma patients are given systemic steroids preoperatively, their risk of having perioperative or postoperative bronchospasm was not zero.

Another dramatic change in the management of asthmatic patients has been the increased use of inhaled corticosteroids (ICSs) for disease maintenance. Unfortunately, there are no data with regard to the use of ICSs in asthmatic patients undergoing surgery or any comparisons with the use of systemic corticosteroids in terms of the risks of pulmonary complications. Furthermore, there are no data with regard to whether preoperative steroids should be used on all asthmatic patients versus only patients with currently active symptoms. Previous studies showed low complication rates in terms of infection, wound healing, and adrenal insufficiency, but these risks must be weighed against the potential benefits of pretreating with corticosteroids. Marked adrenal suppression has been described for doses of 0.75 mg/day of fluticasone propionate.[15] There was a greater potency for dose-related adrenal suppression with fluticasone than with beclomethasone, triamcinolone, or budesonide. Long-term high-dose ICSs have been noted to increase the risk of cataracts, glaucoma, and osteoporosis. There were no significant effects on final adult height based on growth studies.[15] As a general rule, any patient who has received an oral glucocorticoid in doses equivalent to at least 20 mg a day of prednisone for more than 5 days is at risk for adrenal insufficiency,[16] and a stress dose of glucocorticosteroids should be considered.

AREAS OF UNCERTAINTY

The Salmeterol Multicenter Asthma Research Trial has recently raised concern regarding the safety of long-acting beta-adrenergic agonists in the treatment of asthma.[17] In this observational trial, the African-American patients who received salmeterol, a long-acting bronchodilating agent (LABA), had a higher rate of respiratory-related death or life-threatening experiences. This led the Food and Drug Administration (FDA) to change the label information for all long-acting beta-adrenergic bronchodilators (salmeterol and formoterol), which now carry a "black box warning." Although the cause of the increased mortality rate is not clear, most experts agree that monotherapy with an LABA is not appropriate for patients with asthma. There has also been speculation regarding genetic differences in asthma severity in the African-American population of this trial.

Controversy regarding bronchodilators is not new in the asthma literature. There was concern in the 1960s regarding increased mortality rates in asthma with the overuse of short-acting bronchodilators such as isoproterenol. More recently, there has been emerging evidence that beta-2 adrenergic receptor polymorphisms may affect the response to bronchodilators. There is concern that the arg/arg polymorphism at position 16 of the beta-adrenergic receptor may be associated with negative outcomes with the use of short-acting bronchodilators.[18] It is less clear if LABAs affect pulmonary function the same way when used in combination with an inhaled corticosteroid. The consensus in the asthma literature at this time appears to be that if an LABA is prescribed, this should always be in combination with an inhaled corticosteroid.[4]

GUIDELINES

The expert panel report on the guidelines for the diagnosis and management of asthma make some recommendations for patients with asthma undergoing surgery in an effort to reduce complications during and after surgery. They state the importance of a thorough preoperative evaluation (review of symptoms, medication use, and measurement of pulmonary function) and efforts to maximize the pulmonary function (forced expiratory volume in 1 second [FEV$_1$] or peak expiratory flow rate [PEFR]) of the patient before surgery. This may require a short course of oral systemic corticosteroids.

If a patient has received oral systemic corticosteroids during the past 6 months for more than 2 weeks and for selected patients on a long-term high dose of an ICS, consider the administration of 100 mg of hydrocortisone every 8 hours intravenously during the surgical period and reduce the dose rapidly within 24 hours after surgery.

AUTHORS' RECOMMENDATIONS

Patients with asthma should continue previous medications before surgery. For the purposes of perioperative therapy, these patients can be categorized by symptomatology and/or spirometry into four categories: (1) mild disease with either intermittent or persistent symptoms, (2) moderate persistent disease, (3) severe disease, and (4) active wheezing or shortness of breath (Figure 11-1). Patients with controlled moderate persistent to severe persistent disease may benefit from a short course (3 days) of oral corticosteroids. Severe asthmatic patients who are currently on chronic oral corticosteroids or who have recently been on a steroid taper should receive a dose of corticosteroids perioperatively to prevent development of adrenal insufficiency. Patients with difficult-to-control symptoms should receive increased doses of oral corticosteroids and may need to postpone elective surgery until symptoms can be effectively controlled. All patients should be instructed to use their inhalers as previously prescribed on the day of surgery.

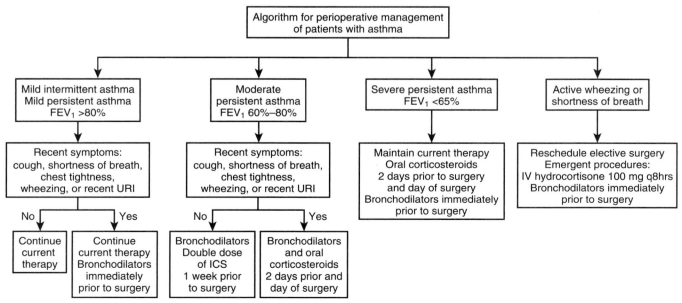

Figure 11-1. Algorithm for Perioperative Management of Patients with Asthma.

REFERENCES

1. Shnider SM, Papper EM: Anesthesia for the asthmatic patient. *Anesthesiology* 1961;22:886-892.
2. Smetana GW: Preoperative pulmonary evaluation. *N Engl J Med* 1999;340(12):937-944.
3. Gold MI, Helrich M: A study of complications related to anesthesia in asthmatic patients. *Anesth Analg* 1963;42:238-293.
4. Expert Panel Report 3 (EPR-3): Guidelines for the diagnosis and management of asthma—summary report 2007. *J Allergy Clin Immunol* 2007;120(5 suppl):S94-S138.
5. Calhoun W et al: Effect of zafirlukast (Accolate) on cellular mediators of inflammation: Bronchoalveolar lavage fluid findings after segmental antigen challenge. *Am J Respir Crit Care Med* 1998;1381-1389.
6. Kingston HG, Hirshman CA: Perioperative management of the patient with asthma. *Anesth Analg* 1984;63(9):844-855.
7. Tonnel AB, Tillie-Leblond I: Omalizumab for asthma. *N Engl J Med* 2006;355(12):1282.
8. Doherty GM et al: Anesthesia and the child with asthma. *Paediatr Anaesth* 2005;15(6):446-454.
9. Forrest JB et al: Multicenter study of general anesthesia. III. Predictors of severe perioperative adverse outcomes. *Anesthesiology* 1992;76(1):3-15.
10. Warner DO et al: Perioperative respiratory complications in patients with asthma. *Anesthesiology* 1996;85(3):460-467.
11. Bishop MJ, Cheney FW: Anesthesia for patients with asthma. Low risk but not no risk. *Anesthesiology* 1996;85(3):455-456.
12. Kabalin CS, Yarnold PR, Grammer LC: Low complication rate of corticosteroid-treated asthmatics undergoing surgical procedures. *Arch Intern Med* 1995;155(13):1379-1384.
13. Pien LC, Grammer LC, Patterson R: Minimal complications in a surgical population with severe asthma receiving prophylactic corticosteroids. *J Allergy Clin Immunol* 1988;82(4):696-700.
14. Su FW et al: Low incidence of complications in asthmatic patients treated with preoperative corticosteroids. *Allergy Asthma Proc* 2004;25(5):327-333.
15. Lipworth BJ: Systemic adverse effects of inhaled corticosteroid therapy: A systematic review and meta-analysis. *Arch Intern Med* 1999;159(9):941-955.
16. Axelrod L: Perioperative management of patients treated with glucocorticoids. *Endocrinol Metab Clin North Am* 2003;32(2):367-383.
17. Nelson HS et al: The Salmeterol Multicenter Asthma Research Trial: A comparison of usual pharmacotherapy for asthma or usual pharmacotherapy plus salmeterol. *Chest* 2006;129(1):15-26.
18. Israel E et al: The effect of polymorphisms of the beta(2)-adrenergic receptor on the response to regular use of albuterol in asthma. *Am J Respir Crit Care Med* 2000;162(1):75-80.

12 Which Patient Should Have a Preoperative Cardiac Evaluation (Stress Test)?

Amy L. Miller, MD, PhD, and Joshua A. Beckman, MD, MS

INTRODUCTION

Preoperative cardiovascular risk assessment attempts to prospectively identify at-risk patients, allowing targeted perioperative management in order to reduce event rates.[1] Perioperative cardiac events include both "demand" events, in which perioperative stress increases myocardial oxygen requirements to a level that cannot be met due to fixed obstructive coronary artery disease (CAD) or low perfusion pressure,[2,3] and true "acute coronary syndromes" (ACSs) with occlusive plaque rupture,[4-6] likely due in part to perioperative inflammation/cytokine response and an associated prothrombotic state.[2] Epicardial obstructive CAD sufficient to cause demand-related biomarker release can be reliably identified by cardiac stress testing and coronary angiography. Consequently, preoperative cardiovascular assessment evolved from risk factor identification to ischemia evaluation, using risk factors to identify at-risk patients, and cardiovascular stress testing (with or without angiography) to identify hemodynamically significant CAD in those patients, who could then be revascularized by percutaneous coronary intervention or coronary artery bypass graft (CABG) surgery.

Revolutionary changes in cardiovascular medical management, particularly the advent of perioperative beta blockade,[7-12] together with advances in surgical and anesthetic technique, have significantly reduced operative morbidity and mortality rates, with event rates decreasing from approximately 10% to 15% in intermediate-risk patients three decades ago[1] to approximately 5% in contemporary "at-risk" patients (i.e., with risk factors for or known CAD) and approximately 1.5% in unselected noncardiac surgery patients.[2] This reduction in risk likely attenuates the benefit of preoperative revascularization. In fact, although retrospective and observational data support the concept of risk reduction by preoperative revascularization,[13] a recent prospective randomized, controlled trial found no risk reduction from revascularization in patients with stable, symptomatic CAD.[14] Consequently, the role of preoperative cardiac stress testing has been reduced to the identification of extremely high-risk patients, for example, with significant left main (LM) disease, for whom preoperative revascularization may provide benefit independent of the operation.

Historically, preoperative cardiovascular risk assessment has lacked widespread standardization or consensus, despite published guidelines. Perceived goals have varied, adherence to recommendations has been poor,[15] and many assessments resulted in no formal recommendations.[16] Furthermore, differing opinions occurred in a majority of cases, and opinions contradicted consensus guidelines in a significant minority.[17] With increasing data to guide the evolution of consensus guidelines into evidence-based guidelines, greater consensus and adherence among practitioners will, it is hoped, follow.

OPTIONS/EVALUATION STRATEGIES

As we integrate new data into our standard practice, the following key issues emerge:

1. Understanding risk factor implications as well as absolute contraindications to elective/urgent surgical procedures
2. Understanding treatment options independent of revascularization that can significantly affect patient outcome
3. Understanding the risks and benefits of revascularization in the preoperative period
4. Appropriate testing—which patients to test and how to test them

EVIDENCE FOR A ROLE OF PERIOPERATIVE RISK STRATIFICATION AND RISK MODIFICATION

Early studies of risk stratification focused primarily on the identification of risk factors predictive of increased event rates,[18] enabling construction of risk indices to prospectively quantify perioperative cardiovascular risk.[19] Current guidelines focus on the Lee Revised Cardiac Risk Index (RCRI; Table 12-1), which divides patients into quartiles of predicted risk.[20] The current American College of Cardiology/American Heart Association (ACC/AHA) guidelines for preoperative cardiac assessment also define four "major" risk factors that preclude nonemergent surgical procedures: active/recent unstable coronary syndrome, decompensated heart failure, significant arrhythmia, and severe valvular disease.[19]

Table 12-1 Revised Cardiac Risk Index*

RCRI Class	RCRI Score	Cardiovascular Event Rate†
Class I	0	0.5 (0.2, 1.1)
Class II	1	1.3 (0.7, 2.1)
Class III	2	3.6 (2.1, 5.6)
Class IV	>2	9.1 (5.5, 13.8)

*Revised Cardiac Risk Index (RCRI) = number of the following risk factors present:
- High-risk surgery
- Ischemic heart disease
- History of cerebrovascular disease
- History of congestive heart failure
- Presence of insulin-requiring diabetes
- Preoperative serum creatinine exceeding 2.0 mg/dL

†Cardiovascular event rates from the derivation patient cohort.
Lee TH et al: Derivation and prospective validation of a simple index for prediction of cardiac risk of major noncardiac surgery. *Circulation* 1999; 100(10):1043-1049.

EVIDENCE THAT SPECIFIC HIGH-RISK MARKERS DEMAND PREOPERATIVE ASSESSMENT AND INTERVENTION

Acute Coronary Syndrome

An active unstable coronary syndrome is, until proven otherwise, an ACS reflecting erosion or rupture of an atherosclerotic plaque. Patients with an ACS are at increased perioperative risk, and in such cases, surgery should be delayed when possible. Retrospective electrocardiogram analysis from the GUSTO-IIb (*global use of strategies to open occluded arteries in acute coronary syndromes*) study demonstrated that mortality rates rise for 20 to 30 days following presentation, after which mortality rates stabilize.[21] As such, current guidelines identify 30 days as the cutoff for a "recent" acute coronary syndrome[19]; further delay in surgery would not be expected to alter risk, in the absence of other confounding issues.

Decompensated Congestive Heart Failure

Although treatments for congestive heart failure have advanced significantly in the past decade, mortality benefits have been more prominent in patients with mild to moderate disease than in those with advanced heart failure.[22] Annual mortality rate in recent randomized trials in Class III/IV heart failure ranges from 18.5% to 73%,[23] whereas the Acute Decompensated Heart Failure National Registry (ADHERE) of decompensated heart failure admissions found an overall in-hospital mortality rate of 4%, with subgroup mortality rates ranging from 2.1% to 21.9%.[24] These rates, which exceed the expected cardiovascular event rates for the vast majority of elective surgical procedures, would almost certainly increase significantly with the hemodynamic and systemic stress of surgery. Early multivariate risk factor analyses confirmed that decompensated heart failure was associated with increased perioperative morbidity and mortality

risk.[1] As such, decompensated congestive heart failure must be treated before surgery.

Arrhythmia

In the perioperative context, "significant" arrhythmia refers to hemodynamically significant rhythm disturbances. However, ventricular arrhythmias are of sufficient threat that even hemodynamically tolerated sustained ventricular arrhythmias should defer anything but emergent surgery. There is no literature characterizing the level of risk that can be ascribed to a preoperative sustained ventricular arrhythmia; given the life-threatening nature of such arrhythmias, to seek to obtain such data would be unethical. In contrast, there is evidence that nonsustained ventricular arrhythmias do not preclude surgical procedures and do not increase perioperative cardiovascular risk.[25,26]

Uncontrolled atrial arrhythmias (i.e., with ventricular response rates exceeding approximately 90 to 100 beats per minute) place patients at increased risk for demand ischemia. Accordingly, rate control should be established before surgery. Although rate-controlled atrial arrhythmias do not preclude surgery, they are associated with an unmodifiable increase in perioperative risk, identifying a sicker cohort of patients. For patients undergoing CABG, preoperative atrial fibrillation (AF) increases length of stay, rehospitalization rate, and long-term mortality rate, but not operative mortality rate.[27] Preoperative AF is associated with increased perioperative cardiovascular mortality rate (adjusted odds rate 4) in noncardiac surgery,[28] but this may reflect unidentified comorbidities that increase both the prevalence of AF and cardiovascular risk, and/or inadequate perioperative rate control.

Finally, there is the ancillary issue of anticoagulation. Rapid postoperative reinstatement of anticoagulation to minimize thromboembolic risk places patients at an increased risk of postoperative bleeding,[29] and may not provide significant benefit.[30] Although patients with AF are, in general, at relatively low short-term risk for thromboembolic events, with age-dependent stroke rates of 1% to 5% per year,[31] the potentially devastating nature of these events makes risk/benefit assessment challenging. Current ACC/AHA guidelines advise that it is reasonable to interrupt anticoagulation for up to a week without "bridge" intravenous therapy,[32] but the available evidence to support or contradict such practice is limited.

Valvular Disease

Valvular disease is the best studied of the four "major" risk factors. In general, regurgitant lesions are not a contraindication to elective surgery, because such lesions are relatively tolerant of perioperative fluid shifts and anesthetic induction. In contrast, symptomatic or severe stenotic lesions are sensitive to changes in both preload and afterload, increasing the risk of perioperative hemodynamic embarrassment.

Although the decreasing incidence of rheumatic heart disease has made mitral valve stenosis a rare clinical finding, aortic stenosis (AS) remains common. Some retrospective surgical series found no increase in perioperative cardiovascular event rates in patients with significant AS,[33] but the majority of studies suggest that morbidity and mortality rates are higher in these patients.[34,35] A recent retrospective case-control analysis supports this contention, with stenosis severity predicting a sevenfold increase in cardiovascular events.[36] Taken together, the available evidence supports the current standard of practice, in which clinically significant AS is addressed before an elective surgical procedure.[19]

EVIDENCE FOR MODIFICATION OF PERIOPERATIVE RISK—ROLE OF MEDICAL TREATMENT

Much of our understanding of relative risk is derived from the Coronary Artery Surgery Study (CASS) registry,[37] in which perioperative cardiovascular morbidity and mortality rates varied as a function of surgical "risk," with the highest risk being associated with vascular surgeries.[37] Based on this registry, we now subdivide surgical procedures into three classes (high, intermediate, and low risk).[19] While much of this information is intuitive, data from the CASS registry codified the stratification of procedural risk. The higher event rates associated with "high-risk" noncardiac surgery (i.e., vascular surgery) have made these procedures the ideal setting in which to explore perioperative risk reduction.

Evidence for Perioperative Beta-Blockade

The role of so-called "demand" perioperative ischemia[2,3] suggests that hemodynamic stress contributes to cardiovascular events. Periods of greatest risk include peri-induction and the immediate postoperative period, presumably as lightened sedation allows increasing sympathetic drive and resultant tachycardia.[3] Sympatholytic therapy with beta-blockade should blunt this response, minimizing myocardial demand.

The first large-scale study of perioperative beta-blockade randomized patients undergoing intermediate- to high-risk surgery to placebo versus atenolol (target heart rate 65 beats per minute), reducing postoperative mortality rate from 8% to 0% by 3 months after surgery.[9] Three years later, the Dutch Echocardiographic Cardiac Risk Evaluation Applying Stress Echocardiography study group (DECREASE) randomized high-risk vascular surgery patients with positive preoperative dobutamine echocardiography to perioperative bisoprolol versus placebo, with a reduction in cardiac death rates from 17% to 3.4% and nonfatal myocardial infarction (MI) rates from 17% to 0%.[10] Subsequent work by the same group demonstrated that maximal beta-blockade dose and heart rate control optimized perioperative protective benefit.[38]

The role, if any, of beta-blockade in low-risk patients remains unclear. In a retrospective analysis of a multicenter cohort (the Premier's Perspective database) undergoing major noncardiac surgery, perioperative mortality rate was lower with beta-blocker use in intermediate- and high-risk patients but showed a trend toward increased mortality rate in low-risk patients.[7] These data are difficult to interpret, because beta-blocker use in these patients may serve as a marker for a negative perioperative event that led to, rather than resulted from, beta-blockade. Although some studies have gone so far as to suggest that beta-blockade is not beneficial even in intermediate-risk patients,[39-42] these results likely reflect methodologic limitations, including underdosing and inadequate duration of beta-blockade,[40-42] as well as dilution with low-risk procedures or patients.[40,41]

In contrast, the DECREASE-2 study randomized a relatively homogenous population of 770 intermediate-risk vascular surgery patients to preoperative stress testing versus no testing; patients with significant stress-induced ischemia could have preoperative revascularization at the discretion of their care team.[43] In this population, of which 8.8% had extensive ischemia (35% of whom were revascularized [50% partial, 50% complete] before vascular surgery), there were no significant differences in death or MI rates. In contrast, heart rate control was significantly correlated with morbidity and mortality rates, with an event rate of 1.7% in patients with a heart rate below 50 beats per minute versus 16.5% in patients with a heart rate exceeding 65 beats per minute. These results suggest that, if adequate beta-blockade can be achieved, preoperative cardiac stress testing has no role in intermediate-risk patients.[43] The weight of evidence supporting perioperative beta-blocker therapy prompted a focused update to the ACC/AHA perioperative guidelines,[44] which advised perioperative beta-blockade in high-risk patients (Class I recommendation for vascular surgery, Class IIa for intermediate- to high-risk surgery), with beta-blockade in low-risk patients receiving a Class IIb recommendation. In the new 2007 guidelines, these recommendations have been broadened to a Class IIA indication encompassing all patients with at least one clinical risk factor and/or with known CAD who are scheduled for intermediate- or high-risk procedures.

Evidence for Other Perioperative Medical Interventions

Invasive monitoring (e.g., pulmonary artery catheters [PACs], arterial lines), cardiac telemetry, and an intensive care unit (ICU) setting have all been proposed to decrease perioperative morbidity. Although there are no randomized controlled trial data examining their role in perioperative cardiovascular risk reduction, cardiac telemetry and ICU admission are widely accepted as cost-effective and beneficial in at least a subset of patients, particularly high-risk patients, as well as those requiring invasive monitoring or frequent titration of hemodynamically active medications.[45] In contrast, the perioperative role of the PAC has decreased in recent years. Observational studies suggest that PAC use *increases* morbidity and mortality rates.[46,47] Although prospective studies of PACs in the perioperative setting have a number of methodologic limitations,[48] the largest randomized controlled study suggests that PACs have insufficient benefit.[49] The PAC has no role in current routine perioperative care, although we cannot exclude the possibility that there does exist a specific subpopulation for which use of the device may be beneficial.

A number of pharmacologic agents, including alpha agonists, nitroglycerin, and diltiazem, have been studied, with only limited evidence of perioperative benefit.[13,50-52]

More recently, HMG CoA reductase inhibitors ("statins"), drugs with recognized pleiotropic therapeutic effects on the cardiovascular system,[53] have been examined. Observational retrospective studies suggest that perioperative statin use is protective,[12,54] and there is a significant body of evidence supporting statin use in vascular surgery patients.[55]

A likely target of future research is aspirin. Although antiplatelet agents were traditionally discontinued perioperatively to minimize bleeding, observational trials demonstrated decreased morbidity and mortality rates in cardiac surgery patients who received perioperative aspirin.[56-58] Although this has not been studied in noncardiac surgery, the need to continue antiplatelet therapy following drug-eluting stent (DES) placement will likely mandate systematic analysis of this issue in the near future. In fact, a recent meta-analysis suggested that the risks of antiplatelet-associated bleeding were less than the risks associated with antiplatelet withdrawal following stenting.[59] Given the still evolving guidelines for antiplatelet therapy after stenting, for any patient with a coronary artery stent, a cardiologist should be consulted before discontinuation of antiplatelet therapy for any procedure.

EVIDENCE FOR MODIFICATION OF PERIOPERATIVE RISK—ROLE OF PREOPERATIVE REVASCULARIZATION

Data defining the role of perioperative revascularization can be temporally stratified by the means of revascularization (CABG, angioplasty, stent, and DES). The CASS database provided the first retrospective evidence of risk reduction with revascularization, with reduced cardiovascular morbidity and mortality rates for at least 6 years following CABG.[37] Importantly, these data predate the use of the left internal mammary artery (LIMA) conduit, which has greater longevity,[60] suggesting that protective effects could be more durable in the current era.

By the mid-1980s, percutaneous transluminal coronary angioplasty (PTCA) was a viable alternative to CABG. Retrospective review suggested that, compared to historical controls, PTCA reduced perioperative cardiovascular morbidity and mortality rates,[61,62] and prospective randomized evaluation found that PTCA was as effective as CABG in lowering perioperative risk.[63,64]

Percutaneous coronary intervention (PCI) employing coronary stents to scaffold open lesions was examined in the coronary-artery revascularization before elective major vascular surgery (Coronary Artery Revascularization Prophylaxis [CARP]) trial.[14] CARP was the first prospective randomized trial to study preoperative revascularization in patients with stable obstructive CAD, enrolling patients scheduled for elective major vascular surgery (abdominal aortic aneurysm [AAA] repair or lower-extremity revascularization) in whom angiography revealed significant CAD amenable to revascularization. Significant (greater than 50%) stenosis of the LM artery was an exclusion criterion, as was a left ventricular ejection fraction (EF) less than 20% or severe AS. The patients, a very high-risk population (67% with multivessel disease; RCRI score of 2 or more in 49% and 3 or more in 13%), were randomized to preoperative revascularization (PCI or CABG) or medical

management. There were no significant differences in short-term (30 day MI rate approximately 13%) or long-term (mortality rate at 2.7 years approximately 22%) morbidity and mortality rates. These moderate rates, in such a high-risk population, illustrate the significant improvement in medical therapy and attendant reduction in mortality rate since the CASS era.

Interestingly, revascularization-related delay in the planned vascular procedure actually resulted in a trend toward increased vascular-related mortality.[14] This is particularly troubling in the context of PCI, particularly with DES. With balloon angioplasty, retrospective analysis found increased event rates for 2 weeks after intervention, suggesting that surgery should be delayed for at least 2 weeks following angioplasty.[65] Although a similar period of increased risk was observed in retrospective and observational analysis with bare-metal stents (BMS), the recommendation with BMS was that surgery be delayed for at least 4 weeks following PCI,[66] although there was some evidence that event rates could be increased for at least 3 months after PCI.[67,68] With the advent of DES, the issue became complicated by longer obligate dual antiplatelet therapy. Although initial guidelines recommended dual antiplatelet therapy for 3 months for a CYPHER (Johnson & Johnson sirolimus-coated) stent and 6 months with a TAXUS (Boston Scientific paclitaxel-coated) stent, current recommendations advise at least 1 year of dual antiplatelet therapy following DES.[69] Retrospective analysis of perioperative event rates following BMS or DES placement reveal no significant differences,[70] but the prolonged antiplatelet regimen for DES is a significant issue for surgeons. Importantly, discontinuation of antiplatelet therapy is the strongest risk factor for cardiovascular events after PCI,[70] underscoring the necessity of cardiologist input before discontinuing antiplatelet therapy in a patient who has had prior PCI.

ASSESSMENT OF ISCHEMIA—WHO AND HOW TO TEST

Functional capacity is predictive of both perioperative and long-term cardiac events,[71] with increased morbidity and mortality rates in patients with less than 4-MET capacity.[72] A simple marker for 4-MET capacity is the ability to walk up two flights of stairs. Patients who can, by history or example, exert themselves to this level do not require stress testing. Surgery can proceed with best medical therapy.

In patients with unclear or poor functional capacity, cardiac stress testing can provide relatively accurate identification and quantification of ischemia, regardless of the mechanism of stress (exercise, pharmacologic stress, or vasodilation) and/or the metric of assessment (electrocardiogram, myocardial perfusion imaging, or echocardiography). Sensitivity and specificity for the detection of significant coronary artery disease are on the order of 70% to 88% across modalities.[73] Modality selection should be guided by local expertise and patient-specific factors, with a preference for exercise over pharmacologic stress whenever possible given the additional functional and hemodynamic information that is obtained with exercise.[71]

For perioperative patients, stress-induced reversible perfusion defects have a positive predictive vale of 2% to 20% for perioperative death or MI; negative predictive value is on the order of 99%.[71] In general, prognostic information is limited to that subset of patients with elevated clinical risk, extensive ischemia, or both.[74,75] Thus, although they have adequate sensitivity and specificity, all modalities have an unacceptably low positive predictive value, and so require a very restrictive criterion for the degree of ischemia that triggers further evaluation. Positive predictive value is expected to further decline with widespread implementation of perioperative beta-blockade, which should further reduce perioperative event rates.

The overarching emphasis of the ACC/AHA guidelines is that preoperative ischemia evaluation is no different than in other elective settings.[19] The fact that a patient is scheduled for surgery, regardless of the degree of surgical risk, does not affect the patient's relative need for assessment and possible revascularization. The recent Clinical Outcomes Utilizing Revascularization and Aggressive Drug Evaluation (COURAGE) trial demonstrated that, for stable CAD, event rates do not differ with the addition of PCI to best medical therapy.[76] This is underscored by the aforementioned results of the CARP trial,[14] which demonstrated that even in patients with clinically stable multivessel disease undergoing high-risk surgery, revascularization has no perioperative mortality benefit.

Taken together, the available evidence suggests that cardiac catheterization is best employed for two purposes: (1) to exclude life-threatening/critical coronary artery disease (e.g., critical LM disease), and (2) relief of refractory symptoms. The former indication is more challenging, as it is difficult to know how broad a net to cast in order to identify those rare patients with critical disease. This was partially addressed by the aforementioned DECREASE-2 study, which demonstrated that with adequate beta-blockade, there was no interval benefit from stress testing with or without revascularization in intermediate-risk vascular surgery patients.[43] These results suggest that preoperative cardiac testing has no role in intermediate-risk patients (RCRI 1-2) for whom adequate perioperative beta-blockade can be provided.[43]

CONTROVERSIES

The role of elective/nonurgent percutaneous revascularization remains a matter of some controversy. As noted previously, COURAGE found no mortality benefit to PCI,[76] and has led to debates regarding the benefit(s) of PCI. Most cardiologists believe that the symptom relief provided by PCI warrants its use in patients with symptoms refractory to best medical therapy. As such, PCI will remain prominent in ischemia management, bringing with it an increase in the difficulty of perioperative care.

Stent selection (BMS versus DES), one of the hottest controversies in cardiovascular medicine, has significant perioperative implications. When the first-generation DES were approved by the Food and Drug Administration (FDA) over 3 years ago, their use rapidly supplanted that of BMS,[77] including off-label use, which, by 2007, made up over half the DES recipient population.[69] With the release of BASKET-LATE (Basel Stent Kosten-Effektivitäts Late Thrombotic Events Trial) and subsequent trials,[78,79] however, it became clear that the current DES platform has intrinsic weaknesses, with the in-stent restenosis reduction counterbalanced in part by a small increase in (potentially fatal) late in-stent thrombosis. Overall, on-label use of DES does provide superior outcomes to BMS.[80,81] However, given the antiplatelet considerations, BMS are preferred for patients with anticipated surgical procedures. Unfortunately, it is easy to see how one's ability to peer into the future may not stretch out to the limits of patients' 1-year required clopidogrel therapy with DES. Consequently, arguments regarding the safety of perioperative antiplatelet therapy will almost certainly continue. It is essential that both prospective randomized trials and registry data examine this issue, particularly in patients with prior coronary artery stents, in order to provide an evidence base on which consensus can be reached.

AREAS OF UNCERTAINTY

The evidence base for cardiovascular risk assessment has developed through the increasing willingness of investigators to randomize patients with an increasing burden of disease. Patients with a significantly reduced EF or LM disease are the two populations perceived to be too high risk for randomization; revascularization in these patients was presumed to be beneficial. Until the CARP trial, however, many investigators would have argued that revascularization of stable multivessel disease was beneficial. The recent DECREASE-V pilot study may herald the next generation of preoperative studies. In it, the previously excluded populations of LM disease and low EF were included in randomization of vascular surgery patients to preoperative revascularization or standard medical management.[82] Of note, 8% of randomized patients had LM disease, and 67% had three-vessel disease. Not surprisingly, given the high-risk characteristics of this population, event rates were high, with 30-day mortality rates of approximately 5% to 10%, and 30-day MI rates of approximately 16%. Revascularization had no statistically significant effect.

DECREASE-V raises more questions than it answers, and will almost certainly lead to a new generation of studies in extremely high-risk patients. If preoperative revascularization in patients with LM or critical three-vessel disease proves ineffective at reducing cardiovascular risk, the role of preoperative stress testing will need to be redefined, if not eliminated.

As the field moves from revascularization toward conservative medical therapy, noninvasive imaging strategies will offer an attractive alternative to the historical stress test/catheterization approach. In particular, computed tomography (CT) can noninvasively evaluate for CAD. For technical reasons, at present, CT can exclude significant obstructive disease, but cannot accurately quantify the degree of disease when present,[83] making it inadequate for preoperative ischemia evaluation, in which the issue is the exclusion of critical disease. Future technical developments will allow CT coronary angiography to provide more physiologically relevant information, which may in turn allow these studies to serve an expanded role in preoperative ischemia evaluation.

GUIDELINES

The ACC/AHA has released new perioperative risk assessment and management guidelines for patients at risk for CAD.[71] These evidence-based guidelines, which reflect the state of our current knowledge base, reserve preoperative cardiac stress testing for patients who meet the following criteria (Figure 12-1):

1. The patient has poor or unknown functional capacity.
   - Adequate functional capacity is a good prognostic indicator. For patients who are able to achieve 4 METS (the equivalent of walking up two flights of stairs), revascularization is unlikely to affect their risk of cardiovascular events.
2. The patient is being considered for a nonemergent surgical procedure of at least intermediate risk.

- Emergent procedures, by definition, do not have the luxury of time to allow ischemia evaluation.
- Low-risk procedures do not require preoperative evaluation.
3. The patient does not have an absolute contraindication/"red flag."
   - Patients with active arrhythmia, unstable coronary syndrome, decompensated heart failure, or significant stenotic valvular lesions should be evaluated and managed by a cardiologist before consideration of surgery.
4. The patient has sufficient clinical risk factors (at least three) to cause concern for LM/multivessel disease.
5. Revascularization would be performed preoperatively if ischemia evaluation were positive (i.e., management of the patient will potentially be altered by the evaluation).

The new ACC/AHA guidelines have also broadened the perioperative beta-blockade recommendations.[71] Although the Class I indication remains unchanged (patients with a nonsurgical beta-blocker indication and high-risk patients scheduled for vascular surgery), the Class IIA indication has been expanded to all patients with at least one clinical risk factor and/or with known CAD who are scheduled for intermediate- or high-risk procedures.

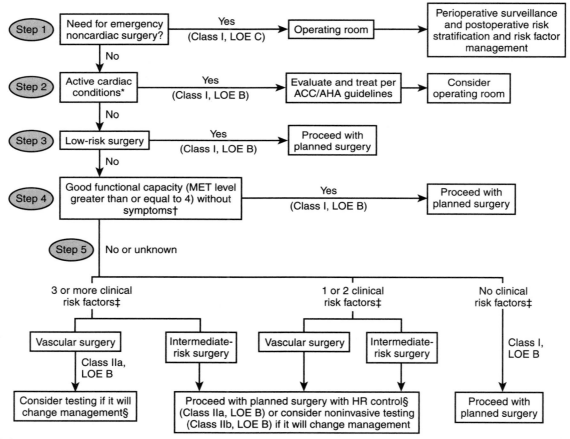

Figure 12-1. Cardiac evaluation and care algorithm for noncardiac surgery based on active clinical conditions, known cardiovascular disease, or cardiac risk factors for patients 50 years of age or greater. Fleisher LA, Beckman JA, Brown KA, et al: ACC/AHA 2007 Guidelines on Perioperative Cardiovascular Evaluation and Care for Noncardiac Surgery—Executive Summary: A Report of the American College of Cardiology/American Heart Association Task Force on Practice Guidelines. (Writing Committee to Revise the 2002 Guidelines on Perioperative Cardiovascular Evaluation for Noncardiac Surgery). *Circulation* 2007, 116:1971-1996.

REFERENCES

1. Goldman L et al: Multifactorial index of cardiac risk in noncardiac surgical procedures. *N Engl J Med* 1977;297(16):845-850.
2. Devereaux PJ et al: Perioperative cardiac events in patients undergoing noncardiac surgery: A review of the magnitude of the problem, the pathophysiology of the events and methods to estimate and communicate risk. *Can Med Assoc J* 2005;173 (6):627-634.
3. Landesberg G: The pathophysiology of perioperative myocardial infarction: Facts and perspectives. *J Cardiothorac Vasc Anesth* 2003;17(1): 90-100.
4. Ellis SG et al: Angiographic correlates of cardiac death and myocardial infarction complicating major nonthoracic vascular surgery. *Am J Cardiol* 1996;77:1126-1128.
5. Libby P: Current concepts in the pathogenesis of the acute coronary syndromes. *Circulation* 2001;104:365-372.
6. Libby P, Theroux P: Pathophysiology of coronary artery disease. *Circulation* 2005;111:3481-3488.
7. Lindenauer PK et al: Perioperative beta-blocker therapy and mortality after major noncardiac surgery. *N Engl J Med* 2005;353 (4):349-361.
8. Schouten O et al: Fluvastatin and bisoprolol for the reduction of perioperative cardiac mortality and morbidity in high-risk patients undergoing non-cardiac surgery: Rationale and design of the DECREASE-IV study. *Am Heart J* 2004;148(6):1047-1052.
9. Mangano DT et al: Effect of atenolol on mortality and cardiovascular morbidity after noncardiac surgery. *N Engl J Med* 1996;335 (23):1713-1720.
10. Poldermans D et al: The effect of bisoprolol on perioperative mortality and myocardial infarction in high-risk patients undergoing vascular surgery. *N Engl J Med* 1999;341:1789-1794.
11. Poldermans D, Boersma E: Beta-blocker therapy in noncardiac surgery. *N Engl J Med* 2005;353(4):412-414.
12. Kertai MD et al: A combination of statins and beta-blockers is independently associated with a reduction in the incidence of perioperative mortality and nonfatal myocardial infarction in patients undergoing abdominal aortic aneurysm surgery. *Eur J Vasc Endovasc Surg* 2004;28(4):343-352.
13. Fleisher LA, Eagle KA: Clinical practice. Lowering cardiac risk in noncardiac surgery. *N Engl J Med* 2001;345(23):1677-1682.
14. McFalls EO et al: Coronary-artery revascularization before elective major vascular surgery. *N Engl J Med* 2004;351(27):2795-2804.
15. Katz RI et al: A survey on the intended purposes and perceived utility of preoperative cardiology consultations. *Anesth Analg* 1998;87(4):830-836.
16. Katz RI, Cimino L, Vitkun SA: Preoperative medical consultations: Impact on perioperative management and surgical outcome. *Can J Anesth* 2005;52(7):697-702.
17. Pierpont GL et al: Disparate opinions regarding indications for coronary artery revascularization before elective vascular surgery. *Am J Cardiol* 2004;94(9):1124-1128.
18. Mangano D et al: Association of perioperative myocardial ischemia with cardiac morbidity and mortality in men undergoing noncardiac surgery. The Study of Perioperative Ischemia Research Group. *N Engl J Med* 1990;323(26):1781-1788.
19. Eagle KA et al: ACC/AHA guideline update for perioperative cardiovascular evaluation for noncardiac surgery—executive summary: A report of the American College of Cardiology/American Heart Association Task Force on Practice Guidelines (Committee to Update the 1996 Guidelines on Perioperative Cardiovascular Evaluation for Noncardiac Surgery). *J Am Coll Cardiol* 2002;39(3):542-553.
20. Lee TH et al: Derivation and prospective validation of a simple index for prediction of cardiac risk of major noncardiac surgery. *Circulation* 1999;100(10):1043-1049.
21. Savonitto S et al: Prognostic value of the admission electrocardiogram in acute coronary syndromes. *JAMA* 1999;281(8):707-713.
22. Teuteberg JJ et al: Characteristics of patients who die with heart failure and a low ejection fraction in the new millennium. *J Card Fail* 2006;12(1):47-53.
23. Yancy CW et al: The second Follow-up Serial Infusions of Nesiritide (FUSION II) trial for advanced heart failure: Study rationale and design. *Am Heart J* 2007;153(4):478-484.
24. Fonarow GC et al: Risk stratification for in-hospital mortality in acutely decompensated heart failure: Classification and regression tree analysis. *JAMA* 2005;293(5):572-580.
25. O'Kelly B et al: Ventricular arrhythmias in patients undergoing noncardiac surgery. The Study of Perioperative Ischemia Research Group. *JAMA* 1992;268(2):217-221.
26. Mahla E et al: Perioperative ventricular dysrhythmias in patients with structural heart disease undergoing noncardiac surgery. *Anesth Analg* 1998;86(1):16-21.
27. Ngaage DL et al: Does preoperative atrial fibrillation influence early and late outcomes of coronary artery bypass grafting? *J Thorac Cardiovasc Surg* 2007;133(1):182-189.
28. Noordzij PG et al: Prognostic value of routine preoperative electrocardiography in patients undergoing noncardiac surgery. *Am J Cardiol* 2006;97(7):1103-1106.
29. Vink R et al: Risk of thromboembolism and bleeding after general surgery in patients with atrial fibrillation. *Am J Cardiol* 2005;96 (6):822-824.
30. Beldi G et al: Prevention of perioperative thromboembolism in patients with atrial fibrillation. *Br J Surg* 2007; 94(11):1351-1355.
31. Frost L et al: Incident stroke after discharge from the hospital with a diagnosis of atrial fibrillation. *Am J Med* 2000;108(1):36-40.
32. Fuster V et al: ACC/AHA/ESC 2006 guidelines for the management of patients with atrial fibrillation—executive summary: A report of the American College of Cardiology/American Heart Association task force on practice guidelines and the European Society of Cardiology committee for practice guidelines (writing committee to revise the 2001 guidelines for the management of patients with atrial fibrillation): Developed in collaboration with the European Heart Rhythm Association and the Heart Rhythm Society. *Circulation* 2006;114(7):700-752.
33. Raymer K, Yang H: Patients with aortic stenosis: Cardiac complications in non-cardiac surgery. *Can J Anaesth* 1998;45(9):855-859.
34. O'Keefe JH Jr, Shub C, Rettke SR: Risk of noncardiac surgical procedures in patients with aortic stenosis. *Mayo Clin Proc* 1989;64 (4):400-405.
35. Torsher LC et al: Risk of patients with severe aortic stenosis undergoing noncardiac surgery. *Am J Cardiol* 1998;81(4):448-452.
36. Kertai MD et al: Aortic stenosis: An underestimated risk factor for perioperative complications in patients undergoing noncardiac surgery. *Am J Med* 2004;116(1):8-13.
37. Eagle KA et al: Cardiac risk of noncardiac surgery: Influence of coronary disease and type of surgery in 3368 operations. CASS Investigators and University of Michigan Heart Care Program. Coronary Artery Surgery Study. *Circulation* 1997;96 (6):1882-1887.
38. Feringa HHH et al: High-dose β-blockers and tight heart rate control reduce myocardial ischemia and troponin T release in vascular surgery patients. *Circulation* 2006;114(1 suppl):I-344-349.
39. Biccard BM, Sear JW, Foex P: Acute peri-operative beta blockade in intermediate-risk patients. *Anaesthesia* 2006;61(10):924-931.
40. Yang H et al: The effects of perioperative β-blockade: Results of the Metoprolol after Vascular Surgery (MaVS) study, a randomized controlled trial. *Am Heart J* 2006;152(5):983-990.
41. Juul AB et al: Effect of perioperative beta blockade in patients with diabetes undergoing major non-cardiac surgery: Randomised placebo controlled, blinded multicentre trial. *BMJ* 2006;332(7556):1482-1485.
42. Powell JT: Perioperative β-blockade (Pobble) for patients undergoing infrarenal vascular surgery: Results of a randomized double-blind controlled trial. *J Vasc Surg* 2005;41(4):602-609.
43. Poldermans D et al: Should major vascular surgery be delayed because of preoperative cardiac testing in intermediate-risk patients receiving beta-blocker therapy with tight heart rate control? *J Am Coll Cardiol* 2006;48(5):964-969.
44. Fleisher LA et al: ACC/AHA 2006 guideline update on perioperative cardiovascular evaluation for noncardiac surgery: Focused update on perioperative beta-blocker therapy: A report of the American College of Cardiology/American Heart Association Task Force on Practice Guidelines (Writing Committee to Update the 2002 Guidelines on Perioperative Cardiovascular Evaluation for Noncardiac Surgery) developed in collaboration with the American Society of Echocardiography, American Society of Nuclear Cardiology, Heart Rhythm Society, Society of Cardiovascular Anesthesiologists, Society for Cardiovascular Angiography

and Interventions, and Society for Vascular Medicine and Biology. *J Am Coll Cardiol* 2006;47(11):2343-2355.

45. Manthous C: Leapfrog and critical care: Evidence- and reality-based intensive care for the 21st century. *Am J Med* 2004;116: 188-193.

46. Connors AF Jr et al: The effectiveness of right heart catheterization in the initial care of critically ill patients. SUPPORT Investigators. *JAMA* 1996;276(11):889-897.

47. Polanczyk CA et al: Right heart catheterization and cardiac complications in patients undergoing noncardiac surgery: An observational study. *JAMA* 2001;286(3):309-314.

48. Hall JB: Searching for evidence to support pulmonary artery catheter use in critically ill patients. *JAMA* 2005;294(13): 1693-1694.

49. Sandham JD et al: A randomized, controlled trial of the use of pulmonary-artery catheters in high-risk surgical patients. *N Engl J Med* 2003;348(1):5-14.

50. Wallace AW et al: Effect of clonidine on cardiovascular morbidity and mortality after noncardiac surgery [see comment]. *Anesthesiology* 2004;101(2):284-293.

51. Stevens RD, Burri H, Tramer MR: Pharmacologic myocardial protection in patients undergoing noncardiac surgery: A quantitative systematic review. *Anesth Analg* 2003;97:623-633.

52. Devereaux PJ et al: Surveillance and prevention of major perioperative ischemic cardiac events in patients undergoing noncardiac surgery: A review. *Can Med Assoc J* 2005;173(7):779-788.

53. Beckman JA, Creager MA: The nonlipid effects of statins on endothelial function. *Trends Cardiovasc Med* 2006;16(5):156-162.

54. Kertai MD et al: Association between long-term statin use and mortality after successful abdominal aortic aneurysm surgery. *Am J Med* 2004;116(2):96-103.

55. Schouten O et al: Statins for the prevention of perioperative cardiovascular complications in vascular surgery. *J Vasc Surg* 2006;44(2):419-424.

56. Mangano DT: Aspirin and mortality from coronary bypass surgery. *N Engl J Med* 2002;347(17):1309-1317.

57. Dacey LJ et al: Effect of preoperative aspirin use on mortality in coronary artery bypass grafting patients. *Ann Thorac Surg* 2000;70:1986-1990.

58. Bybee KA et al: Preoperative aspirin therapy is associated with improved postoperative outcomes in patients undergoing coronary artery bypass grafting. *Circulation* 2005;112:286-292.

59. Burger W et al: Low-dose aspirin for secondary cardiovascular prevention—cardiovascular risks after its perioperative withdrawal versus bleeding risks with its continuation—review and meta-analysis. *J Intern Med* 2005;257(5):399-414.

60. Nwasokwa ON: Coronary artery bypass graft disease. *Ann Intern Med* 1995;123(7):528-533.

61. Gottlieb A et al: Perioperative cardiovascular morbidity in patients with coronary artery disease undergoing vascular surgery after percutaneous transluminal coronary angioplasty. *J Cardiothorac Vasc Anesth* 1998;12(5):501-506.

62. Posner KL, Van Norman GA, Chan V: Adverse cardiac outcomes after noncardiac surgery in patients with prior percutaneous transluminal coronary angioplasty. *Anesth Analg* 1999;89(3): 553-560.

63. Hassan SA et al: Outcomes of noncardiac surgery after coronary bypass surgery or coronary angioplasty in the Bypass Angioplasty Revascularization Investigation (BARI). *Am J Med* 2001;110: 260-266.

64. The Bypass Angioplasty Revascularization Investigation. I. Comparison of coronary bypass surgery with angioplasty in patients with multivessel disease. *N Engl J Med* 1996;335(4):217-225.

65. Brilakis ES et al: Outcome of patients undergoing balloon angioplasty in the two months prior to noncardiac surgery. *Am J Cardiol* 2005;96(4):512-514.

66. Kaluza GL et al: Catastrophic outcomes of noncardiac surgery soon after coronary stenting. *J Am Coll Cardiol* 2000;35(5): 1288-1294.

67. Brichon PY et al: Perioperative in-stent thrombosis after lung resection performed within 3 months of coronary stenting. *Eur J Cardiothorac Surg* 2006;30:793-796.

68. Vicenzi MN et al: Coronary artery stenting and non-cardiac surgery—a prospective outcome study. *Br J Anaesth* 2006;96(6): 686-693.

69. Maisel WH: Unanswered questions—drug-eluting stents and the risk of late thrombosis. *N Engl J Med* 2007;356(10):981-984.

70. Schouten O et al: Noncardiac surgery after coronary stenting: Early surgery and interruption of antiplatelet therapy are associated with an increase in major adverse cardiac events. *J Am Coll Cardiol* 2007;49(1):122-124.

71. Fleisher LA et al: ACC/AHA guideline update for perioperative cardiovascular evaluation for noncardiac surgery—executive summary: A report of the American College of Cardiology/American Heart Association Task Force on Practice Guidelines (Writing Committee to Revise the 2002 Guidelines on Perioperative Cardiovascular Evaluation for Noncardiac Surgery). *Circulation* 2007; 116:1971-1996.

72. Reilly DF et al: Self-reported exercise tolerance and the risk of serious perioperative complications. *Arch Intern Med* 1999;159 (18):2185-2192.

73. Lee TH, Boucher CA: Noninvasive tests in patients with stable coronary artery disease. *N Engl J Med* 2001;344(24):1840-1845.

74. Boersma E et al: Predictors of cardiac events after major vascular surgery: Role of clinical characteristics, dobutamine echocardiography, and β-blocker therapy. *JAMA* 2001;285(14):1865-1873.

75. Etchells E et al: Semiquantitative dipyridamole myocardial stress perfusion imaging for cardiac risk assessment before noncardiac vascular surgery: A metaanalysis. *J Vasc Surg* 2002;36 (3):534-540.

76. Boden WE et al: Optimal medical therapy with or without PCI for stable coronary disease. *N Engl J Med* 2007;356(15):1503-1516.

77. Farb A, Boam AB: Stent thrombosis redux—the FDA perspective. *N Engl J Med* 2007;356(10):984-987.

78. Lagerqvist B et al: Long-term outcomes with drug-eluting stents versus bare-metal stents in Sweden. *N Engl J Med* 2007;356 (10):1009-1019.

79. Pfisterer M et al: Late clinical events after clopidogrel discontinuation may limit the benefit of drug-eluting stents: An observational study of drug-eluting versus bare-metal stents. *J Am Coll Cardiol* 2006;48(12):2584-2591.

80. Kastrati A et al: Analysis of 14 trials comparing sirolimus-eluting stents with bare-metal stents. *N Engl J Med* 2007;356(10): 1030-1039.

81. Stone GW et al: Safety and efficacy of sirolimus- and paclitaxel-eluting coronary stents. *N Engl J Med* 2007;356(10):998-1008.

82. Poldermans D et al: A clinical randomized trial to evaluate the safety of a noninvasive approach in high-risk patients undergoing major vascular surgery: The DECREASE-V pilot study. *J Am Coll Cardiol* 2007;49(17):1763-1769.

83. Di Carli M, Hachamovitch R: New technology for noninvasive evaluation of coronary artery disease. *Circulation* 2007;115: 1464-80.

Should Patients with Stable Coronary Artery Disease Undergo Prophylactic Revascularization before Noncardiac Surgery?

Santiago Garcia, MD, and Edward O. McFalls, MD, PhD

INTRODUCTION

The preoperative assessment of a patient in need of elective noncardiac surgery is often a difficult task. There has been enormous controversy regarding the appropriate strategy to diagnose and manage coronary artery disease before elective noncardiac surgery because of the paucity of clinical trial data. Overall, elective surgical procedures in a population of general medical patients are associated with a very low risk of perioperative cardiac complications with an incidence of either myocardial infarction or death of less than 1%.[1,2] Although the risk increases with the age of the patient, the low risk of perioperative complications does not justify widespread cardiac testing among all groups of surgical patients.

Among patients undergoing vascular surgery, however, the perioperative risk of cardiac complications is high. Although the reasons relate, in part, to the hemodynamic stresses associated with aortic procedures, the prevalence of atherosclerotic heart disease in patients undergoing vascular surgery exceeds 50%,[3] and therefore may require special attention in the preoperative period. Coronary artery disease remains the major cause of death following any vascular operation,[4] and therefore consideration for preoperative coronary artery revascularization has been a justifiable endeavor.

OPTIONS

As outlined by the American College of Cardiology/American Heart Association (ACC/AHA) Task Force recommendations before noncardiac operations,[5] the approach to assessing the potential cardiac risk associated with any patient scheduled for an elective noncardiac operation includes the nature of the operation, the risk of associated coronary artery disease, and the functional capacity of the patient (Figure 13-1). Determining the probability that a patient has severe obstructive coronary artery disease is

one key ingredient of the preoperative risk assessment and should be based initially on the clinical history coupled with the nature of the operation. This entails the understanding that patients with vascular and orthopedic operations have the highest risk of postoperative cardiac complications compared with other noncardiac operations.[6-9] Specifically, individuals in need of a vascular operation involving an abdominal approach for either an expanding abdominal aortic aneurysm or advanced claudication have the highest risk.[2] Although urgent and emergent vascular operations occur in at least 20% of screened patients undergoing vascular operations,[10] these individuals are rarely considered candidates for preoperative coronary angiography and their preoperative risk management will not be addressed. The initial evaluation requires an assessment of a prior history of cardiac problems or risk factors along with either classical angina or unusual symptoms such as shortness of breath or atypical chest pains. Attention should be given to clinical risk variables[2,11] and include age greater than 70 years, angina, history of congestive heart failure, prior myocardial infarction, prior stroke or transient ischemic attack (TIA), history of ventricular arrhythmias, diabetes mellitus (particularly insulin dependent), and abnormal renal function (creatinine greater than 2.0 mg/dL). The physical examination also provides insight into high-risk variables,[5,10] including a chronic debilitated state, increased jugular venous distention, edema, S_3 gallop, and significant aortic stenosis, and the 12-lead electrocardiogram (ECG) provides prognostic information related to the presence of abnormal Q-waves or heart rhythms. Although selected clinical variables do predict perioperative cardiac morbidity and mortality risk, the optimal risk stratification tool for prediction of all complications in the postoperative period is controversial.[9] The final approach, therefore, is to determine whether, despite the absence of unstable clinical variables, there is sufficient concern to justify provocative stress testing preoperatively. Assessing the functional capacity of patients undergoing elective operations is an

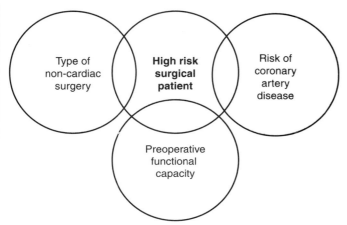

Figure 13-1. Preoperative Assessment.

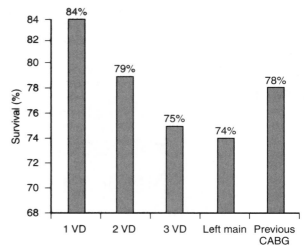

Figure 13-2. Extent of Coronary Artery Disease and Survival 2.5 Years after the Vascular Operation.

important ingredient to determining whether a patient can withstand the rigors of a prolonged operation. In those patients who are unable to achieve a 4-MET demand, a level compatible with routine daily activities, there is increased risk of postoperative events and additional testing may be warranted.[12] Among patients with sufficient exercise capacity and an interpretable ECG, stress testing with an ECG alone may be a cost-effective means of risk-stratifying low-risk patients who do not need additional cardiac workup.[13,14] Among those patients who cannot exercise or who have baseline ECG abnormalities, stress imaging tests have been recommended as the standard alternative for the preoperative detection of multivessel coronary artery disease.[6] The presence of multiple ischemic segments indicative of either multivessel coronary artery disease or left main disease is considered high risk and is associated with an increased risk of perioperative cardiac complications and reduced long-term survival.[15,16] Ultimately, a combined approach of using clinical variables associated with stress imaging tests is most cost-effective.[17] The role of adjuvant pharmacologic therapies cannot be overemphasized[18] and will be addressed in other chapters.

EVIDENCE

Role of Coronary Revascularization

Severe coronary artery disease is common among patients undergoing vascular surgery[3] and is a major determinant of long-term survival following vascular surgery.[4] Thus the role of coronary revascularization in the preoperative management of patients with stable coronary artery disease has been one of the most debated issues in the field of perioperative medicine. As part of the Coronary Artery Revascularization Prophylaxis (CARP) trial, we have learned from the registry and randomized cohorts undergoing preoperative coronary angiography that the extent and severity of coronary artery disease is an identifier of long-term survival following vascular surgery (Figure 13-2).[19] This observation, coupled with outcome data from the CASS trial that suggested better outcomes in patients with vascular disease who underwent coronary artery bypass surgery,[20] would support a plausible

hypothesis that widespread identification and treatment of coronary artery disease should be an essential part of preoperative management. The paucity of prospective randomized data, however, made it difficult for physicians to reach a consensus on the optimal strategy of those patients with coronary artery disease who are scheduled for elective noncardiac surgery. A survey conducted before the publication of the CARP trial showed that recommendations for preoperative revascularization deviated from the guidelines 40% of the time and the chance of widely disparate opinions among the participating cardiologists was 26%.[21] Clearly, a large-scale trial was needed to test the long-term benefit of preoperative coronary artery revascularization before major noncardiac operations.

The CARP trial was the first randomized, multicenter study designed to assess the role of prophylactic revascularization in patients with coronary artery disease undergoing elective vascular operations.[10] Over a 4-year period involving 18 university-affiliated Veterans Affairs medical centers, 510 (9%) of 5859 screened patients were enrolled and randomized to a preoperative strategy of either coronary artery revascularization or no revascularization before elective vascular surgery. The surgical indications were an abdominal aortic aneurysm in 169 (33%) or symptoms of lower-extremity arterial occlusive disease including severe claudication in 189 (37%) and rest pain in 152 (30%). Among the patients randomized to a strategy of preoperative coronary artery revascularization, percutaneous coronary intervention was performed in 141 (59%) and bypass surgery was performed in 99 (41%). The results of the study showed that procedural-related deaths associated with the coronary artery revascularization procedure occurred in only 1.7% of the patients, with no complications related to cerebrovascular events, loss of limb, or dialysis. The median time (interquartiles) from randomization to vascular surgery was 54 (28, 80) days in the coronary revascularization group, however, and 18 (7, 42) days in the no revascularization group ($p < 0.001$). Within 30 days following vascular surgery, the mortality rate was 3.1% in the coronary revascularization group and 3.4% in the no revascularization group ($p = 0.87$). A myocardial infarction, defined by any elevation in troponins following vascular surgery, occurred in 11.6% of the revascularization group and 14.3% of the no revascularization group ($p = 0.37$). At a median time of 2.7 years following randomization, the mortality rate in the revascularization group was 22% and in the no revascularization group was 23% ($p = 0.92$; with relative risk of 0.98, and a 95% confidence interval of 0.70 to 1.37). The conclusions from the CARP study are that among patients undergoing elective vascular surgery, a strategy of preoperative coronary artery revascularization before elective vascular surgery does not improve outcome but rather may delay or even prevent the needed vascular procedure. Based on these data, coronary artery revascularization before elective vascular surgery among patients with stable ischemic heart disease is not supported.[10] Since the CARP trial was published, two other studies have reported outcomes in patients with coronary artery disease undergoing noncardiac surgery[22,23] (Table 13-1).

Landesberg and colleagues[24] have accumulated enormous experience over the past decade and have shown that preoperative stress imaging tests with thallium can identify patients with a worse postoperative outcome. They have also shown the utility of a clinical scoring system that, in conjunction with a high-risk preoperative thallium test, suggests improved outcomes with preoperative coronary artery revascularization.[23] The authors have implicated that the CARP results are not generalizable, because the trial was underpowered for high-risk coronary anatomy due to the low prevalence of patients with triple-vessel coronary artery disease and the exclusion of unprotected left main stenoses from randomization.[23] To address this potential limitation, however, Poldermans and colleagues[22] tested the benefit of a strategy of preoperative coronary artery revascularization in patients with high-risk stress imaging test results who were scheduled for vascular surgery. Their preliminary results showed a borderline unfavorable outcome with revascularization 1 year following vascular surgery (mortality rate at 1 year; revascularization 26.5%, no revascularization 23.1%; $p = 0.58$).

So how should a clinician integrate the findings from these three studies into a unified approach in the preoperative period? Although the findings from Landesberg and colleagues[24] are informative for prognosis, the potential selection bias that favors any decision to undergo coronary artery revascularization in some patients is an important limitation on predicting late outcomes on retrospective analyses. Although the final study results of the DECREASE-V pilot study are unknown, together with the CARP trial results, they do not support an aggressive strategy in the vast majority of patients with stable cardiac symptoms. One important exception to this general rule is worth mentioning. Patients with left main coronary artery disease were excluded from the randomization process in CARP, but their management and outcomes following vascular surgery were captured in the CARP registry.[19] This subset of patients consisted of 48 of 1048 patients undergoing preoperative coronary angiography before their intended vascular surgery (4.6%). Although their long-term survival appears to be improved with preoperative coronary artery revascularization (survival at 2.5 years for surgically and medically treated left main disease was 84% and 52%, respectively; $p < 0.01$), it is uncertain that the prevalence of such a small cohort before vascular surgery warrants widespread screening with expensive stress imaging tests.

AREAS OF UNCERTAINTY

To improve the outcome of high-risk patients undergoing elective operations, we must shift the paradigm from widespread identification and treatment of coronary artery disease in the preoperative phase to a more comprehensive identification and modification of risk factors in the postoperative phase. Among patients undergoing noncardiac operations, postoperative myocardial infarctions occur primarily in those individuals with a prior history of coronary artery disease,[25] and the highest risk is related to surgery for an expanding abdominal aortic aneurysm.[2] Serial troponin assays have become the standard means of surveillance in the postoperative period

Table 13-1   Clinical Studies Assessing the Role of Coronary Revascularization before Major Vascular Surgery

	CARP Trial	DECREASE-V Pilot	Landesberg Study
Study design	Multicenter, prospective	Multicenter, prospective	Single center, retrospective
Treatment allocation	Randomized	Randomized	Nonrandomized
Endpoint	Mortality rate at 2.7 years	Mortality rate at 1 year	Mortality rate at 3 years
Treatment effect	No benefit	No benefit, possible harm	Benefit in intermediate risk
Total patients screened	5859	1880	624
Total patients randomized	510	101	N/A
Patients with three-vessel or left main disease	93	37	73
Mortality rate: no revascularization group	23%	23.1%	21.8%
Mortality rate: revascularization group	22%	26.5%	14.6%

because only a minority of patients with a documented myocardial infarction will have symptoms,[26,27] The cost-effectiveness of widespread measurements of biochemical markers following noncardiac surgery is unclear, but potentially provides a beneficial effect in targeting those individuals with advanced coronary artery disease in need of revascularization. The incidence of perioperative myocardial infarctions among individuals undergoing a vascular operation approaches 20% and can be predicted by abnormalities on preoperative stress imaging with thallium.[27] Among those individuals with a perioperative myocardial infarction, the mortality rate is increased nearly fourfold during a 6-month postoperative follow-up period[28,29] and may predict long-term mortality rate, though this is not certain beyond the first postoperative year.[30] Among those patients undergoing their intended vascular operation within the CARP trial, a perioperative elevation of troponin I above the 99th percentile of normal was most common in patients undergoing abdominal aortic cross-clamp procedures and was associated with a worse long-term outcome.[31] The causative factors that relate to a new myocardial infarction in the postoperative phase are not necessarily related to a severe stenosis within a coronary artery that has not been revascularized. Instead, postoperative ischemic myocardium can be a result of coronary arteries that have been completely occluded with insufficient collateral flow or a new unstable coronary artery lesion.[31] Alternatively, the perioperative phase can be associated with increased myocardial supply-demand mismatch, leading to subendocardial hypoperfusion without any change in the severity of the coronary artery stenoses.[32] Based on pathologic analysis from patients who have died of a perioperative myocardial infarction, advanced coronary artery disease is present in the majority of patients, with only a minority of individuals showing intracoronary artery thrombus.[33,34] Clearly, more studies are needed to understand the biology of acute coronary artery syndromes following noncardiac surgery, as well as determining the optimal timing of revascularization, if that is deemed necessary. Following the operations, it is imperative that therapies directed at secondary prevention be vigorously administered in suitable patients and include antiplatelet agents, statins, beta-blockers, and possibly angiotensin-converting enzyme (ACE) inhibitors. Within the CARP study, the vast majority of patients in both treatment arms were using these medications 2 years following randomization, and this may have contributed to an improved outcome in patients not undergoing an initial strategy of coronary artery revascularization.[9] Other than ischemic heart disease, patients with other modifiable risk characteristics, including congestive heart failure, ventricular arrhythmias,[35] and diabetes, need to be targeted in the postoperative period. Among the nonrandomized patients in the registry of the CARP study, these clinical variables were independent clinical variables that predicted long-term mortality rate.[36]

GUIDELINES

Guidelines published by the American College of Cardiology/American Heart Association (ACC/AHA) on perioperative cardiovascular evaluation and care define recommendations as follows.

Recommendations for Preoperative Coronary Revascularization with Coronary Artery Bypass Grafting or Percutaneous Coronary Intervention

All of the following Class I indications are consistent with the ACC/AHA 2004 Guideline Update for Coronary Artery Bypass Graft Surgery.

CLASS I

- Coronary revascularization before noncardiac surgery is
  - Useful in patients with stable angina who have significant left main coronary artery stenosis. (*LOE: A*)
- Coronary revascularization before noncardiac surgery is
  - Useful in patients with stable angina who have three-vessel disease. (Survival benefit is greater when left ventricular ejection fraction is less than 0.50.) (*LOE: A*)
  - Useful in patients with stable angina who have two-vessel disease with significant proximal left anterior descending stenosis and either ejection fraction less than 0.50 or demonstrable ischemia on noninvasive testing. (*LOE: A*)
  - Recommended for patients with high-risk unstable angina or non–ST-segment elevation myocardial infarction (MI). (*LOE: A*)
  - Recommended in patients with acute ST-segment elevation MI. (*LOE: A*)

CLASS IIa

1. In patients in whom coronary revascularization with percutaneous coronary intervention (PCI) is appropriate for mitigation of cardiac symptoms and who need elective noncardiac surgery in the subsequent 12 months, a strategy of balloon angioplasty or bare-metal stent placement followed by 4 to 6 weeks of dual antiplatelet therapy is probably indicated. (*LOE: B*)
2. In patients who have received drug-eluting coronary stents and who must undergo urgent surgical procedures that mandate the discontinuation of thienopyridine therapy, it is reasonable to continue aspirin if at all possible and restart the thienopyridine as soon as possible. (*LOE: C*)

CLASS IIb

The usefulness of preoperative coronary revascularization is not well established

- In high-risk ischemic patients (e.g., abnormal dobutamine stress echocardiogram with at least 5 segments of wall-motion abnormalities). (*LOE: C*)
- For low-risk ischemic patients with an abnormal dobutamine stress echocardiogram (segments 1 to 4). (*LOE: B*)

CLASS III

1. It is not recommended that routine prophylactic coronary revascularization be performed in patients with stable CAD before noncardiac surgery. (*LOE: B*)
2. Elective noncardiac surgery is not recommended within 4 to 6 weeks of bare-metal coronary stent implantation or within 12 months of drug-eluting coronary stent implantation in patients in whom thienopyridine therapy or aspirin and thienopyridine therapy will need to be discontinued perioperatively. (*LOE: B*)

3. Elective noncardiac surgery is not recommended within 4 weeks of coronary revascularization with balloon angioplasty. (*LOE: B*)

AUTHORS' RECOMMENDATIONS

- To improve the outcomes of high-risk patients, we must shift the paradigm of widespread screening and treatment of coronary artery disease before the operation to a comprehensive strategy for modification of risks in the postoperative period.
- The optimal strategy for identifying and treating high-risk patients before elective noncardiac surgery should underscore the value of a conservative strategy that includes proceeding with a timely operation, if deemed appropriate. It also should ensure use of medical therapies that reduce secondary outcomes in patients with coronary artery disease, particularly regarding therapeutic doses of beta-blockers.
- Patients with an unprotected left main stenosis may be the only subset of patients with multivessel coronary artery disease that need special consideration before a vascular operation. This subset consists of less than 5% of individuals undergoing noncardiac operations and does not justify widespread stress imaging tests preoperatively, to identify such a small subset.
- Those individuals with evidence of a perioperative myocardial infarction, congestive heart failure, ventricular arrhythmias, and diabetes should be targeted and appropriately treated in the postoperative period.

ACKNOWLEDGMENTS

Supported by the Cooperative Studies Program of the Department of Veterans Affairs Office of Research and Development.

REFERENCES

1. Mangano D: Perioperative cardiac morbidity. *Anesthesiology* 1990;72:153-184.
2. Lee T, Marcantonio E, Mangione C, Thomas E, Polanczyk C, Cook E, et al: Derivation and prospective validation of a simple index for prediction of cardiac risk of major noncardiac surgery. *Circulation* 1999;100:1043-1049.
3. Hertzer N, Beven E, Young J, O'Hara P, Ruschhaupt WI, Graor R, et al: Coronary artery disease in peripheral vascular patients: A classification of 1000 coronary angiograms and results of surgical management. *Ann Surg* 1984;199:223-233.
4. Criqui M, Langer R, Fronek A, Feigelson H, Klauber M, McCann T, Browner D: Mortality over a period of 10 years in patients with peripheral arterial disease. *N Engl J Med* 1992;326:381-386.
5. Fleisher LA, Beckman JA, Brown KA, Calkins H, Chaikof E, Fleischmann KE, et al: ACC/AHA 2007 guidelines on perioperative cardiovascular evaluation and care for noncardiac surgery; executive summary: A report of the American College of Cardiology/American Heart Association Task Force on Practice Guidelines. *J Am Coll Cardiol* 2007;50:1707-1732.
6. Goldman L, Caldera D, Nussbaum S, Southwick F, Krogstad D, Murray B, et al: Multifactorial index of cardiac risk in noncardiac surgical procedures. *N Engl J Med* 1977;297:845-850.
7. Detsky A, Abrams H, Forbath N, Scott J, Hilliard J: Cardiac assessment for patients undergoing noncardiac surgery: A multifactorial clinical risk index. *Arch Intern Med* 1986;146: 2131-2134.
8. Ashton C, Petersen N, Wray N, Kiefe C, Dunn J, Wu L, et al: The incidence of perioperative myocardial infarction in men undergoing noncardiac surgery. *Ann Intern Med* 1993;118:504-510.
9. Gilbert K, Larocque B, Patrick L: Prospective evaluation of cardiac risk indices for patients undergoing noncardiac surgery. *Ann Intern Med* 2000;133:356-359.
10. McFalls E, Ward H, Moritz T, Goldman S, Krupski W, Littooy F, et al: Coronary-artery revascularization before elective major vascular surgery. *N Engl J Med* 2004;351:2795-2804.
11. Eagle K, Coley C, Newell J, Brewster D, Darling C, Strauss W, et al: Combining clinical and thallium data optimizes preoperative assessment of cardiac risk before major vascular surgery. *Ann Intern Med* 1989;110:859-866.
12. Reilly D, McNeely M, Doerner D, Greenberg D, Staiger T, Geist M, et al: Self-reported exercise tolerance test and the risk of serious perioperative complications. *Arch Intern Med* 1999;159: 2185-2192.
13. Girish M, Trayner E, Dammann O, Pinto-Plata V, Celli B: Symptom-limited stair climbing as a predictor of postoperative cardiopulmonary complications after high-risk surgery. *Chest* 2001;120:1147-1151.
14. Kertai M, Boersma E, Bax J, Heijenbrok-Kal M, Hunink M, L'Talien G, et al: A meta-analysis comparing the prognostic accuracy of six diagnostic tests for predicting perioperative cardiac risk in patients undergoing major vascular surgery. *Heart* 2003;89:1327-1334.
15. Poldermans D, Arnese M, Fioretti P, Boersma E, Thomson I, Rambaldi R, et al: Sustained prognostic value of dobutamine stress echocardiography for late cardiac events after major noncardiac vascular surgery. *Circulation* 1997;95:53-58.
16. Shaw L, Eagle K, Gersh B, Miller D: Meta-analysis of intravenous dipyridamole-thallium-201 imaging (1985 to 1994) and dobutamine echocardiography (1991 to 1994) for risk stratification before vascular surgery. *J Am Coll Cardiol* 1996;27:787-798.
17. Boersma E, Poldermans D, Bax J, Steyerberg E, Thomson I, Banga J, et al: Predictors of cardiac events after major vascular surgery. Role of clinical characteristics, dobutamine ECHO, and beta-blocker therapy. *JAMA* 2001;285:1865-1873.
18. Stevens R, Burri H, Tramer M: Pharmacologic myocardial protection in patients undergoing noncardiac surgery: A quantitative systematic review. *Cardiovasc Anesth* 2003;97:623-633.
19. Garcia S, Ward H, Pierpont G, Goldman S, Larsen G, Littooy F, et al: Long-term outcomes following vascular surgery in patients with multivessel coronary artery disease: Analysis of randomized and excluded patients from the Coronary Artery Revascularization Prophylaxis (CARP) trial. *Circulation* 2007;16:II-640.
20. Rihal C, Eagle K, Mickel M, Foster E, Sopko G, Gersh B: Surgical therapy for coronary artery disease among patients with combined coronary artery and peripheral vascular disease. *Circulation* 1995;91:46-53.
21. Pierpont G, Moritz T, Goldman S, Krupski W, Littooy F, Ward H, et al: Disparate opinions regarding indications for coronary artery revascularization prior to elective vascular surgery. *Am J Cardiol* 2004;94:1124-1128.
22. Poldermans D, Schouten O, Vidakovic R, Bax J, Thomson I, Hoeks S, et al: A clinical randomized trial to evaluate the safety of a noninvasive approach in high-risk patients undergoing major vascular surgery: The DECREASE-V Pilot Study. *J Am Coll Cardiol* 2007;49:1763-1769.
23. Landesberg G, Berlatzky Y, Bocher M, Alcalai R, Anner H, Ganon-Rozental T, et al: A clinical survival score predicts the likelihood to benefit from preoperative thallium scanning and coronary revascularization before major vascular surgery. *Eur Heart J* 2007;28:533-539.
24. Landesberg G, Mosseri M, Wolf Y, Bocher M, Basevitch A, Rudis E, et al: Preoperative thallium scanning, selective coronary revascularization, and long-term survival after major vascular surgery. *Circulation* 2003;108:177-183.
25. Ashton C, Petersen N, Wray N, Kiefe C, Dunn J, Wu L, et al: The incidence of perioperative myocardial infarction in men undergoing noncardiac surgery. *Ann Intern Med* 1993;118:504-510.
26. Badner N, Knill R, Brown J, Novick V, Gelb A: Myocardial infarction after noncardiac surgery. *Anesthesiology* 1998;88:572-578.
27. Landesberg G, Mosseri M, Shatz V, Akopnik I, Bocher M, Mayer M, et al: Cardiac troponin after major vascular surgery. The role of perioperative ischemia, preoperative thallium scanning and coronary revascularization. *J Am Coll Cardiol* 2004; 44:569-575.

28. Lopez-Jimenez F, Goldman L, Sacks D, Thomas E, Johnson P, Cook E, et al: Prognostic value of cardiac troponin T after noncardiac surgery: 6-month follow-up data. *J Am Coll Cardiol* 1997;29:1241-1245.

29. Kim L, Martainez E, Faraday N, Dorman T, Fleisher L, Perler B, et al: Cardiac troponin I predicts short-term mortality in vascular surgery patients. *Circulation* 2002;106:2366-2371.

30. Filipovic M, Jeger R, Girard T, Probst C, Pfisterer M, Gurke L, et al: Predictors of long-term mortality and cardiac events in patients with known or suspected coronary artery disease who survive major non-cardiac surgery. *Anesthesiology* 2005;60:5-11.

31. McFalls E, Ward H, Moritz T, Apple F, Goldman S, Pierpont G, et al: Predictors and outcomes of a perioperative myocardial infarction following elective vascular surgery in patients with documented coronary artery disease: Results of the Coronary Artery Revascularization Prophylaxis (CARP) trial. *Eur Heart J* 2008;29:394-401.

32. Ellis S, Hertzer N, Young J, Brener S: Angiographic correlates of cardiac death and myocardial infarction complicating major non-thoracic vascular surgery. *Am J Cardiol* 1996;77:1126-1128.

33. Landesberg G: The pathophysiology of perioperative myocardial infarction: Facts and perspectives. *J Cardiothorac Vasc Anesth* 2003;17:90-100.

34. Cohen M, Aretz T: Histological analysis of coronary artery lesions in fatal postoperative myocardial infarction. *Cardiovasc Pathol* 1999;8:133-139.

35. Sprung J, Warner M, Contreras M, Schroeder D, Beighley C, Wilson G, et al: Cardiac arrest during neuraxial anesthesia: frequency and predisposing factors associated with survival. *Anesthesiology* 2003;99:259-69.

36. McFalls E, Ward H, Moritz T, Littooy F, Krupski W, Santilli S, et al: Clinical factors associated with long-term mortality following vascular surgery: Outcomes from the Coronary Artery Revascularization Prophylaxis (CARP) trial. *J Vasc Surg* 2007; 46:694-700.

14 How Long Should You Wait after Percutaneous Coronary Intervention for Noncardiac Surgery?

John G.T. Augoustides, MD, FASE; Hynek Riha, MD, DEAA; and Lee A. Fleisher, MD, FACC, FAHA

INTRODUCTION

Percutaneous coronary intervention (PCI) has revolutionized the management of coronary artery disease (CAD) initially with balloon angioplasty (BA) and subsequently with coronary stenting both with bare-metal stents (BMS) and with drug-eluting stents (DES). The high incidence of coronary restenosis from neointimal coronary endothelial growth after BA prompted the clinical development and introduction of BMS. Although they represented a significant therapeutic advance, they were still associated with coronary restenosis rates of 15% to 30%.[1,2] The second major significant reduction in coronary restenosis after PCI resulted from DES that pharmacologically retard stent endothelialization and neointimal growth with sirolimus or paclitaxel. Due to slow release of these antimitotic agents, the DES are associated with significantly lower coronary restenosis rates of 5% to 10%.[3]

Since the introduction of DES into clinical practice in the last 5 years, more than 5 million of these devices have been implanted worldwide.[4] Coronary stent thrombosis (ST) has been an important clinical concern, particularly before the coronary stent has been coated with endothelium (approximately 4 to 6 weeks for BMS and at least 1 year for DES). As a result, dual antiplatelet therapy with aspirin and clopidogrel has been recommended for at least 1 month after BMS placement and for at least 12 months after DES placement.[5] Although premature discontinuation of antiplatelet therapy is a major risk for ST, there are multiple identified clinical and angiographic risk factors for ST (Table 14-1).[5-7]

The perioperative period qualifies as a major risk factor for ST, since noncardiac surgery (NCS) activates platelets and induces hypercoagulability.[8] The significant risk of perioperative ST for BMS was highlighted in 2000 with a case series ($N = 40$) that documented a 20% mortality rate in NCS soon after BMS deployment.[9] Furthermore, NCS after recent BA is not without risk of myocardial ischemia and perioperative mortality. In a recent case series of 350 patients who had NCS within 2 months after BA, the perioperative mortality rate was 0.9% (95%; confidence interval [CI] 0.2% to 2.5%).[10]

Given that approximately 5% of patients with coronary stents require NCS within 1 year after stenting,[11] the perioperative management of patients with recent PCI (BA, BMS, DES) is important because it not only concerns millions of patients but also entails significant perioperative risk of major myocardial infarction and death. This chapter reviews the options, latest evidence, and current expert recommendations concerning the perioperative risk of recent PCI in NCS.

OPTIONS TO MINIMIZE STENT THROMBOSIS AFTER RECENT PCI AND NONCARDIAC SURGERY

The perioperative options for limiting coronary thrombosis after recent PCI are presented in Table 14-2.[12] The evidence for each option will be presented and expert recommendations will be reviewed and ranked according to the schema of the American Heart Association (AHA) and American College of Cardiology (ACC), as outlined in Tables 14-3A (classes of recommendations) and 14-3B (levels of evidence). The expert recommendations and corresponding levels of evidence have been summarized in Table 14-4 (class I recommendations), Tables 14-5A and 14-5B (classes IIA and IIB recommendations), and Table 14-6 (class III recommendations).[12,13] The recent AHA/ACC guidelines on perioperative cardiovascular evaluation and care for NCS surgery are available at www.americanheart.org (section on statements and practice guidelines; accessed July 10, 2008).

EVIDENCE

Minimize Preoperative Percutaneous Coronary Intervention

Patients with CAD will often not benefit from coronary revascularization with PCI before noncardiac surgery.

Table 14-1	Identified Risk Factors for Coronary Stent Thrombosis

Clinical Risk Factors	Angiographic Risk Factors
Premature interruption of antiplatelet therapy	Long stents
Advanced age	Multiple lesions
Diabetes	Overlapping stents
Low ejection fraction	Ostial lesions
Renal failure	Small-caliber coronary vessels
Acute coronary syndrome	Suboptimal stent deployment
Perioperative period	Bifurcation lesions

Table 14-2	Options for Limiting Coronary Thrombosis after Noncardiac Surgery and Recent Percutaneous Coronary Intervention (PCI)

Options	Considerations within the Option
Minimize preoperative PCI	1. Limit preoperative PCI in stable coronary disease 2. PCI for unstable coronary syndromes
Consider stent type	1. Balloon angioplasty 2. Bare-metal stents 3. Drug-eluting stents
Optimize antiplatelet therapy	1. Continue aspirin and clopidogrel 2. Continue aspirin only 3. Stop clopidogrel for limited period 4. Perioperative intravenous platelet blockade
Education and collaboration	1. Surgeon 2. Cardiologist 3. Surgery at center with primary PCI availability

Table 14-3A	Definition of Classification Scheme for Clinical Recommendations

Clinical Recommendations	Definition of Recommendation Class
Class I	The procedure/treatment should be performed (benefit far outweighs the risk)
Class IIa	It is reasonable to perform the procedure/treatment (benefit still clearly outweighs risk)
Class IIb	It is not unreasonable to perform the procedure/treatment (benefit probably outweighs the risk)
Class III	The procedure/treatment should not be performed because it is not helpful and may be harmful (risk may outweigh benefit)

Taken from the American Heart Association/American Council of Cardiology Manual for Guideline Writing Committees at http://circ.ahajournals.org/manual_IIstep6.shtml (accessed February 25, 2008).

Table 14-3B	Definition of Classification Scheme for Supporting Evidence for Clinical Recommendations

Level of Evidence	Definition of Recommendation Class
Level A	Sufficient evidence from multiple randomized trials or meta-analyses
Level B	Limited evidence from a single randomized trial or multiple nonrandomized studies
Level C	Case studies and expert opinion

Taken from the American Heart Association/American Council of Cardiology Manual for Guideline Writing Committees at http://circ.ahajournals.org/manual_IIstep6.shtml (accessed February 25, 2008).

The Coronary Artery Revascularization Prophylaxis (CARP) trial randomized 510 patients with angiographically proven CAD to coronary revascularization or medical management before elective major vascular surgery (33% abdominal aortic aneurysm repair; 67% infrainguinal vascular bypass).[14] The exclusion criteria included significant left main coronary stenosis, unstable CAD syndromes, aortic stenosis, and severe cardiomyopathy defined as an ejection fraction less than 20%. Coronary revascularization was achieved surgically in 41% and with PCI in 59% of enrolled subjects. Patients with or without preoperative revascularization developed a similar incidence of postoperative myocardial infarction (8.4% versus 8.4%, $p = 0.99$) and a similar 27-month survival rate (78% versus 77%, $p = 0.98$). Therefore this landmark study suggests that preoperative PCI for stable CAD may not be required before NCS.

The DECREASE-II trial evaluated preoperative cardiac testing in major vascular surgical patients who had intermediate cardiac risk factors and who received adequate beta-blocker therapy.[15] This trial demonstrated that preoperative coronary revascularization did not significantly improve the 30-day outcome in patients with extensive ischemia.

The DECREASE-V pilot study randomized 101 vascular surgical patients with extensive ischemia (defined as five or more ischemic segments during dobutamine stress echocardiography or at least three ischemic segments identified by dipyrimadole perfusion scintigraphy) to preoperative coronary revascularization versus best medical therapy.[16] Coronary revascularization was achieved surgically in 35% and with PCI in 65% of enrolled subjects.

Table 14-4	Class I Recommendations for Percutaneous Coronary Intervention (PCI) and Noncardiac Surgery

Recommendation	Class and Evidence
PCI before noncardiac surgery is indicated in appropriate patients with stable angina who have two-vessel disease with significant proximal left anterior descending artery (LAD) stenosis and either an ejection fraction less than 50% or demonstrable ischemia on noninvasive testing.	I (level A)
PCI before noncardiac surgery is recommended for appropriate patients with high-risk unstable angina or non–ST-segment elevation myocardial infarction.	I (level A)
PCI before noncardiac surgery is recommended in appropriate patients with ST-segment elevation myocardial infarction.	I (level A)

Adapted from the following guideline: Fleisher LA, Beckman JA, Brown KA, et al: ACC/AHA guidelines on perioperative cardiovascular evaluation and care for noncardiac surgery. Executive summary: A report of the American College of Cardiology/American Heart Association Task Force on Practice Guidelines (Writing Committee to revise the 2002 Guidelines on Perioperative Cardiovascular Evaluation for Noncardiac Surgery). Developed in collaboration with the American Society of Echocardiography, American Society of Nuclear Cardiology, Heart Rhythm Society, Society of Cardiovascular Anesthesiologists, Society for Cardiovascular Angiography and Interventions, Society for Vascular Medicine and Biology, and Society for Vascular Surgery. *Circulation* 2007;116:1971-1996.

Table 14-5A	Class IIa Recommendations for Percutaneous Coronary Intervention (PCI) and Noncardiac Surgery

Recommendation	Class and Evidence
In patients who require PCI to alleviate myocardial ischemia and who require elective noncardiac surgery in the following 12 months, the recommended strategy is balloon angioplasty or bare-metal stent placement followed by 4-6 weeks of dual antiplatelet therapy (aspirin and clopidogrel).	IIa (level B)
In patients who have drug-eluting coronary stents and who require emergency noncardiac surgery that mandates discontinuation of clopidogrel, it is reasonable to continue aspirin therapy and restart clopidogrel as soon as clinically possible.	IIa (level C)

Adapted from the following guideline: Fleisher LA, Beckman JA, Brown KA, et al: ACC/AHA guidelines on perioperative cardiovascular evaluation and care for noncardiac surgery. Executive summary: A report of the American College of Cardiology/American Heart Association Task Force on Practice Guidelines (Writing Committee to revise the 2002 Guidelines on Perioperative Cardiovascular Evaluation for Noncardiac Surgery). Developed in collaboration with the American Society of Echocardiography, American Society of Nuclear Cardiology, Heart Rhythm Society, Society of Cardiovascular Anesthesiologists, Society for Cardiovascular Angiography and Interventions, Society for Vascular Medicine and Biology, and Society for Vascular Surgery. *Circulation* 2007;116:1971-1996.

The composite primary outcome (perioperative death and myocardial infarction) was similar between study groups (43% for revascularization versus 33% for medical therapy; odds ratio [OR] 1.4; 95% CI, 0.7 to 2.8; $p = 0.30$). The incidence of death and myocardial infarction at 1 year was high at 47% but similar in both groups (49% for revascularization and 44% for medical therapy; OR 1.2; 95% CI, 0.7 to 2.3; $p = 0.48$).

Taken together, these three important clinical trials (CARP, DECREASE-II, and DECREASE-V) point to a more limited role for PCI in stable CAD before NCS. Their cumulative evidence forms the basis of the expert recommendations relating to PCI before elective NCS in stable CAD (see Tables 14-4 to 14-6).

In unstable angina or myocardial infarction, PCI is indicated in appropriate patients for management of the acute coronary syndrome in its own right. First, PCI before NCS surgery is recommended for appropriate patients with high-risk unstable angina or non–ST-segment elevation myocardial infarction (class I recommendation; level A evidence). Second, PCI before NCS surgery is also recommended in appropriate patients with ST-segment elevation myocardial infarction (class I recommendation; level A evidence).

In the setting of stable CAD, PCI has a more limited role, as explained earlier. Routine PCI in patients with stable CAD is not recommended before NCS (class III recommendation; level B evidence). The benefit of PCI before

Table 14-5B	Class IIb Recommendations for Percutaneous Coronary Intervention (PCI) and Noncardiac Surgery

Recommendation	Class and Evidence
The benefit of PCI before noncardiac surgery is not established in high-risk ischemic patients (e.g., 5 or more wall motion abnormalities during dobutamine stress echocardiography).	IIb (level C)
The benefit of PCI before noncardiac surgery is not established in low-risk ischemic patients (e.g., 1-4 wall motion abnormalities during dobutamine stress echocardiography)	IIb (level B)

Adapted from the following guideline: Fleisher LA, Beckman JA, Brown KA, et al: ACC/AHA guidelines on perioperative cardiovascular evaluation and care for noncardiac surgery. Executive summary: A report of the American College of Cardiology/American Heart Association Task Force on Practice Guidelines (Writing Committee to revise the 2002 Guidelines on Perioperative Cardiovascular Evaluation for Noncardiac Surgery). Developed in collaboration with the American Society of Echocardiography, American Society of Nuclear Cardiology, Heart Rhythm Society, Society of Cardiovascular Anesthesiologists, Society for Cardiovascular Angiography and Interventions, Society for Vascular Medicine and Biology, and Society for Vascular Surgery. *Circulation* 2007;116:1971-1996.

Table 14-6	Class III Recommendations for Percutaneous Coronary Intervention (PCI) and Noncardiac Surgery	
Recommendation	**Class and Evidence**	
Routine PCI in patients with stable coronary artery disease is not recommended before noncardiac surgery.	III (level B)	
Elective noncardiac surgery that requires perioperative discontinuation of clopidogrel or aspirin and clopidogrel is not recommended within 4-6 weeks of bare-metal coronary stent deployment.	III (level B)	
Elective noncardiac surgery that requires perioperative discontinuation of clopidogrel or aspirin and clopidogrel is not recommended within 12 months of drug-eluting coronary stent deployment.	III (level B)	
Elective noncardiac surgery is not recommended within 4 weeks of coronary revascularization with balloon angioplasty.	III (level B)	

Adapted from the following guideline: Fleisher LA, Beckman JA, Brown KA, et al: ACC/AHA guidelines on perioperative cardiovascular evaluation and care for noncardiac surgery. Executive summary: A report of the American College of Cardiology/American Heart Association Task Force on Practice Guidelines (Writing Committee to revise the 2002 Guidelines on Perioperative Cardiovascular Evaluation for Noncardiac Surgery). Developed in collaboration with the American Society of Echocardiography, American Society of Nuclear Cardiology, Heart Rhythm Society, Society of Cardiovascular Anesthesiologists, Society for Cardiovascular Angiography and Interventions, Society for Vascular Medicine and Biology, and Society for Vascular Surgery. *Circulation* 2007;116:1971-1996.

NCS is not established in high-risk ischemic patients, for example, five or more wall motion abnormalities during dobutamine stress echocardiography (class IIb recommendation; level C evidence). The benefit of PCI before NCS is also not established in low-risk ischemic patients, for example, one to four wall motion abnormalities during dobutamine stress echocardiography (class IIb recommendation; level B evidence). PCI before NCS surgery, however, is indicated in appropriate patients with stable angina who have two-vessel disease with significant proximal left anterior descending artery (LAD) stenosis and either an ejection fraction less than 50% or demonstrable ischemia on noninvasive testing (class I recommendation; level A evidence).

Type of Percutaneous Coronary Intervention

Balloon Angioplasty

Seven retrospective studies have examined cardiovascular outcome following coronary BA before NCS. The main features of these studies are summarized in Table 14-7.[10,17-22] Five of the seven studies are limited by factors such as a small sample size, a long interval between coronary angioplasty and surgery, or a control group with coronary stents.[17-19,21,22] The remaining two studies suggest that NCS after BA is safe, particularly

if surgery occurs at least 2 weeks after coronary intervention.[10,20] This minimum time period allows the coronary injury at the balloon angioplasty site to heal and thus not be at risk for perioperative thrombosis.

Thus it appears that the 2- to 4-week period after balloon angioplasty minimizes the incidence of an acute coronary syndrome after NCS. However, if surgery occurs more than 8 weeks after coronary BA, significant restenosis at the angioplasty site might cause perioperative myocardial ischemia. The expert recommendation specifies that elective NCS is not recommended within 4 weeks of coronary revascularization with BA (class III recommendation; level B evidence). Daily aspirin therapy should be maintained perioperatively, unless the bleeding risk is deemed too high.

Bare-Metal Coronary Stents

The retrospective study by Kaluza and colleagues[9] ($n = 40$) documented a 20% perioperative mortality rate in patients who had NCS less than 6 weeks after coronary stenting with BMS. A second retrospective study by Wilson and colleagues[23] ($n = 207$) demonstrated a 3% perioperative mortality rate in patients with BMS who underwent NCS within 6 weeks of coronary stenting. A third report by Reddy and Vaitkus[24] ($n = 56$) revealed a 38% incidence of ST or cardiovascular death in patients who had undergone NCS within 14 days of BMS deployment. No patient who had NCS more than 6 weeks after BMS suffered cardiovascular complications. In a fourth study by Sharma and colleagues[25] ($n = 47$), perioperative mortality rate was 26% in the setting of NCS less than 3 weeks after BMS placement as compared with a 5% mortality rate in the setting of NCS more than 3 weeks after BMS placement. This study also documented in the early surgery group an 85.7% (6 of 7) mortality rate in patients who had stopped thienopyridine therapy.

The collective findings from this set of studies can be interpreted with respect to the cellular process that lines BMS with coronary endothelium. Endothelialization of BMS takes about 4 to 6 weeks, after which the risk of BMS thrombosis is extremely unlikely. During the process of stent endothelialization, dual antiplatelet therapy with aspirin and clopidogrel is recommended to minimize the risk of stent thrombosis. The clopidogrel is no longer required after 6 weeks when endothelialization is typically adequate. Thereafter, aspirin therapy is recommended indefinitely and should be continued perioperatively, unless the bleeding risk is judged to be prohibitive.

As a result, the expert recommendation is that elective NCS which requires perioperative discontinuation of clopidogrel is not recommended within 4 to 6 weeks of bare-metal coronary stent deployment (class III recommendation; level B evidence).

Drug-Eluting Stents

Drug-eluting stents revolutionized PCI because they have significantly reduced the rate of coronary restenosis due to retardation of coronary endothelial growth from slow release of paclitaxel or sirolimus.[26] As a consequence, ST with DES remains an ongoing risk due to the lack of endothelial covering: in this generation of coronary stents, thrombosis has replaced restenosis as the major clinical concern.

Table 14-7 Outcomes with Coronary Balloon Angioplasty (CBA) before Noncardiac Surgery

Clinical Study	Sample Size	Time from CBA to Surgery	Mortality Rate	Myocardial Infarction	Comment
Allen et al. (1991)[17]	148	Mean of 338 days	2.7%	0.7%	Long interval to surgery
Huber et al. (1992)[18]	50	Mean of 9 days	1.9%	5.6%	Small study; no control group
Elmore et al. (1993)[19]	14	Mean of 10 days	0%	0%	Very small study
Gottlieb et al. (1998)[20]	194	Mean of 11 days	0.5%	0.5%	Only vascular surgeries
Posner et al. (1999)[21]	686	Median of I year	2.6%	2.2%	Long interval to surgery
Brilakis et al. (2005)[10]	350	Within 2 months	0.3%	0.6%	All events occurred after surgery within 2 weeks after CBA
Leibowitz et al. (2006)[22]	216	Early (0-14 days) Late (15-62 days)	11% 20%	7.2% 16.8%	56% CBA; 44% stents Similar outcomes

Adapted from the following guideline: Fleisher LA, Beckman JA, Brown KA, et al: ACC/AHA guidelines on perioperative cardiovascular evaluation and care for noncardiac surgery. Executive summary: A report of the American College of Cardiology/American Heart Association Task Force on Practice Guidelines (Writing Committee to revise the 2002 Guidelines on Perioperative Cardiovascular Evaluation for Noncardiac Surgery). Developed in collaboration with the American Society of Echocardiography, American Society of Nuclear Cardiology, Heart Rhythm Society, Society of Cardiovascular Anesthesiologists, Society for Cardiovascular Angiography and Interventions, Society for Vascular Medicine and Biology, and Society for Vascular Surgery. *Circulation* 2007;116:1971-1996.

A recent systematic review of perioperative ST included 10 studies (1995 to 2006) for a sum total of 980 patients who had NCS after placement of either BMS or DES.[27] The median interval between stent deployment and NCS was 13 to 284 days, and the majority of the pooled cohort had BMS. The perioperative rates of myocardial infarction and death were 2% to 28% and 3% to 20%, respectively. Despite the limitations of the included studies, two perioperative factors significantly increased perioperative cardiovascular risk: (1) discontinuation of dual antiplatelet therapy (i.e., aspirin and clopidogrel); and (2) surgery within 6 to 12 weeks after stent deployment. These collated findings from the literature were confirmed in a subsequent study by the same investigators ($n = 192$).[28]

These findings from systematic review do not specifically apply to DES, since the pooled study population included BMS as well as DES. The Swedish Coronary Angiography and Angioplasty Registry (SCAAR) studied 6033 patients treated with DES and 13,738 patients treated with BMS with a 3-year follow-up.[29] The relative rate of clinical coronary restenosis was 60% lower in the DES group. However, in the DES group, there was an incremental absolute risk of death of 0.5% per year and an incremental absolute risk of death or myocardial infarction of 0.5% to 1.0% per year after the initial 6 months. The adverse long-term events with DES are principally related to the risk of ST. The multiple risk factors for ST are summarized in Table 14-1.[5-7]

The persistent risk of ST with DES prompted an ACC/AHA expert guideline that focused on the prevention of premature discontinuation of dual antiplatelet therapy in patients with coronary artery stents, especially DES.[5]

The ACC/AHA ecommendation is that elective NCS which requires perioperative discontinuation of clopidogrel is not recommended within 12 months of DES deployment (class III recommendation; level B evidence). Furthermore, in patients who have DES and who require emergency NCS that mandates discontinuation of clopidogrel, it is reasonable to continue aspirin therapy and restart clopidogrel as soon as clinically possible after surgery (class IIa recommendation; level C evidence).

Perioperative Antiplatelet Therapy

In the presence of BMS and/or DES, acute withdrawal of antiplatelet therapy is a major risk factor for perioperative ST.[5-9] The options for perioperative platelet blockade to maintain stent patency and to minimize perioperative ST include the following:

1. Continue dual antiplatelet therapy during and after surgery.
2. Discontinue clopidogrel but bridge the patient to surgery by using short-acting intravenous platelet blockade, and then restarting clopidogrel as soon as possible after surgery.[30]
3. Continue aspirin perioperatively but discontinue clopidogrel preoperatively and restart it as soon as possible after surgery.

Option I: Dual Antiplatelet Therapy during and after Surgery

This option maintains standard double platelet blockade perioperatively and so has a very low incidence of ST. The perioperative team must weigh the risks of bleeding associated with the particular surgical procedure versus the life-threatening consequences of ST. In procedures such as dental extractions,[31] cataract surgery,[32] and routine dermatologic surgery,[33] bleeding can almost always be controlled locally even in the presence of dual platelet blockade. In surgical procedures with a higher bleeding risk, surgeons can often be persuaded to continue both aspirin and clopidogrel when reminded that ST often results in death or significant myocardial infarction.[34] However, this strategy is not appropriate in circumstances where excess bleeding can be catastrophic, such as neurosurgery[35] or retinal surgery.[36]

Option II: Discontinue Clopidogrel and Bridge with Intravenous Anticoagulation

Platelet inhibition due to clopidogrel is irreversible. Clopidogrel must be discontinued for 5 to 10 days before normal hemostasis is achieved from the production and release of new platelets. If NCS is required early after stent placement and clopidogrel must be stopped (e.g., craniotomy for tumor resection), it is not unreasonable to bridge the patient with short-acting intravenous anticoagulation. Since stent thrombosis is primarily due to platelet aggregation, it is logical that an intravenous antiplatelet agent such as tirofiban would be important. Tirofiban is a short-acting intravenous platelet receptor IIb/IIIa blocker that is well tolerated.

This bridging approach is exemplified in a recent case series of three patients with DES undergoing NCS.[37] The clopdogrel was discontinued 5 days before surgery. Each patient was admitted to hospital 3 days before surgery for commencement of tirofiban and heparin infusions. These dual anticoagulant infusions were discontinued 6 hours before surgery. On the first postoperative day, a loading dose of clopidogrel was started followed by maintenance dosage thereafter. Aspirin therapy was continued throughout the perioperative period. Although these patients had no perioperative ST, this case series is proof-of-concept only. Further trials are required to verify the safety and efficacy of this perioperative approach. In concept, it already has a clinical precedent in the preparation of a patient with a mechanical heart valve for NCS. This patient at risk for valve thrombosis is admitted to hospital for discontinuation of Coumadin with interim heparinization as a bridge to surgery.

Option III: Discontinue Clopidogrel Preoperatively and Restart after Surgery

This approach is logical if the coronary stent is fully endothelialized with a low risk of perioperative ST (4 to 6 weeks for BMS and 12 months for DES). However, there is variability in the rate of stent endotheliazation, especially for DES. Consequently, the risk for stent thrombosis may persist in a subset of patients beyond 1 year.[38,39] When clopidogrel is begun postoperatively, it is prudent to give a loading dose as there is post-surgical platelet activation and many patients are hyporesponsive to clopidogrel.[40] Aspirin therapy should be continued throughout the perioperative period.[41] In patients who have DES and who require emergency NCS surgery that mandates discontinuation of clopidogrel, it is reasonable to continue aspirin (class IIa recommendation; level C evidence).

EDUCATION AND COLLABORATION

The severe morbidity and mortality rates associated with perioperative ST mandates a collaborative approach among surgeons, anesthesiologists, and cardiologists.

In a survey of anesthesiologists, 63% were not aware of recommendations about timing of NCS after BMS or DES.[42] Anesthesiologists and surgeons should have a collaborative approach to patients with coronary stents.[43] This approach could include the following aspects:

1. Determination of all stent details such as stent type(s), coronary locations, date(s) of implantation, and duration and type of antiplatelet therapy
2. Consultation with a cardiologist, preferably the patient's cardiologist
3. A joint decision with input from the anesthesiologist, surgeon, and cardiologist about the timing of NCS and the perioperative anticoagulation plan with special emphasis on platelet blockade
4. Performance of the NCS in a medical center that has 24-hour interventional cardiology coverage for prompt therapy of ST, if it occurs

MANAGEMENT OF PERIOPERATIVE STENT THROMBOSIS

Stent thrombosis most often manifests as an ST-segment elevation myocardial infarction and requires early reperfusion. Thrombolytic therapy is contraindicated in this setting due to the risk of severe bleeding after recent surgery. Furthermore, it is less effective than primary PCI. An early invasive strategy for acute myocardial infarction after NCS was still associated with a 35% mortality rate ($n = 48$).[44] Although this is a high perioperative mortality rate, it was in patients who often were treated after cardiac arrest or in cardiogenic shock.

AREAS OF UNCERTAINITY

The natural history of perioperative ST after DES implantation requires further investigation to confirm incidence, determine contemporary perioperative outcome, and assess best perioperative anticoagulant practice. Furthermore, the current problem of ST with DES has prompted the development of bioabsorbable drug-elutng stents in an effort to deal effectively with not only restenosis but also thrombosis.[45,46] Although this next generation of coronary stents has demonstrated clinical equivalency in initial clinical evaluation, long-term large-scale studies are required to assess their efficacy and safety compared with first-generation DESs, including with respect to the perioperative period.

GUIDELINES AND AUTHORS' RECOMMENDATIONS

The options and evidence concerning the perioperative risks and management of recent PCI before NCS have been discussed. This topic is important because it is common and serious. This author supports the expert recommendations on this topic from the recent AHA/ACC guidelines on perioperative cardiovascular evaluation and care for NCS surgery.[5,13] These recommendations are summarized for rapid review and quick reference in Tables 14-4 through 14-6.

REFERENCES

1. Moses JW, Leon MB, Popma JJ, et al: Sirolimus-eluting stents versus standard stents in patients with stenosis in a native coronary artery. *N Engl J Med* 2003;349:1315-1323.
2. Spaulding C, Henry P, Teiger E, et al: Sirolimus-eluting versus uncoated stents in acute myocardial infarction. *N Engl J Med* 2006;355:1093-1104.
3. Metzler H, Huber K, Kozek-Langenecker S: Anaesthesia in patients with drug-eluting stents. *Curr Opin Anaesthesiol* 2008;21:55-59.
4. Schuchman M: Trading restensosis for thrombosis? New questions about drug-eluting stents. *N Engl J Med* 2006;355:1949-1952.
5. Grines CL, Bonow RO, Casey DE, et al: Prevention of premature discontinuation of dual antiplatelet therapy in patients with coronary artery stents. A science advisory from the American Heart Association, American College of Cardiology, Society for Cardiovascular Angiography and Interventions, American College of Surgeons, and American Dental Association, with representation from the American College of Physicians. *J Am Coll Cardiol* 2007;49:734-739.
6. Iakovou I, Schmidt T, Bonnizzoni E, et al: Incidence, predictors and outcome of thrombosis after successful implantation of drug-eluting stents. *JAMA* 2005;2126-2130.
7. Riddell JW, Chiche L, Plaud B, et al: Coronary stents and noncardiac surgery. *Circulation* 2007;116:e378-e382.
8. Schouten O, Bax JJ, Poldermans D: Management of patients with cardiac stents undergoing noncardiac surgery. *Curr Opin Anaesthesiol* 2007;20:274-278.
9. Kaluza GL, Joseph J, Lee JR, et al: Catastrophic outcomes of noncardiac surgery soon after coronary stenting. *J Am Coll Cardiol* 2000;35:1288-1294.
10. Brilakis ES, Orford JL, Fasseas P, et al: Outcome of patients undergoing balloon angioplasty in the 2 months prior to noncardiac surgery. *Am J Cardiol* 2005;96:512-514.
11. Vicenzi MN, Meislitzer T, Heitzinger B, et al: Coronary artery stenting and noncardiac surgery—a prospective outcome study. *Br J Anaesth* 2006;96:686-693.
12. Brilakis ES, Banerjee S, Berger PB: Perioperative management of patients with coronary stents. *J Am Coll Cardiol* 2007;49:2145-2150.
13. Fleisher LA, Beckman JA, Brown KA, et al: ACC/AHA guidelines on perioperative cardiovascular evaluation and care for noncardiac surgery. Executive summary: A report of the American College of Cardiology/American Heart Association Task Force on Practice Guidelines (Writing Committee to revise the 2002 Guidelines on Perioperative Cardiovascular Evaluation for Noncardiac Surgery). Developed in collaboration with the American Society of Echocardiography, American Society of Nuclear Cardiology, Heart Rhythm Society, Society of Cardiovascular Anesthesiologists, Society for Cardiovascular Angiography and Interventions, Society for Vascular Medicine and Biology, and Society for Vascular Surgery. *Circulation* 2007;116:1971-1996.
14. McFalls EO, Ward HB, Moritz TE, et al: Coronary-artery revascularization before elective major vascular surgery. *N Engl J Med* 2004;351:2795-2804.
15. Poldermans D, Bax JJ, Schouten O, et al: Should major vascular surgery be delayed because of preoperative cardiac testing in intermediate-risk patients receiving beta-blocker therapy with tight heart rate control? *J Am Coll Cardiol* 2006;48:964-969.
16. Poldermans D, Schouten O, Vidakovic R, et al (DECREASE Study Group): A clinical randomized trial to evaluate the safety of a noninvasive approach in high-risk patients undergoing major vascular surgery: The DECREASE-V pilot study. *J Am Coll Cardiol* 2007;49:1763-1769.
17. Allen JR, Helling TS, Hartzler GO: Operative procedures not involving the heart after percutaneous transluminal coronary angioplasty. *Surg Gynecol Obstet* 1991;173:285-288.
18. Huber KC, Evans MA, Bresnahan JF, et al: Outcome of noncardiac operations in patients with severe coronary artery disease successfully treated preoperatively with coronary angioplasty. *Mayo Clin Proc* 1992;67:15-21.
19. Elmore JR, Hallett JW Jr, Gibbons RJ, et al: Myocardial revascularization before abdominal aortic aneurysmorrhaphy: Effect of coronary angioplasty. *Mayo Clin Proc* 1993;68:637-641.
20. Gottlieb A, Banoub M, Sprung J, et al: Perioperative cardiovascular morbidity in patients with coronary artery disease undergoing vascular surgery after percutaneous transluminal coronary angioplasty. *J Cardiothorac Vasc Anesth* 1998;12:501-506.
21. Posner KL, Van Norman GA, Chan V: Adverse cardiac outcomes after noncardiac surgery in patients with prior percutaneous transluminal coronary angioplasty. *Anesth Analg* 1999;89:553-560.
22. Leibowitz D, Cohen M, Planer P, et al: Comparison of cardiovascular risk of noncardiac surgery following coronary angioplasty with versus without stenting. *Am J Cardiol* 2006;97;1188-1191.
23. Wilson SH, Fasseas P, Oxford JL, et al: Clinical outcome of patients undergoing non-cardiac surgery in the two months following coronary stenting. *J Am Coll Cardiol* 2003;42:234-240.
24. Reddy PR, Vaitkus PT: Risks of noncardiac surgery after coronary stenting. *Am J Cardiol* 2005;95:755-757.
25. Sharma AK, Ajani AE, Hamwi SM, et al: Major noncardiac surgery following coronary stenting: When is it safe to operate? *Cathet Cardiovasc Interv* 2004;63:141-145.
26. Serruys PW, Kutryk MJB, Ong ATL: Coronary-artery stents. *N Engl J Med* 2006;354:483-495.
27. Schouten O, Bax JJ, Damen J, et al: Coronary artery stent placement immediately before noncardiac surgery: A potential risk? *Anesthesiology* 2007;106:1067-1069.
28. Schouten O, van Domburg RT, Bax JJ, et al: Noncardiac surgery after coronary stenting: Early surgery and interruption of antiplatelet therapy are associated with an increase in major adverse cardiac events. *J Am Coll Cardiol* 2007;49:122-124.
29. Lagerqvist B, James SK, Stenestrand U, et al: Long-term outcomes with drug-eluting stents versus bare-metal stents in Sweden. *N Engl J Med* 2007;356:1009-1019.
30. Augoustides JG: Perioperative thrombotic risk of coronary stents: Possible role of intravenous platelet blockade. *Anesthesiology* 2007;107:516.
31. Valerin M, Brennan M, Noll J, et al: Relationship between aspirin use and postoperative bleeding from dental extractions in a healthy population. *Oral Surg Oral Med Oral Pathol Oral Radiol Endod* 2006;32:1022-1025.
32. Kumar N, Jivan S, Thomas P, et al: Sub-Tenon's anesthesia with aspirin, warfarin and clopidogrel. *J Cataract Refract Surg* 2006;32:1022-1025.
33. Alam M, Goldberg LH: Serious adverse vascular events associated with perioperative interruption of antiplatelet and anticoagulant therapy. *Dermatol Surg* 2002;28:992-998.
34. Orford JL, Lennon NR, Melby S, et al: Frequency and correlates of coronary stent thrombosis in the modern era: Analysis of a single center registry. *J Am Coll Cardiol* 2002;40:1567-1572.
35. Caird J, Chukwunyerenwa C, Ali Z, et al: Craniotomy with prosthetic heart valves: A clinical dilemma. *Br J Neurosurg* 2006;20:40-42.
36. Herbert EN, Mokete B, Williamson TH, et al: Haemorrhagic vitreoretinal complications associated with combined antiplatelet agents. *Br J Opthalmol* 2006;90:1209-1210.
37. Broad L, Lee T, Conroy M, et al: Successful management of patients with a drug-eluting coronary stent presenting for elective, non-cardiac surgery. *Br J Anaesth* 2007;98:19-22.
38. McFadden EP, Stabile E, Regar E, et al: Late thrombosis in drug-eluting coronary stents after discontinuation of antiplatelet therapy. *Lancet* 2004;364:1519-1521.
39. de Souza DG, Baum V, Ballert NM: Late thrombosis of a drug-eluting stent presenting in the perioperative period. *Anesthesiology* 2007;106:1057-1059.
40. Barone-Rochette G, Ormezzano O, Polack B, et al: Resistance to platelet antiaggregants: An important cause of very late thrombosis of drug-eluting stents? Observations from five cases. *Arch Cardiovasc Dis* 2008;101:100-107.

41. Bertrand ME: When and how to discontinue antiplatelet therapy. *Eur Heart J* 2008;10:A35-A4.

42. Patterson L, Hunter D, Mann A: Appropriate waiting time for noncardiac surgery following coronary stent insertion: Views of Canadian anesthesiologists. *Can J Anaesth* 2005;52:440-441.

43. Albaladejo P, Marret E, Piriou V, et al: Perioperative management of antiplatelet agents in patients with coronary stents: Recommendations of a French task force. *Br J Anaesth* 2006;97: 580-585.

44. Berger PB, Bellot V, Bell MR, et al: An immediate invasive strategy for the treatment of acute myocardial infarction early after noncardiac surgery. *Am J Cardiol* 2001;87:1100-1102.

45. Steffel J, Eberli FR, Luscher TF, et al: Drug-eluting stents—what should be improved? *Ann Med* 2008;40:242-252.

46. Ormiston JA, Serruys PW, Regar E, et al: A bioabsorbable everolimus-eluting coronary stent system for patients with single de-novo coronary artery lesions (ABSORB): A prospective open-label trial. *Lancet* 2008;371:899-907.

15 How Should We Prepare the Patient with a Pacemaker/Implantable Cardioverter-Defibrillator?

Marc A. Rozner, PhD, MD

INTRODUCTION

Battery-operated pacemakers (PMs) revolutionized the treatment of fatal electrical conduction abnormalities in 1958, just a few years after the invention of the transistor. As this science has matured, PMs have been designed to provide atrioventricular synchronization, improve the quality of life for the chronotropically incompetent patient, and reduce ventricular contractile dissymmetry in the presence of cardiomyopathy. This science has been extended to treat both atrial and ventricular tachyarrhythmias (in addition to bradyarrhythmia issues) with antitachycardia pacing or shock in the form of implantable cardioverter-defibrillators (ICDs), which were first demonstrated in 1980 and approved by the U.S. Food and Drug Administration (FDA) in 1985. Current ICDs represent extensions and advancement of PM technology, so every ICD implanted today, in addition to antitachycardia therapy, also provides the entire functional set found in a PM.

These devices are no longer confined to keeping the heart beating between a minimum rate (pacing function) and a maximum rate (ICD functions), as they are now employed as therapy to improve the failing heart. Electronic miniaturization of PMs and ICDs has permitted the design and use of sophisticated electronics in patients who need artificial pacing or automated cardioversion/defibrillation of their heart (or both).

Coupled with population aging, continued enhancements and new indications for implantation of pacemakers or cardioverter-defibrillators will lead to increased numbers of patients with these devices. Safe and efficient clinical management of these patients depends on our understanding of implantable systems, indications for their use, and the perioperative needs that they create.

However, the increasing specialization, the proprietary nature of developments, and the complexity of cardiac generators limit generalizations that can be made about the perioperative care of these patients. Additionally, the absence of published trials, the misinterpretation of adverse events in published literature, and the lack of formal perioperative guidelines add to the difficulties in taking care of these patients.

These issues led the American Society of Anesthesiologists (ASA) to publish a Practice Advisory for these patients.[1] Other guidelines have been published as well,[2-5] although not all authors recommend ICD disablement in the perioperative period.[6]

EVIDENCE

Whether PM or ICD patients have increased perioperative morbidity or mortality risk remains an area ripe for investigation. Levine and colleagues[7] previously reported increases in pacing thresholds (i.e., the amount of energy required to depolarize the myocardium) in some thoracic operations. In 1995, Badrinath and colleagues[8] retrospectively reviewed ophthalmic surgery cases in one hospital in Madras, India, from 1979 through 1988 (14,787 cases) and wrote that the presence of a pacemaker significantly increased the probability of a mortal event within 6 weeks postoperatively, regardless of the anesthetic technique. Pili-Floury and colleagues[9] reported that 2 of 65 pacemaker patients (3.1%) undergoing significant noncardiac surgery died postoperatively of cardiac cause across a 30-month study period. They also reported that 12% and 7.8% of patients required preoperative and postoperative modification of pacemaker programming, respectively.[9] In abstract form, Rozner and colleagues[10] reported a 2-year retrospective review of 172 PM patients treated at a preoperative anesthesia clinic, showing that 27 of 172 (16%) needed a preoperative intervention (9 of 27 were generator replacement for battery depletion). Additionally, follow-up of the 149 patients who underwent an open surgical procedure showed 5 ventricular pacing threshold increases, 1 atrial pacing threshold increase, and 1 PM electrical reset,[10] all of which took place in patients undergoing nonthoracic surgery. All of these cases involved electromagnetic interference (EMI) from monopolar electrosurgical unit (ESU), and one large ventricular pacing threshold was observed after a significant fluid and blood resuscitation following the loss of 2500 mL of blood in a 45-year-old woman.

For the patient with ventricular tachycardia (VT) or ventricular fibrillation (VF), ICDs clearly reduce deaths, and they remain superior to antiarrhythmic drug therapy.[11] Further, studies suggesting prophylactic placement in patients *without* evidence of tachyarrhythmias (Multicenter Automatic Defibrillator Implantation Trial–II [MADIT-II]—ischemic cardiomyopathy, ejection fraction less than 0.30;[12] and Sudden Cardiac Death–Heart Failure Trial [SCD-HeFT]—any cardiomyopathy, ejection fraction less than 0.35[13]) have significantly increased the number of patients for whom ICD therapy is indicated.

ICD advancements have a number of important results. First, all ICDs have brady-pacing capability, and the presence of pacing artifacts on an electrocardiogram (ECG) might lead a practitioner to mistake an ICD for a (non-ICD) pacemaker. If ECGs are routinely collected from patients with "pacemakers" using a magnet, some ICDs from Boston Scientific/Guidant/CPI might be permanently deactivated with magnet placement.[14] Second, ICD brady-pacing is *never* converted to asynchronous mode with magnet placement; thus, for many ICDs, confirmation of appropriate magnet placement is absent. Third, ICDs respond to, and process, EMI differently than a pacemaker.

This field is further complicated by the nature of electronics, silent device malfunction, and outright device failure. (A "silent" device failure is one that does not immediately lead to patient symptoms. For example, a patient with a pacemaker set to 70 beats per minute with AV delay of 180 ms but who has an underlying sinus rhythm at 57 beats per minute with a PR interval of 230 ms will probably fail to notice a complete system failure.) Although pacemakers and ICDs are more reliable than almost any other technology, some devices fail prematurely. Maisel and colleagues[15] searched the FDA database for the years 1990–2002; they found that 4.6 PMs and 20.7 ICDs per 1000 implants had been explanted for failures other than battery depletion. For the study period, 2.25 million PMs and 415,780 ICDs were implanted with 30 PM and 31 ICD patients who died as a direct result of device malfunction.[15] Currently, alerts exist for premature ICD lead failure, which can result in inappropriate shock or failure of shock.[16,17] A number of PMs and ICDs remain on "alert" for silent, premature battery failure (Medtronic issues,[18-20] Guidant issues[21-26]). One entire Guidant product line of 46,000 ICDs has their magnet mode permanently disabled because of a switch malfunction.[27]

PACEMAKER AND ICD MECHANICS

PM and ICD implant indications are shown in Tables 15-1A and 15-1B. These systems consist of an impulse generator and lead(s). Leads can have one (unipolar), two

Table 15-1A   Permanent Pacemaker Indications
Sinus node disease
Atrioventricular (AV) node disease
Long Q-T syndrome
Hypertrophic obstructive cardiomyopathy (HOCM)
Dilated cardiomyopathy (DCM)

Table 15-1B   Implantable Cardioverter-Defibrillator Indications
Ventricular tachycardia
Ventricular fibrillation
Post–myocardial infarction patients with ejection fraction (EF) ≤30% (MADIT II)
Cardiomyopathy from any cause with EF ≤35% (SCD-HeFT)
Hypertrophic cardiomyopathy
Awaiting heart transplant
Long Q-T syndrome
Arrhythmogenic right ventricular dysplasia
Brugada syndrome (right bundle branch block, S-T segment elevation in leads V1-V3)

(bipolar), or multiple (multipolar) electrodes with connections in multiple chambers. In unipolar pacing, as well as defibrillation, the generator case serves as an electrode, and tissue contact in a PM has been disrupted by pocket gas.[28] Pacing in a unipolar mode (unusual in an ICD system) produces larger "spikes" on an analog-recorded ECG, and unipolar sensing is more sensitive to EMI. Most pacemaking systems use a bipolar pacing/sensing configuration, because bipolar pacing usually requires less energy and bipolar sensing is more resistant to interference from muscle artifacts or stray electromagnetic fields. Often, bipolar electrodes can be identified on the chest film because they have a ring electrode 1 to 3 cm proximal to the lead tip. ICDs can be distinguished from conventional PMs by the presence of a shock coil on the right ventricular lead (Figure 15-1).

Finally, devices resembling cardiac pulse generators are being implanted at increasing rates for pain control, thalamic stimulation to control Parkinson's disease, phrenic nerve stimulation to stimulate the diaphragm in paralyzed patients, and vagus nerve stimulation to control epilepsy and possibly obesity.[29] These devices can be, and have been, confused with a cardiac generator as well.

The nature of programming, which is unique to each device, necessitates a preoperative evaluation with a pacemaker/ICD programmer. With this interrogation, one can identify programmed parameters, battery longevity (voltage and impedance), lead integrity (impedance), safety margins for sensing underlying rhythm signals (signal amplitude and channel sensitivity), and safety margins for pacing in each chamber (pacing threshold and pacing output), as well as retrieve information about the patient's rhythm behavior since the last time the generator memory was reset. For ICDs (and many PMs), rhythm abnormalities (atrial fibrillation, supraventricular tachycardia, ventricular tachycardia, and ventricular fibrillation) are stored as well.

Pacemaker and ICD programming are described using the Pacemaker (NGB) or Defibrillator (NBD) codes (Tables 15-2A and 15-2B). Since all ICDs perform brady-pacing, the most robust ICD description would include the first three characters of the NBD, followed by a dash ("-"), then the five character PM NBG. As an example, in Figure 15-1, the ICD was configured as VVE-DDDRV (ventricular shock capable, ventricular antitachycardia

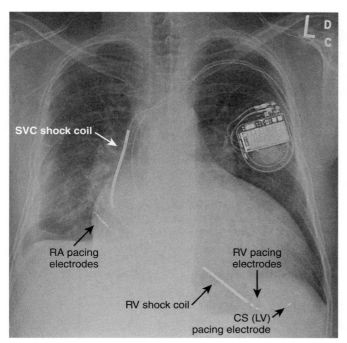

Figure 15-1. A Defibrillator System with Biventricular (BiV) Antibradycardia Pacemaker Capability. This chest film was taken from a 50-year-old man with head and neck cancer, coronary artery disease, and ischemic cardiomyopathy with ejection fraction of 15%. The ICD generator is in the left pectoral position with three leads: a conventional, bipolar lead to the right atrium, a quadripolar lead to the right ventricle (RV), and a unipolar lead to the coronary sinus (CS). This system is designed to provide "resynchronization (antibradycardia) therapy" in the setting of a dilated cardiomyopathy with a prolonged QRS (and frequently with a prolonged P-R interval as well). The bipolar lead in the right atrium will perform both sensing and pacing functions. The lead in this RV is a true bipolar lead with ring and tip electrodes for pacing and sensing. The presence of a "shock" conductor (termed a *shock coil*) on the RV lead in the right ventricle distinguishes a defibrillation system from a conventional pacemaking system. The lead in the CS depolarizes the left ventricle, and the typical current pathway includes the anode (ring electrode) in the right ventricle. Because of the typically wide QRS complex in a left bundle branch pattern, failure to capture the left ventricle can lead to ventricular oversensing (and inappropriate antitachycardia therapy) in an ICD system. Many defibrillation systems (including this one) also have a shock coil in the superior vena cava, which usually is electrically identical to the defibrillator case (called the "can"). When the defibrillation circuit includes the ICD case, it is called an "active can configuration."

pace capable, electrogram detection, plus atrioventricular pacing in a dual chamber [atrial tracking] mode, with rate responsiveness, and multisite ventricular pacing). In the United States, the two most common pacing modes are VVI (single chamber ventricular pacing in the absence of a native ventricular event) and DDD (atrioventricular pacing that forces tracking of the atrial activity, whether sensed or paced).

"Conventional wisdom" regarding care of PM or ICD patients somehow has become "just put a magnet on it." This behavior seems to have originated with the incorrect belief that magnet application to a PM always produces asynchronous pacing and that a magnet on an ICD always inhibits antitachycardia therapy. Thus many physicians mistakenly believe that magnet application will prevent signal oversensing from the "Bovie" ESU, which can result in no pacing; after all, any electrical signal on the ventricular lead is interpreted by the generator as ventricular activity, which then "inhibits" pacing output. For ICDs, the electrical noise (electromagnetic interference [EMI]) can precipitate shocks. However, many PMs and ICDs can have their magnet mode altered by programming, and for some PMs, the default magnet setting does not include sustained, asynchronous behavior. Table 15-3 shows default magnet behavior for many PMs and ICDs.

Preoperative management of the patient with a pacemaker includes evaluation and optimization of coexisting disease(s). For the patient with cardiomyopathy, the perioperative physician(s) should ensure appropriate pharmacologic therapy (beta-blockade, afterload reduction, diuretics where indicated, and antiarrhythmics or other special drugs for late-stage disease).[30] In fact, initiation of beta-blocker therapy produces benefit to the cardiomyopathic patient within 10 to 14 days,[31] so delaying an elective case to institute beta-blocker therapy might be prudent. No special laboratory tests or x-rays are needed for the patient with a conventional pacemaker. A patient with a BiV pacer (or ICD) might need a chest film to document the position of the coronary sinus (CS) lead, especially if central line placement is planned, because spontaneous CS lead dislodgement can occur.[32,33] Central line placement in the thorax should not be performed without electrocardiographic monitoring (PM or ICD), and the ICD (if present) should be disabled to antitachycardia therapy, because patient injury from inappropriate shock has been reported.[34]

Table 15-2A	**NASPE/BPEG Generic Pacemaker Code (NBG) [Revised 2002]**			
Position I	**Position II**	**Position III**	**Position IV**	**Position V**
Chambers Paced	*Chambers Sensed*	*Response to Sensing*	*Programmability*	*Multisite Pacing*
O = None	**O** = None	**O** = None	**O** = None	**O** = None
A = Atrium	**A** = Atrium	**I** = Inhibited	**R** = Rate Modulation	**A** = Atrium
V = Ventricle	**V** = Ventricle	**T** = Triggered		**V** = Ventricle
D = Dual (A+V)	**D** = Dual (A+V)	**D** = Dual (T+I)		**D** = Dual (A+V)

BPEG, British Pacing and Electrophysiology Group; *NASPE,* North American Society of Pacing and Electrophysiology (now the Heart Rhythm Society).

Table 15-2B NASPE/BPG Generic Defibrillator Code (NBD)

Position I	Position II	Position III	Position IV (or use Pacemaker Code)
Shock Chambers	*Antitachycardia Pacing Chambers*	*Tachycardia Detection*	*Antibradycardia Pacing Chambers*
O = None	O = None	E = Electrogram	O = None
A = Atrium	A = Atrium	H = Hemodynamic	A = Atrium
V = Ventricle	V = Ventricle		V = Ventricle
D = Dual (A+V)	D = Dual (A+V)		D = Dual (A+V)

BPEG, British Pacing and Electrophysiology Group; *NASPE*, North American Society of Pacing and Electrophysiology (now the Heart Rhythm Society).

Current North American Society of Pacing and Electrophysiology (NASPE) and Medicare guidelines for PM include telephonic (magnet) evaluation every 4 to 12 weeks (depending on device type and age) and a comprehensive device interrogation with a programmer at least once per year.[35] Currently, no published and agreed standard has been set for ICDs, but the manufacturer documents recommend device evaluation at least every 4 months, with more frequent checks for ICD and lead systems on alert or recall. Some ICDs can now be

Table 15-3 Usual (or Default) Effects of Appropriate Magnet Placement for Most Devices

Manufacturer	Pacemaker	ICD
Biotronik	PROGRAMMABLE • Battery OK: 10 AS events at 90 beats/min, then original programmed mode without rate responsiveness • Battery not OK: 10 AS events at 80 beats/min, then 11% below LRL	NONPROGRAMMABLE NO confirmation • Disables tachy therapies
ELA Medical (Sorin)	NONPROGRAMMABLE • Asynchronous pacing at 96 beats/min gradually declining to 80 beats/min at ERI. After magnet removal, 8 additional asynchronous pacing cycles (the final 2 cycles are at LRL with long atrioventricular delay).	NONPROGRAMMABLE Confirmation: Pacing rate (but not mode) changes to • Battery OK: 90 beats/min • ERI: 80 beats/min • Disables tachy therapy
Guidant (also CPI) now Boston Scientific	PROGRAMMABLE OFF MODE • Battery OK: AS pacing at 100 beats/min • ERI: AS pacing at 85 beats/min	PROGRAMMABLE OFF MODE Confirmation: short beep with each detected heartbeat [CAUTION]**
Medtronic Corporation	NONPROGRAMMABLE • Battery OK: AS pacing 85 beats/min • ERI: AS single-chamber pacing at 65 beats/min	NONPROGRAMMABLE NO confirmation • Disables tachy therapy
Pacesetter (owned by St. Jude Medical)	PROGRAMMABLE OFF (and VARIO*) MODE • Battery OK: AS pacing depends on model • ERI: AS pacing below 90 beats/min	PROGRAMMABLE OFF MODE NO confirmation • Disables tachy therapy
St. Jude Medical	PROGRAMMABLE OFF MODE • Battery OK: AS pacing 98 beats/min gradually declining over life of battery • ERI: AS pacing below 87 beats/min	PROGRAMMABLE OFF MODE NO confirmation • Disables tachy therapy

*VARIO mode: 32 asynchronous events—the first 16 between 100 and 85 beats/min (ERI) to indicate battery performance; the next 15 at 119 beats/min with gradually declining ventricular pacing output to demonstrate capture threshold. The final pace is no output to clearly demonstrate no capture. This sequence repeats as long as the magnet is in place.

**If the "Change Tachy Mode with Magnet" feature also is programmed "ON," after 30 seconds of continuous magnet application the tachy mode changes, i.e., it will switch from enabled (in absence of magnet, beeping) to permanently disabled (constant tone) or vice versa. Any CPI/Guidant ICD that does not emit sound when a magnet is applied should undergo an immediate device interrogation and the patient should be electrocardiographically monitored until the interrogation is complete.

AS, asynchronous; *ERI*, elective replacement indicated—the device is reporting the need for generator replacement due to battery depletion; *LRL*, lower rate limit—the minimum programmed rate for the device.

CAUTION: This table is not meant to be complete. It lists the default (or out-of-box) settings for appropriate magnet placement. Only an interrogation of the generator will reveal the true settings for any programmable device. The term "PROGRAMMABLE OFF MODE" indicates that the magnet response can be eliminated in the generator by programming.

For CPI/Guidant ICDs, if magnet mode is programmed to "ON," appropriate magnet placement immediately disables tachy detection and therapy, and tachy therapies remain disabled for as long as the magnet remains appropriately applied. If each heartbeat produces a "beep," the device will be enabled for tachy therapy on magnet removal provided it is not damaged by electromagnetic interference while the magnet is applied. If the device emits a constant tone with a magnet applied, tachy therapy is disabled whether or not a magnet is present.

evaluated using telephonic checks; however, since pacing thresholds cannot be determined at this time, in-office evaluation with the programmer remains the test of choice.

For some patients, appropriate reprogramming (Table 15-4) is the safest way to avoid intraoperative problems, especially if monopolar ESU will be used. Many pacemaker manufacturers stand ready to assist with this task; however, any industry-employed allied professional (i.e., the manufacturer representative, or "rep") should be supervised by an appropriately trained physician.[36] Reprogramming the PM to asynchronous pacing at a rate greater than the patient's underlying rate usually ensures that no oversensing or undersensing from EMI will take place. However, setting a device to asynchronous mode has the potential to create a malignant rhythm in the patient with structurally compromised myocardium.[37] Reprogramming a device will *not* protect it from internal damage or reset caused by EMI. In general, rate responsiveness and "enhancements" (dynamic atrial overdrive, hysteresis, sleep rate, intrinsic atrio-ventricular activity (A-V) search, etc.) should be disabled by programming because many of these features can mimic pacing dysfunction.[38,39] Note that for many Guidant and CPI devices, Guidant Medical recommends increasing the pacing voltage to "5 volts or higher" when monopolar electrosurgery will be used. Few cardiologists follow this recommendation, but there are reports of threshold changes during both intrathoracic[7] and nonchest surgery.[40] Recently, pacing threshold was shown to be increased by some disease states.[41] Special attention must be given to any device with a minute ventilation (bioimpedance) sensor (Table 15-5)[42] because inappropriate tachycardia has been observed secondary to mechanical ventilation,[43,44] monopolar ("Bovie") electrosurgery,[43,45,46] and connection to an ECG monitor with respiratory rate monitoring.[42,47-51] Sometimes, inappropriate therapy producing life-threatening results has been delivered in these settings.[44,52]

Table 15-4   Pacing Function Reprogramming Possibly Needed

Any rate-responsive device—problems are well known and have been misinterpreted with potential for patient injury; the Food and Drug Administration has issued an alert regarding devices with minute ventilation sensors
Special pacing indication (hypertrophic cardiomyopathy, dilated cardiomyopathy, pediatrics)
Pacemaker-dependent patient
Major procedure in the chest or abdomen
Rate enhancements are present that should be disabled
Special procedures
  Lithotripsy
  Transurethral or hysteroscopic resection
  Electroconvulsive therapy
  Succinylcholine use
  Magnetic resonance imaging (MRI) (usually contraindicated by device manufacturers, although now possible in some patients)

Table 15-5   Pacemakers with Minute Ventilation Sensors

ELA Medical (Sorin)	Symphony, Brio (212, 220, 222)
	Opus RM (4534)
	Chorus RM (7034, 7134)
	Talent (130, 213, 223)
Guidant Medical (and/ or Boston Scientific/ Guidant/CPI)	Pulsar (1172, 1272)
	Pulsar Max (1170, 1171, 1270)
	Pulsar Max II (1180, 1181, 1280)
	Insignia Plus (1194, 1297, 1298)
Medtronic Telectronics/St. Jude	Kappa 400 series (401, 403)
	Meta (1202, 1204, 1206, 1230, 1250, 1254, 1256), Tempo (1102, 1902, 2102, 2902)

CONTROVERSIES

The principle issues surrounding PM and ICD patient care involve the following:

1. *Preoperative device interrogation*: According to guidelines from the American College of Cardiology,[2] as well as the Practice Advisory from the American Society of Anesthesiologists,[1] a recent preoperative interrogation of the PM or ICD remains the procedure of choice for these patients. Not specified is the interval between the last interrogation and the surgery, although the ACC/AHA guidelines suggest that up to 6 months might be acceptable.

2. *Perioperative reprogramming*: In the 2007 ACC/AHA guidelines,[2] perioperative reprogramming was not part of the recommendations. However, a PM or an ICD with a mechanical rate sensor might increase the paced heart rate when pressure is applied over the generator or the chest wall is manipulated, such as during a skin preparation, and certain programming features designed to reduce ventricular pacing (such as the managed ventricular pacing mode present in many Medtronic generators) or increase battery life (such as pacing rate hysteresis) might masquerade as pacing system malfunction.

3. *Disabling of antitachycardia therapy for ICD patients*: Most experts continue to recommend that ICD shock or antitachycardia pacing be disabled for the operating room. Some experts recommend the use of the magnet for this issue. However, application of a magnet to an ICD does not guarantee the deactivation of antitachycardia therapy; some ICDs have no magnet mode due to programming, and only ICDs from Boston Scientific/ Guidant/CPI emit tones (provided the magnet mode is enabled) to indicate appropriate magnet placement. Unfortunately, some ICDs from Boston Scientific/ Guidant/CPI continue to allow permanent deactivation by magnet placement for over 30 seconds.[14]

4. *Postoperative device interrogation*: EMI, regardless of the site or source, has the potential to injure a generator or cause a reset. Nevertheless, economic, personnel, and time pressures can hinder a timely postoperative interrogation of the generator.

AUTHOR'S RECOMMENDATIONS

Table 15-6 shows perioperative guidelines adapted from a number of sources.

Specific recommendations regarding the aforementioned controversies include the following:

1. *Preoperative device interrogation*: Preoperatively, all PMs and ICDs should undergo a comprehensive in-office interrogation not more than 30 days before the surgery/anesthetic. Particular attention should be given to patients in whom a previous problem was discovered, if a generator or lead is on alert or recall, if there is a change in patient symptomatology or condition, or if the patient gets frequent antitachycardia therapy from his or her ICD.
2. *Perioperative reprogramming*: In general, rate enhancements as well as rate responsiveness should be disabled for the intraoperative period to prevent unnecessary (and possibly dangerous) therapy, especially if minute ventilation sensing is present. The patient who demonstrates pacing system dependence might need reprogramming to asynchronous pacing or the placement (and testing, which will likely require reprogramming) of a temporary pacing device for surgery superior to the umbilicus if monopolar ESU use is planned. Consideration should be given to raising the lower paced rate to ensure adequate oxygen delivery in patients undergoing significant surgery.
3. *Disabling of antitachycardia therapy for ICD patients*: In general, most ICDs should have antitachycardia therapy deactivated for surgical procedures, especially if monopolar ESU use is planned. Deactivation by programming is more reliable than magnet placement. In fact, a magnet should be used only after consultation with an ICD expert and a stable and appropriate position of the magnet can be regularly verified during the case. Any patient who undergoes ICD disablement or magnet placement without prior verification of magnet behavior should be kept in a monitored environment until the ICD is interrogated and found to be working appropriately. For cases where there is no generator or lead alert/recall, no monopolar ESU for the case, no planned blood transfusions, and limited fluid administration (which is not

well defined) expected for the case, and no issues discovered at the preoperative ICD interrogation, this author's practice includes no deactivation of the ICD for the case, although magnet placement (assuming prior verification of magnet function) can be acceptable to prevent inappropriate ICD discharge.[53]
4. *Postoperative device interrogation*: In general, a postoperative device check ensures that no issues arose during the case. It also allows any data (such as noise that gets interpreted as an arrhythmia or lead problem) to be cleared from the generator memory. It is required in any case wherein an ICD was disabled to tachyarrhythmia therapy by programming, and it should be the standard of care for any patient exposed to EMI. For any case where no monopolar ESU was used, no blood was transfused, limited fluid was administered for the case, and no issues were identified during the case, this author's practice includes no postoperative generator check.[53]
5. *The monopolar electrosurgery current return pad*: Although no controversy has been described, common practice among operating room personnel involves the placement of this pad on the patient's thigh, regardless of the surgical site. For monopolar ESU use superior to the umbilicus, this placement creates an ESU current path that can include the generator, leads, or both. Strong EMI from the ESU remains the principle enemy of an implanted generator, and the current return pad should be placed to prevent induced current in the leads. As a result, for surgery in the head and neck area, the pad should be placed on the posterior-superior shoulder contralateral to the site of the generator. This shoulder site is acceptable for surgery on the chest wall (such as mastectomy) contralateral to the generator as well. For surgery on the chest wall ipsilateral to the generator, the pad should be placed on the ipsilateral arm and the return wire should be prepped into the field, if necessary, with a sterile, occlusive covering. This sterile wire can then be run superiorly along the arm to the shoulder, made stationary, and then run to the ESU generator.

Table 15-6   Perioperative Guidelines for the Patient with a Cardiac Generator

PREOPERATIVE KEY POINTS

- Have the pacemaker or defibrillator interrogated by a competent authority shortly before the anesthetic.
- Obtain a copy of this interrogation. Ensure that the device will pace the heart with appropriate safety margins.
- Consider replacing any device near its elective replacement period in a patient scheduled to undergo either a major surgery or surgery within 25 cm of the generator.
- Determine the patient's underlying rhythm/rate to determine the need for backup pacing support.
- Identify the magnet rate and rhythm, if a magnet mode is present and magnet use is planned.
- Program minute ventilation rate responsiveness off, if present.
- Program all rate enhancements off.
- Consider increasing the pacing rate to optimize oxygen delivery to tissues for major cases.
- Disable antitachycardia therapy if a defibrillator.

INTRAOPERATIVE KEY POINTS

- Monitor cardiac rhythm/peripheral pulse with pulse oximeter or arterial waveform.
- Disable the "artifact filter" on the ECG monitor.
- Avoid use of monopolar electrosurgery (ESU).
- Use bipolar ESU if possible; if not possible, "pure cut" (monopolar ESU) is better than "blend" or "coag."
- Place the ESU current return pad in such a way as to prevent electricity from crossing the generator-heart circuit, even if the pad must be placed on the distal forearm and the wire covered with sterile drape.
- If the ESU causes ventricular oversensing, pacer quiescence, or tachycardia, limit the period(s) of asystole or reprogram the cardiac generator.

POSTOPERATIVE KEY POINTS

- Have the device interrogated by a competent authority postoperatively. Some rate enhancements can be reinitiated, and optimum heart rate and pacing parameters should be determined. The ICD patient must be monitored until the antitachycardia therapy is restored.

REFERENCES

1. Practice advisory for the perioperative management of patients with cardiac rhythm management devices: Pacemakers and implantable cardioverter-defibrillators: A report by the American Society of Anesthesiologists Task Force on Perioperative Management of Patients with Cardiac Rhythm Management Devices. *Anesthesiology* 2005;103(1):186-198.
2. Fleisher LA, Beckman JA, Brown KA, et al: ACC/AHA 2007 guidelines on perioperative cardiovascular evaluation and care for noncardiac surgery. A report of the American College of Cardiology/American Heart Association Task Force on practice guidelines (writing committee to revise the 2002 guidelines on perioperative cardiovascular evaluation for noncardiac surgery). Published Sept 27, 2007. Available at http://circ.ahajournals.org/cgi/content/abstract/CIRCULATIONAHA.107.185699v1 (accessed Jan 8, 2008).
3. Goldschlager N, Epstein A, Friedman P, Gang E, Krol R, Olshansky B: Environmental and drug effects on patients with pacemakers and implantable cardioverter/defibrillators: A practical guide to patient treatment. *Arch Intern Med* 2001;161(5):649-655.
4. Pinski SL, Trohman RG: Interference in implanted cardiac devices, part I. *Pacing Clin Electrophysiol* 2002;25:1367-1381.
5. Pinski SL, Trohman RG: Interference in implanted cardiac devices, part II. *Pacing Clin Electrophysiol* 2002;25(10):1496-1509.
6. Stevenson WG, Chaitman BR, Ellenbogen KA, et al: Clinical assessment and management of patients with implanted cardioverter-defibrillators presenting to nonelectrophysiologists. *Circulation* 2004;110(25):3866-3869.
7. Levine PA, Balady GJ, Lazar HL, Belott PH, Roberts AJ: Electrocautery and pacemakers: Management of the paced patient subject to electrocautery. *Ann Thorac Surg* 1986;41(3):313-317.
8. Badrinath SS, Bhaskaran S, Sundararaj I, Rao BS, Mukesh BN: Mortality and morbidity associated with ophthalmic surgery. *Ophthalmic Surg Lasers* 1995;26(6):535-541.
9. Pili-Floury S, Farah E, Samain E, Schauvliege F, Marty J: Perioperative outcome of pacemaker patients undergoing noncardiac surgery. *Eur J Anaesthesiol* 2008;25:514-516.
10. Rozner MA, Roberson JC, Nguyen AD: Unexpected high incidence of serious pacemaker problems detected by pre- and postoperative interrogations: A two-year experience. *J Am Coll Cardiol* 2004;43(5):113A.
11. Buxton AE, Lee KL, Fisher JD, Josephson ME, Prystowsky EN, Hafley G: A randomized study of the prevention of sudden death in patients with coronary artery disease. Multicenter Unsustained Tachycardia Trial Investigators. *N Engl J Med* 1999;341(25):1882-1890.
12. Moss A, Zareba W, Hall W, et al: Prophylactic implantation of a defibrillator in patients with myocardial infarction and reduced ejection fraction. *N Engl J Med* 2002;346(12):877-883.
13. Bardy GH, Lee KL, Mark DB, et al: Amiodarone or an implantable cardioverter-defibrillator for congestive heart failure. *N Engl J Med* 2005;352(3):225-237.
14. Rasmussen MJ, Friedman PA, Hammill SC, Rea RF: Unintentional deactivation of implantable cardioverter-defibrillators in health care settings. *Mayo Clin Proc* 2002;77(8):855-859.
15. Maisel WH, Moynahan M, Zuckerman BD, et al: Pacemaker and ICD generator malfunctions: Analysis of Food and Drug Administration annual reports. *JAMA* 2006;295(16):1901-1906.
16. Medtronic. Urgent medical device information: Sprint Fidelis® lead patient management recommendations. Published Oct 15, 2007. Available at http://www.medtronic.com/fidelis/physician-letter.html (accessed Oct 19, 2007).
17. Ellenbogen KA, Wood MA, Shepard RK, et al: Detection and management of an implantable cardioverter defibrillator lead failure: Incidence and clinical implications. *J Am Coll Cardiol* 2003;41(1):73-80.
18. Medtronic: ICD recall. Published Feb 10, 2005. Available at http://www.plaintiffsadvocate.com/marquis/recall.pdf.
19. Medtronic: Important patient management information (Sigma series pacemakers). Published Nov 2005. Available at http://www.medtronic.com/crmLetter.html (accessed Oct 19, 2007).
20. Medtronic: Prodigy pacemaker information and programming guide. St Paul, MN, 1995.
21. Guidant: Urgent medical device safety information and corrective action (PDM Pacemakers). Published July 18, 2005. Available at http://www.guidant.com/physician_communications/PDM.pdf (accessed Jan 1, 2007).
22. Guidant: Urgent medical device safety information and corrective action (Insignia Pacemakers). Published Sept 22, 2005. Available at http://www.guidant.com/physician_communications/insignia-nexus.pdf (accessed Jan 1, 2007).
23. Guidant: Urgent medical device safety information and corrective action (AVT ICDs). Published July 22, 2005. Available at http://www.guidant.com/physician_communications/AVT_2.pdf (accessed Jan 1, 2007).
24. Guidant: Urgent medical device safety information and corrective action (Contak Renewal [H135, H155] ICD). Published June 17, 2005. Available at http://www.guidant.com/physician_communications/RENEWAL_RENEWAL2.pdf (accessed Jan 1, 2007).
25. Guidant: Urgent medical device safety information and corrective action (Prizm 2 [1861] ICD). Published June 17, 2005. Available at http://www.guidant.com/physician_communications/RENEWAL3_RENEWAL4.pdf (accessed Jan 1, 2007).
26. Guidant: Urgent medical device safety information and corrective action (Vitality ICD). Published July 22, 2006. Available at http://www.bostonscientific.com/templatedata/imports/HTML/PPR/files/physician/vit_he_renewal.pdf (accessed Jan 1, 2007).
27. Guidant: Urgent medical device safety information and corrective action (Contak Renewal [3,4,RF] ICD [magnet switch]). Published June 23, 2005. Available at http://www.bostonscientific.com/templatedata/imports/HTML/PPR/ppr/support/current_advisories.pdf.
28. Lamas GA, Rebecca GS, Braunwald NS, Antman EM: Pacemaker malfunction after nitrous oxide anesthesia. *Am J Cardiol* 1985;56(15):995.
29. Kazatsker M, Kusniek J, Hasdai D, Battler A, Birnbaum Y: Two pacemakers in one patient: A stimulating case. *J Cardiovasc Electrophysiol* 2002;13(5):522.
30. Hunt SA: ACC/AHA 2005 guideline update for the diagnosis and management of chronic heart failure in the adult: A report of the American College of Cardiology/American Heart Association Task Force on Practice Guidelines (Writing Committee to Update the 2001 Guidelines for the Evaluation and Management of Heart Failure). *J Am Coll Cardiol* 2005;46(1):1116-1143.
31. Krum H, Roecker EB, Mohacsi P, et al: Effects of initiating carvedilol in patients with severe chronic heart failure: Results from the COPERNICUS Study. *JAMA* 2003;289(6):712-718.
32. Valls-Bertault V, Mansourati J, Gilard M, Etienne Y, Munier S, Blanc JJ: Adverse events with transvenous left ventricular pacing in patients with severe heart failure: Early experience from a single centre. *Europace* 2001;3(1):60-63.
33. Alonso C, Leclercq C, d'Allonnes FR, et al: Six-year experience of transvenous left ventricular lead implantation for permanent biventricular pacing in patients with advanced heart failure: Technical aspects. *Heart* 2001;86(4):405-410.
34. Varma N, Cunningham D, Falk R: Central venous access resulting in selective failure of ICD defibrillation capacity. *Pacing Clin Electrophysiol* 2001;24(3):394-395.
35. Bernstein AD, Irwin ME, Parsonnet V, et al: Report of the NASPE Policy Conference on antibradycardia pacemaker follow-up: Effectiveness, needs, and resources. North American Society of Pacing and Electrophysiology. *Pacing Clin Electrophysiol* 1994;17(11 pt 1):1714-1729.
36. Hayes JJ, Juknavorian R, Maloney JD: The role(s) of the industry employed allied professional. *Pacing Clin Electrophysiol* 2001;24(3):398-399.
37. Preisman S, Cheng DC: Life-threatening ventricular dysrhythmias with inadvertent asynchronous temporary pacing after cardiac surgery. *Anesthesiology* 1999;91(3):880-883.
38. Andersen C, Madsen GM: Rate-responsive pacemakers and anaesthesia. A consideration of possible implications. *Anaesthesia* 1990;45(6):472-476.
39. Levine PA: Response to "Rate-adaptive cardiac pacing: Implications of environmental noise during craniotomy." *Anesthesiology* 1997;87(5):1261.

40. Rozner MA, Nguyen AD: Unexpected pacing threshold changes during non-implant surgery. *Anesthesiology* 2002;96:A1070.

41. Levine PA: Clinical utility of automatic capture algorithms. In: The XII World Congress on Cardiac Pacing and Electrophysiology. Edited by Tse H-F, Lee K LF, Lau C-P. Medimond International Proceedings, Bologna, Italy, pages 601-608, 2003.

42. Interaction between minute ventilation rate-adaptive pacemakers and cardiac monitoring and diagnostic equipment. Center for Devices and Radiologic Health. Published Oct 14, 1998. Available at http://www.fda.gov/cdrh/safety/minutevent.html (accessed Jan 1, 2007).

43. Madsen GM, Andersen C: Pacemaker-induced tachycardia during general anaesthesia: A case report. *Br J Anaesth* 1989;63 (3):360-361.

44. von Knobelsdorff G, Goerig M, Nagele H, Scholz J: [Interaction of frequency-adaptive pacemakers and anesthetic management. Discussion of current literature and two case reports]. *Anaesthesist* 1996;45(9):856-860.

45. Van Hemel NM, Hamerlijnck RP, Pronk KJ, Van der Veen EP: Upper limit ventricular stimulation in respiratory rate responsive pacing due to electrocautery. *Pacing Clin Electrophysiol* 1989;12 (11):1720-1723.

46. Wong DT, Middleton W: Electrocautery-induced tachycardia in a rate-responsive pacemaker. *Anesthesiology* 2001;94(4):710-711.

47. Chew EW, Troughear RH, Kuchar DL, Thorburn CW: Inappropriate rate change in minute ventilation rate responsive pacemakers due to interference by cardiac monitors. *Pacing Clin Electrophysiol* 1997;20(2 pt 1):276-282.

48. Rozner MA, Nishman RJ: Pacemaker-driven tachycardia revisited. *Anesth Analg* 1999;88(4):965.

49. Wallden J, Gupta A, Carlsen HO: Supraventricular tachycardia induced by Datex patient monitoring system. *Anesth Analg* 1998;86(6):1339.

50. Southorn PA, Kamath GS, Vasdev GM, Hayes DL: Monitoring equipment induced tachycardia in patients with minute ventilation rate-responsive pacemakers. *Br J Anaesth* 2000;84(4):508-509.

51. Rozner MA, Nishman RJ: Electrocautery-induced pacemaker tachycardia: Why does this error continue? *Anesthesiology* 2002;96(3):773-774.

52. Lau W, Corcoran SJ, Mond HG: Pacemaker tachycardia in a minute ventilation rate-adaptive pacemaker induced by electrocardiographic monitoring. *Pacing Clin Electrophysiol* 2006;29(4): 438-440.

53. Rozner MA: Management of implanted cardiac defibrillators during eye surgery. *Anesth Analg* 2008;106(2):671-672.

16 When Should Pulmonary Function Tests Be Performed Preoperatively?

Anthony N. Passannante, MD, and Peter Rock, MD, MBA

INTRODUCTION

Pulmonary complications remain common after many surgical procedures, particularly those involving the upper abdomen or thorax.[1] Research concerning the diagnosis and prevention of perioperative cardiac complications after anesthesia and surgery has led to evidence-based intervention strategies such as widespread implementation of perioperative beta-blocker administration.[2] The situation regarding pulmonary complications is different. Many of the preoperative factors that make pulmonary complications more likely are known. A recent comprehensive review breaks down risk factors into those associated with the patient and those associated with the surgical procedure. Patient-associated risk factors include advanced age, American Society of Anesthesiologists (ASA) class 2 or higher, functional dependence, chronic obstructive pulmonary disease, smoking, and congestive heart failure. Surgical procedures associated with increased risk of pulmonary complications include aortic aneurysm repair, thoracic surgery, abdominal surgery, neurosurgery, emergency surgery, head and neck surgery, vascular surgery, and prolonged surgery.[3] Unfortunately, most of these risk factors are not modifiable in the preoperative period. Smoking cessation can safely be encouraged, but acute benefits from cessation are small.[4]

Perioperative care has changed significantly in the past 10 years, with the time between preoperative evaluation and surgery now often very brief. Surgical interventions themselves have changed significantly, often in ways that presumably reduce the likelihood of postoperative pulmonary complications. For example, the widespread application of laparoscopic techniques for many abdominal procedures may improve postoperative pulmonary function,[5] and the introduction and widespread application of video-assisted thoracic surgery and lung-volume reduction surgery has transformed patients who would have been previously told that their pulmonary function was "too bad" for surgery into operative candidates. In addition, the move toward very rapid ambulation and discharge from the hospital has ramifications that may positively affect those patients whose pulmonary function is improved by rapid resumption of the upright posture, and have negative implications for those who clear their secretions poorly at home.

Unfortunately, there is no standard definition of what constitutes a postoperative pulmonary complication. This hinders comparison of historical case series. Reported rates of pulmonary complications vary widely depending on the patient population studied and the surgical intervention studied.[3,6,7] The most important complications are those that cause significant morbidity such as pneumonia or respiratory failure. Preoperative pulmonary function tests have not been useful in performing better than clinical predictors in identifying patients who go on to develop clinically significant pulmonary complications.[3]

These issues, coupled with the relative insensitivity of pulmonary function testing in identifying patients who are going to experience complications, have resulted in more restrictive indications for preoperative pulmonary function testing than 20 years ago. An economic analysis entitled "Blowing Away Dollars" cast significant doubt on the practice of routine spirometric analysis before abdominal surgery.[8] However, it is clear that the incidence of pulmonary complications is increased in patients with preexisting pulmonary disease.[9] It is also clear that the physical examination is not very sensitive in detecting mild to moderate pulmonary disease.[10] Likewise, clinicians are not particularly accurate in estimating the severity of an exacerbation of chronic obstructive pulmonary disease (COPD).[11] There has been a significant shift away from ordering spirometry except in very specific circumstances (thoracic surgery and severe COPD). It may be that it is too much to expect a simple diagnostic test such as spirometry to result in improved outcome when outcome is, in reality, such a complex endpoint.

Some would argue that the ready availability of therapeutic options for bronchospasm may minimize the benefit of preoperative knowledge of the presence and severity of chronic or episodic pulmonary disease. These developments may be tied to the decline in use of preoperative pulmonary function tests, but it is more likely that as the use of spirometry to determine who was eligible or ineligible for surgical intervention went out of vogue (due largely to poor correlation between predicted postoperative forced expiratory volume in 1 second [FEV_1] and measured postoperative FEV_1), the enthusiasm clinicians felt toward ordering and interpreting the tests diminished.

As there are no meta-analyses or modern randomized, placebo-controlled therapeutic trials to review concerning preoperative pulmonary function tests, this chapter will review the evidence that does exist, and suggest a rational strategy for the utilization of preoperative pulmonary function tests. The fact that a noninvasive diagnostic test such as spirometry has not been shown to improve clinical outcome does not mean that it should never be ordered.

PULMONARY FUNCTION TESTING AND THERAPEUTIC OPTIONS

The term *pulmonary function test* is very broad. Examples of pulmonary function tests include measures of anatomic volumes, resistance to airflow, reversibility of increased airway resistance, and assessment of pulmonary reserve. Available tests include spirometry, flow volume loops, assessment of membrane surface area available for gas transport via diffusion capacity of the lung for carbon monoxide (DLCO), assessment of cardiopulmonary reserve by exercise testing, ventilation-perfusion scintigraphy, and split-function lung studies. For most clinical situations an anesthesiologist encounters, the pertinent tests will be spirometry and exercise testing. Patients about to undergo pulmonary resection may require more extensive evaluation, depending on the severity of their lung disease and on the magnitude of the planned pulmonary resection.[12] Reviews of individual tests are readily available for additional detail.[13-20]

Spirometry is a very low-risk, effort-dependent test that can be performed in a physician's office. Spirometric measurements such as the forced expiratory volume in 1 second (FEV_1), vital capacity (VC), and forced vital capacity (FVC) are well known to many clinicians. Spirometry is sensitive and specific for the accurate diagnosis of obstructive respiratory disease, and it may allow estimation of the effectiveness of bronchodilators in an individual patient. Diagnosis of restrictive lung disease requires measurement of lung volumes.

The second set of options that must be discussed are the therapeutic options. Pulmonary function tests allow accurate categorization of a patient's pulmonary disease. Accurate diagnosis should allow for effectively targeted preoperative therapy. The therapeutic options available for pulmonary disease are well described. Antibiotics can effectively treat pulmonary infection, bronchodilators (both beta-agonists and anticholinergics) can effectively treat bronchoconstriction, and steroid therapy may be helpful for subgroups of patients with asthma and COPD. Aggressive treatment with mechanical measures such as incentive spirometry can help minimize the frequency of postoperative pulmonary complications after abdominal surgery, but perhaps not after coronary artery bypass grafting.[7,21-23] A recent review of strategies to reduce postoperative pulmonary complications finds good evidence to support the postoperative use of lung expansion interventions (incentive spirometry, deep-breathing exercises, continuous positive airway pressure), fair evidence to support the selective use of nasogastric tubes after abdominal surgery and the use of short-acting neuromuscular blockers intraoperatively, and conflicting evidence concerning smoking cessation, epidural analgesia or anesthesia, and the use of laparoscopic surgical techniques.[24] Specific pulmonary rehabilitation programs have proven beneficial in improving cardiopulmonary capacity and may be useful in preparing patients for surgical intervention.[25]

EVIDENCE

There is no evidence of a beneficial effect from preoperative pulmonary function testing in asymptomatic patients having nonthoracic surgery. There is evidence that abnormal pulmonary function tests identify a group of patients who have a higher incidence of postoperative pulmonary complications.[9,26-29] Although historically pulmonary function testing was used to identify patients who were thought to be at excessive risk, recent experience shows that some patients with chronic hypercapnia (often used as a marker signifying inoperability) can safely undergo lung-volume reduction surgery.[30] As surgical practice has become more aggressive in patients with emphysema, it has become clear that removing a nonfunctional segment of pulmonary parenchyma can be surprisingly well tolerated.[31] However, there is also evidence that low FEV_1, in combination with knowledge of the homogeneity of emphysema or an estimate of carbon monoxide diffusing capacity, identifies patients at prohibitive risk from lung-volume reduction surgery.[32] There is also evidence that a surprisingly high percentage, 37% in one series, of patients may still be denied potentially curative lung cancer resection for non–small cell lung cancer on the basis of poor preoperative pulmonary function tests.[33]

Exercise testing is useful for examining cardiopulmonary integration and reserve, and it may allow identification of patients who are more likely to survive major thoracic surgical procedures.[34,35] Although formal exercise testing remains the gold standard for assessment of the maximal rate of total body oxygen consumption (VO_2max) and cardiopulmonary function, it is expensive, it is labor intensive, and it is not necessary in patients who can give a clear history of adequate exercise tolerance. If a patient cannot walk more than 2000 feet in 6 minutes, the patient's VO_2max is likely to be less than 15 mL/kg/min.[36] Exercise oximetry also shows promise in identifying patients who are at high risk of adverse outcomes.[37] A predicted postoperative VO_2max of less than 10 mL/kg/min may be one of the few remaining contraindications to pulmonary resection, because the reported mortality rate in this group of patients was 100% in one study.[38] Additional research is necessary to refine recommendations for preoperative estimation of cardiopulmonary reserve, but it appears that physiologic testing may offer advantages over simple spirometry in identifying patients at very high risk.[37,39] A recent study suggests that poor performance on exercise testing predicts patients who will experience extended stays after thoracic surgery.[40] The overall strength of the respiratory musculature is doubtless important as well, and efforts to increase the strength of the respiratory musculature may be helpful.[41]

There is now evidence that a rigorous preoperative pulmonary rehabilitation program directed at increasing exercise ability can improve patient well-being before surgery, may increase the number of frail patients with pulmonary disease who can reasonably undergo potentially curative thoracic surgery, and decrease postoperative pulmonary complications after cardiac surgery.[42-44]

AREAS OF UNCERTAINTY

There are many areas of uncertainty regarding when pulmonary function tests should be ordered preoperatively. In the absence of controlled clinical trials that demonstrate that pulmonary function testing is associated with improved outcome, it is difficult to recommend pulmonary function tests as a necessary prerequisite for any patient or surgical procedure. However, spirometry is inexpensive to obtain, very low risk, and accurate in diagnosing what may be clinically occult pulmonary disease. Although abnormal spirometry allows identification of a group of patients at elevated risk of pulmonary complications, it is poor at attempting to stratify risk among the patients at elevated risk.

GUIDELINES

The American College of Physicians offered the following guidelines in 1990, and they continue to be widely cited and followed. Patients undergoing lung resection may benefit from pulmonary function testing (in order, and as necessary, spirometry and arterial blood gas analysis, split perfusion lung scanning or exercise testing, and right-sided heart catheterization) as such testing may allow risk assessment. With regard to cardiac and upper abdominal surgery, it may be prudent to do preoperative arterial blood gas analysis and spirometry in patients with a history of tobacco use and dyspnea. However, the recent evidence-based guidelines published by the ACP do not recommend arterial blood gases.[24] For lower abdominal surgery, preoperative spirometry may be indicated for patients with uncharacterized pulmonary disease, particularly if the surgical procedure will be prolonged or extensive. For other types of surgery, pulmonary function tests might be useful for patients in whom uncharacterized pulmonary disease is present, particularly in those who might require strenuous postoperative rehabilitation programs.[45]

A set of guidelines aimed at reducing perioperative pulmonary complications in patients undergoing non-cardiothoracic surgery was published by the American College of Physicians in 2006. The six recommendations include screening for the patient-specific and procedure-specific risk factors listed in the introduction section of this chapter, screening for low serum albumin (an albumin less than 35 g/L predicts an increased risk of postoperative pulmonary complications), and the use of postoperative lung expansion maneuvers and indicated postoperative nasogastric tubes. The fifth recommendation states clearly that preoperative spirometry and chest radiography should not be used routinely for predicting postoperative pulmonary

risk. The last recommendation is that right-sided heart catheterization and total parenteral nutrition should not be used solely to attempt to reduce pulmonary complications from noncardiothoracic surgery.[46]

AUTHORS' RECOMMENDATIONS

It is clear that pulmonary function tests are not indicated in patients with a normal history and physical examination undergoing nonthoracic surgery. At the other extreme, it is clear that a wide variety of pulmonary function tests are useful in patients with chronic pulmonary disease undergoing lung volume reduction surgery, or a patient with marginal pulmonary function who has a thoracic malignancy. The authors believe that there has been an excessive shift against ordering and interpreting pulmonary function tests in patients between these two extremes. After all, the only accurate way to assess blood pressure is to measure it, and the only accurate way to identify obstructive or restrictive ventilatory impairments is to measure them with pulmonary function tests.[47] When there is doubt about the presence or absence of pulmonary disease, pulmonary function testing can end the doubt with little or no risk to the patient. Clinicians should not feel compelled to avoid pulmonary function testing when there is legitimate diagnostic uncertainty present after a thorough history and physical examination (Table 16-1).

Table 16-1 Evidence on Pulmonary Function Testing

Preoperative spirometry is not useful if the preoperative history and physical is normal.

Preoperative spirometry can classify undiagnosed lung disease accurately.

Preoperative pulmonary function testing allows clinicians to accurately assess the severity of lung disease in a patient with known preexisting lung disease.

Preoperative pulmonary function testing is well established in the preoperative workup of patients about to undergo pulmonary resection.

Preoperative spirometry should not be used in isolation to declare a patient ineligible for potentially curative surgical intervention, but can be used as a first step in an evaluation that includes a more global assessment of cardiopulmonary function, such as formal or informal exercise testing.

The evaluation of patients undergoing lung-volume reduction surgery is evolving. These patients are at very high risk, and it is likely that sophisticated anatomic, radiographic, and physiologic testing will be necessary to guide medical decision making in this patient group.

REFERENCES

1. Ferguson MK: Preoperative assessment of pulmonary risk. *Chest* 1999;115(5 suppl):58S-63S.
2. Poldermans D et al: Bisoprolol reduces cardiac death and myocardial infarction in high-risk patients as long as 2 years after successful major vascular surgery. *Eur Heart J* 2001;22(15): 1353-1358.

3. Smetana GW, Lawrence VA, Cornell JE: Preoperative pulmonary risk stratification for noncardiothoracic surgery: Systematic review for the American College of Physicians. *Ann Intern Med* 2006;144(8):581-595.

4. Barrera R et al: Smoking and timing of cessation: Impact on pulmonary complications after thoracotomy. *Chest* 2005;127(6):1977-1983.

5. Frazee RC et al: Open versus laparoscopic cholecystectomy. A comparison of postoperative pulmonary function. *Ann Surg* 1991;213(6):651-653, discussion 653-654.

6. Stephan F et al: Pulmonary complications following lung resection: A comprehensive analysis of incidence and possible risk factors. *Chest* 2000;118(5):1263-1270.

7. Celli BR, Rodriguez KS, Snider GL: A controlled trial of intermittent positive pressure breathing, incentive spirometry, and deep breathing exercises in preventing pulmonary complications after abdominal surgery. *Am Rev Respir Dis* 1984;130(1):12-15.

8. De Nino LA et al: Preoperative spirometry and laparotomy: Blowing away dollars. *Chest* 1997;111(6):1536-1541.

9. Kroenke K et al: Postoperative complications after thoracic and major abdominal surgery in patients with and without obstructive lung disease. *Chest* 1993;104(5):1445-1451.

10. Badgett RG et al: Can moderate chronic obstructive pulmonary disease be diagnosed by historical and physical findings alone? *Am J Med* 1993;94(2):188-196.

11. Emerman CL, Lukens TW, Effron D: Physician estimation of FEV_1 in acute exacerbation of COPD. *Chest* 1994;105(6):1709-1712.

12. Martin J: Lung resection in the pulmonary-compromised patient. *Thorac Surg Clin* 2004;14(2):157-162.

13. Cain H: Bronchoprovocation testing. *Clin Chest Med* 2001;22(4):651-659.

14. Crapo RO, Jensen RL, Wanger JS: Single-breath carbon monoxide diffusing capacity. *Clin Chest Med* 2001;22(4):637-649.

15. Culver BH: Preoperative assessment of the thoracic surgery patient: Pulmonary function testing. *Semin Thorac Cardiovasc Surg* 2001;13(2):92-104.

16. Flaminiano LE, Celli BR: Respiratory muscle testing. *Clin Chest Med* 2001;22(4):661-677.

17. Gibson GJ: Lung volumes and elasticity. *Clin Chest Med* 2001;22(4):623-635, vii.

18. Pride NB: Tests of forced expiration and inspiration. *Clin Chest Med* 2001;22(4):599-622, vii.

19. Weisman IM, Zeballos RJ: Clinical exercise testing. *Clin Chest Med* 2001;22(4):679-701, viii.

20. Mazzone PJ, Arroliga AC: Lung cancer: Preoperative pulmonary evaluation of the lung resection candidate. *Am J Med* 2005;118(6):578-583.

21. Morran CG et al: Randomized controlled trial of physiotherapy for postoperative pulmonary complications. *Br J Anaesth* 1983;55(11):1113-1117.

22. Stock MC et al: Prevention of postoperative pulmonary complications with CPAP, incentive spirometry, and conservative therapy. *Chest* 1985;87(2):151-157.

23. Freitas E et al: Incentive spirometry for preventing pulmonary complications after coronary artery bypass graft. *Cochrane Database Syst Rev* 2007(3):CD004466.

24. Lawrence VA, Cornell JE, Smetana GW: Strategies to reduce postoperative pulmonary complications after noncardiothoracic surgery: Systematic review for the American College of Physicians. *Ann Intern Med* 2006;144(8):596-608.

25. Ries AL et al: The effects of pulmonary rehabilitation in the national emphysema treatment trial. *Chest* 2005;128(6):3799-3809.

26. Kanat F et al: Risk factors for postoperative pulmonary complications in upper abdominal surgery. *Aust N Z J Surg* 2007;77(3):135-141.

27. Poe RH et al: Can postoperative pulmonary complications after elective cholecystectomy be predicted? *Am J Med Sci* 1988;295(1):29-34.

28. Barisione G et al: Upper abdominal surgery: Does a lung function test exist to predict early severe postoperative respiratory complications? *Eur Respir J* 1997;10(6):1301-1308.

29. Fuso L et al: Role of spirometric and arterial gas data in predicting pulmonary complications after abdominal surgery. *Respir Med* 2000;94(12):1171-1176.

30. Wisser W et al: Chronic hypercapnia should not exclude patients from lung volume reduction surgery. *Eur J Cardiothorac Surg* 1998;14(2):107-112.

31. Lederer DJ et al: Lung-volume reduction surgery for pulmonary emphysema: Improvement in body mass index, airflow obstruction, dyspnea, and exercise capacity index after 1 year. *J Thorac Cardiovasc Surg* 2007;133(6):1434-1438.

32. National Emphysema Treatment Trial Research Group: Patients at high risk of death after lung-volume-reduction surgery. *N Engl J Med* 2001;345(15):1075-1083.

33. Baser S et al: Pulmonary dysfunction as a major cause of inoperability among patients with non-small-cell lung cancer. *Clin Lung Cancer* 2006;7(5):344-349.

34. Walsh GL et al: Resection of lung cancer is justified in high-risk patients selected by exercise oxygen consumption. *Ann Thorac Surg* 1994;58(3):704-710, discussion 711.

35. Win T et al: Cardiopulmonary exercise tests and lung cancer surgical outcome. *Chest* 2005;127(4):1159-1165.

36. Cahalin L et al: The relationship of the 6-min walk test to maximal oxygen consumption in transplant candidates with end-stage lung disease. *Chest* 1995;108(2):452-459.

37. Rao V et al: Exercise oximetry versus spirometry in the assessment of risk prior to lung resection. *Ann Thorac Surg* 1995;60(3):603-608, discussion 609.

38. Bolliger CT et al: Lung scanning and exercise testing for the prediction of postoperative performance in lung resection candidates at increased risk for complications. *Chest* 1995;108(2):341-348.

39. Wang JS, Abboud RT, Wang LM: Effect of lung resection on exercise capacity and on carbon monoxide diffusing capacity during exercise. *Chest* 2006;129(4):863-872.

40. Weinstein H et al: Influence of preoperative exercise capacity on length of stay after thoracic cancer surgery. *Ann Thorac Surg* 2007;84(1):197-202.

41. Nomori H et al: Preoperative respiratory muscle training. Assessment in thoracic surgery patients with special reference to postoperative pulmonary complications. *Chest* 1994;105(6):1782-1788.

42. Takaoka ST, Weinacker AB: The value of preoperative pulmonary rehabilitation. *Thorac Surg Clin* 2005;15(2):203-211.

43. Jones LW et al: Effects of presurgical exercise training on cardiorespiratory fitness among patients undergoing thoracic surgery for malignant lung lesions. *Cancer* 2007;110(3):590-598.

44. Erik HJ, Hulzebos PT: Preoperative intensive inspiratory muscle training to prevent postoperative pulmonary complications in high-risk patients undergoing CABG surgery. *JAMA* 2006;296:1851-1857.

45. ACP: Preoperative pulmonary function testing. *Ann Intern Med* 1990;112:793-794.

46. Qaseem A et al: Risk assessment for and strategies to reduce perioperative pulmonary complications for patients undergoing noncardiothoracic surgery: A guideline from the American College of Physicians. *Ann Intern Med* 2006;144(8):575-580.

47. Petty TL: The forgotten vital signs. *Hosp Pract (Off Ed)* 1994;29(4):11-12.

PERIOPERATIVE MANAGEMENT

17 Does the Airway Examination Predict Difficult Intubation?

Satyajeet Ghatge, MD, and Carin A. Hagberg, MD

INTRODUCTION

Difficult airway management is one of the most challenging tasks for anesthesiologists. Recent data from the American Society of Anesthesiologists (ASA) Management Closed Claims Project, specifically those findings related to the difficult airway, demonstrate that the percentage of claims resulting from adverse respiratory events, though on the decline (42% in the 1980s to 32% in the 1990s),[1] continue to constitute a large source of injury. A closed claims analysis of the management of the difficult airway published in 2005 showed that out of the 179 claims made between 1985 and 1999 (n = 179), 87% (n = 156) of claims came from the perioperative period. More recent closed claims analyses demonstrated that claims resulting in death and brain damage from difficult airway management were associated with induction of anesthesia but not other phases of anesthesia decreased from 1993 to 1999, as compared to 1985 to 1992.[2] In 2006, a closed claims analysis of trends in anesthesia-related death and brain damage showed an overall reduction in claims for death or brain damage between 1975 and 2000 (odds ratio [OR] 0.95 per year; 95% confidence interval [CI], 0.94 to 0.96, $p <0.01$). Out of all the respiratory events (n = 503) responsible for death or brain damage, difficult intubation (n = 115), inadequate oxygenation (n = 111) and esophageal intubation (n = 66) were the top three causes.[3]

Of the three types of adverse respiratory events reported, claims for inadequate ventilation and esophageal intubation decreased significantly in the 1990s (9% as compared with 25% of claims for death and brain damage in the 1980s), possibly as a result of pulse oximetry and end-tidal carbon dioxide monitoring. Yet the proportion of claims for difficult intubation (a technical act, uninfluenced by monitoring) and other respiratory events leading to death or brain damage remained relatively stable between the 1980s and 1990s (9% and 8%, respectively). Of the adverse respiratory events, three quarters were judged to be preventable. Thus it is *possible* that better prediction of and preparation for difficult airway management might lead to a reduction in these numbers.

Anesthesiologists are confronted daily with the difficult task of determining whether or not a patient will present increased difficulty for endotracheal intubation. Preoperative evaluation of the airway can be accomplished by a thorough history and physical examination, as related to the airway, and various measurements of anatomic features and noninvasive clinical tests can be performed to enhance this assessment. Nonetheless, several reports have questioned whether true prediction is possible.[4-6]

DESCRIPTION OF TERMS

Four terms are important to a review and analysis in this area: *failed intubation, difficult intubation, difficult laryngoscopy,* and *difficult mask ventilation.* The ASA Task Force on Management of Difficult Airway suggests the following descriptions:[7]

Failed intubation, or the inability to place the endotracheal tube (ET) after multiple intubation attempts, is a clear-cut endpoint. Thus there is a fairly uniform reported incidence of approximately 0.05% or 1:2230 of surgical patients, and of approximately 0.13% to 0.35% or 1:750 to 1:280 of obstetric patients.[8,9]

Difficult tracheal intubation (DI) is described as intubation when tracheal intubation requires multiple attempts, in the presence or absence of tracheal pathology. The incidence of DI is higher than failed intubation and has been reported as 1.2% to 3.8 %.[10-13]

Difficult laryngoscopy (DL) is described as not being able to visualize any portion of the vocal cords after multiple attempts at conventional laryngoscopy, and many investigators include grades III and IV or grade IV alone, according to the Cormack-Lehane original grading of the rigid laryngoscopic view[14] (Figure 17-1). According to these definitions, the incidence of difficult direct laryngoscopy varies from 1.5% to 13% in patients undergoing general surgery.[8,15-21]

Difficulty in performing endotracheal intubation is the end result of difficulty in performing laryngoscopy, which depends on the operator's level of expertise, patient characteristics, and circumstances. Thus it has been suggested that the definition of difficult intubation be based on a uniform understanding of the *best* attempt at performing laryngoscopy/intubation and should use the number of attempts and time as boundaries only.[22] The best attempt should incorporate the effect of changing the patient's position; the effect of changing the length or type of laryngoscope blade; and the effect of simple maneuvers, such as conventional cricoid pressure, backward, upward, rightward pressure (BURP), and optimal external laryngeal manipulation (OELM).

Original Cormack-Lehane system	I Full view of the glottis	II Partial view of the glottis or arytenoids		III Only epiglottis visible	IV Neither glottis nor epiglottis visible
View at laryngoscopy	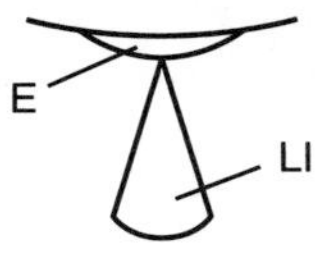 E ⟍⟋ LI	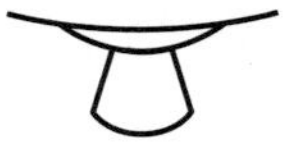	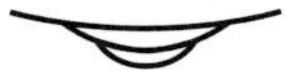	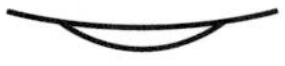	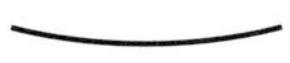
Modified system Cormack-Lehane	I As for original Cormack- Lehane above	IIa Partial view of the glottis	IIb Arytenoids or posterior part of the vocal cords only just visible	III As for original Cormack- Lehane above	IV As for original Cormack- Lehane above

Figure 17-1. Cormack-Lehane Original Grading System Compared with a Modified Cormack-Lehane System (MCLS) *E*, epiglottis; *LI*, laryngeal inlet. *Reproduced with permission from Yentis SM, Lee DJH: Evaluation of an improved scoring system for the grading of direct laryngscopy. Anesthesia 1998;53:1041-1044.*

Difficult mask ventilation (DMV) is a condition in which it is not possible for the anesthesiologist to provide adequate face mask ventilation due to one or more of the following problems: inadequate mask seal, excessive gas leak, or excessive resistance to the ingress or egress of gas.[23] It is clear from clinical experience that there are grades of difficulty, similar to difficult intubation. The incidence of DMV also varies in the literature from 0.01% to 5%.[12,13,24,25]

Difficult laryngeal mask airway ventilation (DLMAV) is a situation in which difficulty is experienced in ventilating and oxygenating a patient on a laryngeal mask airway (LMA). Even though not defined by ASA, researchers have defined this as inability to place the LMA in a satisfactory position within three attempts to allow adequate ventilation and airway patency. Indices of clinically adequate ventilation are generally expired tidal volume greater than 7 mL/kg and leak pressure greater than 15 to 20 cm H_2O. Verghese and Brimacombe,[26] in their study of more than 11,000 patients, had a failure rate of 0.16%.

Descriptive Terms Used for Predicting Difficult Airway

Five terms are commonly used to analyze the usefulness of predictive tests.[27]

Sensitivity: Identifies all difficult intubations as being difficult. A sensitivity of 90% indicates that 90% of difficult intubations will be identified as difficult and 10% will be missed and falsely stated as not difficult/ normal. Ideally, sensitivity should be 100%.

Specificity: Identifies all normal intubations as being normal. A sensitivity of 90% indicates that 90% of normal patients will be identified as normal and 10% will be falsely identified as difficult. Ideally, specificity should be 100%.

Positive predictive value (PPV): The percentage of patients who are true difficult intubations from all those predicted by the test to be difficult intubations. If the test predicts 20 difficult intubations and only 4 are actually difficult, the PPV for the test is 20%. Even though PPV is a useful test, it is limited by the fact that it is dependent on the prevalence of difficult intubation in the sample group.

Likelihood ratio (LR): This is a useful term and can be calculated very quickly using sensitivity and specificity only. It is the chance of a positive test if the person is a difficult intubation divided by the chance of a positive test if the patient was normal. LR is sensitivity/1 − specificity. It can be seen as a factor that links pretest probability to posttest probability of difficult intubation using a nomogram.

Receiver operating characteristic curves (ROCs): These help in determining the best predictive scores. The ROC has sensitivity on the *y*-axis and 1 − specificity on the *x*-axis. The test with greatest area under the curve is the better one.

PREDICTION OF THE DIFFICULT AIRWAY: THE PROBLEM

There has been a heightened awareness of and a steady rise in the amount of literature being published on the recognition and prediction of the difficult airway. To evaluate the evidence supporting the various methods of prediction of the difficult airway, it is important to realize the actual endpoints and their effect on patient outcome, in terms of mortality or brain death. The frequency of airway difficulty varies according to the population studied and the definition of difficult intubation used.[13] There is no universally accepted definition of difficult intubation. Most of the larger studies concentrate on difficult intubation, broadly defined by difficult rigid laryngoscopic view (Cormack-Lehane grades III and IV or grade IV only), *without* the best attempt used. To be useful, a classification of laryngeal view should predict difficulty (or ease) of tracheal intubation, requiring the views to be associated with increasing degrees of intubation difficulty. Yet, in a study of 1200 patients, Arne and colleagues[10] found that there was a significant difference between the incidence of Cormack-Lehane grades III and IV laryngoscopic view and the occurrence of difficult intubation in the general population, as many of the grade III and IV views were actually easy intubations. Thus one of the problems in the prediction of the difficult airway is that a difficult intubation is often not identified until laryngoscopy is performed and, as mentioned previously, there are discrepancies in the literature as to what defines difficulty.

Several authors have suggested the modification of the four-grade Cormack-Lehane scoring system[21,28,29] (see Figure 17-1), which classifies the laryngeal view during laryngoscopy. This widely adopted classification system was described to allow simulated difficult intubation, yet it is applied inaccurately by the majority.[30] Yentis and Lee[29] modified this scoring system by subdividing a grade II laryngoscope view into IIa (partial view of glottis visible) and IIb (only arytenoids visible). This five-grade classification is referred to as the modified Cormack-Lehane system (MCLS) and allows refining the definition of difficult laryngoscopy as including IIb, III, and IV[29] (Figure 17-2). Koh and colleagues[30] found that this system better delineated the difficulty experienced during laryngoscopy and intubation than the four-grade Cormack-Lehane system. Thus the true incidence of difficult laryngoscopy may be underestimated, because it excludes a subgroup of the original grade II (IIb), which may be difficult to manage.

Cook[32] further divided the Yentis and Lee modified systems into 3a (epiglottis can be seen and lifted) and 3b (epiglottis visualized but cannot be lifted); thus it consists of six grades, divided into three functional classes: easy, restricted, and difficult. *Easy* views were defined as when the laryngeal inlet is visible and thus suitable for intubation under direct vision (grades 1 and 2a). *Restricted* views were defined as when the posterior glottic structures (posterior commissure or any arytenoid cartilages) are visible or the epiglottis is visible and can be lifted (grades 2b and 3a). These views are likely to benefit from indirect intubation methods (e.g., gum elastic bougie). *Difficult* views were defined as when the epiglottis cannot be lifted or when no laryngeal structures are visible, which are likely to need specialist methods for intubation and may need to be performed blindly (grades 3b and 4). Cook proposes that this three-category classification system is of more practical value and has greater discrimination than Cormack-Lehane's. He found that an easy view predicts easy intubation in 95% of cases and has less than 3% need of any intubation adjuncts. A difficult view is associated with difficult intubation in three quarters of cases, and specialist intubation techniques are likely to be required. Between these extremes, a restricted view is likely to require the use of a gum bougie, but no other adjuncts.

It would be useful to predict difficult intubation before it occurs, but no preoperative test has adequate sensitivity to identify most cases without substantial false positives.[33]

Several prospective studies have identified various individual characteristics, which have significant association with laryngoscopic or intubation difficulties.[9,13,18,20,34-38] Sensitivity and positive predictive values (PPVs) of these individual variables are low, ranging from 33% to 71% for specificity. Several combinations of these variables have been shown to be more effective predictors of difficult intubation.

To make a meaningful evaluation of the available literature, it is important to make an assumption about a reasonable level of expectancy in terms of sensitivity and specificity of the tests used for prediction of difficult intubation. Thus, in order to predict at least 9 out of 10 difficult intubations, a sensitivity of 90% will be required. And, if we assume that one false alarm a week is acceptable, in a hypothetical practice of 10,000 cases a year, it would correspond to a specificity of 99.5%.[39] A number of investigators have attempted to achieve the goal of predicting difficult laryngoscopy or difficult intubation, or both, by combining different predictors and deriving multivariate indices so that the occurrence of false negatives is decreased and the PPVs are increased.[10,12,25] Yet, to date, no single multifactorial index can be applied to all of the various surgical populations. Also, most, with the exception of Wilson's index, have not been validated prospectively.[19,21]

New investigative modalities, including x-rays, ultrasound, and three-dimensional computed tomography (CT) scans of the airway, have been proposed to help predict a difficult airway.[32,40] A recent review performed by Sustic[41] suggests that ultrasound can be used to assess anatomy of the upper respiratory organs and possibly assist in various applications of airway management.

The Upper Lip Bite Test (ULBT),[42] a new, simple clinical bedside test performed by having the patient attempt to bite his or her own upper lip, has recently been suggested to aid in the prediction of difficulty with intubation. A recent external prospective evaluation of the reliability and validity of ULBT demonstrated that the interobserver reliability was better than the Modified Mallampati Score (Mallampati classification, as modified by Samsoon and Young[9]). They also found that they could not use the test on edentulous patients (11% of total 1425 patients), and concluded that like the Modified Mallampati Score, the ULBT was a *poor* predictor when used as a single screening test.[43]

Additionally, advanced computing techniques over the last decade have improved statistical analysis, allowing improved testing of variables for successful prediction of the difficult airway.[23] Nonetheless, given the low incidence of difficult intubation and the wide variation in acceptable definitions of airway terms, it is difficult to compare different studies and perform a meta-analysis of the predictors of difficult airway management.

EVIDENCE

History

After thorough review of the literature, there is insufficient published evidence to evaluate the effect of either a bedside medical history or of reviewing prior medical

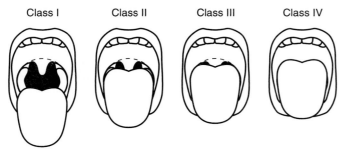

Figure 17-2. Modified Mallampati Classification.

Class I   Class II   Class III   Class IV

records on predicting the presence of a difficult airway. According to the ASA Task Force, there is *suggestive* evidence (as defined by the ASA that there is enough information from case reports and descriptive studies to provide a directional assessment of the relationship between a clinical intervention and a clinical outcome) that some features of both *may be* related to the likelihood of encountering a difficult airway.[7]

Many congenital and acquired syndromes are associated with difficult airway management, some of which are listed in Table 17-1. Also, certain disease states, such as obstructive sleep apnea[44] and diabetes,[45] have been suggested to correlate with an increased risk of difficult intubation. Trauma to the airway, either caused by external forces or iatrogenic from routine endotracheal intubation, may also be associated with difficult airway management. Recently, Tanaka and colleagues[46] demonstrated increased airflow resistance attributable to intraoperative swelling of the laryngeal soft tissues in patients who were normal (easy) airways and underwent routine tracheal intubation. Others have observed serious laryngeal injuries (e.g., vocal cord paralysis, arytenoid cartilage subluxation, laryngeal granulomas, and scars) following short-term intubation and anesthesia.[47] Additionally, the ASA Task Force found that a previous history of difficult airway management offers clinically suggestive evidence that difficulty may recur.[7]

Physical Examination

Single Predictors of Difficult Laryngoscopy/ Intubation

The ability of a specific test to predict a difficult intubation is decreased by the variability of definitions of difficult laryngoscopy and intubation and the inherent inaccuracy of numeric grading systems.[30] Nonetheless, several investigations have identified anatomic features that have unfavorable influences on the mechanics of direct laryngoscopy and endotracheal intubation (Table 17-1). The majority of anesthesiologists rely on predicting difficult intubation mainly as a result of several preoperative bedside screening tests.

Mallampati Classification. The Mallampati classification (MPT)[48] focuses on the relative visibility of oropharyngeal structures when the patient is examined in the sitting position with the mouth fully opened, the tongue fully extended, and without phonation. Samsoon and Young[9] modified (MMP) the originally proposed three oropharyngeal classes to four classes (see Figure 17-2), yet Ezri[49] and Maleck[50] further suggest adding a fifth class, class 0, defined as the ability to visualize any part of the epiglottis on mouth opening and tongue protrusion. Samsoon and Young's method is by far the most widely investigated method of airway evaluation and its association with difficult intubation. The practical value of this method lies in its ease of application, yet practitioners often perform this examination in the supine position with or without phonation. A wide range of observations shows that this method is subject to significant interobserver variability. Overall, the literature suggests that the true sensitivity of the Mallampati classification, as modified by Samsoon and Young, is most likely between 60% and 80% and the

true specificity between 53% and 80%, with a PPV of approximately 20%. A recent meta-analysis of the accuracy of Mallampati classification found substantial differences and variabilities in reported sensitivity and specificity values. Overall accuracy of the test was poor to good and depended on which version of the test and reference tests were used.[51] The meta-analysis also suggested that the Mallampati test was a poor predictor of difficult mask ventilation.[51]

Krobbuaban and colleagues[52] found that Mallampati Class III and IV had a sensitivity of 70% and specificity of 60% with a PPV of 20.

Additionally, a recent study suggested that the best way to perform Mallampati classification was by placing the patient in the sitting position, with the patient's head in full extension, tongue protruded, and *with* phonation, yet phonation did not influence the overall accuracy of this classification.[53]

Mashour and Sandberg[54] evaluated 60 patients first with the Modified Mallampati (MMP) test and then repeated the examination with craniocervical extension. They found that by including craniocervical extension, the MMP scores were reduced. Class 2 MMP became Class 1.6, Class 3 became 2.6, and Class 4 became 3.5. The sensitivity remained the same but the specificity improved from 70% to 80%. The PPV increased from 24% to 31% and negative predictive value (NPP) increased marginally from 97% to 98%.[54]

A recent study of 1956 patients determined that the Mallampati classification is insufficient in predicting difficult intubation on its own.[55]

Thyromental Distance. The concept of thyromental distance (TMD), noted as the distance between the chin and the notch of the thyroid cartilage, was described by Patil and associates in 1983.[23] They proposed that this distance should be 6.5 cm in the normal adult and that if this distance is less than 6 cm, there may be intubation difficulties. Among all the morphometric measurements, TMD has been questioned the most for its value in predicting difficult intubation.[56] The sensitivity of this test is between 60% and 80% with a specificity of 80% to 90% in some studies.[9,13,31,32] Arne and colleagues[10] and El-Ganzouri and colleagues[25] found the test to be highly insensitive (sensitivity 16% to 17%), but very specific (specificity 95% to 99%) with a PPV of 12% to 16%, if a more stringent definition of difficult intubation involving best attempt (with OELM) is applied.

Recently, the role of TMD has been challenged by some authors.[5,6] Chou and Wu[6] suggest that the receding mandible, one of the two components of a micrognathic mandible, is not the real cause for difficult laryngoscopy in these patients, thus TMD is irrelevant. Wong and Hung[57] studied TMD, along with the Mallampati classification and atlanto-occipital extension (AOE), and demonstrated the limitation of absolute anatomic measurements in their study involving Chinese women. The optimal TMD criterion was 5.5 cm in this study, to achieve a sensitivity of 71% and specificity of 83%, yet the PPV was only 7.5%.[57] Schmitt and colleagues[58] attempted to adjust this measurement to the patient's size and proposed the ratio of the patient's height to thyromental distance. Using the receiver operating characteristic curve, they found a cutoff

Table 17-1 Evidence of Single Predictors of Difficult Intubation

Predictors	Study	# Patients	Incidence (%)	Sensitivity (%)	Specificity (%)	Positive Predictive Value (%)	Negative Predictive Value (%)	Definition of Difficult Intubation*	Best Attempt	Population
	Arne, 1998[10]	1200	4	78	85	19	99	4	+	General + ENT
	Savva, 1994[20]	355	1.14	64.7	66.1	8.9		1, 3 and 4	+	General + OB (10%)
	Oates et al., 1991[19]	675	1.8	42	84	4			-	General
	Butler & Dhara, 1992[15]	220	8.2	56	81	21			-	General
	Frerk, 1991[16]	244	4.5	81	82	17			-	General
	Rose & Cohen, 1994[13]	18558	1.8	Relative Risk - 4.5				3 > 2 attempts	-	General
Mallampatti III or IV	Voyagis, 1998[69]	1833	8.3	88.1 / 86.8		37.2 / 50	Original** / Modified**	1	-	Obese / General
	Bergler et al., 1997[44]	91	10	60	72				-	General + ENT
	Brodsky, 2002[72]	100	12	58.3	70.5			1 & 3	-	Morbidly Obese
	Khan et al., 2003[42]	300	5.7	82.4	66.8	13	98.4	1	-	General
	Yamamoto et al., 1997[81]	3680	1.3	67.9	52.5	2.2		1	+	General
	El-Ganzouri et al., 1996[25]	10507	1	44.7 / 59.8	89	21 / 4.4	96.1	1 / 2	+	General
	Wong et al., 1999[57]	411	1.99	85.7	62.6	3.8	99.6	1	-	Chinese ♀
IV Only	Savva, 1994[20]	355	1.14	52.9		87		1, 3 & 4	+	General + OB (10%)
	Wong et al., 1999[57]			28.6	98.3	22.2	98.8	1	-	Chinese ♀
TMD										
<6	Butler & Dhara, 1992[15]	220	8.2	62	25	16			-	General

Continued

Table 17-1   Evidence of Single Predictors of Difficult Intubation—Cont'd

Predictors	Study	# Patients	Incidence (%)	Sensitivity (%)	Specificity (%)	Positive Predictive Value (%)	Negative Predictive Value (%)	Definition of Difficult Intubation*	Best Attempt	Population
<6	El Ganzouri, 1996[25]	10507	1	7	99.2	38.5	94.3	1	+	
				16.8	99	15.4	99.1	2		General
<6.5	Savva, 1994[20]	355	1.14	65	81	15		1, 3 & 4	+	General + OB (10%)
<6.5	Arne, 1998[10]	1200	4	16	95	12	96	4	+	General + ENT
<7	Frerk, 1991[16]	244	4.5	91	82	19			–	General
<7	Schmitt, 2002[58]	270	5.9	81	73			1	+	General
RHTMD										
25	Schmitt, 2002[58]	270	5.9	81	91			1	+	General
SMD	Savva, 1994[20]	355	1.14	82.4	88.6	26.9		1, 3 & 4	+	General + OB (10%)
<12.5										
NECK MOVEMENT										
<80°	El-Ganzouri, 1996[25]	10137	1	10.4	98.4	29.5	94.4	1		General
				16.78		7.9		2		
<90°	Arne, 1998[10]	1200		54	85	14	98			General + ENT
AOE										
<35°	Wong, 1999[57]	411		85	70	4.8		1	–	Chinese ♀
Obesity										
BMI > 30 kg/m²	Voyagis, 1998[69]	1833	8.3	88.9		66.7				Obese

*Definition of Difficult Intubation:
1) Cormack and Lehane Grade III or IV
2) Cormack and Lehane Grade IV only
3) # of attempts
4) Special Techniques and Others
**Original = tongue-protruded by the patient
Modified = tongue-actively pulled out by anesthesiologist

TMD = Thyromental distance
RHTMD = Ratio
SMD = Sternomental distance
AOE = Atlanto-occipital extension
BMI = Body mass index
ENT = Ears, nose, & throat
OB = Obstetric
♀ = Female

value to be 25 or greater for this ratio to predict difficult laryngoscopy with a reasonable degree of sensitivity (81%) and specificity (90%).

A recent meta-analysis performed by Shiga and colleagues[59] stated, "the diagnostic value of thyromental distance proved unsatisfactory in their analysis." They determined that there was a wide range in the sensitivity, which could possibly be due to different cutoff points (4.0 to 7.0 cm) They also found that the positive likelihood ratio of TMD improved from 3.4 to 4.1 when a more strict cutoff criterion (less than 6.0 cm) was applied.[59]

Recently, Krobbuaban and colleagues[52] conducted a prospective randomized study on 550 consecutive Thai patients. They found that the ratio of height to thyromental distance (RHTMD) had higher sensitivity (77%), higher PPV (24%), and fewer false negatives (16%). They also found that RHTMD greater than or equal to 23.5, neck movement less than 80 degrees, and MMP III-IV were major predictors of difficult laryngoscopy. Rosenstock and colleagues[60] found that the interobserver agreement for TMD and neck mobility was low.

Hyomental Distance. Hyomental distance (HMD), a measurement from the tip of the chin to the hyoid cartilage, has also been considered one of the predictors of difficult intubation. Both TMD and HMD give an idea of the available space for the tongue during laryngoscopy. In an investigation involving 12 cadavers and 334 patients, Turkan and colleagues[4] found that mean HMDs were less than the stated limit of 7 cm[61] and that HMD was the only objective variable not affected by age, by using cervical spine radiographs of patients in the neutral position. However, both McIntyre[62] and Randall[56] demonstrated that radiologic measurements have not been able to provide sensitive criteria for prediction of difficult intubation, and that radiographic studies were, at best, regarded valuable in understanding problems encountered during laryngoscopy.

Sternomental Distance. Sternomental distance (SMD), a measurement from the tip of the chin to the sternal notch, normally greater than 12.5 cm, was suggested by Savva[20] to predict difficult intubation if less than 12 cm with maximal head extension. Savva[20] found this measurement to be both more sensitive and more specific than TMD and that this measurement may give a more accurate estimate of head extension. This measure functionally "added" the atlanto-occipital joint into the physical evaluation of the airway.[63] Ramadhani and colleagues[64] suggested that SMD was a superior measurement, as compared to others, by showing that SMD had an increased sensitivity (71.1%) and specificity (66.7%) for predicting subsequent difficult laryngoscopy and it was unaffected by age. However, the patient group in their study was limited to women of childbearing age only. Turkan and colleagues,[4] on the other hand, demonstrated that SMD measurements were affected both by age and gender, as both younger (20 to 30 years) and male patients had longer SMD measurements.

In their meta-analysis, Shiga and colleagues[59] found that SMD yielded moderate sensitivity and specificity. It also yielded a high positive likelihood ratio and diagnostic odds ratio.[59] The negative likelihood ratio for SMD was the lowest, suggesting that it could be the best single test for ruling out difficult intubation. Nonetheless, their study was based on only three studies that included SMD.[59]

Neck Movement and Mouth Opening. Neck movement and mouth opening have also been considered as variables in predicting difficult intubation. El-Ganzouri and colleagues[25] demonstrated that three single variables, such as restricted head and neck movement, including flexion and especially extension capability (less than 80°[23] or less than 90°[8]), along with restricted mouth opening (less than 4 cm[23] or less than 5 cm[8]) and inability to protrude the mandible have a significant association with difficult intubation. The accuracy of the estimation of AOE using the Bellhouse test has been questioned, and similar to other clinical methods, is subject to wide interobserver variability.[65]

Individual examinations and tests are subject to wide interobserver variability, thus any evidence needs to be evaluated accordingly. In a study involving 59 patients, Karkouti and colleagues[66] found that mouth opening and chin protrusion had *excellent* interobserver reliability, whereas seven tests (TMD, mandible subluxation, AOE and angle, profile classification, ramus length, oropharyngeal best view) were only *moderately* reliable between observers, and that the Mallampati technique of assessing oropharyngeal view had *poor* interobserver reliability.[67]

Rosenstock and colleagues[60] evaluated the interobserver reliability of the Simplified Airway Risk Index (SARI). The parameters used in SARI include mouth opening, TMD, ability to protrude mandible, Mallampati score, head and neck mobility, and body weight. Two pairs of assessors (two specialists and two residents) performed the assessment. They used five tests (out of a total of seven) from SARI and evaluated 120 normal patients and 16 documented difficult intubation patients. They found good interobserver agreement with mouth opening, Mallampati class, and mandibular protrusion, whereas TMD and neck movement had low levels of interobserver agreement.[60]

In Yildiz and colleagues'[68] multicenter study, the most sensitive criterion when used alone was mouth opening (sensitivity of 43%). In their study, the incidence of difficult intubation was significantly higher in patients with Mallampati class III-IV, a decreased average TMD and SMD, decreased mouth opening, or decreased protrusion of mandible ($p < 0.05$). Combination of the tests did not improve their results.[68]

Rose and Cohen[13] analyzed the data regarding problems and prediction of difficult airway management in 18,500 patients and found that although the most common single abnormalities noted were restricted neck movement (3%) and decreased visualization of the hypopharynx (2.2%), with a relative risk of 3.2 and 4.5, respectively, decreased mouth opening (less than 2 fingers; relative risk 10.3) and shortened TMD (less than 3 fingers; relative risk 9.7) were the best single predictive factors of difficult tracheal intubation.

Weight. Obesity has been studied as isolated body weight (greater than 110 kg)[25] or body mass index (BMI; greater than 30 kg/m²)[69] and shown to be associated with difficult laryngoscopy, especially when accompanied with a large tongue (as assessed by Mallampati classification).

Recently, Juvin and colleagues,[70] in a study involving 134 lean (BMI less than 30 kg/m^2) and 129 obese (BMI 35 kg/m^2 or greater) determined that difficult intubation is more common among obese than nonobese patients by using the Intubation Difficulty Scale (IDS) developed by Adnet and colleagues,[71] which includes both qualitative and quantitative dimensions of difficult intubation. It is an objective scoring system involving seven variables: number of intubation attempts, skill and experience of the operators, alternative intubation techniques, glottic exposure (Cormack-Lehane), lifting force applied to the laryngoscope, application of external laryngeal pressure, and position of the vocal cords at intubation. In this study, they defined two groups of patients according to the IDS values: those with an IDS score less than 5 (easy and slightly difficult) or 5 or greater (difficult). They found that among the classic risk factors for difficult intubation, only a Mallampati score of III or IV is a risk factor for difficult intubation in obese patients (odds ratio, 12.51, specificity of 62%, and PPV of 29%). They also determined that the risk of hypoxemia is higher in obese patients during anesthesia induction, and that further investigation is necessary to identify the risk factors for difficult intubation in this population.[48]

Shiga and colleagues[59] found that the incidence of difficult intubation in obese patients (BMI greater than 30 kg/m^2) was more than three times higher than in normal patients. Also, Cattano and colleagues[55] found that obesity had the highest sensitivity (32%) and PPV of 16 for predicting difficulty of intubation. The same sensitivity (32%) was found with a Mallampati score of class III-IV.

Brodsky and colleagues,[72] on the other hand, studied 100 consecutive morbidly obese subjects (BMI greater than 40 kg/m^2) and concluded that neither absolute body weight (obesity) nor BMI is associated with intubation difficulties. Rather, they found that a *large neck circumference* (measured at the level of the superior border of the cricothyroid cartilage) of 40 cm showed a 5% probability and of 60 cm showed a 35% probability of problematic intubation, and high (III or greater) Mallampati scores are the only predictors of potential intubation problems in this patient population. Thus, whether tracheal intubation is more difficult in obese patients is debatable.

Komatsu and colleagues[73] used ultrasound to quantify anterior neck soft tissue thickness and predict difficult laryngoscopy in 64 morbidly obese patients (BMI ≥35 kg/m^2). They performed an ultrasound scan of the anterior neck soft tissue and measured the distance from the skin to the anterior aspect of the airway at the level of vocal cords. In contrast to Brodsky's findings, they concluded that the thickness of pretracheal soft tissue at the level of vocal cords is *not* a good predictor of difficult laryngoscopy in both Caucasian and African-American obese patients. In contrast, Ezri and colleagues[48] studied Middle Eastern patients and determined that soft tissue in the neck did influence difficulty in intubation.

Additionally, Siegel and colleagues[74] demonstrated that ultrasound of the airway was a reliable, simple, and comfortable method of identifying the mechanism of airway obstruction. The role of preintubation ultrasound assessment elsewhere in the upper airway for the detection of pharyngeal or laryngeal pathology, such as tumors, abscesses, or epiglottitis, has also been studied.[75,76] Because of these discrepancies in the literature, convincing evidence to correlate soft tissue thickness of the neck with difficult intubation does not exist.[73]

Combined Predictors of Difficult Laryngoscopy and Intubation

Although no single factor has been shown to be a predictor of difficult intubation on its own, it has been widely suggested that combinations of factors improve predictability of difficult intubation. Various combinations of individual predictors have been studied and several multivariable indices have been proposed (Table 17-2), but very few have been prospectively evaluated for their efficacy. In his editorial, Wilson[33] concluded that no single test is likely to be a perfect predictor of difficult intubation, and Bainton[77] suggests that the most satisfactory solution would be the "best algebraic sum" of several tests.

Shiga and colleagues'[59] recent study of bedside screening tests for predicting difficult intubation in apparently normal people suggested that by combining the MPT and TMD difficult intubation is predicted more accurately. In their meta-analysis of 35 studies involving 50,760 patients, they found that MPT and TMD combined have the highest discriminative power. Patients with 5% pretest probability of DI showed a 34% risk of DI after a positive result for the combination, 16% risk after a positive result for MPT alone, and 15% risk for TMD alone.[59]

Krobbuaban and colleagues[52] found that RHTMD greater than 23.5 (PPV 24, FN 16), Mallampati class III-IV (PPV 20, FN 21), and neck movement less than 80° (PPV 22, FN 60) were the major factors in predicting difficult laryngoscopy. RHTMD had a higher PPV, higher sensitivity, and fewer false negatives than the other factors. The multivariate analysis odds ratios (95% confidence interval) of the RHTMD, Mallampati class, and neck movement were 6.72 (3.29 to 13.72), 2.96 (1.63 to 5.35), and 2.73 (1.14 to 6.51), respectively. The interincisor gap (less than 3.5 cm) and TMD (less than 6.5 cm) were not recognized as independent variables for difficult laryngoscopy.[52]

Matthew and colleagues[78] found all 22 patients with known difficult intubation to have a TMD less than 6 cm and Mallampati classifications of III or IV, whereas all 22 matched controls (easy intubations) had a TMD greater than 6.5 cm and Mallampati classification of I or II. By prospectively testing this combination in 244 patients, Frerk[16] found a sensitivity of 80% and a specificity of 98%. Wong and Hung,[57] on the other hand, found it to be 71% and 92% in 411 Chinese women, of whom 151 were pregnant. Janssens and Hartstein[79] and Janssens and Lamy[80] recently developed a new scoring system, the Airway Difficulty Score (ADS), for predicting difficult intubation in which a TMD less than 6 cm, Mallampati class greater than 1, mouth opening less than 4 cm, reduced neck mobility, and presence of upper incisors related to airway difficulty. A score between 5 and 15 is given for each patient, and a score of 8 or greater is considered a potentially difficult intubation. When compared to the Intubation Difficulty Scale (IDS), they found a 75% sensitivity,

Table 17-2 Evidence of Multivariate Predictors of Difficult Intubation

Authors/ Reference No.	No. of Patients	Incidence of Difficult Intubation (%)	Sensitivity (%)	Specificity (%)	Positive Predictive Value (%)	Negative Predictive Value (%)	Definition of Difficult Intubation*	Best Attempt	Population Excluded	False Negative (%)	Misclassification Rate (%)	Association with Difficult Intubation
Wong[57]	411	1.54 nonpregnant 1.99 pregnant	71.4	95.5	21.7		1	–	Non-Chinese and Chinese men	+		
Wilson[21]	778	1.5	75	88	9	99	1	–	obstetric (OB) & ears, nose, and throat (ENT)	0.4	12	
Pottecher et al.[39]	663	5.8	70	84	21	98	1	–	ENT	1.8	17	
El Ganzouri et al.[25]	10570	1	65	94	10	99	2	+	OB & ENT	0.3	7	
Arne et al.[10] (gen surg) (simplified score)	717	2.5	94	96	37	99	4	+	ENT/OB	0.2	4	
Arne et al.[10] (global pop.) (simplified score)	1090	3.8	93	93	34	99	4	+	OB	0.3	7	
Naguib[84] (discriminate eqn.) (clinical criteria)	56	42	95.4	91.2	87.5	96.9	1+3	–				
Naguib[84] (discriminate eqn.) (clinical + radiologic)	56	42	95.8	96.9	95.8	96.9	1+3	–				
Oates et al.[19] (Wilson Risk Sum)	675	1.8	42	92	9		1					
Yamamoto et al.[81] (Wilson Risk Sum)	3608	1.3	55.4	86.1	5.9		1	+				

*Definition of difficult intubation:
1.) Cormack-Lehane Grade III or IV
2.) Cormack-Lehane Grade IV only
3.) No. of attempts
4.) Special techniques and others

85.7% specificity, an excellent negative predictive value (NPV) (98.7%), and a low PPV (18.6%). This score allows the clinician to distinguish difficulty in maintaining upper airway patency and the difficulty with alignment of the axes and in visualizing the larynx. Scoring systems, such as the ADS and the IDS,[70] require further investigation and inclusion of more definitive variables.

Recently, Iohom and colleagues,[40] in a study involving 212 nonobstetric patients, found that by combining Mallampati classification of III or IV with either a thyromental distance less than 6.5 cm or a sternomental distance less than 12.5 decreased the sensitivity (from 40% to 25% and 20%, respectively), but maintained an NPV of 93%. The specificity and PPVs increased from 89% and 27%, respectively, for Mallampati alone to 100%. Thus they suggest that the Mallampati classification, in conjunction with measurement of the TMD and SMD, may be a useful routine screening test for preoperative prediction of difficult intubation.[40]

Wilson and colleagues[21] examined a combination of five risk factors (Wilson Risk Sum): weight, head and neck movement, jaw movement, receding mandible, and buck teeth. One of three levels is assigned per risk, with a level of 0 representing no risk for difficult intubation and a level of 2 representing the greatest risk for difficult intubation.[21] Wilson's group suggested that a score of 2 would correspond to a test that had sensitivity of 75% and specificity of 85%, yet this test would not be applicable to children or pregnant women because of the weight classification. Oates and colleagues,[19] on the other hand, found the Wilson Risk Sum to have a sensitivity of 42% and a specificity of 92%, with a PPV of 9%. When compared to the Mallampati classification, they found it to be slightly superior. Yamamoto and colleagues[81] tested the same scoring in 3608 patients and found the sensitivity to be slightly better (55%), but the specificity and PPVs were 86% and 5.5%, respectively.

Wong and Hung[57] derived the following regression equation: DL = 2.73 − 0.1 TMD − (0.01 AOE − 0.1 Mallampati) and concluded that the laryngoscopic grade would be higher (i.e., greater difficulty intubation) if the combination of AOE and Mallampati yielded a more negative value. They termed the combination of AOE and Mallampati, both of which are independent of body build, as the Predictor of Intubation Difficulty (PID) and used a PID of 0 or less as the criterion for prediction of difficult intubation. They found a sensitivity of 71%, a specificity of 95.5%, and a PPV of 21.7%. This study of Chinese women, including pregnant women, was an attempt to neutralize the effect of body build on absolute anatomic measurements and their limitation as predictors of difficult intubation.

Bellhouse and Dore[82] identified radiographic predictors in patients with known difficult airways and suggested three closely corresponding clinical measures: Mallampati classification III or IV, limited AOE, and receding chin. Since there has been no formal prospective evaluation of their findings, the sensitivity and specificity of this combination of predictors are unknown.

Rocke and colleagues,[8] in their rare study involving 1500 obstetric patients, found four predictors of difficult intubation: Mallampati's classification, receding mandible, short neck, and protruding maxillary incisors. Tse and associates[83] evaluated the combination of Mallampati's classification, head extension, and thyromental distance in 471 patients. They found that combinations of mediators generally seemed to improve specificity, thus decreasing the chance of false alarms, but at the cost of sensitivity, which means missing a large proportion of potential difficult intubations.

El-Ganzouri and colleagues[25] prospectively studied 10,507 patients who underwent surgery under general anesthesia to determine what parameters might be associated with difficult intubation. They derived a composite airway risk index with an odds ratio used to weigh the risk of individual parameters, including mouth opening, Mallampati classification, neck mobility, ability to protrude the mandible, body weight, and a history of difficult intubation. By retrospectively applying a simplified risk index (0 = low, 1 = medium, 2 = high), they found a sensitivity of 65%, a specificity of 94%, and a PPV of 10%, which corresponded to a 1% incidence of difficult intubation (defined as laryngoscopic view of IV alone), as assessed by an experienced anesthesiologist after the best attempt.

Arne and colleagues[10] performed a prospective analysis of 1200 ear, nose, and throat (ENT) and general surgical patients in order to develop and validate a predictive clinical multifactorial risk index aimed at predicting difficult tracheal intubation. They identified seven criteria as independent predictors of difficult intubation, defined as the need to use special techniques as assessed by two senior anesthesiologists, after their *best* attempts in performing endotracheal intubation. A simplified risk index was formulated using regression coefficients as the relative weight of individual predictors. The best predictive threshold for the sum was chosen as 11 using the receiver operating characteristic curve. This scoring system was then prospectively evaluated in a population of 1090 consecutive patients. The sensitivity and specificity were 94% and 96% in general surgery, 90% and 93% in noncancer ENT surgery, and 92% and 66% in ENT cancer surgery, respectively. They claim that the index is investigator-independent, with a 7% misclassification rate. The population studied included only a small number of patients with cervical spine pathology, and patients with a history of spondylosis, rheumatoid arthritis. or occipital atlanto-axial diseases were not included.

Naguib and colleagues[84] evaluated 24 patients in whom unanticipated difficult intubation occurred, along with a control group of 32 patients in whom intubation was easily accomplished, using clinical and radiologic data. They identified four clinical risk factors: thyromental distance, thyrosternal distance, neck circumference, and Mallampati classification. Using both clinical and radiologic data, discriminant analysis identified five risk factors: TMD, thyrosternal distance, Mallampati classification, depth of the second cervical vertebrae spinous process, and the angle at the most antero-inferior point of the upper central incisor tooth. Although a PPV of 95.8% in a study population with an incidence of difficult intubation of 42% is not realistic, the possible role of advanced radiologic techniques such as three-dimensional computer imaging in the prediction of difficult intubation cannot be ignored.

Cattano and colleagues[55] demonstrated that the MPT versus Cormack-Lehane linear correlation index was 0.904. A Mallampati class III correlated with a Cormack-Lehane grade 2 (0.94), and a Mallampati class IV correlated with Cormack-Lehane grade 3 (0.85) and Cormack-Lehane 4 (0.80).[55]

Difficult Mask Ventilation

Although failure to intubate may not necessarily lead to hypoxia and hypoxemia, failure to ventilate *will* cause these adverse consequences. Interestingly, the majority of the literature on prediction of the difficult airway does not include factors predicting difficult mask ventilation (DMV). Williamson and colleagues[85] analyzed 2000 incident reports and indicated a 15% incidence of DMV in patients who had difficult or failed intubation. El-Ganzouri and colleagues[25] found an incidence of 0.08% in their study of 10,507 patients and determined that approximately 100,000 patients would be required to apply a multivariate analysis. They defined DMV as the inability to obtain chest excursion sufficient to maintain a clinically acceptable capnogram waveform despite optimal head and neck positioning, use of muscle paralysis, use of an oral airway, and optimal application of a face mask. Langeron and colleagues[12] observed a 5% incidence of DMV, defined as the inability of an unassisted anesthesiologist to maintain oxygen saturation greater than 92% or to prevent or reverse signs of inadequate ventilation during positive-pressure mask ventilation under general anesthesia. In their study of 1502 patients that excluded ENT, obstetric, and emergency patients, they found five criteria (age more than 55 years, BMI greater than 26 kg/m^2, lack of teeth, presence of a beard, history of snoring) to be independent risk factors for DMV, with two of these criteria indicating a high likelihood of DMV (sensitivity of 72%; specificity of 73%). Lower rates of DMV have been reported in prospective studies by Asai and colleagues[24] (1% to 4%), Rose and Cohen[13] (0.9%), and El-Ganzouri and colleagues,[25] as mentioned earlier. Obviously, there is a lack of a standardized definition for DMV, which could explain the variation in the incidence.

Kheterpal and colleagues[86] found 37 cases (0.16%) of grade 4 MV (impossible to ventilate) and 313 cases (1.4%) of grade 3 MV (difficult to ventilate) out of 22,660 cases. They used a grade 1 to 4 classification, in which grade 1 was easy to ventilate by mask, grade 2 was able to ventilate by mask but with an oral airway/adjuvant with or without muscle relaxant, grade 3 was difficult ventilation (inadequate/unstable or requiring two providers) with or without muscle relaxant, and grade 4 was unable to ventilate with or without muscle relaxant. Out of the 37 cases of grade 4 MV, 1 required an emergency cricothyrotomy, 10 were difficult intubations, and 26 were easy intubations. They identified six predictors for grade 3 MV: BMI greater than 30 kg/m^2, beard, Mallampati class III-IV, age 57 years or older, reduced jaw protrusion, and snoring. Of these

six predictors, the only modifiable predictor was the presence of a beard. They could identify only two predictors for grade 4 MV: snoring and TMD less than 6 cm. They also found that 84 patients with grade 3 or 4 MV were difficult to intubate (0.37%). They suggested that the mandibular protrusion test or UBLT may be an essential element of airway assessment.[86]

Airway Assessment and LMA Use

McCrory and colleagues[87] studied 100 patients by assessing their airway with the original Mallampati classification (MPT) and then placing an LMA. Adequate ventilation was possible in 98 patients, and in 2 patients LMA insertion was abandoned and anesthetic was continued with guedel airway and facemask ventilation. They performed fiber-optic laryngoscopy to view the laryngeal inlet and found that seating of the LMA was suboptimal in 30 patients and that there was no view of laryngeal inlet in 7 patients. All of these 7 patients were Mallampati class III. They concluded that an increasing occlusion of laryngeal inlet and increasing difficulty of LMA insertion occurred with Mallampati classes II and III. They also found that the number of attempts needed for LMA insertion increased with Mallampati classes II and III. Eighteen patients with Mallampati class II needed two attempts, and in Mallampati III, 5 patients needed two attempts and 3 patients needed three attempts. In 2 patients with Mallampati class III, LMA insertion was abandoned (failed insertion after three attempts). The limitation of this study was that there was a small number of Mallampati class III patients ($n = 10$), in 7 of whom there was no view of vocal cords on fiber-optic laryngoscopy and in 2 of whom LMA placement was abandoned.

Intubatability versus Ventilatability—"Can't Intubate, Can't Oxygenate" (CICO)

"Can't intubate, can't oxygenate" (CICO) is a clinical situation in which the anesthesiologist is unable to intubate or perform effective ventilation. Hypoxemia and death can occur quickly unless emergency transtracheal oxygenation is provided.[27] Nonetheless, it is evident that in a number of situations when facemask ventilation fails and intubation is difficult, the laryngeal mask can provide a satisfactory airway. Although a CICO situation is rare in elective patients, guidelines have been established (see www.das.uk.com).

AREAS OF UNCERTAINTY

Preoperative evaluation is important in the detection of patients at risk of difficult airway management, noting any anatomic features and clinical factors associated with the difficult airway,[4,8,10,11,13,14,88] but it is still uncertain whether true prediction is possible[11,23,83,89-91] and which variables should be chosen.[7] The majority of individual predictors appear to have a strong association with the occurrence of difficult intubation, but none of the combinations previously discussed has provided satisfactory results in terms of sensitivity and specificity. The reasons could be the low incidence of the end result (e.g., difficult intubation) and the conflicting inverse relationship between sensitivity and specificity, especially because of the critical nature of the outcome (i.e., death or brain damage). Nonetheless, false positives are clearly less dangerous than false negatives and every patient undergoing anesthetic intervention is subject to the possibility of the occurrence of problems with airway management. Difficult airway management in specific patient populations, including pregnant, obese, pediatric, and those undergoing surgery involving the airway, may require unique considerations. Further investigation of the supraglottic ventilatory devices (e.g., Laryngeal Mask Airway, Esophageal Tracheal Combitube, etc.), as well as the flexible or rigid fiber-optic laryngoscopes, and predictions for difficulty in their use, or how their use can overcome difficult intubation, despite unfavorable traditional predictors for difficult intubation, is necessary. Last, the integration of practice guidelines, as outlined in the next section, into clinical practice is difficult to monitor, making it difficult to directly evaluate their utility regarding patient outcome.

GUIDELINES

There are current guidelines published by national[7] and international[85,86,89] societies that address the issue of interventions in order to reduce perioperative airway complications during management of the difficult airway.

The ASA appointed a task force to develop the ASA's "Practice Guidelines for Management of the Difficult Airway," which were first adopted by the ASA in 1992 and recently revised.[7] The purpose of these guidelines is to facilitate the management of the difficult airway and to reduce the likelihood of adverse outcomes.

These guidelines include the following recommendations:

1. History

An airway history should be conducted, whenever feasible, before the initiation of anesthetic care and airway management in all patients. The intent of the airway history is to detect medical, surgical, and anesthetic factors that may indicate the presence of a difficult airway. Examination of previous anesthetic records, if available in a timely manner, may yield useful information about airway management.

2. Physical Examination

An airway physical examination should be conducted, whenever feasible, before the initiation of anesthetic care and airway management in all patients. The intent of this examination is to detect physical characteristics that may indicate the presence of a difficult airway. Multiple airway features should be assessed, as in Table 17-3.

3. Additional Evaluation

Additional evaluation may be indicated in some patients to characterize the likelihood or nature of the anticipated airway difficulty. The findings of the airway history and physical examination may be useful in guiding the selection of specific diagnostic tests and consultation.

Table 17-3 Components of the Preoperative Airway Physical Examination

	Airway Examination Component	Nonreassuring Findings
1	Length of upper incisors	Relatively long
2	Relation of maxillary and mandibular incisors during normal jaw closure	Prominent "overbite" (maxillary incisors anterior to mandibular incisors)
3	Relation of maxillary and mandibular incisors during voluntary protrusion of the lower jaw	Patient cannot bring mandibular incisors anterior to (in front of) maxillary incisors
4	Interincisor distance	Less than 3 cm
5	Visibility of uvula	Not visible when tongue is protruded with patient in sitting position (e.g., Mallampati class greater than II)
6	Shape of palate	Highly arched or very narrow
7	Compliance of mandibular space	Stiff, indurated, occupied by mass, or nonresilient
8	Thyromental distance	Less than three ordinary finger breadths
9	Length of neck	Short
10	Thickness of neck	Thick
11	Range of motion of head and neck	Patient cannot touch tip of chin to chest or cannot extend neck

AUTHORS' RECOMMENDATIONS

Based on the evidence from randomized controlled trials and the vast body of literature regarding methods for airway evaluation, airway examination does *not* predict difficult intubation. Nonetheless, although current tests are not foolproof, a careful, systematic approach to a historical and physical evaluation of the airway in each patient should be performed.

The following suggestions should serve as a guide to aid clinical judgment and help guide anesthesiologists' decisions about airway management techniques with both patients and surgeons.

1. Use a list of individual predictors (Table 17-4) to separate out patients for further evaluation.
2. Determine whether there are any combinations of individual predictors that may lead to difficulty.
3. Perform any additional testing, including radiographic or endoscopic evaluation, or both, and obtain a preoperative consultation with other specialists (otolaryngologist, pulmonologist, oncologist, thoracic surgeon) in patients with a known or clinically suspicious difficult airway.
4. Review of the above information (suggestions 1 through 3) by an expert or team of experts to consider factors predicting difficult mask ventilation, difficult laryngoscopy, difficult intubation, and difficulty in the performance of a surgical airway, and together formulate a plan, as well as alternative plans, for airway management.

5. Finally, the practitioner should always be prepared by having a difficult airway cart ready and available, and practicing difficult airway drills, as well as special techniques that are helpful in the management of the patient with a difficult airway.[39]

Being able to more accurately predict DMV, difficult laryngoscopy, difficult intubation, and difficulty in the performance of fiber-optic intubation or a surgical airway should, in all likelihood, reduce the number of adverse outcomes and improve the safety of airway management. At least for now, reliable prediction of a difficult intubation remains an unsolved problem and is likely to remain a decision based on clinical judgment.

Table 17-4   **Suggested Contents of the Portable Storage Unit for Difficult Airway Management**

1 Rigid laryngoscope blades of alternate design and size from those routinely used; this may include a rigid fiber-optic laryngoscope
2 Tracheal tubes of assorted sizes
3 Tracheal tube guides. Examples include (but are not limited to) semirigid stylets, ventilating tube changer, light wands, and forceps designed to manipulate the distal portion of the tracheal tube
4 Laryngeal mask airways of assorted sizes; this may include the intubating laryngeal mask airway and the *LMA-Proseal* (LMA North America, Inc., San Diego, CA)
5 Flexible fiber-optic intubation equipment
6 Retrograde intuabtion equipment
7 At least one device suitable for emergency noninvasive airway ventilation. Examples include (but are not limited to) an esophageal tracheal Combitube (Kendall-Sheridan Catheter Corp., Argyle, NY), a hollow jet ventilation stylet, and a transtracheal jet ventilator
8 Equipment suitable for emergency invasive airway access (e.g., cricothyrotomy)
9 An exhaled CO_2 detector

REFERENCES

1. Cheney FW: Changing trends in anesthesia-related death and permanent brain damage. ASA Closed Claims Project. *ASA Newsletter* 2002;66:6-8.
2. Peterson GN, Domino KB, Kaplan RA, Posner KL, Lee LA, Cheney FW: Management of the difficult airway. A closed claims analysis. *Anesthesiology* 2005;103:33-39.
3. Cheney FW, Posner KL, Lee LA, Kaplan RA, Domino KB: Trends in anesthesia-related death and brain damage. *Anesthesiology* 2006;105:1081-1086.
4. Turkan S, Ates Y, Cuhruk H, Tekdemir I: Should we reevaluate the variables for predicting the airway in anesthesiology? *Anesth Analg* 2002;94:1340-1344.
5. Jacobsen J, Jensen E, Waldan T, Poulsen TD: Preoperative evaluation of intubation conditions in patients scheduled for elective surgery. *Acta Anaesthesiol Scand* 1996;40:421-424.
6. Chou HC, Wu TL: Thyromental distance—shouldn't we redefine its role in the prediction of difficult laryngoscopy? *Acta Anaesthesiol Scand* 1998;42:136-137 (letter).
7. Practice guidelines for management of the difficult airway: An updated report by the American Society of Anesthesiologists Task Force on management of the difficult airway. *Anesthesiology* 2003;98:1269-1277.
8. Rocke DA, Murray WB, Rout CC, Gouws E: Relative risk analysis of factors associated with difficult intubation in obstetric anesthesia. *Anesthesiology* 1992;77:67-73.
9. Samsoon GL, Young JRB: Difficult tracheal intubation: A retrospective study. *Anaesthesia* 1987;42:487-490.
10. Arne J, Descoins P, Fusciardi J, et al: Preoperative assessment for difficult intubation in general and ENT surgery: Predictive value of a clinical multivariate risk index. *Br J Anaesth* 1998;80:140-146.
11. Cattano D, Pescini A, Paolicchi A, Giunta F: Difficult intubation: An overview on a cohort of 1327 consecutive patients. *Minerva Anestesiol* 2001;67:45.
12. Langeron O, Mazzo E, Huraux C, et al: Prediction of difficult mask ventilation. *Anesthesiology* 2000;92:1229-1236.
13. Rose DK, Cohen MM: The airway: Problems and prediction in 18,500 patients. *Can J Anaesth* 1994;41:372-383.
14. Cormack RS, Lehane J: Difficult tracheal intubation in obstetrics. *Anaesthesia* 1984;39:1105-1111.
15. Butler PJ, Dhara SS: Prediction of difficult laryngoscopy: An assessment of thyromental distance and Mallampati predictive tests. *Anaesth Intensive Care* 1992;20:139-142.
16. Frerk CM: Predicting difficult intubation. *Anaesthesia* 1991;46:1005-1008.
17. Lewis M, Keramati S, Benumof JL, Berry CC: What is the best way to determine oropharyngeal classification and mandibular space length to predict difficult laryngoscopy? *Anesthesiology* 1994;81:69-75.
18. Mallampatti SR, Gatt SP, Gugino LD, et al: A clinical sign to predict difficult tracheal intubation: A prospective study. *Can Anaesth Soc J* 1985;32:429-434.
19. Oates JDL, Macleod AD, Oates PD, et al: Comparison of two methods for predicting difficult intubation. *Br J Anaesth* 1991;66:305-309.
20. Savva D: Prediction of difficult tracheal intubation. *Br J Anaesth* 1994;73:149-153.
21. Wilson ME, Spiegelhalter D, Robertson JA, Lesser P: Predicting difficult intubation. *Br J Anaesth* 1988;61:211-216.
22. Benumof JL: The difficult airway. In Benumof JL, editor: *Airway management principles and practice.* St. Louis, Mosby–Year Book, 1996, p 121.
23. Patil VU, Stehling LC, Zauder HL: Predicting the difficulty of intubation utilizing an intubation guide. *Anesthesiol Rev* 1983;10:32.
24. Asai T, Koga K, Vaughan RS: Respiratory complications associated with tracheal intubation and extubation. *Br J Anaesth* 1998;80:767-775.
25. El-Ganzouri AR, McCarthy RJ, Tuman KJ, Tanck EN, Ivankovich AD: Preoperative airway assessment: Predictive value of a multivariate risk index. *Anesth Analg* 1996;82:1197-1204.
26. Verghese C, Bricacombe JR: Survey of LMA usage in 11910 patients: Safety and efficacy for conventional and unconventional usage. *Anesth Analg* 1996;82:129-133.
27. Pearce A: Evaluation of the airway and preparation for difficulty. *Best Practice and Research Clinical Anaesthesiology* 2005;19(4):559-579.
28. Takahata S, Kubota M, Mamiya K, et al: The efficacy of the "BURP" maneuver during a difficult laryngoscopy. *Anesth Analg* 1997;84:419-421.
29. Yentis SM, Lee DJH: Evaluation of an improved scoring system for the grading of direct laryngoscopy. *Anaesthesia* 1998;53:1041-1044.
30. Cohen AM, Fleming BG, Wace JR: Grading of direct laryngoscopy. A survey of current practice. *Anaesthesia* 1994;49:522-525.
31. Koh LD, Kong CF, Ip-Yam PC: The modified Cormack-Lehane score for the grading of direct laryngoscopy: Evaluation in the Asian population. *Anaesth Intensive Care* 2002;30:48-51.
32. Cook TM: A new practical classification of laryngeal view. *Anaesthesia* 2000;55:274-279.
33. Wilson ME: Predicting difficult intubation. *Br J Anaesth* 1993;71:333-334 (editorial).
34. Block C, Brechner VL: Unusual problems in airway management. *Anesth Analg* 1971;50:114-123.
35. Brechner VL: Unusual problems in the management of airways: Flexion-extension mobility of the cervical vertebrae. *Anesth Analg* 1968;47:362-373.

36. Calder I, Calder J, Crockard HA: Difficult direct laryngoscopy in patients with cervical spine disease. *Anaesthesia* 1995;50: 756-763.
37. Cass NM, James NR, Lines V: Difficult direct laryngoscopy complicating intubation for anaesthesia. *BMJ* 1956;3:488-489.
38. Chou HC, Wu TL: Mandibulohyoid distance in difficult laryngoscopy. *Br J Anaesth* 1993;71:335-339.
39. Wheeler M, Ovassapian A: Prediction and evaluation of the difficult airway. In Hagberg CA, editor: *Handbook of difficult airway management.* Philadelphia, Churchill Livingstone, 2000, pp 15-30.
40. Iohom G, Ronayne M, Cunningham AJ: Prediction of difficult tracheal intubation. *Eur J Anaesthesiol* 2003;20:31-36.
41. Sustic A: Role of ultrasound in the airway management of critically ill patients. *Crit Care Med* 2007;35(suppl 5):S173.
42. Khan ZH, Kashfi A, Ebrahimkhani E: A comparison of the upper lip bite test (a simple new technique) with modified Mallampati classification in predicting difficulty in endotracheal intubation: A prospective blinded study. *Anesth Analg* 2003;96:595-599.
43. Eberhart LHJ, Arndt C, Cierpka T, Schwanekamp J, Wulf H, Putzke C: Reliability and validity of the upper lip bite test compared with the Mallampati classification to predict difficult laryngoscopy: An external prospective evaluation. *Anesth Analg* 2005;101(1):284-289.
44. Shapiro BA, Glassenberg R, Panchal S: The incidence of failed or difficult intubation in different surgical populations. *Anesthesiology* 1994;81:A1212 (abstract).
45. Nadal JLY, Fernandez BG, Escobar IC, et al. The palm print as a sensitive predictor of difficult laryngoscopy in diabetics. *Acta Anaesthesiol Scand* 1998;42:199-203.
46. Tanaka A, Isono S, Ishikawa T, Sato J, Nishino T: Laryngeal resistance before and after minor surgery: Endotracheal tube versus laryngeal mask airway. *Anesthesiology* 2003;99:252-258.
47. Komron RM, Smoth CP: Laryngeal injury with short term anesthesia. *Laryngoscope* 1983;83:683-690.
48. Mallampati SR: Clinical sign to predict difficult tracheal intubation (hypothesis). *Can Anaesth Soc J* 1983;30:316.
49. Ezri T, Cohen Y, Geva D, Szmuk P: Pharyngoscopic views. *Anesth Analg* 1998;87:748 (letter).
50. Maleck W, Koetter K, Less S: Pharyngoscopic views. *Anesth Analg* 1999;89:256-257 (letter).
51. Lee A, Fan LTY, Karmakar MK, Ngan Kee WD: A systematic review (meta-analysis) of the accuracy of the Mallampati tests to predict difficult airway. *Anesth Analg* 2006;102 (6):1867-1878.
52. Krobbuaban B, Diregpoke S, Kumkeaw S, Tanomsat M: The predictive value of the height ratio and thyromental distance: Four predictive tests for difficult laryngoscopy. *Anesth Analg* 2005;101 (5):1542-1545.
53. Reed MJ, Dunn MJG: Can airway assessment score predict difficulty at intubation in the emergency department? *Emerg Med J* 2005;22:99-102.
54. Mashour GA, Sandberg S: Craniocervical extension improves the specificity and predictive value of the Mallampati airway evaluation. *Anesth Analg* 2006;103(5):1256-1259.
55. Cattano D, Panicucci E, Paolicchi A, Forfori F, Giunta F, Hagberg C: Risk factor assessment of the difficult airway: An Italian survey of 1956 patients. *Anesth Analg* 2004;99(6):1774-1779.
56. Randall T: Prediction of difficult intubation. *Acta Anaesthesiol Scand* 1996;40:1016-1023.
57. Wong SHS, Hung CT: Prevalence and prediction of difficult intubation in Chinese women. *Anaesth Intensive Care* 1999;27: 49-52.
58. Schmitt HJ, Kirmse M, Radespiel-Troger M: Ratio of patient's height of thyromental distance improves prediction of difficult laryngoscopy. *Anaesth Intensive Care* 2002;30:763-765.
59. Shiga T, Wajima Z, Inoue T, Sakamoto A: Predicting difficult intubation in apparently normal patients. *Anesthesiology* 2005;103(2):429-437.
60. Rosenstock C, Gillesberg I, Gatke MR, Levin D, Kristensen MS, Rasmussen LS: Inter-observer agreements of tests used for prediction of difficult laryngoscopy tracheal intubation. *Acta Anaesthesiol Scand* 2005;49(8):1057-1062.
61. Morgan AE, Mikhail MS, editors: *Clinical anesthesiology.* New York, Appleton-Lange, 1996, pp 50-72.
62. McIntyre JWR: The difficult tracheal intubation: Continuing medical education article. *Can J Anaesth* 1987;30:204-213.
63. Rosenblatt WH: Airway management. In Barash PG, Cullen BF, Stoelting RK, editors: Clinical anesthesia. Philadelphia, Lippincott Williams & Wilkins, 2001, pp 595-638.
64. Ramadhani SAL, Mohammed LA, Roche DA, et al: Sternomental distance as the sole predictor of difficult laryngoscopy in obstetric anesthesia. *Br J Anaesth* 1996;77:312-316.
65. Urakami Y, Takenaka I, Nakamura M, et al: The reliability of the Bellhouse test for evaluating extension capacity of the occipito-atlantoaxial complex. *Anesth Analg* 2002;95:1437-1441.
66. Karkouti K, Rose DK, Ferris LE, et al: Inter-observer reliability of ten tests used for predicting difficult tracheal intubation. *Can J Anesth* 1996;43:541-543.
67. White A, Kander PL: Anatomical factors in difficult direct laryngoscopy complicating intubation for anaesthesia. *BMJ* 1956;1:488.
68. Yildiz TS, Korkmaz F, et al: Prediction of difficult tracheal intubation in Turkish patients: A multi-center methodological study. *Eur J Anaesthesiol* 2007;7:1-7.
69. Voyagis GS, Kyriakis KP, Dimitriou V, Vrettou I: Value of oropharyngeal Mallampati classification in predicting difficult laryngoscopy among obese patients. *Eur J Anaesthesiol* 1998;15: 330-334.
70. Juvin P, Lavaut E, Dupont H, et al: Difficult tracheal intubation is more common in obese than in lean patients. *Anesth Analg* 2003;97:595-600.
71. Adnet F, Boron SW, Racine SX et al: The Intubation Difficulty Scale (IDS). *Anesthesiology* 1997;87:1290-1297.
72. Brodsky JB, Lemmens HJM, Brock-Utne JG, Vierra M, Saidman LJ: Morbid obesity and tracheal intubation. *Anesth Analg* 2002;94:732-736.
73. Komatsu R, Sengupta P, Wadhwa A, Akca O, Sessler D I, Ezri T: Ultrasound quantification of anterior soft tissue thickness fails to predict difficult laryngoscopy in obese patients. *Anaesth Intensive Care* 2007;35(1):32-37.
74. Siegel HE, Sonies BC, Vega-Bermudez F, et al: The use of simultaneous ultrasound and polysomnography for diagnosis of obstructive sleep apnea. *Neurology* 1999;52(suppl 2): A1110-A1111.
75. Bohme G: Clinical contribution to ultrasound diagnosis of the larynx (echolaryngography). *Laryngorhinootologie* 1989;68: 504-508.
76. Hatfield A, Bodenham A: Ultrasound: An emerging role in anaesthesia and intensive care. *Br J Anaesth* 1999;83:789-800.
77. Bainton CR: Difficult intubation—what's the best test? *Can J Anaesth* 1996;43:541-543 (editorial).
78. Matthew M, Hanna LS, Aldree JA: Preoperative indices to anticipate the difficult tracheal intubation. *Anesth Analg* 1989;68:S187 (abstract).
79. Janssens M, Hartstein G: Management of difficult intubation. *Eur J Anaesthesiol* 2001;18:3-12.
80. Janssens M, Lamy M: Airway Difficult Score (ADS): A new score to predict difficulty in airway management. *Eur J Anaesthesiol* 2000;17:A113.
81. Yamamoto K, Tsubokawa T, Shibata K, et al: Predicting difficult intubation with indirect laryngoscopy. *Anesthesiology* 1997;86: 316-321.
82. Bellhouse CP, Dore C: Criteria for estimating likelihood of difficulty of endotracheal intubation with the Macintosh laryngoscope. *Anaesth Intensive Care* 1988;16:329.
83. Tse JC, Rimm EB, Hussain A: Predicting difficult endotracheal intubation in surgical patients scheduled for general anesthesia: A prospective blind study. *Anesth Analg* 1995;81:254.
84. Naguib M, Malabarey T, AlSatli RA, Al Damegh S, Samarkandi AH: Predictive models for difficult laryngoscopy and intubation. A clinical, radiologic and three-dimensional computer imaging study. *Can J Anesth* 1999;46:748-759.
85. Williamson JA, Webb RK, Szekely S, et al: The Australian incident monitoring study: Difficult intubation: An analysis of 2000 incident reports. *Anaesth Intensive Care* 1993;21:602.

86. Kheterpal S, Han R, Tremper KK, Shanks A, Tait AR, Michael O'Reilly, Ludwig TA: Incidence and predictors of difficult and impossible mask ventilation. *Anesthesiology* 2006;105(5): 885-891.
87. McCrory CR, Moriarty DC: Laryngeal mask positioning is related to Mallampati grading in adults. *Anesth Analg* 1995;81:1001-1004.
88. Crosby ET, Cooper RM, Douglas MJ, et al: The unanticipated difficult airway with recommendation for management. *Can J Anaesth* 1998;45:757-776.
89. AARC clinical practice guideline. Management of airway emergencies. *Respir Care* 1995;40:749-760.
90. The SIAARTI (Italian Society of Anaesthesia Analgesia and Intensive Care) task force on guidelines for management of difficult airway in adults. *Minerva Anestesiol* 1998;64:361-371.
91. The SFAR (French Society of Anaesthesia and Intensive Care) task force on guidelines for management of difficult airway. *Ann Fr Anesth Reanim* 1996;15:207-214.

18 Should Regional or General Anesthesia Be Used for Cases in Which the Patient Has an Anticipated Difficult Airway?

Seth Akst, MD, MBA, and Lynette Mark, MD

Airway management is the essence of the practice of clinical anesthesiology. Preoperative assessment of the patient's airway is the first step in the evaluation and planning of a safe, appropriate anesthetic plan. For the majority of patients, this can be readily achieved with a brief systematic history and physical examination and does not require additional diagnostic evaluation.

Some patients may be anticipated to be difficult to intubate, based on a history of difficult intubation or clinical predictors of difficult intubation. The American Society of Anesthesiologists' (ASA) "Practice Guidelines for Management of the Difficult Airway" reviews some of the historical and physical examination findings possibly suggestive of a difficult intubation.[1] Some of these predictors of anticipated difficulty with conventional direct laryngoscopy (MAC/Miller) include a large overbite, large tongue, narrow mouth opening, or short chin. Various prediction models, such as correlation with Mallampati oral view I-IV to the Cormack-Lehane laryngoscopic view grades I to IV, have been proposed, but none offers 100% sensitivity for prediction of a difficult airway.[2] Despite such an evaluation, an estimated 1% to 3% of patients in to the operating room have an unanticipated difficult airway with conventional direct laryngoscopy.[3]

In addition to this 1% to 3% incidence of patients with an unanticipated difficult airway, there are cohorts of patients with specific pathologic conditions that are known to prove difficult with conventional laryngoscopy. These patients may require more complex or multispecialty clinician airway management that may only be readily or immediately available in specialty or tertiary care centers.

The ASA's "Practice Guidelines for Management of the Difficult Airway" encourages all practitioners to review the airway algorithm presented in the document and provides resources for the creation of difficult airway management carts that can be readily mobilized for elective and emergency airway management.

The goal, then, of the preoperative airway evaluation is to categorize the patient into one of two categories: (1) not difficult with conventional MAC/Miller direct laryngoscopy; or (2) anticipated to be difficult with conventional MAC/Miller direct laryngoscopy. In either category, unanticipated difficulty with the chosen airway management technique is a reality.

Of the patients who have an anticipated difficult airway, a certain percentage will be scheduled for surgical procedures that are amenable to regional anesthesia as the primary anesthetic or for postoperative pain management. For example, many orthopedic limb cases, lower abdominal surgeries, and urologic procedures can be performed with a regional technique and without anticipated airway management.

In these instances, regional anesthesia can be an attractive option for some clinicians when faced with a patient with anticipated difficult intubation who is scheduled for an appropriate surgery and who does not have other contraindications to regional anesthesia. However, if, during the procedure, the regional technique needs to be converted to a general airway-controlled anesthetic and there are adverse outcomes related to an urgent nature of the airway management, many clinicians are quick to criticize the role of regional anesthesia in these patients as a primary anesthetic. They advocate that in the case of the anticipated difficult airway, the patient's airway must be electively controlled at the beginning of the case, with regional anesthesia being a component of a combined regional/general technique.

This chapter reviews the evidence supporting the decision to initiate a regional or general anesthetic in patients with anticipated difficult airways who are scheduled for appropriate surgical procedures. Patients in whom difficulty with airway management is not anticipated preoperatively and patients undergoing surgical procedures not amenable to regional anesthesia alone (e.g., intrathoracic or intracranial surgery) are not addressed in this chapter.

ALTERNATIVES

The appeal of choosing a primary regional anesthesia technique is that airway management and the potential complications in these complex patients may be able to be avoided. The ability to provide safe and adequate anesthesia without instrumenting the airway can be a relief to both the patient and the anesthesiologist. The need to address issues of extubation of the difficult airway and postoperative care can also be avoided.

Depending on the surgical case, as well as the patient's preferences, many different regional anesthetics may be appropriate. Neuraxial techniques, such as spinal or epidural anesthesia, as well as regional blocks such as brachial plexus, lumbar plexus, and specific nerve blocks, can provide excellent anesthesia, with or without concomitant sedation. Indwelling catheter techniques, such as for epidural or some extremity blocks, also allow postoperative pain to be managed successfully in certain cases.

The potential downfall of the regional anesthesia alternative is that the regional technique may be technically difficult, may be incomplete, or may fail, necessitating the conversion to a general anesthetic with or without intubation/protected airway. The likelihood of failure of the regional technique cannot be predicted because it depends on the skill and experience of the anesthesiologist performing the neuraxial or nerve block. In addition, patient-specific factors, such as inability to tolerate being awake or minimally sedated (so as to avoid respiratory depression), may require conversion to general anesthesia. Finally, surgical considerations such as extension of the procedure may require a change from regional to general anesthesia.

Conversion from a regional to a general anesthetic may be required at a time when the patient's airway is relatively less accessible to the anesthesiology team, as well as at a time when deteriorating patient condition mandates hastening the ventilation and intubation process. It is important to recognize, in the words of Benumof,[4] "Use of regional anesthesia in the patient with a recognized difficult airway does not solve the problem of the difficult airway; it is still there."[4]

On the other hand, the appeal of a planned general anesthetic is that the airway can be approached in a controlled and measured fashion. This chapter does not provide an in-depth review of airway management techniques, but basic considerations include choosing between surgical and nonsurgical approaches, asleep versus awake techniques, and spontaneously ventilating or apneic patients. Specific intubating methods could include direct laryngoscopy, rigid or flexible fiberoptic laryngoscopy, or placement of a laryngeal mask airway (LMA) as a bridge toward definitive control of the airway, among many other possible forms of intubation (Figure 18-1).

A third alternative is the combined general with regional approach to anesthesia. In such circumstances, the regional anesthetic technique is used primarily for intraoperative and potentially postoperative analgesia, while the airway is intubated in a controlled fashion in the beginning of the case. Because the combined alternative leads to airway management in the beginning of the case, it will be considered as part of the general anesthesia option for the purposes of this chapter. In the cases of combined regional with general anesthesia, it can be the contribution of the regional anesthesia that facilitates successful extubation of the patient with an anticipated difficult airway (Figure 18-2).

EVIDENCE

The endpoint of greatest importance when comparing regional versus general anesthesia for the patient with an anticipated difficult airway would be patient mortality. Given the obvious ethical problems posed by comparing two techniques that are alternatives to avoiding significant risk of patient morbidity or mortality, it is not surprising that no randomized control trial has been performed that addresses this issue. In the absence of any randomized control trials, prospective and retrospective data reviews are the next level of evidence that one could look for. These authors are not aware of any paper that directly compares regional versus general anesthesia in regard to airway outcomes. The desire to avoid publication of adverse events and the relative infrequency of lost airways combine to make literature on this topic scarce.

There are several papers that do compare general anesthesia directly against regional anesthesia, but these papers focus on cardiovascular morbidity and mortality.[5-7] Other papers that compare regional versus general anesthesia examine other variables such as return of bowel function or postoperative pain control. A good overview of the state of outcomes research with regard to regional anesthesia has been written by Wu and Fleisher.[8] Airway management is notably absent from their discussion because no evidence has been published regarding the issue of regional versus general anesthesia, particularly for the patient with an anticipated difficult airway.

It is tempting to extrapolate some numbers from a striking paper written by Hawkins and colleagues[9] that examines the relationship between anesthetic choice and maternal mortality rate for obstetric care. This study calculated the rates of death in obstetric patients receiving anesthesia in two time periods, 1979–1984 and 1985–1990. The authors found that obstetric patients receiving general anesthesia had a mortality rate of 20 per million anesthetics in the earlier period and that this rate increased to 32.3 deaths per million general anesthetics in the later period. They contrast these data to patients receiving regional obstetric anesthesia, for whom the mortality rate decreased from 8.6 deaths per million to 1.9 deaths per million. Thus both the absolute numbers and the trends seem to favor regional anesthetic techniques as significantly safer in this population.

However, these data are difficult to interpret. The percentage of regional anesthetics requiring emergent conversion to general anesthetics is not addressed, and it is not clear within what group patients were accounted for in whom death occurred as a result of failed intubation during an attempted conversion from regional to general anesthesia. The apparent increased mortality rate associated with general anesthesia could be the result of failed regional blocks requiring conversion to general with uncontrolled conditions. The internal validity of the data is suspect because the accompanying editorial questions the assumptions used in calculating the mortality rates.[10] Furthermore, the external validity of this study is circumspect because the urgency of many obstetric surgical procedures and the different airway challenges that parturient patients represent (e.g., aspiration risk, edematous pharyngeal

DIFFICULT AIRWAY ALGORITHM

1. Assess the likelihood and clinical impact of basic management problems:
   A. Difficult ventilation
   B. Difficult intubation
   C. Difficulty with patient cooperation or consent
   D. Difficult tracheostomy
2. Actively pursue opportunities to deliver supplemental oxygen throughout the process of difficult airway management
3. Consider the relative merits and feasibility of basic management choices:

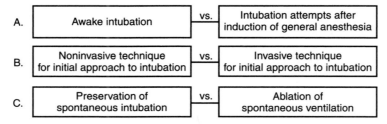

A. | Awake intubation | vs. | Intubation attempts after induction of general anesthesia |

B. | Noninvasive technique for initial approach to intubation | vs. | Invasive technique for initial approach to intubation |

C. | Preservation of spontaneous intubation | vs. | Ablation of spontaneous ventilation |

4. Develop primary and alternative strategies:

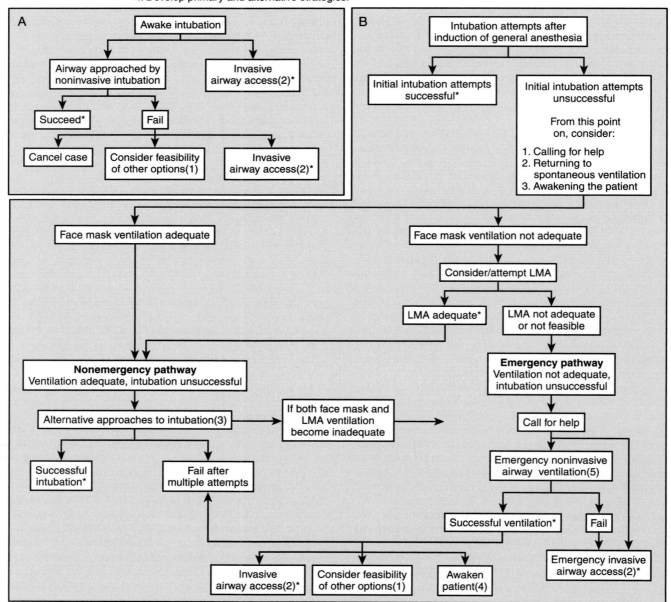

*Confirm ventilation, tracheal intubation, or LMA placement with exhaled CO_2.

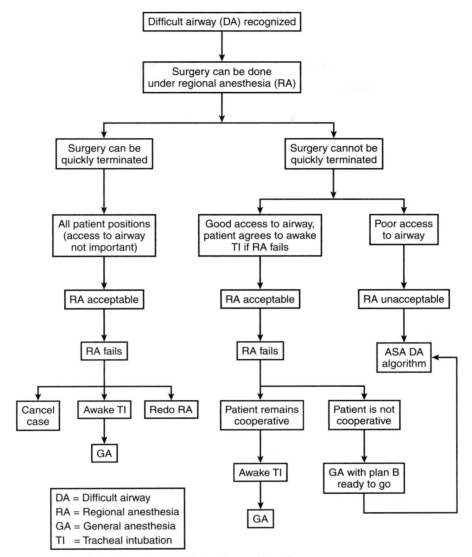

Figure 18-2. Regional Anesthesia and the Recognized Difficult Airway Algorithm.

tissue, decreased functional residual capacity, increased oxygen consumption) may be nonapplicable to our group of interest, which is nonpregnant patients with an anticipated difficult airway undergoing elective surgery.

As discussed earlier, the likelihood of converting from regional to general anesthesia cannot be predicted due to various anesthesiologist-, patient-, and procedure-specific factors. Therefore in the absence of reliable published data, historical institution-specific data may be the most useful for framing the question of regional versus general anesthesia for the patient with an anticipated difficult airway. The Johns Hopkins Hospital Department of Anesthesiology keeps patient data concerning adverse events as an internal database for morbidity and mortality review. Such databases, although not predictive of each new case, can help provide institutional experience in addition to an anesthesiologist's personal experience when making this choice.

Figure 18-1. Difficult Airway Algorithm. *1,* Other options include (but are not limited to) the following: surgery using face mask or LMA anesthesia, local anesthesia infiltration, or regional nerve blockade. Pursuit of these options usually implies that mask ventilation will not be problematic. Therefore these options may be of limited value if this step in the algorithm has been reached via the Emergency Pathway. *2,* Invasive airway access includes surgical or percutaneous tracheostomy or cricothyrotomy. *3,* Alternative noninvasive approaches to difficult intubation include (but are not limited to) the following: use of different laryngoscope blades, LMA as an intubation conduit (with or without fiberoptic guidance), fiberoptic intubation, intubating stylet or tube changes, light wand, retrograde intubation, and blind oral or nasal intubation. *4,* Consider repreparation of the patient for awake intubation or canceling surgery. *5,* Options for emergency noninvasive airway ventilation include (but are not limited to) the following: rigid bronchoscope, esophageal-tracheal combitube ventilation, or transtracheal jet ventilation.

GUIDELINES

The American Society of Anesthesiologists' "Practice Guidelines for Management of the Difficult Airway"[1] should be familiar to every anesthesiologist. Although these guidelines do not specifically address the issue of regional anesthesia as an alternative to general anesthesia with a protected airway, subsequent "New Thoughts and Concepts" published by Benumof in the ASA Refresher Course book specifically address the role of regional anesthesia in anticipated difficult airway patients.[11] He states that use of regional anesthesia in a patient with a known difficult airway requires a high degree of judgment and concludes that it is unacceptable to do regional anesthesia with a known difficult airway when surgery cannot be terminated rapidly and there is poor access to the patient's head. In *Airway Management: Principles and Practice,* Benumof[4] provides clinicians with an algorithm for the use of regional anesthesia and the recognized difficult airway that complements the ASA Difficult Airway Algorithm.

AUTHORS' RECOMMENDATIONS

- Regional anesthesia may provide a reasonable alternative to providing an anesthetic for a patient with an anticipated difficult airway in certain circumstances. However, many surgical cases and many patients present contraindications to regional anesthesia.
- If regional anesthesia were to fail for anesthetic-, patient-, or surgical-related issues, intubation might then have to occur under suboptimal conditions. It is reasonable to assume that an airway will be more easily secured when approached in a controlled fashion in the beginning of the case than in an urgent manner with possibly compromised access to the patient—with fewer adverse outcomes.[12,13]
- Therefore it is mandatory that every anesthesiologist be familiar with the ASA's "Practice Guidelines for Management of the Difficult Airway"[1] and subsequent updates/recommendations. Review of Benumof's algorithm for the use of regional anesthesia and the anticipated difficult airway patient is recommended.
- Anesthesiologists must be comfortable with the preoperative assessment of patients, with appropriate consultation from colleagues with specialties in complex airway management. When appropriate, this multispecialty team must be immediately available to the patient at the time of the surgical procedure.
- Anesthesiologists must be facile with multiple approaches and techniques to airway management and understand the limitations of various techniques.
- It is recommended that a plan for general anesthesia be prepared for every patient with an anticipated difficult airway, and appropriate equipment and supporting clinicians/staff are immediately available to the patient, even if regional anesthesia will be the primary and first choice of anesthesia

for the patient. Dr. Martin Norton states, "The obligation to guarantee airway control is not obviated by epidural, spinal, or regional techniques."[14]
- Discussion of a primary regional anesthetic plan with the patient and surgeon must include a realistic approach to the incidence of failed regional techniques or complications of regional anesthesia and a plan for airway management if required. Regional anesthesia is an acceptable primary anesthetic only if the practitioner is comfortable with his or her ability to secure the airway at any potential time during the surgical case. If there is any doubt about the ability to secure the patient's airway once the surgery is under way, airway management at the beginning of the case is recommended.
- Sedation as a supplement to regional anesthesia must be discussed at the time of evaluation with both the patient and surgeon. Vigilance about ensuring airway access and state of consciousness is essential.

REFERENCES

1. Practice guidelines for management of the difficult airway: An updated report by the American Society of Anesthesiologists Task Force on Management of the Difficult Airway. *Anesthesiology* 2003;98:1269-1277.
2. Mallampati SR: Recognition of the difficulty airway. In Benumof JL, editor: *Airway management: Principles and practice.* St. Louis, Mosby, 1996, pp 126-142.
3. Rose DK, Cohen MM: The airway: Problems and predictions in 18,500 patients. *Can Anaesth Soc J* 1994;41:361-365.
4. Benumof JL: The American Society of Anesthesiologists' management of the difficult airway algorithm and explanation-analysis of the algorithm. In Benumof JL, editor: *Airway management: Principles and practice.* St. Louis, Mosby, 1996, p 150..
5. Christopherson R: Perioperative morbidity in patients randomized to epidural or general anesthesia for lower extremity vascular surgery. Perioperative Ischemia Randomized Anesthesia Trial Study Group. *Anesthesiology* 1993;79:422-434.
6. Bode RH Jr: Comparison of general and regional anesthesia. *Anesthesiology* 1996;84:3-13.
7. Christopherson R, Norris EJ: Regional versus general anesthesia. *Anesthesiol Clin North Am* 1997;15:37-49.
8. Wu CL, Fleisher LA: Outcomes research in regional anesthesia and analgesia. *Anesth Analg* 2000;91:1232-1242.
9. Hawkins JL, Koonin LM, Palmer SK, Gibbs CP: Anesthesia-related deaths during obstetric delivery in the United States, 1979-1990. *Anesthesiology* 1997;86:277-284.
10. Chestnut DH: Anesthesia and maternal mortality. *Anesthesiology* 1997;86:273-276.
11. Benumof JL: The ASA difficult airway algorithm: New thoughts/considerations. *ASA Annual Refresher Course Lectures* 1997;1-7.
12. Mark L, Schauble J, Turley S, et al: The Medic Alert national difficult airway/intubation registry: Technology that pays for itself. Presented at the annual meeting of the Society for Technology in Anesthesia, 1995 (abstract).
13. Gibby GL, Mark L, Drake J: Effectiveness of Teleforms scan-based input tool for difficult airway registry: Preliminary results. Presented at the annual meeting of the Society for Technology in Anesthesia, 1995 (abstract).
14. Norton ML: The difficult airway. In Norton ML, editor: *Atlas of the difficult airway,* ed 2. St. Louis, Mosby, 1996, p 5.

19 Is There a Best Approach to Induction of Anesthesia in Emergent Situations?

Richard P. Dutton, MD, MBA

INTRODUCTION

Most anesthesiologists will take care of emergency patients at some point in their career. Whether dealing with a surgical crisis in the operating room (OR) or a trauma patient in the emergency department (ED), the anesthesiologist must have a plan for rapid and safe induction of general anesthesia. Table 19-1 is a list of some of the potential pitfalls that can be encountered in the emergency situation. Whereas elective patients have a known medical history, optimized medications, hemodynamic stability, and an empty stomach, emergent patients may lack all of these things. Indeed, an older trauma patient brought to the ED with severe injuries might present anatomic challenges to intubation, might be hypovolemic, might have limited cardiac reserve, might be taking unknown chronic medications, has a potentially full stomach, and has a potentially unstable cervical spine. Induction of general anesthesia and successful endotracheal intubation will be critical to the long-term survival of this patient, but how are these best accomplished?

OPTIONS/THERAPIES

By definition, emergency induction is needed when the acuity of the patient's presentation does not allow for the normal preoperative anesthetic assessment. Nonetheless, the anesthesiologist must take advantage of every opportunity to learn about the patient's condition while formulating a plan for his or her care. Table 19-2 is a list of suggested questions. At a minimum, the anesthesiologist should determine why the patient requires emergent induction (e.g., urgent surgery for hemorrhage, airway protection or ventilatory support, septic shock) and as much as time allows about the patient's history. Usually this information can be gleaned from the physicians or nurses already caring for the patient. If possible, these providers should be asked whether the patient has any allergies, and what medications the patient is taking. A quick look at the medical record may be helpful. Any recent anesthetic record is especially useful, as it will provide information about the ease of intubation and

the patient's tolerance of medications. A brief survey of relevant laboratory values can also help to avoid pitfalls: hematocrit (hemodynamic stability), creatinine (acute or chronic renal failure), arterial blood gas (ventilatory difficulties, acidosis), serum potassium (potential for hyperkalemia), and coagulation studies (potential for bleeding).

Physical examination of the patient must be abbreviated, but is still important. It takes only seconds to assess the patient's level of consciousness by asking the patient to extend his or her neck and open the mouth, also providing valuable insight into the airway anatomy and potential for a difficult intubation. Vital signs should be noted. New sources of pain, external hemorrhage, or visible deformity should also be recorded.

Once this brief survey is accomplished, the anesthesiologist is ready to consider various options. Table 19-3 lists a number of important questions that should be addressed. The first has to do with optimizing the emergency induction. If the patient is not in the OR, success can sometimes be improved by moving there, assembling more equipment, or calling for assistance, but only if the benefit of doing so will outweigh the risk of delay to the patient. The second consideration is the manner of anesthetic induction and the technique for securing a definitive airway. While a rapid-sequence approach leading to direct laryngoscopy and endotracheal intubation will most often be correct,[1] there are situations where a more gradual induction or even awake fiberoptic intubation may be more appropriate. Finally, the anesthesiologist must consider the medications to be used, and the dose of each.

EVIDENCE

There is substantial evidence available to support the use of rapid-sequence intubation in most cases in which emergency induction is required. Neuromuscular blockade provides the best intubating conditions on the first approach to the airway, and leads to the highest "first pass" success rate.[2] A rapid transition from awake to anesthetized reduces the patient's exposure to intermediate stages of anesthesia in which complications such as

Table 19-1	Potential Difficulties Posed by the Need for Emergency Induction of General Anesthesia

Table 19-1	Potential Difficulties Posed by the Need for Emergency Induction of General Anesthesia

- Unknown medical history:
  Limited cardiac reserve
  Preexisting neurologic conditions
  Chronic diseases with anesthetic implications (e.g., amyotrophic lateral sclerosis)
- Untested airway, with limited chance for examination and inability to tolerate awake intubation
- Hemodynamic instability:
  Hemorrhage (e.g., trauma, gastrointestinal bleeding)
  Cardiac disease (e.g., recent myocardial infarction)
  Dehydration (e.g., small bowel obstruction)
  Uncontrolled hypertension or diabetes
- Untested cervical spine stability after trauma
- Presumed full stomach

Table 19-2	Suggested Questions, in Approximate Order of Importance, for Assessing the Emergency Patient

- Why is this an emergency?
- Does the patient have any major medical problems?
- What medications/intoxicants has the patient taken recently?
- Is the patient allergic to any medications?
- Has the patient any history of problems with anesthesia?
- Is there a history of neurologic deficit?
- When did the patient last eat?
- Are there any abnormal laboratory values?
- What does the electrocardiogram show?
- Are there any other positive diagnostic tests?

Answers should be sought from the most efficient and knowledgeable source among the patient, the patient's caregivers, and the medical record.

Table 19-3	Questions to Determine the Anesthetic Plan

- Is this the right location to induce anesthesia?
- Do I have the necessary equipment?
- Are the right people here?
- Is this patient hemodynamically stable?
- Is there likely to be an airway difficulty?
- Are there patient factors I should take into account?
- Does this patient have a full stomach?
- Is the cervical spine stable?
- Is the intravenous access adequate?

laryngospasm, pain, hemodynamic lability, combative behavior, and aspiration are most likely to occur. Several large case series have examined the use of neuromuscular blockade to facilitate rapid-sequence intubation outside of the OR, with highly favorable results.[3-5] A recent retrospective study from the author's institution documented the need for surgical airway salvage in only 21 of 6088 patients who underwent rapid-sequence induction within 1 hour of hospital arrival, a rate of 0.3%.[6]

The choice of neuromuscular blocking agent is largely determined by the clinical situation. Succinylcholine is the most commonly used medication for rapid-sequence intubation because it produces the most rapid onset of paralysis and thus the best intubating conditions in the shortest amount of time. Succinylcholine also has the advantage of being short acting, with return of neuromuscular function in approximately 10 minutes after usual doses. In the elective situation when a difficult airway is unexpectedly encountered, this may be beneficial to allow the patient to wake up and resume spontaneous ventilation while other plans are considered. This will seldom be an advantage during emergency induction, however, because the conditions creating the emergency will still be present. Rapid resolution of paralysis following succinylcholine may enable subsequent neurologic assessment. Succinylcholine is contraindicated in patients with neuromuscular conduction abnormalities (e.g., spinal cord injury, amyotrophic lateral sclerosis, Guillain-Barré syndrome) of greater than 24 hours' duration and in patients with recent severe burns. Excessive numbers of postsynaptic choline receptors can cause a fatal hyperkalemia in these patients.[7] Though at least one paper has downplayed the potential for succinylcholine to trigger malignant hyperthermia in susceptible patients,[8] the catastrophic nature of this complication makes it prudent to avoid the use of succinylcholine in patients potentially at risk. Succinylcholine will also produce transient elevation of intracranial and intraocular pressure.[9] This has the theoretic potential to put some patients at risk, although this has never been proven in any large clinical series. In reality, avoidance of succinylcholine may contribute to hypoxia during induction and intubation that is of far more relevance.

Rapid-acting nondepolarizing neuromuscular blocking agents can produce intubating conditions almost as good as succinylcholine, almost as quickly.[10,11] The use of high-dose rocuronium or vecuronium is appropriate when contraindications to succinylcholine exist, accepting the fact that the patient will remain paralyzed for a longer period of time. In most emergent situations this is not a major concern.

Although complete neuromuscular blockade is the key to a rapid transition to mechanical ventilation, and should be used in almost all emergency inductions, the use of sedative/hypnotic agents should be approached on a case-specific basis. Amnesia to the events of induction and intubation is desirable, as is prevention of extreme sympathetic stimulation in response to airway manipulation. Some degree of sedation is therefore appropriate in almost all emergency inductions, yet careful titration is required. Patients in shock have increased sensitivity to the central effects of sedative agents: less medication is required to achieve a similar depression in awareness.[12] Hypovolemic patients are especially problematic. Reduction in compensatory sympathetic outflow, reduced cardiac filling in association with positive pressure ventilation, and the direct vasodilatory and negative inotropic effects of sedative agents may all lead to profound hemodynamic instability and cardiac arrest following normal induction doses of thiopentol, propofol, or midazolam.[1]

There have been a number of recent reports advocating the use of etomidate for induction of anesthesia in emergency situations, because it is not a vasodilator or negative inotrope.[13] As with ketamine, however, a normal induction dose of etomidate may still lead to profound hypotension in patients in hypovolemic shock, due to interruption of sympathetic outflow. Several recent reports have also described the subsequent development of adrenal insufficiency in patients receiving even single doses of etomidate for emergency induction.[14]

The choice of induction agent is thus less important than the dose selected. In general, the least amount consistent with amnesia is appropriate, unless there is reason to be concerned about a hypertensive response to intubation (e.g., the patient with an isolated traumatic brain injury and the potential for increased intracranial hemorrhage). Additional doses can always be given if the first dose is well tolerated. Familiarity with the medication chosen is also important, enabling greater precision in titration. For example, deaths attributed to the use of sodium thiopental in soldiers injured at Pearl Harbor were the result of unfamiliarity with the drug, rather than with its specific function.[15]

CONTROVERSIES

There are a few situations in which securing the airway before induction of anesthesia is appropriate: significant upper airway trauma, known instability of the cervical spine, and a strong suspicion (by history or examination) of a difficult airway. In these situations the use of a fiberoptic bronchoscope, after appropriate topical anesthesia of the upper airway, can provide important diagnostic information and the safest route to a secure airway. This technique requires both time and expertise, however, and is not recommended in uncooperative or hemodynamically unstable patients. Although most trauma patients will be brought to the ED with a cervical collar and backboard in place, the incidence of unstable spinal cord injury is low, and the potential for aggravating an injury during laryngoscopy and intubation is even lower.[16] Several large series have examined the use of manual in-line stabilization of the cervical spine during emergency intubation and have demonstrated the safety of this practice.[17] Rapid-sequence intubation thus remains the preferred approach in trauma patients with "uncleared" cervical spines, unless there is a known or strongly suspected injury.

Awake fiberoptic intubation would be a diagnostic luxury in many patients with face or airway trauma, but this approach is seldom feasible. Bleeding or foreign bodies in the airway will usually make the patient agitated, and will necessitate a faster and more direct approach. A rapid-sequence intubation attempt is appropriate, with immediate progression to a surgical airway as needed.

Surprisingly, massive facial trauma patients are often easy to intubate immediately after injury, because fracture of the facial bones removes a barrier to direct laryngoscopy. Any delay, however, will allow for tissue swelling and distortion that will completely obscure the upper airway.[1]

A final area of controversy surrounds the presence of a full stomach, and the risk of passive reflux and aspiration during the induction of anesthesia. Paralytic ileus is common after trauma and in association with major medical disease, so that delaying anesthesia to allow the stomach to empty is unlikely to work.[18] Instead, measures should be taken to reduce the risk of aspiration while otherwise proceeding with emergent induction. In cooperative patients not otherwise at risk, the use of a nonparticulate antacid such as bicitrate is appropriate before induction.[19] The use of cricoid pressure—the Sellick maneuver—has long been a staple during rapid-sequence induction.[20] The value of this approach in occluding the esophagus and preventing passive regurgitation has been called into question recently,[21] but the maneuver itself is free and easy to perform and the technique may confer other benefits than esophageal occlusion. Posterior displacement of the larynx can improve the view of the vocal cords and facilitate intubation, particularly in trauma patients who are being intubated in the presence of manual in-line cervical stabilization, while palpation of the larynx during intubation can help to confirm successful tube placement. If overzealous application of cricoid pressure is obscuring the laryngeal view, it can always be removed.

AREAS OF UNCERTAINTY

Most likely to change the approach to emergency induction of anesthesia in the near future is the widespread adaptation of video indirect laryngoscopy.[22] Tools such as the Glidescope will potentially improve the safety of emergency intubation, reducing manipulation of the cervical spine and making an asleep rapid-sequence approach even more favored in emergency patients.

Improved markers and monitors of the patient's hemodynamic condition will allow for greater precision in dosing induction drugs in the future. Further development of neuromuscular blocking agents may eventually lead to a better replacement for succinylcholine than the agents now available, while the development of sugammadex as an instantaneous reversal agent may allow more widespread use of rocuronium and vecuronium.[23] It is unlikely, however, that the basic concept of rapid-sequence induction will change.

GUIDELINES

The most comprehensive review and guidelines for emergency airway management were published in 2002 by the Eastern Association for the Surgery of Trauma (EAST), as the result of a guidelines working group.[24] This document includes a discussion of all aspects of emergency airway management, and concludes with the recommended approach seen in Figure 19-1.

PROCEDURAL OPTIONS FOR TRAUMA PATIENTS
NEEDING EMERGENCY TRACHEAL INTUBATION

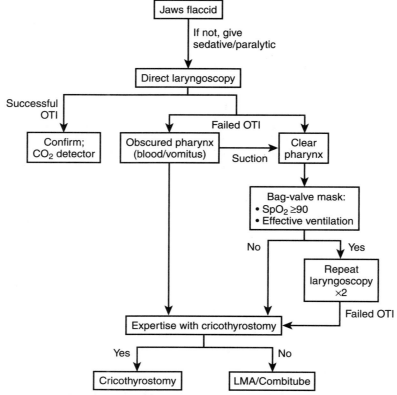

Laryngotracheal injury (severe neck injury): partial airway obstruction → OTI;
severe airway obstruction → surgical airway (cricothyrostomy/tracheostomy)

Figure 19-1. Procedural Options for Trauma Patients Needing Emergency Tracheal Intubation.

AUTHOR'S RECOMMENDATIONS

A recommended "best practice" for induction of anesthesia in emergency situations consists of the following key steps:

1. Pre-crisis preparation, including training of personnel and availability of equipment.
2. Rapid assessment and optimization of the patient and environment, consistent with the time available.
3. Preoxygenation, cricoid pressure, and manual in-line cervical stabilization (if indicated).
4. Induction of anesthesia (carefully titrated dosing) and rapid deep paralysis (succinylcholine).
5. Direct laryngoscopy and intubation, facilitated by an intubating stylet (gum elastic bougie) if needed.
6. Confirmation of successful intubation with capnometry.
7. If intubation cannot be accomplished, rescue with a laryngeal mask airway.
8. Rapid progression to a surgical airway, as needed.
9. Circulatory support following intubation. Gentle application of positive pressure ventilation and upward titration of sedative medications as tolerated by the patient.

REFERENCES

1. Dutton RP, McCunn M: Anesthesia for trauma. In Miller RD, editor: *Miller's anesthesia*, ed 6. Philadelphia, Elsevier Churchill Livingstone, 2005.

2. Bozeman WP, Kleiner DM, Huggett V: A comparison of rapid-sequence intubation and etomidate-only intubation in the prehospital air medical setting. *Prehosp Emerg Care* 2006;10:8-13.
3. Rotondo MF, McGonigal MD, Schwab CW, et al: Urgent paralysis and intubation of trauma patients: Is it safe? *J Trauma* 1993;34:242-246.
4. Stene JK, Grande CM, Barton CR: Airway management for the trauma patient. In Stene JK, Grande CM: *Trauma anesthesia*. Baltimore, Williams & Wilkins, 1991.
5. Talucci RC, Shaikh KA, Schwab CW: Rapid sequence induction with oral endotracheal intubation in the multiply injured patient. *Am Surg* 1988;54:185-187.
6. Stephens CT, Kahntroff S, Dutton RP: Success of emergency endotracheal intubation at a major trauma referral center. Abstract presented at the American Society of Anesthesiologists Annual Meeting (poster #A1298), San Francisco, CA, 2007.
7. Gronert GA, Theye RA: Pathophysiology of hyperkalemia induced by succinylcholine. *Anesthesiology* 1975;43:89-99.
8. Hopkins PM: Malignant hyperthermia: Advances in clinical management and diagnosis. *Br J Anaesth* 2000;85:118-28.
9. Kelly RE, Dinner M, Turner LS, et al: Succinylcholine increases intraocular pressure in the human eye with the extraocular muscles detached. *Anesthesiology* 1993;79:948-952.
10. Sluga M, Ummenhofer W, Studer W, Siegemund M, Marsch SC: Rocuronium versus succinylcholine for rapid sequence induction of anesthesia and endotracheal intubation: A prospective, randomized trial in emergent cases. *Anesth Analg* 2005;101: 1356-1361.
11. Di Filippo A, Grechi S, Rizzo L, Benvenuti S, Novelli GP: High dose vecuronium in "open-eye" emergency surgery. *Minerva Anestesiol* 1995;61:457-462.
12. Johnson KB, Egan TD, Kern SE, et al: Influence of hemorrhagic shock followed by crystalloid resuscitation on propofol: A pharmacokinetic and pharmacodynamic analysis. *Anesthesiology* 2004;101:647-659.

13. Oglesby AJ: Should etomidate be the induction agent of choice for rapid sequence intubation in the emergency department? *Emerg Med J* 2004;21:655-659.
14. Zed PJ, Mabasa VH, Slavik RS, Abu-Laban RB: Etomidate for rapid sequence intubation in the emergency department: Is adrenal suppression a concern? *CJEM* 2006;8:347-350.
15. Bennetts FE: Thiopentone anaesthesia at Pearl Harbor. *Br J Anaesth* 1995;75:366-368.
16. Turkstra TP, Craen RA, Pelz DM, et al: Cervical spine motion: A fluoroscopic comparison during intubation with lighted stylet, GlideScope, and Macintosh laryngoscope. *Anesth Analg* 2005;101:910-915, table.
17. Manoach S, Paladino L: Manual in-line stabilization for acute airway management of suspected cervical spine injury: Historical review and current questions. *Ann Emerg Med* 2007;50:236-245.
18. Nguyen NQ, Ng MP, Chapman M, Fraser RJ, Holloway RH: The impact of admission diagnosis on gastric emptying in critically ill patients. *Crit Care* 2007;11:R16.
19. Søreide E, Holst-Larsen H, Steen PA: Acid aspiration syndrome prophylaxis in gynaecological and obstetric patients. A Norwegian survey. *Acta Anaesthesiol Scand* 1994;38:863-868.
20. Sellick BA: Cricoid pressure to control regurgitation of stomach contents during induction of anaesthesia. *Lancet* 1961;2:404-406.
21. Butler J, Sen A: Best evidence topic report. Cricoid pressure in emergency rapid sequence induction. *Emerg Med J* 2005;22:815-816.
22. Cooper RM, Pacey JA, Bishop MJ, et al: Early clinical experience with a new videolaryngoscope (GlideScope) in 728 patients. *Can J Anaesth* 2005;52:191-198.
23. de Boer HD, Driessen JJ, Marcus MA, Kerkkamp H, Heeringa M, Klimek M: Reversal of rocuronium-induced (1.2 mg/kg) profound neuromuscular block by sugammadex: A multicenter, dose-finding and safety study. *Anesthesiology* 2007;107:239-244.
24. EAST practice management guidelines for emergency tracheal intubation immediately following trauma. 2002. Available at http://www.east.org/tpg/intubation.pdf (accessed April 4, 2008).

20 Do Inhalational Agents Have Beneficial or Harmful Effects?

Stefan G. De Hert, MD, PhD

INTRODUCTION

The answer to the question of whether inhalational anesthetics are beneficial or harmful has evolved over the years. The initially introduced inhalational compounds had a very small therapeutic window and were associated with an important number of adverse events. Over the years, safer drugs were developed, resulting in lower morbidity and mortality rates associated with their administration. Nevertheless, even these compounds shared a common important depressant effect on the cardiovascular system, for which reason most anesthesiologists were reluctant to use them in patients with cardiac disease or compromised cardiac function. Indeed, for many years the use of inhalational anesthetics has been abandoned in favor of intravenous drugs in this subset of patients. In the 1980s, several studies have indicated that, in patients undergoing elective coronary artery surgery, the choice of the primary anesthetic agents did not result in different outcome.[1,2] However, starting in the 1990s, it appeared that the development of fast-track anesthetic techniques has helped to decrease intensive care unit and hospital length of stay with lower resource utilization and cost without adversely affecting mortality and morbidity rates.[3-5] Fast-track anesthetic protocols were mainly based on the use of short-acting intravenous drugs. Compared to the previously used large-dose opioid techniques, fast-track protocols had a shorter recovery time, which has led to a significant reduction in tracheal intubation time, and hence a decrease in intensive care unit length of stay.[3-7] Although inhalation-based techniques could also be suitable for early extubation protocols,[8] it was suggested that especially patients with impaired left ventricular function would not tolerate inhaled anesthetic-induced reduction in myocardial function.[5]

In recent years, however, new experimental and clinical evidence has indicated that the newer inhalational anesthetics might instead have a beneficial effect on the cardiovascular system. Since cardiovascular complications still represent a significant health risk to both the cardiac and the noncardiac surgical population,[6] any measure that may help reduce these adverse events should be part of the perioperative treatment of patients, especially those patients that are at increased risk for developing perioperative myocardial ischemia.

DO INHALATIONAL ANESTHETICS DECREASE THE EXTENT OF MYOCARDIAL DAMAGE IN THE PRESENCE OF MYOCARDIAL ISCHEMIA?

Prevention of ischemia is traditionally focused on maintaining the balance between myocardial oxygen supply and demand.[7] It is well known that all inhalational anesthetics decrease myocardial loading conditions and contractility. Even the newer compounds such as desflurane and sevoflurane demonstrate a similar dose-dependent depression of myocardial function.[8] These depressant effects decrease myocardial oxygen demand and may therefore have a beneficial role on the myocardial oxygen balance during myocardial ischemia. In addition to these *indirect* protective effects, inhalational anesthetics also have *direct* protective properties against reversible and irreversible ischemic myocardial damage. These properties have been related to a direct ischemic preconditioning-like effect, known as pharmacologic preconditioning induced by anesthetics (anesthetic preconditioning). Furthermore, volatile anesthetics applied during myocardial ischemia appear to suppress inflammatory responses that cause myocardial dysfunction. In addition, volatile anesthetics also decrease the extent of reperfusion injury when they are administered early during the reperfusion period. These properties have been summarized in different recent review articles.[9,10] The implementation of the cardioprotective effects of inhalational anesthetic agents during surgery may therefore provide an additional tool in the treatment and the prevention of ischemic cardiac dysfunction in the perioperative period.

Evidence

Experimental studies have indicated that inhalational anesthetic agents protect against the reversible but also the irreversible consequences of myocardial ischemia, as evidenced by a better recovery of myocardial function and a smaller myocardial infarction size after myocardial ischemia in the presence of various inhalational administration protocols.[11-14] In contrast with the large amount of data obtained in the experimental setting, only a limited number of studies have addressed the potential cardioprotective properties of volatile anesthetics in the clinical practice. This is mainly because the experimental protocol necessitates myocardial ischemia to be instituted in a standardized and reproducible way. This situation is normally not present in clinical practice, where all efforts are directed toward the prevention of myocardial ischemia to occur. The clinical situation that most closely resembles the sequence of standardized myocardial ischemia and reperfusion is the setting of coronary artery surgery. This type of surgery therefore allows us to transpose the experimental setting of preconditioning and postconditioning protocols into a clinical protocol sequence.

The clinical studies mainly involved either preconditioning protocols (i.e., administration of the inhalational agent before the institution of myocardial ischemia (aortic cross-clamping) or a protocol in which the inhalational agent was administered throughout the entire operative period. It is of interest to note that, whereas the experimental anesthetic preconditioning protocols consistently showed a beneficial effect on extent of myocardial damage and dysfunction after ischemia, this cardioprotective effect was not as obvious in the clinical situation. A number of studies did indeed report a beneficial effect on markers of myocardial damage or of hemodynamic function,[15-21] but this was not confirmed in other studies.[22,23] Taken together, it seems that the available clinical data do not indicate that administration of an inhalational anesthetic agent in a preconditioning protocol will result in a straightforward beneficial effect on the extent of myocardial damage after ischemia. On the contrary, in the studies where the inhalational anesthetic agent was administered throughout the entire procedure, a consistent cardioprotective effect was observed with less evidence of myocardial damage and a better preservation of myocardial function after ischemia.[24-30]

Anesthetic Cardioprotection in Clinical Practice

From the literature, it appeared that not all clinical anesthetic preconditioning protocols were associated with a protective action against the consequences of myocardial ischemia. Several reasons can be invoked for this phenomenon. In experimental protocols both duration of the preconditioning stimulus and duration of the ischemic period are highly standardized. This is not exactly true in clinical protocols where total duration of ischemia, the possible occurrence of ischemic events before the observation period, and also the modalities of the anesthetic preconditioning period vary greatly between studies. It seems that the extent of clinical cardioprotective effects critically depends on the modalities of administration of the inhalational anesthetic agents, such as the frequency and duration of the anesthetic preconditioning, the duration of the washout period, and the inspired concentration of the volatile anesthetic agent. In addition, inhalational anesthetic agents were also shown to be cardioprotective when administered during the period of myocardial ischemia[31,32] and during the reperfusion period.[33] Taken together it seems that a clinically significant cardioprotective effect of inhalational agents is most obvious in protocols where the agent is given throughout the entire procedure: before (preconditioning), during, and after myocardial ischemia (postconditioning).[33]

Clinical Relevance

Cardioprotective effects of inhalational anesthetic agents were apparent from the preservation of variables of myocardial function, and the lower release of markers of myocardial damage or dysfunction. However, at this moment it is unclear whether these effects also result in a decreased incidence of hard outcome variables such as perioperative morbidity and mortality rates. Although some studies have observed trends such as a shorter intensive care unit and hospital length of stay,[34] a lower incidence of postoperative atrial fibrillation,[35] and even an improved 1-year cardiovascular outcome after coronary surgery[36] with a volatile anesthetic regimen, these studies were severely underpowered to address this issue.

A recent retrospective study on data from 10,535 cardiac surgical procedures retrieved from a National Danish registry from 1999 to 2005 compared cardiac outcome between patients anesthetized with propofol and sevoflurane. No difference in postoperative 30-day mortality rate was observed in patients with preoperative unstable angina and/or a recent myocardial infarction. However, in the group of patients without these characteristics, mortality rate was lower in the group anesthetized with the inhalational agent (2.28 versus 3.14; $p = 0.015$).[37] There are also a few meta-analyses that have been performed on this subject (Table 20-1).[38-40] The meta-analysis by Yu and Beattie[38] included 32 trials on the subject with a total of 2841 patients. The meta-analysis of Symons and Miles[39] included 27 trials with a total of 2979 patients. In both these meta-analyses, no differences were observed in perioperative mortality and myocardial infarction rates between patients anesthetized with a volatile or an intravenous anesthetic regimen. However, it should be noted that these two reports also included studies in which halothane, enflurane, and isoflurane were used as inhalational anesthetics. On the contrary, a more recent meta-analysis including only studies with the newer inhalational anesthetics desflurane and sevoflurane (22 trials with a total of 1922 patients) observed a lower incidence of postoperative mortality (Odds ratio = 0.35; 95% confidence intervals: 0.14 to 0.90) and postoperative myocardial infarction (Odds ratio = 0.53; 95% confidence intervals: 0.32 to 0.86) with the use of an inhalational anesthetic regimen.[40]

The majority of data on the perioperative cardioprotective properties of inhalational anesthetic agents have been obtained in the setting of coronary artery surgery. It is unclear whether such an effect is also present in other types of surgery. One study reported similar cardioprotective effects of an inhalational anesthetic regimen in patients undergoing aortic valve surgery.[41] In patients undergoing mitral valve surgery, the situation seems to be more complex. Data from a recent study indicated that application of a desflurane preconditioning protocol in patients undergoing isolated mitral valve surgery demonstrated that the postoperative troponin release was not decreased. However, in patients undergoing a combined mitral valve and coronary artery surgery procedure, the application of desflurane preconditioning was associated with less myocardial damage.[42] These observations seem to indicate that the occurrence and the extent of inhalational-induced

Table 20-1	Summary of Meta-analyses on the Effects of Inhalational Anesthetic Agents on Perioperative Mortality and Perioperative Myocardial Infarction (PMI) Rates				
Study (Year)	Number of Trials	Number of Patients	Inhalational Agents Included	Incidence of Outcome	
				Inhalational Mortality PMI	**Intravenous Mortality PMI**
Yu & Beattie (2006)[38]	32 trials	2841 patients	Halothane Enflurane Isoflurane/sevoflurane Esflurane	18/1156 54/1402	30/1222 62/1459
Symons & Myles (2006)[39]	27 trials	2979 patients	Halothane Enflurane Isoflurane Sevoflurane Desflurane	No difference (data not reported) 51/1569	No difference (data not reported) 28/840
Landoni et al (2007)[40]	22 trials	1922 patients	Sevoflurane Desflurane	4/977 24/979	14/872 45/874

cardioprotection may depend on specific clinical conditions.

No data on cardioprotective effects in other types of surgery are currently available. Although it can be expected from a pathophysiologic point of view that the cardioprotective properties of inhalational anesthetic agents will also have beneficial effects in patients at risk for perioperative myocardial ischemia undergoing noncardiac surgery, the unequivocal evidence for such a clinical effect may be difficult to obtain. Indeed, it seems that the extent of cardioprotection depends on specific clinical variables such as the occurrence of perioperative myocardial ischemia. Because both the occurrence of perioperative myocardial ischemia and its extent and duration may vary greatly in patients undergoing noncardiac surgery, the potential beneficial effects of an inhalational anesthetic regimen may be blunted.

Another question is whether the protective effects against the consequences of ischemia observed at the level of the myocardium also extend to other organ systems. Although some experimental data have reported protective effects at the level of the spinal cord and the brain,[43,44] the endothelium,[45] the lungs,[46,47] and the kidneys and liver,[48,49] other reports fail to demonstrate such an effect.[50,51] Differences in experimental protocols have been invoked to explain the apparent discrepancies in the results.[52] In addition, even more than is the case for the myocardium, the ability of biochemical markers or measures of organ function to genuinely reflect changes in organ function is a point of debate. These concerns also apply when looking at the scarce clinical data available on protective properties of inhalational anesthetics on other organ function. The use of sevoflurane has been associated with a lower release of tumor necrosis factor α in cardiac surgery patients. It was hypothetized that part of the cytoprotective effects of volatile anesthetics could be due to a reduction in circulating concentrations of this element and its subsequent deleterious effects on different body organs.[53] However, since there seems to be a lack of consistent response with regard to the release of tumor necrosis factor α after various stimuli, it was suggested that tumor necrosis factor α alone may be a poor marker of outcome.[54] Data from a recent study in healthy volunteers indicated that the peri-ischemic administration of sevoflurane improved the postocclusive hyperemic reaction, suggesting a protective effect against the consequences of ischemia at the level of the endothelium.[55] Finally, another recent study in coronary artery surgery patients observed lower postoperative levels of serum glutamic oxaloacetic transaminase, glutamate pyruvate transaminase, and lactate dehydrogenase in patients anesthetized with an inhalational anesthetic regimen.[56] However, it could not be concluded from this study whether the beneficial effect on biochemical markers of hepatic dysfunction was related to a direct protective effect on hepatic function or whether this effect was merely the consequence of a better perioperative organ perfusion due to the preservation of cardiac function.

AREAS OF UNCERTAINTY

Although several studies have indicated that inhalational anesthetic agents may have a beneficial action to decrease the harmful effects of myocardial ischemia, controversies remain with regard to these reported properties. These controversies focus mainly around two topics: (1) the reliability of the phenomenon of anesthetic preconditioning in the clinical setting and (2) the concern about the clinical relevance of the reported cardioprotective properties, as discussed previously.

GUIDELINES

Current strategies on the prevention of adverse perioperative cardiovascular events mainly focus on the preservation of a beneficial myocardial oxygen balance and the application of therapies assumed to modulate plaque stabilization and the inflammatory response. Although these issues have been largely explored, no definitive conclusions with regard to their effectiveness in preventing perioperative morbidity have yet unequivocally been established.[57,58] With regard to the potential benefits of the use of an inhalational anesthetic regimen to decrease the incidence of perioperative cardiovascular events, conclusions are even less established. Indeed, there are no formal guidelines with regard to the use of a specific type of anesthetic agent in the management of patients at risk for developing perioperative myocardial ischemia. Although a number of randomized controlled trials suggest a protective action, all of the studies published until now were severely underpowered to address outcome issues. The results of recent meta-analyses also do not allow us to draw straightforward conclusions. Only in the most recent meta-analysis including the studies comparing the newer volatile anesthetics desflurane and sevoflurane to a total intravenous anesthetic regimen (22 trials with a total of 1922 patients), a lower incidence of perioperative mortality and myocardial infarction was reported.[40] Currently, the American Heart Association (American College of Cardiology/American Heart Association 2007 Guidelines on Perioperative Cardiovascular Evaluation and Care for Noncardiac Surgery) advocates the use of volatile anesthetic agents during noncardiac surgery for the maintenance of general anesthesia in hemodynamically stable patients at risk for myocardial ischemia.[59]

AUTHOR'S RECOMMENDATIONS

Based on the available data and keeping in mind that the suggestions derived from these data do not represent clinical guidelines or a consensus statement and should not replace individual clinical judgment, a number of recommendations may serve as a guide to help anesthesiologists make a rational decision in the care of patients at risk for developing perioperative myocardial ischemia.

- Experimental data have clearly indicated that the use of an inhalational anesthetic regimen protects against the functional and morphologic consequences of myocardial ischemia.
- This protective effect has also been demonstrated in clinical studies in patients undergoing cardiac surgery, with a better preservation of myocardial function and less myocardial damage with the use of an inhalational anesthetic regimen.
- In the clinical setting, the cardioprotective effect of an inhalational anesthetic regimen is most consistently present when the agent is given throughout the entire operative period: before ischemia, during ischemia, and during reperfusion.
- Although no dose-response data are available, the different clinical protocols used suggest that the protective effects are already present at doses of 0.5 MAC sevoflurane or desflurane.
- Although none of the studies performed so far was sufficiently powered to address outcome issues, a first meta-analysis including data from 1922 patients seems to indicate that the use of a volatile anesthetic regimen with the newer agents sevoflurane and desflurane is associated with a lower perioperative mortality rate and a lower incidence of perioperative myocardial infarction.
- Thus far, no data are available on the potential cardioprotective properties of inhalational agents in noncardiac surgery. However, the putative underlying pathophysiologic mechanisms involved in their cardioprotective action in the presence of myocardial ischemia and the clinical evidence from the cardiac surgical setting provide circumstantial evidence that these agents may provide an additional way to protect the myocardium in any patients at risk for developing perioperative myocardial ischemia.

REFERENCES

1. Slogoff S, Keats AS: Randomized trial of primary anesthetic agents on outcome of coronary bypass operations. *Anesthesiology* 1989;70:179-188.
2. Tuman KJ, McCarthy RJ, Spiess BD, Davalle M, Dabir R, Ivankovich AD: Does choice of anesthetic agent significantly affect outcome after coronary surgery? *Anesthesiology* 1989;70:189-198.
3. Cheng DCH, Karski J, Peniston C, Raveendran G, Asokumar B, Carroll J, et al: Early tracheal extubation after coronary artery bypass graft surgery reduces costs and improves resource use: A prospective randomized controlled trial. *Anesthesiology* 1996;85:1300-1310.
4. Cheng DCH, Karski J, Peniston C, Asokumar B, Raveendran G, Carroll J, et al: Morbidity outcome in early versus conventional tracheal extubation after coronary artery bypass grafting: A prospective randomized controlled trial. *J Thorac Cardiovasc Surg* 1996;112:755-764.
5. Myles PS, Buckland MR, Weeks AM, Bujor MA, McRae R, Langley M, et al: Hemodynamic effects, myocardial ischemia, and timing of tracheal extubation with propofol-based anesthesia for cardiac surgery. *Anesth Analg* 1997;84:12-19.
6. Mangano DT: Perioperative cardiac morbidity. *Anesthesiology* 1990;72:153-184.
7. Warltier DC, Pagel PS, Kersten JR: Approaches to the prevention of perioperative myocardial ischemia. *Anesthesiology* 2000;92:253-259.
8. De Hert SG, Van der Linden PJ, ten Broecke PW, Vermeylen KT, Rodrigus IE, Stockman BA: Effects of desflurane and sevoflurane on length-dependent regulation of myocardial function in coronary surgery patients. *Anesthesiology* 2001;95:357-363.
9. Tanaka K, Ludwig LM, Kersten JR, Pagel PS, Warltier DC: Mechanisms of cardioprotection by volatile anesthetics. *Anesthesiology* 2004;100:707-721.
10. De Hert SG, Turani F, Mathur S, Stowe DF: Cardioprotection with volatile anaesthetics: Mechanisms and clinical implications. *Anesth Analg* 2005;100:1584-1593.
11. Kersten JR, Orth KG, Pagel PS, Mei DA, Gross GJ, Warltier DC: Role of adenosine in isoflurane-induced cardioprotection. *Anesthesiology* 1997;86:1128-1139.
12. Toller WG, Kersten JR, Pagel PS, Hettrick DA, Warltier DC: Sevoflurane reduces myocardial infarction size and decreases the time threshold for ischemic preconditioning in dogs. *Anesthesiology* 1999;91:1437-1446.
13. Preckel B, Schlack W, Comfere T, Obal DH, Thamer V: Effects of enflurane, isoflurane, sevoflurane and desflurane on reperfusion injury after regional myocardial ischemia in the rabbit heart in vivo. *Br J Anaesth* 1998;81:905-912.
14. Ebel D, Preckel B, You A, Mullenheim J, Schlack W, Thamer V: Cardioprotection by sevoflurane against reperfusion injury after cardioplegic arrest in the rat is independent of three types of cardioplegia. *Br J Anaesth* 2002;88:828-835.
15. Belhomme D, Peynet J, Louzy M, Launay JM, Kitakaze M, Menasché P: Evidence for preconditioning by isoflurane in coronary artery bypass graft surgery. *Circulation* 1999;100:340-344.
16. Penta de Peppo A, Polisca P, Tomai F, De Paulis R, Turani F, Zupancich E, et al: Recovery of LV contractility in man is enhanced by preischemic administration of enflurane. *Ann Thorac Surg* 1999;68:112-118.
17. Tomai F, De Paulis R, Penta de Peppo A, Colagrande L, Caprara E, Polisca P, et al: Beneficial impact of isoflurane during coronary bypass surgery on troponin I release. *G Ital Cardiol* 1999;29:1007-1014.
18. Haroun-Bizri S, Khoury SS, Chehab IR, Kassas CM, Baraka A: Does isoflurane optimize myocardial protection during cardiopulmonary bypass? *J Cardiothorac Vasc Anesth* 2001;15:418-421.
19. Julier K, da Silva R, Garcia C, Bestmann L, Frascarolo P, Zollinger A, et al: Preconditioning by sevoflurane decreases biochemical markers for myocardial and renal dysfunction in coronary artery bypass graft surgery: A double-blinded, placebo-controlled, multicenter study. *Anesthesiology* 2003;98:1315-1327.
20. Forlani S, Tomai F, De Paulis R, Turani F, Colella DF, Nardi P, et al: Preoperative shift from glibenclamide to insulin is cardioprotective in diabetic patients undergoing coronary artery bypass surgery. *J Cardiovasc Surg (Torino)* 2004;45:117-122.

21. Lee MC, Chen CH, Kuo MC, Kang PL, Lo A, et al: Isoflurane-preconditioning-induced cardioprotection in patients undergoing coronary artery bypass grafting. *Eur J Anaesthesiol* 2006;23: 841-847.

22. Pouzet B, Lecharny JB, Dehoux M, Paquin S, Kitakaze M, Mantz J, et al: Is there a place for preconditioning during cardiac operations in humans? *Ann Thorac Surg* 2002;73:843-848.

23. Fellahi JL, Gue X, Philippe E, Riou B, Gerard JL: Isoflurane may not influence postoperative cardiac troponin I release and clinical outcome in adult cardiac surgery. *Eur J Anaesthesiol* 2004;21: 688-693.

24. De Hert SG, ten Broecke PW, Mertens E, Van Sommeren EW, De Blier IG, Stockman BA, et al: Sevoflurane but not propofol preserves myocardial function in coronary surgery patients. *Anesthesiology* 2002;97:42-49.

25. De Hert SG, Cromheecke S, ten Broecke PW, Mertens E, De Blier IG, Stockman BA, et al: Effects of propofol, desflurane, and sevoflurane on recovery of myocardial function after coronary surgery in elderly high-risk patients. *Anesthesiology* 2003;99:314-323.

26. Conzen PF, Fisher S, Detter C, Peter K: Sevoflurane provides greater protection of the myocardium than propofol in patients undergoing off-pump coronary artery bypass surgery. *Anesthesiology* 2003;99:826-833.

27. Bein B, Renner J, Caliebe D, Scholz J, Paris A, Fraund S, et al: Sevoflurane but not propofol preserves myocardial function during minimally invasive direct coronary artery bypass surgery. *Anesth Analg* 2005;100:610-616.

28. Guarracino F, Landoni G, Tritapepe L, Pompei F, Leoni A, Aletti G, et al: Myocardial damage prevented by volatile anesthetics: A multicenter randomised controlled study. *J Cardiothorac Vasc Anesth* 2006;20:477-483.

29. Kawamura T, Kadosaki M, Nara N, Kaise A, Suzuki H, Endo S, et al: Effects of sevoflurane on cytokine balance in patients undergoing coronary artery bypass graft surgery. *J Cardiothorac Vasc Anesth* 2006;20:503-508.

30. Tritapepe L, Landoni G, Guarracino F, Pompei F, Crivellari M, Maselli D, et al: Cardiac protection by volatile anaesthetics: A multicentre randomized controlled study in patients undergoing coronary artery bypass grafting with cardiopulmonary bypass. *Eur J Anaesthesiol* 2007;24:323-331.

31. Nader ND, Li CM, Khadra WZ, Reedy R, Panos AL: Anesthetic myocardial protection with sevoflurane. *J Cardiothorac Vasc Anesth* 2004;18:269-274.

32. Nader ND, Karamanoukian HL, Reedy RC, Salehpour F, Knight PR: Inclusion of sevoflurane in cardioplegia reduces neutrophil activity during cardiopulmonary bypass. *J Cardiothorac Vasc Anesth* 2006;20:57-62.

33. De Hert SG, Van der Linden PJ, Cromheecke S, Meeus R, Nelis A, Van Reeth V, et al: Cardioprotective properties of sevoflurane in patients undergoing coronary surgery with cardiopulmonary bypass are related to the modalities of its administration. *Anesthesiology* 2004;101:299-310.

34. De Hert SG, Van der Linden PJ, Cromheecke S, Meeus R, ten Broecke PW, De Blier IG, et al: Choice of primary anesthetic regimen can influence intensive care unit length of stay after coronary surgery with cardiopulmonary bypass. *Anesthesiology* 2004;101:9-20.

35. Cromheecke S, ten Broecke PW, Hendrickx E, Meeus R, De Hert SG: Atrial fibrillation after coronary surgery: Can choice of the anesthetic regimen influence the incidence? *Acta Anaesthesiol Belg* 2005;56:147-154.

36. Garcia C, Julier K, Bestmann L, Zollinger A, von Segesser LK, Pasch T, et al: Preconditioning with sevoflurane decreases PECAM-1 expression and improves one-year cardiovascular outcome in coronary artery bypass graft surgery. *Br J Anaesth* 2005;94:159-165.

37. Jakobsen CJ, Berg H, Hindsholm KB, Faddy N, Sloth E: The influence of propofol versus sevoflurane anesthesia on outcome in 10,535 cardiac surgical procedures. *J Cardiothorac Vasc Anesth* 2007;21:664-671.

38. Yu CH, Beattie WS: The effects of volatile anesthetics on cardiac ischemic complications and mortality in CABG: A meta-analysis. *Can J Anesth* 2006;53:906-918.

39. Symons JA, Myles PS: Myocardial protection with volatile anaesthetic agents during cardiopulmonary bypass surgery: A meta-analysis. *Br J Anaesth* 2006;97:127-136.

40. Landoni G, Biondi-Zoccai GCL, Zangrillo A, Elena B, D'Aviola S, Marchetti C, et al: Desflurane and sevoflurane in cardiac surgery: A meta-analysis of randomized clinical trials. *J Cardiothorac Vasc Anesth* 2007;21:502-511.

41. Cromheecke S, Pepermans V, Hendrickx E, Lorsomradee S, ten Broecke PW, Stockman BA, et al: Cardioprotective properties of sevoflurane in patients undergoing aortic valve replacement with cardiopulmonary bypass. *Anesth Analg* 2006;103:289-296.

42. Landoni G, Calabro MG, Marchetti C, Bignami E, Scandroglio AM, Dedola E, et al: Desflurane vs propofol in patients undergoing mitral valve surgery. *J Cardiothorac Vasc Anesth* 2007;21:672-677.

43. Sang H, Cao L, Qiu P, Xiong L, Wang R, Yan G: Isoflurane produces delayed preconditioning against spinal cord ischemic injury via release of free radicals in rabbits. *Anesthesiology* 2006;105:953-960.

44. Sakai H, Sheng H, Yates RB, Ishida K, Pearlstein RD, Warner DS: Isoflurane provides long-term protection against focal cerebral ischemia in the rat. *Anesthesiology* 2007;106:92-99.

45. de Klaver MJM, Manning L, Palmer LA, Rich GF: Isoflurane pretreatment inhibits cytokine-induced death in cultured rat smooth muscle cells and human endothelial cells. *Anesthesiology* 2002;97:24-32.

46. Reutershan J, Chang D, Hayes JK, Ley K: Protective effects of isoflurane pre-treatment in endotoxin-induced lung injury. *Anesthesiology* 2006;104:511-517.

47. Suter D, Spahn DR, Blumenthal S, Reyes L, Booy C, et al: The immunomodulatory effect of sevoflurane in endotoxin-injured alveolar epithelial cells. *Anesth Analg* 2007;104:638-645.

48. Hashiguchi H, Morroka H, Miyoshi H, Matsumoto M, Koji T, Sumikawa K: Isoflurane protects renal function against ischemia and reperfusion through inhibition of protein kinases, JNK and ERK. *Anesth Analg* 2005;101:1584-1589.

49. Lee HT, Emala CW, Joo JD, Kim M: Isoflurane improves survival and protects against renal and hepatic injury in murine septic peritonitis. *Shock* 2007;27:373-379.

50. Kawaguchi M, Kimbro JR, Drummond JC, Cole DJ, Kelly PJ, Patel PM: Isoflurane delays but does not prevent cerebral infarction in rats subjected to focal ischemia. *Anesthesiology* 2000;92: 1335-1342.

51. Obal D, Dettwiler S, Favoccia C, Rasher K, Preckel B, Schlack W: Effect of sevoflurane preconditioning on ischaemia/reperfusion injury in the rat kidney in vivo. *Eur J Anaesthesiol* 2006;23:319-326.

52. Pickler PE, Patel PM: Anesthetic neuroprotection: Some things do last. *Anesthesiology* 2007;106:8-10.

53. El Azab SR, Rosseel PM, De Lange JJ, Groeneveld ABJ, Van Strik R, et al: Effect of sevoflurane on the ex vivo secretion of TNF-α during and after coronary artery bypass surgery. *Eur J Anaesthesiol* 2003;20:380-384.

54. Royston D, Kovesi T, Marczin N: The unwanted response to cardiac surgery: Time for a reappraisal? *J Thor Cardiovasc Surg* 2003;125:32-35.

55. Lucchinetti E, Ambrosio S, Aguirre J, Herrmann P, Härter L, et al: Sevoflurane inhalation at sedative concentrations provides endothelial protection against ischemia-reperfusion injury in humans. *Anesthesiology* 2007;106:262-268.

56. Lorsomradee S, Cromheecke S, Lorsomradee SR, De Hert SG: Effects of sevoflurane on biomechanical markers of hepatic and renal dysfunction after coronary artery surgery. *J Cardiothorac Vasc Anesth* 2006;20:684-690.

57. Devereaux PJ, Beattie WS, Choi PTL, Guyatt GH, Villar JC, et al: How strong is the evidence for the use of perioperative β blockers in non-cardiac surgery? Systematic review and meta-analysis of randomized controlled trials. *BMJ*, doi:10.1136/bmj.38503.623646.8F (published July 4, 2005).

58. Kapoor AS, Kanji H, Buckingham J, Devereaux PJ, McAlister FA: Strength of evidence for perioperative use of statins to reduce cardiovascular risk: Systematic review of controlled studies. *BMJ*, doi:10.1136/bmj.39006.531146.BE (published Nov 6, 2006).

59. Fleisher LA, Beckman JA, Brown KA, Calkins H, Chaikof E, et al: ACC/AHA 2007 guidelines on perioperative cardiovascular evaluation and care for noncardiac surgery: A report of the American College of Cardiology/American Heart Association Task Force on Practice Guidelines (Writing Committee to Revise the 2002 Guidelines on Perioperative Cardiovascular Evaluation for Noncardiac Surgery). *J Am Coll Cardiol* 2007;50:e159-241.

21 Is One General Anesthetic Technique Associated with Faster Recovery?

Ralph Gertler, MD, and Girish P. Joshi, MBBS, MD, FFARCSI

INTRODUCTION

The current health care environment of cost containment and efficient resource utilization increasingly emphasizes the need for a rapid postoperative recovery and early discharge. With the availability of shorter-acting anesthetic drugs, which allow rapid emergence, the need for postanesthesia care unit (PACU) stay is also questioned.[1-3] Although local and regional anesthesia techniques allow a quicker recovery, general anesthesia remains the most commonly used technique.[4] There is evidence that the choice of general anesthetic technique is associated with faster recovery, particularly immediate emergence from anesthesia and early recovery.[1,2] The modern general anesthetic technique consists of the use of a combination of drugs to achieve amnesia, analgesia (or hemodynamic stability), and patient immobility (or muscle relaxation). The skillful use of multiple anesthetic drugs is preferable in providing adequate anesthesia and surgical conditions while allowing for rapid recovery. The most important aspect of an anesthetic technique is its ability to consistently achieve rapid recovery after termination of surgery.

OPTIONS/EVIDENCE

Premedication

Benzodiazepines are often used to provide preoperative anxiolysis and reduce the incidence of intraoperative awareness.[5] Although some older studies did not observe a delay in recovery with the use of preoperative benzodiazepines,[6,7] recent evidence suggests that recovery, particularly in the elderly, may be prolonged.[8] Therefore it might be prudent to avoid preoperative benzodiazepines if possible. Because significant reduction in stress-hormone levels have been observed after diazepam premedication,[9] benzodiazepine premedication might be beneficial in a high-risk population (e.g., cardiac patients) undergoing ambulatory surgery.

Induction of Anesthesia

Either propofol or sevoflurane can be used for the induction of anesthesia. A study comparing induction with propofol and sevoflurane followed by sevoflurane for maintenance of anesthesia reported that the time to emergence (i.e., eye opening to command) was shorter in patients with sevoflurane induction (5.2 minutes versus 7 minutes).[10] However, the incidence of postoperative nausea and vomiting (PONV) was higher after sevoflurane induction. Because propofol induction is associated with higher perioperative patient satisfaction,[11] sevoflurane should be reserved for selected patients (Table 21-1).

Maintenance: Inhalation Anesthesia versus Total Intravenous Anesthesia with Propofol

Ease of titratability and a rapid emergence from anesthesia favor inhaled anesthetic techniques. In addition, inhaled anesthetics potentiate neuromuscular blockade,[12] thereby reducing the requirements of muscle relaxants and subsequent complications of residual paralysis (e.g., visual disturbances, inability to sit up without assistance, facial weakness, and generalized weakness).[13] Compared with isoflurane, the newer shorter-acting inhaled anesthetics (e.g., desflurane and sevoflurane) allow for a more rapid emergence from anesthesia.[14]

Song and colleagues[15] measured recovery times and ability to fast-track with desflurane, sevoflurane, or propofol. Anesthesia with an inhaled anesthetic resulted in shorter times to awakening, tracheal extubation, and orientation, compared with propofol total intravenous anesthesia (TIVA). A considerably larger percentage of patients who received desflurane for maintenance were considered fast-track eligible compared with sevoflurane and propofol (90% versus 75% and 26%, respectively). However, there was no difference between the groups with respect to the times to oral intake and home-readiness. Earlier emergence with desflurane, compared with sevoflurane and propofol, was also reported when bispectral index (BIS) monitoring was used to titrate the hypnotic agents.[16,17] Use of BIS monitoring reduced the emergence times by 30% to 55%,[17,18] However, this effect of BIS was not reproducible in a study of elderly (greater than 65 years old) outpatients in which the use of BIS during shorter procedures (less than 30 minutes) reduced the opioid requirements, but did not improve early recovery.[19] Postural stability is achieved earlier after desflurane anesthesia than after propofol.[20] Similarly, emergence from anesthesia is faster with sevoflurane, compared to propofol and isoflurane.[21-23] Nonetheless, this does not translate into an earlier discharge from the PACU or earlier time to achieve home-readiness.[21,22,24,25]

Juvin and colleagues[25] evaluated the recovery of morbidly obese patients receiving desflurane, isoflurane, and propofol anesthetized to maintain similar BIS values. Immediate recovery occurred faster and was more consistent and oxygen saturations were higher after desflurane than after propofol or isoflurane; however, these differences persisted only in the early recovery phase (up to 2 hours after surgery). Similar results were seen in elderly patients.[26,27] Again, the need for PACU interventions was significantly less with desflurane.

A recent study evaluated the ability to swallow water without coughing or drooling after desflurane and sevoflurane anesthesia and found that patients receiving desflurane were able to swallow water without coughing or drooling significantly earlier.[28] Based on these findings the authors concluded that desflurane allowed an earlier return of protective airway reflexes.

Although propofol TIVA is consistently associated with a lower incidence of PONV as compared with inhaled anesthetic technique,[22,29-33] PONV incidence is equivalent when prophylactic antiemetics are used with inhalation anesthesia and N_2O.[29] Studies using BIS monitoring to titrate hypnotic-sedatives and prophylactic antiemetics have not observed any difference in the incidence of PONV between the different general anesthetic techniques.[17,25,34] Titration of inhaled anesthetic using BIS monitoring has been shown to further reduce the incidence of postoperative vomiting in the phase II area.[35] Nevertheless, propofol TIVA is preferable in patients at very high risk of PONV.

In summary, the newer shorter-acting inhaled anesthetics (e.g., desflurane and sevoflurane) allow for an earlier emergence from anesthesia compared with older inhaled anesthetics (e.g., halothane and isoflurane) (Table 21-1 and Table 21-2). Although xenon is not yet commercially available, emergence of anesthesia appears to be faster with desflurane and xenon.[36] Rapid recovery reduces the risks of postoperative complications, including airway obstruction and hypoxemia.[27,37] In addition, faster emergence allows for fast-tracking (i.e., bypassing the PACU). Interestingly, recent studies suggest a gender difference in recovery, with women recovering faster from general anesthesia than men.[38] This is probably due to the influence of female sex hormones and their role on the modulation of anesthetic action.

Brain function monitors may improve titration of inhaled and intravenous sedative-hypnotic drugs, allow faster emergence, and improve quality of recovery (reduced drowsiness, dizziness, fatigue, nausea, and vomiting). However, these monitors do not influence phase II recovery and home-readiness. Furthermore, these monitors may have limited benefits in patients breathing spontaneously or undergoing shorter surgical procedures.[39]

Nitrous Oxide

Because of its amnestic and analgesic properties, as well as its capability to lower the requirements of costly anesthetic drugs, nitrous oxide (N_2O) is commonly used as part of a balanced anesthesia technique. In addition to reducing the induction time or dose of the inducing agent, the use of N_2O results in smoother induction. It allows for a faster return to spontaneous breathing after equi-MAC (1.3 MAC with or without N_2O) regimens of sevoflurane.[40] N_2O is rapidly eliminated, resulting in a faster recovery even with the use of inhaled anesthetics with higher lipid solubility (e.g., isoflurane) in short procedures (less than 60 minutes) in elderly patients.[24]

Although some studies have reported a higher incidence of PONV with the use of N_2O, a meta-analysis of randomized controlled trials found that the emetic effect of N_2O is not significant.[41] A large study of 740 women undergoing outpatient gynecologic surgery compared the incidence of PONV and the time to home-readiness with a propofol-N_2O–based and a propofol-alone anesthetic technique.[42] In this high-risk population the use of N_2O reduced propofol requirements by 20% to 25% without increasing the incidence of adverse events or the time to home-readiness. Interestingly, most studies assessing the feasibility of fast-tracking after outpatient surgery have used N_2O as a part of their anesthetic technique.[42-44] Overall, there is no convincing evidence to avoid N_2O.[45]

Supralaryngeal Airway Devices

Supralaryngeal airway devices (e.g., laryngeal mask airway [LMA]) have gained widespread popularity as general-purpose airway devices and are increasingly used for routine elective surgical procedures. They do not require the use of neuromuscular blockade and are generally tolerated at lower anesthetic levels than a tracheal tube. With the patient breathing spontaneously, opioid requirements can be based on the respiratory rate, and dosing requirements of hypnotic anesthetics (intravenous or inhaled) can be based on brain function monitors or end-tidal concentrations of inhaled anesthetics. This allows earlier emergence from anesthesia and improved perioperative efficiency.[46] Newer trends may also favor the use of supralaryngeal airway devices in previously excluded areas such as outpatient laparoscopy and controlled mechanical ventilation.[47,48]

Because desflurane has irritant properties, sevoflurane, which is nonpungent, is generally considered the drug of choice for patients breathing spontaneously. However, recent studies suggest that desflurane can also be safely used in patients breathing spontaneously through an LMA.[49-52] Maintenance of anesthesia with desflurane, isoflurane, and propofol in patients breathing spontaneously through a supralaryngeal airway device is considered equally effective and safe. The incidence of respiratory complications was similar between the three groups; however, purposeful movement was significantly more common with propofol TIVA compared with isoflurane or desflurane (63% versus 23% and 7%, respectively).[49] Furthermore, desflurane reduces the time to emergence, home-readiness,[51] and return to normal daily activities without an increase in airway problems.[50]

Opioids

Opioids continue to play an important role in anesthesia practice; however, opioid-related side effects, including nausea, vomiting, and sedation, may contribute to a delayed recovery and discharge home. Therefore opioids should be used sparingly in patients undergoing ambulatory surgery, and analgesia should be provided using nonopioid analgesics. However, if nonopioid analgesic techniques are not used, inadequate intraoperative opioid dose may result in a higher incidence of severe pain in the PACU.[53] Remifentanil is rapidly metabolized and therefore has a very short duration of action independent of the duration of infusion. Studies have reported a reliable and rapid emergence with the use of remifentanil.[54-56] In addition, functional activities are regained significantly faster after remifentanil than after a fentanyl-based anesthetic.[55] Immediate and intermediate recovery criteria are consistently met earlier in remifentanil-treated patients.[55-58] It is suggested that the use of remifentanil allows the administration of lower concentrations of inhaled anesthetics, which may lead to faster recovery.[57] However, because of its short duration of action, it is necessary to plan for postoperative pain relief with longer-acting analgesics before discontinuation of remifentanil. The use of longer-acting opioids at the end of the surgery may increase the incidence of opioid-related adverse side effects in the postoperative period. Therefore the benefits of remifentanil may only be realized if a nonopioid analgesic technique can be used.

It is generally believed that morphine should not be used in ambulatory surgery patients because of the concerns of increased PONV. However, use of fentanyl in the PACU might lead to recurrence of pain in the phase II unit, and delay discharge home and increase the need for hospitalization, particularly if oral analgesics are not administered or are not tolerated.[59]

AREAS OF UNCERTAINTY

The following areas of uncertainty exist:

1. Does the use of a small dose (2 mg) of midazolam provide protection against awareness or delay recovery from anesthesia?
2. Does the use of nitrous oxide reduce intraoperative and/or postoperative opioid requirements?
3. Is there a role for xenon in clinical practice?
4. Are longer-acting opioids (e.g., morphine and hydromorphone) suitable for current ambulatory anesthesia practice, particularly with more extensive surgical procedures on an outpatient basis?

Table 21-1	Summary of Meta-analysis on General Anesthetic Techniques			
Author	**Number of Trials**	**Intervention**	**Control**	**Outcomes**
Joo[11]	12	Sevoflurane	Propofol	Sevoflurane and propofol had similar efficacy for anesthetic induction. Propofol may still be the preferred induction anesthetic because of its favorable induction of anesthesia characteristics, high patient satisfaction, and lower incidence of postoperative nausea and vomiting.
Gupta[14]	58	Propofol, isoflurane, sevoflurane, desflurane		Postoperative recovery after propofol-, isoflurane-, desflurane-, and sevoflurane-based anesthesia in adults demonstrated that early recovery was faster in the desflurane and sevoflurane groups. The incidence of nausea and vomiting was less frequent with propofol.
Robinson[23]	18	Sevoflurane, isoflurane	Propofol	Sevoflurane is associated with a more rapid recovery from anesthesia than either isoflurane or propofol.
Sneyd[30]	80	Propofol	Inhalation agents	Maintenance of anesthesia with propofol had a significantly lower incidence of postoperative nausea and vomiting in comparison with inhalation agents regardless of induction agent, choice of inhalation agent, presence/absence of N_2O, age of patient, or use of opiate.
Tramer[31]	84 ($n = 6069$)	Propofol	Other anesthetic agents	The NNT to prevent early nausea with propofol was 4.7, vomiting 4.9, and any emetic event 4.9. Of five patients treated with propofol for maintenance of anesthesia, one will not vomit or be nauseated who would otherwise have vomited or been nauseated. In all other situations the difference was of doubtful clinical relevance.
Tramer[41]	24 ($n = 2478$)	GA with N_2O	GA omitting N_2O	Omitting N_2O had no effect on complete control of emesis or nausea. The NNT for intraoperative awareness with an N_2O-free anesthetic was 46 compared with anesthetics where N_2O was used. This clinically important risk of major harm reduces the usefulness of omitting N_2O to prevent postoperative emesis.

GA, General anesthesia; *NNT*, number needed to treat.

Table 21-2 Summary of Randomized Controlled Trials

Author	n	Intervention	Control	Outcome
Apfel[29]	5199	Six prophylactic interventions for PONV: ondansetron, dexamethasone, droperidol, propofol, or a volatile anesthetic; nitrogen or N_2O; and remifentanil or fentanyl.		The safest or least expensive should be used first. Prophylaxis is rarely warranted in low-risk patients, moderate-risk patients may benefit from a single intervention, and multiple interventions should be reserved for high-risk patients.
Arellano[42]	1490	N_2O 65% + oxygen	Air + oxygen	No significant differences between groups in home-readiness and the frequency of adverse events for 24 hr
Ashworth[49]	90	Desflurane	Isoflurane or propofol	Purposeful movement with propofol in 63% without recall. Desflurane and propofol have no clinically significant advantage over isoflurane in patients with LMA and spontaneous ventilation.
Bekker[57]	60	Isoflurane-remifentanil-N_2O	Isoflurane-fentanyl-N_2O	Maintenance of anesthesia with remifentanil-N_2O can shorten postoperative recovery of cognitive function in a geriatric population, but did not shorten the overall length of stay in the postanesthesia care unit.
Camci[16]	50	Desflurane-remifentanil-N_2O, BIS guided	Propofol-remifentanil-N_2O, BIS guided	Home-readiness did not differ between the groups. Desflurane is an alternative to propofol for BIS-guided ambulatory anesthesia. The higher frequency of emetic symptoms with desflurane diminished the success of its fast-track eligibility.
Claxton[59]	58	Fentanyl	Morphine	Morphine produced a better quality of analgesia but was associated with an increased incidence of nausea and vomiting, the majority of which occurred after discharge.
Duggan[9]	61	Diazepam 0.1 mg/kg 60 or 90 min preoperatively	Placebo	The reduction in stress hormones following diazepam premedication in patients undergoing day-case surgery may support the role for benzodiazepine premedication.
Einarsson[40]	24	Sevoflurane	Sevoflurane + N_2O	Return to spontaneous breathing and extubation earlier with sevoflurane/N_2O vs. sevoflurane
Fredman[21]	146	Propofol induction + sevoflurane + N_2O	Propofol induction + sevoflurane + N_2O; sevoflurane + N_2O for induction and maintenance	Faster induction with propofol. Similar recovery. More PONV with sevoflurane.
Fredman[26]	90	TIVA vs. desflurane + N_2O vs. isoflurane + N_2O titrated to BIS 60-65		Fast-track eligibility earlier with desflurane compared to isoflurane and propofol (73% vs. 43% and 44%).
Gan[18]	302	Propofol TIVA + BIS monitoring to 45-60, increasing to 60-75 during the final 15 min	TIVA	BIS monitoring decreased propofol requirements, allowed earlier extubation, increased the percentage of patients oriented on arrival to PACU, had better PACU nursing assessments, and resulted in patients being eligible for discharge sooner.

(Continued)

Table 21-2   Summary of Randomized Controlled Trials—Cont'd

Author	n	Intervention	Control	Outcome
Georgiou[37]	50	TIVA with propofol	Isoflurane + N_2O	At least one hypoxemic event in 16.7% in the TIVA group vs. 42.3% in the inhalation anesthesia group.
Juvin[27]	45	Desflurane	Isoflurane or propofol for maintenance	Immediate recovery times shorter with desflurane vs. isoflurane or propofol. Intermediate recovery and time to discharge from PACU similar in the three groups.
Juvin[25]	36	Desflurane	Isoflurane or propofol for maintenance	Immediate recovery occurred faster after desflurane, SpO_2 values were higher, patients were more mobile after desflurane. Beneficial effects for at least 2 hours.
Larsen[58]	60	Remifentanil-propofol	Desflurane-N_2O, or sevoflurane-N_2O, fentanyl	Emergence and return of cognitive function was faster after remifentanil-propofol compared with desflurane and sevoflurane.
Loop[56]	120	Remifentanil with sevoflurane, desflurane, or propofol	Thiopental-alfentanil-isoflurane-N_2O	Remifentanil enables fast and smooth early recovery. Late recovery was comparable among the remifentanil combination groups and the control group.
Mahmoud[50]	60	Desflurane + N_2O	Sevoflurane + N_2O	Time to eye opening and orientation significantly faster with desflurane than sevoflurane group. Home-readiness earlier with desflurane. Desflurane group returned earlier to normal activity.
McKay[28]	64	Sevoflurane	Desflurane	Desflurane allows an earlier return of protective airway reflexes.
Nelskyla[35]	62	Sevoflurane in 65% N_2O titrated to maintain the BIS between 50 and 60.	Sevoflurane adjusted to keep hemodynamic variables within 25% of control values	Orientation and ability to drink were achieved earlier in the BIS group, which also achieved better psychomotor recovery. Less vomiting in BIS group. No differences in time to achieve home-readiness.
Raeder[22]	161	Propofol induction with 60% N_2O through an LMA and sevoflurane	Anesthesia maintained with 60% N_2O through an LMA and TIVA	Faster emergence from sevoflurane anesthesia. Perioperative bradycardia, nausea and vomiting, and late postoperative dizziness were more common in sevoflurane group. No difference between sevoflurane and propofol groups in pain, eligibility for recovery room discharge, or home-readiness.
Saros[52]	70	Sevoflurane	Desflurane	Desflurane is associated with a faster emergence with no differences during the postoperative course except a somewhat higher incidence of airway irritation.
Smith[33]	61	Propofol target of 8 mcg/mL, reduced to 4 mcg/mL after LMA insertion and subsequently titrated to clinical signs	Sevoflurane 8%, reduced to 3% after laryngeal mask insertion and subsequently titrated to clinical signs	Emergence was faster after sevoflurane, but was associated with more nausea and vomiting.

(Continued)

Table 21-2	**Summary of Randomized Controlled Trials—Cont'd**			
Author	**n**	**Intervention**	**Control**	**Outcome**
Song[20]	120	Desflurane	Propofol	Desflurane-based anesthetic was associated with better postural control than the propofol-based anesthetic in the early recovery period after outpatient gynecologic laparoscopic procedures.
Song[17]	60	Desflurane or sevoflurane with 65% N_2O and fentanyl. Volatile anesthetics were titrated to maintain the BIS value at 60	Volatile anesthetics were administered according to standard clinical practice	BIS values were lower in the control groups compared with the BIS-titrated groups. The volatile anesthetic usage in the BIS-titrated groups was 30%-38% lower compared with the control groups. Times to verbal responsiveness were 30%-55% shorter in the BIS-titrated groups.
Song[15]	120	Desflurane or sevoflurane in 60% N_2O	TIVA 60% N_2O	Times to awakening and a recovery score of 10 were significantly shorter, and the percentage of patients judged fast-track eligible on arrival in the PACU was significantly higher, in the desflurane and sevoflurane groups.
Tang[51]	140	Propofol for induction followed by TIVA or sevoflurane with N_2O 67%	Anesthesia was induced and maintained with sevoflurane in N_2O 67%	Compared with sevoflurane-N_2O, use of propofol-N_2O for office-based anesthesia was associated with an improved recovery profile, greater patient satisfaction, and lower costs.
Tang[44]	75	TIVA, BIS index value between 55 and 65	Desflurane with N_2O 67%, BIS index value between 55 and 65	Early recovery times were shorter in the desflurane group. Fast-track criteria were met earlier in the desflurane (versus propofol) group. Use of desflurane reduced the time to standing up and ambulating. During the 24 hr follow-up period, PONV was not significantly different between the two groups with triple antiemetic.
Tang[34]	69	TIVA	TIVA with N_2O 65% in oxygen.	Early and late recovery variables were similar. Propofol anesthesia with administration of N_2O decreased the anesthetic requirement without increasing PONV.
Thwaites[10]	108	Induction with propofol then 2% sevoflurane	Induction with inhalation of sevoflurane 8%	Emergence from anesthesia induced with sevoflurane occurred significantly earlier compared with propofol, but significantly more patients rated induction with sevoflurane as unpleasant.
Visser[32]	2010	Isoflurane-N_2O	TIVA	Propofol TIVA results in a clinically relevant reduction of postoperative nausea and vomiting compared with isoflurane-N_2O anesthesia (NNT = 6). Both anesthetic techniques were otherwise similar.
Zohar[19]	30	Propofol-fentanyl-sevoflurane, BIS guided	Propofol-fentanyl-sevoflurane	Use of BIS monitoring for titrating sevoflurane failed to improve the early recovery process for short procedures in elderly patients.

BIS, bispectral index; *LMA*, laryngeal mask airway; *PONV*, postoperative nausea and vomiting; *TIVA*, total intravenous anesthesia.

GUIDELINES

There are currently no guidelines on the choice of anesthesia for faster recovery.

AUTHORS' RECOMMENDATIONS

Although intravenous induction with propofol and inhalational induction with sevoflurane are both suitable techniques for outpatients, intravenous induction is preferable. Maintenance of anesthesia with the newer shorter-acting inhaled anesthetics (i.e., desflurane and sevoflurane) provides for a rapid emergence as compared with propofol TIVA, while allowing easy titratability of anesthetic depth. However, no differences have been demonstrated with respect to late recovery (e.g., PACU stay and home-readiness). Furthermore, titration of hypnotic-sedatives using electroencephalogram-based brain function monitoring may reduce the time to awakening and thereby may facilitate fast-tracking (i.e., bypassing the PACU). Although clinical differences between desflurane and sevoflurane appear to be small, desflurane may be associated with faster emergence, particularly in elderly and morbidly obese patients. Balanced anesthesia with intravenous propofol induction and inhalation anesthesia with N₂O for maintenance, and a supralaryngeal airway device, may be an optimal technique for ambulatory surgery.

Based on the evidence from randomized controlled trials and the vast body of literature, induction of anesthesia with propofol and maintenance with newer shorter-acting inhaled anesthetics allows for an early emergence, but there is no difference in the late recovery. Furthermore, propofol TIVA may be beneficial in patients at very high risk of PONV.

REFERENCES

1. Joshi GP, Twersky RS: Fast tracking in ambulatory surgery. *Ambul Surg* 2000;8(4):185-190.
2. Joshi GP: Fast-tracking in outpatient surgery. *Curr Opin Anaesthesiol* 2001;14(6):635-639.
3. Apfelbaum JL, Walawander CA, Grasela TH, et al: Eliminating intensive postoperative care in same-day surgery patients using short-acting anesthetics. *Anesthesiology* 2002;97(1):66-74.
4. Joshi GP: Recent developments in regional anesthesia for ambulatory surgery. *Curr Opin Anaesthesiol* 1999;12(6):643-647.
5. Miller DR, Blew PG, Martineau RJ, Hull KA: Midazolam and awareness with recall during total intravenous anaesthesia. *Can J Anaesth* 1996;43(9):946-953.
6. White PF: Comparative evaluation of intravenous agents for rapid sequence induction—thiopental, ketamine, and midazolam. *Anesthesiology* 1982;57(4):279-284.
7. Beechey AP, Eltringham RJ, Studd C: Temazepam as premedication in day surgery. *Anaesthesia* 1981;36(1):10-15.
8. Smith AF, Pittaway AJ: Premedication for anxiety in adult day surgery. *Cochrane Database of Systematic Reviews (Online)* 2003(1): CD002192.
9. Duggan M, Dowd N, O'Mara D, Harmon D, Tormey W, Cunningham AJ: Benzodiazepine premedication may attenuate the stress response in daycase anesthesia: A pilot study. *Can J Anaesth* 2002;49(9):932-935.
10. Thwaites A, Edmends S, Smith I: Inhalation induction with sevoflurane: A double-blind comparison with propofol. *Br J Anaesth* 1997;78(4):356-361.
11. Joo HS, Perks WJ: Sevoflurane versus propofol for anesthetic induction: A meta-analysis. *Anesth Analg* 2000;91(1):213-219.
12. Eriksson LI: The effects of residual neuromuscular blockade and volatile anesthetics on the control of ventilation. *Anesth Analg* 1999;89(1):243-251.
13. Kopman AF, Yee PS, Neuman GG: Relationship of the train-of-four fade ratio to clinical signs and symptoms of residual paralysis in awake volunteers. *Anesthesiology* 1997;86(4):765-771.
14. Gupta A, Stierer T, Zuckerman R, Sakima N, Parker SD, Fleisher LA: Comparison of recovery profile after ambulatory anesthesia with propofol, isoflurane, sevoflurane and desflurane: A systematic review. *Anesth Analg* 2004;98(3):632-641, table of contents.
15. Song D, Joshi GP, White PF: Fast-track eligibility after ambulatory anesthesia: A comparison of desflurane, sevoflurane, and propofol. *Anesth Analg* 1998;86(2):267-273.
16. Camci E, Koltka K, Celenk Y, Tugrul M, Pembeci K: Bispectral index-guided desflurane and propofol anesthesia in ambulatory arthroscopy: Comparison of recovery and discharge profiles. *J Anesth* 2006;20(2):149-152.
17. Song D, Joshi GP, White PF: Titration of volatile anesthetics using bispectral index facilitates recovery after ambulatory anesthesia. *Anesthesiology* 1997;87(4):842-848.
18. Gan TJ, Glass PS, Windsor A, et al: Bispectral index monitoring allows faster emergence and improved recovery from propofol, alfentanil, and nitrous oxide anesthesia. BIS Utility Study Group. *Anesthesiology* 1997;87(4):808-815.
19. Zohar E, Luban I, White PF, Ramati E, Shabat S, Fredman B: Bispectral index monitoring does not improve early recovery of geriatric outpatients undergoing brief surgical procedures. *Can J Anaesth* 2006;53(1):20-25.
20. Song D, Chung F, Wong J, Yogendran S: The assessment of postural stability after ambulatory anesthesia: A comparison of desflurane with propofol. *Anesth Analg* 2002;94(1):60-64, table of contents.
21. Fredman B, Nathanson MH, Smith I, Wang J, Klein K, White PF: Sevoflurane for outpatient anesthesia: A comparison with propofol. *Anesth Analg* 1995;81(4):823-828.
22. Raeder J, Gupta A, Pedersen FM: Recovery characteristics of sevoflurane- or propofol-based anaesthesia for day-care surgery. *Acta Anaesthesiol Scand* 1997;41(8):988-994.
23. Robinson BJ, Uhrich TD, Ebert TJ: A review of recovery from sevoflurane anaesthesia: Comparisons with isoflurane and propofol including meta-analysis. *Acta Anaesthesiol Scand* 1999;43(2):185-190.
24. Mahajan VA, Ni Chonghaile M, Bokhari SA, Harte BH, Flynn NM, Laffey JG: Recovery of older patients undergoing ambulatory anaesthesia with isoflurane or sevoflurane. *Eur J Anaesthesiol* 2007;24(6):505-510.
25. Juvin P, Vadam C, Malek L, Dupont H, Marmuse JP, Desmonts JM: Postoperative recovery after desflurane, propofol, or isoflurane anesthesia among morbidly obese patients: A prospective, randomized study. *Anesth Analg* 2000;91(3):714-719.
26. Fredman B, Sheffer O, Zohar E, et al: Fast-track eligibility of geriatric patients undergoing short urologic surgery procedures. *Anesth Analg* 2002;94(3):560-564.
27. Juvin P, Servin F, Giraud O, Desmonts JM: Emergence of elderly patients from prolonged desflurane, isoflurane, or propofol anesthesia. *Anesth Analg* 1997;85(3):647-651.
28. McKay RE, Large MJ, Balea MC, McKay WR: Airway reflexes return more rapidly after desflurane anesthesia than after sevoflurane anesthesia. *Anesth Analg* 2005;100(3):697-700, table of contents.
29. Apfel CC, Korttila K, Abdalla M, et al: A factorial trial of six interventions for the prevention of postoperative nausea and vomiting. *N Engl J Med* 2004;350(24):2441-2451.
30. Sneyd JR, Carr A, Byrom WD, Bilski AJ: A meta-analysis of nausea and vomiting following maintenance of anaesthesia with propofol or inhalational agents. *Eur J Anaesthesiol* 1998;15(4):433-445.
31. Tramer M, Moore A, McQuay H: Propofol anaesthesia and postoperative nausea and vomiting: Quantitative systematic review of randomized controlled studies. *Br J Anaesth* 1997;78(3):247-255.
32. Visser K, Hassink EA, Bonsel GJ, Moen J, Kalkman CJ: Randomized controlled trial of total intravenous anesthesia with propofol versus inhalation anesthesia with isoflurane-nitrous oxide: Postoperative nausea with vomiting and economic analysis. *Anesthesiology* 2001;95(3):616-626.
33. Smith I, Thwaites AJ: Target-controlled propofol vs. sevoflurane: A double-blind, randomised comparison in day-case anaesthesia. *Anaesthesia* 1999;54(8):745-752.
34. Tang J, White PF, Wender RH, et al: Fast-track office-based anesthesia: A comparison of propofol versus desflurane with

antiemetic prophylaxis in spontaneously breathing patients. *Anesth Analg* 2001;92(1):95-99.

35. Nelskyla KA, Yli-Hankala AM, Puro PH, Korttila KT: Sevoflurane titration using bispectral index decreases postoperative vomiting in phase II recovery after ambulatory surgery. *Anesth Analg* 2001;93(5):1165-1169.
36. Coburn M, Baumert JH, Roertgen D, et al: Emergence and early cognitive function in the elderly after xenon or desflurane anaesthesia: A double-blinded randomized controlled trial. *Br J Anaesth* 2007;98(6):756-762.
37. Georgiou LG, Vourlioti AN, Kremastinou FI, Stefanou PS, Tsiotou AG, Kokkinou MD: Influence of anesthetic technique on early postoperative hypoxemia. *Acta Anaesthesiol Scand* 1996;40(1):75-80.
38. Buchanan FF, Myles PS, Leslie K, Forbes A, Cicuttini F: Gender and recovery after general anesthesia combined with neuromuscular blocking drugs. *Anesth Analg* 2006;102(1):291-297.
39. White PF: Use of cerebral monitoring during anaesthesia: Effect on recovery profile. *Best Practice and Research* 2006;20(1):181-189.
40. Einarsson S, Bengtsson A, Stenqvist O, Bengtson JP: Decreased respiratory depression during emergence from anesthesia with sevoflurane/N$_2$O than with sevoflurane alone. *Can J Anaesth* 1999;46(4):335-341.
41. Tramer M, Moore A, McQuay H: Omitting nitrous oxide in general anaesthesia: Meta-analysis of intraoperative awareness and postoperative emesis in randomized controlled trials. *Br J Anaesth* 1996;76(2):186-193.
42. Arellano RJ, Pole ML, Rafuse SE, et al: Omission of nitrous oxide from a propofol-based anesthetic does not affect the recovery of women undergoing outpatient gynecologic surgery. *Anesthesiology* 2000;93(2):332-339.
43. Johnson GW, St John Gray H: Nitrous oxide inhalation as an adjunct to intravenous induction of general anaesthesia with propofol for day surgery. *Eur J Anaesthesiol* 1997;14(3):295-299.
44. Tang J, Chen L, White PF, et al: Use of propofol for office-based anesthesia: Effect of nitrous oxide on recovery profile. *J Clin Anesth* 1999;11(3):226-230.
45. Smith I: Nitrous oxide in ambulatory anaesthesia: Does it have a place in day surgical anaesthesia or is it just a threat for personnel and the global environment? *Curr Opin Anaesthesiol* 2006;19(6):592-596.
46. Joshi G: The use of laryngeal mask airway devices in ambulatory anesthesia. *Seminars in Anesthesia, Perioperative Medicine, and Pain* 2001(20):257-263.
47. Goulson DT: Anesthesia for outpatient gynecologic surgery. *Curr Opin Anaesthesiol* 2007;20(3):195-200.
48. Miller DM, Camporota L: Advantages of ProSeal and SLIPA airways over tracheal tubes for gynecological laparoscopies. *Can J Anaesth* 2006;53(2):188-193.
49. Ashworth J, Smith I: Comparison of desflurane with isoflurane or propofol in spontaneously breathing ambulatory patients. *Anesth Analg* 1998;87(2):312-318.
50. Mahmoud NA, Rose DJ, Laurence AS: Desflurane or sevoflurane for gynaecological day-case anaesthesia with spontaneous respiration? *Anaesthesia* 2001;56(2):171-174.
51. Tang J, Chen L, White PF, et al: Recovery profile, costs, and patient satisfaction with propofol and sevoflurane for fast-track office-based anesthesia. *Anesthesiology* 1999;91(1):253-261.
52. Saros GB, Doolke A, Anderson RE, Jakobsson JG: Desflurane vs. sevoflurane as the main inhaled anaesthetic for spontaneous breathing via a laryngeal mask for varicose vein day surgery: A prospective randomized study. *Acta Anaesthesiol Scand* 2006;50(5):549-552.
53. Chung F, Ritchie E, Su J: Postoperative pain in ambulatory surgery. *Anesth Analg* 1997;85(4):808-816.
54. Twersky RS, Jamerson B, Warner DS, Fleisher LA, Hogue S: Hemodynamics and emergence profile of remifentanil versus fentanyl prospectively compared in a large population of surgical patients. *J Clin Anesth* 2001;13(6):407-416.
55. Fleisher LA, Hogue S, Colopy M, et al: Does functional ability in the postoperative period differ between remifentanil- and fentanyl-based anesthesia? *J Clin Anesth* 2001;13(6):401-406.
56. Loop T, Priebe HJ: Recovery after anesthesia with remifentanil combined with propofol, desflurane, or sevoflurane for otorhinolaryngeal surgery. *Anesth Analg* 2000;91(1):123-129.
57. Bekker AY, Berklayd P, Osborn I, Bloom M, Yarmush J, Turndorf H: The recovery of cognitive function after remifentanil-nitrous oxide anesthesia is faster than after an isoflurane-nitrous oxide-fentanyl combination in elderly patients. *Anesth Analg* 2000;91(1):117-122.
58. Larsen B, Seitz A, Larsen R: Recovery of cognitive function after remifentanil-propofol anesthesia: A comparison with desflurane and sevoflurane anesthesia. *Anesth Analg* 2000;90(1):168-174.
59. Claxton AR, McGuire G, Chung F, Cruise C: Evaluation of morphine versus fentanyl for postoperative analgesia after ambulatory surgical procedures. *Anesth Analg* 1997;84(3):509-514.

22 Does the Choice of Muscle Relaxant Affect Outcome?

Ashish C. Sinha, MD, PhD

Neuromuscular blocking agents (NMBAs), colloquially known as muscle relaxants, play a critical role in the operative setting. By functioning as acetylcholine inhibitors, NMBAs create a state of reversible paralysis, helping in intubation and assisting abdominal surgery, by relaxation of muscle tone during surgery.

Originating with the purification of d-tubocurarine, by Dr. Harold King, from a sample of curare stored in a test tube (thereby the name) in the British Museum, NMBAs have developed significantly over the years.[1] Tubocurarine was first used in 1942 at the Homeopathic Hospital in Montreal by Harold Griffith and Enid Johnson in a patient having an appendectomy. The credit for introducing neuromuscular blockade in the surgical setting therefore belongs to them.[2]

NMBAs act in a competitive or noncompetitive manner to inhibit the translation of neurotransmitter release into muscle impulse. Structurally similar in functional groups and stereochemistry to acetylcholine, NMBAs often contain both the ester group and the quaternary amino group and are therefore able to interact and bind with the nicotinic α, δ, and ε -subunits. As competitive inhibitors to acetylcholine, NMBAs depend for their effectiveness on the local concentration of blocking agent within the synaptic volume relative to the natural neurotransmitter. This relative rather than absolute concentration dependence has an important impact on both the onset and reversal of paralysis.

Pharmacokinetics are the major determinant in the selection of an NMBA, including the speed of onset and the duration of effect, coupled with careful consideration of elimination and side effects. The optimal NMBA will have a fast onset and offset, with minimal cardiovascular effects, and be easily eliminated by the body, even in patients with compromised renal or hepatic function.

Muscle response to NMBAs is not homogeneous because of variation in blood flow and motor plate receptor density. Diaphragm muscles, for example, exhibit greater resistance to blocking agents than peripheral muscles and thus require higher dosages, but at the same time respond with a quicker onset of paralysis.

NMBAs can be divided into two categories, based on the biochemical effect on the muscle: depolarizing and nondepolarizing agents. In addition, their pharmacologic impact can be distinguished clinically through the use of neuromuscular monitoring.

DEPOLARIZING AGENTS

Succinylcholine, the only clinically used depolarizing NMBA, is structurally similar to a dimer of acetylcholine. The conditions of intubation provided by succinylcholine are rapid but not optimal. Bucx and colleagues[3] showed that at least in pediatric patients, the upper airway muscle tone increases after succinylcholine administration irrespective of presence of a volatile agent. The force applied for laryngoscopy using succinylcholine is more than that needed with vecuronium.[3] This may be attributed partly to an increase in masseteric tone that succinylcholine can cause.

NONDEPOLARIZING AGENTS

Nondepolarizing NMBAs function as competitive antagonistic inhibitors. By occupying the α-subunit of the nicotinic receptors, NMBA molecules preclude acetylcholine binding and cause paralysis by preventing the depolarization of the muscle membrane. The reversal of neuromuscular blockade is usually achieved by using an acetylcholinesterase inhibitor, along with an anticholinergic to counteract the cholinergic side effects of the acetylcholinesterase inhibitor, especially the serious bradycardia that this drug class can produce. These drugs are usually paired based on onset and offset times, neostigmine with glycopyrrolate and edrophonium with atropine. In the future this kind of reversal may be completely avoided by using a cyclodextrin[4] (Tables 22-1 and 22-2).

EVIDENCE

Neuromuscular block monitoring and pharmacologic reversal of blockade with an anticholinesterase drug have both decreased the incidence of residual block in patients receiving nondepolarizing neuromuscular blocking drugs.[5] There is evidence supporting the use of intermediate-lasting agents causing less residual neuromuscular block than long-lasting agents, that is, vecuronium is better than pancuronium.[6] Gender may also affect recovery from neuromuscular blockade, with women recovering faster than men.[7] In terms of age, evidence suggests that the elderly have a faster onset with vecuronium than cisatracurium.[8,9]

Table 22-1	Dosing Recommendations for Neuromuscular Blocking Agents (NMBAs)					
					PROLONGED SURGERY	
Duration	**NMBA**	**Intubating Dose, mg/kg**	**Onset, min**	**Duration, min**	**Repeat dose, mg/kg**	**Infusion Rate (Range)**
Ultrashort	Succinylcholine	0.6 (0.3-1.1)	1	4-6	0.04-0.07	2.5-4.0 mg/min (0.5-10)
Intermediate	Atracurium	0.4-0.5	3-5	20-35	0.08-0.1	5-9 mcg/kg/min (2-15)
	Cis-atracurium	0.15-0.2	1.5-2	55-61	0.03	1-2 mcg/kg/min (1-3)
	Rocuronium	0.6 (0.45-1.2)	1-3	22-67	0.1-0.2	10-12 mcg/kg/min (4-16)
	Vecuronium	0.1-0.28	2.5-3	25-30	0.01-0.015	1 mcg/kg/min (0.8-1.2)
Long	Pancuronium	0.06-0.1	2-4	60-100	0.01-0.06	0.01-0.02 mg/kg/hr

Table 22-2	Commonly Used Drugs' Interactions with Neuromuscular Blocking Agents (NMBAs)	
Class of Drugs	**Effect on Neuromuscular Blockade**	**Dosing and Monitoring**
Antiarrhythmics	Enhanced neuromuscular blocking activity	Monitor response and use lowest possible dose to achieve adequate blockade.
Antibiotics (amino glycosides, macrolides, and lincosamides)	Possible excessive blockade and respiratory depression	Monitor for residual blockade following NMBA administration.
Antiepileptics	Shortened blockade	Monitor response; higher or more frequent dosing.
Aprotinin	Prolonged neuromuscular blocking activity	Monitor response and use lowest possible dose to achieve adequate blockade.
Azathioprine	Enhanced blockade with depolarizer and decreased with nondepolarizers	Monitor response and use lowest possible dose to achieve adequate blockade.
Calcium channel blockers	Enhanced neuromuscular blocking activity	Monitor response and use lowest possible dose to achieve adequate blockade.
Corticosteroids	Enhanced blockade with depolarizer and decreased with nondepolarizers	Monitor response and use lowest possible dose to achieve adequate blockade.
Cyclophosphamide	Prolonged apnea with succinylcholine?	Monitor response and use lowest possible dose to achieve adequate blockade.
Digoxin	Increased rate of cardiac arrhythmias	With succinylcholine, cardiac monitoring is recommended.
Inhalation anesthetics	Enhanced neuromuscular blocking activity	Monitor response and use lowest possible dose to achieve adequate blockade.
Lithium	Protracted neuromuscular blocking activity	Monitor response and use lowest possible dose to achieve adequate blockade.
Magnesium	Enhanced neuromuscular blocking activity	Monitor response and use lowest possible dose to achieve adequate blockade.
Metoclopramide	Extended neuromuscular blocking activity	Monitor response and use lowest possible dose to achieve adequate blockade.
Oral contraceptives	Extended neuromuscular blocking activity with depolarizer	Monitor response and use lowest possible dose to achieve adequate blockade.
Oxytocin	Enhanced neuromuscular blocking activity	Monitor response and use lowest possible dose to achieve adequate blockade.
Terbutaline	Enhanced neuromuscular blocking activity	Monitor response and use lowest possible dose to achieve adequate blockade.
Tricyclic antidepressants	Risk of cardiac arrhythmias	Cardiac monitoring is essential.

SIGNIFICANT DISEASE STATE INTERACTIONS

The situations in which potential clinical effects of NMBAs are potentiated or antagonized are described next. Common neuromuscular diseases that accentuate blockade are myasthenia gravis and Eaton-Lambert syndrome. Hypermagnesemia, hypocalcemia, hypokalemia, and hyponatremia can cause a similar effect. Other conditions that prolong blockade with NMBAs are atypical plasma cholinesterase and, depending on the metabolic route of elimination, liver (rocuronium and vecuronium) or kidney (pancuronium) disease. Because a state of acidosis will prolong metabolism, it also potentiates blockade.

Similarly, demyelinating diseases, peripheral neuropathies and hemiparesis (for many months after a significant burn injury), hypercalcemia, and alkalosis will all attenuate neuromuscular blockade.

The risks of arrhythmias secondary to increase in plasma potassium by succinylcholine can be severe enough to cause cardiac arrest in certain situations. This is secondary to extrajunctional receptors that appear after major burns, multiple trauma (especially crush injury), spinal cord injury, or skeletal muscle denervation. Preexisting hyperkalemia and digitalis toxicity also predispose to fatal arrhythmias with the use of succinylcholine. Even small doses of succinylcholine (approximately 20 mg) can cause increased release of potassium as early as 2 to 4 days after denervating injury. The duration of risk is unclear but probably decreases within 6 months of injury. It would then seem prudent to avoid administration of succinylcholine to any patient more than 24 hours after a burn injury, extensive trauma, or spinal cord transection. Avoidance should continue for 6 months at least, but 1 year is probably safer.

Physiologic changes of pregnancy influence pharmacokinetics and pharmacodynamics of NMBAs. Clinical action of vecuronium is significantly enhanced, rocuronium is either enhanced or prolonged, and atracurium and mivacurium are either unchanged or only slightly prolonged.[10] This makes the latter two the optimal choices for neuromuscular blockade in pregnancy. Magnesium, often used in the preeclampsia setting in pregnancy, significantly increases the block of mivacurium, rocuronium, and vecuronium.[10] This implies that anesthetic care would involve careful dosing and continuous monitoring of the state of paralysis. Blockade induced by succinylcholine is unchanged in the pregnant patient at a 1 mg/kg dose. A dose greater than 1.7 mg/kg may demonstrate an increased block.[10] To prevent effects on the newborn, minimal dosing, along with monitoring and preferential use of short-acting drugs, is probably prudent.

ANAPHYLAXIS WITH NMBAs

The most common pharmacologic cause of perioperative anaphylaxis is muscle relaxants.[11] The French Perioperative Anaphylactoid Reactions Study Group reported that over 60% of anaphylactic reactions were caused by muscle relaxants.[12] The potential for cross reactivity exists because of the common tertiary and quaternary ammonium groups, though very few patients are allergic to all nondepolarizing drugs.[13,14] There was some concern in the last decade about an increased rate of anaphylaxis with regard to use of rocuronium,[15-18] based on reports out of Denmark and Norway[19] and France.[20] According to Bhananker and colleagues,[21] there is no significant difference between the incidence of anaphylaxis with rocuronium or vecuronium, with both being in the one-in-a-million vial range.

AREAS OF UNCERTAINTY

All currently used NMBAs have some limitations and drawbacks, and therefore the quest for the optimal NMBA continues. This drug should have the following qualities: it should have an extremely fast onset, be noncumulative, be metabolized independently of renal or hepatic function, be easily and rapidly reversed, and have few or no contraindications and side effects. Research on this front continues, and new nondepolarizing agents that show promise are being developed as derivatives of tropinyl diesters and bis-tetrahydroquinolinium chlorofumarates.

The most noteworthy occurrence in the field of neuromuscular blockade since the withdrawal of rapacuronium in March 2001 is the development of the reversal agent sugammadex. Sugammadex is a γ-cyclodextrin that forms water-soluble complexes with the steroidal neuromuscular blocking drugs.[4] It can reverse even very profound blockade before the start of spontaneous recovery. When used with rocuronium in a rapid-sequence induction situation, it is even faster than succinylcholine with regard to onset-offset. This kind of reversal eliminates the need for additional anticholinesterase or anticholinergic drugs, and their attendant side effects, thereby making neuromuscular blockade and its reversal safer.[4] Sugammadex allows not just the rescue of patients in "cannot intubate, cannot ventilate" scenarios, but also would allow a rapid reversal in cases requiring profound blockade until the very end of surgery, without waiting for some spontaneous recovery of neuromuscular function.

GUIDELINES

It is possible that sugammadex, if it lives up to its promise and potential, may become part of the guidelines in neuromuscular blockade usage in the future. Food and Drug Administration warnings exist about the use of succinylcholine in pediatric patients for the fear of unmasking preexisting myopathy. Partly because of this, rocuronium has increasingly become the drug of choice in the pediatric population.

Rapid control of airway, even in the adult patient, can be achieved with a larger dose of rocuronium (0.9 mg/kg) in case succinylcholine is contraindicated for any reason. The time for readiness for intubation is comparable, and in the 60-second range.

AUTHOR'S RECOMMENDATIONS

The choice of neuromuscular blocking drug will affect outcomes in anesthesia. The choice will depend on patient factors such as time since last meal, pregnancy, mental status, diseases such as myasthenia gravis, patient or family history of malignant hyperthermia (MH), type of surgery, perceived difficulty of intubation, availability and familiarity of the practitioner with the drug, and cost considerations. The potent drugs have a slower onset and the less potent have a quicker onset secondary to the amount of drug used; higher numbers of drug molecules are able to attach to the neuromuscular junction (NMJ) quicker, to create paralysis.

- If rapid onset of paralysis is required and there are no contraindications to succinylcholine, it is the obvious choice. If myalgia is a concern, as in the muscular patient, a small defasciculation dose of an intermediate-acting NMBA should be considered.
- Alternatively, rocuronium, at the higher dose of 0.9 mg/kg, can achieve intubating conditions in 60 seconds in most patients, which compares favorably to succinylcholine. In my practice I use either of these drugs at induction.
- Continuous following of trend of neuromuscular blockade and trying to keep the patient at one or two twitches out of four with either a small dose each time or an infusion is probably ideal.
- The risk of anaphylaxis is equivalent in most intermediate- and long-acting NMBAs and therefore is probably a nonconsideration for drug choice.
- Residual blockade is a definite consideration and underscores the impact that residual blockade can have on outcomes. Full dose reversal, after the initiation of some spontaneous reversal, should be the common practice. The hesitation of reversal derives from expected side effects of drug combinations used for reversal. This is where my enthusiasm about the development of sugammadex, the specific chelating agent for rocuronium, comes from.
- Sugammadex effectively reverses deep and prolonged neuromuscular block induced by rocuronium. The effective reversal dose appears to be 2 to 4 mg/kg. This reversal can be accomplished any time after the drug is administered, allowing an escape from the "cannot intubate, cannot ventilate" situation.

REFERENCES

1. King H: Curare alkaloids: 1, tubocurarine. *J Chem Soc* 1935:1381-1389.
2. Griffith HR, Johnson GE: The use of curare in general anaesthesia. *Anesthesiology* 1942;3:418-420.
3. Bucx MJ, Van Geel RT, Meursing AE, Stujnen T, Sheck PA: Forces applied during laryngoscopy in children. Are volatile anaesthetics essential for suxamethonium-induced muscle rigidity? *Acta Anaestheisol Scand* 1994;38(5):448-452.
4. Naguib M. Sugammadex: Another milestone in clinical neuromuscular pharmacology. *Anesth Analg* 104:575-581.
5. Baillard C, Clec'h J, Salhi F, Gehan G, Cupa M, Samama CM: Postoperative residual neuromuscular block: A survey of management. *Br J Anaesth* 2005;95:622-626.
6. Ghosh-Karmarkar S, Divatia JV, Kulkarni AP, Patil VP, Mehta P: Residual neuromuscular blockade in the recovery room: Does the choice of muscle relaxant matter? *J Anaesth Clin Pharmacol* 2006;22 (1):29-34.
7. Buchanan FF, Myles PS, Leslie K Forbes A, Cicuttini F: Gender and recovery after general anesthesia combined with neuromuscular blocking drugs. *Anesth Analg* 2006;102:291-297.
8. Pleym H, Spigset O, Kharasch ED, Dale O: Gender differences in drug effects: Implications for anesthesiologists. *Acta Anesthesiol Scand* 2003;47:241-259.
9. Keles GT, Yentur A, Cavus Z, Sakarya M: Assessment of neuromuscular and haemodynamic effects of cisatracurium and vecuronium under sevoflurane-remifentanil anaesthesia in elderly patients. *Eur J Anesth* 2004;21:877-881.
10. Guay J, Grenier Y, Varin F: Clinical pharmacokinetics of neuromuscular relaxants in pregnancy. *Clin Pharmacokinet* 1998;34(6):483-496.
11. Matthey P, Wang P, Finegan BA, Donnelly M: Rocuronium anaphylaxis and multiple neuromuscular blocking drug sensitivities. *Can J Anesth* 2000;47(9):890-893.
12. Laxenaire MC: Epidemiology of anesthetic anaphylactoid reactions. Fourth multicenter survey (July 1994-December 1996). *Ann Fr Anesth Reanim* 1999;18:796-809.
13. Moneret-Vautrin DA, Guéant JL, Kamel L, Laxenaire MC, El Kholty S, Nicolas JP: Anaphylaxis to muscle relaxants: Cross sensitivity studied by radioimmunoassay compared to intradermal tests in 34 cases. *J Allerg Clin Immunol* 1988;82:745-752.
14. Sabah A: Apropos of drug allergy. *Allerg Immunol (Paris)* 1996;28:230-233.
15. Mirakhur RK: Safety aspects of non-depolarising neuromuscular blocking agents with special reference to rocuronium bromide. *Eur J Anesthesiol* 1994;11(suppl 9):133-140.
16. Fisher MM: Anaphylaxis to muscle relaxants: Cross sensitivity between relaxants. *Anaesth Intensive Care* 1980;8:211-213.
17. Joint Task Force on Practice Parameters, American Academy of Allergy, Asthma and Immunology, American College of Allergy, Asthma and Immunology, and the Joint Council of Allergy, Asthma and Immunology: The diagnosis and management of anaphylaxis. *J Allergy Clin Immunol* 1998;101:S482-S484, S512-S515.
18. Moneret-Vautrin DA, Laxenaire MC: Anaphylaxis to muscle relaxants: Predictive tests (Letter). *Anaesthesia* 1990;45:246-247.
19. Guttorsen AB: Allergic reactions during anaesthesia: Increased attention to the problem in Denmark and Norway. *Acta Anaesthesiol Scand* 2001;45:1189-1190.
20. Mertes PM, Laxenaire MC, Alla F: Anaphylactic and anaphylactoid reactions occurring during anesthesia in France in 1999-2000. *Anesthesiology* 2003;99:536-545.
21. Bhananker SM, O'Donnell JT, Salemi JR, Bishop MJ: The risk of anaphylactic reactions to rocuronium in the United States is comparable to that of vecuronium: An analysis of Food and Drug Administration reporting of adverse events. *Anesth Analg* 2005;101:819-822.

23 Does Anesthetic Choice Affect Surgical and Recovery Times?

Anil Gupta, MD, FRCA, PhD

General anesthesia is common for operations during ambulatory surgery in most centers in the Western world. Outcome following surgery and anesthesia is an important aspect that should be considered when deciding on the choice of general anesthetic for ambulatory surgical procedures. Although mortality rates are extremely low following general anesthesia in the ambulatory setting,[1] minor morbidity in the form of postoperative pain, nausea and vomiting, fatigue, shivering, headache, and drowsiness continues to affect a large number of patients.[2] With the continuing emphasis on expansion of ambulatory surgery and the inclusion of elderly and sicker patients onto operating lists, it is likely that both mortality and morbidity rates will increase in the future. Although some systematic reviews have been published in the literature comparing general with regional anesthesia for major surgery with focus on outcome, the choice of anesthetic agents for general anesthesia in the ambulatory setting remains controversial. Specifically, the choice of anesthetic in terms of outcome following ambulatory surgery remains poorly explored.

OPTIONS

Two commonly used methods for general anesthesia for ambulatory surgery are total intravenous anesthesia (TIVA) and inhalation anesthesia. Although propofol is practically the only anesthetic used for TIVA, many inhalation anesthetics are available today, and the choice of these agents has been the subject of many published studies and a great deal of controversy. Surprisingly, there are only two systematic reviews published on this interesting subject,[3,4] which included both inpatients and outpatients. A recent review of the literature did not reveal many new publications in the last 5 years on this subject. In this chapter, the evidence is derived from well-performed prospective studies combined with the author's own experience, as well as data from two currently unpublished systematic reviews in adults.

ENDPOINTS OF INTEREST IN AMBULATORY SURGERY

To analyze the benefits of one anesthetic over another, it is important to be able to define the endpoints that are of interest to the patient and the hospital. One easily defined endpoint that is of interest both to the patient and hospital

is mortality risk following ambulatory surgery. However, the mortality rate is extremely low in this group of patients,[1] and therefore it would be difficult to confirm that the choice of anesthetic has any significant effect on perioperative mortality risk during ambulatory surgery. Another endpoint of importance, which is less well defined, is major morbidity. However, effect of the choice of anesthetic agent on this important outcome remains unclear.

A differentiation must be made between measuring "true outcomes" and "surrogate outcomes."[5] Examples of true outcomes include discharge times, return to work, admission and readmission, and patient satisfaction; examples of surrogate outcomes include incidence of pain, time to first analgesic consumption, early recovery (response to commands) following anesthesia, and nausea and vomiting. Surrogate measures should be accepted only if they yield the same conclusions as their nonsurrogate endpoints.[5] True outcomes such as patient satisfaction are probably the most important factors from the patient's perspective but remain poorly defined and poorly studied. Because most patients have not undergone the same operation twice using different anesthetics, gathering of evidence is restricted to asking patients whether they were satisfied with the anesthetic. Most patients usually answer "yes" to this question, but the answer is of limited value to the researcher. Studies for which the authors have interviewed patients about the preference of inhalation induction compared with intravenous induction (sevoflurane or desflurane versus propofol) have usually preferred propofol to sevoflurane.[6] This could be because of the mood elevation following propofol anesthesia that has been suggested by many authors but the mood elevation effect has never been shown to be the case.

The following endpoints of quality have been evaluated in this chapter to provide the evidence for the selection of the best maintenance agent during ambulatory surgery: "early" recovery ("time to open eyes" and "time to obey commands"); "intermediate" recovery ("time to transfer from phase I to phase II," "home-readiness," and "home discharge"); and minor in-hospital complications, including "pain," "nausea or vomiting," "antiemetics" used, "dizziness/giddiness," "drowsiness/somnolence," "headache," "shivering," and "coughing." Patient satisfaction has been excluded because it is a crude indicator of the evidence for the choice of anesthetic for ambulatory surgery, as discussed earlier. "Pain" as a postoperative complication has not been addressed because of the different ways in which it has been measured and the complexity of its interpretation. Not only do the visual analog scales (VAS) for pain vary between authors, but the time to pain assessment differs, the analgesics used vary considerably between studies, and not all authors present data as VAS, preferring to present data as "time to first analgesic requirement" or "the number of patients requesting analgesics." In addition, because of the variable nature of surgery and consequently postoperative pain, I believe that the data could be incorrectly interpreted, leading to false conclusions. Therefore data have not been extracted on pain intensity or analgesic requirements in this review.

EVIDENCE FOR TOTAL INTRAVENOUS OR INHALATION ANESTHESIA

Two systematic reviews published in the literature comparing inhalation versus intravenous anesthesia have included both inpatients and outpatients,[3,4] which somewhat limits the scope of the findings. Therefore we performed a systematic review of the literature using Medline via PubMed, and 42 articles were extracted addressing aspects of recovery following ambulatory surgery.[7] Halothane and enflurane were not taken into consideration in this review because these agents are rarely used during ambulatory surgery today. A summary of the findings is given as follows.

Propofol versus Isoflurane

A total of 18 studies were found that had data that could be extracted in the postoperative period. No differences were found between propofol and isoflurane in early recovery or transfer from phase I to phase II, but there was significant heterogeneity between groups in all these parameters (Table 23-1). However, home discharge was significantly earlier in the propofol group (15 minutes, confidence interval [CI] 8 to 23 minutes). There was a greater relative risk for postoperative complications, including nausea (number needed to treat [NNT] 8), vomiting (NNT 10), and headache (NNT 22) in the isoflurane group (see Table 23-1). The use of antiemetics (relative risk [RR] 2.7, CI 1.7 to 4.2) was also more common in the isoflurane group. The relative risk for postoperative nausea and vomiting after 24 hours was also significantly higher in the isoflurane group versus the propofol group (see Table 23-1).

Propofol versus Sevoflurane

We found a total of 11 studies with extractable data that compared sevoflurane with propofol in an ambulatory surgical setting. No difference was found in the time to open eyes between the sevoflurane and propofol groups, but time to obey commands was faster in the sevoflurane group (1.6 minutes, CI 0.3 to 3.0), with significant heterogeneity between groups (see Table 23-1). No significant difference

Table 23-1	Postoperative Recovery Profiles and Minor Complications Associated with Propofol Compared with the Inhaled Anesthetics		
Endpoint	**Propofol vs. Isoflurane**	**Propofol vs. Desflurane**	**Propofol vs. Sevoflurane**
Time to open eyes (min)	0.2 (-1.6 to 1.3)[§]	1.3 (0.4 to 2.2)[§†] (D)	0.9 (-2.2 to 0.5)[§]
Time to obey commands (min)	0.5 (-1.0 to 1.9)[§]	1.3 (0.4 to 2.3)[§†] (D)	1.6 (0.3 to 3.0)[§*] (S)
Time to transfer from phase 1 to phase 2 (min)	4.3 (-5.4 to 14.1)[§]	NR	3.6 (-13.5 to 6.4)[§]
Time to home-readiness (min)	9.3 (-17 to 36)[§]	3.1 (-7.7 to 1.5)	5.6 (-3.4 to 14.5)[§]
Time to home discharge (min)	15 (8 to 23)[†] (P)	3.9 (-9.3 to 1.5)	10.3 (3.9 to 16.6)[†] (P)
Postoperative nausea (PON)	2.0 (1.6-2.5)[†] (P), NNH = 8	2.0 (1.4 to 2.8)[†] (P), NNH = 7	1.6 (1.2-2.0)[†] (P), NNH = 11
Postoperative vomiting (POV)	3.2 (1.3-7.5)[†] (P), NNH = 10	2.6 (1.4 to 4.8)[†] (P), NNH = 10	2.0 (1.3-3.0)[†] (P), NNH = 15
Postoperative drowsiness	NR	NR	0.9 (0.1-5.9)[§]
Postoperative dizziness	NR	NR	1.4 (0.8-2.3)
Postoperative shivering	0.8 (0.6-1.3)	1.5 (0.4-5.4)[§]	0.8 (0.5-1.3)
Postoperative headache	3.3 (1.1-9.6)* (P), NNH = 22	3.5 (0.6-19.8)	1.0 (0.2-7.1)
Antiemetics given	2.7 (1.7-4.2)[†] (P), NNH = 8.5	3.3 (1.8-6.0)[†] (P), NNH = 8	4.5 (1.5-14.0)[†] (P), NNH = 11
Postdischarge nausea (PDN)	1.8 (1.3-2.5)[†] (P), NNH = 8	1.2 (0.7-2.1)	1.3 (0.7-2.3)
Postdischarge vomiting (PDV)	2.5[‡] (1.6-4.1) (P), NNH = 9	2.6 (0.1-62.7)	NR

All results are shown as weighted mean difference (WMD) or relative risk (mean and 95% confidence intervals).
*$P < 0.05$.
[†]$P < 0.01$.
[‡]$P < 0.001$.
Significant results are shown in favor of the following: S = sevoflurane, I = isoflurane, D = desflurane, and P = propofol when significant.
[§]Significant heterogeneity; NR = not reported (or reported in only one study); NNH = numbers needed to harm for significant differences.
From: Gupta A, Zuckerman R, Stierer T, et al: *Anesthesia and Analgesia* 2004;98:632-641.

was found in the time to home-readiness between the groups, but with significant heterogeneity between the groups. The time to home discharge was earlier in the propofol group than in the sevoflurane group (10.3 minutes, CI 3.9 to 16.6). The relative risk for postoperative complications, including postoperative nausea (NNT 11) and vomiting (NNT 15), was significantly greater in the sevoflurane group versus the propofol group, but with significant heterogeneity between the groups (see Table 23-1). The need for antiemetics in the postoperative period was significantly greater in the sevoflurane group (RR 4.5, CI 1.5 to 14.0). No other significant differences were seen between the groups.

Propofol versus Desflurane

Thirteen studies had extractable data that were included in the meta-analysis. Time to open eyes was significantly faster in the desflurane group versus propofol (1.3 minutes, CI 0.4 to 2.2) ($p = 0.004$), as was the time to obey commands (1.3 minutes, CI 0.4 to 2.3) ($p = 0.007$), with significant heterogeneity between the groups (see Table 23-1). No differences were found in home-readiness or home discharge between the groups. The relative risk for postoperative complications, including postoperative nausea (NNT 7) and vomiting (NNT 10), was significantly greater in the desflurane group versus the propofol group (see Table 23-1), and the need for antiemetics was also higher in the desflurane group (RR 3.3, CI 1.8 to 6.0) ($p = 0.0001$). No other differences were seen between the groups with respect to postoperative complications.

Summary

Although early recovery (time to open eyes and obey commands) was quicker in the sevoflurane and desflurane groups versus the propofol group, the mean differences were small (1 to 2 minutes). On the other hand, propofol (TIVA) had some important benefits in terms of home discharge and postoperative side effects, specifically nausea and vomiting up to 24 hours.

Early recovery, characterized by time to open eyes and obey commands, is faster following desflurane and sevoflurane anesthesia compared with propofol anesthesia. Intermediate recovery, characterized by home discharge (but not home-readiness), is fastest in patients anesthetized with propofol compared with sevoflurane and isoflurane, but not desflurane. Postoperative complications, specifically nausea and vomiting, are lowest in the propofol group compared with desflurane, sevoflurane, or isoflurane. The choice of anesthetic for maintenance of anesthesia should be guided by the training and experience of the individual physician, as well as the routines and equipment available in the hospital, because choice of anesthetic agents appears to play a minor role in outcome following ambulatory surgery.

EVIDENCE FOR ISOFLURANE, DESFLURANE, OR SEVOFLURANE ANESTHESIA

Until the early 1990s the inhalation agents used were isoflurane, halothane, and enflurane. With the introduction of desflurane and subsequently sevoflurane, the popularity of enflurane and even halothane has dwindled and these agents are now rarely used. Despite the large number of articles published in the literature comparing isoflurane, desflurane, and sevoflurane, recovery following ambulatory surgery is, at best, poorly studied. We were able to extract data from only 16 studies and 1219 patients in which the authors had compared these three agents in randomized prospective studies during ambulatory surgery. The results from these studies are presented next.

Isoflurane versus Desflurane

A total of four studies compared isoflurane with desflurane in the ambulatory setting. In all, 277 patients undergoing different ambulatory surgical procedures were included in these studies. Muscle relaxants were used during surgery in two studies, and nitrous oxide in all studies. A statistically significant difference was found in time to open eyes ($p < 0.004$) and time to obey commands ($p < 0.01$) but in no other parameter of recovery (Table 23-2). The weighted mean differences in the recovery indices between desflurane and isoflurane were modest (4 to 5 minutes), all in favor of desflurane. A higher overall incidence of shivering postoperatively was seen in the desflurane-treated patients compared with isoflurane (see Table 23-2). No other differences were found in the incidence of postoperative complications between these groups.

Isoflurane versus Sevoflurane

Six studies could be included, with relevant data examining a total of 634 patients undergoing a variety of ambulatory surgical procedures. Nitrous oxide was used in all studies, although four studies used muscle relaxants during surgery and the others did not. Statistically significant differences were found in the time to open eyes, time to obey commands, time to transfer from phase I to phase II, home-readiness ($p < 0.00001$), and home discharge ($p = 0.05$) (see Table 23-2). The results of the latter are, however, based on two studies that could be identified with relevant data. The weighted mean differences in the recovery indices between sevoflurane and isoflurane were small, but all in favor of sevoflurane. Drowsiness was more frequent in the isoflurane group versus sevoflurane in the postoperative period ($p = 0.03$) (see Table 23-2).

Sevoflurane versus Desflurane

In all, six studies compared sevoflurane with desflurane, with a total of 246 patients. A majority of studies examined patients undergoing gynecologic laparoscopy, and nitrous oxide was used in all but one study. Muscle relaxants were used during anesthesia in four studies. Recovery parameters, including time to open eyes, were found to be statistically significant ($p < 0.005$), as well as time to obey commands ($p < 0.00001$), oth in favor of desflurane (see Table 23-2). The weighted mean differences in these recovery indices between the groups were minor and in favor of desflurane. The time to transfer from phase I to phase II was, however, found to be earlier in the sevoflurane group versus the desflurane group ($p < 0.00001$) (weighted mean difference 6 minutes). No other significant differences were found between the two anesthetic agents

Table 23-2	Postoperative Recovery Profiles and Minor Complications Associated with Different Inhaled Anesthetic Regimens		
Endpoint	**Isoflurane vs. Desflurane**	**Isoflurane vs. Sevoflurane**	**Sevoflurane vs. Desflurane**
Time to open eyes (min)	NR	2.4 (1.8 to 2.9)[†] (S)	1.4 (-0.1 to 2.9)[‡]
Time to obey commands (min)	4.6 (1.1 to 8.2)[†] (D)	2.4 (1.8 to 2.9)[†] (S)	2.7 (1.2 to 4.1)[†] (D)
Time to transfer from phase 1 to phase 2 (min)	1.3 (-10 to 8)	8.2 (5.7 to 10.6)[†] (S)	6.4 (3.7 to 9.0)[†] (S)
Time to home-readiness (min)	6.4 (-8.7 to 21.5)	5.1 (2.8 to 7.4)[†] (S)	2.0 (-16 to 12)
Time to home discharge (min)	NR	25 (0.4 to 50)* (S)	2.1 (-18 to 13)
Postoperative nausea (PON)	1.7 (1.0-3.1)	1.2 (0.8-1.9)[‡]	0.7 (0.4-1.2)
Postoperative vomiting (POV)	0.8 (0.3-1.6)	0.9 (0.6-1.4)	0.7 (0.2-1.8)
Postoperative drowsiness	NR	0.6 (0.4-1.0)* (S), NNH = 9.5	1.0 (0.6-1.6)
Postoperative dizziness	NR	0.8 (0.4-1.5)	NR
Postoperative shivering	NR	NR	NR
Postoperative headache	NR	NR	NR
Antiemetics given	NR	1.0 (0.7-1.4)	NR
Postdischarge nausea (PDN)	NR	0.4 (0.3-0.7)[†] (S), NNH = 7.2	0.8 (0.4-1.7)
Postdischarge vomiting (PDV)	NR	0.8 (0.4-1.6)	NR

All results are shown as weighted mean difference (WMD) or relative risk (mean and 95% confidence intervals).
*P <0.05.
[†]P <0.01.
Significant differences are shown in favor of the following: S = sevoflurane, I = isoflurane, and D = desflurane when significant.
[‡]Significant heterogeneity; NR = not reported (or reported in only one study), NNH = numbers needed to harm for significant differences.
From: Gupta A, Zuckerman R, Stierer T, et al: *Anesthesia and Analgesia* 2004;98:632-641.

in recovery indices. No differences were found in the incidence of postoperative complications between the sevoflurane and desflurane groups (see Table 23-2).

Summary

Minor differences were found in the time to early recovery (in favor of desflurane and sevoflurane compared with isoflurane), but no differences were found between the inhalation agents in the intermediate recovery indices (home-readiness or home discharge). In addition, minor complications occurred with all agents, some of which favored one agent whereas others favored another agent, with only minor differences between the inhalation agents.

CONCLUSIONS

In this meta-analysis of the literature in patients undergoing ambulatory surgery, we found that early recovery was faster in desflurane versus sevoflurane, which in turn was faster than isoflurane. Intermediate recovery was faster in the sevoflurane versus the isoflurane groups, and apart from minor differences in postoperative complications (e.g., drowsiness), no other differences were found between these inhalation anesthetics. In general, the differences were small in magnitude, and the clinical relevance of this is very likely minimal. The choice of inhalation agent for maintenance of anesthesia appears to play a minor role for outcome following ambulatory surgery.

AREAS OF UNCERTAINTY

Although every effort was made to search the literature for articles meeting our inclusion criteria, some studies with relevant data may have been missed, and this remains a problem with any systematic analysis. We searched only literature in English, which could be considered a bias because many excellent studies have been published in non-English journals. Some authors did not clearly state whether the data presented applied to inpatients or outpatients. This has been a source of frustration and limits our conclusions from studies that provided data for outpatients alone. One other problem was that authors had used different terminology to define a similar event. Thus some authors used "time to eye-opening" whereas others used "time to awakening"; similarly, some authors used "time to response to commands" whereas others used "time to orientation"; "dizziness" and "giddiness" were used to mean (we believe) the same thing, as were "drowsiness" and "somnolence." We agreed to make a distinction between "home-readiness" and "home discharge" because these are two different parameters. Universal agreement on many of these ill-defined parameters could be an advantage for the purpose of research in future studies. Finally, the data presented here are based on 2 to 15 studies in each group, which is a severe limitation to the conclusions, and therefore more studies, with well-defined objectives and comparing a similar group of patients undergoing ambulatory surgery, are needed in the literature.

GUIDELINES

Formal guidelines regarding the choice of anesthetic agents for ambulatory surgery do not exist because of the minor differences between agents, and also because of the lack of outcome data to conclude the superiority of one agent over another. The largest trials have often concluded that choice of anesthetic agent plays a minor role (if any) in morbidity and mortality risk following ambulatory surgery. Even the crude indicators of recovery following anesthesia, including early and intermediate recovery, as well as home-readiness and home discharge, have minimal clinical significance in efficient day surgical units. Local practices, including physician or patient preferences, availability of equipment (vaporizers and infusion pumps), and staffing patterns, would dictate the anesthetic agents that should be used for ambulatory surgery. Although a greater number of patients can probably be "fast-tracked" using the newer inhalation agents such as desflurane and sevoflurane versus propofol, the overall advantage to the patient, or even the health care system, is probably minimal in terms of cost savings. In an excellent article published in 2002,[8] it was shown clearly that it is the efficient organization of an ambulatory surgical unit, rather than anesthetic drugs, that plays a key role in patient satisfaction.

AUTHOR'S RECOMMENDATIONS

Taking into consideration the remarks made earlier, and in view of the limited information available on many aspects of these anesthetic agents, as well as from the evidence available in the literature on aspects of recovery, we offer the following suggestions on the use of anesthetic agents in a day surgical unit:

- *Induction of anesthesia:* Whenever intravenous access is available in adult patients, propofol offers a definite and clear advantage over thiopentone during ambulatory surgery. Even when compared with inhalation agents such as sevoflurane, propofol offers advantages in better and smoother induction of anesthesia and greater patient satisfaction with earlier recovery and therefore should be the natural choice in all but the most exceptional circumstances.
- *Maintenance of anesthesia:* Early recovery may be delayed by 1 to 2 minutes following propofol infusion compared with sevoflurane or desflurane. However, the overall advantages of propofol in terms of reduced incidence of postoperative nausea and vomiting, as well as earlier home discharge, would favor the latter.
- *Choice of inhalation agent:* Early recovery is faster using desflurane versus sevoflurane or isoflurane. However, the time to transfer to phase II is earlier in sevoflurane, and minor complications appear to be equally distributed among the three agents. Therefore factors other than recovery and minor postoperative complications should be considered when determining the inhalation agent of choice in the day surgical unit.

REFERENCES

1. Warner MA, Shields SE, Chute CG: Major morbidity and mortality within one month of ambulatory surgery and anesthesia. *JAMA* 1993;270(12):1437-1441.
2. Wu CL, Berenholtz SM, Pronovost PJ, Fleisher LA: Systematic review and analysis of postdischarge symptoms after outpatient surgery. *Anesthesiology* 2002;96:994-1003.
3. Dexter F, Tinker JH: Comparisons between desflurane and isoflurane or propofol on time to following commands and time to discharge: A meta-analysis. *Anesthesiology* 1995;83:77-82.
4. Robinson BJ, Uhrich TD, Ebert TJ: A review of recovery from sevoflurane anaesthesia: Comparisons with isoflurane and propofol including meta-analysis. *Acta Anaesthesiol Scand* 1999;43:185-190.
5. Fisher D: Surrogate outcomes: Meaningful not! *Anesthesiology* 1999;90:355-356.
6. Thwaites A, Edmends S, Smith I: Inhalation induction with sevoflurane: A double-blind comparison with propofol. *Br J Anaesth* 1997;78:356-361.
7. Gupta A, Zuckerman R, Stierer T, Sakima N, Parker S, Fleisher LA: Comparison of recovery profile after ambulatory anesthesia with propofol, isoflurane, sevoflurane and desflurane: A systematic review. *Anesth Analg* 2004;98:632-641.
8. Apfelbaum JL, Walawander CA, Grasela TH, et al: Eliminating intensive postoperative care in same-day surgery patients using short-acting anesthetics. *Anesthesiology* 2002;97:66-74.

24 What Are the Benefits of Different Ventilatory Techniques?

Maurizio Cereda, MD

OUTLINE

Introduction

A broad variety of techniques and modes of mechanical ventilation are now available to physicians, thanks to improvements in technology. For the most part, the design of these techniques is based on sound physiologic principles. However, there is limited evidence that ventilatory techniques and modes affect hard outcomes. Additionally, the existing randomized controlled trials (RCTs) do not indicate the superiority of any specific mode but they only support certain general strategies for mechanical ventilation, such as tidal volume (TV) limitation and the use of ventilator liberation protocols. It can be argued that clinicians should choose only those modes and techniques that are time honored and have been used in the few existing positive RCTs. Although this approach will benefit a broad population, it is common experience that many patients require a more articulated strategy. In these cases, knowledge of the benefits of the different ventilatory techniques helps the clinician to individualize respiratory care, using the available modes within a general strategy that is supported by solid evidence.

Options—Description of Ventilatory Modes

Assist Control Ventilation

During assist control ventilation (ACV), the ventilator delivers a mandatory breath every time the patient initiates an inspiration. A backup respiratory rate is set to guarantee that the patient always receives a minimal number of breaths, even in the absence of spontaneous inspiratory activity. Mandatory breaths can be delivered with either volume or pressure control. During ACV, the inspiratory time is preset and invariable.

Pressure Support Ventilation

Pressure support ventilation (PSV) assists each inspiratory attempt by the patient with a pressure-limited breath, thus partitioning the work of breathing (WOB) between patient and ventilator.[1,2] The patient maintains partial control of TV and respiratory rate; the operator allows the patient to perform more or less WOB by modifying the level of inspiratory pressure.[3] PSV differs from ACV for the lack of a backup rate and for the fact that, during PSV, inspirations have variable duration and are terminated when inspiratory flow decreases below a predetermined threshold value.

Synchronized Intermittent Mandatory Ventilation

Synchronized intermittent mandatory ventilation (SIMV) assists with a mandatory breath only an adjustable fraction of patient's inspiratory attempts. Unlike ACV, additional inspirations are either unassisted or partially assisted with PSV. During SIMV, higher mandatory rates are used for patients who require higher levels of ventilatory assistance and are progressively decreased during the weaning process, allowing the patient to accomplish more unsupported breaths.

Proportional Assist Ventilation

Proportional assist ventilation (PAV) is characterized by the delivery of a variable airway pressure that is continuously adjusted throughout each breath to match patient's inspiratory effort.[4] Patient's effort is estimated using the continuous measurement of inspired flow and volume in relation to respiratory system compliance and resistance.[5] The use of PAV has been limited so far by the lack of a reliable method to frequently measure respiratory mechanics variables at the bedside, but these measurements are now available thanks to a recent addition to the PAV software.[6-8]

Airway Pressure-Release Ventilation and Biphasic Positive Airway Pressure

Airway pressure-release ventilation (APRV) is a mode of ventilatory support in which the patient breathes spontaneously at a high level of continuous airway pressure, with periodic releases to a low positive end-expiratory pressure (PEEP). CO_2 exchange is partly accomplished by the patient's activity and partly by exhalations during pressure releases.[9] The volume exhaled during releases depends on patient's mechanics and on the difference between the high pressure and the PEEP. The release time is typically maintained lower than 1.5 seconds and PEEP is usually very low or zero. Biphasic positive airway pressure (BiPAP) is a variant of APRV in which a nonnegligible PEEP is applied during releases, which are of longer duration.[10] During BiPAP, patient's inspiratory activity occurs also at PEEP.

High-Frequency Oscillatory Ventilation

High-frequency oscillatory ventilation (HFOV) is a mode of ventilatory support in which small TVs are delivered at a very high rate, in the range of 3 to 15 Hz. During HFOV, gas runs continuously through the ventilator tubing and is oscillated by a piston placed within the circuit. The oscillations are thus transmitted to the patient's lungs, producing cyclic, rapid inflations and deflations. The clinician adjusts the amplitude of the oscillations, their frequency, and the continuous gas flow rate to modulate CO_2 exchange. Arterial oxygenation is proportional to mean airway pressure, which is regulated by a valve placed on the exhaust port of the circuit. The main advantage of HFOV is that it allows the delivery of TVs that, although not negligible,[11] are still lower than with any other modes of ventilation, thus minimizing alveolar overdistention. The fact that normal blood gases can be attained also at very low TVs has been explained using nonbulk, alternative models of gas exchange.[12]

Evidence

Lung Protective Strategy

The choice between modes of mechanical ventilation is probably less important than the adoption of certain general ventilatory strategies. Among these, the use of lung protection is the one that is supported by the strongest evidence. In fact, three RCTs have suggested that the use of small TVs relative to ideal body weight (6 to 8 mL/kg) improve outcomes of acute lung injury (ALI) and acute respiratory distress syndrome (ARDS) compared with larger TVs.[13-15] This research was prompted by animal studies showing that alveolar overdistention causes a mechanical and inflammatory injury called ventilator-induced lung injury (VILI).[16,17] In many patients, the use of low TVs will result in impaired CO_2 clearance and permissive hypercapnia may be necessary. The benefits of hypercapnia in ALI/ARDS have only been suggested by descriptive studies[18] and by a secondary analysis of data from an RCT.[19] However, TV reduction should take precedence over the goal of normalizing arterial PCO_2 in ALI/ARDS patients. In fact, there is currently no evidence that moderate hypercapnia and acidosis are harmful to patients who do not have specific conditions such as intracranial hypertension and severe pulmonary hypertension.[20] Many clinicians treat ALI/ARDS patients with volume-controlled ACV because volume limitation guarantees the delivery of TV values within the range of a lung-protective strategy. However, one RCT did not detect outcome differences between volume- and pressure-controlled ACV[21] (Table 24-1).

Use of Partial Ventilatory Support

The main goal of mechanical ventilation is to support CO_2 excretion and can be accomplished either by having the ventilator substituting for the patient's inspiratory muscles (total ventilatory support) or by letting the patient and the ventilator share the effort of breathing (partial support). Although there is no RCT suggesting a superiority of either strategy, it is currently accepted that partial support is more desirable. In fact, total ventilatory support invariably requires deep sedation and often muscle relaxants. It is now recognized that minimization of sedatives is beneficial. This is based on results of RCTs where protocols to decrease sedation improved clinical outcomes compared with standard management.[22,23] Additionally, prolonged muscle relaxation is known to be harmful, and complete suppression of inspiratory activity has been shown to be associated with diaphragm dysfunction in animal models.[24-26] A recent study showed a pattern of diaphragm myofiber atrophy in organ donors ventilated for longer than 18 hours.[27]

PSV has been in circulation for more than 20 years and is probably one of the simplest ways to provide partial ventilatory support. However, its use is still relatively limited, as shown by a large prospective cohort study,[28] and is mainly relegated to the weaning process in patients who do not have severe oxygenation impairment. However, PSV can be used more broadly: in an observational prospective study, PSV was tolerated by a majority of patients with ALI.[29] In this study, failure of PSV was related to impaired respiratory mechanics and elevated dead space, rather than to poor oxygenation.

SIMV was an early form of partial ventilatory support and is still widely used, both for weaning and as a primary mode of ventilation for patients who require high-level support.[28] However, the advantages of SIMV over other modes are unclear and not demonstrated. The rationale for using SIMV is to alternate spontaneous inspirations with mechanical breaths during which the patient's respiratory muscles are allowed to rest. However, it has

Table 24-1	Highest Level of Evidence for Ventilatory Strategies in Different Groups of Patients		
Patient Group	**Strategy**	**Level of Evidence**	**Comments**
ALI/ARDS	TV limitation	A[13-15]	
	Use of partial support modes	D[24-27]	Avoidance of diagram atrophy
	Open lung approach	A[13,14,82]	Discrepancies between different studies
	Permissive hypercapnia	B[18,19]	No RCT on effects of permissive hypercapnia
	Ventilator liberation protocols	A[39,40]	
Non-ALI/ARDS	TV limitation	B[76,77]	Possible benefit in patients at risk for ALI
	Ventilator liberation protocols	A[39,40]	
COPD/asthma	Ventilator liberation protocols	A[39,40]	
	NIV	A[73,74]	Standard of care for COPD exacerbations
	Permissive hypercapnia	B[69]	Only one study available in status asthmaticus
	PEEP	C[70,71]	Matches inspiratory threshold load of intrinsic PEEP

been demonstrated that this rationale is largely flawed. In fact, WOB performed by the patient does not differ between unsupported and supported breaths[30] because the respiratory centers do not have time to adapt to the new loading conditions when a mandatory breath is delivered.[31] Although the total amount of patient WOB does decrease as the number of mandatory breaths is increased, patient unloading is less efficient during SIMV than during PSV.[32]

APRV, BiPAP, and PAV are newer modalities of partial ventilatory support. Because of its features, PAV provides a level of support that is adjustable and always proportional to patient's inspiratory drive[4] and mechanical load, adapting to acute changes in clinical conditions.[33,34]

Liberation from the Ventilator

It is widely recognized that early liberation from mechanical ventilation is a very desirable target to decrease the rate of complications and the costs of medical care.[35] A large research effort has been made in evaluating strategies for ventilator weaning,[36] but studies have failed to clearly identify an ideal ventilator mode for this purpose. When PSV is used for weaning, inspiratory pressure is decreased progressively, allowing the patient to gradually resume WOB. It is still unclear whether or not this strategy accelerates the liberation from the ventilator, compared with the other commonly used strategy consisting of daily repetitions of spontaneous breathing trials. Two RCTs performed in difficult-to-wean patients provided discordant answers to this question, which was likely due to methodologic differences.[37,38] However, the results of both studies suggested that SIMV is not the best choice for ventilator liberation, although this mode is frequently used for this purpose. In fact, SIMV was associated with delayed liberation from the ventilator, compared with PSV and with spontaneous breathing trials.[37,38]

Two RCTs have demonstrated that the process of liberation from the ventilator is shortened by the use of protocols that identify and liberate patients who are able to tolerate a spontaneous breathing trial.[39,40] Adherence to such ventilator liberation pathways is probably more important than the choice of mode of ventilation used in the process.

Patient-Ventilator Interaction

A considerable amount of research effort has been dedicated to improving the interaction between the patient and the ventilator, with the goal of optimizing patient comfort and decreasing sedation requirements. ACV is often suboptimal under this aspect. In fact, during volume-controlled ACV the patient may accomplish undesired WOB when the ventilator does not match the patient's flow and volume demands.[41,42] This is due to the fact that the patient's inspiratory effort does not cease after triggering the ventilator but continues throughout the mandatory breath.[43] This problem is particularly relevant during a lung-protective strategy, as suggested by the detection of high WOB in ALI patients ventilated with TV of 5 to 6 mL/kg.[44] It is common opinion that these

settings can lead to discomfort, although retrospective analyses of existing RCTs have not proven that TV limitation results in increased need of sedation.[45,46] Additionally, during ACV the inspiratory time is preset and invariable, which often results in patient-ventilator asynchrony.[47] This phenomenon occurs when the patient's neural inspiratory time differs from the inspiratory time set on the ventilator, causing patient discomfort or alveolar hyperinflation.[47]

PSV is characterized by a high level of adaptability to patient demands. However, in certain conditions the mechanical breath may not finish exactly at the end of the patient's neural inspiratory time, causing asynchrony, hyperinflation, and discomfort.[47] In newer ventilators, the flow threshold that ends inspiration is adjustable, allowing one to prolong or shorten inspiratory duration to better match the patient's timing.[48] Another frequently encountered problem with PSV is overassistance, which occurs when inspiratory pressure is too high.[49] This may result in excessive TV and hypocapnia, thus causing central apnea episodes.[50] In fact, PSV is associated with more apneas and sleep disruptions than ACV, probably because the latter mode has fixed TV and a backup rate.[51] Ventilator settings may be important contributors in the genesis of sleep deprivation and disruption in critically ill patients,[52] and it has been suggested that PSV should be avoided altogether during sleep.[53]

Because of its algorithm, PAV improves the matching between neural and machine inspiratory times,[49] which should translate into improved patient comfort and better tolerance of the ventilator. In a group of mechanically ventilated patients recovering from acute respiratory failure, a decreased frequency of patient-ventilator asynchronies with PAV translated into diminished sleep fragmentation, compared with PSV.[54] To date, there are no outcome studies showing the superiority of PAV to other modes of ventilation.

Use of Alternative Modes

APRV and BiPAP are used in many centers for patients with severe hypoxemia because they allow one to maintain alveolar recruitment and oxygenation while avoiding alveolar overdistention, possibly decreasing VILI. In fact, APRV has been shown to achieve similar or better gas exchange at lower peak inspiratory pressures, compared with other modes of ventilation.[55-57] Another advantage of APRV and BiPAP is that the presence of spontaneous breathing has been shown to improve gas exchange.[58] This effect seems to be related to improved diaphragmatic motion causing alveolar recruitment in the dorso-basal regions of the lung.[59,60] Additional benefits of APRV that are related to spontaneous breathing are improvements in hemodynamics,[57,58] renal function,[61] and visceral perfusion.[62]

The ability to allow unsupported breathing renders APRV and BiPAP useful to limit sedative doses in patients who require high-level ventilatory support. APRV was associated with decreased sedation needs and earlier liberation from ventilation in two RCTs: one performed in patients recovering from cardiac surgery[63] and one in patients with ALI and trauma.[64] However, the ability to extrapolate from the results of the latter study is hindered by the fact that the control group was receiving muscle relaxants, a rare practice in modern days. Although APRV and BiPAP have gained popularity, further research should clarify whether they have outcome advantages over modes that are routinely used. In the meantime, APRV and BiPAP should be considered only in patients who require high airway pressures to maintain gas exchange. Care should be taken to ensure that TVs and peak alveolar distention are compatible with a lung-protective strategy. Because of the short release time, APRV should be avoided in patients with COPD or asthma because of the risk of air trapping.

HFOV is also used in patients with severe, refractory hypoxemia, with the rationale of providing high mean airway pressures while minimizing alveolar distention and possibly VILI. HFOV has been extensively studied in the pediatric population, and two large RCTs have been performed in newborns.[65,66] Of these two studies, only one had positive results with HFOV, with shorter time to extubation and lower rates of chronic lung disease compared with SIMV.[66] The results of this study may be explained by the selection of patients with higher risk caused by their very low birth weight. In the adult population, two small RCTs found no significant effects of HFOV on outcomes of patients with ARDS, compared with conventional mechanical ventilation.[67,68] In one of these studies, a trend toward improved survival was detected with HFOV, although this study was underpowered to detect survival differences.[68] The main disadvantage of HFOV is the requirement for deep sedation and, often, muscle paralysis. Until more RCTs become available in adults, HFOV should be used in selected patients who fail to achieve acceptable oxygenation while on conventional modes of ventilation.

Management of Obstructive Lung Disease

The ventilatory management of patients with asthma and chronic obstructive pulmonary disease (COPD) is supported by a large number of physiologic studies, but few outcome trials are available. In these patients, the general goal of ventilation is to avoid hyperinflation and intrinsic PEEP. For this purpose, permissive hypercapnia is routinely practiced, but its use is supported only by an observational study on patients with status asthmaticus.[69] However, there is consensus that the adoption of this strategy has contributed to improved survival in these patients. Although once considered contraindicated, PEEP is commonly used to decrease the inspiratory threshold load of intrinsic PEEP.[70,71]

Noninvasive ventilation (NIV) is currently considered a standard treatment in COPD exacerbation.[72] This is based on strong clinical evidence from RCTs that demonstrated improved outcomes and decreased rates of intubation from its early use.[73,74] A systematic review of existing RCTs suggested that NIV might also be beneficial in other forms of hypoxemic respiratory failure, although the studies had conflicting results due to population heterogeneity.[75] Therefore NIV cannot be recommended for routine use in non-COPD patients with acute respiratory failure but should only be considered in selected cases.

AREAS OF UNCERTAINTY

Although with a certain delay, the use of low-TV ventilation has become common in the treatment of ALI/ARDS. Recent evidence suggests that this approach may also benefit certain patients who did not have these conditions. Two recent observational studies documented an association between early use of high TV and later development of ALI in patients who do not have this syndrome initially.[76,77] Until RCTs are available, it is probably prudent to avoid high TV at least in those patients who are at risk for developing ALI and who do not have contraindications to TV limitation.

It is still unclear how PEEP should be set in ALI/ARDS. PEEP is usually titrated to counteract hypoxemia, but its selection is complicated by the fact that it is still unclear what the target arterial oxygenation in ALI/ARDS should be: data suggest that improved oxygenation is not necessarily associated with better outcomes.[15] It has been hypothesized that the use of high PEEP may positively affect outcomes because of an effect of recruitment and stabilization of collapsed alveoli (open lung strategy).[78,79] This strategy is physiologically sound and is based on good-quality animal studies suggesting that VILI can also be caused by intermittent alveolar collapse and that it can be prevented by PEEP.[80,81] However, the available RCTs in ALI/ARDS had discordant findings regarding the effects of PEEP on outcomes. In three RCTs, survival was not different between groups treated with high or lower PEEP levels.[82-84] However, in the two most recent of these trials secondary outcomes, such as ventilator-free days and rate of refractory hypoxemia, were improved by the use of higher PEEP. Finally, two other studies showed improved survival with the combined use of a low TV and a high PEEP that was chosen based on mechanical evidence of alveolar recruitment, compared with a high TV and low PEEP strategy.[13,14] These findings suggested that high PEEP selection may be beneficial only if titrated on individual patients' mechanical characteristics. In the absence of clearer evidence, clinicians should continue to set ventilation aiming to improve oxygenation while minimizing the harmful effects of PEEP. In patients who seem to favorably respond to PEEP and alveolar recruitment attempts, maintenance of higher PEEP is probably not harmful based on the existing evidence, as long as alveolar overdistention is avoided.

During spontaneous breathing trials, it is common to use low-level PSV, as opposed to simply connecting the patient to a T-piece.[28] The rationale of this use is to provide enough support to compensate for the WOB imposed by the resistance of the endotracheal tube,[85] thus simulating loading conditions after extubation. In fact, an observational study suggested that endotracheal tube resistance may cause failure to succeed a spontaneous breathing trial in patients who would otherwise tolerate extubation.[86] However, another study showed that WOB did not change before and after extubation,[87] suggesting that a T-piece trial adequately reflects WOB after extubation. Outcomes of spontaneous breathing trials are not different whether a T-piece or low-level PSV is used.[88]

GUIDELINES

There are currently no guidelines on the selection of ventilatory modes. A 1999 international consensus conference on ventilator-associated lung injury stated that TV limitation may be beneficial in patients with ALI/ARDS.[89] This statement has not yet been updated, but similar recommendations were included in the 2008 Surviving Sepsis Campaign guidelines, also including a suggestion to use adequate PEEP to avoid extensive alveolar collapse.[90] In 2007, an international task force emphasized the use of spontaneous breathing trials and of organized protocols to facilitate the process of liberation from the ventilator.[91] The 2004 American Thoracic Society guidelines for the management of COPD recommended the use of NIV as initial treatment in COPD exacerbations with respiratory failure.[72]

AUTHOR'S RECOMMENDATIONS
• Consider a trial of NIV before intubation, particularly in COPD patients.
• Start ventilation using ACV, then reassess patients' response based on blood gases and respiratory mechanics.
• Use low TV and limit peak alveolar pressures in ALI/ARDS patients.
• Use lower TV in non-ALI patients if clinically reasonable.
• Tolerate hypercapnia in ALI/ARDS and in COPD/asthma patients, unless contraindicated.
• Select a mode of partial ventilatory support as soon as clinically feasible, and avoid muscle relaxants.
• Frequently assess patient-ventilator interaction, and adjust settings/mode as needed to optimize comfort.
• Frequently assess sedation level, and follow protocols to minimize sedative doses.
• Consider alternative modes of ventilation (APRV/HFOV) if patients need high PEEP to maintain acceptable oxygenation.
• Continuously attempt to deescalate ventilator settings as patient conditions improve.
• Perform daily spontaneous breathing trials in eligible patients, and promptly extubate patients who succeed.
• Avoid SIMV in difficult-to-wean patients.

Table 24-2 Characteristics, Advantages, and Disadvantages of Different Ventilatory Modes

Mode	Type of Support	Characteristics	Advantages	Disadvantages	Uncertainties
ACV	Total/partial	Assists each inspiration with volume or pressure-limited breath	Provides backup rate Guarantees safe TV (volume limited) Improves sleep	May cause patient/ventilator asynchrony Causes excessive WOB at low TV	Might increase sedation requirements at lower TV
SIMV	Partial	Assists only a fraction of inspirations with mandatory breaths	Allows unsupported breathing Provides backup rate when used with PSV	Does not unload patient WOB efficiently Delays liberation from the ventilator	Unclear role in current respiratory care
PSV	Partial	Assists each inspiration with a pressure-limited breath Ends inspiration when flow threshold is reached	Level of support is easily adjustable Improves patient-ventilator interaction Shortens weaning compared with SIMV	Lacks a backup rate May cause patient/ventilator asynchrony and overassistance May cause central apneas and sleep fragmentation	Might prolong weaning compared with spontaneous breathing trials
APRV BiPAP	Partial	Spontaneous, unassisted breaths at two levels of continuous airway pressure High levels of airway pressure are maintained for prolonged time	Improves oxygenation at lower peak inspiratory pressures Spontaneous breathing improves gas exchange Might decrease sedation needs	Risk of hyperinflation in COPD patients	Does not guarantee safe TV delivery
PAV	Partial	Pressure assistance matches inspiratory effort	Improves patient/ventilator interaction Adjustable patient WOB Responds to changes in patient conditions Improves sleep quality	Does not guarantee TV Requires frequent measurements of respiratory mechanics	No outcome studies are available
HFOV	Total	Small TVs at very high rates	Improves oxygenation and alveolar recruitment Decreases alveolar overdistention	Requires deep sedation, muscle paralysis, or both	Improves outcomes in very-low-birth-weight newborns Uncertain effects on outcome in adult population

REFERENCES

1. MacIntyre NR: Respiratory function during pressure support ventilation. *Chest* 1986;89:677-683.
2. Brochard L, Pluskwa F, Lemaire F: Improved efficacy of spontaneous breathing with inspiratory pressure support. *Am Rev Respir Dis* 1987;136:411-415.
3. Brochard L, Harf A, Lorino H, Lemaire F: Inspiratory pressure support prevents diaphragmatic fatigue during weaning from mechanical ventilation. *Am Rev Respir Dis* 1989;139:513-521.
4. Younes M: Proportional assist ventilation, a new approach to ventilatory support theory. *Am Rev Respir Dis* 1992;145:114-120.
5. Grasso S, Ranieri VM: Proportional assist ventilation. *Respir Care Clin North Am* 2001;7:465-473, ix-x.
6. Younes M, Kun J, Masiowski B, Webster K, Roberts D: A method for noninvasive determination of inspiratory resistance during proportional assist ventilation. *Am J Respir Crit Care Med* 2001;163:829-839.
7. Younes M, Webster K, Kun J, Roberts D, Masiowski B: A method for measuring passive elastance during proportional assist ventilation. *Am J Respir Crit Care Med* 2001;164:50-60.
8. Kondili E, Prinianakis G, Alexopoulou C, Vakouti E, Klimathianaki M, Georgopoulos D: Respiratory load compensation during mechanical ventilation-proportional assist ventilation with load-adjustable gain factors versus pressure support. *Intensive Care Med* 2006;32:692-699.
9. Stock MC, Downs JB, Frolicher DA: Airway pressure release ventilation. *Crit Care Med* 1987;15:462-466.
10. Hormann C, Baum M, Putensen C, Mutz NJ, Benzer H: Biphasic positive airway pressure (BiPAP)—a new mode of ventilatory support. *Eur J Anaesthesiol* 1994;11:37-42.
11. Sedeek KA, Takeuchi M, Suchodolski K, Kacmarek RM: Determinants of tidal volume during high-frequency oscillation. *Crit Care Med* 2003;31:227-231.
12. Chang HK: Mechanisms of gas transport during ventilation by high-frequency oscillation. *J Appl Physiol* 1984;56:553-563.
13. Amato MB, Barbas CS, Medeiros DM, et al: Effect of a protective-ventilation strategy on mortality in the acute respiratory distress syndrome. *N Engl J Med* 1998;338:347-354.
14. Villar J, Kacmarek RM, Perez-Mendez L, Aguirre-Jaime A: A high positive end-expiratory pressure, low tidal volume ventilatory strategy improves outcome in persistent acute respiratory distress syndrome: A randomized, controlled trial. *Crit Care Med* 2006;34:1311-1318.
15. Ventilation with lower tidal volumes as compared with traditional tidal volumes for acute lung injury and the acute respiratory distress syndrome. The Acute Respiratory Distress Syndrome Network. *N Engl J Med* 2000;342:1301-1308.
16. Dreyfuss D, Soler P, Basset G, Saumon G: High inflation pressure pulmonary edema. Respective effects of high airway pressure, high tidal volume, and positive end-expiratory pressure. *Am Rev Respir Dis* 1988;137:1159-1164.
17. Tsuno K, Prato P, Kolobow T: Acute lung injury from mechanical ventilation at moderately high airway pressures. *J Appl Physiol* 1990;69:956-961.
18. Hickling KG, Walsh J, Henderson S, Jackson R: Low mortality rate in adult respiratory distress syndrome using low-volume, pressure-limited ventilation with permissive hypercapnia: A prospective study. *Crit Care Med* 1994;22:1568-1578.
19. Kregenow DA, Rubenfeld GD, Hudson LD, Swenson ER: Hypercapnic acidosis and mortality in acute lung injury. *Crit Care Med* 2006;34:1-7.
20. Laffey JG, O'Croinin D, McLoughlin P, Kavanagh BP: Permissive hypercapnia—role in protective lung ventilatory strategies. *Intensive Care Med* 2004;30:347-356.
21. Esteban A, Alia I, Gordo F, et al: Prospective randomized trial comparing pressure-controlled ventilation and volume-controlled ventilation in ARDS. For the Spanish lung failure collaborative group. *Chest* 2000;117:1690-1696.
22. Brook AD, Ahrens TS, Schaiff R, et al: Effect of a nursing-implemented sedation protocol on the duration of mechanical ventilation. *Crit Care Med* 1999;27:2609-2615.
23. Kress JP, Pohlman AS, O'Connor MF, Hall JB: Daily interruption of sedative infusions in critically ill patients undergoing mechanical ventilation. *N Engl J Med* 2000;342:1471-1477.
24. Anzueto A, Peters JI, Tobin MJ, et al: Effects of prolonged controlled mechanical ventilation on diaphragmatic function in healthy adult baboons. *Crit Care Med* 1997;25:1187-1190.
25. Sassoon CS, Caiozzo VJ, Manka A, Sieck GC: Altered diaphragm contractile properties with controlled mechanical ventilation. *J Appl Physiol* 2002;92:2585-2595.
26. Le Bourdelles G, Viires N, Boczkowski J, Seta N, Pavlovic D, Aubier M: Effects of mechanical ventilation on diaphragmatic contractile properties in rats. *Am J Respir Crit Care Med* 1994;149:1539-1544.
27. Levine S, Nguyen T, Taylor N, et al: Rapid disuse atrophy of diaphragm fibers in mechanically ventilated humans. *N Engl J Med* 2008;358:1327-1335.
28. Esteban A, Anzueto A, Frutos F, et al: Characteristics and outcomes in adult patients receiving mechanical ventilation: A 28-day international study. *JAMA* 2002;287:345-355.
29. Cereda M, Foti G, Marcora B, et al: Pressure support ventilation in patients with acute lung injury. *Crit Care Med* 2000;28:1269-1275.
30. Marini JJ, Smith TC, Lamb VJ: External work output and force generation during synchronized intermittent mechanical ventilation. Effect of machine assistance on breathing effort. *Am Rev Respir Dis* 1988;138:1169-1179.
31. Imsand C, Feihl F, Perret C, Fitting JW: Regulation of inspiratory neuromuscular output during synchronized intermittent mechanical ventilation. *Anesthesiology* 1994;80:13-22.
32. Leung P, Jubran A, Tobin MJ: Comparison of assisted ventilator modes on triggering, patient effort, and dyspnea. *Am J Respir Crit Care Med* 1997;155:1940-1948.
33. Ranieri VM, Giuliani R, Mascia L, et al: Patient-ventilator interaction during acute hypercapnia: Pressure-support vs. proportional-assist ventilation. *J Appl Physiol* 1996;81:426-436.
34. Grasso S, Puntillo F, Mascia L, et al: Compensation for increase in respiratory workload during mechanical ventilation. Pressure-support versus proportional-assist ventilation. *Am J Respir Crit Care Med* 2000;161:819-826.
35. MacIntyre NR: Evidence-based ventilator weaning and discontinuation. *Respir Care* 2004;49:830-836.
36. Tobin MJ: Remembrance of weaning past: The seminal papers. *Intensive Care Med* 2006;32:1485-1493.
37. Brochard L, Rauss A, Benito S, et al: Comparison of three methods of gradual withdrawal from ventilatory support during weaning from mechanical ventilation. *Am J Respir Crit Care Med* 1994;150:896-903.
38. Esteban A, Frutos F, Tobin MJ, et al: A comparison of four methods of weaning patients from mechanical ventilation. Spanish lung failure collaborative group. *N Engl J Med* 1995;332:345-350.
39. Kollef MH, Shapiro SD, Silver P, et al: A randomized, controlled trial of protocol-directed versus physician-directed weaning from mechanical ventilation. *Crit Care Med* 1997;25:567-574.
40. Ely EW, Baker AM, Dunagan DP, et al: Effect on the duration of mechanical ventilation of identifying patients capable of breathing spontaneously. *N Engl J Med* 1996;335:1864-1869.
41. MacIntyre NR, McConnell R, Cheng KC, Sane A: Patient-ventilator flow dyssynchrony: Flow-limited versus pressure-limited breaths. *Crit Care Med* 1997;25:1671-1677.
42. Marini JJ, Capps JS, Culver BH: The inspiratory work of breathing during assisted mechanical ventilation. *Chest* 1985;87:612-618.
43. Flick GR, Bellamy PE, Simmons DH: Diaphragmatic contraction during assisted mechanical ventilation. *Chest* 1989;96:130-135.
44. Kallet RH, Campbell AR, Dicker RA, Katz JA, Mackersie RC: Effects of tidal volume on work of breathing during lung-protective ventilation in patients with acute lung injury and acute respiratory distress syndrome. *Crit Care Med* 2006;34:8-14.
45. Cheng IW, Eisner MD, Thompson BT, Ware LB, Matthay MA, Acute Respiratory Distress Syndrome Network: Acute effects of tidal volume strategy on hemodynamics, fluid balance, and sedation in acute lung injury. *Crit Care Med* 2005;33:63-70 discussion 239-240.
46. Kahn JM, Andersson L, Karir V, Polissar NL, Neff MJ, Rubenfeld GD: Low tidal volume ventilation does not increase sedation use in patients with acute lung injury. *Crit Care Med* 2005;33:766-771.
47. Kondili E, Prinianakis G, Georgopoulos D: Patient-ventilator interaction. *Br J Anaesth* 2003;91:106-119.

48. Chiumello D, Pelosi P, Taccone P, Slutsky A, Gattinoni L: Effect of different inspiratory rise time and cycling off criteria during pressure support ventilation in patients recovering from acute lung injury. *Crit Care Med* 2003;31:2604-2610.

49. Giannouli E, Webster K, Roberts D, Younes M: Response of ventilator-dependent patients to different levels of pressure support and proportional assist. *Am J Respir Crit Care Med* 1999;159:1716-1725.

50. Meza S, Mendez M, Ostrowski M, Younes M: Susceptibility to periodic breathing with assisted ventilation during sleep in normal subjects. *J Appl Physiol* 1998;85:1929-1940.

51. Parthasarathy S, Tobin MJ: Effect of ventilator mode on sleep quality in critically ill patients. *Am J Respir Crit Care Med* 2002;166:1423-1429.

52. Weinhouse GL, Schwab RJ: Sleep in the critically ill patient. *Sleep* 2006;29:707-716.

53. Toublanc B, Rose D, Glerant JC, et al: Assist-control ventilation vs. low levels of pressure support ventilation on sleep quality in intubated ICU patients. *Intensive Care Med* 2007;33: 1148-1154.

54. Bosma K, Ferreyra G, Ambrogio C, et al: Patient-ventilator interaction and sleep in mechanically ventilated patients: Pressure support versus proportional assist ventilation. *Crit Care Med* 2007;35:1048-1054.

55. Cane RD, Peruzzi WT, Shapiro BA: Airway pressure release ventilation in severe acute respiratory failure. *Chest* 1991;100: 460-463.

56. Varpula T, Valta P, Niemi R, Takkunen O, Hynynen M, Pettila VV: Airway pressure release ventilation as a primary ventilatory mode in acute respiratory distress syndrome. *Acta Anaesthesiol Scand* 2004;48:722-731.

57. Sydow M, Burchardi H, Ephraim E, Zielmann S, Crozier TA: Long-term effects of two different ventilatory modes on oxygenation in acute lung injury. Comparison of airway pressure release ventilation and volume-controlled inverse ratio ventilation. *Am J Respir Crit Care Med* 1994;149:1550-1556.

58. Putensen C, Mutz NJ, Putensen-Himmer G, Zinserling J: Spontaneous breathing during ventilatory support improves ventilation-perfusion distributions in patients with acute respiratory distress syndrome. *Am J Respir Crit Care Med* 1999;159:1241-1248.

59. Neumann P, Wrigge H, Zinserling J, et al: Spontaneous breathing affects the spatial ventilation and perfusion distribution during mechanical ventilatory support. *Crit Care Med* 2005;33: 1090-1095.

60. Wrigge H, Zinserling J, Neumann P, et al: Spontaneous breathing with airway pressure release ventilation favors ventilation in dependent lung regions and counters cyclic alveolar collapse in oleic-acid-induced lung injury: A randomized controlled computed tomography trial. *Crit Care* 2005;9:R780-R789.

61. Hering R, Peters D, Zinserling J, Wrigge H, von Spiegel T, Putensen C: Effects of spontaneous breathing during airway pressure release ventilation on renal perfusion and function in patients with acute lung injury. *Intensive Care Med* 2002;28: 1426-1433.

62. Hering R, Viehofer A, Zinserling J, et al: Effects of spontaneous breathing during airway pressure release ventilation on intestinal blood flow in experimental lung injury. *Anesthesiology* 2003;99:1137-1144.

63. Rathgeber J, Schorn B, Falk V, Kazmaier S, Spiegel T, Burchardi H: The influence of controlled mandatory ventilation (CMV), intermittent mandatory ventilation (IMV) and biphasic intermittent positive airway pressure (BIPAP) on duration of intubation and consumption of analgesics and sedatives. A prospective analysis in 596 patients following adult cardiac surgery. *Eur J Anaesthesiol* 1997;14:576-582.

64. Putensen C, Zech S, Wrigge H, et al: Long-term effects of spontaneous breathing during ventilatory support in patients with acute lung injury. *Am J Respir Crit Care Med* 2001;164:43-49.

65. Johnson AH, Peacock JL, Greenough A, et al: High-frequency oscillatory ventilation for the prevention of chronic lung disease of prematurity. *N Engl J Med* 2002;347:633-642.

66. Courtney SE, Durand DJ, Asselin JM, et al: High-frequency oscillatory ventilation versus conventional mechanical ventilation for very-low-birth-weight infants. *N Engl J Med* 2002;347: 643-652.

67. Bollen CW, van Well GT, Sherry T, et al: High frequency oscillatory ventilation compared with conventional mechanical ventilation in adult respiratory distress syndrome: A randomized controlled trial [ISRCTN24242669]. *Crit Care* 2005;9:R430-R439.

68. Derdak S, Mehta S, Stewart TE, et al: High-frequency oscillatory ventilation for acute respiratory distress syndrome in adults: A randomized, controlled trial. *Am J Respir Crit Care Med* 2002;166:801-808.

69. Darioli R, Perret C: Mechanical controlled hypoventilation in status asthmaticus. *Am Rev Respir Dis* 1984;129:385-387.

70. Guerin C, Milic-Emili J, Fournier G: Effect of PEEP on work of breathing in mechanically ventilated COPD patients. *Intensive Care Med* 2000;26:1207-1214.

71. MacIntyre NR, Cheng KC, McConnell R: Applied PEEP during pressure support reduces the inspiratory threshold load of intrinsic PEEP. *Chest* 1997;111:188-193.

72. Celli BR, MacNee W, ATS/ERS Task Force: Standards for the diagnosis and treatment of patients with COPD: A summary of the ATS/ERS position paper. *Eur Respir J* 2004;23:932-946.

73. Brochard L, Mancebo J, Wysocki M, et al: Noninvasive ventilation for acute exacerbations of chronic obstructive pulmonary disease. *N Engl J Med* 1995;333:817-822.

74. Plant PK, Owen JL, Elliott MW: Early use of non-invasive ventilation for acute exacerbations of chronic obstructive pulmonary disease on general respiratory wards: A multicentre randomised controlled trial. *Lancet* 2000;355:1931-1935.

75. Keenan SP, Sinuff T, Cook DJ, Hill NS: Does noninvasive positive pressure ventilation improve outcome in acute hypoxemic respiratory failure? A systematic review. *Crit Care Med* 2004;32:2516-2523.

76. Gajic O, Dara SI, Mendez JL, et al: Ventilator-associated lung injury in patients without acute lung injury at the onset of mechanical ventilation. *Crit Care Med* 2004;32:1817-1824.

77. Mascia L, Zavala E, Bosna K, et al: High tidal volume is associated with the development of acute lung injury after severe brain injury: An international observational study. *Crit Care Med* 2007.

78. Lachmann B: Open up the lung and keep the lung open. *Intensive Care Med* 1992;18:319-321.

79. Papadakos PJ, Lachmann B: The open lung concept of mechanical ventilation: The role of recruitment and stabilization. *Crit Care Clin* 2007;23:241-250, ix-x.

80. Muscedere JG, Mullen JB, Gan K, Slutsky AS: Tidal ventilation at low airway pressures can augment lung injury. *Am J Respir Crit Care Med* 1994;149:1327-1334.

81. Webb HH, Tierney DF: Experimental pulmonary edema due to intermittent positive pressure ventilation with high inflation pressures. Protection by positive end-expiratory pressure. *Am Rev Respir Dis* 1974;110:556-565.

82. Brower RG, Lanken PN, MacIntyre N, et al: Higher versus lower positive end-expiratory pressures in patients with the acute respiratory distress syndrome. *N Engl J Med* 2004;351:327-336.

83. Mercat A, Richard JC, Vielle B, et al: Positive end-expiratory pressure setting in adults with acute lung injury and acute respiratory distress syndrome: A randomized controlled trial. *JAMA* 2008;299:646-655.

84. Meade MO, Cook DJ, Guyatt GH, et al: Ventilation strategy using low tidal volumes, recruitment maneuvers, and high positive end-expiratory pressure for acute lung injury and acute respiratory distress syndrome: A randomized controlled trial. *JAMA* 2008;299:637-645.

85. Brochard L, Rua F, Lorino H, Lemaire F, Harf A: Inspiratory pressure support compensates for the additional work of breathing caused by the endotracheal tube. *Anesthesiology* 1991;75: 739-745.

86. Kirton OC, DeHaven CB, Morgan JP, Windsor J, Civetta JM: Elevated imposed work of breathing masquerading as ventilator weaning intolerance. *Chest* 1995;108:1021-1025.

87. Straus C, Louis B, Isabey D, Lemaire F, Harf A, Brochard L: Contribution of the endotracheal tube and the upper airway to breathing workload. *Am J Respir Crit Care Med* 1998;157:23-30.

88. Esteban A, Alia I, Gordo F, et al: Extubation outcome after spontaneous breathing trials with T-tube or pressure support ventilation. The Spanish lung failure collaborative group. *Am J Respir Crit Care Med* 1997;156:459-465.

89. International Consensus Conferences in Intensive Care Medicine: Ventilator-associated lung injury in ARDS. This official conference report was cosponsored by the American Thoracic Society, the European Society of Intensive Care Medicine, and the Societe de Reanimation de Langue Francaise, and was approved by the ATS board of directors, July 1999. *Am J Respir Crit Care Med* 1999;160:2118-2124.

90. Dellinger RP, Levy MM, Carlet JM, et al: Surviving sepsis campaign: International guidelines for management of severe sepsis and septic shock: 2008. *Crit Care Med* 2008;36:296-327.

91. Boles JM, Bion J, Connors A, et al: Weaning from mechanical ventilation. *Eur Respir J* 2007;29:1033-1056.

25 Is There an Optimal Perioperative Hemoglobin?

Jeffrey L. Carson, MD, and Barbara Armas, MD

Blood transfusions are common. In 2001, approximately 13.9 million units of red blood cells were transfused in the United States.[1] Between 60% and 70% of all red blood cell units are transfused in the perioperative setting.[2-5] Surgical patients are frequently anemic from the underlying disease, from the injury leading to the need for surgery, and from the blood loss associated with the surgical procedure.

Over the past 20 years, there has been a trend toward using lower hemoglobin concentration as a transfusion trigger. The main motivation has been concern about blood safety prompted by the human immunodeficiency virus (HIV) epidemic in the 1980s. Fortunately, the risks of transmitting viral infections have become extremely low. The most recent estimates of the risk of residual units of infected blood donated by repeat donors were 1 per 1,935,000 for hepatitis C virus and 1 per 2,135,000 for HIV.[6] New risks from infections may emerge, such as West Nile virus.[7,8] Concerns about the rare transmission of variant Creutzfeldt-Jakob disease[9] have led to the increasing use of leuko-reduced blood and, in the United States, the elimination of donors who lived in the United Kingdom and Europe.[10,11] The result of new testing and donor policies is a blood supply that is so safe that it is difficult to measure changes in markers of disease after policy changes.[12] However, newly identified noninfectious risks such as transfusion-related acute lung injury (TRALI) and the infrequently reported transfusion-associated circulatory overload may be even more common than previously appreciated.[13]

With the improvement in safety and the potential for blood shortage, it is timely to evaluate the evidence that documents when blood transfusion should be administered in the perioperative time period.

OPTIONS/THERAPIES

The indications for red blood cell transfusion are controversial. Most recommendations suggest that the decision to transfuse should be based on individual assessment of signs and symptoms of anemia. However, in practice, most clinicians transfuse at a specific hemoglobin concentration such as 8 g/dL.[14] Opinions on the indications for transfusion of predeposit autologous transfusion also vary. Some clinicians argue that the indications should be the same as for allogeneic blood cells, whereas others

suggest that because the risk of transfusion is less, autologous blood should be given at higher transfusion thresholds.

EVIDENCE

Several critical lines of evidence are needed to guide transfusion decisions. First, it is necessary to understand the risks associated with different levels of anemia in the perioperative time period. Second, randomized clinical trials and observational studies are needed to document that transfusion improves outcome. Third, as previously described, the risks of allogeneic and autologous transfusion must also be taken into account. The current data suggest that allogeneic blood transfusion is extremely safe.[6] To determine the efficacy of transfusion, we need to know at what point the risks of anemia increase and whether transfusions will eliminate or reduce the risks.

Risks Associated with Anemia

Studies in patients who refuse blood transfusion for religious reasons provide insights into the risks of anemia during the perioperative time period. The largest study included 1958 patients undergoing surgery in the operating room.[15] Mortality rates rose as the preoperative hemoglobin levels fell. Patients with underlying cardiovascular disease, who had a hemoglobin level of 10 g/dL or less, had a higher risk of death than patients without underlying cardiovascular disease (Figure 25-1). An analysis of patients from the same cohort with postoperative hemoglobin levels lower than 8 g/dL found that mortality rate rose when the postoperative hemoglobin was less than 7 g/dL and became extremely high with postoperative hemoglobin levels below 5 g/dL.[16] These results are consistent with an analysis of mortality and morbidity rates from case reports in Jehovah's Witness patients.[17]

Studies in volunteers who underwent isovolemic reduction of hemoglobin levels to 5 g/dL also provide insight into the risks of anemia. Two studies found that most transient and asymptomatic electrocardiogram changes occurred in 5 of 87 volunteers when their heart rates were faster and their hemoglobin level was between 5 and 7 g/dL.[18,19] Other studies in young, healthy volunteers under age 35 have identified subtle and reversible cognitive changes at hemoglobin levels between 5 and

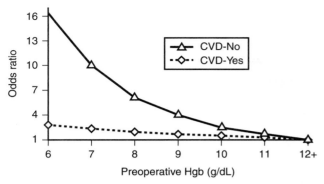

Figure 25-1. Risk of Death in Patients with and without Cardiovascular Disease (CVD). *From Carson JL et al: Effect of anaemia and cardiovascular disease on surgical mortality and morbidity.* Lancet 1996;348 (9034):1055-1066.

7 g/dL and increased fatigue at hemoglobin levels below 7 g/dL.[20] It is uncertain how to apply these results to older patients, though we can surmise that these changes might occur at higher hemoglobin levels.

Clinical Trials Evaluating Transfusion in Adults

A total of 1780 patients have entered trials evaluating transfusion thresholds, although only one is adequately powered to detect important differences in outcomes. The most important trial is the Transfusion Requirement in Critical Care (TRICC) trial.[21,22] In this study, 838 volume-resuscitated intensive care unit (ICU) patients were randomized to a either a "restrictive" or "liberal" transfusion strategy. The "restrictive" group received allogeneic red blood cell transfusions at hemoglobin levels of 7 g/dL (and were maintained between 7 and 9 g/dL), and the "liberal" group received red blood cells at 10 g/dL (and were maintained between 10 and 12 g/dL).[21] The restrictive group had lower average hemoglobin levels (8.5 versus 10.7 g/dL) and fewer transfusions (2.6 versus 5.6) compared with the liberal group. The 30-day mortality rate was slightly lower in the restrictive transfusion group (18.7% versus 23.3%), although the finding was not statistically significant ($p = 0.11$). The risk of clinically recognized myocardial infarction (0.07% versus 2.9%; $p = 0.02$) and congestive heart failure (5.3% versus 10.7%; $p < 0.001$) also occurred less frequently in the restrictive transfusion group.[21] In two subanalyses, patients randomized to the restrictive transfusion group who were less than 50 years of age, and less ill as defined by APACHE score, had a significantly lower mortality rate than patients in the liberal group.[21] In another subanalysis of patients with cardiovascular disease, there were no significant differences in mortality rate, although the confidence intervals were wide (adjusted odds ratio 1.26; 95% confidence interval 0.70 to 2.24).[23] This trial contributed 47% of the patients and 82% of the recorded deaths among all the patients entered into all the trials.

Eight other randomized clinical trials have evaluated the effects of different transfusion thresholds (Table 25-1).[21,22,24-31] The clinical settings and outcomes were different among the studies. The transfusion thresholds varied and overlapped among the "conservative" or "liberal" strategy.

Only two other trials in adults evaluating different transfusion thresholds have included more than 100 patients. Neither found any difference in outcomes. In the trial by Bracey and colleagues,[30] 428 patients undergoing elective coronary artery bypass surgery were randomized to transfusion thresholds of 9 g/dL or 8 g/dL. The differences between perioperative hemoglobin concentrations were small, and the event rates were very low. There were no differences in any outcome. The second trial included 127 patients undergoing knee arthroplasty. Patients were randomized to either receive autologous blood only if the hemoglobin level fell below 9 g/dL or to be transfused immediately after surgery regardless of the hemoglobin level.[31] The difference in postoperative hemoglobin concentration was about 0.7 g/dL, and there were no differences in outcomes.

Only one trial has involved a transfusion strategy that included patient assessment for symptoms.[29] In this trial (a pilot study), 84 hip fracture patients who underwent surgical repair were randomized to a 10 g/dL threshold or to transfusion for symptoms. Transfusion was permitted in the latter group if the hemoglobin level was less than 8 g/dL, even if there were no symptoms. There were no statistically significant differences in any outcomes, including functional recovery, mortality rate, and morbidity. However, at 60 days after surgery, there were 5 deaths in the symptomatic group and 2 deaths in the 10 g/dL group. In all these trials (and the other five trials listed in Table 25-1), the numbers of patients were much too small to evaluate the effect of lower transfusion triggers on clinically important outcomes such as mortality rate, morbidity, and functional status.

A meta-analysis was performed by combining data from trials that compared restrictive with liberal transfusion strategies.[32,33] The analysis of the pooled data found that a restrictive transfusion trigger reduced the proportion of patients receiving red blood cell transfusion by 42% and by 0.93 units of red blood cells per transfused patient. The restrictive group had a 5.6% lower mean hematocrit level than patients who were assigned to the more liberal transfusion group. There were no differences in length of hospital stay or frequency of cardiac events in the two groups. The TRICC trial contributed over 80% of the deaths in the mortality analysis. Mortality rate was not increased in patients assigned to the restrictive transfusion group (Figure 25-2).

Anemia might also impair functional recovery. Only one small study evaluated the effect of red blood cell transfusion on functional ability in anemic patients but was underpowered to detect differences in outcomes.[29] Most of the other evidence that evaluates the relationship between anemia and functional status comes from trials in which recombinant human erythropoietin was administered in patients with cancer or end-stage renal disease.[34] The data are limited but suggest that an increase in hemoglobin concentration improves exercise tolerance. How high the hemoglobin level needs to be awaits further study.

Table 25-1   Results of the Randomized Controlled Trials in Adults

Study (Year)	Setting	Subjects: Eligibility and Comparability	Transfusion Strategy	Blood Usage Units/pt Mean (SD)	Proportion Transfused (%) (n)	Hb/Hct Levels mean (SD)
Topley[24] (1956)	Trauma (n = 22)	>1 L blood loss; considered to be at no clinical risk in raising blood volume ≥100% of normal, or allowing it to reach 30% below normal	Liberal: to achieve RBC volume ≥100% of normal Restrictive: maintain RBC volume 70%-80% of normal	11.3 (6.9) 4.8 (6.7)	100 (10) 67 (8)	Lowest Hb: (15.6 ± 2.0) g/dL Lowest Hb: (11.3 ± 0.7) g/dL
Blair[25] (1986)	GI bleeding (n = 50)	Acute severe upper gastrointestinal hemorrhage	Liberal: patients received at least 2 units of PRBCs immediately on admission to hospital Restrictive: patients were not transfused PRBCs during the first 24 hr unless Hb <8.0 g/dL or shock persisted after initial resuscitation with colloid	4.6 (1.5) 2.6 (3.1)	100 (24) 19.2 (5)	Admission Hct: 28 (5.9%) Discharge Hct: 37.0 (7.8%) Admission Hct: 29 (8.2%) Discharge Hct: 37.0 (7.1%)
Fortune[26] (1987)	Trauma/ acute hemorrhage (n = 25)	Patients who had sustained a Class III or Class IV hemorrhage and had clinical signs of shock	Liberal: Hct was brought up to 40% slowly over period of several hours by infusion of PRBCs Restrictive: Hct was kept close to 30% by administration of PRBCs	—	—	Average Hct for 3-day period: 38.4 (2.1%) Average Hct for 3-day period: 29.7 (1.9%)
Johnson[27] (1992)	Cardiac surgery (n = 38)	Patients undergoing elective coronary revascularization and able to donate at least three units of packed cells preoperatively	Liberal: patients received blood transfusion to achieve Hct value of 32% so long as autologous blood was available Restrictive: patients received transfusion only if Hct value fell below 25%	2.05 (0.93) 1.0 (0.86)	100 (18) 75 (15)	Hct at 4 hr postoperative: 31.3% Hct at 4 hr postoperative: 28.7%
Hebert[22] (1995)	Critical care (n = 69)	Critically ill patients admitted to one of five tertiary-level ICUs with normovolemia after initial treatment who had Hb concentrations <9.0 g/dL within 72 hr	Liberal: patients were transfused PRBCs if their Hb concentration maintained at 10.0-12.0 g/dL Restrictive: patients were transfused PRBCs only if their Hb 7.0-7.5 g/dL; Hb concentration maintained at 7.0-9.0 g/dL	Mean units per patient: 4.8 Total units: 174 Mean units per patient: 2.5 Total units 82	—	Admission Hb: 9.3 (1.3) g/dL Average daily Hb: 10.9 g/dL Admission Hb: 9.7 (1.4) g/dL Average daily Hb: 9.0 g/dL
Bush[28] (1997)	Vascular surgery (n = 99)	Patients undergoing elective aortic and infrainguinal arterial reconstruction	Liberal: transfused with PRBCs to maintain Hb >10.0 g/dL Restrictive: transfused only if Hb level fell below 9.0 g/dL	Total units: 3.7 (3.5) Intraoperative: 2.4 (2.5) blood usage units/ patient Transfused total units 80 (40) Intraoperative: 1.5 (1.7)	88 (43) 28 (3.1)	Hb during 42-hr postoperative period: 11.0 (1.2) g/dL Proportion Hb/Hct levels Hb during 48-hr postoperative period: 9.8 (1.3) g/dL

Study	Surgery (n)	Patient population	Transfusion protocol			
Carson[29] (1998)	Orthopedic surgery (n = 84)	Hip fracture patients undergoing surgical repair who had postoperative Hb levels less than 10.0 g/dL	Liberal: patients received 1 U PRBCs at the time of random assignment and then as needed to maintain Hb >10.0 g/dL Restrictive: transfusion was delayed until patient developed symptoms or consequences of anemia, or Hb value <8.0 g/dL in absence of symptoms	Total median 1 (1-2) Total median 0 (0-2)	98.8 (83) 45.2 (38)	Lowest Hb: 9.4 (1.0) g/dL Lowest Hb: 8.8 (1.2) g/dL
Hebert[21] (1999)	Critical care (n = 838)	Critically ill patients admitted to 1 of 22 tertiary-level and 3 community ICUs with normovolemia after initial treatment who had Hb concentrations <9.0 g/dL within 72 hr	Liberal: patients were transfused with PRBCs to maintain Hb concentration at 10.0-12.0 g/dL Restrictive: Patients were transfused to maintain Hb concentration maintained between 7.0 and 9.0 g/dL	Total 5.6 (5.3) Total 2.6 (4.1)	100 (420)	Hb (mean daily): 10.7 (0.7) g/dL Hb (mean daily): 8.5 (0.7) g/dL
Bracey[30] (1999)	Cardiac surgery (n = 428)	Patients undergoing first-time elective coronary revascularization	Liberal: received RBC transfusions per individual physicians, who considered clinical assessment of patient and institutional guidelines, which propose Hb level <9.0 g/dL as postoperative threshold for RBC transfusion Restrictive: received RBC transfusion in postoperative period for Hb level <8.0 g/dL, unless patient experienced blood loss >750 mL since last transfusion; hypovolemia with hemodynamic instability, and excessive acute blood loss, acute respiratory failure, or inadequate cardiac output and oxygenation; or hemodynamic instability requiring vasopressors	Postoperative: 1.4 (1.8) Total: 2.5 (2.6) Postoperative: 0.9 (1.5) Total: 2.0 (2.2)	Postoperative: 48 (104) Total: 2.5 (2.6) Postoperative: 35 (74) Total: 60 (127)	Hb (g/dL) mean net reduction in Hb (admission to discharge): 4.2 (1.9) g/dL Hb (g/dL); mean net reduction in Hb (admission to discharge) 4.2 (1.7)
Lotke[31] (1999)	Orthopedic surgery (n = 127)	Patients undergoing primary total knee arthroplasty who were able to donate 2 U autologous blood preoperatively	Liberal: received their autologous blood immediately after surgery, the first unit in recovery room and the second unit delivered on return to the ward Restrictive: Received all autologous blood (PAD) if Hb level had fallen below 9.0 g/dL	—	Postoperative: 100 (65) Postoperative: 26 (16)	Mean postoperative Hb (g/dl): Day 1: 11.4 Day 3: 10.7 Mean postoperative Hb (g/dl): Day 1: 10.6 Day 3: 10.0

GI, Gastrointestinal; *Hb*, hemoglobin; *Hct*, hematocrit; *ICU*, intensive care unit; *PRBC*, packed red blood cell; *pt*, patient; *SD*, standard deviation.

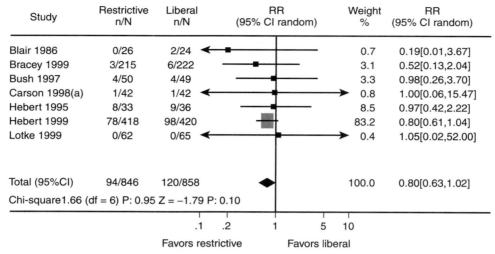

Figure 25-2. Meta-analysis of Transfusion Trials on All-Cause Mortality Rates. *From Carson JL et al:* Transfus Med Rev *2002;16:187-199; Hill SR et al:* Cochrane Database Syst Rev *2002(2);CD002042.*

Observational Studies Evaluating Transfusion in Adults

Many observational studies have evaluated the impact of transfusion on morbidity and mortality rates. However, in general, it is not possible to obtain unbiased assessment of blood transfusion in observational studies. The decision to transfuse a patient is often correlated with illness burden of the patient, and this may not be adequately adjusted for in these studies. This lack of complete adjustment for underlying disease and severity of illness might explain the variation in results of studies evaluating the impact of transfusion in patients with cardiovascular disease.[35-38]

Clinical Trials Evaluating Transfusion in Children

There have been three clinical trials evaluating transfusion triggers in children. The first trial evaluted 100 preterm infants weighing between 500 and 1300 grams.[39] The patients were randomly allocated to a restrictive or liberal transfusion algorithm that considered respiratory status and hematocrit. The restrictive group was transfused 2 fewer red blood cell units than the liberal group. None of the 15 endpoints were designated as the primary outcome. Overall, there were no differences in endpoints, with the exception that the restrictive group had more frequent apneic spells and neurologic events than the liberal group.

The second trial enrolled 451 infants with gestational age less than 31 weeks, age less than 2 days, and weight less than 1000 grams.[40] Similar to the first study, transfusion thresholds varied by amount of respiratory support. The composite primary endpoint was death, severe retinopathy, bronchopulmonary dysplasia, or brain injury. The primary outcome occurred with similar frequency in the two groups: restrictive group 74% and liberal group 69.7%.

The most recent trial recruited 637 children admitted to a pediatric intensive care unit and randomly allocated

to 7 g/dL or 9.5 g/dL thresholds.[41] Red blood cell transfusion was administered to 46% of patients in the restrictive group and 98% in the liberal group. The primary outcome (new or progressive multiorgan dysfunction) was nearly identical in both groups. Overall, the results of the three trials in children suggest that a restrictive transfusion trigger is safe[42] (Table 25-2).

AREAS OF UNCERTAINTY

There remains great uncertainty on the proper indications for red blood cell transfusion, especially in the perioperative period. The only adequately powered randomized trial was performed in ICU patients, and it is unclear if the results of that study should be applied to patients during the perioperative time period. The trials in surgical patients were underpowered or had important limitations in study design. There is some evidence that patients with underlying cardiovascular disease should be transfused at higher hemoglobin levels than patients without cardiovascular disease. However, no randomized clinical trials exist in surgical patients with underlying cardiovascular disease undergoing noncardiac surgery. The results from the ongoing FOCUS trial should inform this issue and be available in 2009.[29]

GUIDELINES

Before the late 1980s, the standard of care was to administer a perioperative transfusion whenever the hemoglobin level fell below 10 g/dL and the hematocrit level fell below 30% (the "10/30 rule"). In 1988, a National Institutes of Health consensus conference on perioperative red blood cell transfusions concluded that there was no evidence to support a single criterion.[43] Because of the paucity of clinical trials, older guidelines relied heavily on expert opinion, which, in general, emphasized the risks of transmission of serious viral illnesses such as HIV and hepatitis C.[44] The American Society of

Table 25-2   Results of the Randomized Controlled Trials in Children

Study (Year)	Setting N	Subjects: Eligibility and Comparability	Transfusion Strategy	Blood Usage Units/pt Mean (SD)	Proportion Transfused (%) (N)	Hb/Hct Levels Mean (SD)	Outcome
Bell[39] (2005)	100	Hospitalized preterm infants 500-1300 grams	Restrictive versus liberal transfusion based on respiratory status and hematocrit	Liberal 5.2 ($\pm$4.5) Restrictive 3.3 ($\pm$2.9)	Liberal 12% (6) Restrictive 10% (5)	Not reported	No difference in 15 outcomes including survival except restrictive group had more frequent apneic spells (0.84 versus 0.42 per day) and intraparenchymal brain hemorrhage, or periventricular leukomalacia (6 versus 0) versus the liberal group.
Kirpalani[40] (2006)	451	Birth weight <1000 grams, gestational age <31 weeks and <48 hours old	Restrictive versus liberal transfusion based on hemoglobin and amount of respiratory support	Liberal 5.7 (5.0) Restrictive 4.9 (4.2)	Liberal 95% Restrictive 89%	About 1 g/dL difference	Primary outcome death or any of severe retinopathy, bronchopulmonary dysplasia, or brain injury or cranial ultrasound. Liberal: 69.7%; restrictive: 74.0% (NS). None of secondary outcomes signficant.
Lacroix[41] (2007)	637	Stable critically ill children with hemoglobin <9.5 g/dL with 7 days of admission to ICU	Liberal 9.5 g/dL Restrictive 7 g/dL	Liberal 1.7 (2.2) Restrictive 0.9 (2.6)	Liberal 98% Restrictive 46%	2.1 g/dL difference	Primary outcome: new or progressive multiorgan dysfunction syndrome Liberal 12% Restrictive 12%

pt, Patient.

Anesthesiologists guidelines are the most rigorously published set of recommendations, and these were updated in 1996.[45] The American Society of Anesthesiologists Task Force advised against a "transfusion trigger," although it concluded that transfusion is rarely indicated when the hemoglobin level is greater than 10 g/dL and is almost always required when the hemoglobin level is below 6 g/dL. In patients with hemoglobin concentrations between 6 and 10 g/dL, transfusion decisions should be guided by risk of or actual bleeding, patient's volume status, cardiopulmonary reserve, and patient's risk of complications of inadequate oxygenation. Another guideline for perioperative blood transfusion and blood conservation in cardiac surgery emphasized use of multiple interventions to reduce blood loss and institution-specific blood transfusion algorithms.[45] These guidelines suggest that the decision to administer red blood cells should be based on a patient's risk for complications from inadequate oxygenation, and important physiologic and surgical factors. They also concluded that the indications for autologous transfusion may be more liberal than for allogeneic transfusion.

AUTHORS' RECOMMENDATIONS

There are no adequately powered clinical trials that examine different transfusion thresholds in the perioperative setting. Published clinical trials have focused on mortality rate but have not evaluated other important outcomes, such as myocardial infarction and functional recovery. Patients with underlying cardiac disease may be more vulnerable to the consequences of anemia. In the absence of good evidence, it is necessary to rely on clinical judgment. The only adequately powered randomized clinical trial found that it is safe to withhold blood until the hemoglobin level falls below 7 g/dL in ICU patients. Although it is uncertain if these results should be applied to surgical patients, our opinion is that in asymptomatic patients without cardiovascular disease, a transfusion trigger of 7 g/dL should be used. In preoperative patients, enough blood should be transfused to anticipate operative blood loss. In patients with cardiovascular disease, the optimal threshold is unknown. We currently favor using a higher transfusion threshold such as 9 to 10 g/dL. Patients with symptoms of anemia should be transfused as needed. Ultimately, careful clinical assessment with thoughtful consideration of risks and benefits should guide the transfusion decision, not a specific hemoglobin concentration. No set of guidelines will apply to every patient.

REFERENCES

1. Sullivan MT, Cotten R, Read EJ, Wallace EL: Blood collection and transfusion in the United States in 2001. *Transfusion* 2007;47: 385-394.
2. Friedman EA, Burns TL, Shork MA: *A study of national trends in transfusion practice.* Springfield, VA, National Technical Information Service, 1980.
3. Cook SS, Epps J: Transfusion practice in central Virginia. *Transfusion* 1991;31:355-360.
4. Lenfant C: Transfusion practice should be audited for both undertransfusion and overtransfusion [letter]. *Transfusion* 1992;32:873-874.
5. Eisenstaedt RS: Modifying physicians' transfusion practice. *Transfusion Medicine Reviews* 1997;11:27-37.
6. Dodd RY, Notari EP, Stramer SL: Current prevalence and incidence of infectious disease markers and estimated window-period risk in the American Red Cross blood donor population. *Transfusion* 2002;42:975-979.
7. Investigations of West Nile virus infections in recipients of blood transfusions. *MMWR Morb Mortal Wkly Rep* 2002;51: 973-974.
8. West Nile virus activity—United States, October 10-16, 2002, and update on West Nile virus infections in recipients of blood transfusions. *MMWR Morb Mortal Wkly Rep* 2002;51:929-931.
9. Llewelyn CA, Hewitt PE, Knight RS, et al: Possible transmission of variant Creutzfeldt-Jakob disease by blood transfusion. *Lancet* 2004;363:417-421.
10. Drohan WN, Cervenakova L: Safety of blood products: Are transmissible spongiform encephalopathies (prion diseases) a risk? *Thromb Haemost* 1999;82:486-493.
11. Food and Drug Administration: *Revised preventive measures to reduce the possible risk of transmission of Creutzfeldt-Jakob (CJD) disease and variant Creutzfeldt-Jakob disease (vCJD) by blood and blood products.* 2002. Available at http://www.fda.gov/cber/gdlns/cjducjdg&a.htm.
12. Klein HG: Will blood transfusion ever be safe enough? *JAMA* 2000;284:238-240.
13. Popovsky MA: Pulmonary consequences of transfusion: TRALI and TACO. *Transfus Apher Sci* 2006;34:243-244.
14. Vincent JL, Baron JF, Reinhart K, et al: Anemia and blood transfusion in critically ill patients. *JAMA* 2002;288:1499-1507.
15. Carson JL, Duff A, Poses RM, et al: Effect of anaemia and cardiovascular disease on surgical mortality and morbidity. *Lancet* 1996;348:1055-1060.
16. Carson JL, Noveck H, Berlin JA, Gould SA: Mortality and morbidity in patients with very low postoperative Hb levels who decline blood transfusion. *Transfusion* 2002;42:812-818.
17. Viele MK, Weiskopf RB: What can we learn about the need for transfusion from patients who refuse blood? The experience with Jehovah's Witnesses. *Transfusion* 1994;34:396-401.
18. Leung JM, Weiskopf RB, Feiner J, et al: Electrocardiographic ST-segment changes during acute, severe isovolemic hemodilution in humans. *Anesthesiology* 2000;93:1004-1010.
19. Weiskopf RB, Viele MK, Feiner J, et al: Human cardiovascular and metabolic response to acute, severe isovolemic anemia. *JAMA* 1998;279:217-221.
20. Toy P, Feiner J, Viele MK, et al: Fatigue during acute isovolemic anemia in healthy, resting humans. *Transfusion* 2000;40: 457-460.
21. Hebert PC, Wells G, Blajchman MA, et al: A multicenter, randomized, controlled clinical trial of transfusion requirements in critical care. Transfusion Requirements in Critical Care Investigators, Canadian Critical Care Trials Group [see comments]. *N Engl J Med* 1999;340:409-417.
22. Hebert PC, Wells G, Marshall J, et al: Transfusion requirements in critical care. A pilot study. Canadian Critical Care Trials Group. *JAMA* 1995;273:1439-1444 [erratum: *JAMA* 1995;274(12):944].
23. Hebert PC, Yetisir E, Martin C, et al: Is a low transfusion threshold safe in critically ill patients with cardiovascular diseases? *Crit Care Med* 2001;29:227-234.
24. Topley E, Fischer MR: The illness of trauma. *Br J Clin Pract* 1956;1:770-776.
25. Blair SD, Janvrin SB, McCollum CN, Greenhalgh RM: Effect of early blood transfusion on gastrointestinal haemorrhage. *Br J Surg* 1986;73:783-785.
26. Fortune JB, Feustel PJ, Saifi J, et al: Influence of hematocrit on cardiopulmonary function after acute hemorrhage. *J Trauma* 1987;27:243-249.
27. Johnson RG, Thurer RL, Kruskall MS, et al: Comparison of two transfusion strategies after elective operations for myocardial revascularization. *J Thorac Cardiovasc Surg* 1992;104:307-314.
28. Bush RL, Pevec WC, Holcroft JW: A prospective, randomized trial limiting perioperative red blood cell transfusions in vascular patients. *Am J Surg* 1997;174:143-148.
29. Carson JL, Terrin ML, Barton FB, et al: A pilot randomized trial comparing symptomatic vs. hemoglobin-level-driven red blood cell transfusions following hip fracture. *Transfusion* 1998;38: 522-529.
30. Bracey AW, Radovancevic R, Riggs SA, et al: Lowering the hemoglobin threshold for transfusion in coronary artery bypass procedures: Effect on patient outcome. *Transfusion* 1999;39: 1070-1077.
31. Lotke PA, Barth P, Garino JP, Cook EF: Predonated autologous blood transfusions after total knee arthroplasty: Immediate versus delayed administration. *J Arthroplasty* 1999;14:647-650.
32. Carson JL, Hill S, Carless P, et al. Transfusion triggers: A systematic review of the literature. *Transfus Med Rev* 2002;16: 187-199.
33. Hill SR, Carless PA, Henry DA, et al: Transfusion thresholds and other strategies for guiding allogeneic red blood cell transfusion. *Cochrane Database Syst Rev* 2002;CD002042.
34. Carson JL, Terrin ML, Jay M: Anemia and postoperative rehabilitation. *Can J Anesth* 2003;50:S60-S64.
35. Carson JL, Duff A, Berlin JA, et al: Perioperative blood transfusion and postoperative mortality. *JAMA* 1998;279:199-205.
36. Wu WC, Rathore SS, Wang Y, et al: Blood transfusion in elderly patients with acute myocardial infarction. *N Engl J Med* 2001;345:1230-1236.
37. Rao SV, Jollis JG, Harrington RA, et al: Relationship of blood transfusion and clinical outcomes in patients with acute coronary syndromes. *JAMA* 2004;292:1555-1562.
38. Sabatine MS, Morrow DA, Giugliano RP, et al: Association of hemoglobin levels with clinical outcomes in acute coronary syndromes. *Circulation* 2005;111:2042-2049.
39. Bell EF, Strauss RG, Widness JA, et al: Randomized trial of liberal versus restrictive guidelines for red blood cell transfusion in preterm infants. *Pediatrics* 2005;115:1685-1691.
40. Kirpalani H, Whyte RK, Andersen C, et al: The Premature Infants in Need of Transfusion (PINT) study: A randomized, controlled trial of a restrictive (low) versus liberal (high) transfusion threshold for extremely low birth weight infants. *J Pediatr* 2006;149: 301-307.
41. Lacroix J, Hebert PC, Hutchison JS, et al: Transfusion strategies for patients in pediatric intensive care units. *N Engl J Med* 2007;356:1609-1619.
42. Corwin HL, Carson JL: Blood transfusion—when is more really less? *N Engl J Med* 2007;356:1667-1669.
43. Consensus Conference: Perioperative red blood cell transfusion. *JAMA* 1988;260:2700-2703.
44. Hebert PC, Schweitzer I, Calder L, et al: Review of the clinical practice literature on allogeneic red blood cell transfusion. *Can Med Assoc J* 1997;156:S9-S26.
45. American Society of Anesthesiologists Task Force on Blood Component Therapy: Practice guidelines for blood component therapy. *Anesthesiology* 1996;84:732-747.

26 When Are Platelet/Plasma Transfusions Indicated?

Gregory A. Nuttall, MD

INTRODUCTION/BACKGROUND

A large percentage of platelet concentrates and plasma transfusions are given to surgical patients in the operating room and the intensive care unit to treat or prevent bleeding, especially to cardiac surgery and liver transplant patients.[1,2] As a result of the aging of the population in the United States, demand for blood and blood components will rise and supply will decrease.[3,4] Therefore shortages of blood and blood components will become more common. The increased use of antiplatelet agents and potentially oral antithrombin agents[5] will further aggravate the demand for platelet and plasma to rapidly reverse these agents for surgery. As a result, appropriate use of platelet and plasma transfusions will become even more important in the future to preserve an increasingly scarce resource. Further, platelet and plasma transfusions can result in some well-known adverse effects such as bacterial contamination, venous thromboembolism, allergic reactions, transfusion-related acute lung injury, and transfusion-related circulatory overload.

To better understand when platelet concentrates and plasma are indicated, we need to understand what they are and how they affect the coagulation system. Transfusion of platelet concentrates was first demonstrated to reduce mortality rate from bleeding in acute leukemia patients in the 1950s.[6,7] Use of platelet concentrates has steadily grown since that time. Platelet concentrates are generally produced in two ways, either from whole blood by differential centrifugation (whole blood–derived platelet concentrates) or by plateletpheresis (apheresis-derived platelet concentrates). Each unit of whole blood–derived platelet concentrates contains approximately 5×10^8 platelets in 50 to 70 mL of plasma. Generally between 5 and 10 units of buffy coat–derived platelet concentrates may be pooled together in a single component bag. For each unit of apheresis-derived platelet concentrate, a single donor donates the equivalent of 3 to 5×10^9 or 4 to 6 units of platelets suspended in a volume of 200 to 400 mL of plasma. One unit of apheresis-derived platelet concentrate or a pool of 4 to 6 buffy coat–derived platelet concentrates increases the platelet count by approximately 30 to 50×10^{10}/L in the average adult. In the 1970s and 1980s, the use of whole blood–derived platelet concentrates greatly exceeded that of apheresis-derived platelet concentrates. Since the beginning of the 1990s, apheresis-derived platelet concentrates have made up more than half of all transfused platelets.[8]

The use of plasma in the United States has steadily increased every year.[9] Why the use of plasma has continued to rise is not known. An audit of transfusion requests at Massachusetts General Hospital in Boston found that the most frequent reason to request plasma outside of the operating room was "Before procedure with elevated INR."[10] There has been a large increase in the number of bedside invasive procedures and the practice of transfusing plasma before procedures in patients with abnormal coagulation test results.[9,11] Plasma is derived by the removal of red blood cells from the whole blood by differential centrifugation; the remaining platelet-rich plasma is then further centrifuged to separate the platelets from the plasma. The remaining plasma contains all the blood coagulation factors, fibrinogen, antithrombin, and other plasma proteins in a volume of 170 to 250 mL.[12] The plasma is then frozen within 8 hours of donation to prevent complete inactivation of temperature-sensitive ("labile") coagulation factors V and VIII, which is then called fresh frozen plasma (FFP). If the FFP is stored at temperatures colder than $-18°C$, the FFP can be stored for up to 1 year with minimal loss of coagulant activity. Plasma may also be obtained by plasmapheresis. Before administration, FFP must be thawed in a water bath at $37°C$, which takes approximately 30 minutes. Since bleeding and prolongation of coagulation tests occur when the coagulation factor concentrations are less than 30% of normal,[13,14] FFP should be administered in a dose calculated to achieve this level as a minimum. The volume of FFP that will increase coagulation proteins by 25% to 30% in most patients is 10 to 15 mL/kg. A smaller dose of 5 to 8 mL/kg may be adequate to urgently reverse warfarin anticoagulation, though this may vary based on the initial levels of the vitamin K–dependent coagulation factors.[15]

PATHOPHYSIOLOGY/MECHANISM OF ACTION

Platelets are administered to correct a deficiency in either platelet number (thrombocytopenia) or platelet function (thrombocytopathy or qualitative platelet disorders). Thrombocytopenia can result from massive transfusion.

When crystalloid, colloid, or red blood cells are used to replace lost volume in a severely bleeding patient, coagulation defects develop not only from dilution of platelets but also coagulation factors.[16] Coagulopathy associated with massive transfusion and other clinical situations is characterized by the presence of microvascular bleeding or oozing from the wound and puncture sites. It is for this reason that visual assessment of the surgical field is standard practice in the determination of the need for platelet or plasma transfusions. Impaired platelet function can result from multiple disease states and special surgical techniques such as cardiopulmonary bypass (CPB). Further, multiple drugs have been developed that impair different aspects of platelet function. Aspirin and the thienopyridines are oral antiplatelet agents that interfere with platelet activation in complementary, but different, pathways. The thienopyridines (ticlopidine, clopidogrel) are thought to induce irreversible alteration of the platelet receptor P2Y12 that mediates the inhibition of stimulated adenylyl cyclase activity by adenosine diphosphate (ADP), resulting in platelet function inhibition.[17] Combination therapy of aspirin with other antiplatelet agents has demonstrated a benefit for the management of acute coronary syndrome (ACS). Another class of drugs that have been very beneficial for the management of ACS is the platelet GP IIb/IIIa inhibitors (abciximab, eptifibatide, and tirofiban), which are used routinely to prevent recurrent ischemic events after percutaneous coronary revascularization with or without stent placement.[18] GP IIb/IIIa is the platelet receptor for fibrinogen that mediates platelet aggregation. GP IIb/IIIa receptor blockade prevents the binding of fibrinogen and thus clot formation since the platelets cannot aggregate together.

As noted previously, 1 unit of apheresis-derived platelet concentrate or a pool of 4 to 6 buffy coat–derived platelet concentrates will increase the platelet count by about 30 to 50 $\times$ 10^9/L in the average adult. How active are the platelets that are administered? In patients with chemotherapy-induced thrombocytopenia, platelet transfusion causes an immediate increase in platelet count number and platelet function as measured by agonist-induced whole blood impedance aggregometry and dense granule release of adenosine triphosphate, which is independent of storage time.[19] Clopidogrel administration before cardiac surgery with CPB is associated with increased bleeding and transfusion requirements.[20] In an ex vivo model, administration of platelet transfusions normalized platelet function as measured by platelet-rich plasma aggregometry in volunteers who have ingested clopidogrel and aspirin.[21]

The majority of plasma units are given either prophylactically to prevent bleeding or to manage active microvascular bleeding. Plasma is transfused to correct congenital and acquired deficiencies in coagulation factors in the surgical and nonsurgical patient. Deficiencies in coagulation factors are frequently diagnosed by a prolongation of either the activated partial thromboplastin time (aPTT) or prothrombin time (PT) or a coagulation factor assay of less than 25%.[12] Warfarin is a common anticoagulant that inhibits the vitamin K–dependent gamma-carboxylation of coagulation factors II, VII, IX, and X such that there is the synthesis of immunologically detectable but biologically inactive forms of these coagulation proteins. Since this results in inhibition of the extrinsic pathway, there is a prolongation of the PT and the international normalization ratio (INR). The level of factors II, VII, IX, and X will influence both the PT and aPTT when sufficiently low. The PT prolongs first because of the short half-life of factor VII. It also corrects first because of the short half-life of factor VII. The aPTT is vitally important in evaluating adequacy of hemostasis and is too often overlooked. In emergent situations, plasma transfusions have been used to reverse the effect of warfarin before surgery or during active bleeding episodes.

EVIDENCE

Historically, platelet transfusions were given to patients undergoing chemotherapy for hematologic malignancies or to patients with aplastic anemia with platelets being administered prophylactically when a patient's platelet count fell below 20 $\times$ 10^9/L.[22] In 1991, Gmur and colleagues[23] recorded evidence of only three fatal hemorrhages in their 10-year transfusion study in 103 leukemic patients, suggesting that the traditional transfusion trigger of 20 $\times$ 10^9/L platelets could be safely decreased to 10 $\times$ 10^9/L in stable patients with cancer or blood disorders. Several other prospective and retrospective studies have subsequently confirmed these findings, and this value is now widely adopted in clinical practice.[24–29]

Platelets are also used in treating patients with accelerated platelet destruction or decreased production, platelet dysfunction, and for various surgical indications as noted previously. The literature supporting these indications is listed in Table 26-1. There are no prospective randomized trials for these indications.

It should be noted that platelet transfusion should be avoided if at all possible in thrombotic thrombocytopenic purpura–hemolytic uremic syndrome. In this setting, platelet transfusion can lead to new or worsening neurologic symptoms and to acute renal failure, presumably because of new or expanding thrombi as the infused platelets are consumed.[30,31] There are similar considerations in the situation of heparin-induced thrombocytopenia.

The indications for plasma transfusion are for correction of bleeding caused by excess warfarin, vitamin K deficiency, deficiency of multiple coagulation factors, or treatment of thrombotic thrombocytopenic purpura–hemolytic uremic syndrome. Deficiency of multiple coagulation factors can result from disseminated intravascular coagulation, liver disease or failure, or dilutional coagulopathy caused by massive bleeding without hemostatic factor replacement. The literature supporting these indications is listed in Table 26-2. There are no prospective randomized trials for these indications.

Since a large percentage of allogeneic blood is transfused in the operating room, especially to cardiac surgery and liver transplant patients,[1,2,32] coagulation

Table 26-1	Evidence for Platelet Transfusion, Both Indications and Contraindications	
Indication	**Clinical Use**	**Evidence**
Platelet transfusion indicated	To prevent spontaneous bleeding in severe thrombocytopenia ($\leq 10 \times 10^9$/L)	Evidence based in oncology patients only[23-29]
	Active bleeding with thrombocytopenia ($<50 \times 10^9$/L)	No formal studies; expert opinion and experience
	To prevent bleeding before invasive procedure with thrombocytopenia ($<50 \times 10^9$/L)	No formal studies; expert opinion and experience
	Bleeding with known or suspected platelet dysfunction	No formal studies; expert opinion and experience
Platelet transfusion contraindicated	Thrombotic thrombocytopenic purpura and heparin-induced thrombocytopenia	Evidence based[30,31]
	Lumbar puncture in children with platelet count $>10 \times 10^9$/L	Evidence based in oncology patients only[49]

Table 26-2	Evidence for Plasma Transfusion, Both Indications and Contraindications	
Indication	**Clinical Use**	**Evidence**
Plasma transfusion indicated	Active bleeding with multiple coagulation factor deficiencies	No formal studies; expert opinion and experience
	To prevent bleeding before invasive procedure with multiple coagulation factor deficiencies	Not evidence based
	Rapid reversal of warfarin	One formal study,[50] expert opinion, and experience
Plasma transfusion contraindicated	To prevent spontaneous bleeding with multiple coagulation factor deficiencies	No benefit in severe liver disease[51-55] and cardiac surgery[56-60]
	Multiple red blood cell transfusions without evidence of coagulopathy	Not evidence based
	Volume replacement	Not evidence based

test–based transfusion algorithm studies have been performed in this population. Six prospective randomized trials have compared the use of transfusion algorithms versus clinical judgment for administration of non–red blood cell components in cardiac surgery.[33-38] Though each study used different algorithms with different coagulation tests, five of the six studies demonstrated reduction of allogeneic blood exposure with the use of a transfusion algorithm. Two of the studies demonstrated a reduction of blood loss in the intensive care unit in addition to reduced allogeneic blood exposure.[33,35]

Aside from the platelet count (greater than 10×10^9/L) needed to prevent spontaneous bleeding in severe thrombocytopenia in oncology patients, there are no prospective randomized trials for the indications for transfusion of platelets and plasma. The majority of guidelines are based on expert opinion and clinical experience.

CONTROVERSIES

In a patient who is massively transfused, clinical bleeding from coagulation factor deficiencies is unlikely until factor levels fall below 30% of normal. Based on studies performed in the trauma and cardiac surgical settings, this usually does not occur until greater than one blood volume has been replaced and the PT and aPTT are greater than 1.5 to 1.8 times control values.[14,39-41] Recently, several studies have suggested that a rise in the PT may be a "late" marker in a trauma patient with massive bleeding that the patient is developing a severe dilutional coagulopathy resulting from inadequate replacement of coagulation factors.[42-44] These studies suggest that plasma should be given much sooner to massively bleeding trauma patients to avoid potential dilutional coagulopathy despite a normal PT value.

Plasma is frequently given to patients with an abnormal INR or aPTT before an invasive procedure to prevent bleeding from the procedure.[9] This transfusion behavior rests on two assumptions. The first assumption is that abnormal coagulation test results identify patients at increased risk of procedure-related bleeding. The second assumption is that transfusion of plasma will reduce the risk of procedure-related bleeding. Recent literature documents that mild to moderate abnormalities of the INR and the aPTT do not predict which patients will have procedure-related bleeding, and therefore these tests should not be used to make decisions about prophylactic preprocedure plasma transfusions.[45] The procedures that have been studied include central line placement, thoracentesis, paracentesis, organ biopsies, angiography, and lumbar puncture. The second assumption of preprocedure plasma transfusion is that the infusing plasma will correct the coagulopathy documented by the abnormal coagulation test. For mild to moderate prolongation of the INR, there is very little evidence to support this assumption. In one study, 179 patients with prolonged INR results were given FFP for a variety of indications. The effect of the FFP transfusions on the INR was determined.[46] The decrease in INR with plasma transfusion reached zero or no effect when the pretransfusion INR was 1·7 or less. For patients with INR values greater than 2, the correction of INR was modest and incomplete. These results were supported by another study in which 121 adult patients with a pretransfusion INR of 1·6 or less were given 1 to 4 units of FFP; the posttransfusion INR corrected to within the normal range in only two patients.[47] It should be noted that in both of these studies the doses or volume of FFP transfused may have been inadequate to replace coagulation factor levels above 30% of normal.

GUIDELINES

There have been multiple consensus conferences and specialty society task forces convened to publish recommendations for the transfusion of different blood components. These include those by the National Institutes of Health, the American College of Obstetricians and Gynecologists, the American Association of Blood Banks, the American College of Physicians, the College of American Pathologists, and the American Society of Anesthesiologists. The most recent published recommendations for the transfusion of different blood components are the practice guidelines for blood component therapy reported by the "American Society of Anesthesiologists practice guidelines for perioperative blood transfusion and adjuvant therapies," and Society of Thoracic Surgeons Blood Conservation Guideline Task Force published in 2006 and 2007.[15,48] In the "ASA Practice guidelines for perioperative blood transfusion and adjuvant therapies,"[15] the task force recommended that "a visual assessment of the surgical field should be jointly conducted by the anesthesiologist and surgeon to determine whether excessive microvascular bleeding (i.e., coagulopathy) is occurring." The Society of Thoracic Surgeons Blood Conservation Guideline Task Force has recommended that transfusion of hemostatic allogeneic blood products after cardiac

surgery should be based on the existence of microvascular bleeding and laboratory parameters that are measured as part of a transfusion algorithm.[48] Clinical and physiologic parameters should also be used for transfusion decisions.

AUTHOR'S RECOMMENDATIONS

- Transfusion of platelets can increase the platelet count and improve platelet function test results when there is platelet dysfunction caused by drugs, disease, or CPB. Transfusion of plasma can result in improved coagulation factor levels and improved coagulation test results if sufficient plasma is given.
- In surgical patients, a visual assessment of the surgical field should be conducted to determine whether excessive microvascular bleeding indicating a coagulopathy is occurring.
- Transfusion of platelets and plasma should ideally be guided by coagulation test results.
- The consequence of bleeding such as bleeding into a confined space (e.g., brain, spinal cord or eye) needs to be included in the decision to transfuse platelets and plasma.
- Prophylactic platelet transfusions are indicated in patients undergoing chemotherapy for hematologic malignancies or to patients with aplastic anemia when a patient's platelet count falls below 10×10^9/L.
- In surgical or obstetric patients with normal platelet function, platelet transfusion is rarely indicated if the platelet count is greater than 100×10^9/L; the presence of excessive bleeding is indicated when the count is below 50×10^9/L.
- Transfusion of platelets is indicated if there is microvascular bleeding and known or suspected platelet dysfunction.
- Transfusion of plasma is not indicated if PT, INR, and aPTT are normal or solely for augmentation of plasma volume or albumin concentration.
- Transfusion of plasma is indicated to correct microvascular bleeding in the presence of a PT greater than 1.5 times normal or an INR greater than 1.8, or an aPTT greater than 1.8 times normal; correct microvascular bleeding secondary to coagulation factor deficiency in patients who are massively transfused, such as more than one blood volume (approximately 70 mL/kg); and urgently reverse warfarin therapy.

REFERENCES

1. Goodnough LT, Johnston MF, Toy PT: The variability of transfusion practice in coronary artery bypass surgery. *JAMA* 1991;265:86-90.
2. Stover EP, Siegel LC, Parks R, Levin J, Body SC, Maddi R, et al: Variability in transfusion practice for coronary artery bypass surgery persists despite national consensus guidelines: A 24-institution study. Institutions of the Multicenter Study of Perioperative Ischemia Research Group. *Anesthesiology* 1998;88: 327-333.
3. Simon T: Where have all the donors gone? A personal reflection on the crisis in American volunteer blood program. *Transfusion* 2003;43:273-278.
4. Vamvakas EC, Taswell HF: Epidemiology of blood transfusion. *Transfusion* 1994;34:464-470.
5. Desai SS, Massad MG, DiDomenico RJ, Abdelhady K, Hanhan Z, Lele H, et al: Recent developments in antithrombotic therapy: Will sodium warfarin be a drug of the past? *Recent Patents Cardiovasc Drug Discov* 2006;1:307-316.
6. Hersh EM, Bodey GP, Nies BA, Freireich EJ: Causes of death in acute leukemia: A ten-year study of 414 patients from 1954–1963. *JAMA* 1965;193:105-109.

7. Freireich EJ: Supportive care for patients with blood disorders. *Br J Haematol* 2000;111:68-77.

8. Bock M, Rahrig S, Kunz D, Lutze G, Heim MU: Platelet concentrates derived from buffy coat and apheresis: Biochemical and functional differences. *Transfus Med* 2002;12:317-324.

9. Dzik WH: The James Blundell Award Lecture 2006: Transfusion and the treatment of haemorrhage: Past, present and future. *Transfus Med* 2007;17:367-374.

10. Dzik W, Rao A: Why do physicians request fresh frozen plasma? *Transfusion* 2004;44:1393-1394.

11. Dzik WH: Predicting hemorrhage using preoperative coagulation screening assays. *Curr Hematol Rep* 2004;3:324-330.

12. Miller R: *Transfusion therapy*, ed 5. Philadelphia, Churchill Livingstone, 2000.

13. Reiss R: Hemostatic defects in massive transfusion: Rapid diagnosis and management. *Am J Crit Care* 2000;9:158-165.

14. Despotis GJ, Santoro SA, Spintznagel E, Kater KM, Barnes P, Cox JL, Lappas DG: On-site prothombin time, activated partial thromboplastin time, and platelet count. A comparison between whole blood and laboratory assays with coagulation factor analysis in patients presenting for cardiac surgery. *Anesthesiology* 1994;80:338-351.

15. Practice guidelines for perioperative blood transfusion and adjuvant therapies: An updated report by the American Society of Anesthesiologists Task Force on Perioperative Blood Transfusion and Adjuvant Therapies. *Anesthesiology* 2006;105:198-208.

16. Hardy JF, de Moerloose P, Samama CM: Massive transfusion and coagulopathy: Pathophysiology and implications for clinical management. *Can J Anaesth* 2006;53:S40-S58.

17. Antithrombotic Trialists' Collaboration: Collaborative meta-analysis of randomised trials of antiplatelet therapy for prevention of death, myocardial infarction, and stroke in high risk patients. *BMJ* 2002;324:71-86.

18. Singh S, Gopal A, Bahl V: Glycoprotein IIb/IIIa receptor antagonists: Are we ignoring the evidence? *Indian Heart J* 2005;57:201-209.

19. Rosenfeld BA, Herfel B, Faraday N, Fuller A, Braine H: Effects of storage time on quantitative and qualitative platelet function after transfusion. *Anesthesiology* 1995;83:1167-1172.

20. Tanaka K, Szlam F, Kelly A, Vega J, Levy J: Clopidogrel (Plavix) and cardiac surgical patients: Implications for platelet function monitoring and postoperative bleeding. *Platelets* 2004;15:325-332.

21. Vilahur G, Choi BG, Zafar MU, Viles-Gonzalez JF, Vorchheimer DA, Fuster V, Badimon JJ: Normalization of platelet reactivity in clopidogrel-treated subjects. *J Thromb Haemost* 2007;5:82-90.

22. Stroncek DF, Rebulla P: Platelet transfusions. *Lancet* 2007;370:427-438.

23. Gmur J, Burger J, Schanz U, Fehr J, Schaffner A: Safety of stringent prophylactic platelet transfusion policy for patients with acute leukaemia. *Lancet* 1991;338:1223-1226.

24. Gil-Fernandez JJ, Alegre A, Fernandez-Villalta MJ, Pinilla I, Gomez Garcia V, Martinez C, et al: Clinical results of a stringent policy on prophylactic platelet transfusion: Non-randomized comparative analysis in 190 bone marrow transplant patients from a single institution. *Bone Marrow Transplant* 1996;18:931-935.

25. Heckman KD, Weiner GJ, Davis CS, Strauss RG, Jones MP, Burns CP: Randomized study of prophylactic platelet transfusion threshold during induction therapy for adult acute leukemia: 10,000/microL versus 20,000/microL. *J Clin Oncol* 1997;15:1143-1149.

26. Rebulla P, Finazzi G, Marangoni F, Avvisati G, Gugliotta L, Tognoni G, et al: The threshold for prophylactic platelet transfusions in adults with acute myeloid leukemia. Gruppo Italiano Malattie Ematologiche Maligne dell'Adulto. *N Engl J Med* 1997;337:1870-1875.

27. Lawrence JB, Yomtovian RA, Hammons T, Masarik SR, Chongkolwatana V, Creger RJ, et al: Lowering the prophylactic platelet transfusion threshold: A prospective analysis. *Leuk Lymphoma* 2001;41:67-76.

28. Strauss RG: Pretransfusion trigger platelet counts and dose for prophylactic platelet transfusions. *Curr Opin Hematol* 2005;12:499-502.

29. Wandt H, Frank M, Ehninger G, Schneider C, Brack N, Daoud A, et al: Safety and cost effectiveness of a $10 \times 10(9)/L$ trigger for prophylactic platelet transfusions compared with the traditional $20 \times 10(9)/L$ trigger: A prospective comparative trial in 105 patients with acute myeloid leukemia. *Blood* 1998;91:3601-3606.

30. Harkness DR, Byrnes JJ, Lian EC, Williams WD, Hensley GT: Hazard of platelet transfusion in thrombotic thrombocytopenic purpura. *JAMA* 1981;246:1931-1933.

31. Lind SE: Thrombocytopenic purpura and platelet transfusion. *Ann Intern Med* 1987;106:478.

32. Goodnough LT, Soegiarso RW, Birkmeyer JD, Welch HG: Economic impact of inappropriate blood transfusion in coronary artery bypass graft surgery. *Am J Med* 1993;94:509-514.

33. Despotis GJ, Grishaber JE, Goodnough LT: The effect of an intraoperative treatment algorithm on physicians' transfusion practice in cardiac surgery. *Transfusion* 1994;34:290-296.

34. Shore-Lesserson L, Manspeizer H, DePerio M, Francis S, Vela-Cantos F, Ergin M: Thromboelastography-guided transfusion algorithm reduces transfusions in complex cardiac surgery. *Anesth Analg* 1999;88:312-319.

35. Nuttall GA, Oliver WC, Santrach PJ, Bryant S, Dearani JA, Schaff HV, Ereth MH: Efficacy of a simple intraoperative transfusion algorithm for nonerythrocyte component utilization after cardiopulmonary bypass. *Anesthesiology* 2001;94:773-781.

36. Capraro L, Kuitunen A, Salmenpera M, Kekomaki R: On-site coagulation monitoring does not affect hemostatic outcome after cardiac surgery. *Acta Anaesthesiol Scand* 2001;45:200-206.

37. Royston D, von Kier S: Reduced haemostatic factor transfusion using heparinase-modified thrombelastography during cardiopulmonary bypass. *Br J Anaesth* 2001;86:575-578.

38. Avidan M, Alcock E, Da Fonseca J, Ponte J, Desai J, Despotis G, Hunt B: Comparison of structured use of routine laboratory tests or near-patient assessment with clinical judgement in the management of bleeding after cardiac surgery. *Br J Anaesth* 2004;92:178-186.

39. Murray D, Pennel B, Weinstein S, Olson J: Packed red cells in acute blood loss: Dilutional coagulopathy as a cause of surgical bleeding. *Anesth Analg* 1995;80:336-342.

40. Murray D, Olson J, Strauss R, Tinker J: Coagulation changes during packed red cell replacement of major blood loss. *Anesthesiology* 1988;69:839-845.

41. Ciavarella D, Reed R, Counts R, Baron L, Pavlin E, Heimbach D, Carrico C: Clotting factor levels and the risk of diffuse microvascular bleeding in the massively transfused patient. *Br J Haematol* 1987;67:365-368.

42. Hirshberg A, Dugas M, Banez EI, Scott BG, Wall MJ Jr, Mattox KL: Minimizing dilutional coagulopathy in exsanguinating hemorrhage: A computer simulation. *J Trauma* 2003;54:454-463.

43. Gonzalez EA, Moore FA, Holcomb JB, Miller CC, Kozar RA, Todd SR, et al: Fresh frozen plasma should be given earlier to patients requiring massive transfusion. *J Trauma* 2007;62:112-119.

44. Ho AM, Dion PW, Cheng CA, Karmakar MK, Cheng G, Peng Z, Ng YW: A mathematical model for fresh frozen plasma transfusion strategies during major trauma resuscitation with ongoing hemorrhage. *Can J Surg* 2005;48:470-478.

45. Segal JB, Dzik WH: Paucity of studies to support that abnormal coagulation test results predict bleeding in the setting of invasive procedures: An evidence-based review. *Transfusion* 2005;45:1413-1425.

46. Holland LL, Brooks JP: Toward rational fresh frozen plasma transfusion: The effect of plasma transfusion on coagulation test results. *Am J Clin Pathol* 2006;126:133-139.

47. Abdel-Wahab OI, Healy B, Dzik WH: Effect of fresh-frozen plasma transfusion on prothrombin time and bleeding in patients with mild coagulation abnormalities. *Transfusion* 2006;46:1279-1285.

48. Ferraris V, Ferraris S, Saha S, Hessel E, Haan C, Royston B, et al: Society of Thoracic Surgeons Blood Conservation Guideline Task Force and Society of Cardiovascular Anesthesiologists Special Task Force on Blood Transfusion. Perioperative blood transfusion and blood conservation in cardiac surgery: The Society of Thoracic Surgeons and the Society of Cardiovascular Anesthesiologists clinical practice guideline. *Ann Thorac Surg* 2007;83 (5 suppl):S27-S86.

49. Howard SC, Gajjar A, Ribeiro RC, Rivera GK, Rubnitz JE, Sandlund JT, et al: Safety of lumbar puncture for children with

acute lymphoblastic leukemia and thrombocytopenia. *JAMA* 2000;284:2222-2224.

50. Boulis NM, Bobek MP, Schmaier A, Hoff JT: Use of factor IX complex in warfarin-related intracranial hemorrhage. *Neurosurgery* 1999;45:1113-1118, discussion 1118-1119.

51. Beck KH, Mortelsmans Y, Kretschmer VV, Holtermann W, Lukasewitz P: Comparison of solvent/detergent-inactivated plasma and fresh frozen plasma under routine clinical conditions. *Infusionsther Transfusionsmed* 2000;27:144-148.

52. Lerner RG, Nelson J, Sorcia E, Grima K, Kancherla RR, Zarou-Naimo CM, Pehta JC: Evaluation of solvent/detergent-treated plasma in patients with a prolonged prothrombin time. *Vox Sang* 2000;79:161-167.

53. Williamson LM, Llewelyn CA, Fisher NC, Allain JP, Bellamy MC, Baglin TP, et al: A randomized trial of solvent/detergent-treated and standard fresh-frozen plasma in the coagulopathy of liver disease and liver transplantation. *Transfusion* 1999;39:1227-1234.

54. Mannucci PM, Franchi F, Dioguardi N: Correction of abnormal coagulation in chronic liver disease by combined use of fresh-frozen plasma and prothrombin complex concentrates. *Lancet* 1976;2:542-545.

55. Gazzard BG, Henderson JM, Williams R: Early changes in coagulation following a paracetamol overdose and a controlled trial of fresh frozen plasma therapy. *Gut* 1975;16:617-620.

56. Kasper SM, Giesecke T, Limpers P, Sabatowski R, Mehlhorn U, Diefenbach C: Failure of autologous fresh frozen plasma to reduce blood loss and transfusion requirements in coronary artery bypass surgery. *Anesthesiology* 2001;95:81-86, discussion 6A.

57. Wilhelmi M, Franke U, Cohnert T, Weber P, Kaukemuller J, Fischer S, et al: Coronary artery bypass grafting surgery without the routine application of blood products: Is it feasible? *Eur J Cardiothorac Surg* 2001;19:657-661.

58. Oliver WC Jr, Beynen FM, Nuttall GA, Schroeder DR, Ereth MH, Dearani JA, Puga FJ: Blood loss in infants and children for open heart operations: Albumin 5% versus fresh-frozen plasma in the prime. *Ann Thorac Surg* 2003;75:1506-1512.

59. Trimble AS, Osborn JJ, Kerth WJ, Gerbode F: The prophylactic use of fresh frozen plasma after extracorporeal circulation. *J Thorac Cardiovasc Surg* 1964;48:314-316.

60. Menges T, Rupp D, van Lessen A, Hempelmann G: Measures for reducing the use of homologous blood. Effects on blood coagulation during total endoprosthesis. *Anaesthesist* 1992;41:27-33.

27 What Drugs Decrease Postoperative Bleeding?

Veena Guru, MD, and Stephen E. Fremes, MD

INTRODUCTION

The risks associated with transfusion of blood products, especially in the setting of intractable surgical bleeding, are measurable, and this has led to a search for therapies to reduce postoperative blood loss. A number of clinical trials have been completed in the field of cardiac surgery to reduce postoperative bleeding analyzing outcomes such as the amount of blood loss, rates of transfusion, and rates of reoperation for bleeding. In the case of cardiac surgery, reexploration for bleeding has correlated with increased surgical mortality rate up to threefold, as well as other significant complications.[1] Fortunately, with the advent of comprehensive screening processes, blood transfusion risks have been reduced. The risks associated with blood transfusion include the transmission of human immunodeficiency virus (HIV) (2 cases/million units transfused), hepatitis C virus (10 cases/million units transfused), and hepatitis B virus (16 cases/million units transfused).[2] Other complications associated with blood product usage involve incorrect labeling, contamination, and overtransfusion. Noninfectious complications such as transfusion reactions are more common and are proportional to the number of units to which a patient is exposed.[3] The complications with massive transfusion can be lethal and include transfusion-related lung injury in which patients develop an acute respiratory distress syndrome.[4,5] The cost of blood products is also significant, with an average cost of $250 per unit of blood.[6] Patients with specific religious beliefs (e.g., Jehovah's Witnesses) or patient preferences may preclude the use of blood products. Many strategies are employed to try to reduce the use of blood products for patients undergoing surgical procedures with an expected significant blood loss. Many of the trials have focused on reducing transfusion rates rather than accurately measuring the total amount of blood loss. There are also challenges in accurately estimating blood loss both intraoperatively and postoperatively. The randomized trials discussed here involve pharmacologic strategies to reduce postoperative blood loss and avoid transfusion.

OVERVIEW OF NONDRUG OPTIONS TO AVOID POSTOPERATIVE BLOOD PRODUCT TRANSFUSION

Preoperative management of antithrombotic medications can help reduce the rate of postoperative blood product transfusion. Antiplatelet agents such as aspirin and clopidogrel can increase intraoperative blood loss and, if clinical risks associated with discontinuation are low, should be discontinued approximately 1 week before surgery (i.e., their effect lasts for the duration of a platelet life: 7 to 10 days). Nonsteroidal antiinflammatory drugs can also cause platelet dysfunction; however, because their action is reversible they may be continued until 1 day before surgery. Warfarin should be discontinued 3 to 5 days before surgery if clinical risks with a normal international normalization ratio (INR) are high and should be replaced with therapeutic anticoagulation either with unfractionated or fractionated heparin.

Intraoperative techniques, including mode of surgery (i.e., off-pump coronary artery bypass surgery versus on-pump coronary artery bypass surgery), and the systematic attention to hemostasis can significantly influence the rates of postoperative blood product usage. For example, the use of fibrin sealant as a hemostatic intraoperative adjunct has been shown to be effective in helping to reduce postoperative blood loss and transfusion with a meta-analysis showing a relative risk ratio of 0.4 (95% confidence interval [CI] 0.26 to 0.61).[7] The maintenance of intraoperative normothermia can prevent blood loss, as studies have shown even mild hypothermia (less than 1°C) increases the relative risk for transfusion by 22% (3% to 37%).[8]

A meta-analysis demonstrated that the intraoperative use of cell salvage (collection and transfusion of blood that has been lost in the operative field) reduced the rate of exposure to allogeneic red blood cell transfusion by a relative risk (RR) of 0.61 (95% CI 0.52 to 0.71) with a large absolute reduction in risk of 23% (95% CI 16% to 30%).[9] This benefit varied according to the type of operative procedure, with orthopedic procedures having more benefit (i.e., RR of exposure to red cell transfusion was 0.42, 95% CI 0.32 to 0.54) and cardiac procedures having less benefit (RR 0.77, 95% CI 0.68 to 0.87).[9] There were no adverse outcomes with the use of cell salvage.[9] The trials included in this review, however, had poor methodologic quality because they were unblinded and had inadequate concealment of treatment allocation, which may have biased the providers' decisions to transfuse patients based on whether cell salvage had been employed.[9]

Autologous blood donation has been used as a strategy to decrease the requirement of perioperative allogeneic blood transfusion. A systematic review of autologous blood donation in adult patients scheduled for elective surgery showed a relative risk of allogeneic blood transfusion of 0.37 (95% CI 0.26, 0.54), with an absolute risk reduction of 43.8% (26.8% to 60.7%).[10] Unfortunately, autologous blood transfusion appears to increase the risk of requiring either an allogeneic or autologous (or both) blood transfusion (RR = 1.29; 95% CI 1.12, 1.48).[10] There is controversy regarding whether autologous blood transfusion is safer considering the increased transfusion rate. Transfused autologous blood has similar noninfectious complications as allogeneic blood. Unfortunately, the trial designs of studies in this review were not ideal and at present the best evidence does not conclusively indicate whether autologous blood donation is beneficial or harmful.[10]

Acute normovolemic hemodilution (ANH, defined as whole blood withdrawn on the day of surgery and replaced with crystalloid or colloid solution) has also been employed to reduce perioperative blood loss.[11] A systematic review suggests that ANH reduced the likelihood of exposure to allogeneic blood with an odds ratio (OR) of 0.31 (95% CI 0.15 to 0.62) but failed to reduce the likelihood of transfusion (OR 0.64, 95% CI 0.31 to 1.31).[11] Poor trial design could have biased the results of this review.[11,12] ANH has been found to decrease the allogeneic transfusion rate in patients of ASA I or II status, undergoing major liver resections.[13] Erythropoetin (Epo) has also been used and shown to decrease the need for perioperative blood transfusion in cardiac and orthopedic procedures. A systematic review was completed for Epo use in patients requiring orthopedic or cardiac surgery with or without autologous blood availability.[14] The odds ratio for requiring allogeneic blood transfusion in addition to autologous transfusion was 0.42 (95% CI 0.28 to 0.62) for orthopedic surgery and 0.25 (95% CI 0.08 to 0.82) for cardiac surgery.[14] The odds ratio for Epo alone for allogeneic blood transfusion was 0.36 (95% CI 0.24 to 0.56) in orthopedic surgery and 0.25 (95% CI 0.06 to 1.04) in cardiac surgery.[14] This indicates that Epo significantly decreased the exposure to perioperative allogeneic blood transfusion in cardiac

and orthopedic surgery.[14-17] One trial demonstrated that perioperative intravenous iron with erythropoietin in patients with gastrointestinal tract cancer and preoperative mild anemia reduced the postoperative transfusion rate.[18] Another strategy for reducing perioperative blood loss includes the use of recombinant activated factor VII. Limited evidence has shown that the use of factor VIIa may be effective in patients undergoing major surgery (i.e., in this trial it was retropubic prostatectomy) even in the absence of coagulopathy or intractable bleeding.[19]

It has also been shown that low hemoglobin levels themselves are not immediately life threatening and in fact may be the right option in critically ill patients (transfusion threshold of approximately 7 g/dL).[20] The threshold for perioperative patients, however, has not been extensively investigated. Transfusion triggers in trials involving antifibrinolytic therapy have varied widely, including thresholds such as hemoglobin levels from 5 to 10 g/dL or hematocrit levels of 18% to 30%.[2]

DRUG THERAPIES AVAILABLE TO REDUCE POSTOPERATIVE BLOOD LOSS

The medications available to reduce the need for allogeneic blood transfusion include antifibrinolytic drugs such as aprotonin (AP), tranexamic acid (TA), and epsilon aminocaproic acid (EACA). Randomized trials for the effectiveness of antifibrinolytics have been most extensively explored both in adult and pediatric cardiac surgery. Trials have been completed in noncardiac surgery associated with excessive blood loss, including hip and knee replacement surgery, orthotopic liver transplantation, vascular surgery, and liver resection. The dosage ranges for various antifibrinolytics employed have also varied greatly between trials (Table 27-1). Desmopressin (DDAVP) has been investigated in reducing perioperative

Table 27-1	Adult Dosage Ranges Previously Used in Trials for Perioperative Antifibrinolytic Therapy		
Agent	**Dose Strategy**	**Loading Dose**	**Continuous Infusion**
Aprotinin	High dose or full Hammersmith regimen	1. IV 2 million kallikrein inactivator units (KIU) (280 mg) over 20-30 min at induction 2. 2 million KIU (280 mg) is added to the pump prime of the cardiopulmonary bypass unit	IV 500,000 KIU/hr (70 mg/hr), during surgery
Aprotinin	Low-dose or half Hammersmith regimen	1. IV 1 million KIU (140 mg) over 20-30 min 2. 1 million KIU (140 mg) is added to the pump prime of the cardiopulmonary bypass unit	IV 250,000 KIU/hr (35 mg/hr), during surgery
Aprotinin	Pump prime dose	1. 500,000 to 2 million KIU (70-280 mg) is added to the prime of the cardiopulmonary bypass unit	
Tranexamic acid (TA)		IV 2.5-100 mg/kg over 20-30 min	IV 0.25-4 mg/kg/hr over 1-12 hr
Epsilon aminocaproic acid (EACA)		IV 80 mg-15 g	IV 1-2 g/hr over various time periods
Desmopressin (DDAVP)		IV 0.3 mcg/kg	
Dipyridamole (DIP)		PO 100 mg QID for 1.5 days preoperatively	IV 0.24 mg/kg/hr from anesthetic induction to 1 hr postoperative[28]

blood loss. Dipyridamole (DIP) has been studied specifically for reducing blood loss following cardiac surgery.

Mechanism of Hemostatic Drugs (Figure 27-1) and Side Effects

AP is a serine proteinase inhibitor derived from bovine lung that prevents fibrinolysis by forming enzyme complexes that deactivate human trypsin, plasmin, plasma kallikrein, and tissue kallikrein.[21] It also acts by minimizing contact phase activation of coagulation and, in the case of cardiopulmonary bypass, foreign surface activation. AP may preserve platelet function through these mechanisms during cardiopulmonary bypass.[21] AP can cause a hypersensitivity reaction, especially after repeated exposures. In the most comprehensive systematic review, no increase in adverse effects was seen in the use of AP, including the risk of myocardial infarction (MI) (RR 0.92, 95% CI 0.72 to 1.18), stroke (RR 0.76, 95% CI 0.35 to 1.64), renal dysfunction (RR 1.16, 95% CI 0.79 to 1.70), or overall mortality rate (RR 0.90, 95% CI 0.67 to 1.20).[2] The analyses of MI and death appear not to have been biased by underreporting; however, renal events may not have been consistently tracked, which could explain how this differs from the results of recently published nonrandomized studies.[2,22,23] Recent retrospective studies suggest that patients undergoing coronary artery bypass surgery had an increased risk of renal failure requiring dialysis (odds ratio 2.34, 95% CI 1.27 to 4.31), 55% increase in risk of myocardial infarction or heart failure, 181% increase in risk of stroke or encephalopathy, and increased risk of 5-year mortality with a hazard ratio of 1.48 (95% CI 1.19 to 1.85).[22,23]

The IMAGE trial was specifically designed to examine these adverse effects of AP, including graft patency, MI rates, and postoperative blood loss in primary coronary surgery. Although blood loss and transfusion requirements were reduced, there was a higher rate of saphenous vein graft occlusions at mean time of 11 days following surgery in the AP group as compared with controls (15.4% versus 10.9%).[24] This effect was negated when there was adjustment for risk factors for vein graft occlusion (e.g., female gender, lack of aspirin use, small and poor distal vessels, and possible use of AP blood for vein graft dilation).[24] In subgroup analyses, the difference in bypass patency existed in patients who were operated on in non-U.S. centers.[24]

EACA and TA are synthetic derivatives of the amino acid lysine that act as effective inhibitors of fibrinolysis. EACA and TA bind reversibly to plasminogen and block the binding of plasminogen to fibrin, and therefore block the activation and transformation to plasmin. TA is about 10 times more potent than EACA because it has stronger binding to both the strong and weak sites of the plasminogen molecule in a ratio corresponding to the difference in potency between the compounds. Both of these compounds have side effects that are dose dependent and that usually involve the gastrointestinal tract (nausea, vomiting, diarrhea, abdominal pain). There is no evidence of increased risk of thromboembolic events in the latest meta-analysis.[25] However, there are case reports that attribute thrombi to these drugs.

DDAVP is a vasopressin analog that increases the circulating levels of coagulation factor VIII and von Willebrand factor by two to four times their baseline levels. Repeated doses can lead to tachyphylaxis. The side effects associated with DDAVP infusion include mild vasodilation and hypotension, hyponatremia, and decreased urine output.[26]

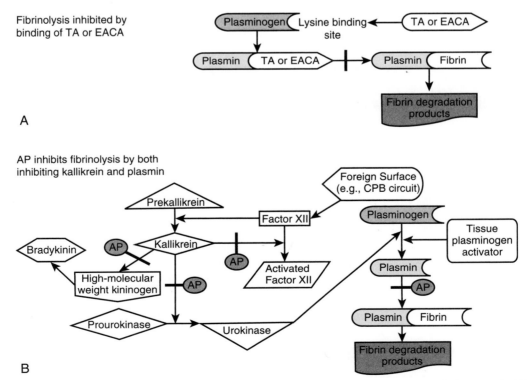

Figure 27-1. Mechanisms of Hemostatic Drugs. Tranexamic acid (TA) or epsilon aminocaproic acid (EACA); aprotinin (AP).

DIP is a pyrido-pyrimidine agent that prevents platelet activation by inhibiting platelet phosphodiesterase activity, aggregation, and granular release.[27] These properties can allow this agent to preserve platelet counts during cardiopulmonary bypass.[28] Adverse reactions associated with DIP include nausea, phlebitis with intravenous infusion, and urticarial skin reactions.[29]

Evidence of Effectiveness of Drug Treatments to Reduce Perioperative Blood Loss

There is strong evidence summarized by a comprehensive meta-analysis for the use of antifibrinolytic therapy in the setting of adult elective surgical procedures involving significant blood loss. Antifibrinolytics that have been shown in a systematic review to be effective include AP ($n = 116$ of 211 trials included in the review), TA ($n = 45$), and EACA ($n = 11$) in reducing allogeneic blood transfusions as summarized in Table 27-2.[2,25] The meta-analysis mainly reviewed trials involving cardiac surgery (147 of 211 trials included in the review) but also included a minority of trials involving elective adult orthopedic procedures ($n = 42$), liver surgery ($n = 14$), vascular surgery ($n = 4$), thoracic surgery ($n = 2$), neurosurgery ($n = 1$), and orthognathic surgery ($n = 1$).[2] This meta-analysis separated out the effect of each agent analyzed by surgical subtype.[2] AP was found to reduce the exposure to allogeneic blood transfusions for cardiac surgery (RR 0.66, 95% CI 0.61 to 0.71), orthopedic surgery (RR 0.69, 95% CI 0.56 to 0.85), thoracic surgery (RR 0.28, 95% CI 0.11 to 0.74), and liver surgery (RR 0.58, 95% CI 0.37 to 0.90).[2] TA was found to be effective in lowering allogeneic blood transfusions for patients undergoing cardiac surgery (RR 0.69, 95% CI 0.60 to 0.79) and orthopedic surgery (RR 0.44, 95% CI 0.33 to 0.60).[2] EACA significantly lowered the transfusion of allogeneic blood products only in cardiac surgery (RR 0.65, 95% CI 0.47 to 0.91).[2] There was no statistical

difference in transfusion rates between cardiac surgery patients receiving TA or EACA versus AP (see Table 27-2).[2]

DDAVP does not show a trend toward a net reduction in blood loss as compared with placebo and no difference in the requirement for blood transfusion.[30] DIP has been shown through a small randomized trial to reduce blood loss as compared with placebo by 46% and reduce red cell transfusions by 44% (1.5 units of packed red cells).[29] DIP has been shown through another randomized trial to be more effective in combination with high-dose AP in reducing postoperative blood loss.[28]

Systematic reviews completed before the comprehensive Cochrane review have shown similar results as summarized here. One systematic review on DDAVP in adult cardiac surgery patients showed no difference in transfusion requirements but did show a 34% reduction in blood loss in the subgroup of patients with the highest net blood loss (defined as greater than 1 L).[31] A total of four other previous systematic reviews regarding hemostatic drug prophylaxis have been completed in cardiac surgery. Two of these systematic reviews indicate a significant reduction in transfusion requirements as well as blood loss when using AP, TA, or EACA, but not with DDAVP.[32,33] Another review demonstrated a mortality benefit for both AP (OR 0.55) and TA or EACA (OR 0.78) but showed an increased risk of MI with DDAVP (OR 2.4).[33] The recent BART trial comparing AP with TA or EACA in high-risk cardiac surgical patients was halted prematurely after recruitment of 2331 patients because of increased 30-day all-cause mortality in the AP arm of the trial.[34] At 30 days, all-cause mortality was 6.0% in the AP patients, as compared with 3.9% with TA (relative risk, 1.55; 95% CI 0.99 to 2.42) and 4.0% with EACA (relative risk, 1.52; 95% CI 0.98 to 2.36). Deaths attributed to cardiac causes were increased in the AP study patients, whereas deaths attributed to other causes were similar in the three arms. There was only modest evidence of

Table 27-2 Meta-analyses That Outline the Evidence for the Use of Drug Therapy to Minimize Perioperative Blood Transfusion in Patients Undergoing Adult Elective Surgery

| Agent | No. of Trials (Patients) | NEED FOR BLOOD TRANSFUSION (95% CONFIDENCE INTERVAL) | | | REOPERATION FOR BLEEDING |
		Relative Risk	Absolute Risk	Savings	Relative Risk
The Cochrane Database of Systematic Reviews[2,30] *2006*					
Desmopressin (DDAVP)	18 trials (1295 patients) no reduction in risk	0.95 (0.86-1.06)			0.69 (0.26-1.83) no reduction in risk
Aprotinin (AP)	98 trials (10,144 patients)	0.66 (0.61-0.71)	21% (17%-25%)	Average saving of 1.1 units of blood	0.48 (0.35-0.68)
Tranexamic acid (TA)	53 trials (3836 patients)	0.61 (0.54-0.69)	17.2% (8.7%-25.7%)	Average saving of 1.1 units of blood	0.67 (0.41-1.09)
Epsilon aminocaproic acid (EACA)	14 trials (801 patients)	0.75 (0.58-0.96)		Average saving of 1.8 units of blood	0.35 (0.11-1.17)
TA or EACA versus AP	17 trials (2170 patients)	0.83 (0.69-0.99) AP superior			

superior efficacy with respect to massive bleeding composite outcome (RR 0.79, 95% CI 0.59 to 1.05). AP is currently released on a compassionate-use basis.

EVIDENCE FOR SPECIFIC SURGICAL PROCEDURES

Orthotopic Liver Transplantation

This procedure is associated with great losses of blood and massive transfusion requirements caused by a combination of the magnitude of the surgical procedure and preexisting coagulopathy secondary to liver insufficiency. One study has shown that high-dose AP reduced transfusion requirements by 37%.[35] A second trial has found that TA is more effective than EACA in reducing intraoperative transfusion requirements.[36] A trial comparing the relative efficacy of AP against TA showed no difference between the two agents.[37]

Hepatic Resections

TA was effective in reducing the volume of operative blood loss and need for transfusion in elective hepatic tumor resections.[38]

Total Hip Replacement

TA has been shown to reduce postoperative bleeding when given preoperatively with an infusion as opposed to postoperatively.[39-42] One small randomized trial did have a conflicting result where the TA arm had a greater number of patients requiring transfusion.[43] EACA as compared with control patients undergoing primary total hip replacement surgery resulted in a 27% lower mean postoperative blood loss and 11% reduction in allogeneic blood transfusion.[44,45] AP has also been shown to be effective in reducing blood loss in this group of surgical patients.[46]

Total Knee Replacement

TA has been shown to reduce postoperative blood loss by 32% and to reduce transfusion requirements with repeated preoperative and postoperative doses as compared with controls, normovolemic hemodilution, or desmopressin.[47-51] The average total blood loss in these studies ranged from approximately 40 to 3000 mL.[47] One study found that neither AP nor TA was effective in reducing blood loss or transfusion requirements; interestingly, the total blood loss was much lower than previous trials with a mean of 150 mL intraoperatively and 810 mL postoperatively.[52] It was advocated that the use of bone cement and excellent surgical hemostasis can avoid significant blood loss.[52]

Spinal Fusion

In a trial of AP and EACA versus controls in patients having complex spinal fusions, a significant reduction in blood loss and transfusion requirements occurred using half-dose AP as opposed to the EACA or control groups.[53] Further to this, one small trial has shown that

aminocaproic acid as compared with controls was effective in reducing blood loss and transfusion in surgery for idiopathic scoliosis.[54]

SPECIFIC SURGICAL CANDIDATES NOT COVERED IN META-ANALYSES

Cardiac Surgery in Pediatric Patients

AP has been investigated in pediatric patients undergoing cardiac surgery with conflicting results. One trial advocated that use should be restricted to reoperations, arterial switches, and those operations with a high likelihood of hemorrhage.[55] EACA and low-dose AP have been found to be equally effective in reducing postoperative blood loss and blood product transfusion in children with congenital cyanotic heart disease having surgery.[56] The use of TA in pediatric patients undergoing redo cardiac surgery using two 100 mg/kg boluses followed by a 10 mg/kg/hr infusion was evaluated in children and showed a 24% reduction in total blood loss, and reduced transfusion requirements.[57] Avoidance of blood transfusion in pediatric cardiac surgical patients is especially important because this group tends to require multiple staged operations over several years and can be exposed to multiple units of blood products in the process. It appears that the benefit with TA may be greater in those pediatric patients with cyanotic congenital heart disease.[58]

Orthopedic Surgery in Pediatric Patients

AP and TA have also been used in pediatric patients who undergo scoliosis surgery, which often requires multiple blood transfusions with a loss of one or more blood volumes.[44] A small trial in this setting has shown that the total amount of blood transfused is reduced by 28% with the use of TA.[44] This study tried to standardize perioperative care except for the unrestricted use of cell-saved blood, which was similar in both groups.[44] Another small trial demonstrated that both blood loss and transfusion requirements were significantly reduced with AP use.[59]

INTRACTABLE POSTOPERATIVE BLEEDING WITH OR WITHOUT INHERITED COAGULOPATHY

Recombinant factor VIIa has been used in patients with acquired bleeding disorders such as hemophilia to allow completion of surgery.[60] It has been successfully used in pediatric patients with bleeding disorders undergoing surgical procedures, trauma patients with intractable bleeding, and cardiac surgery patients with intractable bleeding.[61-63] Factor VIIa (NovoSeven) is given as 90 to 100 mcg/kg bolus doses every 2 hours, and two or three repeated doses may be required for hemophiliacs with moderate bleeding, though even more may be required for severe bleeding.[60] AP, EACA, and TA given only postoperatively have been found to be ineffective in preventing further significant blood loss.[41,64]

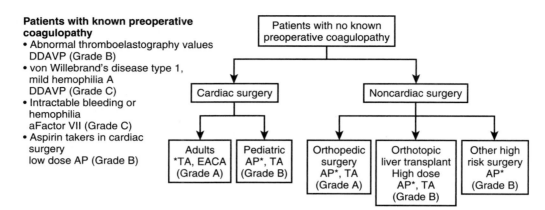

Patients with known preoperative coagulopathy
- Abnormal thromboelastography values DDAVP (Grade B)
- von Willebrand's disease type 1, mild hemophilia A DDAVP (Grade C)
- Intractable bleeding or hemophilia aFactor VII (Grade C)
- Aspirin takers in cardiac surgery low dose AP (Grade B)

Grade A evidence: there is good evidence through randomized clinical trials of efficacy and safety
Grade B evidence: there is fair evidence through clinical trials of some efficacy and safety
Grade C evidence: there is poor evidence through studies or case series of efficacy and safety
*There has been some recent major concern from retrospective data and one large randomized trial regarding the safety of AP in adult cardiac surgery—AP is only available on a compassionate use basis. The use of TA (or EACA) may be safer than AP in other high risk situations, although studies with EACA are lacking.

Figure 27-2. Algorithm for Grade of Evidence for the Use of Hemostatic Drugs.

AREAS OF UNCERTAINTY

Trials are under way evaluating hemostatic drugs in a wider range of noncardiac surgical specialities. The heterogeneity of completed trials, including such variables as type of surgery, transfusion thresholds, and outcomes measured, makes it hard to draw conclusions even with systematic reviews.[25] The best evidence for the use of antifibrinolytic therapy applies to adult, elective cardiac surgery where the amount of blood loss can be large. More research is required for noncardiac surgery involving significant blood loss. DDAVP has demonstrated conflicting results in reducing the risk of allogeneic blood transfusion and has been found to be associated with no benefit in multiple meta-analyses.[65]

GUIDELINES (FIGURE 27-2)

Antifibrinolytic drugs demonstrate effectiveness in reducing blood loss and the need for transfusion and reoperation for bleeding. This is especially true of AP and TA in the context of adult, elective cardiac surgery. These results may translate into benefits for other surgical procedures with similar risk of blood loss, though more research is required in this area. A recent retrospective study suggests that AP may have adverse effects in cardiac surgery, including renal dysfunction, thromboembolic events, and death.[22,23] The BART trial demonstrated that the use of AP is associated with a greater mortality risk than either TA or EACA for high-risk cardiac surgery. The trials to date have been heterogeneous both in cohort selection and in the evaluation of outcomes, with less data for EACA, a significantly less expensive agent. In developed countries, the adverse risks associated with blood transfusion are low; the cost-effectiveness of such blood conservation strategies may differ in developing countries where the risk of acquiring HIV through transfusion is high.

AUTHORS' RECOMMENDATIONS

Trial evidence suggests that antifibrinolytic therapy with the use of either AP, TA, or EACA reduces perioperative transfusion of blood products. AP seems to be the most effective hemostatic drug considering the best current evidence available; however, recent concerns regarding the safety of this drug have emerged, particularly since the publication of the BART trial. AP is currently available only on a compassionate-use basis, and it is very likely that its use will be significantly curtailed. TA and EACA are more cost-effective and show similar statistical efficacy in reducing transfusion rates as compared with AP. Our recommendations include TA or EACA because the results are similar to AP and the costs are much lower (e.g., in the case of cardiac surgery the highest dose range is approximately $235) and the two agents appear to be much safer. The BART investigators could not identify any patient group that had better outcomes with AP, although certain relevant patient groups were not studied (primary isolated coronary artery bypass graft with recent clopidogrel, and Jehovah's Witness patients were ineligible). The greatest benefit of antifibrinolytic therapy is experienced by patients at high risk of significant hemorrhage from a surgical procedure. Such high-risk patients include those on preoperative antiplatelet or thrombolytic therapy, or those undergoing various procedures such as reoperative cardiac surgery, orthotopic liver transplantation, and aortic surgery. Conversely, low-risk surgery would include procedures such as isolated coronary artery bypass surgery.

REFERENCES

1. Moulton MJ, Creswell LL, Mackey ME, Cox JL, Rosenbloom M: Reexploration for bleeding is a risk factor for adverse outcomes after cardiac operations. *J Thorac Cardiovasc Surg* 1996;111 (5):1037-1046.
2. Henry DA, Carless PA, Moxey AJ, et al: Anti-fibrinolytic use for minimising perioperative allogeneic blood transfusion. *Cochrane Database Syst Rev* 2007(4):CD001886.
3. Sazama K: Reports of 355 transfusion-associated deaths: 1976 through 1985. *Transfusion* 1990;30(7):583-590.

4. Phillips GR 3rd, Kauder DR, Schwab CW: Massive blood loss in trauma patients. The benefits and dangers of transfusion therapy. *Postgrad Med* 1994;95(4):61-62, 67-72.

5. Dry SM, Bechard KM, Milford EL, Churchill WH, Benjamin RJ: The pathology of transfusion-related acute lung injury. *Am J Clin Pathol* 1999;112(2):216-221.

6. Despotis GJ, Filos KS, Zoys TN, Hogue CWJr, Spitznagel E, Lappas DG: Factors associated with excessive postoperative blood loss and hemostatic transfusion requirements: A multivariate analysis in cardiac surgical patients. *Anesth Analg* 1996;82 (1):13-21.

7. Carless PA, Anthony DM, Henry DA: Systematic review of the use of fibrin sealant to minimize perioperative allogeneic blood transfusion. *Br J Surg* 2002;89(6):695-703.

8. Rajagopalan S, Mascha E, Na J, Sessler DI: The effects of mild perioperative hypothermia on blood loss and transfusion requirement. *Anesthesiology* 2008;108(1):71-77.

9. Carless PA, Henry DA, Moxey AJ, O'Connell DL, Brown T, Fergusson DA: Cell salvage for minimising perioperative allogeneic blood transfusion. *Cochrane Database Syst Rev* 2006(4): CD001888.

10. Henry DA, Carless PA, Moxey AJ, et al: Pre-operative autologous donation for minimising perioperative allogeneic blood transfusion. *Cochrane Database Syst Rev* 2002(2):CD003602.

11. Bryson GL, Laupacis A, Wells GA: Does acute normovolemic hemodilution reduce perioperative allogeneic transfusion? A meta-analysis. The International Study of Perioperative Transfusion. *Anesth Analg* 1998;86(1):9-15.

12. Kumar R, Chakraborty I, Sehgal R: A prospective randomized study comparing two techniques of perioperative blood conservation: Isovolemic hemodilution and hypervolemic hemodilution. *Anesth Analg* 2002;95(5):1154-1161, table of contents.

13. Matot I, Scheinin O, Jurim O, Eid A: Effectiveness of acute normovolemic hemodilution to minimize allogeneic blood transfusion in major liver resections. *Anesthesiology* 2002;97(4): 794-800.

14. Laupacis A, Fergusson D: Erythropoietin to minimize perioperative blood transfusion: A systematic review of randomized trials. The International Study of Peri-operative Transfusion (ISPOT) Investigators. *Transfus Med* 1998;8(4):309-317.

15. Alghamdi AA, Albanna MJ, Guru V, Brister SJ: Does the use of erythropoietin reduce the risk of exposure to allogeneic blood transfusion in cardiac surgery? A systematic review and meta-analysis. *J Card Surg* 2006;21(3):320-326.

16. Sonzogni V, Crupi G, Poma R, et al: Erythropoietin therapy and preoperative autologous blood donation in children undergoing open heart surgery. *Br J Anaesth* 2001;87(3):429-434.

17. Deutsch A, Spaulding J, Marcus RE: Preoperative epoetin alfa vs autologous blood donation in primary total knee arthroplasty. *J Arthroplasty* 2006;21(5):628-635.

18. Kosmadakis N, Messaris E, Maris A, et al: Perioperative erythropoietin administration in patients with gastrointestinal tract cancer: Prospective randomized double-blind study. *Ann Surg* 2003;237(3):417-421.

19. Friederich PW, Henny CP, Messelink EJ, et al: Effect of recombinant activated factor VII on perioperative blood loss in patients undergoing retropubic prostatectomy: A double-blind placebo-controlled randomised trial. *Lancet* 2003;361(9353):201-205.

20. Hebert PC, Wells G, Blajchman MA, et al: A multicenter, randomized, controlled clinical trial of transfusion requirements in critical care. Transfusion Requirements in Critical Care Investigators, Canadian Critical Care Trials Group. *N Engl J Med* 1999;340 (6):409-417.

21. Tabuchi N, De Haan J, Boonstra PW, Huet RC, van Oeveren W: Aprotinin effect on platelet function and clotting during cardiopulmonary bypass. *Eur J Cardiothorac Surg* 1994;8(2):87-90.

22. Mangano DT, Tudor IC, Dietzel C: The risk associated with aprotinin in cardiac surgery. *N Engl J Med* 2006;354(4):353-365.

23. Mangano DT, Miao Y, Vuylsteke A, et al: Mortality associated with aprotinin during 5 years following coronary artery bypass graft surgery. *JAMA* 2007;297(5):471-479.

24. Alderman EL, Levy JH, Rich JB, et al: Analyses of coronary graft patency after aprotinin use: Results from the International Multicenter Aprotinin Graft Patency Experience (IMAGE) trial. *J Thorac Cardiovasc Surg* 1998;116(5):716-730.

25. Henry DA, Moxey AJ, Carless PA, et al: Anti-fibrinolytic use for minimising perioperative allogeneic blood transfusion. *Cochrane Database Syst Rev* 2001(1):CD001886.

26. Reich DL, Hammerschlag BC, Rand JH, et al: Desmopressin acetate is a mild vasodilator that does not reduce blood loss in uncomplicated cardiac surgical procedures. *J Cardiothorac Vasc Anesth* 1991;5(2):142-145.

27. Best LC, McGuire MB, Jones PB, et al: Mode of action of dipyridamole on human platelets. *Thromb Res* 1979;16(3-4):367-379.

28. Cohen G, Ivanov J, Weisel RD, Rao V, Mohabeer MK, Mickle DA: Aprotinin and dipyridamole for the safe reduction of postoperative blood loss. *Ann Thorac Surg* 1998;65(3):674-683.

29. Teoh KH, Christakis GT, Weisel RD, et al: Dipyridamole preserved platelets and reduced blood loss after cardiopulmonary bypass. *J Thorac Cardiovasc Surg* 1988;96(2):332-341.

30. Carless PA, Henry DA, Moxey AJ, et al: Desmopressin for minimising perioperative allogeneic blood transfusion. *Cochrane Database Syst Rev* 2004(1):CD001884.

31. Cattaneo M, Harris AS, Stromberg U, Mannucci PM: The effect of desmopressin on reducing blood loss in cardiac surgery—a meta-analysis of double-blind, placebo-controlled trials. *Thromb Haemost* 1995;74(4):1064-1070.

32. Fremes SE, Wong BI, Lee E, et al: Metaanalysis of prophylactic drug treatment in the prevention of postoperative bleeding. *Ann Thorac Surg* 1994;58(6):1580-1588.

33. Levi M, Cromheecke ME, de Jonge E, et al: Pharmacological strategies to decrease excessive blood loss in cardiac surgery: A meta-analysis of clinically relevant endpoints. *Lancet* 1999;354 (9194):1940-1947.

34. Fergusson DA, Hébert PC, Mazer CD, et al: A comparison of aprotinin and lysine analogues in high-risk cardiac surgery. *N Engl J Med* 2008;358(22):2319-2331.

35. Porte RJ, Molenaar IQ, Begliomini B, et al: Aprotinin and transfusion requirements in orthotopic liver transplantation: A multicentre randomised double-blind study. EMSALT Study Group. *Lancet* 2000;355(9212):1303-1309.

36. Dalmau A, Sabate A, Acosta F, et al: Tranexamic acid reduces red cell transfusion better than epsilon-aminocaproic acid or placebo in liver transplantation. *Anesth Analg* 2000;91(1):29-34.

37. Ickx BE, van der Linden PJ, Melot C, et al: Comparison of the effects of aprotinin and tranexamic acid on blood loss and red blood cell transfusion requirements during the late stages of liver transplantation. *Transfusion* 2006;46(4):595-605.

38. Wu CC, Ho WM, Cheng SB, et al: Perioperative parenteral tranexamic acid in liver tumor resection: A prospective randomized trial toward a "blood transfusion"-free hepatectomy. *Ann Surg* 2006;243(2):173-180.

39. Claeys MA, Vermeersch N, Haentjens P: Reduction of blood loss with tranexamic acid in primary total hip replacement surgery. *Acta Chir Belg* 2007;107(4):397-401.

40. Ekback G, Axelsson K, Ryttberg L, et al: Tranexamic acid reduces blood loss in total hip replacement surgery. *Anesth Analg* 2000;91 (5):1124-1130.

41. Benoni G, Lethagen S, Nilsson P, Fredin H: Tranexamic acid, given at the end of the operation, does not reduce postoperative blood loss in hip arthroplasty. *Acta Orthop Scand* 2000;71(3):250-254.

42. Yamasaki S, Masuhara K, Fuji T: Tranexamic acid reduces blood loss after cementless total hip arthroplasty—prospective randomized study in 40 cases. *Int Orthop* 2004;28(2):69-73.

43. Garneti N, Field J: Bone bleeding during total hip arthroplasty after administration of tranexamic acid. *J Arthroplasty* 2004;19 (4):488-492.

44. Neilipovitz DT, Murto K, Hall L, Barrowman NJ, Splinter WM: A randomized trial of tranexamic acid to reduce blood transfusion for scoliosis surgery. *Anesth Analg* 2001;93(1):82-87.

45. Harley BJ, Beaupre LA, Jones CA, Cinats JG, Guenther CR: The effect of epsilon aminocaproic acid on blood loss in patients who undergo primary total hip replacement: A pilot study. *Can J Surg* 2002;45(3):185-190.

46. Ray M, Hatcher S, Whitehouse SL, Crawford S, Crawford R: Aprotinin and epsilon aminocaproic acid are effective in reducing blood loss after primary total hip arthroplasty—a prospective randomized double-blind placebo-controlled study. *J Thromb Haemost* 2005;3(7):1421-1427.

47. Jansen AJ, Andreica S, Claeys M, D'Haese J, Camu F, Jochmans K: Use of tranexamic acid for an effective blood conservation strategy after total knee arthroplasty. *Br J Anaesth* 1999;83 (4):596-601.

48. Zohar E, Fredman B, Ellis M, Luban I, Stern A, Jedeikin R: A comparative study of the postoperative allogeneic blood-sparing effect of tranexamic acid versus acute normovolemic hemodilution after total knee replacement. *Anesth Analg* 1999;89(6): 1382-1387.

49. Zohar E, Fredman B, Ellis MH, Ifrach N, Stern A, Jedeikin R: A comparative study of the postoperative allogeneic blood-sparing effects of tranexamic acid and of desmopressin after total knee replacement. *Transfusion* 2001;41(10):1285-1289.

50. Veien M, Sorensen JV, Madsen F, Juelsgaard P: Tranexamic acid given intraoperatively reduces blood loss after total knee replacement: A randomized, controlled study. *Acta Anaesthesiol Scand* 2002;46(10):1206-1211.

51. Camarasa MA, Olle G, Serra-Prat M, et al: Efficacy of aminocaproic, tranexamic acids in the control of bleeding during total knee replacement: A randomized clinical trial. *Br J Anaesth* 2006;96(5):576-582.

52. Engel JM, Hohaus T, Ruwoldt R, Menges T, Jurgensen I, Hempelmann G: Regional hemostatic status and blood requirements after total knee arthroplasty with and without tranexamic acid or aprotinin. *Anesth Analg* 2001;92(3):775-780.

53. Urban MK, Beckman J, Gordon M, Urquhart B, Boachie-Adjei O: The efficacy of antifibrinolytics in the reduction of blood loss during complex adult reconstructive spine surgery. *Spine* 2001;26 (10):1152-1156.

54. Thompson GH, Florentino-Pineda I, Poe-Kochert C: The role of amicar in decreasing perioperative blood loss in idiopathic scoliosis. *Spine* 2005;30(17 suppl):S94-S99.

55. Davies MJ, Allen A, Kort H, et al: Prospective, randomized, double-blind study of high-dose aprotinin in pediatric cardiac operations. *Ann Thorac Surg* 1997;63(2):497-503.

56. Chauhan S, Kumar BA, Rao BH, et al: Efficacy of aprotinin, epsilon aminocaproic acid, or combination in cyanotic heart disease. *Ann Thorac Surg* 2000;70(4):1308-1312.

57. Reid RW, Zimmerman AA, Laussen PC, Mayer JE, Gorlin JB, Burrows FA: The efficacy of tranexamic acid versus placebo in decreasing blood loss in pediatric patients undergoing repeat cardiac surgery. *Anesth Analg* 1997;84(5):990-996.

58. Zonis Z, Seear M, Reichert C, Sett S, Allen C: The effect of preoperative tranexamic acid on blood loss after cardiac operations in children. *J Thorac Cardiovasc Surg* 1996;111(5):982-987.

59. Cole JW, Murray DJ, Snider RJ, Bassett GS, Bridwell KH, Lenke LG: Aprotinin reduces blood loss during spinal surgery in children. *Spine* 2003;28(21):2482-2485.

60. Hedner U: Recombinant factor VIIa (NovoSeven) as a hemostatic agent. *Semin Hematol* 2001;38(4 suppl 12):43-47.

61. Lynn M, Jeroukhimov I, Klein Y, Martinowitz U: Updates in the management of severe coagulopathy in trauma patients. *Intensive Care Med* 2002;28(suppl 2):S241-S247.

62. O'Connell N, Mc Mahon C, Smith J, et al: Recombinant factor VIIa in the management of surgery and acute bleeding episodes in children with haemophilia and high responding inhibitors. *Br J Haematol* 2002;116(3):632-635.

63. Hendriks HG, van der Maaten JM, de Wolf J, Waterbolk TW, Slooff MJ, van der Meer J: An effective treatment of severe intractable bleeding after valve repair by one single dose of activated recombinant factor VII. *Anesth Analg* 2001;93(2):287-289, 2nd contents page.

64. Ray MJ, Hales MM, Brown L, O'Brien MF, Stafford EG: Postoperatively administered aprotinin or epsilon aminocaproic acid after cardiopulmonary bypass has limited benefit. *Ann Thorac Surg* 2001;72(2):521-526.

65. Henry DA, Moxey AJ, Carless PA, et al: Desmopressin for minimising perioperative allogeneic blood transfusion. *Cochrane Database Syst Rev* 2001(2):CD001884.

28 Does Perioperative Hyperglycemia Increase Risk? Should We Have Aggressive Glucose Control Perioperatively?

Stanley Rosenbaum, MA, MD, and Sherif Afifi, MD, FCCM, FCCP

INTRODUCTION

The body of clinical evidence suggesting that surgery elicits a stress response, which manifests as hyperglycemia in the early postoperative period, has been well corroborated by studies on both inflammation and immunomodulation. Recent literature has redefined the prevalence of hyperglycemia according to narrower ranges of serum glucose and in relation to the rising epidemic of diabetes mellitus (DM) in the world. DM affects more than 170 million individuals worldwide, and approximately 18 million in the United States (approximately 6.3% of the population).[1] Furthermore, age-adjusted mortality rates among adults with diabetes is twice that of those without the disease.[2]

Over the past few years, significant changes in the practice of perioperative glycemic surveillance and control have been influenced by many interventional investigations. The response to surgery has varied between diabetic and nondiabetic patients. Based on clinical outcomes favoring the maintenance of tight perioperative euglycemia with insulin therapy, the incidence of complications varied between surgical and medical critically ill patients. Finally, the impact of various types of anesthetic regimens on the stress response to surgery is only at the cusp of investigations. This chapter will display the stress response to surgery, demonstrate the disadvantages of perioperative hyperglycemia, review the favorable effect of perioperative euglycemia, and survey the impact of anesthetic management on both perioperative glycemic control and patient outcome.

OPTIONS

The goal for all patients in the perioperative period is to keep metabolism as nearly normal as possible. This cannot be overemphasized for diabetic patients undergoing major cardiovascular or abdominal surgery. Methods to achieve normoglycemia in diabetic patients are a matter of physician preference, with only subtle differences between approaches to manage patients with insulin-dependent diabetes mellitus (IDDM) and those with non–insulin-dependent diabetes mellitus (NIDDM).

In any case, failure to maintain physiologic control subjects patients to a wide range of metabolic disturbances and renders them vulnerable to complications. Essential to any method is frequent and accurate blood glucose monitoring because it is crucial to adjustment of insulin doses for restoration and maintenance of normoglycemia.

Recent large-scale outcome studies have defined intraoperative and perioperative glucose control regimens in terms of favorable outcome in the short-term and long-term postoperative periods. The common denominators of any regimen is that it should

1. Maintain good glycemic control to avoid excessively high or low glucose levels.
2. Prevent other metabolic disturbances.
3. Apply to a variety of situations (operating room, recovery room, and general medical and surgical wards).
4. Be relatively easy to understand with clear end-goals of therapy.

Glucose Control Regimens

A survey of anesthesiologists compared their strategies for perioperative management of diabetic patients in 1993 with those in 1985[3] and found that a greater proportion of anesthesiologists tend to maintain the perioperative blood glucose concentration of their diabetic patients at less than 180 mg/dL. Anesthesiologists are also more likely to be interventional in their management of diabetic patients than in the past, and the methods used have changed in relative popularity. In 1993 diabetic patients undergoing major surgery were most commonly managed with separate infusions of insulin and glucose, whereas in 1985 the combined infusion of glucose, insulin, and potassium was the most popular technique. The use of protocols in hospitals may increase the degree of uniformity of practice between anesthesiologists.

Although several glucose control regimens are outlined in this chapter, there is no substitute for the safe guideline of emphasizing frequent monitoring of blood glucose levels and intervening with appropriate individualized amounts of insulin rather than relying on prescheduled doses.

Intravenous Infusion of Insulin

Intravenous delivery of insulin is widely preferred because of ease in administration, quick dose adjustment, and uninterrupted metabolic control during unanticipated changes in scheduling of surgical procedures.[4]

The role of intraoperative glycemic control with a standardized insulin protocol to modulate outcomes was investigated in a prospective observational study of patients with DM undergoing coronary artery bypass graft (CABG) surgery. Although postoperative blood glucose was similar, those patients who achieved tight control of blood glucose concentrations intraoperatively demonstrated decreased morbidity and mortality rates compared with patients whose blood glucose was poorly controlled (defined as four consecutive blood glucose measurements exceeding 200 mg/dL despite insulin therapy).[5]

Glucose-Insulin-Potassium (GIK) Infusion

Thirty percent dextrose in water, potassium, and 80 mEq/L of regular insulin, 50 units, are given intravenously at 1 mL/kg per hour after induction of anesthesia.

Studies with glucose-insulin-potassium (GIK) solutions have shown that treatment of hyperglycemia has direct metabolic effects and can enhance myocardial performance when blood glucose concentrations were well controlled,[6,7] but not when blood glucose levels were inadequately controlled.[8] An ensuing DIGAMI 2 study[9] compared three treatment strategies in patients with acute myocardial infarction (MI): group 1 received acute insulin-glucose infusion followed by insulin-based long-term glucose control; group 2 received insulin-glucose infusion followed by standard glucose control; and group 3 received routine metabolic management in accordance with local practice. Unfortunately, this study did not reach recruitment goals and showed no treatment differences. Moreover, the primary treatment target of a fasting blood glucose level of 90 to 126 mg/dL for those in group 1 was never achieved. Mean fasting blood glucose levels (149 mg/dL) and hemoglobin A_{1c} (6.8%) were similar among the three study groups. Thus, if glycemia is predictive of outcomes, no differences would have been expected—and no differences were observed. Another large multicenter study, the Clinical Trial of Metabolic Modulation in Acute Myocardial Infarction Treatment Evaluation (CREATE-ECLA), failed to show benefit from glucose-insulin-potassium infusions on mortality rate.[10]

The benefit of glucose-insulin-potassium to produce cardioprotection is controversial and may not be similar to the use of insulin to specifically control blood glucose concentration. Conclusions from the DIGAMI 2 and CREATE-ECLA studies strongly suggest that insulin infusion in the absence of blood glucose lowering has no effect on outcomes.

EVIDENCE

Effect of Stress-related Hormonal Changes on Metabolic Changes in Diabetic and Nondiabetic Patients

Surgical stress was reported to cause hyperglycemia and hyperinsulinemia in nondiabetic patients,[11] whereas it caused hyperglycemia and even hypoinsulinemia in some diabetic patients.[12] Perioperative hyperglycemia is believed to be the result of stress-related hormonal changes that induce a number of metabolic changes in both nondiabetic and diabetic patients.

The nociceptive signals produced during operative manipulation evoke responses from the hypothalamic nuclei, which prompt release of several endogenous hormones.[13-16] The hormones exert their effects on different organs that result in overall hyperglycemia. The increase in glucose levels results from either direct stimulation of glucose-producing pathways or indirectly through stimulating biochemical pathways that increase formation of products that are incorporated in glucose formation. The pathways that directly increase glucose production and storage are gluconeogenesis and glycogenolysis. Glycogenolysis takes place in the liver and skeletal muscles, whereas gluconeogenesis occurs in the liver only. Proteolysis, glycolysis, and lipolysis produce glycerol, pyruvate, and amino acids, all of which are substrates for gluconeogenesis in the liver.

The endocrine response to stressful stimuli consists of activation of the hypothalamo-adrenal and the sympatho-adrenal axes, which, in turn, increase endogenous catecholamines and glucocorticoids. The result is hyperglycemia.[17] At the same time, the release of catabolic hormones (cortisol, glucagon, and growth hormone) accelerates gluconeogenesis, whereas glycogenolysis and lipolysis are inhibited. In the liver, catecholamines increase gluconeogenesis, whereas corticotrophins, glucagons, and growth hormone (GH) inhibit glycogenesis, but promote glycogenolysis.[9] The net effect in the liver is increased glucose stores.

The degree of hyperglycemia occurring in the early postoperative period was found to be proportional to the degree of stress during surgery. The work of Chernow and colleagues[18] confirmed the relationship between the intensity of surgical stress and the hormonal response contributing to the elevation of blood glucose. Clarke[19] reported the production of mild hyperglycemia after minor or uncomplicated operations. Compared with minor procedures such as inguinal herniorrhaphy, the severe surgical stress of cholecystectomy or subtotal colectomy resulted in significant elevation of catabolic hormone levels starting at 1 hour after surgery and persisted to the fifth postoperative day (Figure 28-1).

Effect of Perioperative Hyperglycemia on Wound Healing and Postoperative Infections

Perioperative hyperglycemia leads to delayed wound healing. Evidence to support the rationale for control of

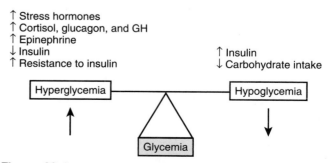

Figure 28-1. Factors Affecting Blood Glucose Levels.

perioperative blood glucose levels is twofold. One line of investigations has demonstrated the beneficial effects of insulin, and another group of studies has shown that blocking the action of insulin impaired wound healing. A deficiency of insulin in the early postoperative period leads to impaired hydroxyproline accumulation into the structure of healing wounds.[20] The beneficial effects of glycemic control with insulin on wound healing were proven in several investigations. In one study, Yue and colleagues[21] showed that in diabetic animals treated with insulin, the repaired tissue could withstand three times the mechanical force that separated the incision of non–insulin-treated animals. Conversely, Weringer and colleagues[22] demonstrated that blocking insulin activity inhibited DNA and protein synthesis in wounds, with resultant reductions in capillary proliferation, fibroblast activation, and collagen synthesis.

Perioperative Hyperglycemia and Infectious Outcomes

It is well established that individuals with diabetes are at a higher risk than their nondiabetic counterparts for a variety of bacterial infections such as cystitis, pneumonia, cellulitis, and postoperative wound infections.[23] In one study, diabetic patients undergoing elective vascular or abdominal procedures had a higher rate of nosocomial infections (pneumonia, bacteremia, and surgical wound infection) when blood glucose was greater than 220 mg/dL.[24] Another study found a strong graded relationship between wound infection risk and the mean concentration of blood glucose on the first postoperative day (the incidence of wound infection was 1.3% among patients with glucose levels 100 to 150 mg/dL versus 6.7% among patients with glucose levels 250 to 300 mg/dL).[25] In a prospective study of a cohort of diabetic patients undergoing coronary artery surgery, those with mean glucose concentrations greater than 200 mg/dL within the first 36 postoperative hours were more likely to develop infectious complications (pneumonia, urinary tract infections, infections of the leg, and chest wounds) than their counterparts who were under better glycemic control. In a prospective study of 2467 diabetic cardiac surgery patients, continuous insulin infusion induced a significant decrease in perioperative blood glucose levels (less than 200 mg/dL), which led to a significant reduction in the incidence of sternal wound infection to 0.8% versus 2.0% in patients with hyperglycemia.[26] All these studies concluded that perioperative hyperglycemia is an independent risk factor for the development of infectious complications after surgery.[27]

Perioperative Hyperglycemia and Outcome after Cardiovascular Surgery

Cardiac surgery introduces unique challenges to the maintenance of perioperative euglycemia. Without careful management during cardiopulmonary bypass (CPB), postoperative serum glucose concentrations often become elevated far above the normal range, even in nondiabetic patients. The multifactorial surgical stress response previously described tends to be profound during cardiovascular surgery, where acute glucose intolerance in the

form of insulin suppression, stress hormone-induced gluconeogenesis, and impaired glucose excretion resulting from enhanced renal tubular resorption are all encountered.[28,29] This is further aggravated by insulin resistance persisting after CPB[30] and resulting in carbohydrate metabolism being restricted in myocardial and peripheral musculature.

Investigations have consistently reaffirmed evidence that the resulting hyperglycemia is an independent risk factor that predicts an increase in short-term and long-term morbidity and mortality rates after cardiovascular surgery. Many retrospective analyses conducted in patients undergoing coronary artery surgery indicated that increased blood glucose concentration was an important predictor of morbidity and mortality. These results were confirmed by a prospective randomized clinical trial of critically ill patients (63% cardiac surgical patients) admitted to a surgical intensive care unit (ICU) who received intensive treatment with intravenous insulin to control blood glucose concentrations between 80 and 110 mg/dL, who were compared with conventionally treated patients who received insulin only if blood glucose exceeded 215 mg/dL. Aggressively treated patients with a prolonged length of stay in the ICU demonstrated significant decreases in morbidity and mortality rates.

In a single-center observational study of 1157 CABG surgery patients older than 75 years of age, one significant predictor of postoperative mortality was postoperative plasma glucose greater than 300 mg/dL.[31] The evidence further suggests that hyperglycemic damage during cardiovascular surgery can sometimes occur at glucose concentrations that are not much higher than the normal range.

The detriment of hyperglycemia in the cardiovascular surgical patient is related to the cerebral ischemia encountered during these surgeries, where hyperglycemia was proven to further exacerbate neurologic injury. There appear to be several different mechanisms by which hyperglycemia can give rise to increased neuronal injury in the presence of cerebral ischemia,[32] including intracellular lactic acidosis caused by anaerobic glycolysis[33] and microvascular dysregulation.[34] Furthermore, decreased glutamine transport resulting in endothelial swelling, and microvascular plugging[35] and hemorrhagic transformation of ischemic infarcts[36] can also be factors. Finally, significant reduction in blood-brain barrier transport and in regional cerebral blood flow demonstrated with hyperglycemia could further exacerbate neuronal injury in the presence of ischemia.[37]

Glycemic Control in the Setting of Acute Myocardial Infarction

The acute myocardial ischemia that usually precedes emergent revascularization has also been shown to be independently associated with the stress response. In patients with acute MI, elevated glucose levels are a predictor of mortality in patients with and without diabetes.[38,39] Furthermore, hyperglycemia was associated with larger infarct size in patients without a prior history of diabetes who were being treated with perfusion therapy for ST-segment elevation MI.[40] A meta-regression analysis of data published in 20 studies of more than

95,000 patients showed a similar relationship between fasting blood glucose concentration and the relative risk of sustaining a cardiovascular event.[41]

Once more, not only was hyperglycemia associated with unfavorable outcome in the setting of acute MI, but treatments to maintain euglycemia in acute coronary syndromes proved to be beneficial to patient outcome. Glycemic control interventions were related to the outcome after acute myocardial infarction in diabetic patients. The Diabetes and Insulin-Glucose Infusion in Acute Myocardial Infarction (DIGAMI) study addressed prognostic factors and the effect of conventional or aggressive treatment of hyperglycemia initiated within 24 hours of MI on mortality rate in patients with diabetes.[42] The study found that intensive insulin treatment during MI reduces the deleterious effect of poor metabolic control on the subsequent incidence of death.

Perioperative Hyperglycemia and the Outcome of Critically Ill Patients

Hyperglycemia associated with insulin resistance is common in critically ill patients, even if they have not previously had diabetes.[43-45] It has been reported that pronounced hyperglycemia might lead to complications in such patients.[46-48] For example, preoperative hyperglycemia was shown to increase the risk of renal failure (highest relative risk of 3.7) in critically ill patients in a prospective observational multicenter study of 2222 patients undergoing elective CABG surgery.[49]

Intensive insulin therapy to maintain blood glucose at or below 110 mg/dL was proven to reduce morbidity and mortality rates among critically ill patients after surgery, regardless of whether they had a history of diabetes. A large-scale prospective, randomized, controlled study was conducted on critically ill adults admitted to a surgical ICU to assess the effect of glycemic control on the outcome of such patients.[50] On admission, patients were randomly assigned to receive "intensive" insulin therapy (maintenance of blood glucose at a level between 80 and 110 mg/dL) or "conventional" treatment (infusion of insulin only if the blood glucose level exceeded 215 mg/dL and maintenance of glucose at a level between 180 and 200 mg/dL). Intensive insulin therapy reduced mortality rate during intensive care from 8% with conventional treatment to 4.6%. The benefit of intensive insulin therapy was attributable to its effect on mortality rate among patients who remained in the ICU for more than 5 days (20.3% versus 10.6% conventional versus intensive insulin therapy). The greatest reduction in mortality rate involved deaths that were due to multiple-organ failure with a proven septic focus. Intensive insulin therapy also reduced overall in-hospital mortality rate by 34%, bloodstream infections by 46%, acute renal failure requiring dialysis or hemofiltration by 41%, and critical-illness polyneuropathy by 44%. Patients receiving intensive therapy were less likely to require prolonged mechanical ventilation and intensive care.

Tight glycemic control in the medical ICU, similarly, showed improved outcome in patients who required a prolonged ICU stay (longer than 3 days). Results included reduced measures of morbidity (such as renal dysfunction and prolonged mechanical ventilation); however, mortality rate was not significantly reduced with intent to treat analysis of data (40% versus 37.3% in conventional compared with tight glycemic therapy). Surprisingly, among patients who had a short ICU stay (less than 3 days), mortality rate was higher in the tight glycemic therapy group (26.8% versus 18.8% in intensively and conventionally treated groups, respectively). After adjustment for baseline characteristics, including Acute Physiologic Assessment and Chronic Health Evaluation (APACHE 2) score, this difference was not statistically significant. The increased early mortality rate, albeit not statistically significant, will necessitate further investigations.

Perioperative Hyperglycemia and Neurologic Outcome after Brain Injury

The prognostic value of hyperglycemia as a reflection of the extent of brain damage has been elucidated in patients with cerebral infarction, intracerebral hemorrhage, subarachnoid hemorrhage, and traumatic head injury. A multivariate regression analysis showed a strong correlation between blood glucose (within 24 hours of a cerebrovascular accident) and outcome in 1259 patients with acute ischemic stroke and confirmed that hyperglycemia may worsen the clinical outcome in nonlacunar (atheroembolic, cardioembolic) stroke.[51] Hemorrhagic extension of ischemic stroke has also been strongly correlated both in frequency and extent with hyperglycemia in various clinical series, as well as in experimental studies.[52]

Hyperglycemia after subarachnoid hemorrhage proved to be associated with serious hospital sequelae, including increased ICU stay, increased mortality rate, and severe disability.[53] Hyperglycemia has also been shown to worsen neurologic outcome after traumatic brain injury,[54,55] where brain injury is associated with an acute sympatho-adrenomedullary response characterized by an increase in the blood levels of catecholamines. The increase in circulating catecholamines causes intracranial hypertension,[56] a hyperdynamic cardiovascular response,[57] increased brain oxygen requirements,[58] and a rise in serum glucose levels.[59]

AREAS OF UNCERTAINTY

A few areas in clinical hyperglycemia and its intervention need further research, including further elucidation of the mechanism of exacerbation of hyperglycemia, development of complications from hyperglycemia, and variables that improve on perioperative glycemic control.

1. Central mechanisms underlying exacerbation of hyperglycemia and its complications
   a. Counterregulatory hormones
   b. Decreased glucose utilization (insulin resistance)
   c. Role of inflammatory response (cytokines)
   d. Glycemic variability and increased free radical production

2. Improving glycemic control
   a. Refinement and standardization of insulin protocols and serum glucose monitoring
   b. Optimal glycemic targets for medical ICUs
   c. Role of various anesthetic regimens and agents on glycemic control
   d. Impact of intraoperative intensive insulin therapy on perioperative outcome

Although intensive glycemic control has been strongly advocated by many, some authors have argued that strict glycemic control may pose the risk of significant hypoglycemia in some patients.[1] The study by Chaney and colleagues[59a] documented that attempting to maintain normoglycemia during CPB with insulin may initiate postoperative hypoglycemia in nondiabetic patients. Moreover, the recommended ranges for safe glucose levels after surgery varied widely from one study to another, with the proposed threshold being sometimes as low as 100 mg/dL and other times as high as 200 mg/dL.

To date, there is no general consensus on the pathophysiologic mechanism whereby hyperglycemia increases the risk of perioperative infectious complications. Most authors agree that if the increased risk of postoperative infection in diabetic individuals is related to short-term effects of hyperglycemia, strict perioperative glycemic control might reduce this risk. On the other hand, many argue that if the risk is related indirectly to glycemic control via its long-term connection with microvascular disease, the disadvantages of strict glycemic control (i.e., increased risk of significant hypoglycemia, added costs related to monitoring) might outweigh any potential benefits.

GUIDELINES

Although clinical trials demonstrated the deleterious effects of perioperative hyperglycemia, the ideal target for and cardiovascular benefit of intraoperative and postoperative glycemic control are not entirely clear. Results of regression analyses suggest that blood glucose concentrations controlled to less than 150 mg/dL in the perioperative period may improve outcome and minimize the risk of severe hypoglycemia in anesthetized patients.

The American College of Endocrinology recently published a position statement recommending that preprandial glucose concentration should be less than 110 mg/dL, with maximal glucose not to exceed 180 mg/dL in hospitalized patients, and that blood glucose concentration should be controlled to less than 110 mg/dL in the ICU.

The use of intravenous insulin therapy to maintain glycemic control in the perioperative period was recommended.

Guidelines for the perioperative care of patients with diabetes have recommended levels of glycemic control high enough to avoid hypoglycemia, but low enough to avoid excess catabolism, ketoacidosis, and hyperosmolarity.[60,61]

AUTHORS' RECOMMENDATIONS

For elective cases, preoperative preparation is the general preamble of practice. Diabetic patients should achieve adequate glycemic control preoperatively, where most favorable outcomes were associated with a preoperative glycosylated hemoglobin level of 7.4% or less.

A balanced approach of maintaining normoglycemia and intensive insulin therapy is probably warranted. Initially, it is important to attempt to establish normal blood glucose levels by prophylactic means:

- Avoid glucose-containing solutions.
- Minimize glucose load during cardiac surgery in CPB prime and cardioplegia solutions.
- Anticipate hyperglycemia associated with starting exogenous catecholamine infusions.

Blood glucose levels should have targeted control during the perioperative period, particularly in certain higher-risk patient populations, which include the following:

- Patients with diabetes mellitus
- Patients who are at high risk of myocardial ischemia
- Patients who undergo vascular surgical procedures
- Patients who undergo major or prolonged noncardiac surgical procedures
- Patients who are admitted to the ICU in the perioperative period
- Patients who have acute hyperglycemia postoperatively
- Patients who have neurosurgical procedures for traumatic brain injury

Most important, once insulin therapy is implemented, the key to minimizing the risk/benefit ratio of interventional therapy is frequent blood glucose monitoring.

REFERENCES

1. Centers for Disease Control and Prevention: *National diabetes fact sheet: General information and national estimates on diabetes in the United States.* Atlanta, US Dept of Health and Human Services, Centers for Disease Control and Prevention, 2003.
2. Engelgau MM, Geiss LS, Saaddine JB, et al: The evolving diabetes burden in the United States. *Ann Intern Med* 2004;140: 945-950.
3. Perioperative management of diabetic patients. Any changes for the better since 1985? *Anaesthesia* 1996;51:45-51.
4. Schade DS: Surgery and diabetes. *Med Clin North Am* 1988;72: 1531-1543.
5. Gandhi GY, Nuttall GA, Abel MD, Mullany CJ, Schaff HV, O'Brien PC, et al: Intensive intraoperative insulin therapy versus conventional glucose management during cardiac surgery—a randomized trial. *Ann Intern Med* 2007;146:233-243.
6. Lazar HL: Enhanced preservation of acutely ischemic myocardium and improved clinical outcomes using glucose-insulin-potassium (GIK) solutions. *Am J Cardiol* 1997;80:90A-93A.
7. Lazar HL, Chipkin SR, Fitzgerald CA, Bao Y, Cabral H, Apstein CS: Tight glycemic control in diabetic coronary artery bypass graft patients improves perioperative outcomes and decreases recurrent ischemic events. *Circulation* 2004;109:1497-1502.
8. Lell WA, Nielsen VG, McGiffin DC, Schmidt FEJ, Kirklin JK, Stanley AWJ: Glucose-insulin-potassium infusion for myocardial protection during off-pump coronary artery surgery. *Ann Thorac Surg* 2002;73:1246-1251.
9. Malmberg K, Ryden L, Wedel H, et al (DIGAMI 2 Investigators): Intense metabolic control by means of insulin in patients with diabetes mellitus and acute myocardial infarction (DIGAMI 2): Effects on mortality and morbidity. *Eur Heart J* 2005;26:650-661.

10. Mehta SR, Yusuf S, Diaz R, et al (CREATE-ECLA Trial Group Investigators): Effect of glucose-insulin-potassium infusion on mortality in patients with acute ST-segment elevation myocardial infarction: The CREATE-ECLEA randomized controlled trial. *JAMA* 2005;293:437-446.

11. Giddings AEB, Mangnall D, Rowlands BJ, Clark RG: Early changes due to operation in the insulin response to glucose. *Ann Surg* 1977;681-686.

12. Yki-Jarvinen H, Helve E, Koivisto VA: Hyperglycemia decreases glucose uptake in type I diabetes. *Diabetes* 1987;36:892-896.

13. Yaksh TL, Hammond DL: Peripheral and central substrates involved in the rostrad transmission of nociceptive information. *Pain* 1982;13:1-85.

14. Allison SP, Tomlin PI, Chamgerlain MJ: Some effects of anaesthesia and surgery on carbohydrate and fat metabolism. *Br J Anaesth* 1969;41:588-593.

15. Ichikawa Y, Kawagoe M, Nishikai M, Hoshida K, Homma M: Plasma corticotropin (ACTH), growth hormone (GH) and 11-OHCS (hydroxycorticosteroid) response during surgery. *J Lab Clin Med* 1971;33:481-487.

16. Newsome HH, Rose JC: The response of human adrenocorticotrophic hormone and growth hormone to surgical stress. *J Clin Endocrinol Metab* 1971;78:881-887.

17. McCowen KC, Malhotra A, Bistrian BR: Stress-induced hyperglycemia. *Crit Care Clin* 2001;17:107-124.

18. Chernow B, Alexander R, Smallridge RC, et al: Hormonal responses to graded surgical stress. *Arch Intern Med* 1987; 147:1273-1278.

19. Clarke RS: The hyperglycaemic response to different types of surgery and anaesthesia. *Br J Anaesth* 1970;42:45-53.

20. Goodson W, Hunt T: Studies of wound healing in experimental diabetes mellitus. *J Surg Res* 1977;22:221-227.

21. Yue DK, Swanson B, McLennan S, Marsh M, Spaliviero J, Delbridge L, et al: Abnormalities of granulation tissue and collagen formation in experimental diabetes, uraemia and malnutrition. *Diabetic Medicine* 1986;3(3):221-225.

22. Weringer EJ, Kelso JM, Tamai IY, Arquilla ER: Effects of insulin on wound healing in diabetic mice. *Acta Endocrinologica* 1982;99 (1):101-108.

23. Bokyo EJ, Lipsky BA: Infection and diabetes. In Harris MI, Cowie CC, Stern MP, Bokyo EJ, Reiber GE, Bennet PH, editors: *Diabetes in America*, ed 2. NIH pub no 95-1468. Washington, DC, US Government Printing Office, 1995, pp 485-499.

24. Pomposelli JJ, Baxter JK, Babineau TJ, Pomfret EA, Driscoll DF, Forse A, Bistrian BR: Early postoperative glucose control predicts nosocomial infection rate in diabetic patients. *J Parent Enteral Nutrition* 1998;22:77-81.

25. Zerr K, Furnary A, Grunkemeier G, Bookin S, Kanhere V, Starr A: Glucose control lowers the risk of wound infection in diabetes after open heart operations. *Ann Thorac Surg* 1997;63:356-361.

26. Furnary AP, Zerr KJ, Grunkemcier GL, Starr A: Continuous intravenous insulin infusion reduces the incidence of deep sternal wound infection in diabetic patients after cardiac surgical procedures. *Ann Thorac Surg* 67:352-360, 1999.

27. Golden SH, Peart-Vigilance C, Kao L, Brancati FL: Perioperative glycemic control and the risk of infectious complications in a cohort of adults with diabetes. *Diabetes Care* 1999;22(9): 1408-1413.

28. Werb MR, Zinman B, Teasdale SJ, et al: Hormonal and metabolic responses during coronary artery bypass surgery: Role of infused glucose. *J Clin Endocrinol Metab* 1989;69:1010-1018.

29. Braden H, Cheema-Dhadli S, Mazer CD, et al: Hyperglycemia during normothermic cardiopulmonary bypass: The role of the kidney. *Ann Thorac Surg* 1998;65:1588-1593.

30. Svensson S, Ekroth R, Milocco I, et al: Glucose and lactate balances in heart and leg after coronary surgery: Influence of insulin infusion. *Scand J Thorac Cardiovasc Surg* 1989;23:145-150.

31. Rady MY, Ryan T, Starr NJ: Perioperative determinants of morbidity and mortality in elderly patients undergoing cardiac surgery. Crit Care Med 1998;26:225-235.

32. Wass CT, Lanier WL: Glucose modulation of ischemic brain injury: Review and clinical recommendations. *Mayo Clinic Proc* 1996;71:801-812.

33. Davies MG, Hagen PO: Alterations in venous endothelial cell and smooth muscle cell relaxation induced by high glucose concentrations can be prevented by aminoguanidinie. *J Surg Res* 1996;63:474-479.,

34. Li PA, Siesjo BK: Role of hyperglycaemia-related acidosis in ischaemic brain damage. *Acta Physiol Scand* 1997;161:567-580.

35. Kawai N, Stummer W, Ennis SR, et al: Blood-brain barrier glutamine transport during normoglycemic and hyperglycemic focal cerebral ischemia. *J Cereb Blood Flow Metab* 1999;19:79-86.

36. Broderiick JP, Hagen T, Brott T, Tomsick T: Hyperglycemia and hemorrhagic transformations of cerebral infarcts. *Stroke* 1995;26:484-487.

37. Kawai N, Keep RF, Betz Al, Nagao S: Hyperglycemia induces progressive changes in the cerebral micro-vasculature and blood-brain barrier transport during focal cerebral ischemia. *Acta Neurochir* 1998;71:219-221.

38. Sala J, Masia R, Gonzalez de Molina FJ, et al (REGICOR Investigators): Short-term mortality of myocardial infarction patients with diabetes or hyperglycaemia during admission. *J Epidemiol Community Health* 2002;56:707-712.

39. Kosiborod M, Rathore SS, Inzucchi SE, et al Admission glucose and mortality in elderly patients hospitalized with acute myocardial infarction: Implications for patients with and without recognized diabetes. *Circulation* 2005;111:3078-3086.

40. Timmer JR, van der Horst IC, Ottervanger JP, et al (Zwolle Myocardial Infarction Study Group): Prognostic value of admission glucose in non-diabetic patients with myocardial infarction. *Am Heart J* 2004;148:399-404.

41. Coutinho M, Gerstein HC, Wang Y, Yusaf S: The relationship between glucose and incident cardiovascular events: A meta-regression analysis of published data from 20 studies of 95,738 individuals followed for 12.4 years. *Diabetes Care* 1999;22: 233-240.

42. Malmberg K, Norhammar A, Wedel H, Ryden L: Glycometabolic state at admission: Important risk marker in mortality in conventionally treated patients with diabetes mellitus and acute myocardial infarction: Long-term results from the DIGAMI Study. *Circulation* 1999;99:2626-2632.

43. Wolfe RR, Allsop JR, Burke JE: Glucose metabolism in man: Responses to intravenous glucose infusion. *Metabolism* 1979;28:210-220.

44. Wolfe RR, Herndon DN, Jahoor P, NEyoshi H, Wolfe M: Effect of severe burn injury on substrate cycling by glucose and fatty acids. *N Engl J Med* 1987;317:403-408.

45. Krinsley S: Effect of intensive glucose management protocol on the mortality of critically ill adult patients. *Mayo Clin Proc* 2004;79:992-1000.

46. Mizock RA: Alterations in carbohydrate metabolism during stress: A review of the literature. *Am J Med* 1995;98:75-84.

47. McCowen KC, Malhotra A, Bistrian BR: Stress-induced hyperglycemia. *Crit Care Clin* 2001;17:107-124.

48. Scott JF, Robinson GM, French JM, O'Connell JE, Alberti KG, Gray CS: Glucose potassium insulin infusions in the treatment of acute stroke patients with mild to moderate hyperglycemia: The Glucose Insulin in Stroke Trial (GIST). *Stroke* 1999;30: 793-799.

49. Mangano CM, Diamondstone LS, Ramsay JG, et al: Renal dysfunction after myocardial revascularization: Risk factors, adverse outcomes, and hospital resource utilization. The Multi-center Study of Perioperative lschemia Research Group. *Ann Intern Med* 1998;128:194-203.

50. Van den Berghe G, Wouters P, Weekers F, et al: Intensive insulin therapy in critically ill patients. *N Engl J Med* 2001;345:1359-1367.

51. Bruno A, Biller J, Adams HP Jr, et al: Acute blood glucose level and outcome from ischemic stroke: Trial of ORG 10172 in Acute Stroke Treatment (TOAST) investigators. *Neurology* 1999;52:280-284.

52. de Courten-Meyers G, Meyers Re, Schoofield L: Hyperglycemia enlarges infarct size in cerebrovascular occlusion in cats. *Stroke* 1988;19:623-630.

53. Rontera J, Fernandez A, Claassen J, Schmidt M, Schumacher C, Wartenberg K, et al: Hyperglycemia after SAH. Predictors, associated complications, and impact on outcome. *Stroke* 2006; 37:1-6.

54. Jeremitsky E, Omert LA, Dunham CM, Wilberger J, Rodriguez A: The impact of hyperglycemia on patients with severe brain injury. *J Trauma* 2005;58:47-50.

55. Carlson AP, Schermer CR, Lu SW: Retrospective evaluation of anemia and transfusion in traumatic brain injury. *J Trauma* 2006;61(3):567-571.
56. Langfitt TW, Weinstein JD, Kassell NF: Cerebral vasomotor paralysis produced by intracranial hypertension. *Neurology* 1965;15:622-641.
57. Clifton GL, Ziegler MG, Grossman RG: Circulating catecholamines and sympathetic activity after head injury. *Neurosurgery* 1981;8:10-13.
58. Rosner MJ, Newsome HH, Becker DP: Mechanical brain injury: The sympathoadrenal response. *J Neurosurg* 1984;61:76-86.
59. De Salles AAF, Muizelaar JP, Young HF: Hyperglycemia, cerebrospinal fluid lactic acidosis, and cerebral blood flow in severely head-injured patients. *Neurosurgery* 1987;21:45-50.
59a. Chaney MA, Nikolov MP, Blakeman BP, Bakhos M. Attempting to maintain normoglycemia during cardiopulmonary bypass with insulin may initiate postoperative hypoglycemia. *Anesth Analg* 1999;89:1091-1095.
60. Hirsch I, Paauw D: Inpatient management of adults with diabetes. *Diabetes Care* 1995;18:870-878.
61. Alberti KGMM: Diabetes and surgery. In Porte D Jr, Sherwin R, editors: *Ellenberg and Rifkin's diabetes mellitus*, ed 5. Stamford, CT, Appleton & Lange, 1997, pp 875-878.

29 When Should Perioperative Glucocorticoid Replacement Be Administered?

Diane E. Head, MD; Aaron Joffe, DO; and Douglas B. Coursin, MD

Glucocorticoids were introduced into clinical practice in 1949 with the release of a purified preparation known as cortisone. The treatment was revolutionary for patients suffering from adrenal insufficiency (AI) and for the management of other acute and chronic diseases such as rheumatoid arthritis and systemic lupus erythematosus. Shortly after the introduction of cortisone, two case reports were published describing surgical patients on chronic glucocorticoid treatment whose treatment was held in the perioperative period. The first involved a 34-year-old man who had cortisone therapy (25 mg twice daily) discontinued 48 hours before surgery. His subsequent death was attributed to acute AI caused by abrupt withdrawal of glucocorticoids. However, there were extenuating circumstances that may have contributed to his death.[1,2] The second case involved a 20-year-old woman who had been taking 62.5 to 100 mg of cortisone daily for approximately 4 months. She died less than 6 hours after surgery, with autopsy findings confirming bilateral adrenal hemorrhages and cortical atrophy indicative of AI.[2,3] From these case reports came the conventional wisdom to supplement patients receiving exogenous steroids with large "stress doses" throughout the perioperative period. This practice has come under scrutiny over the past decade because of questions about efficacy and concern about side effects from excessive doses.

Endogenous glucocorticoids are cholesterol derivatives produced in the zona fasciculata of the adrenal cortex. Their release is controlled by a feedback mechanism known as the hypothalamic-pituitary-adrenal (HPA) axis. Corticotropin-releasing hormone (CRH), released by the hypothalamus, acts on the pituitary gland to initiate the production of adrenocorticotropic hormone (ACTH or corticotropin). ACTH then stimulates the adrenal glands to produce cortisol, which acts as negative feedback for CRH in the hypothalamus. Glucocorticoids are integral factors in normal cellular homeostasis and metabolism. Cortisol potentiates production of catecholamines and regulates the synthesis, responsiveness, coupling, and regulation of beta-adrenergic receptors. Glucocorticoids also regulate the normal metabolism of carbohydrates, proteins, and lipids. Glucocorticoid hormones modulate cardiovascular function and wound healing and have numerous other important metabolic functions.[4-6]

Daily endogenous glucocorticoid secretion is estimated to be between 5 and 10 mg/m². This corresponds to 5 to 7 mg/day of oral prednisone or 20 to 30 mg/day of hydrocortisone. Cortisol synthesis can increase under conditions of stress to 100 mg/m²/day.[7-16]

Deficiencies of glucocorticoid production result in AI, which can be classified as a primary, secondary, or tertiary process with acute and chronic forms (Table 29-1). Primary AI occurs in patients who have destruction of greater than 90% of the adrenal glands by hemorrhage, tumor, infection, or an inflammatory process. This results in deficient production of both mineralocorticoids and glucocorticoids. Primary AI is relatively rare, most often resulting from autoimmune destruction of the adrenal glands. In developing regions of the world, it is most commonly due to tuberculous destruction of the adrenals. Secondary AI is also relatively uncommon and results from insufficient production of ACTH resulting from destruction or dysfunction of the pituitary gland itself.[7,17]

Tertiary, or iatrogenic, AI is the most commonly encountered type. Tertiary AI results from the suppression of the HPA axis over time, as a result of the administration of exogenous glucocorticoids. Chronic ACTH suppression from steroid treatment leads to adrenal atrophy. This can result in a potentially harmful situation if exogenous glucocorticoids are discontinued, because the adrenals can no longer produce adequate cortisol.[18] Many trials have evaluated the need for glucocorticoids to protect patients from acute AI in the perioperative period. The use of steroids to modulate life-threatening illnesses such as sepsis and the acute respiratory distress syndrome (ARDS) in the critically ill is a common focus of investigation.[6]

In this chapter, evidence supporting the need for perioperative glucocorticoid supplementation is reviewed along with appropriate dosing of glucocorticoids to protect patients from acute, stress-induced AI. Current evidence-based indications for steroid treatment in severe sepsis, ARDS, meningitis, acute spinal cord injury, and traumatic brain injury are also reviewed.

EVIDENCE FOR PERIOPERATIVE STEROID REPLACEMENT

Most of the clinical data on adrenal replacement therapy in the perioperative period are based on case series or drawn from clinical experience. Glucocorticoid replacement has often been done on an empiric basis with little regard to

Table 29-1	Characteristics of Adrenal Insufficiency (AI)		
Type	**Features**	**Incidence**	**Etiologies**
Primary	ACTH independent Adrenal gland dysfunction, destruction, or replacement; requires >90% loss of adrenal tissue Loss of mineralocorticoid and glucocorticoid production Increased ACTH production Requires lifetime therapy	Prevalence: 40-110 cases/million Incidence: 6 cases/million per year	Autoimmune (70%-90% of U.S. cases) frequently associated with a polyglandular deficiency syndrome HIV infection is most common infectious cause in the United States AI develops in 30% of patients with advanced AIDS Tuberculosis is most common infectious cause worldwide Inflammation Cancer (breast, lung, melanoma most common) Acute infectious Addisonian crisis (meningococcemia, purpua fulminans, stress, hemorrhage, shock)
Secondary	ACTH dependent Signs and symptoms usually caused by loss of glucocorticoid function Usually have intact mineralocorticoid function Rarely hypovolemic, more commonly hypoglycemic	Uncommon	Decreased or absent ACTH (may be panhypopituitary or anterior pituitary dysfunction) Pituitary depression, dysfunction/damage Tumor, postpartum Hypothalamic failure or dysfunction
Tertiary	Caused by hypothalamic/pituitary depression or absence	Most common form	Usually from iatrogenic corticosteroid therapy and suppression of the HPA axis

From Coursin DB, Wood KE: *JAMA* 2002;287:236-240; Orth DS, Kovas J: In Wilson JD, Foster DW, et al: *Williams textbook of endocrinology*, ed 9, Philadelphia, WB Saunders, 1998; Oelkers W: *N Engl J Med* 1996;335:1206-1212.
ACTH, adrenocorticotropic hormone (corticotropin); *AIDS,* acquired immunodeficiency syndrome; *HIV,* human immunodefiency virus; *HPA axis,* hypothalamic-pituitary-adrenal axis.

the duration of dosing, total daily dose, stress of the surgery, or the ability to evaluate the HPA axis and cortisol production. In 1953 Lewis and colleagues[3] proposed the first treatment guidelines for patients taking exogenous glucocorticoids. These guidelines, which recommended large perioperative increases in glucocorticoids, became the standard of therapy despite being based on limited anecdotal experience. There are few well-designed, prospective, randomized, blinded clinical trials investigating optimal perioperative steroid supplementation. As well, future studies investigating optimal perioperative steroid use are unlikely because of cost, logistical problems, and enrollment limitations.

EVIDENCE THAT SURGERY-INDUCED ACUTE ADRENAL INSUFFICIENCY IS HARMFUL

The case reports from Fraser and colleagues[1] and Lewis and colleagues[3] were sufficient to convince the medical community that acute AI from perioperative glucocorticoid withdrawal had the potential to cause serious morbidity and mortality risks. In 1976 Kehlet[19] produced an extensive review of 57 case reports from 1952 to 1973 documenting perioperative shock or death in patients taking glucocorticoids. In all cases, adverse outcomes were suspected to be secondary to stress-induced AI. The interval between surgery and shock or death ranged from preoperatively to 48 hours postoperatively. Interestingly, only 3 cases out of the 57 displayed hypotension and low plasma cortisol levels to suggest acute AI. The remainder of the cases were inconclusive or had no evidence to link the outcomes to AI.[19]

In contrast, two large studies by Mohler and colleagues[20] and Alford and colleagues[21] support the rarity of acute AI secondary to inadequate perioperative glucocorticoid coverage. Mohler and colleagues[20] performed a retrospective review of 6947 urologic procedures in glucocorticoid-treated patients. Only one case of perioperative AI was identified (0.01% of patients).[20,22] Alford and colleagues[21] performed a similar review of 4346 cardiothoracic surgeries and confirmed only 5 cases of AI (0.1% of patients). These reviews support the fact that surgically induced AI can occur, though it is a relatively rare occurrence.

One group of patients that may deserve special consideration is elderly surgical patients. To determine the incidence and outcome of AI in elderly patients having high-risk surgery, Rivers and colleagues[23] performed a prospective, observational case study. One hundred four adult patients who required vasopressor therapy postoperatively despite adequate volume resuscitation received a cosyntropin (synthetic ACTH) stimulation test with plasma cortisol measurements at 30 and 60 minutes. Empiric hydrocortisone (100 mg intravenously [IV] for three doses) was given at the discretion of the primary team. Adrenal dysfunction (defined as serum cortisol less than 20 mg/dL with change in cortisol of less than 9 mg/dL after ACTH) or functional hypoadrenalism (serum cortisol less than 30 mg/dL with change in cortisol of less than 9 mg/dL after ACTH) was found in 32.7% of patients. Mortality rate was significantly lower in the hydrocortisone-treated patients with AI (21% versus 45%, p <0.01). This incidence of relative AI is higher than would be expected for both the general surgical population and for those on chronic steroid treatment.

WHICH PATIENTS SHOULD BE TREATED?

For many years, surgical patients on glucocorticoids were placed on a standardized "set" dose of supplementary steroid throughout the perioperative period. This method eventually came under question because of the deleterious effects of large doses of steroids, including poor wound healing, inadequate glucose control, fluid retention, hypertension, electrolyte imbalances, immunosuppression, gastrointestinal bleeding, and untoward psychologic effects.[2] There was a call for a replacement regimen that would approximate the duration and magnitude of the normal surgical stress response while minimizing excess steroid exposure and avoiding untoward side effects.

In a 1994 review, Salem and colleagues[8] concluded as follows:

1. Clinicians need to replace glucocorticoids only in an amount equivalent to the normal physiologic response to surgical stress,[24-26]
2. The risk of anesthetizing and operating on unsupplemented glucocorticoid treated patients (prolonged use preoperatively, but none given intraoperatively) is dependent on the duration and severity of the surgery.[8]

They further recommended that the amount and duration of the steroid therapy take into account the preoperative dose and duration of glucocorticoid treatment.[8]

WHAT IS THE NORMAL RESPONSE TO SURGICAL STRESS?

In the work of Salem and colleagues,[8] seven prospective analyses from 1957 to 1975 examining cortisol secretion after major surgery were reviewed. The combined number of subjects in all of the investigations was 40. None of the patients in the studies were adrenally insufficient or taking glucocorticoids. The range of 24-hour cortisol secretion was wide, varying from 60 mg/24 hours to 310 mg/24 hours. In 1973 Kehlet and Binder[12] found a cortisol secretion rate of 10 mg/hr immediately postoperatively, which decreased to 5 mg/hr by 24 hours following surgery. Wise and colleagues' work[11] in 1972 found 24-hour cortisol secretion to be only 60 mg.[8-15] Nevertheless, it is generally accepted that most healthy, non–steroid-dependent patients will secrete somewhere between 75 and 150 mg of cortisol in the first 24 hours after major surgery or up to 100 mg/m.[2,7,27]

INTEGRITY OF THE HYPOTHALAMIC-PITUITARY-ADRENAL AXIS IN PATIENTS TAKING CHRONIC STEROIDS

Several studies have confirmed that patients on small doses of steroids have normal responses to HPA testing.

La Rochelle and colleagues[28] prospectively observed the integrity of the HPA axis in patients receiving chronic low-dose prednisone. They selected 50 steroid-dependent patients receiving no more than 10 mg/day of prednisone for a mean duration of 41 months. The patients were then given a rapid cosyntropin stimulation test with 250 mcg of cosyntropin. All the patients receiving less than 5 mg/day had a normal cortisol response to cosyntropin. Those receiving between 5.5 and 6.8 mg/day displayed an intermediate response, and those with means above 6.8 mg/day displayed a suppressed response to ACTH stimulation.

In 1995 Friedman and colleagues[29] prospectively evaluated 28 patients on chronic glucocorticoid therapy undergoing a total of 35 major orthopedic surgeries, including total hip and knee replacements. The mean dose of prednisone was 10 mg/day with a mean duration of therapy of 7 years. No perioperative stress doses of steroids were administered, though baseline therapy was continued. Patients were observed for changes in blood pressure, fever, serum electrolytes, and other clinical variables. In addition, 24-hour urinary-free cortisol was measured to identify normal levels and increases reflecting production of endogenous glucocorticoids. Despite the lack of "stress"-dose corticosteroids, there were no significant changes in clinical parameters indicative of perioperative glucocorticoid deficiency. In addition, biochemical markers revealed a normal endogenous response to stress despite chronic steroid use.

In 1973 Kehlet and Binder[16] performed a prospective case-control study to determine if patients on chronic glucocorticoid therapy could mount a physiologic response to major surgery if steroids were discontinued perioperatively. With 14 non–steroid-dependent patients undergoing surgery as controls, they followed 74 patients on long-term glucocorticoid therapy undergoing major surgery (prednisone dose 5 to 80 mg/day) and 30 steroid-dependent patients undergoing minor surgery (prednisone dose 5 to 30 mg/day). Glucocorticoids were stopped 36 hours preoperatively and restarted 24 hours postoperatively. Plasma cortisol levels were measured for the first 24 hours postoperatively. Approximately 30% of the glucocorticoid-treated patients exhibited a blunted adrenocortical response to surgery, but only one patient showed any clinical signs or symptoms of AI. Interestingly, the majority of the controls in the minor surgery category showed little or no cortisol response to surgery. The researchers concluded that impaired adrenal responses were more prevalent in patients taking higher doses and for those taking steroids for longer durations. Patients who received more than 12.5 mg of prednisone for more than 6 months, more than 10 mg of prednisone for more than 2 years, or more than 7.5 mg of prednisone for more than 5 years all showed an impaired adrenocortical response. The one patient who was symptomatic had no detectable plasma cortisol, but was treated without resultant morbidity. From this study, it can be hypothesized that even an impaired ACTH response may be somewhat protective and that dose and duration of steroid therapy influence cortisol response to stress.

Kenyon and Albertson[30] performed a prospective study on 40 patients taking prednisone (doses from

5 to 10 mg/day) who were admitted to the hospital for illness, metabolic abnormalities, or surgery. No stress-dose steroids were given at any time during hospitalization. Over the first 36 hours the authors measured serum cortisol, 24-hour urine cortisol, and ACTH. Once the patients' clinical condition improved, a cosyntropin stimulation test (250 mcg) was repeated. Although the response to the cosyntropin stimulation test was blunted in 63% of the subjects, 97% had normal or increased urinary cortisol concentrations. This implies that despite chronic steroid treatment, adrenal function and endogenous glucocorticoid production were sufficient to meet the stress of illness or surgery.[8,30]

DURATION AND SEVERITY—ADAPTING THE REGIMENS

The routine use of one-dose-fits-all steroid replacement in surgical patients came into question in 1975 when Kehlet suggested that procedures be divided into "major" and "minor" categories. For major surgeries (intrathoracic, major vascular, or major abdominal operations), the recommendation was for hydrocortisone 25 mg IV at induction, followed by hydrocortisone 100 mg IV every 24 hours until the patient was able to resume oral steroid therapy. The goal of this approach was to adequately replace the increased cortisol requirements of 75 to 150 mg in the first 24 hours.[7,16] For minor surgeries (surgeries taking less than 1 hour and those performed under local anesthetic), Kehlet suggested hydrocortisone 25 mg IV at the start of surgery, with oral therapy resuming postoperatively.[27] This recommendation was based on a study showing that normal subjects often do not mount a stress response to minor surgery and at most secrete 50 mg/day of cortisol.[16]

In 1978 Gran and Pahle[31] recommended depot-betamethasone acetate/phosphate as a single intramuscular (IM) injection in perioperative patients receiving glucocorticoids. In a prospective cohort study on 1461 surgical patients on chronic steroid therapy, patients received depot-betamethasone before surgery, 2 mg for major procedures and 1 mg for minor procedures. There were no reports of AI, delayed healing, or gastrointestinal bleeding. The authors contend that ease of administration is a major benefit of this regimen.

Salem and colleagues[8] advised that perioperative supplementation should be individualized and based on prior steroid dose, duration, and degree of anticipated surgical stress. For minor surgeries, 25 mg hydrocortisone or equivalent dose (oral prednisone or a parenteral equivalent) was suggested, with resumption of the chronic dose the day after surgery. For procedures of perceived moderate stress, such as an open cholecystectomy or segmental colon resection, 50 to 75 mg/day of hydrocortisone equivalent oral or parenteral) with a rapid taper over 1 to 2 days was recommended. For major surgery, such as cardiac surgery involving bypass, a target of 100 to 150 mg of hydrocortisone equivalent per day with a rapid taper over 2 to 3 days was advised (see Table 29-3 later in this chapter).

AREAS OF EVOLVING INTEREST AND ONGOING CONTROVERSY

There are several areas of specific interest in the therapeutic administration of glucocorticoids in critically ill patients. These include treatment of patients suffering from severe sepsis and septic shock, ARDS, meningitis, traumatic brain injury (TBI), and acute spinal cord injury (SCI). The use of etomidate in critically ill patients, a topic of renewed interest, is also reviewed.

Severe Sepsis and Septic Shock

Several large prospective studies performed in the 1970s and 1980s using supraphysiologic doses of corticosteroids (e.g., 30 mg/kg methylprednisolone) up to several times per day did not show a survival benefit in patients with septic shock. In some instances morbidity was increased because of secondary infectious complications.[32-37] In recent years, however, there has been renewed interest in low- to moderate-dose ("physiologic") glucocorticoids in the treatment of sepsis. Annane and colleagues[38] reported a prospective, randomized, placebo-controlled trial (RCT) of low-dose corticosteroids in septic shock. In this investigation, 300 patients with septic shock refractory to fluid resuscitation and vasopressors were randomized to receive hydrocortisone 50 mg IV every 6 hours plus oral fludrocortisone 50 mcg daily for 7 days versus placebo. All underwent cosyntropin stimulation testing. In the 229 patients who were nonresponders to ACTH testing (76%), there was a significant reduction in the risk of death in the steroid versus placebo group (53% versus 63%, $p = 0.02$). In addition, the duration of vasopressor therapy was significantly shorter in patients treated with steroids. There were no significant differences in adverse events between groups. This influential study led to renewed interest and widespread clinical use of physiologic supplementation ($\leq$300 mg/day of hydrocortisone or its equivalent) of glucocorticoids in the treatment of septic shock and sepsis-induced hypotension.

In contrast, the recently reported 499-patient Corticosteroid Therapy of Septic Shock (CORTICUS) trial reported no benefit of corticosteroid supplementation on overall survival or reversal of shock.[39] The largest multicenter RCT to date, patients with septic shock unresponsive to fluids and vasopressors were randomized to receive steroids (hydrocortisone 50 mcg every 6 hours for 5 days followed by a 6-day taper) or placebo. All underwent cosyntropin stimulation testing before treatment. In a departure from the study by Annane, there was no difference in mortality rate between the hydrocortisone and placebo groups in those unresponsive to cosyntropin stimulation. In patients whose shock was reversible, reversal occurred more quickly in the hydrocortisone group, though there were more superinfections in the treatment arm. Other side effects noted were hyperglycemia and hypernatremia.

Evidence on steroids in the treatment of sepsis is continually evolving. The most recent 2008 Surviving Sepsis Campaign international guidelines for the management of severe sepsis and septic shock recommend that stress-dose steroid therapy only be given after conventional treatment with fluids and vasopressors has failed to restore adequate perfusion. The guidelines also suggest that cosyntropin stimulation testing not be used to identify those with septic shock who will receive hydrocortisone treatment.[40]

Acute Respiratory Distress Syndrome

Corticosteroids, in doses of 1 mg/kg/day methylprednisolone or equivalent, have been reported to lead to improvement in clearing lung inflammation and lung physiologic parameters.[41] A single-center randomized trial involving 24 patients in the fibroproliferative phase ($\geq$7 days from onset) of ARDS reported improved lung function and survival with moderate-dose, prolonged corticosteroid administration.[42]

However, the ARDSnet Clinical Trial Group study, a 180-patient multicenter RCT of steroids in persistent ARDS, did not report a mortality benefit with steroid treatment.[43] In this study, methylprednisolone (2 mg/kg for one dose, then 0.5 mg/kg every 6 hours for 14 days with an extended taper), was associated with reductions in shock symptoms and ventilator days, improved respiratory system compliance, and reduction in need for vasopressor therapy, but not improved survival. In addition, significantly increased 60- and 180-day mortality rates were identified in steroid-treated patients enrolled greater than 14 days after disease onset. Infectious complications were not increased, but the incidence of neuromuscular weakness was higher in the methylprednisolone-treated patients.

A recently published prospective RCT that administered methylprednisolone by continuous infusion in 91 patients with early ARDS (onset $\leq$72 hours) reported improvements in lung function and extrapulmonary organ function, and reductions in both duration of mechanical ventilation and intensive care unit (ICU) length of stay.[44] It should be noted that strict infection surveillance, tight glucose control, and avoidance of neuromuscular blocking drugs were integral parts of the protocol.

Given the inconsistencies in clinical evidence, the precise role of corticosteroids in ARDS remains elusive and requires further study with multicenter RCTs.

Meningitis, Traumatic Brain Injury, and Acute Spinal Cord Injury

One recent RCT and a systematic review indicate that dexamethasone, administered in conjunction with the first antibiotic dose, significantly reduces mortality rate, severe hearing loss, and neurologic sequelae in adults with community-acquired bacterial meningitis.[45,46]

Despite a significant incidence of hypoadrenalism soon after TBI (25%), there is strong evidence against routine corticosteroid treatment in head-injured patients.[47] In a large multicenter study the risk of death from all causes within 14 days was higher in those patients with TBI who received a 48-hour infusion of corticosteroids when compared with those administered placebo. Furthermore, at 6 months, the relative risk of death or severe disability favored the placebo group.[48,49]

The treatment of acute SCI with steroids is controversial. Evidence from the National Acute Spinal Cord Injury Studies (NASCIS) in the early 1990s supported high-dose methylprednisolone (30 mg/kg with infusion of 5.4 mg/kg/hr for 24 hours) following acute SCI, ideally administered within 8 hours of injury.[50] Based on these initial studies, the treatment was widely adopted and became a standard of care. However, there has been much criticism of the study design and statistical analysis, and other conflicting clinical evidence has emerged, causing some clinicians to abandon use because of an unacceptable risk/benefit ratio.[51-53] A Cochrane review supports methylprednisolone use for SCI, as does a recent retrospective review on the use of steroids in incomplete acute cervical SCI.[54,55] In an investigation by Leypold and colleagues[56] comparing acute SCI lesions by MRI characteristics, patients who received methylprednisolone had significantly less intramedullary spinal cord hemorrhage than those who were not treated.

Indicative of the situation is a recent survey of 305 spine surgeons that found 90% would initiate methylprednisolone, especially if within the 8-hour window. Importantly, many cited institutional protocols and medicolegal reasons as justification for use; only 24% used steroid treatment because of a belief in improved outcomes.[57] An area of ongoing debate, high-dose methylprednisolone may be effective in promoting some degree of neurologic improvement if given early following injury, though more well-designed RCTs are necessary.

Etomidate

There has been increased interest recently in the use of the induction agent etomidate in critically ill patients, in particular to facilitate intubation. An imidazole derivative, etomidate is often a first-line agent for endotracheal intubation or procedural sedation in the critically ill because of its minimal hemodynamic side effects. However, it is known to inhibit the 11β-hydroxylase enzyme responsible for converting 11β-deoxycortisol into cortisol within the adrenal gland. The potent suppression of adrenal steroidogenesis by etomidate was first described in 1984 by Wagner and White.[58] A more contemporary report confirms that AI, defined as an inadequate response to the administration of 250 mcg of cosyntropin, can last for 24 hours in children suffering meningococcal sepsis[59] and for up to 48 hours in critically ill adults.[60] However, a recent publication reported that neither clinical outcome nor therapy was affected when etomidate was used in critically ill patients.[61] The clinical relevance of the effect of etomidate on adrenal function remains open to debate. Until further evidence is available, some authors recommend etomidate be used judiciously in the critically ill, whereas others recommend discontinuing its use altogether, particularly in patients with severe sepsis or septic shock.

GUIDELINES

There are currently limited accepted guidelines on the perioperative use of a glucocorticoid replacement. An ongoing Cochrane analysis on perioperative steroid management for the adrenally insufficient patient is under way.[62]

AUTHORS' RECOMMENDATIONS

- Patients on chronic glucocorticoid therapy of more than 5 mg/day of prednisone or its equivalent (Table 29-2) should receive their daily therapeutic dose either orally or parenterally (especially if there is question of enteral absorption) before a procedure or during an illness. A graduated supplementation schedule of the patient's basic glucocorticoid dose (as outlined in Table 29-3) is advocated for patients sustaining increasingly stressful procedures or illnesses. Supplemental doses should be tapered to baseline relatively quickly (within a day or so) depending on stress of surgery and illness, as well as patient response. Oral medications should be administered when the patient is able to ingest and absorb them. Patients with primary AI usually require both mineralocorticoid and glucocorticoid replacement unless the total hydrocortisone dose is in excess of 50 mg within 24 hours. Most patients with secondary or tertiary AI have intact aldosterone synthesis and usually only require glucocorticoid replacement. Rarely, if ever, do patients require greater than 200 mg/day of hydrocortisone or its equivalent for glucocorticoid replacement or mineralocorticoid supplementation therapy. Although perioperative adrenal crisis is rare, a physiologically based glucocorticoid replacement schedule appears to be efficacious in limiting untoward side effects and avoiding potential compromise secondary to acute AI. The relatively high rate of functional hypoadrenalism in septic patients and the elderly should be appreciated. These patients should receive physiologic perioperative steroid replacement as needed based on the clinical situation and random cortisol measurements.
- Routine use of corticosteroids in patients with septic shock or ARDS is not recommended, but should be used on a case-by-case basis weighing the absolute cortisol level in septic shock patients and the risk/benefit ratio in sepsis or ARDS. Cosyntropin stimulation is not recommended routinely in the evaluation of patients with septic shock.
- A short course of steroids is routinely recommended in the acute treatment of common causes of bacterial meningitis, particularly *Streptococcus pneumoniae*.
- Corticosteroid treatment for acute SCI is controversial, though generally is used if initiated within 8 hours of the injury. Methylprednisolone bolus within 8 hours of injury followed by a 24- to 48-hour infusion is advised when used.
- Steroids are not, however, recommended in the treatment of TBI.
- Etomidate is associated with transient inhibition of adrenal steroidogenesis and should be used judiciously in the critically ill patient.

Table 29-3   Guidelines for Adrenal Supplementation Therapy

Medical or Surgical Stress	Corticosteroid Dosage
MINOR	
Inguinal hernia repair	25 mg of hydrocortisone or 5 mg of methylprednisolone IV day of procedure only
Colonoscopy	
Mild febrile illness	
Mild-moderate nausea/vomiting	
Gastroenteritis	
MODERATE	
Open cholecystectomy	50-75 mg of hydrocortisone or 10-15 mg of methylprednisolone IV day of procedure
Hemicolectomy	
Significant febrile illness	Taper quickly over 1-2 days to usual dose
Pneumonia	
Severe gastroenteritis	
SEVERE	
Major cardiothoracic surgery	100-150 mg of hydrocortisone or 25-30 mg of methylprednisolone IV day of procedure
Whipple procedure	
Liver resection	Rapid taper to usual dose over next 1-2 days
Pancreatitis	

From Coursin DB, Wood KE: *JAMA* 2002;287:236-240.

Table 29-2   Comparative Steroid Potency (mg Basis)*

Steroid Preparation	Glucocorticoid Effect	Mineralocorticoid Effect	Biologic Half-Life (hr)	Formulation
Hydrocortisone	1	1	6-8	PO, IV, IM
Prednisone	4	0.1-0.2	18-36	PO
Methylprednisolone	5	0.1-0.2	18-36	IV
Dexamethasone	30	<0.1	36-54	PO, IV
Fludrocortisone	0	20	18-36	PO

IM, intramuscular; *IV,* intravenous; *NPO,* nil per os (nothing by mouth); *PO,* per os (by mouth).
*Intravenous supplementation is the preferred route for patients who are NPO, have unpredictable or poor absorption of medications, or have major stresses or critical illness. Prednisone is not recommended in patients who are unable to methylate it into an active form.

REFERENCES

1. Fraser CG, Preuss FS, Bigford WD: Adrenal atrophy and irreversible shock associated with cortisone therapy. *JAMA* 1952;149:1542-1543.
2. Nicholson G, Burrin JM, Hall GM: Peri-operative steroid supplementation. *Anaesthesia* 1998;53:1091-1104.
3. Lewis L, Robinson RF, Yee J, Hacker LA, Eisen G: Fatal adrenal cortical insufficiency precipitated by surgery during prolonged continuous cortisone treatment. *Ann Intern Med* 1953;39:116-126.
4. Zaloga GP, Marik P: Hypothalamic-pituitary-adrenal insufficiency. *Crit Care Clin* 2001;17:25-41.
5. Saito T, Takanashi M, Gallagher E, et al: Corticosteroid effect on early beta-adrenergic down-regulation during circulatory shock. *Intensive Care Med* 1995;21:204-210.
6. Coursin DB, Wood KE: Corticosteroid supplementation for adrenal insufficiency. *JAMA* 2002;287:236-240.
7. Orth DS, Kovas WJ: The adrenal cortex. In Wilson JD, Foster DW, Kronenberg HM, Larsen PR, editors: *Williams textbook of endocrinology*, ed 9. Philadelphia, WB Saunders, 1998.
8. Salem M, Tanish RE, Bromberg J, et al: Perioperative glucocorticoid coverage: A reassessment 42 years after emergence of a problem. *Ann Surg* 1994;219:416-425.
9. Hardy JD, Turner MD: Hydrocortisone secretion in man: Studies of adrenal vein blood. *Surgery* 1957;42:194-201.
10. Hume DM, Bell CC, Bartter F: Direct measurement of adrenal secretion during operative trauma and convalescence. *Surgery* 1962;52:174-187.
11. Wise L, Margraf HW, Ballinger WF: A new concept on the pre and postoperative regulation of cortisol secretion. *Surgery* 1972;72:290-299.
12. Kehlet K, Binder C: Value of an ACTH test in assessing hypothalamic-pituitary-adrenocortical function in glucocorticoid-treated patients. *Br Med J* 1973;2:147-149.
13. Peterson RE: The miscible pool and turnover rate of adrenocortical steroids in man. *Recent Prog Hormone Res* 1959;15:231-274.
14. Ichikawa Y: Metabolism of cortisol-4C-14 in patients with infections and collagen diseases. *Metabolism* 1966;15:613-625.
15. Thomas JP, El-Shaboury AH: Aldosterone secretion in steroid-treated patients with adrenal suppression. *Lancet* 1971;I:623-625.
16. Kehlet K, Binder C: Adrenocortical function and clinical course during and after surgery in unsupplemented glucocorticoid-treated patients. *Br J Anesth* 1973;45:1043-1049.
17. Oelkers W: Adrenal insufficiency. *N Engl J Med* 1996;335:1206-1212.
18. Streck WF, Lockwood DW: Pituitary adrenal recovery following short term suppression with corticosteroids. *Am J Med* 1979;66:910-914.
19. Kehlet H: *Clinical course and hypothalamic-pituitary-adrenocortical function in glucocorticoid-treated surgical patients*. Copenhagen, FADL's Forlag, 1976.
20. Mohler JL, Flueck JA, McRoberts JW: Adrenal insufficiency following unilateral adrenal pseudocyst resection. *J Urol* 1986;135:554-556.
21. Alford WC Jr, Meador CK, Mihalevich J, et al: Acute adrenal insufficiency following cardiac surgical procedures. *J Thorac Cardiovasc Surg* 1979;78:489-493.
22. Mohler JL, Michel KA, Freedman AM, et al: The evaluation of postoperative function of the adrenal gland. *Surg Gynecol Obstet* 1985;161:551-556.
23. Rivers EP, Gaspari M, Saad GA, et al: Adrenal insufficiency in high-risk surgical patients. *Chest* 2001;119:889-896.
24. Chernow B, Alexander HR, Thompson WR, et al: The hormonal responses to surgical stress. *Arch Intern Med* 1987;147:1273-1278.
25. Udelsman R, Ramp J, Gallucci WT, et al: Adaptation during surgical stress—a re-evaluation of the role of glucocorticoids. *J Clin Invest* 1986;44:1377-1381.
26. Udelsman R, Goldstein DS, Loriaux DL, Chrousos GP: Catecholamine-glucocorticoid interactions during surgical stress. *J Surg Res* 1987;43:539-545.
27. Kehlet H: A rational approach to dosage and preparation of parenteral glucocorticoid substitution therapy during surgical procedures. *Acta Anesthesiol Scand* 1975;19:260-264.
28. La Rochelle G, La Rochelle AG, Ratner RE, Borenstein DG: Recovery of the hypothalamic-pituitary-adrenal (HPA) axis in patients receiving low-dose prednisone. *Am J Med* 1993;95:258-264.
29. Friedman RJ, Schiff CF, Bromberg JS: Use of supplemental steroids in patients having orthopedic operations. *J Bone Joint Surg* 1995;77A:1801-1806.
30. Kenyon NJ, Albertson TE: Steroids and sepsis: Time for another reevaluation. *J Intensive Care Med* 2002;17:68-74.
31. Gran L, Pahle JA: Rational substitution for steroid-treated patients. *Anaesthesia* 1978;33:59-61.
32. Cronin L, Cook DJ, Cartlet J, et al: Corticosteroid for sepsis: A critical appraisal and meta-analysis of the literature. *Crit Care Med* 1995;23:1430-1439.
33. Veterans Administration Systemic Sepsis Cooperative Study Group: Effect of high-dose glucocorticoid therapy on mortality in patients with clinical signs of systemic sepsis. *N Engl J Med* 1987;317:659-665.
34. Bone RC, Fisher CJ Jr, Clemmer TP, et al: A controlled clinical trial of high-dose methylprednisolone in the treatment of severe sepsis and septic shock. *N Engl J Med* 1987;317:653-658.
35. Bernard GR, Luce J, Sprung CL, et al: High-dose corticosteroids in patients with the adult respiratory distress syndrome. *N Engl J Med* 1987;317:1565-1570.
36. Lefering R, Neugebauer EA: Steroid controversy in sepsis and septic shock: A meta-analysis. *Crit Care Med* 1995;23:1294-1303.
37. Bollaert PE: Stress doses of glucocorticoids in catecholamine dependency: A new therapy for a new syndrome. *Intensive Care Med* 2000;26:3-5.
38. Annane D, Sébille V, Charpentier C, et al: Effect of treatment with low doses of hydrocortisone and fludrocortisone on mortality in patients with septic shock. *JAMA* 2002;288:862-871.
39. Sprung CL, Annane D, Keh D, et al, CORTICUS Study Group: Hydrocortisone therapy for patients with septic shock. *N Engl J Med* 2008;358:111-124.
40. Dellinger RP, Levy MM, Carlet JM, et al: Surviving Sepsis Campaign: International guidelines for management of severe sepsis and septic shock: 2008. *Crit Care Med* 2008;36:296-327.
41. Annane D: Glucocorticoids for ARDS: Just do it! *Chest* 2007;131:945-946.
42. Meduri GU, Headley AS, Golden E, et al: Effect of prolonged methylprednisolone therapy in unresolving acute respiratory distress syndrome: A randomized controlled trial. *JAMA* 1998;280:159-165.
43. Steinberg KP, Hudson LD, Goodman RB, et al; National Heart, Lung, and Blood Institute Acute Respiratory Distress Syndrome (ARDS) Clinical Trials Network: Efficacy and safety of corticosteroids for persistent acute respiratory distress syndrome. *N Engl J Med* 2006;354:1671-1684.
44. Meduri GU, Golden E, Freire AX, et al: Methylprednisolone infusion in early severe ARDS: Results of a randomized controlled trial. *Chest* 2007;131:954-963.
45. van de Beek D, de Gans J, McIntyre P, et al: Corticosteroids for acute bacterial meningitis. *Cochrane Database Syst Rev* 2007;1:CD004405.
46. de Gans J, van de Beek D; European Dexamethasone in Adulthood Bacterial Meningitis Study Investigators: Dexamethasone in adults with bacterial meningitis. *N Engl J Med* 2002;347:1549-1556.
47. Powner DJ, Boccalandro C: Adrenal insufficiency following traumatic brain inury in adults. *Curr Opin Crit Care* 2008;14:163-166.
48. Roberts I, Yates D, Sandercock P, et al; CRASH trial collaborators: Effect of intravenous corticosteroids on death within 14 days in 10,008 adults with clinically significant head injury (MRC CRASH trial): Randomised placebo-controlled trial. *Lancet* 2004;364:1321-1328.
49. Edwards P, Arango M, Balica L, et al; CRASH trial collaborators: Final results of MRC CRASH, a randomised placebo-controlled trial of intravenous corticosteroid in adults with head injury-outcomes at 6 months. *Lancet* 2005;365:1957-1959.
50. Bracken MB, Shepard MJ, Collins WF, et al: A randomized, controlled trial of methylprednisolone or naloxone in the treatment of acute spinal-cord injury. Results of the Second National Acute Spinal Cord Injury Study. *N Engl J Med* 1990;322:1405-1411.

51. Miller SM: Methylprednisolone in acute spinal cord injury: A tarnished standard. *J Neurosurg Anesthesiol* 2008;20:140-142.

52. George ER, Scholten PJ, Buechler CM: Failure of methylprednisolone to improve the outcome of spinal cord injury. *Am Surg* 1995;61:659-663.

53. Pointillart V, Petitjean ME, Wiart L: Pharmacotherapy of spinal cord injury during the acute phase. *Spinal Cord* 2000;38:71-76.

54. Bracken MB: Steroids for acute spinal cord injury. *Cochrane Database Syst Rev* 2002;(3):CD001046.

55. Tsutsumi S, Ueta T, Shiba K, et al: Effects of the Second National Acute Spinal Cord Injury Study of high-dose methylprednisolone therapy on acute cervical spinal cord injury—results in spinal injuries center. *Spine* 2006;31:2992-2996.

56. Leypold BG, Flanders AE, Schwartz ED, et al: The impact of methylprednisolone on lesion severity following spinal cord injury. *Spine* 2007;32:373-378.

57. Eck JC, Nachtigall D, Humphreys SC, et al: Questionnaire survey of spine surgeons on the use of methylprednisolone for acute spinal cord injury. *Spine* 2006;31:E250-253.

58. Wagner RL, White PF: Etomidate inhibits adrenocortical function in surgical patients. *Anesthesiology* 1984;61(6):647-651.

59. den Brinker M, Hokken-Koelega AC, Hazelzet JA, et al: One single dose of etomidate negatively influences adrenocortical performance for at least 24 h in children with meningococcal sepsis. *Intensive Care Med* 2008;34(1):163-168.

60. Vinclair M, Broux C, Faure P, et al: Duration of adrenal inhibition following a single dose of etomidate in critically ill patients. *Intensive Care Med* 2008;34:714-719.

61. Ray DC, McKeown DW: Effect of induction agent on vasopressor and steroid use, and outcome in patients with septic shock. *Crit Care* 2007;11:R56.

62. Yong SL: Supplemental perioperative steroids for surgical patients with adrenal insufficiency. Available at: http://www.cochrane.org/reviews/en/info_547503112316012746.html

30 Does the Choice of Fluid Matter in Major Surgery?

Anthony M. Roche, MBChB, FRCA, MMed; Catherine M.N. O'Malley, MBBS, FCARCSI; and Elliott Bennett-Guerrero, MD

INTRODUCTION

Numerous preparations of intravenous (IV) fluid are available for the replacement of perioperative fluid losses in patients undergoing major surgery. The selection of a specific fluid may be influenced by multiple factors. In the past, this choice may have been governed by variables such as availability, cost, and tradition. Of late, attention has focused on the possible systemic effects of the various fluid preparations. Additionally, there is awareness that particular fluids may not only influence clinical parameters during the intraoperative period but may also affect postoperative outcome. Increasingly, it is the beneficial or detrimental effects of IV fluids, independent of their efficacy as blood volume expanders, that influence clinicians in their choice of fluid replacement therapy for patients undergoing major surgical procedures.

Many clinical and experimental studies have been carried out to determine the potential clinical effects of IV fluids. Unfortunately, there is a paucity of large, prospective, randomized, blinded clinical studies of the effects of the intraoperative administration of IV fluids on clinical outcomes despite the fact that approximately 3 million major surgical procedures are performed annually in the United States alone. However, multiple outcomes have been examined in small investigations in numerous and diverse patient populations and in studies of healthy volunteers. To address the question "Does the choice of fluid matter in major surgery?" we will consider the available data from prospective, clinical studies of intravascular volume replacement in patients undergoing major surgery. In the context of major surgery, it is reasonable to suppose that the administration of a small volume of a particular fluid type is unlikely to have a marked impact on clinical outcome. Presumably, if differences are seen with small volumes of fluids these effects will also be observed when larger volumes are administered. Hence, we will consider clinical studies in which at least 1 L of fluid is administered intraoperatively. The interpretation of studies of IV fluids is somewhat confounded by their size and design. In many cases, only small numbers of patients are studied. These trials may not have sufficient power to detect differences in clinically relevant outcomes, and their results are therefore interpreted with this caveat in mind.

OPTIONS

Traditionally, IV fluids have been classified according to whether they are crystalloid or colloid in nature. Crystalloid fluids comprise electrolyte solutions with or without a bicarbonate precursor such as acetate or lactate. The colloids contain a complex sugar or protein suspended in an electrolyte solution. A further distinction between IV fluid types may be based on the nature of the solution. Preparations based on 0.9% NaCl (normal saline [NS]) (crystalloid or colloid) contain no electrolytes other than sodium and chloride. In contrast, balanced salt–based fluids such as lactated Ringer's solution are those that contain other electrolytes with or without a bicarbonate precursor.

Several types of colloid are available, but three are most commonly used: hydroxyethyl starch, gelatin, and albumin. The hydroxyethyl starch (HES) preparations differ from one another according to their concentration, molecular weight, and extent of hydroxyethylation or substitution, with resultant varying physiochemical properties. HES solutions may be described according to concentration (3%, 6%, 10%), weight-averaged mean molecular weight in kilodaltons (kDa): high molecular weight (450 to 670 kDa), middle molecular weight (200 kDa, 270 kDa), low molecular weight (130 kDa, 70 kDa), and the molar substitution (0.38 to 0.7). HES 450/0.7 is available in a normal saline solution (HES 450/NS) and in a lactated, balanced salt solution (HES 450/BS). Two forms of gelatin are available: modified (succinylated) and the polygelines. Whereas all these colloids are used in Europe, gelatins are not available in the United States and the only hydroxyethyl starch preparations approved by the Food and Drug Administration (FDA) are the 6% high molecular weight (450kDa) formulations.

EVIDENCE

The Impact of Intravenous Fluids on Coagulation

The administration of a large volume of any type of IV fluid will cause dilution of platelets and coagulation factors and may lead to coagulopathy. In addition, fluids can have a direct impact on blood clotting through effects on circulating components of the coagulation cascade or by altering platelet function. Because of the multifactorial etiology of bleeding during surgery it is impossible to know in any given patient whether the type of fluid administered is a cause of bleeding independent of the impact of hemodilution. Only properly designed, randomized, clinical trials can determine fluid-specific effects on bleeding and other clinical outcomes. Although many studies report some clinical outcomes related to bleeding, a large number focus on measurements of markers of coagulation and are not designed to explore outcomes of more clinical relevance such as blood product usage and surgical reexploration for bleeding (Table 30-1).

The gelatins have not been associated, other than on an anecdotal basis, with abnormalities in coagulation or clinically significant perioperative bleeding. Six prospective studies have compared gelatins with a number of HES preparations for intraoperative intravascular volume replacement in cardiac[1] and noncardiac surgical patients.[2-6] The administration of gelatin was not associated with more blood loss or blood or blood product transfusions than any other fluid in these studies.

The effects of the hydroxyethyl starches and 5% albumin on perioperative blood loss and markers of blood clotting have been investigated in a number of clinical trials.[7-17] In a study of 120 major surgical patients, blood loss was greater among patients who received HES 450/NS than in patients who received HES 450/BS.[8] Other small studies have found little difference in clinically relevant bleeding outcomes between 5% albumin and HES 450/NS.[7,9,11,12] However, several retrospective analyses have suggested that HES 450/NS may be associated with more bleeding than other fluids.[17-20]

With regard to coagulation, another potentially relevant variable relates to properties of the starch component of fluids, in particular the mean molecular weight, the degree of molar substitution, and the C_2/C_6 ratio. A hydroxyethyl starch is available in Europe and Canada (Voluven, Fresenius Kabi, Germany) that was designed with a better coagulation profile in mind. It has a mean molecular weight of 130, molar substitution of 0.4, and C_2/C_6 ratio of approximately 9:1.[14,21-23] Several studies demonstrate that Voluven has fewer adverse effects on coagulation compared with the higher molecular weight starches or has an impact on coagulation similar to gelatin.[14,21-24] Voluven has recently become commercially available in the United States. Of note, a recent paper described a study of general surgical patients randomized to administration of a balanced 140/0.4 starch with a saline-based 140/0.4 starch.[25] Another starch that may become available in the United States is Pentalyte, a 6% hetastarch (molecular weight 250,000, degree of substitution 0.45) formulated in a balanced electrolyte solution, containing lactate, K^+, Ca^{2+}, and Mg^{2+}. There are some animal and in vitro data that coagulation effects are more favorable with this medium molecular weight starch.[26,27] Pentalyte has recently undergone phase II testing in the United States.

Some studies suggest that the nature of the solution itself may influence coagulation and bleeding. HES 450/NS may be associated with more bleeding than other fluids, and HES 670 in a balanced salt solution appears to be equivalent to 5% albumin with respect to bleeding

outcomes.[10] Waters and colleagues[28] reported that patients undergoing abdominal aortic aneurysm repair who received lactated Ringer's solution received smaller volumes of platelets and had less blood product exposure than those treated with normal saline. However, other data exist that do not support a beneficial effect of balanced salt–type fluids on coagulation.[16,29]

When differences between fluid types are seen they may be mediated through impaired platelet function, possibly as a consequence of diminished circulating von Willebrand factor (vWF) antigen and vWF: ristocetin cofactor in patients treated with normal saline–based rather than balanced salt–based fluids.[30] A second possible explanation is the lack of calcium in 0.9% NaCl and related fluids. Calcium is a necessary co-factor at several points in the coagulation process. It is necessary for activation of clotting factors, as well as for normal platelet function. In particular, calcium binding is a prerequisite for the stability and function of the platelet GPIIb/IIIa receptor. This receptor binds fibrinogen and vWF with resultant platelet activation and aggregation. With blood loss and IV fluid administration ionized calcium levels may fluctuate, and this variation may affect coagulation. Ionized calcium levels may be lower following administration of normal saline and related fluids rather than balanced salt fluids.[2,8,29,31] The presence of calcium in IV fluids may maintain more constant plasma calcium levels, avoiding the potential detrimental effect of low or fluctuating ionized calcium levels on coagulation.

Many of the clinical studies of coagulation-related effects of IV fluids have focused on bleeding outcomes without examining the possible procoagulant effect of various fluid preparations. It is possible that certain fluids may induce hypercoagulability that may be reflected not only by less bleeding but also by an increased incidence of postoperative thrombotic complications (e.g., deep vein thrombosis, cerebrovascular accident). There are some laboratory data[8,29] to suggest that IV fluid administration may induce a hypercoagulable state, but the clinical significance of this remains to be specifically explored in prospective clinical studies.

The Impact of Intravenous Fluids on Urine Output/Renal Function

There is a growing body of evidence suggesting that the type of fluid administered to a patient can have a significant impact on renal function. The administration of HES to critically ill patients in the intensive care unit (ICU) was associated with the development of renal dysfunction.[32-34] In contrast with this, no difference in renal function was observed in 50 perioperative cardiac surgical patients with known renal dysfunction (serum creatinine 1.5 to 2.5 mmol/L) randomized to either HES 130/NS or 5% albumin solution.[35] Data in patients with normal renal function undergoing major surgery do not demonstrate that HES is detrimental to renal function (Table 30-2). Clinical studies have compared different HES/NS preparations,[4,14,21] HES/NS with gelatin,[1,2,5,36] and HES/NS with 5% albumin.[11,12,37] Only one of these studies noted differences between study groups in reported measures of renal function.[11]

Table 30-1 The Impact of Commonly Used Intravenous Fluids on Coagulation: Prospective, Randomized Clinical Trials of the Intraoperative Administration of ≥1 L of Intravenous Fluid

Author	Fluids Studied	Type of Surgery	Findings
Beyer et al.[2]	HES 200/NS (n = 19), gelatin/NS (n = 22)	Orthopedic	No difference in blood loss or blood product administration
Boldt et al.[29]	LR (n = 21), 0.9% NaCl (n = 21)	Abdominal	No difference in blood loss or blood product administration
Boldt et al.[37]	HES 130 (n = 25), 5% albumin (n = 25)	Abdominal	No difference in blood loss, blood product administration, or coagulation markers
Claes et al.[7]	HES 450/NS (n = 20), 5% albumin/NS (n = 20)	Neurosurgical, abdominal	No difference in blood loss or blood product administration
Gallandat Huet et al.[21]	HES 200/NS (n = 29), HES 130/NS (n = 30)	Cardiac	Greater blood loss in HES 200/NS group No difference in blood product administration, reoperation rate
Gan et al.[8]	HES 450/BS (n = 60), HES 450/NS (n = 60)	Abdominal, gynecologic, orthopedic, urologic	No difference in blood loss or blood product administration
Gandhi et al.[22]	HES 670/BS (n = 51), HES 130/NS (n = 49)	Orthopedic	Similar volumes administered with some differences in some measures of coagulation
Gold et al.[9]	HES 450/NS (n = 20), 5% albumin/NS (n = 20)	Abdominal aortic aneurysm	No difference in blood loss or blood product administration
Haisch et al.[1]	HES 130/NS (n = 21), gelatin/NS (n = 21)	Cardiac	No difference in blood loss or blood product administration
Haisch et al.[3]	HES 130/NS (n = 21), gelatin/NS (n = 21)	Abdominal	No difference in blood loss or blood product administration
Huttner et al.[6]	HES 70/NS (n = 20), HES 200/NS (n = 20), gelatin/NS (n = 20)	Abdominal	No difference in blood loss or blood product administration
Kumle et al.[4]	HES 70/NS (n = 20), HES 200/NS (n = 20), gelatin/NS (n = 20)	Abdominal	No difference in blood loss or blood product administration
Lang et al.[39]	HES 130/NS (n = 21), LR (n = 21)	Abdominal	No difference in blood loss or blood product administration
Langeron et al.[14]	HES 130/NS (n = 52), HES 200/NS (n = 48)	Orthopedic	More allogeneic blood administration in HES 200/NS group
Marik et al.[15]	HES 450/NS (n = 15), LR (n = 15)	Abdominal aortic aneurysm	No difference in blood loss or blood product administration
McFarlane & Lee[40]	Plasmalyte 14 (n = 15), 0.9% NaCl (n = 15)	Hepatobiliary, pancreatic	No difference in blood loss or blood product administration
Mortelmans et al.[5]	HES 200/NS (n = 21), gelatin/NS (n = 21)	Orthopedic	Greater blood loss in HES 200/NS group, more allogeneic blood administration in gelatin group
Petroni et al.[10]	HES 450/BS (n = 14), 5% albumin/BS (n = 14)	Cardiac	No difference in blood loss or blood product administration
Prien et al.[16]	LR (n = 6), 20% albumin/NS (n = 6), 10% HES/NS (n = 6)	Hemipancreato-duodenectomy	More blood administration in LR group
Scheingraber et al.[38]	LR (n = 12), 0.9% NaCl (n = 12)	Gynecologic	No difference in blood loss
Van der Linden et al.[24]	HES 130/NS (n = 64), gelatin/NS (n = 68)	Cardiac surgery	No difference in blood loss or blood product administration
Virgilio et al.[13]	LR (n = 14), 5% albumin/BS (n = 15)	Abdominal aortic surgery	No difference in blood loss or blood product administration
Vogt et al.[11]	HES 200/NS (n = 20), 5% albumin/NS (n = 21)	Orthopedic	No difference in blood loss or blood product administration
Vogt et al.[12]	HES 200/NS (n = 25), 5% albumin/NS (n = 25)	Urologic	No difference in blood loss or blood product administration
Waters et al.[28]	0.9% NaCl (n = 33), LR (n = 33)	Abdominal aortic aneurysm	More platelet administration and blood product exposure in 0.9% NaCl group
Wilkes et al.[31]	HES 450/NS and NS (n = 23), HES 450/BS and LR (n = 24)	Abdominal, orthopedic, genitourinary, plastic surgery	No difference in blood product administration

BS, balanced salt–based solution; HES, hydroxyethylstarch; LR, lactated Ringer's; NS, 0.9% NaCl or normal saline–like solution.

Table 30-2	The Impact of Commonly Used Intravenous Fluids on Renal Function: Prospective, Randomized Clinical Trials of the Intraoperative Administration of $\geq$1 L of Intravenous Fluid		
Author	**Fluids Studied**	**Type of Surgery**	**Findings**
Beyer et al.[2]	HES 200/NS (n = 19), gelatin/NS (n = 22)	Orthopedic	No difference in urine output, serum creatinine
Boldt et al.[29]	LR (n = 21), 0.9% NaCl (n = 21)	Abdominal	No difference in urine output
Boldt et al.[37]	HES 130 (n = 25), 5% Albumin (n = 25)	Abdominal	No difference in urine output or markers of renal injury
Boldt et al.[35]	HES 130/NS (n = 25), 5% Albumin (n = 25)	Cardiac	No difference in urine output or markers of renal injury Increase in NGAL (marker of tubular ischemia) in albumin group
Gallandat Huet et al.[21]	HES 130/NS (n = 30), HES 200/NS (n = 29)	Cardiac	No difference in urine output, serum creatinine
Gan et al.[8]	HES 450/BS (n = 60), HES 450/NS (n = 60)	General, gynecologic, orthopedic, urologic	No difference in urine output
Haisch et al.[1]	HES 130/NS (n = 21), gelatin/NS (n = 21)	Cardiac	No difference in urine output
Haisch et al.[3]	HES 130/NS (n = 21), gelatin/NS (n = 21)	Abdominal	No difference in urine output
Kumle et al.[4]	HES 70/NS (n = 20), HES 200/NS (n = 20), gelatin/NS (n = 20)	Abdominal	No difference in urine output, serum creatinine, creatinine clearance, fractional excretion of sodium
Lang et al.[39]	HES 130/NS (n = 21), LR (n = 21)	Abdominal	Lower urine output in HES 130/NS group
Langeron et al.[14]	HES 130/NS (n = 52), HES 200/NS (n = 48)	Orthopedic	No difference in urine output
Mahmood et al.[36]	HES 200/NS (n = 21), HES 130/NS (n = 21), gelatin/NS (n = 20)	Abdominal aortic aneurysm	No difference in urine output Less derangement in markers or glomerular and tubular function with HES 200/NS and HES 130/NS
Mortelmans et al.[5]	HES 200/NS (n = 21), gelatin/NS (n = 21)	Orthopedic	No difference in urine output
O'Malley et al.[42]	LR (n = 25), 0.9% NaCl (n = 26)	Kidney transplant recipients	No difference in urine output, creatinine clearance, or serum creatinine change Less hyperkalemia and metabolic acidosis in LR-treated patients
Scheingraber et al.[38]	LR (n = 12), 0.9% NaCl (n = 12)	Gynecologic	No difference in urine output
Virgilio et al.[13]	LR (n = 14), 5% albumin/BS (n = 15)	Abdominal aortic surgery	Greater urine output in LR group on postoperative day 2
Vogt et al.[11]	HES 200/NS (n = 20), 5% albumin/NS (n = 21)	Orthopedic	No difference in urine output, creatinine clearance Greater serum creatinine in 5% albumin/NS group 6 hours postoperatively
Vogt et al.[12]	HES 200/NS (n = 25), 5% albumin/NS (n = 25)	Urologic	No difference in urine output, serum creatinine
Waters et al.[28]	0.9% NaCl (n = 33), LR (n = 33)	Abdominal aortic aneurysm	Greater urine output in 0.9% NaCl group, no difference in serum creatinine
Wilkes et al.[31]	HES 450/NS and NS (n = 23), HES 450/BS and LR (n = 24)	Abdominal, orthopedic, genitourinary, plastic surgery	No difference in urine output

BS, balanced salt–based solution; *HES,* hydroxyethylstarch; *LR,* lactated Ringer's; *NS,* 0.9% NaCl or normal saline–like solution.

Several prospective, randomized studies have compared the effects of normal saline–based and balanced salt–based fluids and have observed greater urinary output in patients treated with the balanced salt–type fluid preparations.[8,31,38] In a comparison of lactated Ringer's with HES 130/NS, urine output was lower in the HES 130/NS–treated group.[39] Hyperchloremic metabolic acidosis can occur with the administration of large volumes of 0.9% NaCl and normal saline–based fluids.[11,28,31,38-40] Hyperchloremia may cause renal vasoconstriction and a decrease in glomerular filtration rate,[41] which may explain, in part, the mechanism for the putative normal saline–induced changes in renal performance. Alternatively, the metabolic acidosis itself may induce vasoconstriction and redistribution of intrarenal blood flow with subsequent effects on function.

Other investigators have not noted superior renal function following the administration of balanced salt fluids. Intraoperative urine output was greater in patients who received normal saline than in patients who were given lactated Ringer's solution during abdominal aortic aneurysm repair.[28] However, normal saline–treated patients received a larger volume of fluid than patients in the lactated Ringer's group. In patients undergoing major abdominal surgery, cumulative urine output measured on the second postoperative day was greater in 0.9% NaCl–treated patients than in lactated Ringer's–treated patients, although this difference did not reach statistical significance.[29] In both these studies normal saline–treated patients received significant quantities of sodium bicarbonate intraoperatively for treatment of hyperchloremic metabolic acidosis, suggesting that the prevention or treatment of hyperchloremic metabolic acidosis may have negated the negative impact of normal saline on renal function in some way.

The impact of fluid choice was studied in 51 patients undergoing kidney transplantation.[42] Patients were randomized to receive either 0.9% NaCl or lactated Ringer's for intraoperative fluid resuscitation. Despite each group receiving approximately 6 L of fluid on average, no statistically significant differences were observed in any of the reported measures of renal function, including urine output, 24-hour creatinine clearance, and postoperative change in serum creatinine. It is interesting to note that eight (31%) of patients in the saline group versus zero (0%) patients in the lactated Ringer's group were treated for metabolic acidosis. In addition, five (19%) of patients in the saline group had potassium concentrations greater than 6 mEq/L and were treated for hyperkalemia versus zero in the lactated Ringer's group. This small single-center study alone does not justify a change in practice; however, it does challenge the dogma that saline should be administered to patients with renal failure.

The Impact of Intravenous Fluids on the Gastrointestinal Tract

Splanchnic Perfusion

Considerable evidence supports the role of the gut in the pathogenesis of the systemic inflammatory response syndrome and the multiple organ dysfunction syndrome after major surgery. Two studies have explored the impact of intraoperative fluid replacement on splanchnic perfusion as manifested by gastric tonometric variables. Marik and colleagues[15] measured gastrointestinal pH using saline tonometry in patients undergoing abdominal aortic aneurysm repair. Patients who received HES 450/NS had less splanchnic hypoperfusion, as reflected by a smaller decrease in gastrointestinal pH (pHi), than patients who were given lactated Ringer's solution.[15] The authors suggested that HES somehow protected the gut mucosa from ischemia. Proposed mechanisms included inhibition of endothelial cell activation and limiting fluid extravasation through maintenance of plasma oncotic pressure or augmentation of endothelial cell basement membrane.

Wilkes and colleagues[31] utilized the newer and easier technique of automated air gastric tonometry and measured the gastric-arterial PCO_2 difference (CO_2 gap), which is the most accurate reflection of splanchnic ischemia. Elderly surgical patients were randomized to receive either a combination of HES 450/BS and lactated Ringer's or a combination of HES 450/NS and 0.9% NaCl for intraoperative fluid replacement. In the group treated with balanced salt–based fluids there was a smaller intraoperative increase in CO_2 gap, indicating that balanced salt–based fluids are associated with superior splanchnic perfusion than normal saline–based fluids. It was postulated that impaired gut perfusion or hyperchloremia associated with normal saline–based preparations may have caused an impairment of splanchnic perfusion in the patients who were administered 0.9% NaCl and HES 450/NS. Of note, the poor splanchnic perfusion in patients treated with the normal saline–based regimen may have been mediated by generalized vasoconstriction (perhaps secondary to metabolic acidosis), given that these patients also exhibited other evidence of vasoconstriction, that is, lower urine flow rates and lower peripheral-to-core temperature gradients (reflecting peripheral vasoconstriction).

Gastrointestinal Tract Function

The administration of IV fluids during the perioperative period results in a lower incidence of nausea, vomiting, and antiemetic use after minor or day-case surgery.[43-46] In noncardiac surgical patients the administration of HES 450 (in a balanced salt–based or normal saline–based solution) was associated with less edema, postoperative nausea, vomiting, and antiemetic use than the administration of lactated Ringer's solution (Figure 30-1).[47] The intraoperative administration of a balanced salt–based fluid regimen was associated with a lower incidence of nausea and vomiting and antiemetic use in elderly surgical patients than the administration of a normal saline–based fluid regimen.[31]

Superior gut function in patients who receive HES for intraoperative volume resuscitation might be explained by the presence of less intestinal edema with the starch than with crystalloids or albumin. More severe periorbital edema was observed after the administration of lactated Ringer's than after intraoperative HES administration in patients who underwent major abdominal surgery.[47] It seems likely that edema may also occur in the gastrointestinal tract and that this may influence gut function in patients undergoing gastrointestinal and nongastrointestinal surgery.

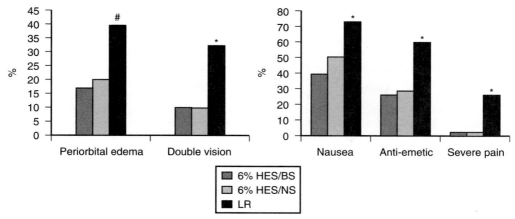

Figure 30-1. Effects of Intravenous Fluids on the Incidence of Nausea, Antiemetic Use, and Edema in Noncardiac Surgical Patients *LR,* lactated Ringer's; *HES 450/NS,* 6% hetastarch in 0.9% NaCl; *HES 450/BS,* 6% hetastarch in balanced salt solution; *p <0.05, # p = 0.08.

Indeed, more intestinal edema was seen in patients undergoing Whipple's operation who received lactated Ringer's solution rather than HES 450/NS or 20% albumin/NS for intraoperative fluid replacement.[16]

The Impact of Intravenous Fluids on Postoperative Pain

Few studies have been designed that explore the impact of IV fluid type on the severity of postoperative pain. However, just as edema may potentially influence gut function, so peripheral or wound edema may affect the occurrence of pain after surgery. Pain after noncardiac surgery was more severe when lactated Ringer's solution was used for intraoperative fluid resuscitation rather than HES 450/NS or HES 450/BS.[47]

The Impact of Intravenous Fluids on Central Nervous System Function

Studies of patients undergoing ambulatory surgery have shown that perioperative IV fluid administration decreases the incidence of dizziness, drowsiness, thirst, and headache.[44,46] It is also interesting to note that in a randomized crossover study of healthy volunteers, subjective deterioration in mental status (lassitude and difficulty in abstract thinking) was reported only by individuals who received 0.9% NaCl and not by those who received lactated Ringer's solution.[48] The possible effect of different IV fluid preparations on central nervous system function has not yet been explored in prospective, randomized clinical studies of patients undergoing major surgical procedures.

The Impact of Intravenous Fluids on Pulmonary Function

The relative impact of crystalloids and colloids on pulmonary function has been the subject of long-standing debate. No difference in postoperative pulmonary function was seen in cardiac surgery patients,[21] orthopedic patients,[11] or urologic surgery patients[12] treated intraoperatively with different colloids. In a number of studies in major surgical patients that compared crystalloid (lactated Ringer's) with colloid (HES 130/NS,[39] HES 450/NS,[15] 5% albumin/BS[13]),

no difference was seen in the incidence or duration of mechanical ventilation or other indices of respiratory function. These studies suggest that the intraoperative administration of crystalloids does not have a detrimental effect on pulmonary function compared with the administration of colloids. In contrast, Rittoo and colleagues[49] randomized 40 patients undergoing elective infrarenal abdominal aortic aneurysm surgery to receive either hydroxyethyl starch (eloHAES 6%, Fresenius Kabi, Germany) or gelatin (Gelofusine 4%, B. Braun, United Kingdom). Several indices of pulmonary function (PaO$_2$/FiO$_2$ ratio, respiratory compliance, lung injury score) were better in patients randomized to hydroxyethyl starch.

The Impact of Intravenous Fluids on the Inflammatory Response

Two recent studies have investigated the role of IV fluid in modulating the inflammatory response in patients.[37,50] In a randomized study of 40 patients receiving either HES 200/NS or a gelatin solution during elective infrarenal aortic aneurysm repair surgery, lower levels of inflammatory markers (C-reactive protein, microalbuminuria, plasma vWF) were observed in the HES-treated group than with the gelatin-treated group after crossclamp removal. A similar picture was observed with 50 elderly patients undergoing elective major abdominal surgery. These patients were randomized to either a human albumin–based fluid regimen or an HES 130/NS–based regimen. Plasma levels of C-reactive protein, interleukin-6, soluble endothelial leukocyte adhesion molecule-1, and soluble intercellular adhesion molecule-1 were lower in the HES-treated group than the human albumin–treated group. These data suggest that HES may mediate the inflammatory response in major vascular and major general surgery; however, these studies were too small to detect any outcome differences, if any existed.

Other Effects of Intravenous Fluids

Hyperamylasemia is associated with the administration of HES but not other fluid types.[2,51] Amylasemia is caused by HES through the formation of an HES-amylase complex with consequent reduction in elimination of amylase by the kidney. This effect is greater with HES 200/NS than with HES 130/NS in cardiac surgical patients[21] and in noncardiac surgical patients,[14] consistent with the pharmacokinetics of different HES preparations. Intraneural deposition of HES has been purported to cause pruritus after HES administration.[52] Small retrospective studies, in a number of patient populations, have reported a high incidence of HES-induced pruritus.[53-55] However, no large epidemiologic studies examining this phenomenon have been performed in patients undergoing major surgery who have received large volumes of fluid. Interestingly, the incidence of postoperative pruritus in a prospective study of 750 surgical patients was similar (10%) in patients who received 500 mL of HES 200/NS and in patients who received 1000 mL of lactated Ringer's.[56] The most important potential adverse effect of IV fluids is the occurrence of possibly life-threatening anaphylactic or anaphylactoid reactions. The incidence of severe anaphylactic reactions is 0.038% to 0.345% with gelatins, 0.0004% to 0.058% with HES administration, and 0.099% in patients who receive albumin.[57]

The Impact of Intravenous Fluids on Resource Utilization

Significant cost reduction (32% to 35%) has been shown when HES was used for intraoperative fluid replacement rather than 5% albumin.[11,12] The clinical studies of IV fluids during major surgery have not been designed to demonstrate differences in outcomes such as intensive care length of stay, hospital length of stay, or mortality rate, and no demonstrable differences in these outcomes have been associated with the administration of any type of IV fluid.[6,13,15,21,28]

LANDMARK STUDIES IN INTENSIVE CARE UNIT PATIENTS

The focus of this review is fluid choice in surgical patients; therefore there is limited discussion of fluid management in ICU patients. Two landmark studies are discussed because of their impact.

The Saline versus Albumin Fluid Evaluation (SAFE) study involved 6997 adult ICU patients at 16 hospitals in Australia.[58] Patients were randomized to either albumin ($n = 3497$) or saline ($n = 3500$). No differences were observed in mortality rate, single organ failure, multiple organ failure, ICU or hospital length of stay, days of mechanical ventilation, or days of renal-replacement therapy. One limitation of the study relates to the "small" volumes of study fluid administered to each group (approximately 2 to 3 L mean volume over 4 days). Therefore it is clear that the choice of fluid may not be critical with smaller infused volumes; however, it is unclear whether the same conclusions would have been reached with larger volumes. In addition, neither of the fluids was a balanced fluid, so the conclusions may only be representative of the comparison of a saline crystalloid with a saline-like colloid fluid. Interestingly, a post hoc subset analysis of patients with traumatic brain injury ($n = 460$) revealed a higher mortality rate in albumin-treated patients (33.2% versus 20.4%).[59]

The other landmark ICU study involved the comparison of two fluid management strategies in acute lung injury.[60] In this large U.S. multicenter trial conducted at 20 centers, 1001 patients with acute lung injury were randomized to "conservative" versus "liberal" fluid management for 7 days. The mean cumulative fluid balance was −136 mL in the conservative group and +6992 mL in the liberal group. There was no difference in 60-day mortality rate between groups. However, oxygenation index, lung injury score, and ICU length of stay were better in patients randomized to the conservative fluid group. These results, while important in ICU patients, must be interpreted with extreme caution in surgical patients. Patients with preexisting acute lung injury (as in this trial) are likely to have capillary leak syndrome and be predisposed to the adverse effects of liberal fluid management. This is not necessarily the case in surgical patients, who may be at greater risk of organ dysfunction from inadequate volume resuscitation, and be at less risk for pulmonary edema.[61]

GUIDELINES

To our knowledge there are no published guidelines from any professional society, consensus group, or federal agency regarding the choice of IV fluid preparation for administration during major surgery. Of note, several authors refer to a dose limit of 20 mL/kg for HES preparations. In fact, manufacturer's guidelines do not assert that there is an upper limit to the volume of HES that should be administered. The package insert states "doses of more than 1500 mL per day for the typical 70 kg patient (approximately 20 mL per kg of body weight) are usually not required, although higher doses have been reported in postoperative and trauma patients where severe blood loss has occurred." This may soon change given the findings of a Food and Drug Administration (FDA) review panel that recommended adding a warning statement to the HES 450/NS label stating that excessive bleeding may occur in cardiac surgical patients who receive HES 450/NS. The FDA panel did not recommend issuing such a warning for HES 450/BS, apparently because of recent evidence demonstrating differences in the effects of the normal saline–based and balanced salt–based HES 450 preparations on coagulation, renal function, and other clinical outcomes.

AREAS OF UNCERTAINTY

It is clear from this review that the evidence regarding the impact of intraoperative IV fluid administration on postoperative clinical outcome in patients undergoing major surgery is limited. The principal constraint is the small number of published studies large enough to detect significant differences in clinically relevant outcome measures. There is an obvious need to conduct large, prospective, randomized, clinical trials to further delineate the effect of intraoperative fluid therapy on clinical outcomes. We have delineated some specific interesting areas that warrant further investigation, such as the impact of IV fluids on the gastrointestinal system and the central nervous system.

The data that are available raise several interesting points. First, it is evident that fluids should no longer be merely classified into crystalloids or colloids. The nature of the solution (i.e., normal saline–based or balanced salt–based fluid) has a bearing on the impact of the fluid on various organ systems. Second, all colloids are not the same. Various colloids, even when prepared in similar solutions, may have different clinical effects. Third, the impact on clinical outcome is dependent on the type of surgery and the clinical condition of the patient. Last, intriguing questions are raised as to the potential mechanisms by which clinical outcomes may be influenced by intraoperative IV fluid administration. Is the putative normal saline–induced renal dysfunction observed in some surgical patients mediated by a similar mechanism, possibly vasoconstriction, as the decrease in splanchnic perfusion observed in elderly surgical patients treated with normal saline–based fluids?[31]

AUTHORS' RECOMMENDATIONS

Does the choice of fluid matter in major surgery? Based on the evidence presented here, we believe that the choice of fluid matters in major surgery, with the caveats stated earlier. Because no single fluid or fluid type is superior in all ways to all others, it may be that best practice involves the administration of combinations of these fluids to attain maximum benefit while minimizing possible adverse effects. HES 450 in normal saline appears to be associated with more bleeding and blood product use than other IV fluids. In patients at risk of bleeding, the intraoperative administration of HES 450/NS should be avoided where possible. This view is supported by the findings of an FDA review panel, which recommends the addition of a warning to the HES 450/NS label stating the risk of bleeding associated with the intraoperative administration of HES 450/NS during cardiac surgery. There is a growing body of evidence that suggests that renal function is adversely affected by 0.9% NaCl. Therefore it seems prudent to avoid the use of large volumes of 0.9% NaCl and normal saline–based fluids in patients who are at risk of renal dysfunction where balanced salt–based fluid preparations are available. The results of an ongoing, prospective, randomized blinded study comparing the impact of intraoperative 0.9% NaCl and lactated Ringer's on renal function after renal transplantation are awaited.

REFERENCES

1. Haisch G, Boldt J, Krebs C, Suttner S, Lehmann A, Isgro F: Influence of a new hydroxyethylstarch preparation (HES 130/0.4) on coagulation in cardiac surgical patients. *J Cardiothorac Vasc Anesth* 2001;15(3):316-321.
2. Beyer R, Harmening U, Rittmeyer O, et al: Use of modified fluid gelatin and hydroxyethyl starch for colloidal volume replacement in major orthopaedic surgery. *Br J Anaesth* 1997;78(1):44-50.
3. Haisch G, Boldt J, Krebs C, Kumle B, Suttner S, Schulz A: The influence of intravascular volume therapy with a new hydroxyethyl starch preparation (6% HES 130/0.4) on coagulation in patients undergoing major abdominal surgery. *Anesth Analg* 2001;92(3):565-571.
4. Kumle B, Boldt J, Piper S, Schmidt C, Suttner S, Salopek S: The influence of different intravascular volume replacement regimens on renal function in the elderly. *Anesth Analg* 1999;89(5):1124-1130.
5. Mortelmans YJ, Vermaut G, Verbruggen AM, et al: Effects of 6% hydroxyethyl starch and 3% modified fluid gelatin on intravascular volume and coagulation during intraoperative hemodilution. *Anesth Analg* 1995;81(6):1235-1242.
6. Huttner I, Boldt J, Haisch G, Suttner S, Kumle B, Schulz H: Influence of different colloids on molecular markers of haemostasis and platelet function in patients undergoing major abdominal surgery. *Br J Anaesth* 2000;85(3):417-423.
7. Claes Y, Van Hemelrijck J, Van Gerven M, et al: Influence of hydroxyethyl starch on coagulation in patients during the perioperative period. *Anesth Analg* 1992;75(1):24-30.
8. Gan TJ, Bennett-Guerrero E, Phillips-Bute B, et al: Hextend, a physiologically balanced plasma expander for large volume use in major surgery: A randomized phase III clinical trial. Hextend Study Group. *Anesth Analg* 1999;88(5):992-998.
9. Gold MS, Russo J, Tissot M, Weinhouse G, Riles T: Comparison of hetastarch to albumin for perioperative bleeding in patients undergoing abdominal aortic aneurysm surgery. A prospective, randomized study. *Ann Surg* 1990;211(4):482-485.
10. Petroni K, Green R, Birmingham S: Hextend is a safe alternative to 5% human albumin for patients undergoing elective cardiac surgery. *Anesthesiology* 2001;95:A198.
11. Vogt NH, Bothner U, Lerch G, Lindner KH, Georgieff M: Large-dose administration of 6% hydroxyethyl starch 200/0.5 total hip arthroplasty: Plasma homeostasis, hemostasis, and renal function compared to use of 5% human albumin. *Anesth Analg* 1996;83 (2):262-268.
12. Vogt N, Bothner U, Brinkmann A, de Petriconi R, Georgieff M: Peri-operative tolerance to large-dose 6% HES 200/0.5 in major urological procedures compared with 5% human albumin. *Anaesthesia* 1999;54(2):121-127.
13. Virgilio RW, Rice CL, Smith DE, et al: Crystalloid vs. colloid resuscitation: Is one better? A randomized clinical study. *Surgery* 1979;85(2):129-139.
14. Langeron O, Doelberg M, Ang ET, Bonnet F, Capdevila X, Coriat P: Voluven, a lower substituted novel hydroxyethyl starch (HES 130/0.4), causes fewer effects on coagulation in major orthopedic surgery than HES 200/0.5. *Anesth Analg* 2001;92(4):855-862.
15. Marik PE, Iglesias J, Maini B: Gastric intramucosal pH changes after volume replacement with hydroxyethyl starch or crystalloid in patients undergoing elective abdominal aortic aneurysm repair. *J Crit Care* 1997;12(2):51-55.
16. Prien T, Backhaus N, Pelster F, Pircher W, Bunte H, Lawin P: Effect of intraoperative fluid administration and colloid osmotic pressure on the formation of intestinal edema during gastrointestinal surgery. *J Clin Anesth* 1990;2(5):317-323.
17. Wilkes MM, Navickis RJ, Sibbald WJ: Albumin versus hydroxyethyl starch in cardiopulmonary bypass surgery: A meta-analysis of postoperative bleeding. *Ann Thorac Surg* 2001;72(2):527-533, discussion 34.
18. Cope JT, Banks D, Mauney MC, et al: Intraoperative hetastarch infusion impairs hemostasis after cardiac operations. *Ann Thorac Surg* 1997;63(1):78-82, discussion 83.
19. Knutson JE, Deering JA, Hall FW, et al: Does intraoperative hetastarch administration increase blood loss and transfusion requirements after cardiac surgery? *Anesth Analg* 2000;90(4):801-807.
20. Villarino ME, Gordon SM, Valdon C, et al: A cluster of severe postoperative bleeding following open heart surgery. *Infect Control Hosp Epidemiol* 1992;13(5):282-287.
21. Gallandat Huet RC, Siemons AW, Baus D, et al: A novel hydroxyethyl starch (Voluven) for effective perioperative plasma volume substitution in cardiac surgery. *Can J Anaesth* 2000; 47(12):1207-1215.
22. Gandhi SD, Weiskopf RB, Jungheinrich C, et al: Volume replacement therapy during major orthopedic surgery using Voluven (hydroxyethyl starch 130/0.4) or hetastarch. *Anesthesiology* 2007;106(6):1120-1127.
23. Jungheinrich C, Sauermann W, Bepperling F, Vogt NH: Volume efficacy and reduced influence on measures of coagulation using hydroxyethyl starch 130/0.4 (6%) with an optimised in vivo molecular weight in orthopaedic surgery: A randomised, double-blind study. *Drugs R D* 2004;5(1):1-9.
24. Van der Linden PJ, De Hert SG, Deraedt D, et al: Hydroxyethyl starch 130/0.4 versus modified fluid gelatin for volume expansion in cardiac surgery patients: The effects on perioperative bleeding and transfusion needs. *Anesth Analg* 2005;101(3):629-634, table of contents.

25. Boldt J, Schollhorn T, Munchbach J, Pabsdorf M: A total balanced volume replacement strategy using a new balanced hydoxyethyl starch preparation (6% HES 130/0.42) in patients undergoing major abdominal surgery. *Eur J Anaesthesiol* 2007;24(3):267-275.

26. Nielsen VG: Effects of PentaLyte and Voluven hemodilution on plasma coagulation kinetics in the rabbit: Role of thrombin-fibrinogen and factor XIII-fibrin polymer interactions. *Acta Anaesthesiol Scand* 2005;49(9):1263-1271.

27. Nielsen VG: Antithrombin efficiency is maintained in vitro in human plasma following dilution with hydroxyethyl starches. *Blood Coagul Fibrinolysis* 2005;16(5):319-322.

28. Waters JH, Gottlieb A, Schoenwald P, Popovich MJ, Sprung J, Nelson DR: Normal saline versus lactated Ringer's solution for intraoperative fluid management in patients undergoing abdominal aortic aneurysm repair: An outcome study. *Anesth Analg* 2001;93(4):817-822.

29. Boldt J, Haisch G, Suttner S, Kumle B, Schellhase F: Are lactated Ringer's solution and normal saline solution equal with regard to coagulation? *Anesth Analg* 2002;94(2):378-384, table of contents.

30. Harrison P, Roche AM, Wilkes NJ, Stephens R, Mythen MG: Comparison of the influence of balanced electrolyte versus saline based intravenous fluids on platelet function within the PFA-100. *Anesthesiology* 2001;95:A184.

31. Wilkes NJ, Woolf R, Mutch M, et al: The effects of balanced versus saline-based hetastarch and crystalloid solutions on acid-base and electrolyte status and gastric mucosal perfusion in elderly surgical patients. *Anesth Analg* 2001;93(4):811-816.

32. Cittanova ML, Leblanc I, Legendre C, Mouquet C, Riou B, Coriat P: Effect of hydroxyethylstarch in brain-dead kidney donors on renal function in kidney-transplant recipients. *Lancet* 1996;348 (9042):1620-1622.

33. Legendre C, Thervet E, Page B, Percheron A, Noel LH, Kreis H: Hydroxyethylstarch and osmotic-nephrosis-like lesions in kidney transplantation. *Lancet* 1993;342(8865):248-249.

34. Schortgen F, Lacherade JC, Bruneel F, et al: Effects of hydroxyethylstarch and gelatin on renal function in severe sepsis: A multicentre randomised study. *Lancet* 2001;357(9260):911-916.

35. Boldt J, Brosch C, Ducke M, Papsdorf M, Lehmann A: Influence of volume therapy with a modern hydroxyethylstarch preparation on kidney function in cardiac surgery patients with compromised renal function: A comparison with human albumin. *Crit Care Med* 2007;35(12):2740-2746.

36. Mahmood A, Gosling P, Vohra RK: Randomized clinical trial comparing the effects on renal function of hydroxyethyl starch or gelatine during aortic aneurysm surgery. *Br J Surg* 2007;94 (4):427-433.

37. Boldt J, Scholhorn T, Mayer J, Piper S, Suttner S: The value of an albumin-based intravascular volume replacement strategy in elderly patients undergoing major abdominal surgery. *Anesth Analg* 2006;103(1):191-199, table of contents.

38. Scheingraber S, Rehm M, Sehmisch C, Finsterer U: Rapid saline infusion produces hyperchloremic acidosis in patients undergoing gynecologic surgery. *Anesthesiology* 1999;90(5):1265-1270.

39. Lang K, Boldt J, Suttner S, Haisch G: Colloids versus crystalloids and tissue oxygen tension in patients undergoing major abdominal surgery. *Anesth Analg* 2001;93(2):405-409, 3rd contents page.

40. McFarlane C, Lee A: A comparison of Plasmalyte 148 and 0.9% saline for intra-operative fluid replacement. *Anaesthesia* 1994;49 (9):779-781.

41. Wilcox CS: Regulation of renal blood flow by plasma chloride. *J Clin Invest* 1983;71(3):726-735.

42. O'Malley CM, Frumento RJ, Hardy MA, et al: A randomized, double-blind comparison of lactated Ringer's solution and 0.9% NaCl during renal transplantation. *Anesth Analg* 2005;100(5):1518-1524, table of contents.

43. Elhakim M, el-Sebiae S, Kaschef N, Essawi GH: Intravenous fluid and postoperative nausea and vomiting after day-case termination of pregnancy. *Acta Anaesthesiol Scand* 1998;42(2):216-219.

44. Keane PW, Murray PF: Intravenous fluids in minor surgery. Their effect on recovery from anaesthesia. *Anaesthesia* 1986;41 (6):635-637.

45. Spencer EM: Intravenous fluids in minor gynaecological surgery. Their effect on postoperative morbidity. *Anaesthesia* 1988;43 (12):1050-1051.

46. Yogendran S, Asokumar B, Cheng DC, Chung F: A prospective randomized double-blinded study of the effect of intravenous fluid therapy on adverse outcomes on outpatient surgery. *Anesth Analg* 1995;80(4):682-686.

47. Moretti EW, Robertson KM, El-Moalem H, Gan TJ: Intraoperative colloid administration reduces postoperative nausea and vomiting and improves postoperative outcomes compared with crystalloid administration. *Anesth Analg* 2003;96(2):611-617, table of contents.

48. Williams EL, Hildebrand KL, McCormick SA, Bedel MJ: The effect of intravenous lactated Ringer's solution versus 0.9% sodium chloride solution on serum osmolality in human volunteers. *Anesth Analg* 1999;88(5):999-1003.

49. Rittoo D, Gosling P, Burnley S, et al: Randomized study comparing the effects of hydroxyethyl starch solution with gelofusine on pulmonary function in patients undergoing abdominal aortic aneurysm surgery. *Br J Anaesth* 2004;92(1):61-66.

50. Rittoo D, Gosling P, Simms MH, Smith SR, Vohra RK: The effects of hydroxyethyl starch compared with gelofusine on activated endothelium and the systemic inflammatory response following aortic aneurysm repair. *Eur J Vasc Endovasc Surg* 2005;30(5):520-524.

51. Kohler H, Kirch W, Weihrauch TR, Prellwitz W, Horstmann HJ: Macroamylasaemia after treatment with hydroxyethyl starch. *Eur J Clin Invest* 1977;7(3):205-211.

52. Metze D, Reimann S, Szepfalusi Z, Bohle B, Kraft D, Luger TA: Persistent pruritus after hydroxyethyl starch infusion therapy: A result of long-term storage in cutaneous nerves. *Br J Dermatol* 1997;136(4):553-559.

53. Morgan PW, Berridge JC: Giving long-persistent starch as volume replacement can cause pruritus after cardiac surgery. *Br J Anaesth* 2000;85(5):696-699.

54. Murphy M, Carmichael AJ, Lawler PG, White M, Cox NH: The incidence of hydroxyethyl starch-associated pruritus. *Br J Dermatol* 2001;144(5):973-976.

55. Kimme P, Jannsen B, Ledin T, Gupta A, Vegfors M: High incidence of pruritus after large doses of hydroxyethyl starch (HES) infusions. *Acta Anaesthesiol Scand* 2001;45(6):686-689.

56. Bothner U, Georgieff M, Vogt NH: Assessment of the safety and tolerance of 6% hydroxyethyl starch (200/0.5) solution: A randomized, controlled epidemiology study. *Anesth Analg* 1998;86 (4):850-855.

57. Ring J, Messmer K: Incidence and severity of anaphylactoid reactions to colloid volume substitutes. *Lancet* 1977;1(8009):466-469.

58. Finfer S, Bellomo R, Boyce N, French J, Myburgh J, Norton R: A comparison of albumin and saline for fluid resuscitation in the intensive care unit. *N Engl J Med* 2004;350(22):2247-2256.

59. Myburgh J, Cooper J, Finfer S, et al: Saline or albumin for fluid resuscitation in patients with traumatic brain injury. *N Engl J Med* 2007;357(9):874-884.

60. Wiedemann HP, Wheeler AP, Bernard GR, et al: Comparison of two fluid-management strategies in acute lung injury. *N Engl J Med* 2006;354(24):2564-2575.

61. Grocott MP, Mythen MG, Gan TJ: Perioperative fluid management and clinical outcomes in adults. *Anesth Analg* 2005;100 (4):1093-1106.

31 What Works in a Patient with Acute Respiratory Distress Syndrome?

Michael G. Fitzsimons, MD, FCCP, and William E. Hurford, MD

INTRODUCTION

Acute respiratory distress syndrome (ARDS) is a phenomenon often encountered by anesthesiologists in the operating room and intensive care unit (ICU) settings. It is also a feared complication of aspiration of gastric contents. ARDS is a syndrome of pathologic changes, caused by a variety of toxic and infectious agents, that evolve over time from endothelial injury and alveolar consolidation to fibroblast proliferation and collagen deposition.[1] In 1994, the American-European Consensus Conference on ARDS (AECC) defined ARDS to include bilateral infiltrates on chest radiograph consistent with pulmonary edema; PaO_2/FiO_2 ratio of less than 200 mm Hg (PaO_2/FiO_2 ratio less than 300 mm Hg defined acute lung injury); and a pulmonary artery occlusion pressure less than or equal to 18 mm Hg, or no evidence of left atrial hypertension.[2] Many mediators have been implicated in its pathophysiology, including complement, cytokines, oxygen radicals, arachidonic acid products, nitric oxide, and proteases. Multiple insults incite the syndrome. Direct causes are those that directly injure the lung, such as aspiration, pneumonia, pulmonary contusion, thermal inhalation, amniotic fluid embolism, and particle inhalation. Indirect causes injure the lung via mediator release and include pancreatitis, sepsis, and bacteremia. The presence of multiple insults increases the risk of ARDS.

The true incidence and mortality rates of ARDS remain somewhat unclear because many studies completed before the AECC did not use a standard definition. A study at Harborview Medical Center in Seattle, Washington, reported an incidence of ARDS of 12.6 per 100,000 per year and an incidence of 18.9 per 100,000 per year for acute lung injury (ALI).[3] The hospital mortality rate has been reported between 40% and 60% in most studies but has decreased over the past three decades.[4] An older age, higher APACHE score, transfusion of blood cells, and the use of steroids before the development of ARDS predict a higher mortality risk.[5]

OPTIONS

Therapeutic interventions either have been directed at a specific phase of the syndrome, or are more general and supportive in nature. Most deaths associated with ARDS are caused by sepsis, rarely from the inability to provide adequate ventilatory support.[4] Here we will discuss the evidence supporting or dismissing certain ventilatory strategies, including low lung volumes, positioning, and oxygenation; antiinflammatory therapies such as corticosteroid administration; hemodynamic management; and other supportive techniques.

Evidence for Lower Tidal Volume Ventilation in ARDS

Traditional ventilatory strategy in ARDS included the use of tidal volumes in the 10 to 15 mL/kg range in an effort to normalize $PaCO_2$ and pH. This mode of ventilation has been implicated as contributing to additional lung injury and multisystem organ failure.[6] The repetitive opening and closing of recruitable alveoli with traditional ventilation may alter endothelial permeability, increase edema, and release inflammatory mediators that may contribute to extrapulmonary organ failure and worsened outcome.

Amato and colleagues[7] randomized 53 patients from December 1990 to July 1995 with ARDS to either a conventional or protective mechanical ventilation strategy. The mortality rate at 28 days was 38% in the protective strategy group and 71% in the conventional mechanical ventilation group. They also found a lower incidence of barotrauma in the protective-ventilation group. The rate of survival to hospital discharge was not different between the groups. The National Heart, Lung, and Blood Institute Acute Respiratory Distress Clinical Trials Network (ARDS Net) studied patients at 10 university centers between 1996 and 1998.[8] Eight-hundred sixty-one patients were enrolled and equally randomized to either traditional (initial tidal volume 12 mL/kg ideal body weight [IBW]) or low tidal volume ventilation (6 mL/kg tidal volume). Mortality rate at 28 days was reduced from 40% to 30%, death rate before hospital discharge was reduced, ventilator-free days were higher, and the number of days without failure of nonpulmonary organs or systems was increased. Interleukin-6 levels were lower, possibly indicating less lung inflammation. Kallet and colleagues[9] applied the ARDS network protocol to 292 patients with acute lung injury of ARDS and found an overall mortality rate of 32% when compared with historical controls (51%).

Permissive hypercapnia is the elevation of $PaCO_2$ to levels above normal in the setting of tidal volume limitation. It is a consequence of ventilation management strategies that permit lower minute volumes in an attempt to reduce ventilator-induced lung injury and generally appears to be well tolerated.[10] Additional work is needed to determine whether permissive hypercapnia is detrimental or perhaps even beneficial.

The ARDS Net compared high levels of positive end-expiratory pressure (PEEP) to lower levels in patients with early ARDS while maintaining a plateau pressure less than 30 mm Hg in both groups. The hypothesis of the study was that higher levels of PEEP would improve oxygenation and decrease ventilator-induced lung injury.[11] No benefit was noted in terms of overall mortality rate, ventilator-free days, ICU-free days, or organ-failure–free days. The conclusion further supported the finding that ventilation with lower tidal volumes and inspiratory pressures improved outcome, and that increasing PEEP levels further added little benefit.

Overall, current evidence supports ventilation strategies that include lower tidal volumes (approximately 6 mL/kg IBW), lower plateau airway pressures (less than 30 cm H_2O), and higher levels of PEEP to maintain alveolar recruitment even at the expense of elevated $PaCO_2$ and decreased pH. Increasing PEEP beyond the recommended levels does not appear to improve outcome (Table 31-1).

Evidence for Additional Respiratory Strategies in ARDS

Multiple other strategies have been suggested as adjuvants to traditional ventilation, including prone positioning, inhaled nitric oxide (iNO), extracorporeal membranous oxygenation (ECMO), recruitment maneuvers, and noninvasive positive pressure ventilation (NIPPV).

Prone and vertical positioning often improve oxygenation.[12,13] The improvement with prone positioning is believed to result from a more uniform distribution of tidal volume and an improvement in ventilation-perfusion matching. The issue is whether a temporary improvement in oxygenation from prone positioning improves overall outcome. Gattinoni and colleagues[14] randomized 304 patients with acute respiratory failure to either intermittent prone positioning or continual supine positioning. The PaO_2 measured each morning was higher in the prone position patients, but no survival benefit was observed at 10 days, at ICU discharge, or after 6 months' follow-up. Although their study indicated that prone positioning can be done safely, the authors cautioned that routine use of the prone position in patients with acute respiratory failure was not justified.[14]

Vertical positioning involves raising the head 45 degrees and lowering the legs by 45 degrees. The PaO_2 increases significantly in a high number of patients and is likely caused by a time-dependent increase in lung volume, suggestive of alveolar recruitment.[13]

iNO has been suggested as an adjunctive therapy for ARDS because of its ability to improve the intrapulmonary right-to-left shunting characteristic of ARDS and decrease pulmonary artery pressure. Multiple trials of iNO have been performed in patients with ARDS; most show a transient but short-lasting improvement in PaO_2 without any outcome benefit.[15-19]

ECMO accompanied by a limited ventilation strategy has been reported as a possible therapeutic modality in severe ARDS.[20] Zapol and colleagues[21] randomized 90 patients to either conventional ventilation or partial veno-arterial bypass. They reported no survival benefit, but did document that ECMO could support respiratory gas exchange in patients with severe acute respiratory failure.[21] An uncontrolled trial by Gattinoni and colleagues[22] reported improved survival in those patients receiving ECMO.[22] A subsequent randomized trial performed by Morris and colleagues,[23] however, failed to show any benefit. ECMO is complicated, labor intensive, not widely available, and of questionable benefit. Its routine use cannot be justified in ARDS, but highly selected patients might be candidates. The results of a large randomized clinical trial may finally resolve this issue.[24]

NIPPV has many benefits compared with traditional intubation for the management of respiratory insufficiency. Benefits include a lower incidence of nosocomial pneumonia, lower intubation rates, less sinusitis, and easier communication with the patient. It is also an alternative for patients who refuse intubation. Disadvantages include increased nursing time, poor airway protection, inability to deliver high levels of PEEP, and difficulty with implementation in the combative or delirious patient. Declaux and colleagues[25] randomized 123 patients (102 with acute lung injury and 21 with cardiac disease) with acute hypoxemic respiratory failure to either continuous positive airway pressure (CPAP) or standard oxygen therapy. They found that subjective responses to treatment were greater with CPAP, but there was no reduction in intubation rate, ICU length of stay, or hospital mortality rate.[25] Antonelli and colleagues[26] studied NIPPV in patients with ARDS and found that early implementation may avoid intubation in up to 54% of the patients. Patients with a higher Simplified Acute Physiology Score (SAPS) and a failure to improve PaO_2/FiO_2 ratio within an hour were more likely to fail the trial and require intubation. Since ARDS is rarely a short-term problem and rarely a single-organ abnormality, it is difficult to recommend NIPPV as a first step in all patients with ARDS, but it may be a viable option in selected patients or when intubation is not desirable.

High-frequency oscillatory ventilation (HFOV) has been suggested as a possible management strategy in ARDS. The advantages of HFOV are lower tidal volumes and higher mean airway pressure for a given peak pressure, minimizing the risk of overdistention and maintaining end-expiratory lung volume and alveolar recruitment. HFOV has been reported to improve clinical outcome in premature infants with respiratory distress syndrome compared with conventional ventilation.[27,28] In adult patients, Carlon and colleagues[29] randomized 309 patients to either volume-cycled ventilation (VCV) or high-frequency jet ventilation (HFJV). They found that VCV provided a slightly improved PaO_2 at equivalent PEEP, but on HFJV, oxygenation and ventilation were maintained with lower peak inspiratory pressures and smaller tidal volumes.

Table 31-1   Ventilator/ECMO/iNO Trials

Parameter	Study (Year)	Type	Results	Outcomes
Extracorporeal membranous oxygenation (ECMO)	Zapol (1979)[21]	Randomized	ECMO can support respiratory gas exchange	No difference in survival
High-frequency jet ventilation (HFJV)	Carlton (1983)[29]	Randomized	Oxygenation, ventilation maintained at lower peak pressure and TV on HFJV	No difference in survival of ICU stay
ECMO	Morris (1994)[23]	Randomized	Survival similar in both groups	Extracorporeal support not recommended in ARDS
High-frequency oscillatory ventilation (HFOV)	Fort (1997)[30]	Prospective, clinical	Improvement in PaO_2/FiO_2 ratio, no change in cardiac output, O_2 delivery	HFOV is safe and effective, additional studies needed
Protective ventilation vs. conventional ventilation	Amato (1998)[7]	Randomized	28-day mortality rate 38% (protective) vs. 71% (conventional), less barotrauma	No difference in survival to discharge
Inhaled nitric oxide (iNO)	Dellinger (1998)[17]	Randomized, double-blind, placebo-controlled	Improvement in oxygenation after 4 hours and at 4 days	No improvement in mortality rate
iNO	Michael (1998)[16]	Randomized	PaO_2/FiO_2 improved at 1 hour, 12 hours, 24 hours	Benefits do not persist, no survival benefit
iNO	Trouncy (1998)[15]	Randomized	Oxygenation improved in first 24 hours	No benefit after 24 hours, similar mortality rate
Lower tidal volume vs. traditional tidal volume	ARDS Network (2000)[8]	Randomized	28-day mortality rate 30%, higher ventilator-free days, lower IL-6, death before hospital discharge reduced	Mortality rate reduced, but long-term benefits need to be studied
Continuous positive airway pressure (CPAP)	Delclaux (2000)[25]	Randomized, concealed, unblinded	Subjective response to CPAP greater than standard O_2	No difference in intubation rate, mortality, ICU stay
Prone position	Gattinoni (2001)[14]	Randomized	Increased PaO_2/FiO_2, similar complication rate	No improvement in survival
Recruitment maneuvers	Oczenski (2004)[34]	Randomized	Recruitment maneuvers improved PaO_2/FiO_2 ratio	Benefits of recruitment did not persist beyond 30 minutes
High vs. lower PEEP	ARDS Network (2004)[11]	Randomized	PaO_2/FiO_2 was higher in the "high PEEP" group	No significant difference in mortality rate, ventilator-free days, or organ-failure-free days
Lower tidal volume ventilation	Kallet (2005)[2]	Retrospective, uncontrolled	Mortality rate lower in ARDS patients subject to ARDS Network protocol (32% vs. 51%)	Adoption of ARDS Network protocol for ALI/ARDS reduced mortality rate compared with historical controls
Lung recruitment	Gattinoni (2006)[33]	Observational study	Percentage of recruitable lung varied among patients On average 24% of the lung could not be recruited Patients with a lower respiratory-system compliance, higher $PaCO_2$, and lower PaO_2:FiO_2 at the beginning demonstrated more recruitability	This observational trial did not address outcome
Inhaled nitric oxide (iNO)	Angus (2006)[19]	Randomized	Hospital costs, length of stay, were similar in the iNO group	No difference in survival at 1 year
iNO	Adhikari (2007)[18]	Meta-analysis	iNO may increase oxygenation until up to 4 days	No overall mortality rate benefit

There was no improvement in overall survival or ICU length of stay.[29] Fort and colleagues[30] performed a prospective clinical study in 1997 on 17 patients with ARDS. They reported that 13 of 17 had an improvement in their PaO_2/FiO_2 ratio, without decrements in blood pressure, cardiac output, or oxygen delivery.[30] A large randomized controlled trial is needed to assess the benefits of HFOV.

Lung collapse is a major contributing factor to the hypoxemia of acute lung injury and ARDS. The repeated cyclic opening and closure of individual alveoli contributes to ventilator-associated lung injury. Recruitment maneuvers involve the application of high levels of PEEP and have been demonstrated in early lung injury and ARDS to reverse hypoxemia.[31] The ability to recruit alveoli has been demonstrated in ARDS caused by both primary pulmonary and secondary pulmonary causes.[32] The percentage of lung tissue that can be "recruited" varies among individual patients, but may sometimes actually be greater in those with more severe lung injury.[33] Unfortunately these maneuvers generally do not result in a sustained improvement in oxygenation.[34] Complications associated with recruitment may include barotrauma and hemodynamic compromise. No study has yet effectively demonstrated long-term benefits attributed to a particular recruitment strategy (Table 31-2).

Evidence for Pharmacologic Strategies in ARDS

The pharmacologic interventions that have been tested in ARDS generally are directed at blocking the inflammatory mediators released after the inciting event has occurred. Interventions have included cytokine blockers, monoclonal antibodies against endotoxins or interleukins, antioxidants, activated protein C, nonsteroidal antiinflammatory drugs, and prostanoids.[35]

Although many of these interventions have shown benefit in initial trials and some animal studies, few benefits have been realized in human trials. Studies of prostaglandin E_1,[36] procysteine,[37] lisophylline,[38] and ketoconazole[39] have not shown a survival benefit.

Reduced surfactant production and function leads to increased surface tension, alveolar collapse, and decreased parenchyma compliance. Airway pressures needed to open these alveoli are exceedingly high. Anzueto and colleagues[40] studied the efficacy of artificial aerosolized surfactant in ARDS patients. They found no improvement in oxygenation, ventilation, or mortality rate.[40] Work continues on improved techniques of surfactant administration; however, it is unclear whether its pulmonary effects would be sufficient to alter clinical outcome[41] (see Table 31-2).

Table 31-2 Pharmacologic/Steroid Trials

Parameter	Study (Year)	Type	Results	Outcomes
Prostaglandin E_1 (PGE$_1$)	Bone (1989)[38]	Randomized, double-blind	PGE$_1$ increased heart rate, stroke volume, and cardiac output	PGE$_1$ did not increase survival
Corticosteroids	Meduri (1991)[54]	Prospective clinical	Improvement in lung injury score, improvement in PaO_2/FiO_2	Larger randomized-controlled trial needed
Corticosteroids	Meduri (1994)[55]	Prospective clinical	Improved lung injury score, decreased PEEP, improved chest x-ray	Larger randomized-controlled trial needed
Aerosolized surfactant	Anzueto (1996)[40]	Randomized, placebo-controlled	No improvement, oxygenation, duration of mechanical ventilation, or survival	Aerosolized surfactant not beneficial in ARDS
Corticosteroids	Meduri (1998)[56]	Randomized, double-blind, placebo-controlled	Lung injury score improved, PaO_2/FiO_2 improved, MODS score improved, mortality rate 12% vs. 62% (control)	Survival improved with methylprednisolone ARDS Network performing larger trial
Ketoconazole	ARDS Network (2000)[39]	Randomized, placebo-controlled	No differences in organ-failure free days, adverse events, or pulmonary function	Ketoconazole did not reduce mortality rate or improve outcome
Lisophylline	ARDS Network (2002)[38]	Randomized, double-blind, placebo-controlled	No difference in organ failure, ventilator-free days, or infections	Lisophylline did not improve mortality rate
Corticosteroids	ARDS Network (2006)[57]	Randomized	Mortality rate 28.6% in placebo group, 29.2% in treated group Higher number of ventilator- and shock-free days in treated group	No improvement in overall mortality rate, possibly higher mortality rate in patients who had steroids started later
Corticosteroids	Meduri (2007)[53]	Randomized, controlled	Mortality rate reduced in treated patients (20.6% vs. 42.9%) Duration of mechanical ventilation and infections reduced	Mortality rate reduced

Evidence for Hemodynamic Manipulation

The goals of hemodynamic management in ARDS are still an area of controversy. The ARDS Net has addressed the benefits of pulmonary versus central venous catheters and "conservative" versus "liberal" fluid management strategies in its Fluid and Catheter Treatment Trial (FACTT).

The Pulmonary Artery Catheter Consensus Conference in 1997 noted that there was inadequate evidence from existing clinical trials and case series to definitively determine benefit or harm from pulmonary artery catheter (PAC) use in patients with respiratory failure.[42] The benefits of PACs were evaluated in 100 patients with acute lung injury through the ARDS Net.[43] Compared to patients managed with a central venous catheter, no difference in lung or renal function, incidence of hypotension, ventilator settings, dialysis rate, or use of vasopressors was noted. Survival was not improved at 60 days. The incidence of complications related to catheterization was higher in the PAC group, particularly concerning ventricular and atrial arrhythmias. The routine use of a PAC for management of patients with ARDS to improve organ function and survival cannot be recommended.

It is clear that the increased permeability is responsible for the accumulation of alveolar fluid in ARDS. This accumulation occurs at lower pulmonary capillary wedge pressures than normal. It has been argued that diuresis and fluid restriction may benefit the ARDS patient by limiting or preventing edema. Mitchell and colleagues[44] studied patients with ARDS who had PACs in place. Those with lower extravascular lung water had shorter periods of mechanical ventilation and shorter ICU stays, but mortality rate was not different.[44] It is unclear, however, whether overly aggressive fluid restriction may worsen extrapulmonary organ failure. The FACTT trial compared "liberal" versus "conservative" fluid management strategies.[45] Patients randomized to the "conservative" arm of the clinical trial received nearly 7 L less fluid in the first 7 days of the study. Benefits were noted in oxygenation, lung injury score, and ventilator-free days without an increase in organ failure or need for dialysis. No difference was noted in 60-day mortality rate. Accordingly, current evidence suggests that clinicians observe a more conservative management strategy for patients with ARDS (Table 31-3).

Evidence for Supportive and Preventive Care

The systemic manifestations of ARDS must not be neglected. Sedation must balance patient comfort and the ability to assess neurologic status. Nutritional needs must be met. Secondary injury to skin and other tissue must be avoided.

Complications of sedation include hypotension, slow ventilator wean, and the inability to assess neurologic

Table 31-3   Nutrition, Position, Sedation, Monitoring, and Fluid Bundle Trials

Parameter	Study (Year)	Type	Results	Outcomes
Enteral feeding with specific nutrients and antioxidants	Gadek (1999)[49]	Prospective, multicenter, double-blind, randomized controlled trial	Deceased number of neutrophils in alveolar tissue, improvement in oxygenation, fewer days of ventilator support, decreased length of ICU stay, lower rate of development of new organ failure	No significant difference in mortality rate
"Sedation vacation" in ventilated patients (not ARDS)	Kress (2000)[46]	Randomized control	Decreased median duration of mechanical ventilation (4.9 days vs. 7.3 days) and duration of ICU stay (6.4 vs. 9.9 days)	No difference in in-hospital mortality rate
Prone position	Gattinoni (2001)[14]	Randomized	Increased PaO_2/FiO_2, similar complication rate	No improvement in survival
Ventilator bundles in ventilated patients	Resar (2005)[50]	Historical control	44.5% reduction in ventilator-associated pneumonia in intubated patients	Increased adherence to ventilator bundle
Vertical positioning	Richard (2006)[13]	Prospective observational physiologic study	Vertical positioning significantly improved PaO_2 and lung recruitment.	Study was not designed to compare outcomes
Conservative vs. liberal fluid management trials	ARDS Network (2006)[45]	Randomized	Patients treated with a conservative fluid management protocol demonstrated improved oxygenation, increased ventilator-free days, and greater number of days out of the intensive care unit	No difference in overall 60-day outcome
Pulmonary artery vs. central venous catheter to guide treatment of acute lung injury (FACTT)	ARDS Network (2006)[43]	Randomized	No significant difference in pulmonary or renal function, rate of hypotension, dialysis, or use of vasopressors	The PAC did not improve clinical outcome and patients had a higher number of complications

status. Complications of the addition of neuromuscular blocking agents include worsening of critical care myopathy. Although no specific sedation technique is clearly superior to another, daily interruption of sedative infusions (stopping an infusion until the patient is awake and then restarting the drug, commonly called a "sedation vacation") has been reported to decrease the duration of mechanical ventilation and length of stay in the ICU.[46] It is recommended that protocols be developed for the sedation of ICU patients requiring mechanical ventilation that address pain control, comfort, and patient safety.

Patients commonly do not receive adequate nutrition in both medical and surgical ICUs.[47] Fortunately, nutritional support protocols increase the proportion of patients adequately fed.[48] Gadek and colleagues[49] demonstrated that enteral feeding with certain nutrients and antioxidants improved gas exchange, lowered the requirement for mechanical ventilation, decreased the length of ICU stay, and reduced the incidence of new organ failure. It is recommended that units implement protocols for the early implementation of enteral feeding in patients with ARDS.

The implementation of a small set of evidence-based interventions referred to as "ventilator bundles" may decease the incidence of complications common in patients receiving mechanical ventilation. These include peptic ulcer disease prophylaxis, deep venous thrombosis (DVT) prophylaxis, elevation of the head of the bed, and a daily interruption of sedative infusions. Implementation of such bundles has been reported to decrease the incidence of ventilator-associated pneumonia[50] (see Table 31-3).

AREAS OF CONTROVERSY

Corticosteroids remain a major area of controversy in the management of both early and late ARDS. Early studies failed to show any benefit from the use of corticosteroids in early ARDS.[51,52] A more recent randomized, double-blind, placebo-controlled trial showed a reduction in mechanical ventilation, ICU stay, and ICU mortality rate in patients receiving methylprednisolone.[53] It has been postulated that corticosteroids may inhibit release of proinflammatory or profibrotic cytokines and reduce collagen deposition and fibrosis in the injured lung. Meduri and colleagues[54] initially studied eight patients with ARDS without an obvious site of infection. Methylprednisolone was administered as a bolus of 2 mg/kg followed by 2 to 3 mg/kg/day divided in every-6-hour

dosing. Six of the eight patients survived to discharge and had lower lung injury scales.[54] A small follow-up study also suggested a survival benefit in those patients treated with steroids.[55,56] The ARDS Net performed a large trial evaluating the effectiveness of methylprednisolone in persistent ARDS.[57] Steroids were initiated 7 to 28 days after the onset of ARDS. Despite improvements in respiratory-system compliance, blood pressure, and ventilator-free days, there was no improvement in overall mortality rate. Indeed, mortality rate at 60 and 180 days was significantly higher in the group receiving steroids compared with the group receiving placebo. Some potential benefit has been shown when steroids are administered to patients with septic shock and adrenal insufficiency,[58] or with sepsis syndrome and adrenal insufficiency associated with ARDS.[59] Overall, however, corticosteroid treatment of ARDS remains controversial at best and may be harmful (see Table 31-2).

AUTHORS' RECOMMENDATIONS

The diagnosis of ARDS should be established. An acute onset of respiratory failure, PaO_2/FiO_2 $\leq$200 mm Hg (300 mm Hg for acute lung injury), bilateral patchy infiltrates on chest radiograph, and no evidence of a cardiogenic etiology of pulmonary edema defines the syndrome.

The original insult responsible for inciting ARDS must be identified and treated. Pneumonia, sepsis, and bacteremia must be treated with antibiotics and surgical drainage when indicated. Further injury must be prevented.

Close monitoring of fluid balance is imperative. The administration of excessive amounts of fluid in attempts to maintain hemodynamic stability imparts no clear outcome benefit. A "conservative" strategy to fluid management may shorten the duration of intubation without contributing to nonpulmonary organ failure.[45]

The adoption of sedation protocols that include a daily "sedation vacation" reduces the duration of mechanical ventilation and allows assessment of neurologic status.

Protocols established for the early initiation of enteral nutrition decrease the rate of underfeeding.

The integration of "ventilator bundles" that routinely provide prophylaxis for peptic ulcer disease and DVT and require elevation of the head of the bed decreases the incidence of ventilator-associated pneumonia.

Mechanical ventilation according to the protocols published by the National Institutes of Health ARDS Clinical Network is recommended.[60] This protocol has become the "gold standard" against which methods of management of ARDS can be tested (Table 31-4).

Table 31-4   ARDS Clinical Network Mechanical Ventilation Protocol Summary

INCLUSION CRITERIA: Acute onset of:

1. $PaO_2/FiO_2 \leq 300$ (corrected for altitude)
2. Bilateral (patchy, diffuse, or homogeneous) infiltrates consistent with pulmonary edema
3. No clinical evidence of left atrial hypertension

PART I: VENTILATOR SETUP AND ADJUSTMENT

1. Calculate predicted body weight (PBW)
Males = 50 + 2.3 [height (inches) - 60]
Females = 45.5 + 2.3 [height (inches) - 60]
2. Select Assist Control Mode
3. Set initial TV to 8 ml/kg PBW
4. Reduce TV by 1 ml/kg at intervals ≤ 2 hours until TV = 6 ml/kg PBW.
5. Set initial rate to approximate baseline VE (not >35 beats/min).
6. Adjust TV and RR to achieve pH and plateau pressure goals below.
7. Set inspiratory flow rate above patient demand (usually >80 L/min)

Oxygenation Goal: PaO_2 55-80 mm Hg or SpO_2 88%-95%

Use incremental FiO_2/PEEP combinations below to achieve goal. Higher PEEP options (lower row) will decrease FiO_2 and may be preferred in patients with high FiO_2 who can tolerate higher PEEP (stable blood pressure, no barotrauma). Survival is similar with both PEEP approaches.

Fio_2	0.3	0.4	0.4	0.5	0.5	0.6	0.7	0.7
PEEP	5 12-14	5 14	8 16	8 16	10 18-20	10 20	10 20	12 20
Fio_2	0.7	0.8	0.9	0.9	0.9	1.0	1.0	1.0
PEEP	14 20	14 20-22	14 22	16 22	18 22	20 22	22 22	24 24

Plateau Pressure Goal: ≤ 30 cm H_2O

Check P_{plat} (0.5 second inspiratory pause), SpO_2, Total RR, TV and pH (if available) at least every 4 hours and after each change in PEEP or TV.
If P_{plat} >30 cm H_2O: decrease TV by 1 mL/kg steps (minimum = 4 mL/kg).
If P_{plat} <25 cm H_2O: TV <6 mL/kg, increase TV by 1 ml/kg until P_{plat} >25 cm H_2O or TV = 6 mL/kg.
If P_{plat} <30 and breath stacking occurs: may increase TV in 1 mL/kg increments (maximum = 8 mL/kg).
pH GOAL: 7.30-7.45
Acidosis Management: (pH <7.30)
If pH 7.15-7.30: Increase RR until pH >7.30 or $PaCO_2$ <25 (maximum RR = 35).
If RR = 35 and $PaCO_2$ <25, may give $NaHCO_3$.
If pH <7.15: Increase RR to 35.
If pH remains <7.15 and $NaHCO_3$ considered or infused, TV may be increased in 1 mL/kg steps until pH >7.15 (P_{plat} target may be exceeded).
Alkalosis Management: (pH >7.45) Decrease vent rate if possible.
I:E RATIO GOAL: 1:1.0 - 1:3 Adjust flow rate to achieve goal. If FiO_2 = 1.0 and PEEP = 24 cm H_2O, may adjust I:E to 1:1.

PART II: WEANING

A. Conduct a CPAP Trial daily when:

1. FiO2 ≤ 0.40 and PEEP ≤ 8 or, if using the higher PEEP scale and FiO_2 ≤ 0.3 and PEEP 12-14, slowly reduce PEEP to 8 and increase FiO_2 to 0.4 for 30 min.
2. PEEP and FiO_2 $\leq$ values of previous day
3. Patient has acceptable spontaneous breathing efforts. (May decrease vent rate by 50% for 5 minutes to detect effort.)
4. Systolic BP ≥ 90 mm Hg without vasopressor support.

CONDUCTING THE TRIAL:

Set CPAP = 5 cm H_2O, FiO_2 = 0.50
If RR ≤ 35 for 5 min: advance to Pressure Support Weaning below:
If RR >35 in <5 min: may repeat trial after appropriate intervention (e.g., suctioning, analgesia, anxiolysis)
If CPAP trial not tolerated: return to previous A/C settings

(Continued)

Table 31-4   ARDS Clinical Network Mechanical Ventilation Protocol Summary—Cont'd

B. PRESSURE SUPPORT (PS) WEANING PROCEDURE
1. Set PEEP = 5, and FiO_2 = 0.50
2. Set initial PS based on RR during CPAP trial:
   a. **If CPAP RR <25:** set PS = 5 cm H_2O and go to step 3d.
   b. **If CPAP RR = 25-35:** set PS =20 cm H_2O then reduce by 5 cm H_2O at ≤5-minute intervals until RR = 26-35 then go to step 3a.
   c. **If initial PS not tolerated:** return to previous A/C settings.
3. **REDUCING PS:** (No reductions made after 1700 hours)
   a. Reduce PS by 5 cm H_2O q1-3h
   b. If PS ≥10 cm H_2O not tolerated, return to previous A/C settings (Reinitiate last tolerated PS level next AM and go to step 3a)
   c. If PS = 5 cm H_2O not tolerated, return to PS = 10 cm H_2O. If tolerated, 5 or 10 cm H_2O may be used overnight with further attempts at weaning the next morning
   d. If PS = 5 cm H_2O tolerated for ≥2 hours assess for ability to sustain unassisted breathing below.
C. UNASSISTED BREATHING TRIAL:
1. Place on T-piece, trach collar, or CPAP ≤5 cm H_2O
2. Assess for tolerance as below for 2 hours.
   a. SpO_2 ≥90: and/or PaO_2 ≥60 mm Hg
   b. Spontaneous TV ≥4 mL/kg PBW
   c. RR ≤35/min
   d. pH ≥7.3
   e. No respiratory distress (distress= 2 or more)
      - HR >120% of baseline
      - Marked accessory muscle use
      - Abdominal paradox
      - Diaphoresis
      - Marked dyspnea
3. If tolerated consider extubation.
4. If not tolerated resume PS 5 cm H_2O.

Reproduced with permission from ARDS Network, http://www.ardsnet.org

REFERENCES

1. Bigatello LM, Zapol WM: New approaches to acute lung injury. *Br J Anaesth* 1996;77:99-109.
2. Bernard GR, Artigas A, Brigham KL Carlet J, et al: The American-European Consensus Conference on ARDS: Definitions, mechanisms, relevant outcomes, and clinical trial coordination. *Am J Respir Crit Care Med* 1994;149:818-824; *J Crit Care* 1994;9:72-81; *Intensive Care Med* 1994;20:225-232.
3. Hudson LD, Steinberg KP: Epidemiology of acute lung injury and ARDS. *Chest* 1999;116:74S-82S.
4. Stapleton RD, Wang BM, Hudson LD, Rubenfeld GD, Caldwell ES, Steinberg KP: Causes and timing of deaths in patients with ARDS. *Chest* 2005;128:525-532.
5. Gong MN, Thompson BT, Williams P, Pothier L, Boyce PD, Christiani DC: Clinical predictors of and mortality in acute respiratory distress syndrome: Potential role of red cell transfusion. *Crit Care Med* 2005;33:1191-1198.
6. Slutsky AS, Tremblay LN: Multiple system organ failure, is mechanical ventilation a contributing factor? *Am J Respir Crit Care Med* 1998;157:1721-1725.
7. Amato MB, Barbas CSV, Medieros DM, Magaldi RB: Effect of protective-ventilation strategy on the mortality in the acute respiratory distress syndrome. *N Engl J Med* 1998;338:347-354.
8. Acute Respiratory Distress Syndrome Network: Ventilation with lower tidal volumes as compared with traditional tidal volumes for acute lung injury and the acute respiratory distress syndrome. *N Engl J Med* 2000;342:1301-1308.
9. Kallet RH, Jasmer RM, Pittet JF, Tang JF, et al: Clinical implementation of the ARDS network protocol is associated with reduced hospital mortality compared with historical controls. *Crit Care Med* 2005;33:925-929.
10. Kacmarek RM, Hickling KG: Permissive hypercapnia. *Resp Care* 1993;38:373-387.
11. Brower RG, Lanken PN, MacIntyre N, Matthay MA, Morris A, Ancukiewicz M, et al, National Heart, Lung, and Blood Institute ARDS Clinical Trials Network: Higher versus lower positive end-expiratory pressures in patients with the acute respiratory distress syndrome. *N Engl J Med* 2004;351:327-336.
12. Douglas WW, Rheder K, Beynen FM, Sessler AD, Marsh HM: Improved oxygenation in patients with acute respiratory failure: The prone position. *Am Rev Respir Dis* 1974;115:559-566.
13. Richard JC, Maggiore SM, Mancebo J, Lemaire F, et al: Effects of vertical positioning on gas exchange and lung volumes in acute respiratory distress syndrome. *Intensive Care Med* 2006;32:1623-1626.
14. Gattinoni L, Tognoni G, Presenti A, Taccone P, et al: Effect of prone positioning on the survival of patients with acute respiratory failure. *N Engl J Med* 2001;345:568-573.
15. Troncy E, Collet J, Shapiro S, Guimond J, et al: Inhaled nitric oxide in acute respiratory distress syndrome, a pilot randomized controlled study. *Am J Respir Crit Care Med* 1998;157: 1483-1488.
16. Michael JR, Barton RG, Saffle JR, Mone M, et al: Inhaled nitric oxide versus conventional therapy, effect on oxygenation in ARDS. *Am J Respir Crit Care Med* 1998;157:1372-1380.
17. Dellinger RP, Zimmermann JL, Taylor RW, Straube RC, et al: Effects of inhaled nitric oxide in patients with acute respiratory distress syndrome: Results of a randomized phase II trial. *Crit Care Med* 1998;26:15-23.
18. Adhikari NK, Burns KE, Friedrich J, Granton JT, et al: Effect of nitric oxide on oxygenation and mortality in acute lung injury: Systemic review and meta-analysis. *BMJ* 2007;334:779.
19. Angus DC, Clermont G, Linde-Zwirble WT, Musthafa AA, et al: Healthcare costs and long-term outcomes after acute respiratory distress syndrome: A phase III trial of nitric oxide. *Crit Care Med* 2006;34:2883-2890.
20. Zapol WM, Snider MT, Schneider RC: Extracorporeal membrane oxygenation for acute respiratory failure. *Anesthesiology* 1977;46:272-285.
21. Zapol WM, Snider MT, Hill JD, Fallat RJ, et al: Extracorporeal membrane oxygenation in severe acute respiratory failure. *JAMA* 1979;242:2193-2196.
22. Gattinoni L, Presenti A, Mascheroni D, Fumagalli R, et al: Low-frequency positive pressure ventilation with extracorporeal CO_2 removal in severe acute respiratory failure. *JAMA* 1986;256: 881-886.

23. Morris AH, Wallace CJ, Menlove RL, Clemmer TP, et al: Randomized clinical trial of pressure-controlled inverse ratio ventilation and extracorporeal CO_2 removal for adult respiratory distress syndrome. *Am J Respir Crit Care Med* 1994;149:295-305.
24. Peek GJ, Clemens F, Elbourne D, Firmin R, et al: CEDAR: Conventional ventilatory support vs extracorporeal membrane oxygenation for severe adult respiratory failure. *BMC Health Sciences Research* 2006;6:163.
25. Declaux CD, Alberti C, Mancebo J, Abroug F, et al: Treatment of acute hypoxemic nonhypercapnic respiratory insufficiency with continuous positive airway pressure delivered by a face mask. A randomized controlled trial. *JAMA* 2000;284:2352-2360.
26. Antonelli M, Conti G, Esquinas A, Montini L, et al: A multicenter survey on the use in clinical practice of noninvasive ventilation as a first-line intervention for acute respiratory distress syndrome. *Crit Care Med* 2007;35:18-25.
27. Clark RH, Gerstmann DR, Null DM, deLemos RA: Prospective randomized comparison of high-frequency oscillatory and conventional ventilation in respiratory distress syndrome. *Pediatrics* 1992;89:5-12.
28. Gerstmann DR, Monton SD, Stoddard RA, Meredith KS, et al: The Provo Multicenter Early High-frequency Oscillatory Ventilation Trial improved pulmonary and clinical outcome in respiratory distress syndrome. *Pediatrics* 1996;98:1044-1057.
29. Carlon GC, Howland WS, Ray C, Miodownik, et al: High-frequency jet ventilation: A prospective randomized evaluation. *Chest* 1983;84:551-559.
30. Fort P, Farmer C, Westerman J, Johannigman, J, et al: High-frequency oscillatory ventilation for adult respiratory distress syndrome—a pilot study. *Crit Care Med* 1997;25:937-947.
31. Borges JB, Okamoto VN, Matos GF, Caramez MP, et al: Reversibility of lung collapse and hypoxemia in early acute respiratory distress syndrome. *Am J Respir Crit Care Med* 2006;174: 268-278.
32. Thile AW, Richard JC, Maggiore SM, Ranieri VM, Brochard L: Alveolar recruitment in pulmonary and extrapulmonary acute respiratory distress syndrome. *Anesthesiology* 2007;106: 212-217.
33. Gattinoni L, Caironi P, Cressoni M, Chiumello D, et al: Lung recruitment in patients with the acute respiratory distress syndrome. *N Engl J Med* 2007;354:1775-1786.
34. Oczenski W, Hormann C, Keller C, Lorenzl N, et al: Recruitment maneuvers after a positive end-expiratory pressure trial do not induced sustained effects in early adult respiratory distress syndrome. *Anesthesiology* 2004;101:620-625.
35. Pittet JF, Mackersie RC, Martin TR, Matthay MA: Biological markers of acute lung injury: Prognostic and pathogenetic significance (state of art). *Am J Respir Crit Care Med* 1997;155: 1187-1205.
36. Bone RC, Slotman G, Maunder R, Silverman H, et al: Randomized double-blind, multicenter study of prostaglandin E_1 in patients with adult respiratory distress syndrome: Prostaglandin E_1 Study Group. *Chest* 1989;96:114-119.
37. Ware LB, Matthay MA: The acute respiratory distress syndrome. *N Engl J Med* 2000;342:1334-1349.
38. ARDS Network: A randomized placebo controlled trial of lisophylline for early treatment of acute lung injury and acute respiratory distress syndrome. *Crit Care Med* 2002;30:1-6.
39. ARDS Network: Ketoconazole for early treatment of acute lung injury and acute respiratory distress syndrome: A randomized controlled trial. *JAMA* 2000;283:1995-2002.
40. Anzueto A, Baughman RP, Guntupalli KK, Weg JG, et al: Aerosolized surfactant in adults with sepsis-induced acute respiratory distress syndrome. *N Engl J Med* 1996;334:1417-1421.
41. Brower RG, Ware LB, Berthiaume Y, Matthay MA: Treatment of ARDS. *Chest* 2001;120:1347-1367.
42. Pulmonary Artery Catheter Consensus Conference: Pulmonary Artery Catheter Consensus Conference: Consensus statement. *Crit Care Med* 1997;25:910-925.
43. The National Heart, Lung, and Blood Institute Acute Respiratory Distress Syndrome (ARDS) Clinical Trials Network: Pulmonary-artery versus central venous catheter to guide treatment of acute lung injury. *N Engl J Med* 2006;354:2213-2224.
44. Mitchell JP, Schuller D, Calandrino FS, Schuster DP: Improved outcome based on fluid management in critically ill patients requiring pulmonary artery catheterization. *Am Rev Respir Dis* 1992;145:990-998.
45. Wiedemann HP, Wheeler AP, Bernard GR, Thompson BT, Hayden D, deBoisblanc B, et al, National Heart, Lung, and Blood Institute Acute Respiratory Distress Syndrome (ARDS) Clinical Trials Network: Comparison of two fluid-management strategies in acute lung injury. *N Engl J Med* 2006;354:2564-2575.
46. Kress JP, Pohlman AS, O'Connor MF, Hall JB: Daily interruption of sedative infustions in critically ill patients undergoing mechanical ventilation. *N Engl J Med* 2000;342:1417.
47. Hise ME, Halterman KH, Gajewski BJ, Parkhurst M, Moncure M, Brown JC: Feeding practices of severely ill intensive care unit patients: An evaluation of energy sources and clinical outcomes. *J Am Diet Assoc* 2007;107:458-465.
48. Mackenzie SL, Zygun DA, Whitmore BL, Doig CJ, Hameed SM: Implementation of a nutritional support protocol increases the proportion of mechanically ventilated patients reaching enteral nutrition targets in the adult intensive care unit. *Journal of Parenteral and Enteral Nutrition* 2005;29:74-80.
49. Gadek JE, DeMichele SJ, Karlstad MD, Pacht ER, et al: Effect of enteral feeding with eicosapentaenoic acid, gamma-linolenic acid, and antioxidants in patients with acute respiratory distress syndrome. *Crit Care Med* 1999;27:1409-1420.
50. Resar R, Pronovost P, Haraden C, Simmonds T, Rainey T, Nolan T: Using a bundle approach to improve ventilator care processes and reduce ventilator associated pneumonia. *Jt Comm J Qual Patient Saf* 2005;31:243-248.
51. Bernard GR, Luce JM, Sprung CL, Rinaldo JE, et al: High-dose corticosteroids in patients with adult respiratory distress syndrome. *N Engl J Med* 1978;317:1565-1570.
52. Luce JM, Montgomery AB, Marks JD, Turner J, Metz CA, Murray JF: Ineffectiveness of high-dose methylprednisolone in preventing parenchymal lung injury and improving mortality in patients with septic shock. *Am Rev Respir Dis* 1988;138: 62-68.
53. Meduri GU, Golden E, Freire AX, Taylor E, et al: Methylprednisolone infusion in early severe ARDS, results of a randomized controlled trial. *Chest* 2007;131:954-963.
54. Meduri GU, Belenchia JM, Estes RJ, Wunderink RG, el Torkey M, Leeper KV: Fibroproliferative phase of ARDS, clinical findings and effects of corticosteroids. *Chest* 1991;100:943-952.
55. Meduri GU, Chinn AJ, Leeper KV, Wunderink RG, et al: Corticosteroid rescue treatment of progressive fibroproliferation in late ARDS. Patterns of response and predictors of outcome. *Chest* 1994;105:1516-1527.
56. Meduri GU, Headley AS, Golden E, Carson SJ, et al: Effect of prolonged methylprednisolone therapy in unresolving acute respiratory distress syndrome. A randomized controlled trial. *JAMA* 1998;280:159-165.
57. Steinberg KP, Hudson LP, Goodman RB, Hough CL, Lanken PN, Hyzy R, et al, National Heart, Lung, and Blood Institute Acute Respiratory Distress Syndrome (ARDS) Clinical Trials Network: Efficacy and safety of corticosteroids for persistent acute respiratory distress syndrome. *N Engl J Med* 2006;354:1671-1684.
58. Annane D, Sebille V, Charpentier C, Bollaert PE, et al: Effect of treatment with low doses of hydrocortisone and fludrocortisone on mortality in patients with septic shock. *JAMA* 2002;288: 862-871.
59. Annane D, Sebille V, Bellissant E, Ger-Inf-05 Study Group: Effect of low doses of corticosteroids in septic shock patients with or without early acute respiratory distress syndrome. *Crit Care Med* 2006;34:22-30.
60. NHLBI ARDS Clinical Network: Available at: http://www.ardsnet.org (accessed June 10, 2007).

32 What Actions Can Be Used to Prevent Peripheral Nerve Injury?

Sanjay M. Bhananker, MBBS, MD, DA, FRCA, and Karen B. Domino, MD, MPH

Perioperative peripheral nerve injury is a significant source of morbidity for patients and the second most frequent cause for professional liability for anesthesiologists, accounting for 16% of claims in the American Society of Anesthesiologists (ASA) closed claims project database.[1] The incidence of postoperative peripheral nerve dysfunction is estimated at 0.1% to 0.15%, or 1 in 1000 to 1500 anesthetics.[2-4]

The etiology of perioperative nerve damage is largely unknown. Injuries to the nerves of the brachial plexus or sciatic nerve may be secondary to stretching and/or compression with malpositioning of the patient. In contrast, ulnar nerve injury may occur despite protective padding and careful positioning. Direct trauma from needles or instruments and chemical toxicity of injected local anesthetics or vasoconstrictors may be implicated in nerve damage following regional anesthetic techniques.[5] However, there are very few prospective studies on the genesis or prevention of perioperative neuropathy. None of these are randomized and blinded. The relationship between conventional perioperative care and development of postoperative neuropathy is poorly understood.

Because of the absence of randomized controlled trials and paucity of epidemiologic studies, the evidence on which practice patterns for prevention of perioperative peripheral neuropathy are based is largely consensus opinion. Using expert consensus, the ASA Task Force on Prevention of Perioperative Peripheral Neuropathies[6] formed guidelines regarding perioperative positioning of the patient, use of protective padding, and avoidance of contact with hard surfaces or supports to reduce perioperative neuropathies (Table 32-1). However, even with close adherence to these recommendations, many peripheral neuropathies, especially those involving the ulnar nerve, are not preventable.

THERAPIES/OPTIONS AVAILABLE TO REDUCE PERIPHERAL NEUROPATHY

Understanding of the etiology and pathogenesis of neuropathy is essential to formulate ways of preventing or minimizing its occurrence. Lack of this understanding with regard to the development of postoperative peripheral nerve dysfunction is the major impediment to developing preventive steps.

Based on the current knowledge of pathogenesis of perioperative neuropathy, several recommendations have been made to prevent its occurrence. These include a preoperative screening to detect any subclinical neuropathy, preoperative history and physical examination directed at defining the comfortable range of stretching and movement at different joints, meticulous attention to avoiding intraoperative compression of superficial nerves, padding of the extremities and points at which nerves may get compressed, measures aimed at reducing the stretching of the nerves, periodic intraoperative checking for optimal positioning of the extremities, and performing regional blocks while awake and with a nerve stimulator. However, there is no definitive scientific evidence that these maneuvers are effective in preventing perioperative neuropathy.

EVIDENCE

In attempting to study the evidence with respect to causation and prevention of peripheral neuropathy, one must consider the different criteria used to diagnose neuropathy in each of the studies. Although transient sensory neurologic dysfunction lasting less than 2 weeks is not uncommon after anesthesia and surgery, permanent disabling nerve injuries are infrequent.

Ulnar Neuropathy

The ulnar nerve is the most common site of postoperative peripheral nerve damage, accounting for 28% of claims for anesthesia-related nerve injuries in the ASA closed claims database.[1] The incidence of ulnar nerve dysfunction is estimated to be between 0.26% and 0.5% in prospective studies of postsurgical patients (Table 32-2).[7,8] Ulnar neuropathy has been documented not only in surgical patients but also in medical inpatients and outpatients,[9] and irrespective of whether general anesthesia, regional anesthesia, or sedation-monitored anesthesia care is administered.[1]

Male gender, extremes of body habitus, and prolonged hospitalization are important risk factors for perioperative ulnar neuropathy.[7,8,10] The male predisposition may be explained by gender-related anatomic variations in the cubital tunnel at the elbow that render the ulnar nerve

Table 32-1   **Summary of Task Force Consensus**

PREOPERATIVE ASSESSMENT

When judged appropriate, it is helpful to ascertain that patients can comfortably tolerate the anticipated operative position.

UPPER EXTREMITY POSITIONING

Arm abduction should be limited to 90 degrees in supine patients; patients who are positioned prone may comfortably tolerate arm abduction greater than 90 degrees.
Arms should be positioned to decrease pressure on the postcondylar groove of the humerus (ulnar groove).
When arms are tucked at the side, a neutral forearm position is recommended.
When arms are abducted on armboards, either supination or a neutral forearm position is acceptable.
Prolonged pressure on the radial nerve in the spiral groove of the humerus should be avoided.
Extension of the elbow beyond a comfortable range may stretch the median nerve.

LOWER EXTREMITY POSITIONING

Lithotomy positions that stretch the hamstring muscle group beyond a comfortable range may stretch the sciatic nerve.
Prolonged pressure on the peroneal nerve at the fibular head should be avoided.
Neither extension nor flexion of the hip increases the risk of femoral neuropathy.

PROTECTIVE PADDING

Padded armboards may decrease the risk of upper extremity neuropathy.
The use of chest rolls in laterally positioned patients may decrease the risk of upper extremity neuropathies.
Padding at the elbow and at the fibular head may decrease the risk of upper and lower extremity neuropathies, respectively.

EQUIPMENT

Properly functioning automated blood pressure cuffs on the upper arms do not affect the risk of upper extremity neuropathies.
Shoulder braces in steep head-down positions may increase the risk of brachial plexus neuropathies.

POSTOPERATIVE ASSESSMENT

A simple postoperative assessment of extremity nerve function may lead to early recognition of peripheral neuropathies.

DOCUMENTATION

Charting specific positioning actions during the care of patients may result in improvements of care by (1) helping practitioners focus attention on relevant aspects of patient positioning and (2) providing information that continuous improvement processes can lead to refinements in patient care.

From *Anesthesiology* 2000;92:1168-1182. Reprinted with permission of the publisher.

Table 32-2   **Ulnar Neuropathy**

Author, Year	Anesthesia Technique	Study Design	Incidence of Neuropathy	Comment
Dhuner, 1950[2]	GA/spinal	Retrospective review of 30,000 cases	Ulnar neuropathy in 8 patients	Transient paresis lasting a few weeks in 7 cases
Alvine, 1987[7]	GA for orthopedic, cardiac, urology, general surgical procedures	Prospective study in 6538 patients	Ulnar neuropathy in 0.26% patients	Subclinical ulnar neuropathy may become symptomatic secondary to perioperative maneuvers and manipulations
Warner, 1994[10]	GA, sedation, regional	Retrospective review of 1,129,692 cases	Ulnar neuropathy in 1 per 2729 patients (0.04%)	No correlation with anesthetic technique or patient position; males, extremes of body habitus, prolonged hospital stay had higher incidence
Warner, 1999[8]	GA, sedation, regional	Prospective study in 1502 patients	Ulnar neuropathy in 7 per 1502 patients (1 in 215 patients) (0.5%)	More frequent in men 50-75 years of age; signs and symptoms develop 2-7 days after surgery
Warner, 2000[9]	Medical inpatients	Prospective study in 986 patients	Ulnar neuropathy in 2 of 986 (0.2% incidence)	Prolonged bed rest in supine position and elbow flexion may be causative
Lee, 2002[14]	GA	Prospective study in 203 orthopedic patients	6 cases (3% incidence) of ulnar neuropathy	Higher incidence in tilted patients in the lowermost adducted arm

GA, general anesthesia.

more sensitive to injury. Men have a 50% larger tubercle of the ulna, thicker retinaculum, and a shallow cubital tunnel, whereas women have 2 to 9 times more fat content in the cubital tunnel.[11] It is speculated that these anatomic differences may predispose the ulnar nerve to ischemia, by either direct compression or a reduction in blood flow by compression of the ulnar collateral artery and vein. Patients with perioperative neuropathy have a high incidence of contralateral nerve conduction dysfunction, suggesting that a subclinical neuropathy may become symptomatic as a result of manipulations during the perioperative period.[7]

The risk of ulnar nerve injury may be increased by flexion of the elbow[12] and pronation of the forearm[12] (see Table 32-2). The ASA Task Force concluded that flexion of the elbow may increase the risk of ulnar neuropathy.[6] This opinion is supported by anatomic evidence of a reduction in the cross-sectional contour of the cubital tunnel and sevenfold increase in pressure within the tunnel, to a range that can compromise the intraneural circulation.[13] Pronation of the forearm increases the pressure over the ulnar groove.[12] Supination of the forearm produces the least amount of pressure, whereas a neutral position results in an intermediate value. Supination also "lifts" the cubital tunnel and ulnar nerve away from a contact surface. Almost half of the men who experience pressure on their nerve sufficient to impair the electrophysiologic function do not perceive symptoms.[12] A higher incidence of ulnar neuropathy is also found in tilted patients in the lowermost adducted arm, speculated as occurring because internal rotation of the shoulder rotates the ulnar nerve toward compressive forces at the elbow.[14]

The ASA Task Force on Prevention of Perioperative Peripheral Neuropathies (see Table 32-1) made the following recommendations to prevent ulnar nerve injury: (1) position arms to decrease pressure on the ulnar groove, (2) use a neutral forearm position when arms are tucked at the sides, (3) use supination or a neutral forearm position when the arms are abducted on armboards, and (4) use padded armboards and padding at the elbow.[6] Periodic checking and documentation were also recommended. Properly functioning blood pressure cuffs on the upper arms do not affect the risk of upper extremity neuropathy.[6]

Despite the theoretical value of these precautions in positioning the arms, there is no evidence that these practices decrease the risk of postoperative ulnar neuropathy. On the contrary, the evidence suggests that ulnar nerve damage may occur despite padding and placement of the patient's arms in supination.[15]

Brachial Plexus Injury

Injury to the brachial plexus is the second most common nerve injury, responsible for 20% of claims for anesthesia-related nerve injuries in the ASA closed claims analysis.[1] The perioperative incidence of brachial plexus neuropathy is estimated at 0.2% to 0.6%.[2,16] Injury to the brachial plexus is most commonly reported after procedures involving median sternotomy, especially with dissection of the internal mammary artery;[17,18] Trendelenburg

position, especially with shoulder braces for support;[2] and after surgery in the prone position.[19]

Most brachial plexus nerve injuries are caused by stretching and traction on the plexus.[2,4,16,19,20] The anatomic features that make the brachial plexus most susceptible to injury include the following: (1) the nerve roots of the brachial plexus run a long, mobile, and superficial course between two firm points of fixation—the intervertebral foramina above and the axillary fascia below; (2) its close anatomic relationships with a number of freely movable bony prominences; and (3) the plexus runs its course through the limited space between the first rib and the clavicle.[19,21] The first two features make the brachial plexus more susceptible to stretch-induced injury, whereas the third one (along with fracture or displacement of the first rib) is generally implicated in direct or compression injury after cardiac surgery.

Arm Position

Brachial plexus neuropathy has been reported after arm abduction equal to or greater than 90 degrees.[2,21] Positions that induce stretching of the brachial plexus include extension and lateral flexion of the head to one side, allowing the arm to sag off the operating table,[2] or use of a shoulder roll or gallbladder rest to "bump" the patient to one side.[20] Contralateral cervical lateral flexion, lateral rotation of the shoulder, fixation of the shoulder girdle in neutral position, and wrist extension also stretch the brachial plexus.[22] Simultaneous application of these positions has a cumulative effect. Ninety-six percent of ASA members believed that limiting the arm abduction to 90 degrees in supine patients may reduce the risk of brachial plexus injury.[6] The ASA Task Force on Prevention of Perioperative Peripheral Neuropathies concluded that arm abduction should be limited to 90 degrees in supine patients (see Table 32-1).[6]

Shoulder Braces

Use of shoulder braces to stop patients from sliding down when placed in a steep Trendelenburg position has been associated with development of postoperative brachial plexus damage.[2,6,16] Shoulder braces can compress the brachial plexus against the numerous bony and rigid structures within the shoulder complex. The danger is even greater when the arm is abducted, causing the brace to act as a fulcrum and stretching the plexus. Fixation of the shoulder (caused by use of shoulder braces even in the recommended position over the acromioclavicular joints) loads the nerves of the upper extremity and reduces the range of elbow extension in the brachial plexus tension test.[22] The ASA Task Force on Prevention of Perioperative Peripheral Neuropathies concurred that shoulder braces in a steep head-down position may increase the risk of brachial plexus neuropathies (see Table 32-1).[6]

Prone Position

Placement of a patient into the prone position can also be accompanied by a stretch injury to the brachial plexus. Once prone position is established, the arms may be positioned either alongside the torso or extended above the head. In the presence of symptoms suggestive of thoracic outlet syndrome (paresthesia, numbness, or pain on raising hands above the head), arms should be restrained by the side of the body to avoid stretching of the brachial plexus.[23] Closure of retroclavicular space in the prone position can occur as a result of dorsal and caudal displacement of the clavicle by the chest roll, causing compression of the brachial plexus between the thorax and clavicle. The ASA Task Force on Prevention of Perioperative Peripheral Neuropathies concluded that patients who are positioned prone may comfortably tolerate arm abduction greater than 90 degrees (see Table 32-1).[6]

Lateral Decubitus Position

Compression of the brachial plexus between the thorax and the head of the humerus of the down-side extremity can also occur in the lateral decubitus position.[16] This can possibly be reduced by placing a roll under the chest wall just caudad to the axilla, with the aim of elevating the rib cage off the table and freeing the dependent shoulder.[6,23] The ASA Task Force on Prevention of Perioperative Peripheral Neuropathies recommended use of chest rolls in laterally positioned patients to reduce the risk of upper extremity neuropathies (see Table 32-1).[6]

Other Upper Extremity Neuropathies

Radial Nerve Injury

The radial nerve is susceptible to compression injury as it passes dorsolaterally around the middle and lower thirds of the humerus in the musculospiral groove. The nerve can be compressed approximately 5 cm above the lateral epicondyle of the humerus between an external object, such as the vertical bar of an anesthesia screen, an improperly positioned tourniquet, or the distal edge of a blood pressure cuff, and the underlying bone.[6,24] The ASA Task Force on Prevention of Perioperative Peripheral Neuropathies recommended that prolonged pressure on the radial nerve in the spiral groove of the humerus should be avoided (see Table 32-1).[6]

Median Nerve Dysfunction

Isolated median nerve damage in the perioperative setting is relatively uncommon, and the mechanism is poorly understood.[1,25] Needle trauma during venipuncture or intravenous cannulation in the antecubital fossa is possible. Median nerve dysfunction is predominantly seen in muscular men, in the 20- to 40-year-old age-group, who are unable to fully extend their elbows because of their large biceps and relatively inflexible tendons. The ASA Task Force on Prevention of Perioperative Peripheral Neuropathies concluded that extension of the elbow beyond a comfortable range may stretch the median nerve (see Table 32-1).[6]

Long Thoracic Nerve Damage

Long thoracic nerve dysfunction is an infrequent neuropathy.[1,26] The absence of any apparent mechanism of injury in most of these injuries has led to the postulation that a coincidental infectious neuropathy may be responsible for the postoperative long thoracic nerve dysfunction.[27]

Lower Extremity Neuropathy

Postoperative nerve lesions in the lower extremity occur infrequently and are poorly studied (Table 32-3).[28-32] In the analysis of closed claims for nerve damage, Cheney

Table 32-3	**Lower Extremity Neuropathy**			
Author, Year	**Study Design**	**Incidence of Neuropathy**	**Comment**	
Burkhart, 1966[34]	Retrospective analysis of 2526 vaginal surgical procedures	0.2% incidence of sciatic neuropathy	Stretch injury and not compression injury	
McQuarrie, 1972[33]	Vaginal hysterectomy in 1000 patients	0.3% incidence of sciatic neuropathy	Sciatic and common peroneal nerves are anatomically fixed at the sciatic notch and neck of fibula, making them susceptible to stretch	
Keykhah, 1979[28]	488 cases of neurosurgery in sitting position	1% incidence of peroneal neuropathy	—	
Warner, 1994[29]	Retrospective review of 198,461 patients in lithotomy position	Persistent motor deficit in lower extremity for >3 mo in 55 patients (1 per 3608 cases)	Association with prolonged duration in lithotomy, very thin body habitus, and smoking in preoperative period	
Nercessian, 1994[30]	7133 consecutive total hip arthroplasties	45 cases (0.63%) of neuropathy, 34 (0.48%) in lower extremity and 11 (0.15%) in upper limb	Common peroneal and ulnar nerves commonly involved; females more likely to develop neuropathy	
Warner, 2000[31]	Prospective study in 991 patients in lithotomy position	Lower extremity neuropathy in 15 patients (1.5% incidence)	Sensory neuropathy, developing within 4 hr, complete recovery within 6 mo, direct correlation with time in lithotomy position	
Anema, 2000[32]	Prospective study in 185 male patients undergoing urethral reconstruction in high lithotomy position	12 cases of neuropathy (6.5% incidence)	Duration of lithotomy position was significant risk factor; height, weight, type of stirrups were not associated with increased risk	

and colleagues[1] reported 23 cases of sciatic nerve injuries, of which 10 were associated with the use of lithotomy position and 2 with frog-leg position for the surgery. Warner and colleagues[31] prospectively studied 991 patients undergoing surgery in lithotomy position and observed a 1.5% incidence of lower extremity neuropathies. Of the 15 patients who developed neuropathies, the obturator nerve was involved, indicating that multiple nerves are affected with similar frequency. All the neuropathies were purely sensory.

The risk of developing lower extremity neuropathy increases with the duration of lithotomy position,[29,31,32] and limiting the duration of lithotomy may decrease the incidence of postoperative lower extremity nerve dysfunction.

Sciatic Neuropathy

Perioperative sciatic nerve injury is relatively uncommon but may occur from stretching, compression, ischemia, or a combination of these mechanisms. Stretch injury to the sciatic nerve could occur if the patient is placed in some variant of the lithotomy position, especially those with simultaneous hyperflexion of the hip and extension of the knee or external rotation of the thigh.[19,33,34] Case reports of left-sided sciatic neuropathy after cesarean section in patients with left lateral tilt[35,36] suggest that pressure on the sciatic nerve in this position may cause sciatic nerve injury. Because the same forces stretch the sciatic nerve and the hamstring group of muscles, eliminating the stretch (tautness) of knee flexor muscles in a surgical position helps reduce the incidence of stretch-related injury to the sciatic nerve.[6,19] The ASA Task Force on Prevention of Perioperative Peripheral Neuropathies recommended that flexion of the hip and extension of the knee should be jointly considered to reduce the amount of stretch on hamstring when positioning a patient in lithotomy (see Table 32-1).[6]

Peroneal Nerve Dysfunction

The common peroneal nerve (common fibular nerve) wraps superficially around the neck of the fibula before dividing into the sensory superficial peroneal nerve and predominantly motor deep peroneal nerve. The common peroneal nerve is vulnerable to compression between the head of the fibula and external hard objects, particularly in the lithotomy and sitting positions[28,29,31] and after hip surgery.[30] Warner and colleagues[31] observed only sensory deficits in their patients who developed peroneal neuropathy after prolonged duration in lithotomy positions, suggesting that only the superficial peroneal nerve was affected either because of compression distal to the fibular head or by stretching secondary to plantar flexion of the foot. The ASA Task Force on Prevention of Perioperative Peripheral Neuropathies recommended use of protective padding at the fibular head to decrease the risk of peroneal neuropathy (see Table 32-1).[6]

Femoral Neuropathy

Postoperative femoral neuropathy is relatively uncommon and is often associated with surgical factors, such as the use of self-retaining retractors for abdominopelvic operations,[37] ischemia after aortic cross-clamp, and compression caused by hematoma.[38] Femoral nerve ischemia may also result from extreme abduction and external rotation of thighs in the lithotomy position.[39]

Obturator Neuropathy

The obturator nerve lies deep within the pelvis and medial thigh and is relatively well protected. The nerve is particularly at risk during total hip arthroplasty and pelvic surgery.[40]

Nerve Damage Following Peripheral Nerve Block

The incidence of persistent neuropathy following peripheral nerve block is estimated at 0.2%, although transient sensory deficits and paresthesia are relatively common, occurring in up to 7% to 14% of patients (Table 32-4).[41-51] In a review of all studies investigating neurologic complications following regional anesthesia, Brull and colleagues[52] found that the rate of transient neuropathy following peripheral nerve blockade was less than 3% and that permanent nerve damage was rare. The etiology of nerve injury is thought to be secondary to needle trauma, local anesthetic neurotoxicity, ischemia, or a combination of these factors.[53] Hematoma, intraneural edema, and direct neuronal toxicity may result in an immediate injury. Formation of perineural edema, inflammation, and microhematoma around the nerve may account for the 2- to 3-week delay sometimes seen from performing a regional block to the onset of neurologic symptoms. A tissue reaction or scar formation in response to mechanical or chemical trauma may also be responsible for delayed neurologic dysfunction.[53]

Risk factors for neurologic dysfunction following peripheral nerve block have been speculated to include elicitation of paresthesia, use of a multiple injection technique, use of a long-bevel needle, use of continuous block techniques, performance of blocks under general anesthesia, and performing regional blocks in anticoagulated patients. The scientific quality of evidence in support of these risk factors is relatively poor, relying mostly on small clinical series, case reports, and editorials. In contrast, tourniquet inflation pressures of greater than 400 mm Hg have been demonstrated to be associated with the development of postoperative neurologic dysfunction.[46]

An analysis of risk factors for the development of neurologic complications following axillary blocks found no association of neuronal dysfunction with elicitation of paresthesia, nerve stimulator response, use of epinephrine, or use of long-beveled needles.[47] The multiple injection technique is also not associated with an increased incidence of postoperative neurologic dysfunction.[46] Continuous nerve block techniques may theoretically increase the risk of nerve injury; however, the risk of neurologic complications with continuous axillary blocks is similar to that of single-dose techniques.[51]

Commonly used endpoints for successful localization of nerve(s) to be blocked include elicitation of paresthesia, motor stimulation of the muscles innervated, and ultrasound guidance. Although early studies suggested that searching for paresthesia increased the incidence of nerve injury,[41] more recent studies have not demonstrated

Table 32-4 Neuropathy Following Regional Nerve Blockade

Author, Year	Anesthesia Technique	Study Design	Incidence of Neuropathy	Comment
Selander, 1979[41]	AxB	Prospective study in 533 patients	Nerve lesions in 10 of 533 patients attributed to block	Searching for paresthesia increased incidence of nerve lesions from 0.8% to 2.8% (not significant statistical difference)
Urban, 1994[42]	AxB and ISB AxB	Prospective study in 508 patients, 242 AxB and 266 ISB	Incidence of paresthesia at 2 wk postblock was 3% with ISB and 7% with AxB	All but one patient in each group made complete recovery in 4 wk with AxB and 6 wk with ISB
Stan, 1995[43]	AxB by transarterial approach	Prospective study in 996 patients	Transient sensory neuropathy in 2 of 996 patients (0.2% incidence)	Direct needle trauma believed to be cause; complete recovery within 1 mo
Giaufre, 1996[44]	Regional anesthetics	Prospective study in pediatric patients	No complications in 4090 peripheral nerve blocks	Demonstrated safety of peripheral nerve blocks over central blocks in pediatric anesthesia
Auroy, 1997[45]	Regional anesthesia	Prospective study, 103,730 regional anesthetics including 21,278 peripheral nerve blocks	Nerve damage in 34 patients	Paresthesia during needle placement or pain during injection in all patients with nerve injury; complete recovery in 19 patients within 3 mo
Fanelli, 1999[46]	Sciatic-femoral, AxB, and ISB using nerve stimulator	Prospective study in 3996 patients, using multiple-injection technique	69 patients (1.7% incidence) developed neurologic dysfunction in the first month	Tourniquet inflation to >400 mm Hg associated with nerve injury; complete recovery in all but one patient in 4-12 wk
Horlocker, 1999[47]	Repeated AxBs	Retrospective study of 1614 AxBs in 607 patients	1.1% incidence of anesthesia-related neurologic dysfunction	Repeated AxBs did not increase risk of neurologic complications
Borgeat, 2001[53]	ISB for shoulder surgery	Prospective study in 520 patients, followed up for 9 mo	Severe long-term complication (persistent dysesthesias at 9 months) rate of 0.2%; no incidence of motor weakness	Need to exclude sulcus ulnaris syndrome, carpal tunnel syndrome, or complex regional pain syndrome in cases of persistent dysesthesias after regional block
Grant, 2001[49]	Continuous peripheral nerve block	Prospective study in 228 patients	No incidence of postoperative neurologic dysfunction	Safety of using insulated Tuohy catheter system for continuous blocks
Klein, 2002[50]	Peripheral nerve blocks	Prospective study of 2382 blocks with ropivacaine	6 cases (0.25% incidence) of paresthesia at 7 days postoperative	Neurologic recovery in all patients over 6 mo
Auroy, 2002[54]	AxB	Prospective study of 11,024 patients	2 cases of neurologic deficits	Follow-up beyond 6 months not available
Auroy, 2002[54]	Femoral nerve block	Prospective study of 10,309 patients	3 cases	Follow-up beyond 6 months not available
Auroy, 2002[54]	Sciatic nerve block	8507 patients	2 cases	Follow-up beyond 6 months not available
Auroy, 2002[54]	ISB	3459 patients	1 case	Follow-up beyond 6 months not available
Bergman, 2003[51]	Continuous AxBs	Retrospective study in 405 patients with axillary catheters	2 cases (0.5% incidence) of anesthesia-related neurologic deficits	Use of continuous axillary blockade does not increase risk of nerve damage

AxB, axillary block; *ISB,* interscalene block.

this relationship.[43,47] Some experts believe that use of a peripheral nerve stimulator reduces the risk of nerve injury, but this claim remains unproven and warrants further study. In a French survey of anesthesiologists, Auroy and colleagues[54] found that a nerve stimulator was used in 9 out of 12 peripheral nerve blocks that resulted in a neurologic complication. Ultrasound guidance for performing peripheral nerve blocks is becoming popular worldwide. Animal studies have shown that ultrasound may prove useful to detect intraneural injection, whereas a motor response above 0.5 mA may not exclude intraneural needle placement.[55] However,

Bigeleisen[56] found that puncturing of the peripheral nerves and apparent intraneural injection during axillary plexus block did not necessarily lead to a neurologic injury. Perlas and colleagues[57] noted that paresthesia was 38.2% sensitive and motor response was 74.5% sensitive for detection of needle-to-nerve contact as detected by ultrasound. Performance of peripheral nerve blocks under general anesthesia is also controversial. No neurologic sequelae were noted in a prospective study of over 4000 peripheral nerve blocks in pediatric patients.[44] Several case reports and editorials point out potentially serious complications of placing nerve blocks in anesthetized patients,[58,59] yet brachial plexus and other blocks are frequently performed in anesthetized patients.

Data on neurologic injury following peripheral nerve blocks in patients receiving anticoagulation therapy are scanty and are in the form of isolated case reports. The consensus statements on neuraxial anesthesia and systemic anticoagulation, including oral anticoagulants, heparin, and thrombolytic-fibrinolytic therapy published by the American Society of Regional Anesthesia,[60] can be applied to any regional anesthetic technique. Placement of blocks and removal of catheters in patients receiving these anticoagulation therapies may increase the risk of hematoma and neurologic dysfunction. Close monitoring of anticoagulated patients undergoing peripheral nerve blocks for early signs of neural compression such as pain, weakness, and numbness may help in early detection and timely intervention to prevent neurologic sequelae from compression caused by hematoma.

AREAS OF UNCERTAINTY

Many peripheral neuropathies occur in the absence of a definite mechanism of nerve injury. Some of the areas of uncertainty with regard to causation and prevention of perioperative peripheral neuropathy are as follows:

1. *Padding of superficial nerves:* Conventional wisdom dictates that the superficial peripheral nerves can be protected from injury by the use of protective padding (e.g., foam sponges, towels, blankets, soft gel pads); however, there are no data to suggest that any of these materials are more protective than the others or that any of them are better than none at all.
2. *Frequent change of position:* Prolonged duration in one position is associated with increased risk of neurologic injury,[29,31] and limiting the time spent in one position decreases this risk.[32] The ASA Task Force on Prevention of Perioperative Peripheral Neuropathies recommended periodic perioperative assessments of the position of extremities to ensure maintenance of desired position and reduce the incidence of neuropathies (see Table 32-1).[6]
3. *Electrophysiologic monitoring:* Electrophysiologic studies, such as somatosensory evoked potentials (SSEP) and electromyography, can detect changes in nerve function in the perioperative period.[61] The nonspecificity and poor sensitivity of SSEP in predicting postoperative neurologic deficits, combined with time, cost, and personnel issues involved in SSEP monitoring, make the role of SSEP questionable as a routine monitor.

4. *Elicitation of paresthesia for regional blocks:* Although early studies suggested an increased risk of postblock neurologic dysfunction with elicitation of paresthesia,[41] this relationship has not been subsequently proven,[43,47] and it requires further study.
5. *Ultrasound guidance for regional blocks:* Ultrasound guidance may be more sensitive than elicitation of paresthesia or obtaining a motor twitch to electrical stimulation when localizing peripheral nerves.[57] Although ultrasound may help in reducing the incidence of intraneural injection, the clinical significance of intraneural injection in causation of nerve dysfunction remains debated.[56]

AUTHORS' RECOMMENDATIONS AND GUIDELINES

A summary of the consensus of the ASA Task Force on Prevention of Perioperative Peripheral Neuropathies is given in Table 32-1.[6] However, the protective effect of these recommendations on the development of postoperative neuropathies reflects the consensus opinion of anesthesiologists, not randomized controlled trials, and remains unproven. At this time, the authors agree with the current ASA Guidelines.

AUTHORS' RECOMMENDATIONS

Many peripheral neuropathies, especially ulnar neuropathy, are not currently preventable. Further scientific research may shed more light on the genesis of postoperative nerve dysfunction and measures aimed at preventing this complication. Based on available evidence, specific steps should be taken to minimize compression, stretching, ischemia, and trauma to the peripheral nerves (see Table 32-1).[6] When positioning and padding the extremities, direct compression of the superficial peripheral nerves should be avoided, and the limbs should be positioned so that any compressive forces that must be placed on the nerves are distributed over as large an area as possible. It is advisable to define the patient's preoperative condition and the normally tolerated limits of stretch in the limbs. Then, avoid any stretching over these limits while the patient is anesthetized. A description of the intraoperative positioning and measures aimed at preventing peripheral nerve dysfunction should be documented in the anesthetic record.

REFERENCES

1. Cheney FW, Domino KB, Caplan RA, Posner KL: Nerve injury associated with anesthesia: A closed claims analysis. *Anesthesiology* 1999;90:1062-1069.
2. Dhuner K: Nerve injuries during operations: A survey of cases occurring during a six-year period. *Anesthesiology* 1950;11:289-293.
3. Eggstein S, Franke M, Hofmeister A, Ruckauer KD: Postoperative peripheral neuropathies in general surgery. *Zentralbl Chir* 2000;125:459-463.
4. Parks BJ: Postoperative peripheral neuropathies. *Surgery* 1973;74:348-357.

5. Sawyer RJ, Richmond MN, Hickey JD, Jarrratt JA: Peripheral nerve injuries associated with anaesthesia. *Anaesthesia* 2000; 55:980-991.
6. Practice advisory for the prevention of perioperative peripheral neuropathies: A report by the American Society of Anesthesiologists Task Force on Prevention of Perioperative Peripheral Neuropathies. *Anesthesiology* 2000;92:1168-1182.
7. Alvine FG, Schurrer ME: Postoperative ulnar-nerve palsy. Are there predisposing factors? *J Bone Joint Surg Am* 1987;69:255-259.
8. Warner MA, Warner DO, Matsumoto JY, Harper CM, Schroeder DR, Maxson PM: Ulnar neuropathy in surgical patients. *Anesthesiology* 1999;90:54-59.
9. Warner MA, Warner DO, Harper CM, Schroeder DR, Maxson PM: Ulnar neuropathy in medical patients. *Anesthesiology* 2000;92: 613-615.
10. Warner MA, Warner ME, Martin JT: Ulnar neuropathy. Incidence, outcome, and risk factors in sedated or anesthetized patients. *Anesthesiology* 1994;81:1332-1340.
11. Contreras MG, Warner MA, Charboneau WJ, Cahill DR: Anatomy of the ulnar nerve at the elbow: Potential relationship of acute ulnar neuropathy to gender differences. *Clin Anat* 1998;11:372-378.
12. Prielipp RC, Morell RC, Walker FO, Santos CC, Bennett J, Butterworth J: Ulnar nerve pressure: Influence of arm position and relationship to somatosensory evoked potentials. *Anesthesiology* 1999;91:345-354.
13. Gelberman RH, Yamaguchi K, Hollstien SB, Winn SS, Heidenreich FP Jr, et al: Changes in interstitial pressure and cross-sectional area of the cubital tunnel and of the ulnar nerve with flexion of the elbow. An experimental study in human cadavera. *J Bone Joint Surg Am* 1998;80:492-501.
14. Lee CT, Espley AJ: Perioperative ulnar neuropathy in orthopaedics: Association with tilting the patient. *Clin Orthop Relat Res* 2002:106-111.
15. Stoelting RK: Postoperative ulnar nerve palsy—is it a preventable complication? *Anesth Analg* 1993;76:7-9.
16. Cooper DE, Jenkins RS, Bready L, Rockwood CA Jr: The prevention of injuries of the brachial plexus secondary to malposition of the patient during surgery. *Clin Orthop Relat Res* 1988; 33-41.
17. Sharma AD, Parmley CL, Sreeram G, Grocott HP: Peripheral nerve injuries during cardiac surgery: Risk factors, diagnosis, prognosis, and prevention. *Anesth Analg* 2000;91:1358-1369.
18. Vahl CF, Carl I, Muller-Vahl H, Struck E: Brachial plexus injury after cardiac surgery. The role of internal mammary artery preparation: A prospective study on 1000 consecutive patients. *J Thorac Cardiovasc Surg* 1991;102:724-729.
19. Warner MA: Perioperative neuropathies. *Mayo Clin Proc* 1998;73:567-574.
20. Kiloh LG: Brachial plexus lesions after cholecystectomy. *Lancet* 1950;1:103-105.
21. Jackson L, Keats AS: Mechanism of brachial plexus palsy following anesthesia. *Anesthesiology* 1965;26:190-194.
22. Coppieters MW, Van de Velde M, Stappaerts KH: Positioning in anesthesiology: Toward a better understanding of stretch-induced perioperative neuropathies. *Anesthesiology* 2002;97:75-81.
23. Nakata DA, Stoelting RK: Positioning the extremities. In Matin JT, Warner MA, editors: *Positioning in anesthesia and surgery,* ed 3. Philadelphia, WB Saunders, 1997.
24. Bickler PE, Schapera A, Bainton CR: Acute radial nerve injury from use of an automatic blood pressure monitor. *Anesthesiology* 1990;73:186-188.
25. Melli G, Chaudhry V, Dorman T, Cornblath DR: Perioperative bilateral median neuropathy. *Anesthesiology* 2002;97:1632-1634.
26. Bizzarri F, Davoli G, Bouklas D, Oncchio L, Frati G, Neri E: Iatrogenic injury to the long thoracic nerve: An underestimated cause of morbidity after cardiac surgery. *Tex Heart Inst J* 2001;28: 315-317.
27. Martin JT: Postoperative isolated dysfunction of the long thoracic nerve: A rare entity of uncertain etiology. *Anesth Analg* 1989;69:614-619.
28. Keykhah MM, Rosenberg H: Bilateral footdrop after craniotomy in the sitting position. *Anesthesiology* 1979;51:163-164.
29. Warner MA, Martin JT, Schroeder DR, Offord KP, Chute CG: Lower-extremity motor neuropathy associated with surgery performed on patients in a lithotomy position. *Anesthesiology* 1994;81:6-12.
30. Nercessian OA, Macaulay W, Stinchfield FE: Peripheral neuropathies following total hip arthroplasty. *J Arthroplasty* 1994;9: 645-651.
31. Warner MA, Warner DO, Harper CM, Schroeder DR, Maxson PM: Lower extremity neuropathies associated with lithotomy positions. *Anesthesiology* 2000;93:938-942.
32. Anema JG, Morey AF, McAninch JW, Mario LA, Wessells H: Complications related to the high lithotomy position during urethral reconstruction. *J Urol* 2000;164:360-363.
33. McQuarrie HG, Harris JW, Ellsworth HS, Stone RA, Anderson AE 3rd: Sciatic neuropathy complicating vaginal hysterectomy. *Am J Obstet Gynecol* 1972;113:223-232.
34. Burkhart FL, Daly JW: Sciatic and peroneal nerve injury: A complication of vaginal operations. *Obstet Gynecol* 1966;28:99-102.
35. Umo-Etuk J, Yentis SM: Sciatic nerve injury and caesarean section. *Anaesthesia* 1997;52:605-606.
36. Roy S, Levine AB, Herbison GJ, Jacobs SR: Intraoperative positioning during cesarean as a cause of sciatic neuropathy. *Obstet Gynecol* 2002;99:652-653.
37. Goldman JA, Feldberg D, Dicker D, Samuel N, Dekel A: Femoral neuropathy subsequent to abdominal hysterectomy. A comparative study. *Eur J Obstet Gynecol Reprod Biol* 1985;20:385-392.
38. Dillavou ED, Anderson LR, Bernert RA, Mularski RA, Hunter GC, Fiser SM, Rappaport WD: Lower extremity iatrogenic nerve injury due to compression during intraabdominal surgery. *Am J Surg* 1997;173:504-508.
39. Tondare AS, Nadkarni AV, Sathe CH, Dave VB: Femoral neuropathy: A complication of lithotomy position under spinal anaesthesia. Report of three cases. *Can Anaesth Soc J* 1983;30:84-86.
40. Sorenson EJ, Chen JJ, Daube JR: Obturator neuropathy: Causes and outcome. *Muscle Nerve* 2002;25:605-607.
41. Selander D, Edshage S, Wolff T: Paresthesia or no paresthesia? Nerve lesions after axillary blocks. *Acta Anaesthesiol Scand* 1979;23:27-33.
42. Urban MK, Urquhart B: Evaluation of brachial plexus anesthesia for upper extremity surgery. *Reg Anesth* 1994;19:175-182.
43. Stan TC, Krantz MA, Solomon DL, Poulos JG, Chaouki K: The incidence of neurovascular complications following axillary brachial plexus block using a transarterial approach. A prospective study of 1,000 consecutive patients. *Reg Anesth* 1995;20: 486-492.
44. Giaufre E, Dalens B, Gombert A: Epidemiology and morbidity of regional anesthesia in children: A one-year prospective survey of the French-Language Society of Pediatric Anesthesiologists. *Anesth Analg* 1996;83:904-912.
45. Auroy Y, Narchi P, Messiah A, Litt L, Rouvier B, Samii K: Serious complications related to regional anesthesia: Results of a prospective survey in France. *Anesthesiology* 1997;87:479-486.
46. Fanelli G, Casati A, Garancini P, Torri G: Nerve stimulator and multiple injection technique for upper and lower limb blockade: Failure rate, patient acceptance, and neurologic complications. Study Group on Regional Anesthesia. *Anesth Analg* 1999;88: 847-852.
47. Horlocker TT, Kufner RP, Bishop AT, Maxson PM, Schroeder DR: The risk of persistent paresthesia is not increased with repeated axillary block. *Anesth Analg* 1999;88:382-387.
48. Borgeat A, Ekatodramis G, Kalberer F, Benz C: Acute and nonacute complications associated with interscalene block and shoulder surgery: A prospective study. *Anesthesiology* 2001;95: 875-880.
49. Grant SA, Nielsen KC, Greengrass RA, Steele SM, Klein SM: Continuous peripheral nerve block for ambulatory surgery. *Reg Anesth Pain Med* 2001;26:209-214.
50. Klein SM, Nielsen KC, Greengrass RA, Warner DS, Martin A, Steele SM: Ambulatory discharge after long-acting peripheral nerve blockade: 2382 blocks with ropivacaine. *Anesth Analg* 2002;94:65-70, table of contents.
51. Bergman BD, Hebl JR, Kent J, Horlocker TT: Neurologic complications of 405 consecutive continuous axillary catheters. *Anesth Analg* 2003;96:247-252, table of contents.
52. Brull R, McCartney CJ, Chan VW, El-Beheiry H: Neurological complications after regional anesthesia: Contemporary estimates of risk. *Anesth Analg* 2007;104:965-974.

53. Borgeat A, Ekatodramis G: Nerve injury associated with regional anesthesia. *Curr Top Med Chem* 2001;1:199-203.
54. Auroy Y, Benhamou D, Bargues L, Ecoffey C, Falissard B, Mercier FJ, Bouaziz H, Samii K: Major complications of regional anesthesia in France: The SOS Regional Anesthesia Hotline Service. *Anesthesiology* 2002;97:1274-1280.
55. Chan VW, Brull R, McCartney CJ, Xu D, Abbas S, Shannon P: An ultrasonographic and histological study of intraneural injection and electrical stimulation in pigs. *Anesth Analg* 2007;104:1281-1284, tables of contents.
56. Bigeleisen PE: Nerve puncture and apparent intraneural injection during ultrasound-guided axillary block does not invariably result in neurologic injury. *Anesthesiology* 2006;105:779-783.
57. Perlas A, Niazi A, McCartney C, Chan V, Xu D, Abbas S: The sensitivity of motor response to nerve stimulation and paresthesia for nerve localization as evaluated by ultrasound. *Reg Anesth Pain Med* 2006;31:445-450.
58. Benumof JL: Permanent loss of cervical spinal cord function associated with interscalene block performed under general anesthesia. *Anesthesiology* 2000;93:1541-1544.
59. Neal JM: How close is close enough? Defining the "paresthesia chad." *Reg Anesth Pain Med* 2001;26:97-99.
60. Wu CL: Regional anesthesia and anticoagulation. *J Clin Anesth* 2001;13:49-58.
61. Hickey C, Gugino LD, Aglio LS, Mark JB, Son SL, Maddi R: Intraoperative somatosensory evoked potential monitoring predicts peripheral nerve injury during cardiac surgery. *Anesthesiology* 1993;78:29-35.

33 When Is Forced-Air Warming Cost-Effective?

Andrea Kurz, MD

INTRODUCTION/BACKGROUND

Core body temperature is one of the most tightly regulated human physiologic parameters. The thermoregulatory system usually maintains core body temperature within 0.2°C to 0.4°C −of "normal" (about 37.8°C in humans).[1] Nonetheless, hypothermia commonly develops in patients during anesthesia and surgery because anesthetics inhibit thermoregulation and patients are exposed to a cold operating-room environment.[1,2] Hypothermia is associated with severe complications, which can be avoided by actively warming patients in the perioperative period. Hypothermia-related complications are associated with significant cost of care. This article reviews anesthesia-related aspects of hypothermia, and evaluates the effectiveness of active warming in the perioperative period.

Anesthetic-induced thermoregulatory inhibition is dose dependent, and it impairs vasoconstriction and shivering. Opioids[3] and the intravenous anesthetic propofol,[4] as well as alpha-2 agonists such as dexmetedomidine, linearly decrease the vasoconstriction and shivering thresholds. In contrast, volatile anesthetics, such as isoflurane[5] and desflurane,[6] decrease cold responses nonlinearly. Typical anesthetic doses increase the interthreshold range (core temperatures not triggering thermoregulatory defenses) approximately twentyfold from its normal value near 0.2°C. As a result, anesthetized patients are poikilothermic over an approximately 4°C range of core temperatures and thus develop hypothermia.

Regional anesthesia impairs both central and peripheral thermoregulatory control. This peripheral inhibition of thermoregulatory defenses is a major cause of hypothermia during regional or combined regional/general anesthesia.[7,8]

OPTIONS

Thermal management can be performed by means of passive methods, which mainly decrease cutaneous heat loss, and active warming methods, which actively transfer heat into the body (Figure 33-1).

Passive Warming

Heat loss through radiation accounts for roughly 60% of the total perioperative heat loss. Operating room temperatures determine the rate at which metabolic heat is lost through radiation and convection from the skin and by evaporation from within surgical incisions. However, room temperatures exceeding 23°C are generally required to maintain normothermia in patients undergoing all but the smallest procedures.[9] Increasing ambient temperature is thus rarely a practical way of keeping surgical patients warm.

Thermal insulators readily available in most operating rooms include cotton blankets, surgical drapes, plastic sheeting, and reflective composites ("space blankets"). A single layer of each reduces heat loss by approximately 30%, and there are no clinically important differences among the insulation types.[10] Passive warming decreases perioperative heat loss, but does not actively transfer heat.

Active Warming

Convective Warming

Forced-air warming is the most common perioperative warming system. The best forced-air systems eliminate loss of metabolic heat and even transfer heat across the skin surface (approximately 50 watts).[11] Forced-air warming usually maintains normothermia even during large operations,[12] and it is superior to circulating-water mattresses placed underneath the patient.[13] It is probably the most cost-efficient warming system that is currently available.

Forced-air warming might be insufficient for maintaining normothermia in very large surgical procedures, notably liver transplantation, off-pump coronary artery bypass (OPCAB) surgery, polytrauma, and major abdominal surgery in lithotomy position.[14,15]

Conductive Warming

Circulating-water mattresses **placed *over* or *around*** patients can almost completely eliminate metabolic heat loss.[11] Recently developed **circulating-water garments,** such as the Allon thermoregulation system and the Arctic Sun temperature-controlling adhesive pad system, transfer large amounts of heat by increasing the warmed surface area or using materials that facilitate conduction.[16,17] **Resistive heating electrical blankets** are reusable blankets driven by carbon fiber warming and are almost as effective as forced-air warming.[14,15]

Conductive warming transfers slightly more heat than convective warming. However, it is associated with greater costs.

219

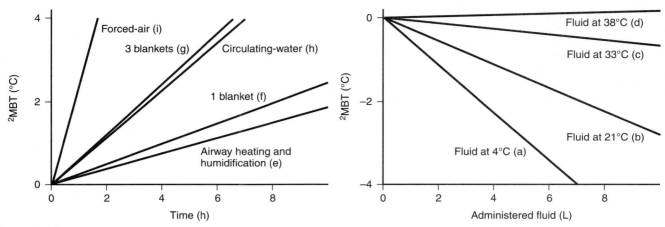

Figure 33-1. Relative Effects of Warming Methods on Mean Body Temperature (ΔMBT) as a Function of Time (Upper Portion) or Administered Fluid (Lower Portion). Mean body temperature (MBT) is the average temperature of body tissues, and is usually somewhat less than core temperature. The calculations assume an undressed 70-kg patient with a metabolic rate of 80 kcal/hr, in thermal steady state with a typical 21°C operating room environment. (a–d) Changes in MBT per liter of administered blood or crystalloid at various fluid temperatures. (e) Inspiring warmed, humidified gas. (f, g) Warmed or unwarmed blankets, with all skin below the neck covered. Savings are similar with a single layer of other passive insulators. (h) Full-length circulating-water mattress. (i) Full-length forced-air warmer. (*From Sessler DI: Consequences and treatment of perioperative hypothermia. Anesth Clin North Am 1994;12:425-456.*)

Endovascular Warming

Internal warming is probably the most efficient heat transfer method because it applies heat directly to the body core. Endovascular warming consists of a heat-exchanging catheter, usually inserted into the inferior vena cava via the femoral vein, and a servo-controller. They transfer heat into and out of the body in the range of 400 to 700 watts and thus are very efficient in warming and cooling patients. However, this warming method is invasive and very expensive and thus should be used only in patients in whom conductive or convective warming is insufficient, such as major trauma.

Core Temperature Monitoring

Whenever cooling or warming is performed in perioperative or critically ill patients it is essential to monitor core temperature. Several recommendations state that core temperature should be monitored whenever anesthesia time exceeds 30 minutes (American Society of PeriAnesthesia Nurses [ASPAN], Italien Guidelines). The most accurate way to monitor core temperature is the pulmonary artery temperature. Because this is a highly invasive and not commonly used monitoring device, esophageal temperature in anesthetized patients and tympanic temperature in awake patients are excellent substitutes. However, even bladder or rectal temperature, as well as oral temperature, can be used, as long as the user is aware of the limitations of such devices. Newer devices such as infrared tympanic thermometers or temporal artery thermometers need to be viewed with caution because of their limited accuracy or user-dependent high variability.

Despite all the available warming and monitoring methods, it remains unknown to what extent thermal management has improved over the past decade or what degree maintenance of perioperative normothermia has actually become part of clinical practice. Ratnaraj and colleagues[16]

evaluated patients' core temperature in the postanesthesia care unit (PACU) and noted that their hypothermia was still commonly observed in the operation room and PACU. Furthermore, a recent survey of 800 European hospitals showed that approximately 40% of patients receive active warming and in only 25% of patients temperature was monitored.[17]

EVIDENCE

Complications of Hypothermia and Economic Aspects

Even mild hypothermia is associated with numerous complications in the perioperative period. However, despite the well-documented ability of forced-air warming to maintain normothermia, it is still debated whether this technique results in a net increase or decrease in costs. Perioperative temperature management deserves the same cost/benefit calculations as other medical treatments. The discussion of costs associated with thermal management has two main components: (1) the cost of active warming and temperature monitoring and (2) the cost savings associated with decreased postoperative complications due to maintenance of perioperative normothermia.

Cost of Active Warming and Temperature Monitoring

The use of forced-air warming is associated with costs for the disposable blankets. In general, costs of disposable warming blankets have decreased over time and are now a few dollars per blanket. Furthermore, reusable warming modalities make active warming of patients even more cost efficient.

Circulating water garments are more expensive as compared with forced-air warming. However, heat transfer is more efficient with these devices and thus the additional costs are probably justified, specifically for extensive surgeries (e.g., cardiac surgery, transplantation, or trauma surgery).

Endovascular warming is probably the most expensive way of warming patients, with unit costs of up to $20,000 and catheter costs of $800 to $1,500. This type of warming transfers up to 600 watts and thus provides the most rapid rewarming technique. Furthermore internal warming does not depend on available surface area and is thus indicated for patients in whom only little skin surface area is available for active warming.

Costs Associated with Hypothermia-related Complications

Many studies have investigated the adverse consequences of perioperative hypothermia such as prolonged drug action, prolonged postoperative recovery, increased duration of hospitalization, increased incidence of postoperative surgical infections, increased perioperative blood loss, and adverse myocardial outcomes (Table 33-1).

All these consequences of hypothermia are associated with increased cost of care. For example, prolonged drug action leads to delayed extubation and also to prolonged duration of postoperative recovery; 2°C of hypothermia increases duration of action of vecuronium by 60%; and

3°C of hypothermia increases propofol plasma levels by 30%. Furthermore, the MAC of inhalational agents decreases by 15% with each degree of hypothermia.

In a prospective cost-finding study, forced-air warming was compared with routine thermal care in 100 patients undergoing general anesthesia. The time from completion of surgical dressing until tracheal extubation was significantly reduced in the forced-air warming group (10 ± 1 minute compared with 14 ± 1 minute; mean ± standard error of mean (SEM); $p < 0.01$).[32] Another study in 50 orthopedic patients compared the effects of passive thermal insulation with forced-air active warming on the efficacy of normothermia maintenance and time for discharging from the recovery room after combined spinal/epidural anesthesia. Core temperatures in actively warmed patients were approximately 1°C higher at the end of surgery. Achievement of both discharging criteria and normothermia required 32 ± 18 minutes in the active group and 74 ± 52 minutes in the passive group ($p < 0.0005$).[33] This study is consistent with a study by Lenhardt and colleagues,[30] who also showed delayed recovery in hypothermic patients undergoing colon surgery. Using a modified Aldrete score (which included core temperature) the authors showed that mean duration in the PACU was approximately 30 minutes in normothermic patients whereas it was 120 minutes in hypothermic patients (Figure 33-2).

Table 33-1	Consequences of Mild Perioperative and Perianesthetic Hypothermia[*]						
Consequence	**Author**	**N**	**ΔT_{core} (°C)**	**Normothermic**	**Hypothermic**	**P**
Surgical wound infection	Kurz et al.[18]	200	1.9	6%	19%	<0.01
Duration of hospitalization	Kurz et al.[18]	200	1.9	12.1 ± 4.4 days	14.7 ± 6.5 days	<0.01
Lymphocyte proliferation at 24 hr postanesthesia	Beilin et al.[19]	60	1.0	4800 CPM	2750 CPM	<0.05
Allogeneic transfusion requirement	Schmied et al.[20]	60	1.6	1 unit	8 units	<0.05
Intraoperative blood loss	Schmied et al.[20]	60	1.6	1.7 ± 0.3 L	2.2 ± 0.5 L	<0.001
Intraoperative blood loss	Winkler et al.[21]	150	0.4	488 mL	618 mL	<0.005
Intraoperative blood loss	Widman et al.[22]	46	0.5	516 ± 272 mL	702 ± 344 ml	<0.05
Intraoperative blood loss	Johansson et al.[23]	50	0.8	665 ± 292 mL	698 ± 314 mL	NS
Urinary excretion of nitrogen	Carli et al.	12	1.5	982 mmol/day	1798 mmol/day	<0.05
Trauma mortality rate at 24 hr	Gentilello et al.[25]	57	1.0-2.0	7%	43%	<0.05
Duration of vecuronium	Heier et al.	20	2.0	28 ± 4 min	62 ± 8 min	<0.001
Keo for vecuronium	Caldwell et al.[27]	12	2.0	0.20 min^{-1}	0.15 min^{-1}	<0.05
Duration of atracurium	Leslie et al.[28]	6	3.0	44 ± 4 min	68 ± 7 min	<0.05
Postoperative shivering	Just et al.	14	2.3	141 ± 9 mL. min^{-1}m^{-2}	269 ± 60 mL min^{-1}m^{-2}	<0.001
Duration of postanesthetic recovery	Lenhardt et al.[30]	150	1.9	53 ± 36 min	94 ± 65 min	<0.001
Thermal discomfort	Kurz et al.	74	2.6	50 ± 10 mm VAS	18 ± 9 mm VAS	<0.001

[*]Only prospective randomized human trials are included. Observers blinded to treatment group and core temperature evaluated subjective responses. N is total number of subjects. ΔT_{core} is difference in core temperature between treatment groups. Outcomes of studies are shown on separate rows. Baroflex sensitivity is defined as the change in the R-R interval of the ECG (ms, milliseconds) per 1 mm Hg change in systolic blood pressure. CPM is counts per minute and measures radioactivity (after addition of titrated thymidine and cell activation, the amount of radioactivity is proportional to the number of dividing cells[19]). VAS is a 100-mm-long visual analog scale (0 mm intense cold, 100 mm intense heat).

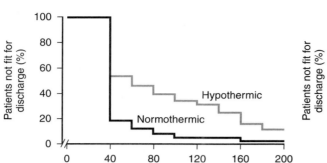

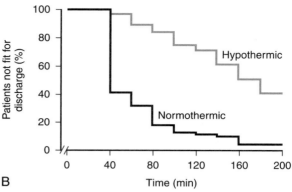

Figure 33-2. Kaplan-Meier "Survival" Analysis (a) Kaplan-Meier "survival" analysis showing the percentage of patients *not* sustaining a recovery score ≥13. The *p* value, using a Wilcoxon analysis, was less than 0.0001. (b) Kaplan-Meier "survival" analysis showing the percentage of patients *not* sustaining a recovery score ≥13 and a core temperature >36°C. The *p* value, using a Wilcoxon analysis, was less than 0.0001.

However, maintenance of normothermia not only affects intraoperative anesthetic factors but even more so postoperative surgical complications, which significantly affect cost of care. Maintenance of normothermia decreases postoperative wound infections by 60%. Wound infections are serious and costly complications of anesthesia and surgery as they might require extra treatment and furthermore can prolong duration of hospitalization.[18,34] Based on recent studies, the number needed to treat in regard to wound infection is eight patients to avoid one infection. Specifically in critical patient populations, such as the morbidly obese, wound infections are a major cause of postoperative morbidity and mortality.

Furthermore, hypothermia increases perioperative blood loss and transfusion requirements. Each degree of hypothermia increases blood loss by approximately 280 mL.[20] A recent meta-analysis shows that hypothermia increases blood loss by approximately 16% and increases perioperative transfusion requirements by 20% (Figure 33-3).[35] In another study blood loss and transfusion requirements were less in the actively warmed patients, who also had a shorter duration of stay in the PACU (94 [SD 42] minutes versus 217 [169] minutes; *p* ≤0.01) and a 24% reduction in

total anesthetic costs.[33] Perioperative transfusions are associated with considerable postoperative morbidity. It is important to recognize that hypothermia adds to the cost of blood products, but more important, it causes blood product–related and costly complications such as postoperative infections, organ failures, cancer recurrence, and increased mortality risk.[36-48]

Even fairly expensive warming therapies, such as the use of a flexible adherent hydrogel matrix combined with a conductive water delivery system to provide uninterrupted skin contact, prove cost efficient in specific patient populations. Several studies have not only shown the effectiveness of these devices in preventing or treating perioperative hypothermia[15,49-54] (Figure 33-4), but also the effect of normothermia on improved outcome. Those devices transfer an enormous amount of heat over small surface areas and are thus helpful in large operations, where little skin surface is available for warming (e.g., cardiovascular operations).

A meta-analysis by Fleisher and colleagues[55] addressed the following questions: (1) Is the difference in adverse patient outcomes between normothermic and mildly hypothermic patient groups significant across studies and

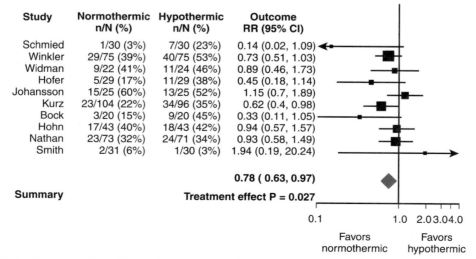

Figure 33-3. Transfusion Meta-analysis and Forest Plot Treatment effect expressed as the relative risk of transfusion in normothermic versus hypothermic patients. Normothermia is associated with 22% less risk of transfusion than hypothermia (95% CI 3%, 37%, *p* = 0.027.)

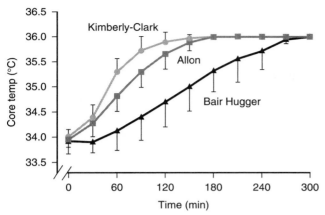

Figure 33-4. Core Temperature (±95% Confidence Intervals) as a Function of Rewarming Time in Seven Healthy Volunteers on Three Separate Study Days, Each with a Different Warming Device. The three warming devices were (1) Kimberly Clark energy transfer pads, (2) Allon circulating-water garment, and (3) Bair Hugger forced-air warming. Even after volunteers reached 36°C on the Kimberly Clark day and the study was stopped, they are shown as continuing at that temperature in the figure.

within studies? (2) What is the magnitude of the difference in adverse patient outcomes across studies? (3) What are the costs resulting from the difference in adverse patient outcomes? (4) Does a significant difference exist in effectiveness of modality for maintaining intraoperative normothermia? The results of this meta-analytic study provide evidence that the difference in adverse patient outcomes between the normothermic and mildly hypothermic patients is significant across studies for all adverse outcomes examined (see Table 33-1). In addition, a significant difference in effectiveness between warming modalities was found. A significant increase in the risk of costly complications occurred when patient temperatures dropped a mean of 1.5°C. For example, patients who become mildly hypothermic are much more likely to receive blood transfusions and to develop infections; both these outcomes result in increased costs. The cost of preventing intraoperative hypothermia is much less than the cost of treating the adverse outcomes that affect patients experiencing intraoperative hypothermia. Meta-analytic results show that hypothermia averaging only 1.5°C less than normal resulted in cumulative adverse outcomes adding between $2,500 and $7,000 per surgical patient to hospitalization costs across a variety of surgical procedures. Intraoperative normothermia in this meta-analysis was maintained most effectively with the use of forced-air warming.[55]

Taken together, many warming devices are available to ensure maintenance of perioperative normothermia. Forced-air warming is the most commonly used warming device because it is efficient, is easy to use, and has been proven to prevent major complications related to perioperative hypothermia. The costs of forced-air warming are negligible as compared with the related complications.

GUIDELINES

Optimization of health care cost and quality is possible. The Premier's Performance Pays study proves that when evidence-based processes are delivered, quality is higher

and costs are lower. Clinical performance measures, such as "maintenance of perioperative normothermia," developed by the American Society of Anesthesiologists and the Physician Consortium for Performance Improvement were designed for individual quality improvement.

Rationale for Maintenance of Normothermia

Anesthetic-induced impairment of thermoregulatory control is the primary cause of perioperative hypothermia. Even mild hypothermia (1°C to 2°C below normal) has been associated in randomized trials with a number of adverse consequences. Several methods to maintain normothermia are available to the anesthesiologist in the perioperative period; various studies have demonstrated the superior efficacy of forced-air warming and warm water garments.

Measuring Maintenance of Normothermia

Percentage of patients, regardless of age, undergoing surgical or therapeutic procedures under general or neuraxial anesthesia of 60 minutes' duration or longer for whom *either* active warming was used intraoperatively for the purpose of maintaining normothermia, *or* at least one body temperature equal to or greater than 36°C (96.8°F) was recorded within the 30 minutes immediately before or the 30 minutes immediately after anesthesia end time. "Active warming" is limited to forced-air warming and warm water garments.

Suggested Preoperative Patient Management

Assessment

Identify the patient's risk factors for unplanned perioperative hypothermia. Measure patient temperature on admission. Determine the patient's thermal comfort level. Assess for other signs and symptoms of hypothermia (shivering, piloerection, and/or cold extremities).

Interventions

Institute preventive warming measures for patients who are normothermic (normothermia is defined as a core temperature range from 36°C to 38°C [96.8°F to 100.4°F]). A variety of measures may be used, unless contraindicated. Passive insulation may include warmed cotton blankets, socks, head covering, limited skin exposure, circulating water mattresses, and increased ambient room temperature (minimum 68°F to 75°F). Institute active warming measures for patients who are hypothermic (defined as a core temperature less than 36°C). Active warming is the application of a forced-air convection warming system. Consider warmed intravenous (IV) fluids.

Intraoperative Patient Management

Assessment

Identify the patient's risk factors for unplanned perioperative hypothermia. Determine the patient's thermal comfort level, if applicable (ask the patient if he or she is cold). Assess for other signs and symptoms of hypothermia (shivering, piloerection, and/or cold extremities). Monitor the patient's temperature intraoperatively.

Intervention

Implement active warming methods. Maintenance of body temperature in a normothermic range is recommended for most procedures other than during periods in which mild hypothermia is intended to provide organ protection (e.g., during high aortic cross-clamping).

AUTHOR'S RECOMMENDATIONS

- Hypothermia is common during anesthesia and surgery.
- Hypothermia develops because of anesthetic-induced impairment of thermoregulatory control paired with cold operating room environment and heat loss via the surgical field.
- Hypothermia-related complications are severe: prolonged drug action, increased blood loss, increased transfusion requirements, wound infections, prolonged duration of hospitalization, and adverse myocardial events.
- All patients having surgery longer than 30 minutes should be actively warmed and core temperature should be measured.
- Active warming with convective and conductive warming maintains perioperative normothermia.

REFERENCES

1. Andrews DT, Leslie K, Sessler DI, et al: The arterial blood propofol concentration preventing movement in 50% of healthy women after skin incision. *Anesth Analg* 1997;85(2):414-419.
2. Vaughan MS, Vaughan RW, Cork RC: Postoperative hypothermia in adults: Relationship of age, anesthesia, and shivering to rewarming. *Anesth Analg* 1981;60:746-751.
3. Kurz A, Go JC, Sessler DI, et al: Alfentanil slightly increases the sweating threshold and markedly reduces the vasoconstriction and shivering thresholds. *Anesthesiology* 1995;83:293-299.
4. Matsukawa T, Kurz A, Sessler DI, et al: Propofol linearly reduces the vasoconstriction and shivering thresholds. *Anesthesiology* 1995;82:1169-1180.
5. Xiong J, Kurz A, Sessler DI, et al: Isoflurane produces marked and non-linear decreases in the vasoconstriction and shivering thresholds. *Anesthesiology* 1996;85:240-245.
6. Annadata RS, Sessler DI, Tayefeh F, et al: Desflurane slightly increases the sweating threshold, but produces marked, non-linear decreases in the vasoconstriction and shivering thresholds. *Anesthesiology* 1995;83:1205-1211.
7. Leslie K, Sessler DI: Reduction in the shivering threshold is proportional to spinal block height. *Anesthesiology* 1996;84:1327-1331.
8. Emerick TH, Ozaki M, Sessler DI, et al: Epidural anesthesia increases apparent leg temperature and decreases the shivering threshold. *Anesthesiology* 1994;81:289-298.
9. Morris RH: Operating room temperature and the anesthetized, paralyzed patient. *Surgery* 1971;102:95-97.
10. Sessler DI, McGuire J, Sessler AM: Perioperative thermal insulation. *Anesthesiology* 1991;74:875-879.
11. Sessler DI, Moayeri A: Skin-surface warming: Heat flux and central temperature. *Anesthesiology* 1990;73:218-224.
12. Hynson J, Sessler DI: Intraoperative warming therapies: A comparison of three devices. *J Clin Anesth* 1992;4:194-199.
13. Kurz A, Kurz M, Poeschl G, et al: Forced-air warming maintains intraoperative normothermia better than circulating-water mattresses. *Anesth Analg* 1993;77:89-95.
14. Negishi C, Hasegawa K, Mukai S, et al: Carbon-fiber and forced-air warming are comparably effective. *Anesth Analg* 2003;96:1683-1687.
15. Hofer CK, Worn M, Tavakoli R, et al: Influence of body core temperature on blood loss and transfusion requirements during off-pump coronary artery bypass grafting: A comparison of 3 warming systems. *J Thorac Cardiovasc Surg* 2005;129(4):838-843.
16. Ratnaraj J, Kabon B, Talcott MR, et al: Supplemental oxygen and carbon dioxide each increase subcutaneous and intestinal intramural oxygenation. *Anesth Analg* 2004;99(1):207-211.
17. Torossian A: Survey on intraoperative temperature management in Europe. *Eur J Anaesthesiol* 2007;24(8):668-675.
18. Kurz A, Sessler DI, Lenhardt RA, et al: Perioperative normothermia to reduce the incidence of surgical-wound infection and shorten hospitalization. *N Engl J Med* 1996;334:1209-1215.
19. Beilin B, Shavit Y, Razumovsky, J, et al: Effects of mild perioperative hypothermia on cellular immune responses. *Anesthesiology* 1998;89(5):1133-1140.
20. Schmied H, Kurz A, Sessler DI, et al: Mild intraoperative hypothermia increases blood loss and allogeneic transfusion requirements during total hip arthroplasty. *Lancet* 1996;347:289-292.
21. Winkler M, Akça O, Birkenberg B, et al: Aggressive warming reduces blood loss during hip arthroplasty. *Anesth Analg* 2000;91(4):978-984.
22. Widman J, Hammarqvist F, Sellden E: Amino acid infusion induces thermogenesis and reduces blood loss during hip arthroplasty under spinal anesthesia. *Anesth Analg* 2002;95(6):1757-1762.
23. Johansson T, Lisander B, Ivarsson I: Mild hypothermia does not increase blood loss during total hip arthroplasty. *Acta Anaesthesiol Scand* 1999;43(10):1005-1010.
24. Carli F, Emery PW, Freemantle CAJ: Effect of perioperative normothermia on postoperative protein metabolism in elderly patients undergoing hip arthroplasty. *Br J Anaesth* 1989;63: 276-282.
25. Gentilello LM, Jurkovich GJ, Stark MS, et al: Is hypothermia in the victim of major trauma protective or harmful? A randomized, prospective study. *Ann Surg* 1997;226(4):439-447, discussion 447-439.
26. Heier T, Caldwell JE, Sessler DI, et al: Mild intraoperative hypothermia increases duration of action and spontaneous recovery of vecuronium blockade during nitrous oxide-isoflurane anesthesia in humans. *Anesthesiology* 1991;74:815-819.
27. Caldwell JE, Heier T, Wright PMC, et al: Temperature-dependent pharmacokinetics and pharmacodynamics of vecuronium. *Anesthesiology* 2000;92:84-93.
28. Leslie K, Sessler DI, Bjorksten AR, et al: Mild hypothermia alters propofol pharmacokinetics and increases the duration of action of atracurium. *Anesth Analg* 1995;80:1007-1014.
29. Just B, Delva E, Camus Y, et al: Oxygen uptake during recovery following naloxone. *Anesthesiology* 1992;76:60-64.
30. Lenhardt R, Marker E, Goll V, et al: Mild intraoperative hypothermia prolongs postanesthetic recovery. *Anesthesiology* 1997; 87:1318-1323.
31. Kurz A, Sessler DI, Narzt E, et al: Postoperative hemodynamic and thermoregulatory consequences of intraoperative core hypothermia. *J Clin Anesth* 1995;7:359-366.
32. Mahoney CB, Odom J: Maintaining intraoperative normothermia: A meta-analysis of outcomes with costs. *AANA J* 1999;67(2): 155-163.
33. Casati A, Fanelli G, Ricci A, et al: Shortening the discharging time after total hip replacement under combined spinal/epidural anesthesia by actively warming the patient during surgery. *Minerva Anestesiol* 1999;65(7-8):507-514.
34. Melling AC, Ali B, Scott EM, et al: Effects of preoperative warming on the incidence of wound infection after clean surgery: A randomised controlled trial. *Lancet* 2001;358(9285):876-880.
35. Rajagopalan S, Mascha E, Na J, et al: The effects of mild perioperative hypothermia on blood loss and transfusion requirement: A meta-analysis. *Anesthesiology* 2008;108:71-77.
36. Leal-Noval SR, Rincon-Ferrari MD, Garcia-Curiel A, et al: Transfusion of blood components and postoperative infection in patients undergoing cardiac surgery. *Chest* 2001;119(5):1461-1468.
37. Chelemer SB, Prato BS, Cox PM Jr, et al: Association of bacterial infection and red blood cell transfusion after coronary artery bypass surgery. *Ann Thorac Surg* 2002;73(1):138-142.
38. Taylor RW, Manganaro L, O'Brien J, et al: Impact of allogenic packed red blood cell transfusion on nosocomial infection rates in the critically ill patient. *Crit Care Med* 2002;30(10): 2249-2254.
39. Schreiber GB, Busch MP, Kleinman SH, et al: The risk of transfusion-transmitted viral infections. The Retrovirus Epidemiology Donor Study. *N Engl J Med* 1996;334(26):1685-1690.

40. Leal-Noval SR, Marquez-Vacaro JA, Garcia-Curiel A, et al: Nosocomial pneumonia in patients undergoing heart surgery. *Crit Care Med* 2000;28(4):935-940.
41. Vamvakas EC: Meta-analysis of randomized controlled trials investigating the risk of postoperative infection in association with white blood cell-containing allogeneic blood transfusion: The effects of the type of transfused red blood cell product and surgical setting. *Transfus Med Rev* 2002;16(4):304-314.
42. Vincent JL, Baron JF, Reinhart K, et al: Anemia and blood transfusion in critically ill patients. *JAMA* 2002;288(12):1499-1507.
43. Michalopoulos A, Tzelepis G, Dafni U, et al: Determinants of hospital mortality after coronary artery bypass grafting. *Chest* 1999;115(6):1598-1603.
44. Engoren MC, Habib RH, Zacharias A, et al: Effect of blood transfusion on long-term survival after cardiac operation. *Ann Thorac Surg* 2002;74(4):1180-1186.
45. Ranucci M, Pavesi M, Mazza E, et al: Risk factors for renal dysfunction after coronary surgery: The role of cardiopulmonary bypass technique. *Perfusion* 1994;9(5):319-326.
46. Zacharias A, Habib RH: Factors predisposing to median sternotomy complications. Deep vs superficial infection. *Chest* 1996;110(5):1173-1178.
47. Moore FA, Moore EE, Sauaia A: Blood transfusion. An independent risk factor for postinjury multiple organ failure. *Arch Surg* 1997;132(6):620-624, discussion 624-625.
48. Malone DL, Dunne J, Tracy JK, et al: Blood transfusion, independent of shock severity, is associated with worse outcome in trauma. *J Trauma* 2003;54(5):898-905, discussion 905-907.
49. Stanley TO, Grocott HP, Phillips-Bute B, et al: Preliminary evaluation of the Arctic Sun temperature controlling system during off pump coronary artery bypass surgery. *Ann Thorac Surg* 2003;75:1140-1144.
50. Grocott HP, Mathew JP, Carver EH, et al: A randomized controlled trial of the Arctic Sun temperature management system versus conventional methods for preventing hypothermia during off-pump cardiac surgery. *Anesth Analg* 2004;98(2):298-302.
51. Bar-Yosef S, Anders M, Mackensen GB, et al: Aortic atheroma burden and cognitive dysfunction after coronary artery bypass graft surgery. *Ann Thorac Surg* 2004;78(5):1556-1562.
52. Woo YJ, Atluri P, Grand TJ, et al: Active thermoregulation improves outcome of off-pump coronary artery bypass. *Asian Cardiovasc Thorac Ann* 2005;13(2):157-160.
53. Janicki PK, Higgins MS, Janssen J, et al: Comparison of two different temperature maintenance strategies during open abdominal surgery: Upper body forced-air warming versus whole body water garment. *Anesthesiology* 2001;95(4):868-874.
54. Nesher N, Wolf T, Kushnir I, et al: Novel thermoregulation system for enhancing cardiac function and hemodynamics during coronary artery bypass graft surgery. *Ann Thorac Surg* 2001;72(3):S1069-1076.
55. Fleisher LA, Metzger SE, Lam J, et al: Perioperative cost-finding analysis of the routine use of intraoperative forced-air warming during general anesthesia. *Anesthesiology* 1998;88(5):1357-1364.

34 What Is the Best Means of Preventing Perioperative Renal Injury?

Vivek Moitra, MD; Alan Gaffney, MBBCh; Hugh Playford, MBBS, FANZCA, FFICANZCA; and Robert N. Sladen, MBChB, MRCP(UK), FRCP(C), FCCM

ACUTE KIDNEY INJURY

Acute kidney injury (AKI) is a clinical syndrome that reflects the clinical manifestation of isolated or multiple insults to the kidney. The degree of renal damage ranges from the trivial, that is, a transient increase in serum creatinine (S_{Cr}) or decrease in urine output, to the profound, that is, established acute renal failure (ARF) requiring renal replacement therapy (RRT). A consensus definition of AKI by a multinational expert panel, the Acute Dialysis Quality Initiative Group (ADQI),[1] attempts to standardize the classification and reporting of AKI (Table 34-1). The classification is based on the degree of elevation of S_{Cr} or calculated glomerular filtration rate (GFR), severity and duration of oliguria, and the requirement for RRT. The acronym RIFLE serves to organize a hierarchy of severity of AKI into risk of injury (R), acute injury (I), established failure (F), sustained loss of function (L), and end-stage renal disease (E).

A consensus definition of ARF in critically ill patients such as RIFLE is long overdue, given that more than 30 different definitions can be found in the literature. However, there are some important caveats. RIFLE does not take into consideration that about three-quarters of ARF is nonoliguric in nature[2]; that acute changes in GFR may not be reflected by rapid changes in S_{Cr}[3]; or that S_{Cr} may increase slowly and subtly in patients with depleted muscle mass.[4] It was also not designed to examine the specific AKI associated with surgery, and may not be as useful for anesthesiologists as a criterion such as peak percentage change in postoperative SCr.[5] Nonetheless, there have been several investigations of the predictive ability, internal validity, robustness, ease of application, and clinical relevance of RIFLE in a variety of settings.[6-12] These retrospective and prospective studies demonstrate a broad correlation between the RIFLE severity and overall mortality rate from AKI. It appears that the RIFLE classification is easy to use; identifies patients with early signs of dysfunction that may progress to more severe renal disease; and can identify patients of different mortality risk. However, the RIFLE criteria have yet to be used in large multicenter randomized controlled clinical trials in a wide variety of patient populations.

Perioperative AKI, characterized by postoperative elevation of S_{Cr}, is generally uncommon. However, it has a predilection for certain surgical procedures, particularly vascular surgery involving aortic manipulation, where the incidence is between 10% and 25%.[13-15] One study demonstrated a relatively static incidence over a 12-year period.[15] The risk of AKI is enhanced by nephrotoxic factors such as obstructive jaundice or exposure to radiocontrast agents (Table 34-2).[16] Regardless of its etiology, pathogenesis, or requirement for RRT, postoperative AKI is associated with increased length of hospital stay, increased mortality rate, and impaired quality of life.[13,14,17-19]

A considerable research effort has been marshaled to evaluate perioperative interventions to protect the kidneys when they are placed at risk by preexisting impairment, nephrotoxins, renal ischemia, and the inflammatory process. Preventive strategies have focused on preoperative optimization of renal function, judicious perioperative fluid balance, and "renoprotective" pharmacologic agents. However, given the wide variety of renal insults that contribute to perioperative AKI, outcome studies of therapeutic interventions have addressed only a limited territory of perioperative renal protection.

These strategies appear to have had some benefit because although the incidence of postoperative AKI has been increasing over the last two decades, the mortality rate of ARF requiring RRT is decreasing. For example, a study on coronary artery bypass grafting (CABG) in a sample of 20% of U.S. hospitals revealed an increase in incidence of postoperative ARF from 1% to 4% between 1988 and 2003.[20] However, the proportion of cases requiring RRT declined from about 16% to less than 9%, and mortality rate declined from nearly 40% to less than 18%. These figures may be influenced by less stringent criteria for the diagnosis of ARF, but the proportion of survivors requiring special care after discharge almost doubled from 35% to 65%, emphasizing the increasing burden of perioperative AKI on our health care system.

Table 34-1	**Risk, Injury, Failure, Loss, and End-stage Kidney (RIFLE) Classification**[1]		
Class	**S_{Cr} Increase**	**GFR Decrease**	**Oliguria (UO <0.5 mL/kg/hr)**
Risk	×1.5	>25%	>6 hours
Injury	×2	>50%	>12 hours
Failure	×3 (or >4 mg/dL, with an acute increase >0.5 mg/dL)	>75%	>24 hours (or anuria >12 hours)
Loss	ARF >4 weeks		
ESRD	ARF >3 months		

ARF, acute renal failure; *GFR*, (calculated) glomerular filtration rate; S_{Cr}, serum creatinine; *UO*, urine output.
RIFLE class is determined based on the worst of either S_{Cr}, GFR, or UO criteria. S_{Cr} change is calculated as an increase of S_{Cr} above baseline S_{Cr}. Acute kidney injury should be both abrupt (within 1-7 days) and sustained (>24 hours). When the baseline S_{Cr} is not known and patients are without a history of chronic kidney insufficiency, it is recommended to calculate a baseline S_{Cr} using the Modification of Diet in Renal Disease (MDRD) equation for assessment of kidney function, assuming a GFR of 75 mL/min/$1.73M^2$. When the baseline S_{Cr} is elevated, an abrupt increase of at least 0.5 mg/dL to >4 mg/dL is all that is required to achieve the class of Failure.

Table 34-2	**Risk Factors for Developing Perioperative Renal Failure**[16]

Cardiac surgery
- Preexisting renal insufficiency
- Emergency procedures
- Sepsis
- Prolonged cardiopulmonary bypass
- Postoperative cardiac dysfunction

Vascular surgery
- Preexisting renal insufficiency
- Postoperative dye studies
- Sepsis
- Aortic cross-clamp
  - Direct renal ischemia
  - Myocardial ischemia, low cardiac output
  - Declamping hypotension
- Renal artery atheromatous embolization
- Ruptured aortic aneurysm
- Biliary tract and hepatic surgery including liver transplantation

Kidney transplantation
Urogenital surgery
Complicated obstetrics
Major trauma
- Direct renal trauma
- Hemorrhagic shock
- Massive blood transfusion
- Elevated intraabdominal pressure
- Rhabdomyolysis
- Sepsis and multiorgan dysfunction syndrome

Perioperative Risk Factors for Acute Kidney Injury

An isolated risk factor or insult rarely induces AKI. Inevitably, AKI is the consequence of the complex, often sequential interaction of multiple factors. Indeed, AKI may be the final common pathway of a confluence of factors such as preexisting renal insufficiency or a genetic predisposition, high-risk surgery, compromised hemodynamic function, nephrotoxic insults, and acute inflammation. It is little wonder that no single intervention has been shown to be the "magic bullet" that prevents AKI.

Patient Factors

Patient factors demonstrated to be associated with an increased risk of the development of postoperative AKI include advanced age, hypertension, diabetes mellitus, ventricular dysfunction, sepsis, hepatic failure, and chronic kidney disease (CKD). Because CKD also has various definitions, the association between preoperative CKD and postoperative AKI is difficult to quantify accurately, but it is strong.[21-23] Poorly controlled diastolic hypertension is an established risk factor for AKI, but wide pulse pressure hypertension (isolated systolic hypertension) is independently associated with worsened renal function after cardiac surgery.[24]

Genetic polymorphisms may also play a role in the predisposition to AKI. The Duke group demonstrated a negative association between possession of the apolipoprotein E4 allele and postoperative increase in S_{Cr} in a prospective study on 564 patients undergoing CABG.[25] This renal protective effect is interesting because the same polymorphism is associated with atherosclerotic disease and an increased risk of perioperative neurologic impairment.[25,26]

Intraoperative Factors

Ischemia and Inflammation. *Ischemia-Reperfusion Injury.* Although the renal medulla receives less than 10% of renal blood flow (RBF), the medullary process of urinary concentration has a high metabolic requirement. Any compromise to RBF increases the regional perfusion imbalance and renders the medulla ischemic. Compromise may result from aortic occlusion, atheromatous embolism, hypotension, low blood flow states, and hypovolemia.

Suprarenal aortic cross-clamping creates an ischemia-reperfusion injury and self-limited acute tubular necrosis (ATN) that takes up to 48 hours to recover.[3] Injury is exacerbated by the proinflammatory cytokine liberation that follows reperfusion. Infrarenal aortic cross-clamping also significantly compromises RBF, most likely through reflex renal vasoconstriction.[27]

Atheromatous renal artery embolism is a devastating complication that may be provoked by trauma as trivial as coughing; aortic and renal angiography; manipulation of the renal arteries by the proximate application of the cross-clamp; or by placement of an endovascular graft. Patchy or confluent renal infarction can occur that is usually irreversible.

The Inflammatory Response. Ischemia-reperfusion injury provokes an inflammatory response that may be more detrimental than the original ischemic insult itself. Major surgery itself provokes inflammation. A cascade of stress responses are elicited, mediated by the release of various cytokines and stress hormones, culminating in the systemic inflammatory response syndrome (SIRS). The kidneys sequester proinflammatory cytokines and may be damaged by them. SIRS is activated to a variable degree in all patients who undergo cardiopulmonary bypass (CPB) and in many who undergo major operations.[28,29]

Gut ischemia and portal endotoxemia frequently complicate major aortic surgery. The insult appears to be more frequent in patients who undergo surgery via the intraperitoneal abdominal aorta than the endovascular approach.[30] Endotoxin and other activated cytokines cause afferent arteriolar constriction, mesangial contraction, and direct tubular injury that diminish RBF, GFR, sodium excretion, and urine flow.[31] Compared with open aortic repair, endovascular techniques require shorter aortic occlusion times and are associated with a diminished acute-phase response and proinflammatory surge.[32]

Glucose Homeostasis. Abnormal glucose homeostasis (hyperglycemia) is characteristic of the acute inflammatory response and is exacerbated by the perioperative administration of high-dose steroids, for example, in patients undergoing transplantation. Strict perioperative glycemic control has been advocated in the intensive care setting on the basis of data indicating improved survival with a concomitant decrease in the incidence of ARF.[33-35] In one study evaluating persistent intraoperative hyperglycemia despite an insulin protocol, hyperglycemia was associated with worsened renal outcomes.[36] However, in another randomized, controlled trial in patients undergoing cardiac surgery, tight glucose control did not reduce the incidence of perioperative ARF.[37] Presently, it is unclear whether intraoperative hyperglycemia is simply a marker of acute illness or whether it is a reversible, treatable, and independent effector of renal outcome.

Nephrotoxins. *Renin-Angiotensin System–Blocking Drugs.* Drugs that block the renin-angiotensin system include the angiotensin-converting enzyme (ACE) inhibitors and the selective angiotensin-II receptor antagonists. These groups of drugs have become well established in the treatment of hypertension and promote beneficial cardiac remodeling in congestive heart failure (CHF). As such, they may prevent the progression of chronic renal disease.

However, angiotensin release is an important protective mechanism that induces efferent renal arteriolar constriction in states of decreased RBF or perfusion pressure. The presence of ACE inhibitors or angiotensin-II receptor antagonists may impair the maintenance of RBF and GFR when renal perfusion is compromised. In one prospective study of 249 patients undergoing aortic surgery, chronic preoperative ACE inhibitor administration was the only factor independently associated with a 20% decline in GFR after surgery.[38]

Aprotinin. Aprotinin is an inhibitor of endogenous serine proteases such as kallikrein and plasmin. Its effectiveness in decreasing bleeding after cardiopulmonary bypass (CPB)—through its antifibrinolytic action and platelet stabilization—was established more than 20 years ago.[39] Numerous observations have suggested that aprotinin administration is associated with elevations in postoperative S_{Cr},[40-42] likely mediated through its effects on kinin pathways and subsequent alteration of intrarenal hemodynamics.[43,44] Aprotinin may cause vasoconstriction of the afferent arteriole, which reduces glomerular perfusion pressure and renal excretory function. Indeed, there may be a deleterious interaction of ACE inhibitors and aprotinin on renal function when neither drug alone has any effect.[45]

Two retrospective observational reports published in 2006 evoked much debate. They indicated that significant increases in adverse postoperative events, including renal failure, occurred with aprotinin, while the reduction in blood loss was no better than simpler, safer antifibrinolytic agents such as episilon aminocaproic acid or tranexamic acid.[46,47] In contrast, meta-analyses of 13 randomized, controlled trials that reported data on AKI published before these observational studies failed to show an adverse effect of aprotinin on renal or other organ function.[48,49] This dichotomy may be resolved by the results of a Canadian study that is the largest blinded, randomized, controlled trial of antifibrinolytic drugs in high-risk cardiac surgery.[50] At the time of writing the study had been halted because of a higher mortality rate in patients randomized to aprotinin, although specific data have not been published, and the U.S. Food and Drug Administration (FDA) has withdrawn the drug from routine use.

Nonsteroidal Antiinflammatory Drugs. Nonsteroidal antiinflammatory drugs (NSAIDs) exert multiple renal effects. Their inhibition of cyclo-oxygenase suppresses the formation of endogenous prostaglandins that induce afferent arteriolar vasodilatation during situations of renal stress. Thus administration of NSAIDs causes little harm when renal circulation is normal,[51] but may exacerbate renal injury during low-flow states or in conjunction with other nephrotoxic agents. Administration of NSAIDs has also been implicated in interstitial and membranous nephritis and minimal change protein leak disease. NSAIDs may be harmful in conditions such as cirrhosis, CKD, and CHF where maintenance of RBF is dependent on precapillary vasodilation.

Calcineurin Inhibitors. In the early 1980s, the introduction of supplemental immunosuppression by the calcineurin phosphatase inhibitor, cyclosporine A, revolutionized solid organ transplantation. It soon became apparent that its benefit was limited by dose-dependent acute nephrotoxicity, induced by afferent arteriolar vasoconstriction.[52] Subsequently, the importance of chronic nephrotoxicity was also appreciated, but the mechanisms are more complex, involving the renin-angiotensin system, endothelin, nitric oxide, and inflammatory activation.[53] Another widely used calcineurin inhibitor, tacrolimus, shares the propensity for nephrotoxicity, and its actions on growth factor may promote fibrogenesis as a component of chronic renal impairment.[54]

Radiocontrast Media. The mechanism of nephrotoxicity of radiocontrast media is multifactorial. They cause direct cytotoxic injury, and their hyperosmolality crenates red cells and causes microcirculatory obstruction. They induce an imbalance of renal oxygen supply and demand, by promoting acute vasoconstriction that impairs renal medullary perfusion, while the osmotic load they induce increases medullary oxygen consumption.[55] Contrast material filtered through the glomerulus precipitates in the renal tubules and liberates damaging free oxygen radicals. The risk of radiocontrast nephropathy (RCN) is greatly exacerbated by dehydration and hypovolemia, and the concomitant administration of other nephrotoxic agents.

Options and Therapies

1. Optimize renal function preoperatively and minimize nephrotoxic insults.
2. Minimize hemodynamic insults to the kidney.
   a. Avoid prolonged aortic cross-clamping.
   b. Maintain renal blood flow and perfusion pressure.
   c. Avoid pharmacologic agents that may compromise renal blood flow or increase the metabolic demand of the kidney.
3. Consider pharmacologic renoprotective strategies.

Evidence

Overall, there are limited studies on prophylactic and therapeutic interventions in patients at high risk for developing perioperative AKI. The majority of studies have concentrated on RCN, and their findings may not be applicable to perioperative AKI. Tables 34-3, 34-4 and 34-5 summarize and grade the evidence using established criteria.[56]

Level	Type of Evidence
1a	Systematic review (with homogeneity*) of RCTs
1b	Individual RCT (with narrow confidence interval)
1c	All or none†
2a	Systematic review (with homogeneity*) of cohort studies
2b	Individual cohort study (including low-quality RCT)
2c	"Outcomes" research
3a	Systematic review (with homogeneity*) of case-control studies
3b	Individual case-control studies
4	Case series (and poor-quality cohort and case-control studies)
5	Expert opinion without explicit critical appraisal, or based on physiology, bench research, or "first principles"

Table 34-3   **Levels of Evidence**[56]

*Homogeneity of both direction and degree of results between the individual studies.

†When all patients developed renal failure before the therapy was available, but now some do not; or when some patients developed renal failure before therapy was available, but now none do.

RCT, randomized, controlled trial.

Grade	Criteria
A	Consistent Level 1 studies
B	Consistent Level 2 or 3 studies *or* extrapolations* from Level 1 studies
C	Level 4 studies *or* extrapolations from Level 2 or 3 studies
D	Level 5 evidence *or* troubling inconsistent or inconclusive studies of any level

Table 34-4   **Grades of Recommendations**[56]

*Extrapolations are from data regarding renal failure obtained from studies with a different clinical focus.

A Cochrane Database review of 37 studies of the protective renal effects of perioperative administration of dopamine, diuretics, calcium channel blockers, ACE inhibitors, or simple hydration concludes that certain interventions show some benefit, but that all the results suffer from significant heterogeneity.[57] The authors deemed the evidence from available literature too unreliable for any conclusions to be drawn about the effectiveness of these interventions in protecting the kidneys from damage during surgery.

Hydration

Hypotheses regarding the impact of hydration on the prevention of perioperative AKI—either a liberal versus conservative strategy, or the superiority of one type of crystalloid or colloid over another—have not been subjected to randomized controlled trials.

However, there is considerable evidence that the single most important protective measure to ameliorate RCN is fluid loading and hydration before intravascular administration of radiocontrast media.[58-63] There is no agreement on the minimal duration, optimal rate, and composition of intravenous fluid administered. Administration of intravenous isotonic saline for several hours before, during, and after radiocontrast media injection is usually advocated. One randomized controlled trial demonstrated a more favorable impact on the incidence of RCN by the infusion of isotonic sodium bicarbonate than sodium chloride.[64]

The mainstay of the prevention of AKI as a consequence of rhabdomyolysis and myoglobinemia is the early, aggressive administration of large quantities of fluids. It is advocated that intravenous access be obtained in the field in cases of traumatic crush injury and saline at 1.5 L/hr be infused.[65] There is animal evidence that alkalinization of the urine to a pH greater than 6.0 prevents the conversion of myoglobin to toxic ferrihematin in the renal tubules and further ameliorates the risk of AKI. There is anecdotal evidence from wartime experience that this approach can yield impressive benefits,[66] but, perhaps not unexpectedly, it has never been subjected to randomized controlled human studies.

Some initial studies suggested that fluid therapy guided by invasive hemodynamic monitoring via a pulmonary artery catheter could provide renal protection during open aortic aneurysm resection[67,68]; however,

Table 34-5 Summary of Renal Protective Strategies in Humans for High-risk Surgery

Study	Level of Evidence (see Table 34-3)	Type of Study	Conclusions
Dopamine, Diuretics, Calcium Channel Blockers, Angiotensin-Converting Enzyme Inhibitors, Hydration Fluids			
Zacharias et al[57]	1a	Systematic review	Cochrane database: 37 studies. The results indicated that certain interventions showed some benefits, but all the results suffered from significant heterogeneity. There is no evidence from this meta-analysis that interventions during surgery thus far studied protect the kidneys from damage.
Dopamine			
Kellum[75]	1a	Systematic review	Routine use of diuretics or dopamine for the prevention of acute renal failure cannot be justified on the basis of available evidence.
Kellum & Decker[76]	1a	Systematic review	No justification for the use of low-dose dopamine for the treatment or prevention of acute renal failure.
Marik[77]	1a	Systematic review	Dopamine demonstrates no renoprotective effect in patients at high risk of developing renal failure.
Bellomo et al.[73]	1b	Critically ill	Large placebo-controlled RCT ($n = 328$) of dopamine in critically ill patients with signs of sepsis. No differences in peak creatinine need for renal replacement therapy or mortality.
Fenoldopam			
Landoni et al.[85]	1a	Meta-analysis	Meta-analysis of 1290 patients from 16 RCTs demonstrated that fenoldopam infusion is associated with decreased risk of AKI, need for RRT, ICU length of stay, and in-hospital mortality rate.
Stone et al.[84]	1b	RCN	Prospective, multicenter, double-blind RCT ($n = 315$) in patients with CrCl <60 mL/min undergoing angiography, comparing fenoldopam to placebo for prevention of RCN (S_{Cr} increase >25%) within 96 hours. There were no significant differences in RCN, 30-day mortality rate, dialysis, or rehospitalization.
Halpenny et al.[79]	2b	Cardiac surgery	Small placebo-controlled RCT ($n = 31$) of fenoldopam during cardiac surgery with CPB. The fenoldopam group was spared decline in postoperative CrCl.
Halpenny et al.[80]	2b	Vascular surgery	Small placebo-controlled RCT ($n = 28$) of fenoldopam in patients undergoing infrarenal cross-clamping. Fenoldopam was associated with postoperative maintenance of CrCl and prevention of deterioration of S_{Cr}.
Dopamine vs. Fenoldopam			
Bove et al[81]	2b	Cardiac surgery	Prospective single-center, double-blind RCT ($n = 80$). Fenoldopam or dopamine after the induction of anesthesia for a 24-hour period. No difference in clinical outcome.
Oliver et al[82]	2b	Vascular surgery	Single-center, double-blind RCT ($n = 60$). Fenoldopam or dopamine with nitroprusside after the induction of anesthesia in patients undergoing aortic cross-clamping. No difference in clinical outcome.
Furosemide			
Kellum[75]	1a	Systematic review	Level 1 evidence exists against the use of diuretics for prevention of perioperative renal failure after vascular surgery.
Lassnigg et al.[86]	1b	Cardiac surgery	Prospective ($n = 126$) RCT of cardiac surgical patients who received either "renal dose" dopamine, or furosemide, or placebo until 48 hours postoperatively. Furosemide infusion was associated with greater deterioration in S_{Cr}, lower CrCl, and greater need for RRT (negative treatment effect).

Mannitol

Reference	Level	Setting	Description
Tiggeler et al.[89]	2b	Renal transplant	Prospective (n = 61) study of cadaveric renal transplant recipients receiving either restricted fluids (1.1 L), or restricted fluids (1.5 L) plus mannitol, or moderate fluids (2.5 L) plus mannitol. The incidence of ATN was 43%, 53%, and 4.8%, respectively.
Nicholson et al.[92]	2b	Vascular surgery	Prospective (n = 28) study of mannitol or placebo for aortic surgery with infrarenal aortic cross-clamping. No differences in BUN, S_{Cr} or CrCl. Mannitol group had lower urinary albumin and N-acetyl glucosaminidase.
Ip-Yam et al.[93]	2b	Cardiac surgery	Prospective (n = 23) study of hypothermic vs. normothermic CPB vs. normothermic CPB plus mannitol in bypass prime. No significant differences between the groups in markers of renal function.
Gubern et al.[95]	2b	Obstructive jaundice	Prospective RCT (n = 31) of mannitol in postoperative patients with obstructive jaundice. Mannitol had no beneficial effects on renal function.
Homsi et al.[94]	4	Rhabdomyolysis	Retrospective case series (n = 24) of saline vs. saline plus bicarbonate plus mannitol for rhabdomyolysis (CPK >500 U/L). No additive benefit with the addition of bicarbonate or mannitol.

Antioxidants (N-Acetylcysteine)

Reference	Level	Setting	Description
Marenzi et al.[101]	1b	RCN after PCI	RCT (n = 354) of N-acetylcysteine vs. placebo in patients with acute myocardial infarction undergoing percutaneous intervention (PCI) with primary angioplasty. Three groups: standard dose (n = 116), 600 mg IV before PCI, then 600 mg PO twice daily for 48 hours; high dose (n = 119), 1200 mg IV before PCI, then 1200 mg PO twice daily for 48 hours; placebo (n = 119 patients). Dose-dependent decrease in RCN: high dose (8%) vs. standard dose (15%) vs. placebo (33%) and in-hospital mortality rate.
Burns et al[102]	1b	Cardiac surgery	Quadruple-blind RCT (n = 295) comparing IV N-acetylcysteine with placebo in patients undergoing CABG over 24 hours. No difference in proportion of patients with postoperative renal dysfunction. Post hoc subgroup analysis (baseline S_{Cr} >1.4 mg/dL) showed a nonsignificant trend toward decreased risk of postoperative renal dysfunction in the N-acetylcysteine group.
Haase et al.[103]	1b	Cardiac surgery	Placebo-controlled RCT (n = 60) of a 24-hour infusion of N-acetylcysteine. No difference in delta or peak S_{Cr}, urine output, or serum cystatin C.
Wijnen et al.[104]	2b	Vascular surgery	Small RCT (n = 44) of standard therapy plus antioxidants (allopurinol, vitamins E and C, N-acetylcysteine, mannitol) vs. standard therapy only. No difference in urine albumin/creatinine ratio but antioxidant group had higher CrCl at POD 2.

Calcium Channel Blockers

Reference	Level	Setting	Description
Shilliday et al.[110]	1a	Renal transplant/ systematic review	Cochrane Database Systematic Review. Ten trials included. Treatment with calcium channel blockers in the peritransplant period was associated with a significant decrease in the incidence of posttransplant and delayed graft. There was no difference between control and treatment groups in graft loss, mortality rate, or requirement for hemodialysis.
van Riemsdijk et al.[109]	2b	Renal transplant	Placebo-controlled RCT (n = 210) of isradipine after renal transplantation. Isradipine was associated with better renal function at 3 and 12 months without changes in acute rejection or delayed graft function.
Antonucci et al.[111]	2b	Vascular surgery	Small RCT (n = 16) of nifedipine or dopamine for aortic surgery with infrarenal cross-clamping. Immediate postoperative GFR was maintained in the nifedipine group (but not the dopamine group).
Young et al.[112]	4	Cardiac surgery	Case series of perioperative diltiazem infusion (n = 271) and control (n = 143). Diltiazem was associated with higher creatinine rise, greater need for dialysis (4.4% vs. 0.7%)

(Continued)

Table 34-5 Summary of Renal Protective Strategies in Humans for High-risk Surgery—Cont'd

Study	Level of Evidence (see Table 34-3)	Type of Study	Conclusions
Natriuretic Peptides			
Mentzer et al.[129]	1b	Cardiac surgery	Multicenter, double-blind RCT (n = 303) of nesiritide infusion (0.01 mcg/kg/min) vs. placebo for 24 to 96 hours after induction of anesthesia in patients with LV dysfunction (EF <40%) undergoing CABG and/or MVR with CPB. Compared with placebo, nesiritide was associated with increased urine output within 24 hours, a significantly attenuated peak increase in SCR and decline in GFR, and decreased hospital stay and 180-day mortality rate.
Sezai et al.[126]	1b	Cardiac surgery	Prospective RCT (n = 150) in patients undergoing CABG with CPB, comparing alpha-human atrial natriuretic peptide (hANP) infusion (200 ng/kg/min) with placebo. Infusion of hANP was associated with significantly lower renin activity, angiotensin-II, and aldosterone during CPB, postoperative ventricular arrhythmias, postoperative peak level of CPK-MB, and BNP at 1 month.
Sward et al[141]	2b	Post-cardiac surgery	Double-blind RCT (n = 61). Patients with normal preoperative renal function suffering from post-cardiac surgical heart randomized to receive recombinant h-ANP (anaritide) or placebo when serum creatinine increased by >50% from baseline. Significant reduction in the proportion of patients requiring dialysis before or at day 21 and significant reduction in the proportion of patients with the composite endpoint of dialysis or death before or at day 21 compared with placebo.
Langrehr et al.[119]	2b	Liver transplant	Placebo-controlled RCT (n = 70) of ularitide immediately after liver transplantation. No difference in course of urea or creatinine. There was no difference in urine flow or need for dialysis. Less diuretic use in the ularitide group.
Wiebe et al.[120]	2b	Cardiac surgery	Small placebo-controlled RCT (n = 14) of 7 days of ularitide in post-cardiac surgical patients with anuric acute renal failure. No ularitide patients needed hemodialysis (compared with 6 of 7 control group).
Brenner et al.[121]	2b	Cardiac surgery	Small placebo-controlled RCT (n = 24) of 6 days of ularitide immediately after cardiac transplantation. Equal numbers of each group (50%) required hemodialysis, although the duration and frequency were less in the ularitide group.
Prostaglandins			
Manasia et al.[132]	2b	Liver transplant	Small (n = 21) placebo-controlled RCT of PGE1 for 5 days immediately after liver transplantation in patients with an immediate postoperative GFR <50 mL/min. No difference in GFR or effective renal plasma flow.
Klein et al.[133]	2b	Liver transplant	Larger (n = 118) placebo-controlled multicenter RCT of PGE1 immediately after liver transplantation. PGE1 associated with lower peak creatinine, "severe renal dysfunction," need for dialysis, and intensive care length of stay.
Abe et al.[135]	2b	Cardiac surgery	Small (n = 20) placebo-controlled RCT of PGE1 during cardiopulmonary bypass. PGE1 group had better results for N-acetyl-glucosaminidase, free water clearance, and beta-2 microglobulin.
Abe et al.[134]	4	Cardiac surgery	Small (n = 10) case-control study of PGE1 during cardiopulmonary bypass. Rise in N-acetyl-glucosaminidase less, and no change in free water clearance in PGE1 group.
Feddersen et al.[136]	4	Cardiac surgery	Small (n = 36) case-control study of prostacyclin during cardiopulmonary bypass. Prostacyclin was associated with a postoperative increase in GFR but more hypotension than control.
Insulin-like growth factor-1 (IGF-1)			
Franklin et al.[140]	2b	Vascular surgery	Small (n = 54) placebo-controlled RCT of 72 hours IGF-1 with primary endpoint as change in creatinine clearance within 72 hours after surgery involving suprarenal aorta or renal arteries. Fewer patients with IGF-1 had postoperative decline in creatinine clearance (22% vs. 33%).

AKI, acute kidney injury; ANP, atrial (A-type) natriuretic peptide; BNP, brain (B-type) natriuretic peptide; CABG, coronary artery bypass graft; CPB, cardiopulmonary bypass; CrCl, creatinine clearance; EF, ejection fraction; GFR, glomerular filtration rate; LV, left ventricular; PCI, percutaneous intervention; RCN, radiocontrast nephropathy; RCT, randomized controlled trial; SCr, serum creatinine.

subsequent controlled studies failed to confirm this benefit.[67-70] On the other hand, mannitol and dopamine appear to be no better than saline hydration in the amelioration of the transient decline in GFR following infrarenal aortic cross-clamping.[71]

Dopaminergic Agents

Dopamine. Dopamine is an endogenous catecholamine with a broad range of activity on dopaminergic, beta-adrenergic, and alpha-adrenergic receptors. "Low dose" dopamine, that is, less than 3 mcg/kg/min, was long considered a useful agent for renal protection by virtue of its dopaminergic actions on the kidney, both in inducing renal vasodilation and in blocking tubular sodium reabsorption (natriuresis). However, the pharmacokinetics of dopamine vary so widely in the general population that there may be a thirtyfold variability in the plasma concentration.[72] This may in part explain why multiple trials have been unable to demonstrate a beneficial effect of prophylactic "low-dose" dopamine on renal outcome, and the consensus today is that it has no role in this regard.[73-78] The impact of therapeutic intervention with dopamine as an inotropic agent to enhance cardiac function and RBF has not been subjected to randomized controlled trials.

Fenoldopam. Fenoldopam is a phenolated derivative of dopamine that has several pharmacologic advantages over the parent compound. It is a selective dopaminergic-1 receptor agonist that induces dose-dependent renal vasodilation, increases in RBF, and natriuresis. Its pharmacokinetics are very predictable and there is a close relationship between dose and plasma concentration. It lacks any beta- or alpha-adrenergic effects that could induce unwanted tachycardia or vasoconstriction and as such is safe to administer by a peripheral catheter.

Preliminary observations suggested a renoprotective effect of fenoldopam infusion during CPB[79] and infrarenal cross-clamping.[80] Infusion of low-dose fenoldopam (0.01 to 0.03 mcg/kg/min) in cardiac surgery patients with preoperative S_{Cr} greater than 1.5 mg/dL was associated with significantly lower postoperative S_{Cr}. However, two other randomized, prospective studies were unable to detect a difference in renal function between fenoldopam and dopamine prophylaxis during cardiac surgery or vascular surgery with aortic cross-clamping.[81,82] After a preliminary study suggested that fenoldopam may confer greater renal protection against RCN than saline,[83] a large, prospective controlled study failed to confirm a benefit over simple hydration.[84]

Despite these somewhat conflicting data, a recent meta-analysis of 1290 patients from 16 randomized studies demonstrated that fenoldopam infusion was associated with decreased risk of AKI, need for RRT, intensive care unit (ICU) length of stay, and in-hospital mortality rate.[85] The authors concluded, appropriately, that large randomized controlled outcome studies are needed to confirm these findings and fully define the role of fenoldopam in protection against AKI.

Loop Diuretics

The so-called loop diuretics include furosemide, bumetanide, torsemide (all structurally related to the sulphonylureas), and ethacrynic acid. They act as potent blockers of active sodium, potassium, and chloride transport at the medullary thick ascending limb (mTAL) of the loop of Henle, causing diuresis and natriuresis. Theoretically, mTAL blockade enhances tubular oxygen balance by decreasing tubular energy requirement and oxygen consumption. However, the loop diuretics also induce renal cortical vasodilation that could "steal" blood flow from the already oligemic medulla, which could undermine this benefit.

There is little or no evidence to support the use of loop diuretics as renoprotective agents, either by bolus or continuous infusion. A systematic review of undifferentiated patients at risk for ARF concluded that the addition of diuretics confers no benefit over fluids alone.[75] In patients with chronic renal impairment, prevention of RCN was accomplished better with saline hydration alone than hydration plus furosemide, which actually appeared to increase the risk of AKI.[63] Diuretic administration that results in intravascular hypovolemia may actually worsen renal function. In an effort to evaluate renal protection during cardiac surgery, a double-blind randomized study was performed on 126 patients who received continuous infusions of dopamine (2 mcg/kg/min), furosemide (0.5 mcg/kg/min, or about 2 mg/hr), or saline placebo from anesthetic induction to 48 hours after surgery. The effect of dopamine was no different than placebo, but patients who received furosemide suffered AKI reflected by increases in S_{Cr} and decreases in creatinine clearance, and two patients required RRT.[86]

Mannitol. Mannitol is an inert sugar that is widely used as an osmotic diuretic. There is considerable experimental evidence in animals that mannitol attenuates ischemia-reperfusion injury by multiple mechanisms, including maintenance of glomerular filtration pressure, preventing tubular obstruction by cellular casts, scavenging hydroxyl free radicals, and prevention of cellular swelling.[87,88]

Although there is a paucity of confirmatory evidence from clinical studies, mannitol has been widely used for renal protection during renal transplantation, CPB, aortic surgery, and rhabdomyolysis. Its routine use (with hydration) in renal transplantation was established by studies showing a renal protective effect more than two decades ago.[89,90] Animal models of suprarenal aortic cross-clamping revealed that neither mannitol nor dopamine, nor both together, prevented a persistent decrease in GFR and RBF after cross-clamp release.[91] Human studies on patients undergoing infrarenal cross-clamping have revealed that infusions of mannitol and/or dopamine induce more diuresis, but are no more effective than saline hydration at attenuating a transient decrease in GFR,[71] although there is evidence of attenuated biochemical glomerular and tubular injury in patients who received mannitol.[92] There is no evidence from randomized controlled trials that mannitol decreases AKI in patients with traumatic rhabdomyolysis or who receive radiocontrast media or undergo CPB, vascular surgery, or biliary tract surgery.[93-96]

Antioxidants. *N*-acetylcysteine (NAC) is an antioxidant that directly scavenges reactive oxygen species and has received intense study as a potential renal protective agent. A seminal study on 83 patients with severe CKD (mean S_{Cr} 2.4 mg/dL) showed a decrease in the incidence of RCN, defined as an S_{Cr} increase of greater than 0.5 mg/dL, from 21% to 2% by the preprocedure administration of 600 mg twice-daily oral NAC.[97] Subsequent larger studies disputed these results, suggesting that the dose of contrast medium is a greater determinant of RCN than NAC administration,[98] or that NAC confers no greater protection than fenoldopam or saline loading.[99] Moreover, there is evidence that NAC administration decreases creatinine production, thus rendering uncertain any studies using S_{Cr} or derived creatinine clearance as endpoints.[100] In contrast, a large prospective placebo-controlled study evaluated NAC in 354 patients with acute myocardial infarction undergoing primary angioplasty.[101] Patients were randomized to standard-dose NAC (600 mg IV bolus before angioplasty and 600 mg orally twice daily for 48 hours), high-dose NAC (1200 mg on an identical regimen), or saline placebo. AKI, defined as greater than 25% increase in S_{Cr}, occurred in 33% of control patients, 15% of patients receiving standard-dose NAC, and 8% after high-dose NAC ($p < 0.001$). Moreover, there was also a significant decrease in in-hospital mortality rate (11%, 4%, and 3%, respectively, $p = 0.02$).

In other settings, notably cardiac surgery with CPB and major vascular surgery, randomized controlled trials have demonstrated no benefit to the perioperative infusion of NAC in the prevention of postoperative AKI.[102-104] In conclusion, although evidence supports the prophylactic administration of NAC for the amelioration of RCN, there is no evidence to recommend NAC outside this setting.

Calcium Channel Blockers. Calcium channel blockers (CCBs) promote renal vasodilation, increase RBF, and increase GFR. They appear to confer protection against intracellular calcium injury in ischemia-reperfusion injury,[105] inhibit angiotensin action in the glomerulus, and decrease circulating interleukin-2 receptors.[106] Their role in treating chronically hypertensive patients with or without CKD appears to be beneficial to the kidney.[107]

CCBs specifically protect the kidney against the nephrotoxic effects of calcineurin inhibitors, cyclosporine and tacrolimus, which induce renal injury in part by causing increased sympathetic tone and renal arteriolar vasoconstriction. In a prospective randomized study in patients undergoing cadaveric kidney transplantation, diltiazem was added to preservative solution and infused into the recipient for 2 days. Patients who received diltiazem had a significantly lower incidence of graft ATN (10% versus 41%) and requirement for postoperative RRT. Moreover, they tolerated higher cyclosporine blood levels with better graft function and fewer episodes of rejection. Diltiazem also appeared to delay cyclosporine elimination, allowing a 30% decrease in dose with comparable immunosuppressive blood levels.

This benefit appears to continue with long-term (5-year) follow-up,[108] but a study with another CCB, the dihydropyridine isradipine, demonstrated improved S_{Cr} without improved early allograft dysfunction.[109] A subsequent systematic review of CCBs in cadaveric kidney transplantation concluded that graft ATN is significantly decreased but there is no significant difference between treatments for graft loss, mortality rate, or postoperative RRT requirement.[110]

Studies on CCBs in other situations have been more equivocal. A small placebo-controlled trial of patients undergoing aortic surgery with infra-aortic cross-clamping showed that nifedipine prevented the postoperative decline in GFR.[111] A retrospective study on cardiac surgical patients suggested that prophylactic diltiazem infusion increased the incidence of AKI,[112] but prospective studies have indicated that it is not harmful and may confer some benefit as evidenced by decreased biochemical urinary markers of tubular injury.[113-115]

Natriuretic Peptides. The natriuretic peptides are a family of endogenous compounds of varying size (28 to 32 amino acids) with a similar active core and actions.[116] They act on specific receptors to induce activation of guanosine cyclase, which converts guanosine triphosphate (GTP) to cyclic guanosine monophosphate (cGMP). Through this pathway, natriuretic peptides oppose the vasoconstrictor, salt-retaining actions of catecholamines and the renin-angiotensin-aldosterone axis. They promote renal afferent arteriolar dilation and thereby increase GFR, as well as natriuresis.

Atrial natriuretic peptide (A-type natriuretic peptide, ANP) is secreted in response to stretching of cardiac atrial cells.[117] Brain natriuretic peptide (B-type natriuretic peptide, BNP) is released by ventricular stretch; C-type natriuretic peptide (CNP) is released from the endothelium of the great vessels; and urodilatin is elaborated in the kidney itself. ANP (anaritide), BNP (nesiritide), and urodilatin (ularitide) have been produced in human recombinant form for IV administration.

In a small series of patients who had heart or liver transplantation or cardiac surgery, it was suggested that ularitide had beneficial effects on urine flow and RBF[118] and decreased requirement for RRT.[118-121] However, in patients with established ARF, ularitide decreased neither RRT requirement nor mortality rate.[122]

Based on animal studies and preliminary human studies, anaritide infusion engendered considerable interest as a "rescue" agent for established ATN.[123] A randomized controlled study of anaritide infusion at 200 ng/kg/min in 504 patients with ATN showed no difference in RRT-free days.[2] However, a subanalysis of the 76% of patients with nonoliguric ATN (greater than 400 mL/day urine) and the 24% of patients with oliguric ATN demonstrated a significant decrease in RRT-free days in the latter group. Subsequently, a prospective study on 222 patients with oliguric ATN showed no benefit on RRT-free days, ICU length of stay, or mortality rate.[124] Of note, patients who received anaritide sustained a significantly greater incidence of systemic hypotension, suggesting that the vasodilatory, hypotensive effects of the natriuretic peptide negated its benefit on renal recovery. This hypothesis is reinforced by a perioperative study on cardiac surgery patients in which a lower dose of anaritide (50 ng/kg/min) resulted in a halving of the RRT-free days and RRT-free survival.[118] Anaritide infusion had previously been shown to prevent elevations in renin, angiotensin II, and aldosterone induced by CPB, and also maintain GFR.[125] Subsequent studies have also indicated that continuous infusion during thoracic aortic surgery with CPB increased urine output and decreased diuretic requirement.[126]

Nesiritide is the only natriuretic peptide approved for clinical use, and it is indicated for the parenteral treatment of patients with acutely decompensated congestive heart failure (ADCHF) who have dyspnea at rest or with minimal activity. Although initial prospective studies revealed no adverse effect in patients with ADCHF and renal insufficiency,[127] a meta-analysis suggested that nesiritide infusion is associated with an increase risk of elevated S_{Cr} in patients with ADCHF.[128] However, a randomized prospective study on 279 patients with ejection fraction less than 40% undergoing cardiac surgery demonstrated that infusion of nesiritide 0.01 mcg/kg/min from anesthetic induction to 24 to 96 hours after surgery was associated with significant decrease in postoperative elevation of S_{Cr}, as well as significantly decreased 6-month mortality rate.[129]

Prostaglandins. Prostaglandins PGE_2, PGD_2, and prostacyclin (PGI_2) are endogenous eicosanoids that act as intrarenal vasodilators. They are released during renal stress and may protect the kidneys by preserving intrarenal hemodynamics and medullary perfusion and increasing natriuresis.[16,130] Alprostadil (synthetic PGE_1), which has been used for many years for ductus arteriosus dilation in the treatment of congenital heart disease, has been evaluated for renal protection. In patients with CKD undergoing radiocontrast angiography, PGE_1 limited the increase in S_{Cr}, but without change in measured creatinine clearance.[131] In studies of PGE_1 infusion after orthotopic liver transplantation, beneficial effects on renal function have been inconsistent.[132,133] In cardiac surgery, PGE_1 and prostacyclin have been infused during CPB only, without any demonstrated renal benefit.[134-136] The limiting factor appears to be prostaglandin-induced hypotension, particularly with the loss of renal autoregulation during anesthesia and hypothermic CPB.

Growth Factors. Growth factors improve regeneration and repair of damaged nephrons in ischemic ATN, and may speed renal recovery after AKI. Acidic fibroblast growth factor-1 (FGF-1) has been protective in an animal model, perhaps mediated by the antiinflammatory and vasodilating effects of nitric oxide.[137] Results with insulin-like growth factor-1 (IGF-1) have been similarly encouraging.[138] In humans with end-stage CKD, administration of IGF-1 improved renal function,[139] and in a small clinical trial, high-risk vascular surgical patients given IGF-1 had less renal dysfunction.[140] However, as yet there is insufficient evidence to recommend IGF-1 for clinical use.

AREAS OF UNCERTAINTY

Although there remain numerous definitions of AKI, and the lack of consensus has hampered research in the area thus far, perioperative AKI is an ominous development for the individual patient. We look forward to the RIFLE criteria being used in perioperative clinical trials. Currently, there are no "magic bullets" to prevent development of ARF and, despite vigorous research, very limited evidence for therapeutic strategies.

GUIDELINES

At present there are no published guidelines of measures to prevent perioperative AKI.

AUTHORS' RECOMMENDATIONS

Table 34-6 outlines our recommendations.

ACKNOWLEDGMENT

The authors acknowledge and thank Sally Kozlik for her invaluable editorial assistance.

Table 34-6 **Authors' Recommendations for Perioperative Interventions**			
Intervention	**Evidence**	**Effect**	**Grade[56]**
Minimize radiocontrast media exposure	Nil		D
Maintain renal blood flow	Nil		D
Maintain renal perfusion pressure	Nil		D
Minimize duration of aortic cross-clamping	Nil		D
Maintain intravascular volume	Extrapolated	Beneficial	C
Avoid perioperative nephrotoxins	Nil		D
Pharmacologic Strategies			
Dopamine	Yes	No benefit	A
Fenoldopam	Some subgroups	May be of benefit	C
Furosemide	Some subgroups	May be harmful	B
Mannitol	Some subgroups	May be of benefit	C
Antioxidants (*N*-acetylcysteine)	Some subgroups	May be of benefit	B
Calcium channel blockers	Some subgroups	May be of benefit	C
Natriuretic peptides	Some subgroups	May be of benefit	B
Prostaglandins	Some subgroups	No benefit	C

REFERENCES

1. Bellomo R, Ronco C, Kellum JA, et al: Acute renal failure—definition, outcome measures, animal models, fluid therapy and information technology needs: The Second International Consensus Conference of the Acute Dialysis Quality Initiative (ADQI) Group. *Crit Care* 2004;8:R204-R212.
2. Allgren RL, Marbury TC, Rahman SN, et al: Anaritide in acute tubular necrosis. Auriculin Anaritide Acute Renal Failure Study Group. *N Engl J Med* 1997;336:828-834.
3. Myers BD, Miller DC, Mehigan JT, et al: Nature of the renal injury following total renal ischemia in man. *J Clin Invest* 1984;73:329-341.
4. Doolan PD, Alpen EL, Theil GB: A clinical appraisal of the plasma concentration and endogenous clearance of creatinine. *Am J Med* 1962;32:65-81.
5. Swaminathan M, McCreath BJ, Phillips-Bute BG, et al: Serum creatinine patterns in coronary bypass surgery patients with and without postoperative cognitive dysfunction. *Anesth Analg* 2002;95:1-8.
6. O'Riordan A, Wong V, McQuillan R, et al: Acute renal disease, as defined by the RIFLE criteria, post-liver transplantation. *Am J Transplant* 2007;7:168-176.
7. Abosaif NY, Tolba YA, Heap M, et al: The outcome of acute renal failure in the intensive care unit according to RIFLE: Model application, sensitivity, and predictability. *Am J Kidney Dis* 2005;46:1038-1048.
8. Bell M, Liljestam E, Granath F, et al: Optimal follow-up time after continuous renal replacement therapy in actual renal failure patients stratified with the RIFLE criteria. *Nephrol Dial Transplant* 2005;20:354-360.
9. Hoste EA, Clermont G, Kersten A, et al: RIFLE criteria for acute kidney injury are associated with hospital mortality in critically ill patients: A cohort analysis. *Crit Care* 2006;10:R73.
10. Kuitunen A, Vento A, Suojaranta-Ylinen R, et al: Acute renal failure after cardiac surgery: Evaluation of the RIFLE classification. *Ann Thorac Surg* 2006;81:542-546.
11. Uchino S, Bellomo R, Goldsmith D, et al: An assessment of the RIFLE criteria for acute renal failure in hospitalized patients. *Crit Care Med* 2006;34:1913-1917.
12. Ahlstrom A, Kuitunen A, Peltonen S, et al: Comparison of 2 acute renal failure severity scores to general scoring systems in the critically ill. *Am J Kidney Dis* 2006;48:262-268.
13. Rectenwald JE, Huber TS, Martin TD, et al: Functional outcome after thoracoabdominal aortic aneurysm repair. *J Vasc Surg* 2002;35:640-647.
14. Huynh TT, Miller CC 3rd, Estrera AL, et al: Determinants of hospital length of stay after thoracoabdominal aortic aneurysm repair. *J Vasc Surg* 2002;35:648-653.
15. Godet G, Fleron MH, Vicaut E, et al: Risk factors for acute postoperative renal failure in thoracic or thoracoabdominal aortic surgery: A prospective study. *Anesth Analg* 1997;85:1227-1232.
16. Sladen RN, Prough DS: Perioperative renal protection. *Problems in Anesthesia* 1997;9:314-331.
17. Hertzer NR, Mascha EJ, Karafa MT, et al: Open infrarenal abdominal aortic aneurysm repair: The Cleveland Clinic experience from 1989 to 1998. *J Vasc Surg* 2002;35:1145-1154.
18. Coselli JS, LeMaire SA, Conklin LD, et al: Morbidity and mortality after extent II thoracoabdominal aortic aneurysm repair. *Ann Thorac Surg* 2002;73:1107-1115, discussion 1115-1116.
19. Crawford ES, Crawford JL, Safi HJ, et al: Thoracoabdominal aortic aneurysms: Preoperative and intraoperative factors determining immediate and long-term results of operations in 605 patients. *J Vasc Surg* 1986;3:389-404.
20. Swaminathan M, Shaw AD, Phillips-Bute BG, et al: Trends in acute renal failure associated with coronary artery bypass graft surgery in the United States. *Crit Care Med* 2007;35: 2286-2291.
21. Vossler MR, Ni H, Toy W, et al: Pre-operative renal function predicts development of chronic renal insufficiency after orthotopic heart transplantation. *J Heart Lung Transplant* 2002;21:874-881.
22. Conlon PJ, Stafford-Smith M, White WD, et al: Acute renal failure following cardiac surgery. *Nephrol Dial Transplant* 1999;14: 1158-1162.
23. Chertow GM, Lazarus JM, Christiansen CL, et al: Preoperative renal risk stratification. *Circulation* 1997;95:878-884.
24. Aronson S, Fontes ML, Miao Y, et al: Risk index for perioperative renal dysfunction/failure: Critical dependence on pulse pressure hypertension. *Circulation* 2007;115:733-742.
25. Chew ST, Newman MF, White WD, et al: Preliminary report on the association of apolipoprotein E polymorphisms, with postoperative peak serum creatinine concentrations in cardiac surgical patients. *Anesthesiology* 2000;93:325-331.
26. Strittmatter WJ, Bova Hill C: Molecular biology of apolipoprotein E. *Curr Opin Lipidol* 2002;13:119-123.
27. Gamulin Z, Forster A, Morel D, et al: Effects of infrarenal aortic cross-clamping on renal hemodynamics in humans. *Anesthesiology* 1984;61:394-399.
28. Wan S, LeClerc JL, Vincent JL: Inflammatory response to cardiopulmonary bypass: Mechanisms involved and possible therapeutic strategies. *Chest* 1997;112:676-692.
29. Gu YJ, Mariani MA, Boonstra PW, et al: Complement activation in coronary artery bypass grafting patients without cardiopulmonary bypass: The role of tissue injury by surgical incision. *Chest* 1999;116:892-898.
30. Lau LL, Halliday MI, Lee B, et al: Intestinal manipulation during elective aortic aneurysm surgery leads to portal endotoxaemia and mucosal barrier dysfunction. *Eur J Vasc Endovasc Surg* 2000;19:619-624.
31. Badr KF: Sepsis-associated renal vasoconstriction: Potential targets for future therapy. *Am J Kidney Dis* 1992;20:207-213.
32. Bolke E, Jehle PM, Storck M, et al: Endovascular stent-graft placement versus conventional open surgery in infrarenal aortic aneurysm: A prospective study on acute phase response and clinical outcome. *Clin Chim Acta* 2001;314:203-207.
33. Furnary AP, Gao G, Grunkemeier GL, et al: Continuous insulin infusion reduces mortality in patients with diabetes undergoing coronary artery bypass grafting. *J Thorac Cardiovasc Surg* 2003;125:1007-1021.
34. Krinsley JS: Effect of an intensive glucose management protocol on the mortality of critically ill adult patients. *Mayo Clin Proc* 2004;79:992-1000.
35. van den Berghe G, Wouters P, Weekers F, et al: Intensive insulin therapy in the critically ill patients. *N Engl J Med* 2001;345: 1359-1367.
36. Ouattara A, Lecomte P, Le Manach Y, et al: Poor intraoperative blood glucose control is associated with a worsened hospital outcome after cardiac surgery in diabetic patients. *Anesthesiology* 2005;103:687-694.
37. Gandhi GY, Nuttall GA, Abel MD, et al: Intensive intraoperative insulin therapy versus conventional glucose management during cardiac surgery: A randomized trial. *Ann Intern Med* 2007;146:233-243.
38. Cittanova ML, Zubicki A, Savu C, et al: The chronic inhibition of angiotensin-converting enzyme impairs postoperative renal function. *Anesth Analg* 2001;93:1111-1115.
39. Royston D, Bidstrup BP, Taylor KM, et al: Effect of aprotinin on need for blood transfusion after repeat open-heart surgery. *Lancet* 1987;2:1289-1291.
40. Blauhut B, Gross C, Necek S, et al: Effects of high-dose aprotinin on blood loss, platelet function, fibrinolysis, complement, and renal function after cardiopulmonary bypass. *J Thorac Cardiovasc Surg* 1991;101:958-967.
41. Cosgrove DM 3rd, Heric B, Lytle BW, et al: Aprotinin therapy for reoperative myocardial revascularization: A placebo-controlled study. *Ann Thorac Surg* 1992;54:1031-1036, discussion 1036-1038.
42. Lemmer JH Jr, Stanford W, Bonney SL, et al: Aprotinin for coronary artery bypass grafting: Effect on postoperative renal function. *Ann Thorac Surg* 1995;59:132-136.
43. Kramer HJ, Moch T, von Sicherer L, et al: Effects of aprotinin on renal function and urinary prostaglandin excretion in conscious rats after acute salt loading. *Clin Sci (Lond)* 1979;56:547-553.
44. Seto S, Kher V, Scicli AG, et al: The effect of aprotinin (a serine protease inhibitor) on renal function and renin release. *Hypertension* 1983;5:893-899.
45. Kincaid EH, Ashburn DA, Hoyle JR, et al: Does the combination of aprotinin and angiotensin-converting enzyme inhibitor cause renal failure after cardiac surgery? *Ann Thorac Surg* 2005;80:1388-1393, discussion 1393.
46. Karkouti K, Beattie WS, Dattilo KM, et al: A propensity score case-control comparison of aprotinin and tranexamic acid in

high-transfusion-risk cardiac surgery. *Transfusion* 2006;46:
327-338.

47. Mangano DT, Tudor IC, Dietzel C: The risk associated with
aprotinin in cardiac surgery. *N Engl J Med* 2006;354:353-365.

48. Henry DA, Moxey AJ, Carless PA, et al: Anti-fibrinolytic use for
minimising perioperative allogeneic blood transfusion. *Cochrane
Database Syst Rev* 2001;CD001886.

49. Sedrakyan A, Treasure T, Elefteriades JA: Effect of aprotinin on
clinical outcomes in coronary artery bypass graft surgery: A systematic review and meta-analysis of randomized clinical trials.
J Thorac Cardiovasc Surg 2004;128:442-448.

50. Mazer D, Fergusson D, Hebert P, et al: Incidence of massive
bleeding in a blinded randomized controlled trial of antifibrinolytic drugs in high risk cardiac surgery [abstract]. *Anesth Analg*
2006;102:SCA95.

51. Lee A, Cooper MC, Craig JC, et al: Effects of nonsteroidal antiinflammatory drugs on post-operative renal function in normal
adults. *Cochrane Database Syst Rev* 2001;CD002765.

52. Myers BD: Cyclosporine nephrotoxicity. *Kidney Int* 1986;30:
964-974.

53. Li C, Lim SW, Sun BK, et al: Chronic cyclosporine nephrotoxicity: New insights and preventive strategies. *Yonsei Med J*
2004;45:1004-1016.

54. Shihab FS, Bennett WM, Tanner AM, et al: Mechanism of fibrosis in experimental tacrolimus nephrotoxicity. *Transplantation*
1997;64:1829-1837.

55. Heyman SN, Reichman J, Brezis M: Pathophysiology of radiocontrast nephropathy: A role for medullary hypoxia. *Invest
Radiol* 1999;34:685-691.

56. Phillips B, Ball C, Sackett D, et al: Levels of evidence and grades
of recommendations. Oxford Centre for Evidence Based Medicine, 2001. Available at www.indigojazz.co.uk/cebm/levels_
of_evidence.asp.

57. Zacharias M, Gilmore IC, Herbison GP, et al: Interventions for
protecting renal function in the perioperative period. *Cochrane
Database Syst Rev* 2005;CD003590.

58. Mueller C, Buerkle G, Buettner HJ, et al: Prevention of contrast
media-associated nephropathy: Randomized comparison of
2 hydration regimens in 1620 patients undergoing coronary
angioplasty. *Arch Intern Med* 2002;162:329-336.

59. Benko A, Fraser-Hill M, Magner P, et al: Canadian Association
of Radiologists: Consensus guidelines for the prevention of contrast-induced nephropathy. *Can Assoc Radiol J* 2007;58:79-87.

60. Briguori C, Tavano D, Colombo A: Contrast agent-associated
nephrotoxicity. *Prog Cardiovasc Dis* 2003;45:493-503.

61. McCullough PA, Wolyn R, Rocher LL, et al: Acute renal failure
after coronary intervention: Incidence, risk factors, and relationship to mortality. *Am J Med* 1997;103:368-375.

62. Baker CS, Baker LR: Prevention of contrast nephropathy after
cardiac catheterization. *Heart* 2001;85:361-362.

63. Solomon R, Werner C, Mann D, et al: Effects of saline, mannitol,
and furosemide to prevent acute decreases in renal function
induced by radiocontrast agents. *N Engl J Med* 1994;331:
1416-1420.

64. Merten GJ, Burgess WP, Gray LV, et al: Prevention of contrast-
induced nephropathy with sodium bicarbonate: A randomized
controlled trial. *JAMA* 2004;291:2328-2334.

65. Nespoli A, Corso V, Mattarel D, et al: The management of shock
and local injury in traumatic rhabdomyolysis. *Minerva Anestesiol*
1999;65:256-262.

66. Better OS, Stein JH: Early management of shock and prophylaxis of acute renal failure in traumatic rhabdomyolysis. *N Engl
J Med* 1990;322:825-829.

67. Bush HL Jr, Huse JB, Johnson WC, et al: Prevention of renal
insufficiency after abdominal aortic aneurysm resection by optimal volume loading. *Arch Surg* 1981;116:1517-1524.

68. Hesdorffer CS, Milne JF, Meyers AM, et al: The value of
Swan-Ganz catheterization and volume loading in preventing
renal failure in patients undergoing abdominal aneurysmectomy. *Clin Nephrol* 1987;28:272-276.

69. Isaacson IJ, Lowdon JD, Berry AJ, et al: The value of pulmonary artery and central venous monitoring in patients undergoing abdominal aortic reconstructive surgery: A comparative
study of two selected, randomized groups. *J Vasc Surg* 1990;
12: 754-760.

70. Joyce WP, Provan JL, Ameli FM, et al: The role of central haemodynamic monitoring in abdominal aortic surgery. A prospective
randomised study. *Eur J Vasc Surg* 1990;4:633-636.

71. Paul MD, Mazer CD, Byrick RJ, et al: Influence of mannitol and
dopamine on renal function during elective infrarenal aortic
clamping in man. *Am J Nephrol* 1986;6:427-434.

72. MacGregor DA, Smith TE, Prielipp RC, et al: Pharmacokinetics
of dopamine in healthy male subjects. *Anesthesiology* 2000;92: 338-346.

73. Bellomo R, Chapman M, Finfer S, et al: Low-dose dopamine in
patients with early renal dysfunction: A placebo-controlled randomised trial. Australian and New Zealand Intensive Care Society (ANZICS) Clinical Trials Group. *Lancet* 2000;356:2139-2143.

74. Chertow GM, Sayegh MH, Allgren RL, et al: Is the administration of dopamine associated with adverse or favorable outcomes
in acute renal failure? Auriculin Anaritide Acute Renal Failure
Study Group. *Am J Med* 1996;101:49-53.

75. Kellum JA: The use of diuretics and dopamine in acute renal failure:
A systematic review of the evidence. *Crit Care (Lond)* 1997;1:53-59.

76. Kellum JA, Decker JM: Use of dopamine in acute renal failure:
A meta-analysis. *Crit Care Med* 2001;29:1526-1531.

77. Marik PE: Low-dose dopamine: A systematic review. *Intensive
Care Med* 2002;28:877-883.

78. Marik PE, Iglesias J: Low-dose dopamine does not prevent acute
renal failure in patients with septic shock and oliguria. NORA-
SEPT II Study Investigators. *Am J Med* 1999;107:387-390.

79. Halpenny M, Lakshmi S, O'Donnell A, et al: Fenoldopam: Renal
and splanchnic effects in patients undergoing coronary artery
bypass grafting. *Anaesthesia* 2001;56:953-960.

80. Halpenny M, Rushe C, Breen P, et al: The effects of fenoldopam
on renal function in patients undergoing elective aortic surgery.
Eur J Anaesthesiol 2002;19:32-39.

81. Bove T, Landoni G, Calabro MG, et al: Renoprotective action of
fenoldopam in high-risk patients undergoing cardiac surgery: A
prospective, double-blind, randomized clinical trial. *Circulation*
2005;111:3230-3235.

82. Oliver WC Jr, Nuttall GA, Cherry KJ, et al: A comparison of
fenoldopam with dopamine and sodium nitroprusside in
patients undergoing cross-clamping of the abdominal aorta.
Anesth Analg 2006;103:833-840.

83. Tumlin JA, Wang A, Murray PT, et al: Fenoldopam mesylate
blocks reductions in renal plasma flow after radiocontrast dye
infusion: A pilot trial in the prevention of contrast nephropathy.
Am Heart J 2002;143:894-903.

84. Stone GW, McCullough PA, Tumlin JA, et al: Fenoldopam
mesylate for the prevention of contrast-induced nephropathy:
A randomized controlled trial. *JAMA* 2003;290:2284-2291.

85. Landoni G, Biondi-Zoccai GG, Tumlin JA, et al: Beneficial
impact of fenoldopam in critically ill patients with or at risk
for acute renal failure: A meta-analysis of randomized clinical
trials. *Am J Kidney Dis* 2007;49:56-68.

86. Lassnigg A, Donner E, Grubhofer G, et al: Lack of renoprotective effects of dopamine and furosemide during cardiac surgery.
J Am Soc Nephrol 2000;11:97-104.

87. Burke TJ, Cronin RE, Duchin KL, et al: Ischemia and tubule
obstruction during acute renal failure in dogs: Mannitol in protection. *Am J Physiol* 1980;238:F305-F314.

88. Schrier RW, Arnold PE, Gordon JA, et al: Protection of mito-
chondrial function by mannitol in ischemic acute renal failure.
Am J Physiol 1984;247:F365-F369.

89. Tiggeler RG, Berden JH, Hoitsma AJ, et al: Prevention of acute
tubular necrosis in cadaveric kidney transplantation by the combined use of mannitol and moderate hydration. *Ann Surg*
1985;201:246-251.

90. Weimar W, Geerlings W, Bijnen AB, et al: A controlled study on
the effect of mannitol on immediate renal function after cadaver
donor kidney transplantation. *Transplantation* 1983;35:99-101.

91. Pass LJ, Eberhart RC, Brown JC, et al: The effect of mannitol and
dopamine on the renal response to thoracic aortic cross-clamping. *J Thorac Cardiovasc Surg* 1988;95:608-612.

92. Nicholson ML, Baker DM, Hopkinson BR, et al: Randomized controlled trial of the effect of mannitol on renal reperfusion injury
during aortic aneurysm surgery. *Br J Surg* 1996;83:1230-1233.

93. Ip-Yam PC, Murphy S, Baines M, et al: Renal function and pro-
teinuria after cardiopulmonary bypass: The effects of temperature and mannitol. *Anesth Analg* 1994;78:842-847.

94. Homsi E, Barreiro MF, Orlando JM, et al: Prophylaxis of acute renal failure in patients with rhabdomyolysis. *Ren Fail* 1997;19:283-288.

95. Gubern JM, Sancho JJ, Simo J, et al: A randomized trial on the effect of mannitol on postoperative renal function in patients with obstructive jaundice. *Surgery* 1988;103:39-44.

96. Beall AC, Holman MR, Morris GC: Mannitol-induced osmotic diuresis during vascular surgery. *Arch Surg* 1963;86.

97. Tepel M, van der Giet M, Schwarzfeld C, et al: Prevention of radiographic-contrast-agent-induced reductions in renal function by acetylcysteine. *N Engl J Med* 2000;343:180-184.

98. Briguori C, Manganelli F, Scarpato P, et al: Acetylcysteine and contrast agent-associated nephrotoxicity. *J Am Coll Cardiol* 2002;40:298-303.

99. Allaqaband S, Tumuluri R, Malik AM, et al: Prospective randomized study of N-acetylcysteine, fenoldopam, and saline for prevention of radiocontrast-induced nephropathy. *Catheter Cardiovasc Interv* 2002;57:279-283.

100. Hoffmann U, Fischereder M, Kruger B, et al: The value of N-acetylcysteine in the prevention of radiocontrast agent-induced nephropathy seems questionable. *J Am Soc Nephrol* 2004;15: 407-410.

101. Marenzi G, Assanelli E, Marana I, et al: N-acetylcysteine and contrast-induced nephropathy in primary angioplasty. *N Engl J Med* 2006;354:2773-2782.

102. Burns KE, Chu MW, Novick RJ, et al: Perioperative N-acetylcysteine to prevent renal dysfunction in high-risk patients undergoing CABG surgery: A randomized controlled trial. *JAMA* 2005;294:342-350.

103. Haase M, Haase-Fielitz A, Bagshaw SM, et al: Phase II, randomized, controlled trial of high-dose N-acetylcysteine in high-risk cardiac surgery patients. *Crit Care Med* 2007; 35:1324-1331.

104. Wijnen MH, Vader HL, Van Den Wall Bake AW, et al: Can renal dysfunction after infra-renal aortic aneurysm repair be modified by multi-antioxidant supplementation? *J Cardiovasc Surg (Torino)* 2002;43:483-488.

105. Schrier RW, Burke TJ: Role of calcium-channel blockers in preventing acute and chronic renal injury. *J Cardiovasc Pharmacol* 1991;18(suppl 6):S38-S43.

106. Neumayer HH, Gellert J, Luft FC: Calcium antagonists and renal protection. *Ren Fail* 1993;15:353-358.

107. Locatelli F, Del Vecchio L, Andrulli S, et al: Role of combination therapy with ACE inhibitors and calcium channel blockers in renal protection. *Kidney Int Suppl* 2002;53–60.

108. Morales JM, Rodriguez-Paternina E, Araque A, et al: Long-term protective effect of a calcium antagonist on renal function in hypertensive renal transplant patients on cyclosporine therapy: A 5-year prospective randomized study. *Transplant Proc* 1994;26:2598-2599.

109. van Riemsdijk IC, Mulder PG, de Fijter JW, et al: Addition of isradipine (Lomir) results in a better renal function after kidney transplantation: A double-blind, randomized, placebo-controlled, multi-center study. *Transplantation* 2000;70:122-126.

110. Shilliday IR, Sherif M: Calcium channel blockers for preventing acute tubular necrosis in kidney transplant recipients. *Cochrane Database Syst Rev* 2005;CD003421.

111. Antonucci F, Calo L, Rizzolo M, et al: Nifedipine can preserve renal function in patients undergoing aortic surgery with infra-renal crossclamping. *Nephron* 1996;74:668-673.

112. Young EW, Diab A, Kirsh MM: Intravenous diltiazem and acute renal failure after cardiac operations. *Ann Thorac Surg* 1998;65:1316-1319.

113. Bergman AS, Odar-Cederlof I, Westman L, et al: Diltiazem infusion for renal protection in cardiac surgical patients with preexisting renal dysfunction. *J Cardiothorac Vasc Anesth* 2002; 16:294-299.

114. Manabe S, Tanaka H, Yoshizaki T, et al: Effects of the postoperative administration of diltiazem on renal function after coronary artery bypass grafting. *Ann Thorac Surg* 2005;79:831-835, discussion 835-836.

115. Piper SN, Kumle B, Maleck WH, et al: Diltiazem may preserve renal tubular integrity after cardiac surgery. *Can J Anaesth* 2003;50:285-292.

116. Baughman KL: B-type natriuretic peptide—a window to the heart. *N Engl J Med* 2002;347:158-159.

117. Espiner EA: Physiology of natriuretic peptides. *J Intern Med* 1994;235:527-541.

118. Sward K, Valson F, Ricksten SE: Long-term infusion of atrial natriuretic peptide (ANP) improves renal blood flow and glomerular filtration rate in clinical acute renal failure. *Acta Anaesthesiol Scand* 2001;45:536-542.

119. Langrehr JM, Kahl A, Meyer M, et al: Prophylactic use of low-dose urodilatin for prevention of renal impairment following liver transplantation: A randomized placebo-controlled study. *Clin Transplant* 1997;11:593-598.

120. Wiebe K, Meyer M, Wahlers T, et al: Acute renal failure following cardiac surgery is reverted by administration of urodilatin (INN: ularitide). *Eur J Med Res* 1996;1:259-265.

121. Brenner P, Meyer M, Reichenspurner H, et al: Significance of prophylactic urodilatin (INN: ularitide) infusion for the prevention of acute renal failure in patients after heart transplantation. *Eur J Med Res* 1995;1:137-143.

122. Meyer M, Pfarr E, Schirmer G, et al: Therapeutic use of the natriuretic peptide ularitide in acute renal failure. *Ren Fail* 1999;21:85-100.

123. Rahman SN, Kim GE, Mathew AS, et al: Effects of atrial natriuretic peptide in clinical acute renal failure. *Kidney Int* 1994;45:1731-1738.

124. Lewis J, Salem MM, Chertow GM, et al: Atrial natriuretic factor in oliguric acute renal failure. Anaritide Acute Renal Failure Study Group. *Am J Kidney Dis* 2000;36:767-774.

125. Sezai A, Shiono M, Orime Y, et al: Low-dose continuous infusion of human atrial natriuretic peptide during and after cardiac surgery. *Ann Thorac Surg* 2000;69:732-738.

126. Sezai A, Shiono M, Hata M, et al: Efficacy of continuous low-dose human atrial natriuretic peptide given from the beginning of cardiopulmonary bypass for thoracic aortic surgery. *Surg Today* 2006;36:508-514.

127. Butler J, Emerman C, Peacock WF, et al: The efficacy and safety of B-type natriuretic peptide (nesiritide) in patients with renal insufficiency and acutely decompensated congestive heart failure. *Nephrol Dial Transplant* 2004;19:391-399.

128. Sackner-Bernstein JD, Skopicki HA, Aaronson KD: Risk of worsening renal function with nesiritide in patients with acutely decompensated heart failure. *Circulation* 2005;111:1487-1491.

129. Mentzer RM Jr, Oz MC, Sladen RN, et al: Effects of perioperative nesiritide in patients with left ventricular dysfunction undergoing cardiac surgery: The NAPA trial. *J Am Coll Cardiol* 2007;49:716-726.

130. Garella S, Matarese RA: Renal effects of prostaglandins and clinical adverse effects of nonsteroidal anti-inflammatory agents. *Medicine (Baltimore)* 1984;63:165-181.

131. Koch JA, Plum J, Grabensee B, et al: Prostaglandin E_1: A new agent for the prevention of renal dysfunction in high risk patients caused by radiocontrast media? PGE$_1$ Study Group. *Nephrol Dial Transplant* 2000;15:43-49.

132. Manasia AR, Leibowitz AB, Miller CM, et al: Postoperative intravenous infusion of alprostadil (PGE$_1$) does not improve renal function in hepatic transplant recipients. *J Am Coll Surg* 1996;182:347-352.

133. Klein AS, Cofer JB, Pruett TL, et al: Prostaglandin E_1 administration following orthotopic liver transplantation: A randomized prospective multicenter trial. *Gastroenterology* 1996;111: 710-715.

134. Abe K, Fujino Y, Sakakibara T: The effect of prostaglandin E_1 during cardiopulmonary bypass on renal function after cardiac surgery. *Eur J Clin Pharmacol* 1993;45:217-220.

135. Abe K, Sakakibara T, Yoshiya I: The effect of prostaglandin E_1 on renal function after cardiac surgery involving cardiopulmonary bypass. *Prostaglandins Leukot Essent Fatty Acids* 1993;49:627-631.

136. Feddersen K, Aren C, Granerus G, et al: Effects of prostacyclin infusion on renal function during cardiopulmonary bypass. *Ann Thorac Surg* 1985;40:16-19.

137. Cuevas P, Martinez-Coso V, Fu X, et al: Fibroblast growth factor protects the kidney against ischemia-reperfusion injury. *Eur J Med Res* 1999;4:403-410.

138. Ding H, Kopple JD, Cohen A, et al: Recombinant human insulin-like growth factor-I accelerates recovery and reduces catabolism in rats with ischemic acute renal failure. *J Clin Invest* 1993;91:2281-2287.
139. Vijayan A, Franklin SC, Behrend T, et al: Insulin-like growth factor I improves renal function in patients with end-stage chronic renal failure. *Am J Physiol* 1999;276:R929-R934.
140. Franklin SC, Moulton M, Sicard GA, et al: Insulin-like growth factor I preserves renal function postoperatively. *Am J Physiol* 1997;272:F257-F259.
141. Sward K, Valsson F, Odencrants P, et al: Recombinant human atrial natriuretic peptide in ischemic acute renal failure: a randomized placebo-controlled trial. *Crit Care Med* 2004;32:1310-1315.

35 Are Alpha-2 Agonists Effective in Reducing Perioperative Cardiac Complications in Noncardiac Surgery?

Douglas C. Shook, MD, and John E. Ellis, MD

INTRODUCTION

Alpha-2 receptor agonists have many desirable effects such as MAC reduction, analgesia, anxiolysis, sedation, and sympatholysis.[1,2] Adding to this list the possibility of perioperative myocardial protection makes the perioperative use of alpha-2 agonists very appealing in patients with known or suspected coronary artery disease. It is well known that drugs that positively affect myocardial oxygen supply and demand are beneficial in the perioperative period for myocardial protection.[3] Perioperative beta-blockade is an excellent example of this.[4,5] The ability of alpha-2 agonists to modulate sympathetic tone may similarly offer perioperative myocardial protection.

OPTIONS/THERAPIES

The most widely studied alpha-2 agonists are clonidine, mivazerol, and dexmedetomidine. Clonidine is available in oral, transdermal, and parenteral forms. It is a partial agonist with an alpha-2 to alpha-1 selectivity ratio of 39:1. Mivazerol is an intravenous alpha-2 agonist with a selectivity ratio of 119:1. Finally, dexmedetomidine is a shorter-acting intravenous alpha-2 agonist with a selectivity ratio of 1300:1 (Table 35-1).[1] All three alpha-2 agonists have been shown to cause dose-dependent sympatholysis, but clonidine and mivazerol have been most extensively studied with regard to perioperative cardiac protection. Unfortunately, mivazerol is not available in the United States.

EVIDENCE

Several studies have been published investigating alpha-2 agonists and their role in perioperative myocardial protection. Many studies have evaluated the hemodynamic stabilizing effects and sympatholysis produced by alpha-2 agonists. It is important to understand the endpoints in these investigations because many used myocardial ischemia as a surrogate marker for myocardial infarction and cardiac death. Although several studies have linked perioperative myocardial ischemia to subsequent increased cardiac morbidity and mortality rates,[6,7] most of the studies to date have not linked the use of perioperative alpha-2 agonists to decreased rates of myocardial infarction and death.

Randomized Controlled Trials—Clonidine

The perioperative use of clonidine for myocardial protection in noncardiac surgery has been studied in three well-designed small, randomized trials. Ellis and colleagues[8] studied the use of transdermal clonidine combined with oral clonidine in a randomized, double-blind, placebo-controlled clinical trial of 61 patients undergoing elective major noncardiac surgery. The treatment group received premedication with the transdermal clonidine system (0.2 mg/day) the night before surgery, which was left in place for 72 hours, and 0.3 mg oral clonidine 60 to 90 minutes before surgery. The incidence of intraoperative electrocardiographic (ECG) ischemia was diminished in the clonidine group (4% versus 21%, $p = 0.05$). There was no difference, however, between the two groups in the incidence of postoperative ischemia. Later, Stuhmeier and colleagues[9] did a randomized, double-blind study looking at 297 patients scheduled for vascular surgery. They evaluated the effect of 2 mcg/kg of oral clonidine 90 minutes before induction of anesthesia. Patients receiving oral clonidine demonstrated a decreased incidence of intraoperative myocardial ischemia (24% versus 39%, $p < 0.01$). However, no statistical difference was noted in the number of patients suffering a nonfatal myocardial infarction or in patients dying from major cardiac events. In 2004 Wallace and colleagues[10] conducted a prospective, double-blind, randomized, clinical trial of 190 patients at risk for coronary artery disease scheduled for noncardiac surgery. All of the patients in the clonidine group ($n = 125$) received 0.2 mg orally the night before and 1 hour before surgery. A transdermal patch (0.2 mg/day) was placed the night before surgery and removed on postoperative day 4. The incidence of myocardial ischemia in the clonidine group was reduced on days 0 to 3 versus the placebo group (14% versus 31%, $p < 0.01$). Long-term follow-up revealed that the clonidine

Table 35-1	Specificity of Alpha-2 Agonists for the Alpha-2 Receptor	
Alpha-2 Agonist	**Alpha-2:Alpha-1 Specificity**
Dexmedetomidine	1300:1
Mivazerol	119:1
Clonidine	39:1

group had a reduced mortality rate at 30 days (0.8% versus 6.5%, $p = 0.048$) and at 2 years (15% versus 29%, $p = 0.035$), but this benefit lost statistical significance after removing all patients who received preoperative or intraoperative beta-blockers.

Randomized Controlled Trials—Mivazerol

Mivazerol, an intravenous alpha-2 agonist administered by continuous infusion, has been studied in larger trials. A European multicenter group studied mivazerol in a phase II, placebo-controlled, double-blind, randomized trial.[11] Three hundred patients with known coronary artery disease (CAD) were placed into three groups: high-dose mivazerol (1.5 mcg/kg/hr), low-dose mivazerol (0.75 mcg/kg/hr), or placebo. High-dose mivazerol had significantly less intraoperative myocardial ischemia versus placebo (20% versus 34%, $p = 0.026$), but no differences were observed for perioperative myocardial infarction or death. In addition, there was no difference in postoperative myocardial ischemia. In 1999 Oliver and colleagues[12] conducted a large double-blind, randomized, placebo-controlled study of 2854 patients (1897 with known CAD and 957 with risk factors for CAD). Patients received perioperative mivazerol at 1.5 mcg/kg/hr for 72 hours or placebo. On subgroup analysis, in the group of 1897 patients with known CAD, there were fewer cardiac deaths in the mivazerol group versus placebo (13 of 956 versus 25 of 941, $p = 0.037$). The rates of myocardial infarction and all-cause deaths were not statistically different between the two groups. In the subgroup of patients undergoing vascular procedures ($n = 904$), mivazerol produced significant myocardial protection. The cardiac death rate was 6% versus 18% ($p = 0.009$), and the combined cardiac death and myocardial infarction rate was 10% versus 14% ($p = 0.02$). Myocardial infarction alone was not significantly different.

Randomized Controlled Trials—Dexmedetomidine

There are no large randomized controlled trials studying the infusion of dexmedetomidine to reduce perioperative cardiac morbidity and mortality rates in noncardiac surgical patients. Dexmedetomidine has been investigated in small studies for its hemodynamic effects. Talke and colleagues[13] evaluated the hemodynamic effects of four different doses of dexmedetomidine in 22 vascular surgery patients at risk for CAD. Although patients at the higher doses of dexmedetomidine appeared to have greater hemodynamic stability (less tachycardia and systolic hypertension), they needed more intraoperative vasopressor

and fluid support. Because of the study size, no statistical significance could be concluded regarding myocardial ischemia and perioperative myocardial infarction. A second study by Jalonen and colleagues[14] looked at 80 patients scheduled for elective coronary artery bypass grafting. Again, dexmedetomidine produced less tachycardia and lower blood pressures, but the study patients needed more fluid challenges and pharmacologic treatment for hypotension. No statistical significance was concluded with respect to myocardial ischemia and infarction. Table 35-2 summarizes all of the randomized controlled trials.

Meta-analysis of Alpha-2 Agonists

A meta-analysis published by Nishina and colleagues[15] in 2002 looked at the efficacy of clonidine for the prevention of perioperative myocardial ischemia. The study systematically reviewed the randomized controlled trials that tested this endpoint. Seven studies were included in the meta-analysis. Two of them were referenced previously,[8,9] and the other five looked at the use of clonidine for the prevention of ischemia in cardiac surgery. The meta-analysis concluded that clonidine in both cardiac surgery patients and noncardiac surgery patients reduced perioperative myocardial ischemia. An attempt was made to form conclusions on preferable endpoints such as myocardial infarction and death, but low statistical power hindered the results. A more comprehensive meta-analysis by Wijeysundera and colleagues[16] investigated the perioperative cardiac effects of all alpha-2 adrenergic agonists studied through 2002. Twenty-three studies were included (cardiac and noncardiac surgical patients), enrolling 3395 patients. The study concluded that alpha-2 agonists significantly reduced overall mortality rate and reported ischemia, but failed to show a statistically significant reduction in myocardial infarctions. In vascular surgery patients, alpha-2 agonists significantly reduced mortality rate and myocardial infarctions, and were associated with a trend toward ischemia reduction. A recent meta-analysis by Biccard and colleagues[17] looked at dexmedetomidine and cardiac protection in noncardiac patients. Twenty studies were included, involving 840 patients. The regimen of dexmedetomidine infusion varied between studies, and most of the studies did not continue the infusion postoperatively. Perioperative cardiac outcomes were not the primary outcome measure in any of the studies included in the analysis. The study concluded that perioperative dexmedetomidine infusion was associated with a trend toward, but did not significantly reduce, cardiac mortality rate, myocardial infarction, or myocardial ischemia. Dexmedetomidine was also associated with more hypotension and bradycardia. Table 35-3 summarizes all the meta-analysis studies.

AREAS OF UNCERTAINTY

The endpoints studied in the majority of the randomized, controlled trials are primarily surrogate endpoints, such as myocardial ischemia, rather than more definitive endpoints such as myocardial infarction or death. Two trials looked specifically at mortality and myocardial infarction rates. Oliver and colleagues[12] evaluated endpoints such

| Table 35-2 | Summary of Randomized Controlled Trials |

Author	Procedure	Number of Subjects	Study Design	Intervention	Ischemia	MI	Cardiac Death
Ellis 1994	Noncardiac	Control 31 Treated 30	Double-blind Placebo	TD clonidine 0.2 mg night prior (72 hr) Clonidine 0.3 mg PO preoperatively	D: 1/28 (4%) C: 5/24 (21%) $p = 0.05$		
Stuhmeier 1996	Vascular	Control 152 Treated 145	Double-blind Placebo	Clonidine 2 mcg/kg PO preoperatively	D: 35/145 (24%) C: 59/152 (39%) $p < 0.01$	D: 0/145 (0%) C: 4/152 (3%) NS	D: 2/145 (1%) C: 1/152 (1%) NS
McSPI 1997	Noncardiac	Control 103 Treated 98	Double-blind Placebo	Mivazerol 1.5 mcg/kg/hr (high dose) Started 20 min before induction Continued for 72 hr	D: 17/87 (20%) C: 34/99 (34%) $p = 0.026$ (high dose only)	D: 2/98 (2%) C: 6/103 (6%) NS (high dose only)	D: 1/98 (1%) C: 1/98 (1%) NS (high dose only)
Oliver 1999	Noncardiac with known CAD	Control 941 Treated 946	Double-blind Placebo	Mivazerol 1.5 mcg/kg/hr Started 20 min before induction Continued for 72 hr		D: 78/946 (8%) C: 79/941 (8%) NS	D: 13/946 (3%) C: 25/941 (1%) $p = 0.037$
Oliver 1999	Vascular	Control 450 Treated 454	Double-blind Placebo	Mivazerol 1.5 mcg/kg/hr Started 20 min before induction Continued for 72 hr		D: 42/454 (9%) C: 53/450 (12%) NS	D: 6/454 (1%) C: 18/450 (4%) $p = 0.009$
Wallace 2004	Noncardiac	Control 65 Treated 125	Double-blind Placebo	TD clonidine 0.2 mg night prior (4 days) Clonidine 0.2 mg PO preoperatively and night prior	D: 18/125 (14%) C: 20/65 (31%) $p = 0.01$	D: 5/125 (4%) C: 3/65 (5%) NS	D: 19/125 (15%) C: 19/65 (29%) $p = 0.035$

C, Control; CAD, coronary artery disease; D, drug; MI, myocardial infarction; NS, no statistical significance; PO, per os (by mouth); TD, transdermal.

| Table 35-3 | Summary of Meta-analysis Studies |

Author	Procedures (Trials)	Number of Trials	Number of Subjects	Perioperative Interventions (Trials)	Outcome
Nishina 2002	Cardiac (5) Noncardiac (2)	7	664	Clonidine	Reduced overall ischemia, OR = 0.49, 95% CI 0.34-0.71
Wijeysundera 2003	Cardiac (10) Noncardiac (11)	23	3395	Clonidine (15) Dexmedetomidine (6) Mivazerol (2)	Reduced mortality rate (overall), RR = 0.64, 95% CI 0.42-0.99 Reduced ischemia (overall), RR = 0.76, 95% CI 0.63-0.91 Reduced mortality rate (vascular), RR = 0.47, 95% CI 0.25-0.90 Reduced MI (vascular), RR = 0.66, 95% CI 0.46-0.94
Biccard 2008	Noncardiac	20	840	Dexmedetomidine	Mortality rate, OR = 0.27, 95% CI 0.01-7.13 (NS) MI, OR = 0.26, 95% CI 0.04-1.60 (NS) Ischemia, OR = 0.65, 95% CI 0.26-1.63 (NS)

CI, Confidence interval; MI, myocardial infarction; NS, no statistical significance; OR, odds ratio; RR, relative risk.

as myocardial infarction and death and found that the group most affected was patients with known CAD and undergoing vascular surgery. The validity of this conclusion is limited in that the effect was not seen in the overall group, as originally intended, but only on subsequent subgroup analysis. Wallace and colleagues[10] concluded that perioperative clonidine reduced episodes of ischemia and, more important, reduced long-term incidence of myocardial infarction and death. Unfortunately, the long-term benefit may have been due to perioperative administration of beta-blockers in both the study and placebo groups.

The studies we reviewed demonstrated less intraoperative ischemia with use of alpha-2 agonists but did not consistently show the ability to continue this protection into the postoperative period. It is possible that the doses needed for postoperative sympatholysis may be higher than those effective during surgery and anesthesia. We also believe that many studies were underpowered to demonstrate outcome differences, if one indeed were to exist. It is widely recognized that the risk of myocardial infarction is greatest over the first 3 postoperative days.[18] Therefore, in addition to questions of dosage, the exact time frame in which to use alpha-2 agonists for myocardial protection remains unclear. No study reviewed continued alpha-2 agonists beyond 72 hours postoperatively. Increasing the preoperative dose of clonidine will invariably increase sympatholysis and decrease heart rate and blood pressure. Unfortunately, the effects of clonidine are long acting and not quickly reversed or stopped if severe hypotension or bradycardia develops. Indeed, several studies suggest increased need for fluid and/or vasopressor support.[9,12-14] Dexmedetomidine, which has a shorter half-life, may be advantageous in this regard. Although evidence supporting the routine use of alpha-2 agonists is not nearly as complete and accepted as that of perioperative beta-blockade, this may change after completion of future large-scale, prospective studies.

GUIDELINES

The American College of Cardiology and American Heart Association updated their practice guidelines in 2007 on perioperative cardiovascular evaluation for noncardiac surgery.[19] As a Class IIb recommendation, alpha-2 agonists for the perioperative control of hypertension may be considered in patients with known CAD or at least one clinical risk factor who are undergoing surgery. Perioperative beta-blockers for similar indications are Class I, IIa, and IIb recommendations because studies of beta-blockade have shown amelioration of clinical endpoints. Similarly designed large-scale, prospective studies of alpha-2 agonists that assess outcomes, not just the surrogate marker of myocardial ischemia, are needed to help further define the role of alpha-2 agonists in the prevention of perioperative cardiac morbidity and mortality.

AUTHORS' RECOMMENDATIONS

- Based on the evidence of randomized, controlled trials and meta-analysis studies, alpha-2 agonists *may* have a role as an adjunct in the prevention of perioperative cardiac morbidity and mortality in patients with known or suspected CAD, especially in patients scheduled for vascular surgical procedures.
- Achieving sympatholysis before induction appears to be optimal. This can be done by a number of means, including oral preparations 60 to 90 minutes before induction, transdermal application the night before surgery, or starting an infusion so as to reach effect before induction. However, this may or may not increase the need for vasopressor support.
- Therapy should probably be continued for at least 72 hours postoperatively.

REFERENCES

1. Khan ZP, Ferguson CN, Jones RM: Alpha-2 and imidazoline receptor agonists. Their pharmacology and therapeutic role. *Anaesthesia* 1999;54:146-165.
2. Kamibayashi T, Maze M: Clinical uses of alpha$_2$-adrenergic agonists. *Anesthesiology* 2000;93:1345-1349.
3. Roizen MF: Should we all have a sympathectomy at birth? Or at least preoperatively? *Anesthesiology* 1988;68:482-484.
4. Mangano DT, Layug EL, Wallace A, Tateo I: Effect of atenolol on mortality and cardiovascular morbidity after noncardiac surgery. Multicenter Study of Perioperative Ischemia Research Group [comment] [erratum appears in *N Engl J Med* 1997;336(14):1039]. *N Engl J Med* 1996;335:1713-1720.
5. Poldermans D, Boersma E, Bax JJ, et al: The effect of bisoprolol on perioperative mortality and myocardial infarction in high-risk patients undergoing vascular surgery. Dutch Echocardiographic Cardiac Risk Evaluation Applying Stress Echocardiography Study Group [comment]. *N Engl J Med* 1999;341:1789-1794.
6. Mangano DT, Browner WS, Hollenberg M, et al: Association of perioperative myocardial ischemia with cardiac morbidity and mortality in men undergoing noncardiac surgery. The Study of Perioperative Ischemia Research Group [comment]. *N Engl J Med* 1990;323:1781-1788.
7. Mangano DT, Browner WS, Hollenberg M, et al: Long-term cardiac prognosis following noncardiac surgery. The Study of Perioperative Ischemia Research Group [comment]. *JAMA* 1992;268:233-239.
8. Ellis JE, Drijvers G, Pedlow S, et al: Premedication with oral and transdermal clonidine provides safe and efficacious postoperative sympatholysis. *Anesth Analg* 1994;79:1133-1140.
9. Stuhmeier KD, Mainzer B, Cierpka J, et al: Small, oral dose of clonidine reduces the incidence of intraoperative myocardial ischemia in patients having vascular surgery. *Anesthesiology* 1996;85:706-712.
10. Wallace AW, Galindez D, Salahieh A, et al: Effect of clonidine on cardiovascular morbidity and mortality after noncardiac surgery. *Anesthesiology* 2004;101:284-293.
11. Perioperative sympatholysis. Beneficial effects of the alpha 2-adrenoceptor agonist mivazerol on hemodynamic stability and myocardial ischemia. McSPI—Europe Research Group. *Anesthesiology* 1997;86:346-363.
12. Oliver MF, Goldman L, Julian DG, Holme I: Effect of mivazerol on perioperative cardiac complications during non-cardiac surgery in patients with coronary heart disease: The European Mivazerol Trial (EMIT). *Anesthesiology* 1999;91:951-961.
13. Talke P, Li J, Jain U, et al: Effects of perioperative dexmedetomidine infusion in patients undergoing vascular surgery. The Study of Perioperative Ischemia Research Group. *Anesthesiology* 1995;82:620-633.
14. Jalonen J, Hynynen M, Kuitunen A, et al: Dexmedetomidine as an anesthetic adjunct in coronary artery bypass grafting. *Anesthesiology* 1997;86:331-345.
15. Nishina K, Mikawa K, Uesugi T, et al: Efficacy of clonidine for prevention of perioperative myocardial ischemia: A critical appraisal and meta-analysis of the literature. *Anesthesiology* 2002;96:323-329.
16. Wijeysundera DN, Naik JS, Beattie WS: Alpha-2 adrenergic agonists to prevent perioperative cardiovascular complications: A meta-analysis. *Am J Med* 2003;114:742-752.
17. Biccard BM, Goga S, de Beurs J: Dexmedetomidine and cardiac protection for non-cardiac surgery: A meta-analysis of randomised controlled trials. *Anaesthesia* 2008;63:4-14.
18. Mangano DT, Hollenberg M, Fegert G, et al: Perioperative myocardial ischemia in patients undergoing noncardiac surgery—I: Incidence and severity during the 4-day perioperative period. The Study of Perioperative Ischemia (SPI) Research Group. *J Am Coll Cardiol* 1991;17:843-850.
19. Fleisher LA, Beckman JA, Brown KA, et al: ACC/AHA 2007 guidelines on perioperative cardiovascular evaluation and care for noncardiac surgery: A report of the American College of Cardiology/American Heart Association Task Force on Practice Guidelines (Writing Committee to Revise the 2002

Guidelines on Perioperative Cardiovascular Evaluation for Noncardiac Surgery) developed in collaboration with the American Society of Echocardiography, American Society of Nuclear Cardiology, Heart Rhythm Society, Society of Cardiovascular Anesthesiologists, Society for Cardiovascular Angiography and Interventions, Society for Vascular Medicine and Biology, and Society for Vascular Surgery. *J Am Coll Cardiol* 2007;50:e159-241.

36 Which Are the Best Techniques for Reducing the Incidence of Postoperative Deep Vein Thrombosis?

Charles Marc Samama, MD, PhD, FCCP

INTRODUCTION

Venous thromboembolism (VTE) is a major public health issue. A survey carried out in 2004–2005 in the United Kingdom showed that VTE accounts for 25,000 deaths per year due to pulmonary embolism.[1] VTE is thus one of the main causes of death. It also causes considerable morbidity as nonfatal pulmonary embolism and deep vein thrombosis (DVT) induce short- and long-term complications.[2,3] In addition, anticoagulant treatment, although effective, may be a potential source of iatrogenic complications.

The benefit-to-risk ratio of widespread postoperative prophylaxis is highly positive, at least in patients at moderate or high risk of DVT. As established over the last 20 years, prophylaxis is increasingly effective. Many evidence-based studies and meta-analyses have indicated that DVT prevention considerably reduces the risk of pulmonary embolism. However, all problems have not yet been solved.

PATHOPHYSIOLOGY AND RISK

Postoperative thromboembolic risk is the result of two risks, namely, patient-related risk and surgical risk.[3]

Patient-related risk increases linearly with age, becoming more marked after 40 years of age, even more so after 60 years of age.[4,5] Obesity is responsible for an increased risk of thrombosis on account of longer immobilization and decreased fibrinolytic activity. Cancer, especially lung, pancreas, colon, or pelvic cancer, increases thromboembolic risk, although surprisingly metastases do not. Cancer-related risk is independent of age. Several other important factors increasing perioperative VTE risk have been reported (Table 36-1).[5]

The surgical risk is usually well established and ranges from low or absent (e.g., hand surgery, osteosynthesis device removal) to high (e.g., surgery for hip fracture, pelvic surgery for cancer) (Table 36-2). However, the risk may also be uncertain as, for instance, for laparoscopy.

Although the minimally invasive nature of laparoscopy might be thought to reduce risk,[6] other aspects—the reverse-Trendelenburg position, gas insufflation (vena cava compression with impaired venous return) and a longer operative time—might increase the risk.

The overall risk combining patient-related risk and surgical risk can be classified into three broad categories: low, moderate, and high, which have not, however, been precisely quantified.[3] The level of risk should be taken into account in the choice of prophylaxis. However, if three moderate risks are summed (e.g., prolonged immobilization, obesity, and age over 60 years), the crucial question is whether the overall risk is significantly increased or not.

Prevention can not only stop the formation of a thrombus but also control its extension.[7] The new generation of antithrombotic agents, which interact with both free and clot-bound thrombin, should prove to be particularly useful in prevention.[8] Procedures for fast-track patient management, increasingly developed by care teams and much appreciated by patients, reduce the duration and invasive nature of surgery, immobilization time, and hospital stay, and thus will probably significantly reduce the VTE risk as compared with earlier methods of management.[9] However, their impact on VTE has not been measured even though it is widely accepted that the incidence of DVT and pulmonary embolism after prophylaxis has decreased regularly over more than 20 years. The rate of symptomatic events at 3 months is now below 1.5% after hip or knee replacement procedures and/or after hip fracture.[10,11]

OPTIONS

The first method of VTE prevention should be early mobilization and ambulation. However, this is not always possible and other techniques are needed. Mechanical and pharmacologic prevention can be proposed either separately or concomitantly, even if chemical prophylaxis appears to be more effective than mechanical prophylaxis, which can be understood as a first-line approach.

| Table 36-1 | **Patient-related Risk Factors for Thrombosis[2-4]** |

- Age over 40 years
- Obesity (BMI >30)
- Cancer and cancer treatment (hormones, chemotherapy, radiotherapy)

and

- History of VTE
- Idiopathic or acquired thrombophilia
- Acute medical illness
- Active heart or respiratory failure
- Severe infection
- Estrogen-containing contraception or hormone replacement therapy
- Selective estrogen response modifiers (SERM)
- Inflammatory bowel disease
- Immobilization, bed rest, limb paralysis
- Nephrotic syndrome
- Myeloproliferative syndrome
- Paroxysmal nocturnal hemoglobinuria
- Smoking
- Varicose veins
- Central venous catheter

BMI, body mass index; *VTE,* venous thromboembolism.

EVIDENCE

Mechanical Prophylaxis

There are two main techniques of mechanical prophylaxis: (1) graduated elastic compression and (2) intermittent pneumatic compression of the leg or venous foot pump.[12] Their aim is to increase venous flux and reduce stasis. Both techniques have proven efficacy, neither increases the risk of bleeding, and there are few contraindications (peripheral arterial occlusive disease, skin lesions). In both cases, the longer compression is kept in place throughout the day and night, the greater the efficacy.

In graduated elastic compression, the stocking exerts graded circumferential pressure on the lower limb (18 mm Hg at the ankle, 14 mm halfway up the calf, 8 mm at the knee, and if the stocking goes right up to the thigh, 10 mm at the lower half of the thigh and 8 mm at the top of

| Table 36-2 | **Risk Categories for Venous Thromboembolism (VTE) Surgery[3]** |

Examples of Surgical Procedures	Risk Category
Varicose vein	Low
Minor abdominal surgery	Low
Knee arthroscopy	Low
Trauma to knee without fracture	Low
Endoscopic prostate surgery	Low
Percutaneous kidney surgery	Low
Diagnostic laparoscopy (<30 mm)	Low
Minor abdominal surgery with extensive and/or bloody dissection, very long operative time, or emergency	Moderate
Fracture of lower extremity	Moderate
Laminectomy	Moderate
Vaginal hysterectomy	Moderate
Breast cancer surgery	Moderate
Major abdominal surgery (even in the absence of cancer)	High
Bariatric surgery	High
Total hip or knee replacement	High
Hip fracture	High
Open kidney surgery	High
Open prostate surgery	High
Prolapse surgery	High
Uterine and ovarian surgery for cancer	High
Lung resection by thoracotomy	High
Intracranial neurosurgery	High

the thigh). Venous flux velocity is increased by 75% (Table 36-3). The 2007 guidelines published by the National Institute for Health and Clinical Excellence (NICE) recommend the systematic use of compression in all patients who have undergone surgery.[4]

In intermittent pneumatic compression, bags wrapped around the calf and/or thigh are intermittently inflated and deflated in order to accelerate venous return. The reduction in risk is 56% for all thromboses and 44% for proximal thromboses.[4] However, the studies are not powerful enough to establish an effect on pulmonary embolism. The results for venous foot compression vary and depend on the indication.

| Table 36-3 | **Effect of Graduated Compression Stockings (GCS) Alone or Combined with Another Prophylactic Method (APM) (GCS + APM) on DVT Prophylaxis[12]** | | | | |

Study, Year	Number of Trials	Number of Subjects (Intervention/No Intervention)	Total DVTs		Odds Ratio
			Intervention	Control	
Cochrane database, 2000	7	1027 (536/491)	GCS alone 81 (15%)	Control 144 (29%)	0.36 *p* <0.00001
	9	1184 (589/595)	GCS + APM 18 (3%)	Control 84 (14%)	0.22 *p* <0.00001

DVT, deep vein thrombosis.

It seems to be more effective in surgery for hip replacements than total knee prostheses but will be recommended in hip replacement surgery only if there is a contraindication to anticoagulants. An effect on proximal thromboses and on pulmonary embolism has not been demonstrated.[2,4]

Pharmacologic Prophylaxis

Three types of anticoagulants—vitamin K antagonists, heparins (unfractionated heparin [UFH], low-molecular-weight-heparin [LMWH]), and fondaparinux—and several new oral antithrombotic agents (anti-IIa and anti-Xa) are currently used or under clinical development for VTE prophylaxis. We will not discuss hirudins, danaparoid, and dextran because they have been the subject of few studies, their efficacy is a matter of debate, and the benefit-to-risk ratio is lower than for the above agents.

Vitamin K Antagonists

The most frequently used vitamin K antagonist is warfarin even though acenocoumarol and fluindione are still often prescribed in Europe and Africa. Vitamin K antagonists inhibit a carboxylation step in the synthesis of factors II, VII, IX, and X by the liver, and by decreasing the levels of these factors, exert powerful anticoagulant activity.[13] They are still widely used postoperatively in North America, but they are gradually being replaced by injectable anticoagulants (LMWH, fondaparinux)[14] and will probably finally disappear when the new oral antithrombotic agents become fully available in the near future.[15] In the recent NICE review, an analysis of 11 pooled studies (1320 patients) found a reduction in risk versus no prophylaxis of 51% for all thromboses, 58% for proximal thromboses, and 82% for pulmonary embolism.[4] The efficacy of oral anticoagulants (OACs) is somewhat counterbalanced by interactions with other drugs and food, and by an increased risk of bleeding (OACs increased the risk of major bleeding by 58%).

Heparins—Fondaparinux

UFH is extracted from pig intestine. It is a mixture of medium-molecular-weight polysaccharides (15,000 daltons) with equivalent antithrombin (IIa) and anti-Xa activity. UFH interacts with antithrombin via a pentasaccharide moiety present in a third of its molecules. It is eliminated by the reticuloendothelial system. Two or three daily subcutaneous injections are usually given to prevent postoperative thromboembolic disease.[16,17]

Even though UFH has uncontested efficacy, it is being replaced by one or two daily subcutaneous injections of LMWH. LMWHs have been marketed in Europe since

1985 and in the United States since 1993.[17] Their anti-Xa activity is two to six times higher than their antithrombin activity. They are eliminated by the kidney. They are more effective than UFH on overall risk of thrombosis and on risk of proximal thrombosis, and better at preventing pulmonary embolism without increasing the risk of bleeding (Table 36-4).[4,17] In addition, the risk of heparin-induced thrombocytopenia is 5 to 10 times lower than with UFH.[18] LMWHs have become the gold standard for the prevention of perioperative VTE and are used as the comparator for all new anticoagulants (e.g., fondaparinux) in clinical trials of superiority or noninferiority.[19]

Fondaparinux—a product of research on LMWH—was put on the market at the end of 2002. The short pentasaccharide moiety of the heparin molecule, fondaparinux, was synthesized. It binds reversibly to antithrombin, inducing powerful anti-Xa activity. It inhibits factor Xa and the subsequent coagulation cascade.[8] Once released from antithrombin, it is recycled two or three times and made reavailable to bind. This attractive mechanism of action explains its high activity at low doses. Currently, it is the most potent injectable anti-Xa available. It was first tested in VTE prevention in orthopedics, then in abdominal surgery. It is effective in preventing asymptomatic DVT, but has a slight but nevertheless significant tendency to increase bleeding complications and transfusion requirements.[19] Safety is of much less concern when it is administered late, that is, 6 to 8 hours (even 24 hours) after surgery. Fondaparinux does not seem to induce thrombocytopenia, unlike UFH and LMWH, but this needs to be confirmed.[20]

New Oral Antithrombotic Agents

This class of drugs has long been awaited because vitamin K antagonists, although oral drugs, are not powerful enough, and LMWHs are safe and highly effective but injectable. Several apparently safe, highly effective, oral drugs are in the advanced stages of development. They are either anti-IIa or anti-Xa agents, with no apparent superiority over each other.[21] They should be used with caution after an initial period of observation because there are no antagonists to these drugs.

- *Dabigatran* is a direct thrombin inhibitor with the following properties: bioavailability is 6% to 8%, peak plasma concentrations are reached within 2 hours, postoperative peak concentrations occur later and are lower, the terminal half-life is 14 to 17 hours, it is given once or twice daily, it has no interactions with food, and it is excreted unchanged via the kidney.[22] Dabigatran was first developed for orthopedic

Table 36-4	Pooled Analysis of Randomized Controlled Trials (RCTs) of LMWH vs. UFH[4]					
			Relative Risk			
Study, Year	Number of RCTs	Number of Subjects	DVT	Proximal DVT	Pulmonary Embolism	Bleeding
NICE, 2007	76	22,574	0.87	0.62	0.66	0.87

LMWH, low-molecular-weight heparin; *UFH,* unfractionated heparin.

surgery. Two large randomized double-blind studies of short-term (10 to 14 days) and long-term (28 days) prophylaxis after, respectively, total knee arthroplasty and total hip replacement found it to be noninferior to enoxaparin (40 mg once daily).[23,24] Dabigatran is about to be approved by the European Medicines Agency (EMEA) and probably will be marketed soon.

- *Rivaroxaban* is an orally active oxazolidone derivative that acts as a potent direct anti-Xa agent.[25] Its oral bioavailability is greater than 70%. It inhibits factor Xa with a Ki of 0.4 nM. It reaches peak concentrations after 2 to 4 hours. Its terminal half-life is close to 9 hours, and it is cleared by the kidneys (two thirds) and the gut (one third). Like other oral compounds, rivaroxaban was first developed for orthopedic surgery where it has been found to be superior to enoxaparin (total knee replacement).[26]
- *Apixaban* is a potent direct reversible anti-Xa inhibitor with the following properties: oral bioavailability of 51% to 85%, inhibition of factor Xa with a Ki of 0.08 nM, terminal half-life of about 10 to 15 hours, renal elimination 25%, nonrenal elimination 75% (hepatic metabolism, biliary and intestinal excretion).[21] Phase III studies are ongoing.

INTERPRETATION OF DATA AND CONTROVERSIES

Clearly, effective prevention is available, but several points are still a matter of debate.

Mechanical prophylaxis is the first-line approach recommended by recent NICE guidelines, but the eighth guidelines of the American College of Chest Physicians (ACCP) are not quite as positive.[2] There is no proof of the efficacy of mechanical prophylaxis on fatal or nonfatal pulmonary embolism. Available studies date back several years and often lack power. Most are not double-blind and are difficult to interpret because of the wide variety of compression modalities used. For instance, should compression be limited to just the calf or be applied to the whole leg even if this is less well tolerated and more difficult to adjust? Are all pneumatic compression devices equally effective? For how long should compression be applied after surgery? The ACCP guidelines therefore recommend the use of mechanical methods in patients at high risk of bleeding or in combination with pharmacologic methods. In practice, mechanical methods are probably sufficient for patients at moderate risk but insufficient for patients at high risk.[2]

The clinical studies of pharmacologic agents (UFH, LMWH, fondaparinux, anti-Xa and anti-IIa agents) have used asymptomatic DVTs assessed by bilateral ascending venography as a surrogate endpoint. The high rate of events observed with this method has meant that the numbers of patients included into phase II and phase III studies have been relatively small. However, although there may be a relationship between venographic and symptomatic thrombosis, it ranges from a factor of 5 for total hip replacement to a factor of 21 for total knee arthroplasty.[27] In addition, the relevance of distal thromboses diagnosed by venography is debatable. The upcoming new guidance from European regulators on outcomes in trials of prophylaxis for venous thromboembolism therefore suggest the use of a combination of three criteria, namely, symptomatic or asymptomatic proximal DVT assessed by ultrasound (or venography), pulmonary embolism, and VTE-related death.[28] If these criteria are used in the development of future molecules, the results will probably better reflect the real-life situation, even if it is necessary to significantly increase the number of patients entered into trials.

The overall safety of the drugs used in prophylaxis is good, but most of the antithrombotic agents used are eliminated via the kidney. There is thus a genuine risk of drug accumulation and increased bleeding in patients with renal insufficiency. Nevertheless, few cases of severe bleeding have been encountered. Starting the administration of the drugs less than 6 hours before or after surgery to obtain better results on venographic asymptomatic distal DVTs has also led to an increase in perioperative bleeding and transfusion requirements (e.g., as found in the fondaparinux and ximelagatran studies). The ACCP and French guidelines do not see any benefit in the preoperative injection of LMWH. The development of all new agents is now based on systematic administration after surgery, sometimes even on the day after surgery. Since efficacy is guaranteed with a rate of thromboembolic events of 1.5% at 3 months, the current emphasis is naturally on safety. In the ESCORTE survey published in 2006 of nearly 7000 hip fractures with prolonged postoperative LMWH prophylaxis, the overall rate of thromboembolic events was 1.34% at 3 months, the rate of severe bleeding was 1.2% at 6 months, the rate of fatal bleeding and also of pulmonary embolism was 0.2%, and the rate of fatal pulmonary embolism was 0.04%.[11]

GUIDELINES

There are many well-conducted studies and several meta-analyses on the prevention of thromboembolic disease. A number of guidelines are available. The ACCP guidelines are updated every 4 years, and the eighth version was published in June 2008.[2] NICE published very detailed guidelines in 2007.[4] French guidelines from the Société Française d'Anesthésie Réanimation (SFAR) were translated into English and published in 2006.[3]

AUTHOR'S RECOMMENDATIONS

- The overall thromboembolic risk is the resultant of patient-related risk and surgical risk. The surgical risk is decreasing, especially with the introduction of new procedures (fast-track surgery).
- The value of prophylaxis has been firmly established.
- Mechanical prophylaxis is to be used as first-line prophylaxis when there is a risk of bleeding. Combining this with drugs increases the antithrombotic efficacy. However, the effectiveness of prophylaxis on pulmonary embolism and mortality risk has not been demonstrated.
- Renal function needs to be evaluated when LMWH, fondaparinux, dabigatran, or rivaroxaban is prescribed. Age over 75

Continued

REFERENCES

1. House of Commons Health Committee: *The prevention of venous thromboembolism in hospitalised patients*. London, Stationery Office Limited, 2005.
2. Geerts WH, Bergqvist D, Pineo GF, et al: Prevention of venous thromboembolism: American College of Chest Physicians Evidence-Based Clinical Practice Guidelines (8th ed.). *Chest* 2008;133(Suppl 6):381S-453S.
3. Samama CM, Albaladejo P, Benhamou D, et al: Venous thromboembolism prevention in surgery and obstetrics: Clinical practice guidelines. *Eur J Anaesthesiol* 2006;23(2):95-116.
4. Hill J, Treasure T: Reducing the risk of venous thromboembolism (deep vein thrombosis and pulmonary embolism) in inpatients having surgery: Summary of NICE guidance. *BMJ* 2007;334(7602):1053-1054.
5. Heit JA: Venous thromboembolism: Disease burden, outcomes and risk factors. *J Thromb Haemost* 2005;3(8):1611-1617.
6. Bergqvist D, Lowe G: Venous thromboembolism in patients undergoing laparoscopic and arthroscopic surgery and in leg casts. *Arch Intern Med* 2002;162(19):2173-2176.
7. Sors H, Safran D, Stern M, Reynaud P, Bons J, Even P: An analysis of the diagnostic methods for acute pulmonary embolism. *Intensive Care Med* 1984;10(2):81-83.
8. Weitz JI, Bates SM: New anticoagulants. *J Thromb Haemost* 2005;3(8):1843-1853.
9. Kehlet H: Future perspectives and research initiatives in fast-track surgery. *Langenbecks Arch Surg* 2006;391(5):495-498.
10. White RH, Zhou H, Romano PS: Incidence of symptomatic venous thromboembolism after different elective or urgent surgical procedures. *Thromb Haemost* 2003;90(3):446-455.
11. Rosencher N, Vielpeau C, Emmerich J, Fagnani F, Samama CM: Venous thromboembolism and mortality after hip fracture surgery: The ESCORTE study. *J Thromb Haemost* 2005;3(9):2006-2014.
12. Amaragiri SV, Lees TA: Elastic compression stockings for prevention of deep vein thrombosis. *Cochrane Database Syst Rev* 2000(3):CD001484.
13. Ansell J, Hirsh J, Poller L, Bussey H, Jacobson A, Hylek E: The pharmacology and management of the vitamin K antagonists: The Seventh ACCP Conference on Antithrombotic and Thrombolytic Therapy. *Chest* 2004;126(3 suppl):204S-233S.
14. Samama CM, Vray M, Barre J, et al: Extended venous thromboembolism prophylaxis after total hip replacement: A comparison of low-molecular-weight heparin with oral anticoagulant. *Arch Intern Med* 2002;162(19):2191-2196.
15. Mismetti P, Laporte S, Zufferey P, Epinat M, Decousus H, Cucherat M: Prevention of venous thromboembolism in orthopedic surgery with vitamin K antagonists: A meta-analysis. *J Thromb Haemost* 2004;2(7):1058-1070.
16. Collins R, Scrimgeour A, Yusuf S, Peto R: Reduction in fatal pulmonary embolism and venous thrombosis by perioperative administration of subcutaneous heparin. Overview of results of randomized trials in general, orthopedic, and urologic surgery. *N Engl J Med* 1988;318(18):1162-1173.
17. Hirsh J, Raschke R: Heparin and low-molecular-weight heparin: The Seventh ACCP Conference on Antithrombotic and Thrombolytic Therapy. *Chest* 2004;126(3 suppl):188S-203S.
18. Warkentin TE, Greinacher A: Heparin-induced thrombocytopenia: Recognition, treatment, and prevention: The Seventh ACCP Conference on Antithrombotic and Thrombolytic Therapy. *Chest* 2004;126(3 suppl):311S-337S.
19. Turpie AG, Bauer KA, Eriksson BI, Lassen MR: Fondaparinux vs enoxaparin for the prevention of venous thromboembolism in major orthopedic surgery: A meta-analysis of 4 randomized double-blind studies. *Arch Intern Med* 2002;162(16):1833-1840.
20. Warkentin TE, Maurer BT, Aster RH: Heparin-induced thrombocytopenia associated with fondaparinux. *N Engl J Med* 2007;356(25):2653-2655, discussion 2655.
21. Weitz JI. Factor Xa or thrombin: Is thrombin a better target? *J Thromb Haemost* 2007;5(suppl 1):65-67.
22. Di Nisio M, Middeldorp S, Buller HR: Direct thrombin inhibitors. *N Engl J Med* 2005;353(10):1028-1040.
23. Eriksson BI, Dahl OE, Rosencher N, et al: Oral dabigatran etexilate versus subcutaneous enoxaparin for the prevention of venous thromboembolism after total knee replacement: The RE-MODEL randomized trial. *J Thromb Haemost* 2007;5:2178-2185.
24. Eriksson BI, Dahl OE, Rosencher N, et al: Dabigatran etexilate versus enoxaparin for prevention of venous thromboembolism after total hip replacement: A randomised, double-blind, non-inferiority trial. *Lancet* 2007;370(9591):949-956.
25. Turpie AG: Oral, direct factor Xa inhibitors in development for the prevention and treatment of thromboembolic diseases. *Arterioscler Thromb Vasc Biol* 2007;27(6):1238-1247.
26. Lassen MR, Ageno W, Borris LC, et al: Rivaroxaban versus enoxaparin thromboprophylaxis after total knee arthroplasty. *N Engl J Med* 2008;358:2776–2786.
27. Quinlan DJ, Eikelboom JW, Dahl OE, Eriksson BI, Sidhu PS, Hirsh J: Association between asymptomatic deep vein thrombosis detected by venography and symptomatic venous thromboembolism in patients undergoing elective hip or knee surgery. *J Thromb Haemost* 2007;5(7):1438-1443.
28. Committee for Medicinal Products for Human Use (CPMP): Guideline on clinical investigation of medicinal products of prophylaxis of high intra- and postoperative venous thromboembolic risk. http://www.emea.europa.eu/pdfs/human/ewp/70798en_fin.pdf.

37 What Is the Optimal Perioperative Management for Latex Allergy?

Robert S. Holzman, MD, FAAP

INTRODUCTION

Anaphylaxis and the first deaths resulting from exposure to latex were reported by Slater in 1989.[1] Rapid recognition of latex allergy and dissemination of information led to numerous case reports, guidelines, and policies that were well meaning and informative, but the evidence linking various latex products with manufacturing techniques, clinical practices, and patient outcome has evolved over the last 20 years. Anesthesiologists have often been on the front lines of latex allergy management and were among the earliest to treat life-threatening latex allergy.[2-7]

Natural rubber latex (NRL) is a complex suspension of polyisoprene, lipids, phospholipids, and proteins. The proteins are found in three physical states: water-soluble, starch-bound, or latex-bound proteins, and there are at least 240 potentially allergenic proteins in the processed latex product. The protein content of latex gloves can vary up to 1000-fold among different lots marketed by the same manufacturer, and 3000-fold between gloves from different manufacturers.[8] A number of chemicals, including preservatives, accelerators, antioxidants, and vulcanizing compounds, are added during the manufacturing process to yield the final product. Finally, cornstarch is commonly used as a lubricant in order to facilitate the donning and removal of surgical gloves. A typical pair of surgical gloves carries as much as 700 mg of cornstarch powder.[9]

Although the Food and Drug Administration (FDA) now requires identification of the latex content of medical equipment, there is no requirement to quantify the allergen level. The misleading label of "hypoallergenic" had been a source of confusion over the years; as of September 30, 1998, the FDA eliminated the term "hypoallergenic" from any product that contains latex. The term "glove powder content" encompasses several particulate components including dusting or donning powder, mold-release compounds, and manufacturing debris. Dusting or donning powder must meet specifications of the United States Pharmacopoeia (USP) to be acceptable for use as a lubricant for medical gloves. Cornstarch is currently the lubricant most commonly used for medical gloves, but calcium carbonate, oat powder, talc, and lycopodium have all been used. The amount of particulate matter on a medium-size powdered glove is 120 to 400 mg. For a manufacturer to make the claim that its gloves are "powder free" or "powderless," they must meet the FDA limit of less than 2 mg per glove. At this time, there are no federal requirements that define acceptable maximum powder levels.

OPTIONS

Latex allergy is now established as a significant health care concern. Several issues are reviewed here in order to better understand the evidence for optimal perioperative management of latex-allergic patients:

1. Avoiding latex exposure from birth in certain high-risk pediatric groups or in anticipation of multiple surgical procedures
2. Engineering a latex-safe perioperative environment
3. The role of chemoprophylaxis
4. Minimizing latex exposure for unaffected as well as affected health care workers
5. Desensitization strategies for short- and long-term care of latex-allergic patients

EVIDENCE

Evidence for Avoiding Latex Exposure from Birth in Certain High-risk Pediatric Groups or in Anticipation of Multiple Surgical Procedures

Degenhardt and colleagues[10] reviewed 86 children (mean age, 10.2 years) who underwent gastrointestinal or urologic surgery in the first year of life. Twenty-seven patients were sensitized to latex (31.4%). Twenty patients were atopic (25.6%). Atopic patients were more often sensitized and provocation positive to latex ($p < 0.01$). Children already operated on in the first year of life ($n = 44$) with a positive provocation showed significantly higher latex-specific immunoglobulin E (IgE) values than individuals with a negative outcome ($p < 0.0001$). More than eight surgical interventions during the first year of life increased the risk of clinical allergy to latex.[10] Nieto and colleagues[11] found that over 6 years, the prevalence of latex sensitization fell from 4 of 15 (26.7%) to 1 of 22 (4.5%) in children with spina bifida treated in a latex-free environment from birth compared with historical controls.

Evidence for the Efficacy of a Latex-safe Perioperative Environment

The notion of a "latex-safe" environment was introduced in 1992.[12] In a case report, Valentino and colleagues[13] described four cases of health care workers with dermatitis and work-related respiratory symptoms. The subjects were diagnosed with latex hypersensitivity after skin prick testing (SPT) and the latex-specific IgE were positive. In addition, changes in methacholine responsiveness took place. In one case, an occupational exposure test was carried out, which resulted in a 24% decrease in the FEV_1 after 25 minutes of inhalation exposure. At least 1 year after the diagnosis, two nurses who had been removed completely from latex exposure experienced no further latex-induced symptoms.[13] In another case report, four health care workers with suspected latex-glove–related respiratory and skin disorders had a positive skin test reaction to the latex extract; specific IgE antibodies were detected in only one subject. The fourth subject had a negative specific inhalation and skin test reaction to the latex extract. Peak expiratory flow monitoring at work and away from work showed a pattern consistent with work-related asthma.[14] In still another case report, four nurses with previous allergic contact urticaria to latex surgical gloves dusted with cornstarch powder were exposed to nonpowdered latex surgical glove extract, powdered latex surgical glove extract, and cornstarch powder extract, respectively. Whereas nebulization of cornstarch powder extract caused no bronchial reaction in the patients, nebulization of nonpowdered latex surgical glove extract as an undiluted solution induced immediate bronchoconstriction in two subjects, and nebulization of powdered latex surgical glove extract induced immediate bronchoconstriction in all subjects at the 1:10 dilution.[15] Protein allergen can be demonstrated to be transferred to the powder in surgical gloves.[16,17]

In a prospective controlled study, Heilman and colleagues[18] showed that rubber gloves are the major contributor to latex aeroallergen levels in the operating room by sampling operating room air on 52 consecutive days, including 33 surgery days and 19 nonsurgery days. On each surgery day all personnel wore either high-allergen gloves ($n = 18$ days) or low-allergen gloves ($n = 15$ days). Latex aeroallergen levels (ng/M^2) and extractable latex glove allergen contents were measured by inhibition immunoassays. Latex aeroallergen levels during low-allergen glove use days were lower than on high-allergen glove use days ($p < 0.001$) but not significantly different from that on nonsurgery days. Latex aeroallergen levels were correlated with the total number of gloves used on designated high-allergen glove days ($r = 0.66$, $p = 0.003$).[18] Liss and colleagues[19] evaluated 2062 hospital employees who regularly used latex gloves. Glove extracts were assayed for antigenic protein, and area and personal air samples were obtained on two occasions (summer and winter) to estimate exposure to airborne latex protein. An interviewer administered a questionnaire on medical and occupational information. SPT was performed with latex reagents, three common inhalants, and six foods. Protein concentrations were 324 (±227) mcg/g in powdered surgical gloves and 198 (±104) mcg/g in powdered

examination gloves. Personal latex aeroallergen concentrations ranged from 5 to 616 ng/M^3. There were a total of 1351 (66%) participants. The prevalence of positive latex skin tests was 12.1%. This prevalence did not vary by sex, age, hospital, or smoking status, but subjects who were latex positive were more likely to be atopic ($p < 0.01$). Participants who were latex positive were also more likely to have positive skin tests to one or more foods. Work-related symptoms were more often reported among latex-positive subjects and included hives (odds ratio [OR] = 6.3), eye symptoms (OR = 1.9), and a wheezy or whistling chest (OR = 4.7). The prevalence of latex sensitivity was highest among laboratory workers (16.9%) and nurses and physicians (13.3%). When the glove consumption per health care worker for each department was grouped into tertiles, the prevalence of latex skin test positivity was greater in the higher tertiles of glove use for sterile (surgical) gloves ($p < 0.005$) but not for examination gloves.[19] In a single-case report, an 8-year-old girl who experienced intraoperative latex anaphylaxis from which she was successfully resuscitated underwent successful surgery 2 weeks later when neoprene surgical gloves were used and all latex products eliminated from the anesthetic equipment.[20] It is ironic that health care workers are surrounded by most antigenic NRL devices; powdered surgical latex gloves, elastic bandages, and Penrose drains contain antigenic concentrations of hevein fractions that are an order of magnitude greater than household rubber gloves, toy balloons, or latex mattresses.[21]

Beezhold and colleagues[22] have shown that a reduction in protein content will lower antigen levels and allergenicity of latex medical gloves. Three types of NRL gloves were manufactured with a common batch of compounded latex and analyzed for total protein and specifically for latex proteins. Allergen levels in the extracts were determined by endpoint titration SPT on patients allergic to NRL. Fifty-eight percent of patients allergic to latex reacted at the 50 mcg/g detection limit allowed by the FDA. The enzyme-linked immunosorbent assay (ELISA) had a good correlation with SPT reactivity ($r = 0.93$) and gloves testing below the ELISA reporting limit (0.06 mcg/mL) had a lower potential for eliciting reactions in patients allergic to latex.[22] Bronchial hyperresponsiveness is degraded with the use of lower-antigen-content gloves. Eight health care workers with latex-induced asthma were exposed to the powdered latex gloves causing asthma at work and various brands of gloves with a lower protein content, whether low-powdered, nonpowdered, or powdered. Exposure to lower-antigen gloves resulted in the absence (in six subjects) or a significant reduction (in two subjects) of bronchial response.[23] Reduction of latex allergen content can also be accomplished in other medical devices. Lundberg and colleagues[24] evaluated three methods (water leaching, chlorination, and treatment with savinase) of protein reduction in medical catheter balloons. All the methods used to reduce the allergen content were effective, and increased leaching stabilized the allergen content at a low level.[24]

Product alternatives and nonallergenic natural latex alternatives exist. Siler and colleagues[25] studied Parthenium argentatum (guayule), an alternative rubber source. IgE antibodies from 62 subjects allergic to Hevea latex

(46 adults and 16 children with spina bifida) and from serum pools of adults allergic to Hevea latex ($n = 183$), pediatric patients ($n = 101$), and patients with spina bifida ($n = 53$), as well as IgG antibodies from hyperimmunized mice, were unable to cross-react with any proteins in guayule by RAST or Western blot analysis. No competitive inhibition of IgE anti-Hevea binding to Hevea solid phase was detected by the preincubation of sera from subjects allergic to Hevea latex with soluble guayule latex before RAST analysis.[25] Antigenic proteins in natural latex sap and latex gloves can be changed by treatment with KOH solution, which is followed by a loss of their capability to bind specific IgE antibodies from most latex-sensitized patients. A KOH concentration, temperature, and time-dependent decrease in allergenicity, finally resulting in complete loss of IgE-binding activity, occurs. Using an SPT, Baur and colleagues[26] found only four weakly positive reactions to proteins extracted from KOH-washed gloves in 30 latex-sensitized patients. Up to 97% of the aqueous extractable protein content can be removed from latex gloves by washing in KOH solution under certain conditions.[26]

Glove powder, specifically cornstarch, promotes latex sensitization as a result of bonding with protein from the latex.[17] Cornstarch particles readily adsorb latex allergens and increase allergenicity of the gloves.[27] This protein-bearing powder is readily aerosolized and can remain suspended in the air for as long as 5 hours and is also easily transferred from the hands of the wearer to items of clothing, other areas such as skin and hair, and inanimate objects such as food and telephones.[28] Additionally, cornstarch carrying the latex allergen is readily aerosolized and has been associated with respiratory allergic symptoms.[29] Air samples have been collected from work sites by using area and personal breathing zone air samplers. Latex aeroallergen concentrations where powdered latex gloves were frequently used ranged from 13 to 208 ng/M^3, and in areas where powdered latex gloves were never or seldom used, concentrations ranged from 0.3 to 1.8 ng/M^3. Installation and use of a laminar flow glove changing station in one work area did not reduce latex aeroallergen levels. Large quantities of allergen were recovered from used laboratory coats and anesthesia scrub suits and from laboratory surfaces. Latex allergen concentrations in personal breathing zone samplers worn by health care workers in areas where powdered gloves were frequently used ranged from 8 to 974 ng/M^3.[28] Airborne latex allergen exposure in the workplace of a hospital laboratory technician with occupational latex sensitization whose coworkers changed to powder-free latex gloves with subsequent resolution of her symptoms was compared with a laboratory still using powdered latex gloves. Levels were below the level of detection (less than 0.02 ng/M^3 of latex allergen) in the laboratory using powder-free latex gloves but ranged from 39 to 311 ng/M^3 in the laboratory using powdered gloves.[30] The use of nonpowdered, low-protein natural rubber latex (NRL) gloves has been shown to reduce respiratory symptoms in latex-allergic individuals. Howell and colleagues[31] have shown that mice demonstrated dose-dependent increases in total serum IgE levels with increased airway hyperreactivity on respiratory

challenge with methacholine (day 60) or nonammoniated latex proteins (day 93).

NRL plungers in syringes and multidose vial stoppers have also come under scrutiny. Jones and colleagues[32] examined extracts of syringe plungers and collagen solutions for latex allergens before and after storage in syringes with NRL plungers. Thirty-nine patients known to be allergic to latex underwent SPT with extracts of the latex plungers, collagen solutions before and after storage in syringes, standard latex skin test reagents, four extracts from commercially available gloves, and positive (histamine) and negative (diluent) control solutions. Thirty-one control patients not known to be latex allergic were similarly tested. No latex proteins were detected using in vitro immunochemical techniques. Only 1 of 39 (2.5%) latex-allergic patients reacted to the syringe extract and the collagen stored in the syringe; no reactions were recorded to collagen that had no contact with latex.[32] Thomsen and colleagues[33] examined the practice of removing natural rubber stoppers on multidose vials as a means of decreasing exposure to latex protein. Twenty samples were prepared in accordance with latex-allergy precaution guidelines to include removal of the stopper; five latex-free samples and one latex-contaminated sample served as negative and positive controls. The conventional method involved swabbing a vial top with an alcohol prep pad, puncturing the dry natural rubber stopper with an 18-gauge needle attached to a latex-free syringe, and withdrawing the contents of the vial into the syringe. The latex-allergy precaution preparation technique was similar, except that the stopper was removed before the vial contents were withdrawn. There was no difference in latex allergen concentrations between the two drug preparation methods. None of the samples prepared with the standard method supported any microbial growth, whereas one sample prepared with the latex-allergy precaution method grew bacteria.[33]

Birmingham and colleagues[34] examined the prevalence of intraoperative allergic reactions in children with spina bifida who underwent 1025 operations in a 36-month period before and after institution of a standardized latex-avoidance protocol. Risk factors for an intraoperative reaction were a history of latex allergy ($p = 0.001$) and surgery performed before institution of the latex-avoidance protocol ($p = 0.01$). The estimate of increased risk for allergic reaction was 3.09 times higher in cases performed without latex avoidance. Recognized violation of the protocol after its institution led to severe allergic reactions in three patients.[34] Potter and colleagues[35] screened 2316 hospital workers for the presence of work-related symptoms. Workers who were symptomatic had RAST or skin-prick tests to confirm latex sensitivity, and latex-avoidance measures were implemented in positive subjects. One hundred symptomatic, sensitized individuals were followed up 3 months after intervention to assess their clinical status, and a cohort of 25 individuals with ongoing nasal symptoms was studied in detail. Sensitized symptomatic workers were more likely to have had a previous history of urticaria ($p < 0.001$), oral allergy syndrome ($p < 0.001$), or allergic conjunctivitis ($p = 0.001$) but not hay fever, perennial rhinitis, eczema, or insect allergies. Ocular and cutaneous symptoms were associated with latex sensitization (p <0.001). After avoidance measures were introduced, ocular symptoms (p <0.001), skin rashes (p <0.001), and wheezing (p = 0.001) reduced significantly. Nasal symptoms did not improve.[35]

Tarlo and colleagues[36] assessed an intervention program to reduce exposure and detect cases of sensitization early among 8000 hospital employees. Using a retrospective review, the annual numbers of employees visiting the occupational health clinic, allergy clinic, or both for manifestations of NRL allergy compared with the timing of introduction of intervention strategies, such as worker education, voluntary medical surveillance, and hospital conversion to low-protein, powder-free NRL gloves was examined. The number of workers identified with NRL allergy rose annually, from 1 in 1988 to 6 in 1993. When worker education and voluntary medical surveillance were introduced in 1994, a further 25 workers were identified. Nonsterile gloves were changed to low-protein, powder-free NRL gloves in 1995. Diagnoses fell to 8 workers that year, and 2 of the 3 nurses who had been off work because of asthma-anaphylaxis were able to return to work with personal avoidance of NRL products. With a change to lower-protein, powder-free NRL sterile gloves in 1997, allergy diagnoses fell to 3, and only 1 new case was identified subsequently.[36] Saary and colleagues[37] used a historical control method to compare sensitization and clinical allergy rates to latex in the student body of a dental school to determine whether a change in glove use from high-protein/powdered to low-protein/powder-free latex gloves reduced the prevalence of NRL sensitivity. A total of 97 subjects (61 students and 36 staff members) completed the questionnaire and underwent SPT; this compared with 131 subjects in 1995. Subjects reporting asthma symptoms, rhinitis or conjunctivitis, urticaria, or pruritis within minutes of NRL exposure were 4%, 7%, 6%, and 8%, respectively; the corresponding percentages in the 1995 survey were 7% (n.s.), 13% (n.s.), 20% (p = 0.004), and 22% (p = 0.005). Results were similar for the subset of senior students, but in addition there were also fewer complaints of rhinoconjunctivitis in 2000 than in 1995 (0% and 12%, respectively; p = 0.007). Of 97 subjects who underwent SPT, 3 (3%) had positive SPT responses of 2+ or greater to NRL; this compared with 13 (10%) of 131 subjects in 1995 (p = 0.03). There were 3 positive SPT responses among staff members in 2000; there were none among students.[37] The long-term outcome at work following a change of gloves in the working environment from high- to low-allergen latex or nonlatex gloves was examined among hospital workers from 1995 to 1996; 160 of 174 adult subjects diagnosed with NRL allergy between 1982 and 1994 were reexamined 3 years after the diagnosis. Special attention was paid to the occurrence of hand eczema. Of 71 health care workers and 89 non–health care workers, 72% and 83% were atopic; 54% and 65% had hand eczema at the time of original diagnosis and 89% and 19% had work-related allergy to NRL, respectively. On reexamination, none of the health care workers had changed work because of NRL allergy, and only 38% had hand eczema. Ninety-eight percent of the non–health care workers (of whom 58% had hand eczema) continued with their previous jobs.[38]

Evidence for the Efficacy of Chemoprophylaxis

One case report has noted the relative inefficacy of chemoprophylaxis in preventing a latex allergy reaction.[39] On the other hand, another case report indicated that in a subsequent anesthetic, a patient who had previously experienced latex anaphylaxis was successfully managed with a preoperative regimen of diphenhydramine, ranitidine, and hydrocortisone, as well as latex avoidance.[7] Holzman[40] reviewed 162 children with latex allergy who underwent 267 anesthetics according to a latex-safe protocol without chemoprophylaxis. One patient of 162 (1 procedure of 267) had an allergic reaction after injection of an epidural catheter with pharmacy-prepared bupivacaine and fentanyl.[40]

Evidence for Minimizing Latex Exposure for Unaffected as well as Affected Health Care Workers

Forty-eight epidemiologic studies of type I latex allergy among health care workers were subjected to meta-analysis and revealed a prevalence of sensitization in health care workers between 0% and 30%; this large variation remains unexplained.[41] Increased risk of sensitization was not clearly associated with the duration of work in health care, the time spent wearing latex gloves, the frequency of exposure, the specific job categories, the use of powdered versus nonpowdered latex gloves, the use of latex versus nonlatex gloves, or any measurements of ambient exposure to latex proteins in the studies cited. The conclusion of this meta-analysis was that epidemiologic studies do not support the notion that health care workers are at clearly increased risk of latex sensitization or type I allergies compared with other occupations in the United States and that the role of latex gloves in causing latex sensitization and type I allergic symptoms remains poorly defined because of the inconsistent results of the earlier studies.[41] On the other hand, LaMontagne and colleagues[42] reviewed eight primary prevention studies where powdered latex gloves were replaced by low-protein, powder-free NRL gloves or latex-free gloves. They found that the glove replacements greatly reduced NRL aeroallergens, NRL sensitization, and NRL asthma in health care workers.[42]

Desensitization Strategies for Short- and Long-term Care of Latex-Allergic Patients

Attention is now being turned to immunotherapy for latex-allergic patients, using the same principles of desensitization that have proven effective for patients with insect allergy. Strategies that have been applied include subcutaneous, percutaneous, and sublingual desensitization.[43,44] Although the latter strategies may generally be safer and more effective, subcutaneous desensitization has been the more standard approach. Nevertheless, at this time, the benefits of immunotherapy include an improvement in cutaneous symptoms with a possible improvement in rhinitis and asthma.[45,46] More important, these efforts may point the way for acute (i.e., within 4 days of surgery) preparation for exposure to a latex-containing environment, as well as a possible solution for occupational exposure on a long-term basis to a latex-containing environment for previously latex-allergic individuals.

CONTROVERSIES

A possible shortcoming of health care workers conducting studies on health care workers is that "occupational myopia" may affect the conclusions. On the other hand, caution in embracing the conclusion of the meta-analysis is warranted, because clinical latex allergy remains a relatively rarely encountered problem. The dearth of prospective, randomized controlled trials relative to the number of case-control or concurrently evaluated clinical reports does not negate the validity of the immunologic findings in clinically affected patients. Because the risks are so significant, vigilance should be maintained until more is understood, particularly the long-term effects of latex exposure in certain occupations and the basic biology of susceptibility to latex allergy in certain populations such as those with spina bifida.

GUIDELINES

The American Society of Anesthesiologists publication "Natural Rubber Latex Allergy: Considerations for Anesthesiologists" (http://www.asahq.org/publications AndServices/latexallergy.html) provides guidelines for management of the latex-allergic patient and health care worker, as well as considerations for health care facilities. These practical guidelines are summarized in Tables 37-1 and 37-2.

Table 37-1 Perioperative Management of Latex-Allergic Patients

PREOPERATIVE

Solicit specific history of latex allergy or risks for latex allergy
    Chronic care with latex products
    History of spina bifida or repeat urologic reconstructive surgery
    History of multiple surgical procedures (e.g., >9)
History of intolerance to latex products: balloons, rubber gloves, condoms, dental dams, rubber urethral catheters

    Allergy to tropical fruits
    Intraoperative anaphylaxis of uncertain etiology
    Health care workers, especially with a history of atopy or hand eczema
    Consider allergy consultation
    Minimize latex exposure for at-risk patients
Latex alert: patients with significant risk factors for latex allergy but no overt signs or symptoms
Latex allergy: patients with or without significant risk factors for latex allergy and positive history, signs, symptoms, and allergy evaluation

Careful and thorough communication between surgical, anesthesia, and nursing teams
    Nonlatex product alternatives
    Scheduling—first case of the day preferable
    Display "Latex Allergy" or "Latex Alert" signs inside and outside the operating room

INTRAOPERATIVE

Anesthesia equipment
    Latex-free gloves, airways, endotracheal tubes
    Masks—polyvinylchloride if available or old, well-washed black rubber masks
    Rebreathing bags—neoprene if available or old, well-washed black rubber bags
Ventilator bellows—neoprene or silicone if available or old, well-washed black rubber bellows
Breathing circuit—disposable, polyvinylchloride, packaged separately from a latex rebreathing bag
    Blood pressure cuffs—if new latex, cover with soft cotton
Ambu-type bag—ensure that bag and valve do not have latex components; alternative is silicone self-inflating bag
Check syringe plungers for latex content

(Continued)

Table 37-1   **Perioperative Management of Latex-Allergic Patients—Cont'd**

SURGICAL EQUIPMENT

Avoid latex surgical gloves
Avoid latex drains (e.g., Penrose)
Avoid latex urinary catheters
Avoid latex instrument mats
Avoid rubber-shod clamps
Avoid latex vascular tags
Avoid latex bulb syringes for irrigation
Avoid rubber bands

POSTOPERATIVE

Medical alert (e.g., Medic Alert) tag
Warning sign posted on chart
Warning sign posted on bed

Table 37-2   **Treatment of Latex-Induced Hypersensitivity Reactions**

INITIAL THERAPY

1. Stop administration/reduce absorption of offending agent
2. Remove all latex from the surgical field
3. Change gloves
4. Discontinue all antibiotic and blood administration
5. Maintain the airway and administer 100% oxygen
6. Intubate the trachea, as indicated
7. Administer 25-50 mL/kg of crystalloid or colloid, as indicated
8. Administer epinephrine:

Intravenous: 0.1 mcg/kg or approximately 10 mcg in an adult
Subcutaneous (in the absence of an IV): 300 mcg (0.3 mg)
Endotracheal: five to 10 times the intravenous dose, or 50-100 mcg in an adult (10 mL of 1:10,000 dilution)

9. Discontinue all anesthetic agents
10. Display prominent signs such as "Latex Allergy" or "Latex Alert" on the inside of the operating room, as well as on the entry doors

SECONDARY THERAPY

1. Administer antihistamine
   Diphenhydramine 1 mg/kg IV or IM (maximum dose 50 mg)
   Ranitidine 1 mg/kg (maximal dose 50 mg)
2. Administer glucocorticoids
   Hydrocortisone 5 mg/kg initially and then 2.5 mg/kg every 4-6 hours
   Methylprednisolone 1 mg/kg initially and 0.8 mg/kg every 4-6 hours
3. Administer aminophylline for bronchospasm (may be ineffective during anesthesia)
   Loading dose 5-6 mg/kg Continuous infusion 0.4-0.9 mg/kg/hr (check blood level)
4. Administer inhaled beta-2 agonists for bronchospasm
5. Administer a continuous catecholamine infusion for blood pressure support

   Epinephrine 0.02-0.05 mcg/kg/min (2-4 mcg/min)
   Norepinephrine 0.05 mcg/kg/min (2-4 mcg/min)
   Dopamine 5-20 mcg/kg/min
   Isoproterenol (same dosing as epinephrine)

6. Administer sodium bicarbonate, as indicated 0.5-1 mg/kg initially, with titration using arterial blood gas analysis

AUTHOR'S RECOMMENDATIONS

- Anesthesiologists should recognize that there are patients who have a higher risk of latex allergy: those with spina bifida, bladder extrophy, and/or multiple surgeries; health care workers; atopic individuals; and workers in the rubber industry.
- Powdered latex gloves are the most important source of sensitization. The risk of NRL allergy appears to be largely linked to occupational exposure by aerosol or cutaneous contact. Airborne NRL is dependent on the use of powdered NRL gloves; conversion to non-NRL or nonpowdered low-allergen NRL substitutes results in predictable rapid disappearance of detectable levels of aeroallergen. After occupational exposure, rates of sensitization and NRL-induced asthma are elevated in individuals using powdered NRL gloves but not in individuals using powder-free low-allergen or non-NRL gloves.
- Preventive measures reduce latex sensitization and reverse allergic reactions. Institution of latex-safe measures is effective in preventing allergic reactions.
- Chemoprophylaxis does not play a significant role in reducing the risk of NRL allergic reactions.
- Avoidance of latex antigen exposure, particularly in populations occupationally or genetically susceptible to sensitization, remains the cornerstone of safe medical management and institutional policy. The specific role of immunotherapy is evolving and requires more research.

REFERENCES

1. Slater JE: Rubber anaphylaxis. *N Engl J Med* 1989;320:1126-1130.
2. Leynadier F, Pecquet C, Dry J: Anaphylaxis to latex during surgery. *Anaesthesia* 1989;44:547-550.
3. Gerber AC, Jorg W, Zbinden S, Seger RA, Dangel PH: Severe intraoperative anaphylaxis to surgical gloves: Latex allergy, an unfamiliar condition. *Anesthesiology* 1989;71:800-802.
4. Moneret-Vautrin DA, Laxenaire MC, Bavoux F: Allergic shock to latex and ethylene oxide during surgery for spinal bifida. *Anesthesiology* 1990;73:556-568.
5. Swartz JS, Gold M, Braude BM, Dolovich J, Gilmour RF, Shandling B: Intraoperative anaphylaxis to latex: An identifiable population at risk. *Can J Anaesth* 1990;37:S131.
6. Holzman R, Pascucci R, Sethna N, Berde C: Hypotension, flushing and bronchospasm in myelodysplasia patients undergoing surgery [abstract]. Section on Anesthesiology, American Academy of Pediatrics, Seattle, 1990.
7. Swartz J, Braude BM, Gilmour RF, Shandling B, Gold M: Intraoperative anaphylaxis to latex. *Can J Anaesth* 1990;37:589-592.
8. Yunginger JW, Jones R, Fransway A: Extractable latex allergens and proteins in disposable medical gloves and other rubber products. *J Allergy Clin Immunol* 1994;93:836-884.
9. Jaffray D, Nade S: Does surgical glove powder decrease the inoculum of bacteria required to produce an abscess? *J R Coll Surg Edinb* 1983;28:219-222.
10. Degenhardt P, Golla S, Wahn F, Niggemann B: Latex allergy in pediatric surgery is dependent on repeated operations in the first year of life. *J Pediatr Surg* 2001;36:1535-1539.
11. Nieto A, Mazon A, Pamies R, Lanuza A, Estornell F, Garcia-Ibarra F: Efficacy of latex avoidance for primary prevention of latex sensitization in children with spina bifida. *J Pediatr* 2002;140:370-372.
12. Holzman R, Sethna N: *A "latex-safe" environment prevents allergic reactions in latex-allergic patients, International Latex Conference: Sensitivity to Latex in Medical Devices*. Baltimore, MD, FDA Center for Devices and Radiological Health, 1992.
13. Valentino M, Pizzichini MA, Monaco F, Governa M: Latex-induced asthma in four healthcare workers in a regional hospital. *Occup Med* 1994;44:161-164.
14. Ho A, Chan H, Tse K, Chan-Yeung M: Occupational asthma due to latex in health care workers. *Thorax* 1996;51:1280-1282.
15. Pisati G, Baruffini A, Bernabeo F, Stanizzi R: Bronchial provocation testing in the diagnosis of occupational asthma due to latex surgical gloves. *Eur Respir J* 1994;7:332-336.
16. Beezhold DH, Kostyal DA, Wiseman J: The transfer of protein allergens from latex gloves. A study of influencing factors. *AORN J* 1994;59:605-613.
17. Tomazic VJ, Shampaine EL, Lamanna A, Withrow TJ, Adkinson NF Jr, Hamilton RG: Cornstarch powder on latex products is an allergen carrier. *J Allergy Clin Immunol* 1994;93:751-758.
18. Heilman D, Jones R, Swanson M, Yunginger J: A prospective, controlled study showing that rubber gloves are the major contributor to latex aeroallergen levels in the operating room. *J Allergy Clin Immunol* 1996;98:325-330.
19. Liss G, Sussman G, Deal K, Brown S, Cividino M, Siu S, et al: Latex allergy: Epidemiological study of 1351 hospital workers. *Occup Environ Med* 1997;54:335-342.
20. Hodgson CA, Andersen BD: Latex allergy: An unfamiliar cause of intra-operative cardiovascular collapse. *Anaesthesia* 1994;49:507-508.
21. Crippa M, Belleri L, Mistrello G, Tedoldi C, Alessio L: Prevention of latex allergy among health care workers and in the general population: Latex protein content in devices commonly used in hospitals and general practice. *Int Arch Occup Environ Health* 2006;79:550-557.
22. Beezhold D, Pugh B, Liss G, Sussman G: Correlation of protein levels with skin prick test reactions in patients allergic to latex. *J Allergy Clin Immunol* 1996;98:1097-1102.
23. Vandenplas O, Delwiche JP, Depelchin S, Sibille Y, Vande Weyer R, Delaunois L: Latex gloves with a lower protein content reduce bronchial reactions in subjects with occupational asthma caused by latex. *Am J Respir Crit Care Med* 1995;151:887-891.
24. Lundberg M, Wrangsjo K, Eriksson-Widblom K, Johansson SG: Reduction of latex-allergen content in Swedish medical catheter balloons—a survey of 3 years' production. *Allergy* 1997;52:1057-1062.
25. Siler D, Cornish K, Hamilton R: Absence of cross-reactivity of IgE antibodies from subjects allergic to Hevea brasiliensis latex with a new source of natural rubber latex from guayule (Parthenium argentatum). *J Allergy Clin Immunol* 1996;98:895-902.
26. Baur X, Rennert J, Chen Z: Latex allergen elimination in natural latex sap and latex gloves by treatment with alkaline potassium hydroxide solution. *Allergy* 1997;52:306-311.
27. Beezhold D, Beck WC: Surgical glove powders bind latex antigens. *Arch Surg* 1992;127:1354-1357.
28. Swanson MC, Bubak ME, Hunt LW, Yunginger JW, Warner MA, Reed CE: Quantification of occupational latex aeroallergens in a medical center. *J Allergy Clin Immunol* 1994;94:445-451.
29. Vandenplas O, Delwiche JP, Evrard G, Aimont P, van der Brempt X, Jamart J, Delaunois L: Prevalence of occupational asthma due to latex among hospital personnel. *Am J Respir Crit Care Med* 1995;151:54-60.
30. Tarlo SM, Sussman G, Contala A, Swanson MC: Control of airborne latex by use of powder-free latex gloves. *J Allergy Clin Immunol* 1994;93:985-989.
31. Howell M, Weissman D, Jean Meade B: Latex sensitization by dermal exposure can lead to airway hyperreactivity. *Int Arch Allergy Immunol* 2002;128:204-211.
32. Jones J, Sussman G, Beezhold D: Latex allergen levels of injectable collagen stored in syringes with rubber plungers. *Urology* 1996;47:898-902.
33. Thomsen DJ, Burke TG: Lack of latex allergen contamination of solutions withdrawn from vials with natural rubber stoppers. *Am J Health Syst Pharm* 2000;57:44-47.
34. Birmingham P, Dsida R, Grayhack J, Han J, Wheeler M, Pongracic J, Cote C, Hall S: Do latex precautions in children with myelodysplasia reduce intraoperative allergic reactions? *J Pediatr Orthop* 1996;16:799-802.
35. Potter P, Crombie I, Marian A, Kosheva O, Maqula B, Schinkel M: Latex allergy at Groote Schuur Hospital—prevalence, clinical features and outcome. *S Afr Med J* 2001;91:760-765.
36. Tarlo S, Easty A, Eubanks K, Parsons C, Min F, Juvet S, et al: Outcomes of a natural rubber latex control program in an Ontario teaching hospital. *J Allergy Clin Immunol* 2001;108.
37. Saary M, Kanani A, Alghadeer H, Holness D, Tarlo S: Changes in rates of natural rubber latex sensitivity among dental school

students and staff members after changes in latex gloves. *J Allergy Clin Immunol* 2002;109:131-135.

38. Turjanmaa K, Kanto M, Kautiainen H, Reunala T, Palosuo T: Long-term outcome of 160 adult patients with natural rubber latex allergy. *J Allergy Clin Immunol* 2002;110:S70-S74.

39. Setlock MA, Cotter TP, Rosner D: Latex allergy: Failure of prophylaxis to prevent severe reaction. *Anesth Analg* 1993;76:650-652.

40. Holzman R: Clinical management of latex-allergic children. *Anesth Analg* 1997;85:529-533.

41. Garabrant D, Schweitzer S: Epidemiology of latex sensitization and allergies in health care workers. *J Allergy Clin Immunol* 2002;110:S82-S95,

42. LaMontagne A, Radi S, Elder D, Abramson M, Sim M: Primary prevention of latex related sensitisation and occupational asthma: A systematic review. *Occup Environ Med* 2006;63:359-364.

43. Nucera E, Schiavino D, Pollastrini E, Rendeli C, Pietrini D, Tabacco F, et al: Sublingual desensitization in children with congenital malformations and latex allergy. *Pediatr Allergy Immunol* 2006;17:606-612.

44. Patriarca G, Nucera G, Pollastrini E, Roncallo C, Buonomo C, Bartolozz F, et al: Sublingual desensitization: A new approach to latex allergy problem. *Anesth Analg* 2002;95:956-960.

45. Leynadier F, Herman D, Vervloet D: Specific immunotherapy with a standardized latex extract versus placebo in allergic healthcare workers. *J Allergy Clin Immunol* 2000;106:585-590.

46. Sastre, J, Fernandez-Nieto M, Rico P: Specific immunotherapy with a standardized latex extract in allergic workers: A double-blind, placebo-controlled study. *J Allergy Clin Immunol* 2003;111:985-994.

38 Are There Special Techniques in Obese Patients?

David M. Eckmann, PhD, MD

INTRODUCTION

The obesity epidemic now affects a significant proportion of the adult population in the United States and throughout developed nations.[1] The body mass index (BMI) is the most widely applied classification used to assess weight status. The BMI is defined as one's weight, measured in kilograms, divided by the square of one's height, measured in meters. Using this system, patients are considered overweight with a BMI between 25 and 29.9 kg/m^2 and obese with a BMI between 30 and 49.9 kg/m^2. Obese classification is further subdivided into class 1 (BMI range 30 to 34.9 kg/m^2), class 2 (35 to 39.9 kg/m^2) and class 3 (40 to 49.9 kg/m^2), based on increasing risk of developing health problems. Patients with a BMI of 50 kg/m^2 or greater are considered superobese.

It is estimated that more than 100,000,000 Americans, or 65% of the U.S. adult population, are overweight or obese. Obesity is often accompanied by multiple comorbid states, including insulin resistance, type 2 diabetes mellitus, obstructive sleep apnea, hypoventilation, cardiovascular disease, hypertension, certain malignancies, and osteoarthritis. Obesity is associated with early death. The rapid increase in the prevalence of both morbid obesity and superobesity, together with the increased risk of early demise within the obese population, has significantly increased the number of bariatric surgical procedures performed annually to enable patients to lose weight. It is estimated that over 175,000 bariatric surgeries were performed in 2006 and that over 200,000 will be performed in 2008 and beyond. Care of obese patients is not limited to obesity surgery, however, because these patients undergo all types of operations.

Obese patients present special challenges for the anesthesiologist in airway management, positioning, monitoring, choice of anesthetic technique and anesthetic agents, pain control, and postoperative care. The most significant and best studied of these are in the areas of endotracheal intubation following careful patient positioning and pulmonary physiology and maintenance of oxygenation and lung volume. There is mounting evidence that specific interventions, techniques, and approaches used in caring for obese patients alter outcomes.

PATIENT POSITIONING AND AIRWAY MANAGEMENT

Laryngoscopy and endotracheal intubation have often been considered more difficult to perform in obese patients than those having a normal BMI. This is usually thought to result from the obese patient having a short, thick neck, large tongue, and significant redundant pharyngeal soft tissue. The correlation between morbid obesity and difficulty with laryngoscopy and intubation is not the universally observed clinical experience, however. In fact, it is also often reported that there is no difference between laryngoscopy and intubation in thin and obese individuals. This is likely to result from a simple, but important, difference in clinical practice. Careful attention to patient positioning before induction of general anesthesia plays an important role in providing optimal conditions for successful placement of the endotracheal tube under direct vision.

PULMONARY PHYSIOLOGY AND MAINTENANCE OF OXYGENATION AND LUNG VOLUME

Obese patients have multiple pulmonary abnormalities, including decreased vital capacity, inspiratory capacity, expiratory reserve volume, and functional residual capacity. Closing capacity in obese individuals is close to, or may fall within, tidal breathing, particularly with patients in supine or recumbent position. The obese patient is likely to undergo rapid oxygen desaturation, particularly during periods of apnea such as occur during induction of general anesthesia, and may derecruit gas exchange units throughout the anesthetic course.[2] A variety of maneuvers have been studied as measures to preserve oxygenation and maintain lung volume specifically in the obese population.

EVIDENCE

A number of studies have been conducted to determine the incidence of difficult laryngoscopy or intubation in the obese population (Table 38-1). However, although many of these studies have demonstrated a significant increase in the incidence of difficult laryngoscopy or intubation in comparison to the general population, some studies have shown no difference whatsoever. One study attempting to associate oropharyngeal Mallampati classification along with BMI as predictors of difficult laryngoscopy found a significantly higher positive predictive value of difficult laryngoscopy using both indices (BMI and Mallampati classification).[3] During laryngoscopy, patients' heads were maintained in optimum sniffing

| | | Table 38-1 | **Summary of Trials for Airway Management** | | | |

Study, Year	Number of Subjects (Intervention/No Intervention)	Study design Double-blind Placebo-controlled	Intervention	Control	Outcomes
Voyagis, 1998	1833 (1733 normal/99 obese)	Unblinded	None	Sniffing position	Increased risk of difficult laryngoscopy with obesity
Brodsky, 2002	100 obese	Unblinded	None	Ramped position	Obesity does not increase intubation difficulty
Juvin, 2003	263 (134 normal/129 obese)	Unblinded	None	Semirecumbent, sniffing position	Increased risk of difficult intubation with obesity
Ezri, 2003	50 obese	Unblinded	None	Sniffing position	Increased risk of difficult laryngoscopy with greater neck soft tissue
Collins, 2004	60 obese (30 ramped/30 sniffing position)	Blinded	Ramped position	Sniffing position	Improved laryngoscopic view in ramped position

position, regardless of BMI. In a study conducted exclusively with obese patients, BMI was not found to be associated with intubation difficulties.[4] A high Mallampati score was identified as a predictor of "potential intubation problems," but intubation by direct laryngoscopy was successful in 99 of 100 patients studied. All patients were positioned with pillows or towels under their shoulders, with the head elevated and neck extended. Another group studied both lean and obese patients and found a Mallampati score of III or IV to be the only independent risk factor for difficult intubation in the obese study group.[5] The authors determined the Mallampati score to have low specificity and positive predictive values (62% and 29%, respectively) for difficult intubation. They concluded that intubation was more difficult in the obese patients. During intubation, patients in this study were placed in a semirecumbent position (30°) with the head in the sniffing position. Another group of authors used ultrasound to quantify the amount of soft tissue between the skin and the anterior aspect of the trachea at the level of vocal cords.[6] They also used classical assessment of difficult intubation, including measurement of thyromental distance, mouth opening, degree of neck mobility, Mallampati score, neck circumference, and presence of sleep apnea. Only the abundance of pretracheal soft tissue measured ultrasonically and neck circumference were positive predictors of difficult intubation. Laryngoscopy was carried out with patients in the sniffing position. A meta-analysis of 35 studies, including the four studies described previously, was conducted to determine the diagnostic accuracy of preinduction tests for predicting difficult intubation in patients having no airway pathology.[7] A major finding was that the incidence of difficult intubation in obese patients was three times the incidence determined in the nonobese population. This may have resulted from suboptimal patient positioning, which was not clearly described in any of the preceding studies to include ramped positioning, or elevating the upper body and head of morbidly obese patients to align the ear with the sternum horizontally, as has been shown to improve

laryngoscopic view.[8] In that study of morbidly obese patients, patients were assigned to be either in sniffing position or ramped position for the laryngoscopy and intubation. The study results showed a statistically significant difference in laryngeal view, with ramped position providing the superior view.

Research has also been conducted to examine the rate of development of hypoxemia in patients during apnea (Table 38-2). In one study patients received 100% oxygen by facemask for denitrogenation before induction of general anesthesia.[2] Apnea was permitted until the SpO_2 fell to 90%. Obese patients reached the endpoint in less than 3 minutes, whereas it took 6 minutes in patients having a normal BMI. Efforts to prevent atelectasis formation and desaturation during induction of general anesthesia in the obese population have included application of continuous positive airway pressure (CPAP) during preoxygenation,[9-11] along with the addition of positive end-expiratory pressure (PEEP) and mechanical ventilation by mask after induction.[11] Application of 10 cm H_2O CPAP during preoxygenation in supine position resulted in a higher PaO_2 after intubation and decreased the amount of atelectasis that developed.[9] The combination of CPAP during preoxygenation and PEEP/mechanical ventilation after induction significantly prolonged the nonhypoxemic apnea duration to 3 minutes from 2 minutes found in controls not receiving CPAP or PEEP. Use of 7.5 cm H_2O CPAP during 3 minutes of preoxygenation while supine, however, did not alter the time required for obese patients to desaturate to an SpO_2 of 90%.[10] Preoxygenation using 25° head-up (i.e., back inclined), as opposed to supine, positioning without positive airway pressure did prolong the time required for anesthetized, apneic, obese individuals to desaturate to an SpO_2 of 92%.[12] The patients in head-up position had a significantly higher PaO_2 after preoxygenation, just before induction. The obesity-associated gas exchange defect was shown to depend on the waist-to-hip ratio, an index of the distribution of adipose tissue surrounding the thorax.[13] This study also demonstrated that morbidly

Table 38-2	Summary of Trials for Oxygenation and Pulmonary Mechanics				
Study, Year	**Number of Subjects (Intervention/No Intervention)**	**Study Design Double-blind Placebo-controlled**	**Intervention**	**Control**	**Outcomes**
Jense, 1991	24 (7 normal/11 obese class 1/6 obese class 3)	Unblinded	None	None	Apneic obese patients desaturated faster than normals.
Boyce, 2003	26 (9 reverse Trendelenburg/9 supine/9 back up)	Unblinded	None	None	Apneic patients in reverse Trendelenburg position desaturated most slowly.
von Ungern-Sternberg, 2004	161 (125 normal/36 obese)	Unblinded	None	Preoperative values	Obese patients had larger decrement in postoperative spirometry values.
Bardoczky, 1995	8	Unblinded	Increasing tidal volume	Baseline tidal volume	Increasing tidal volume increased airway pressures but not oxygenation.
Perilli, 2000	15	Unblinded	Reverse Trendelenburg position	Supine position	Pulmonary mechanics and oxygenation improved.
Cressey, 2001	20 (10 no CPAP/10 CPAP)	Randomized, unblinded	CPAP	No CPAP	Preoxygenation using CPAP increased apneic time to desaturation.
Coussa, 2004	18 (9 CPAP + PEEP/9 no CPAP or PEEP)	Randomized, unblinded	CPAP preinduction, PEEP postintubation	No CPAP or PEEP applied	Positive airway pressure increased oxygenation and decreased atelectasis.
Gander, 2005	27 (12 CPAP and PEEP/15 no CPAP or PEEP)	Randomized, unblinded	CPAP preinduction, PEEP postinduction	No CPAP or PEEP applied	Positive airway pressure increased oxygenation and prolonged apneic time to desaturation.
Dixon, 2005	42 (21 head up/21 supine)	Randomized, unblinded	Head-up position	Supine position	Head-up position increased oxygenation and prolonged apneic time to desaturation.
Sprung, 2003	12 (6 obese, 6 normal)	Unblinded	Alterations in body position, respiratory rate, tidal volume, pneumoperitoneum	Supine position, no pneumoperitoneum, baseline ventilation	Oxygenation is lower in obese patients and independent of body position and ventilatory mode during pneumoperitoneum.
Whalen, 2006	20 (10 recruitment maneuver /10 no maneuver)	Randomized	Sustained lung inflation plus PEEP	No sustained intervention or PEEP	Recruitment maneuver increased oxygenation.
Pelosi, 1999	18 (9 obese/9 normal)	Unblinded	PEEP	No PEEP	PEEP improved pulmonary mechanics and oxygenation of intubated, ventilated obese patients.

obese men are more likely to have poorer pulmonary gas exchange than morbidly obese women. In another study conducted to assess effects of patient positioning on development of hypoxemia in superobese patients during apnea after anesthetic induction and intubation, patients were ventilated with 50% oxygen/50% air mixture for 5 minutes before the ventilator circuit was disconnected.[14] Apnea persisted until the SpO_2 fell to 92% before ventilation resumed. Patients in the supine position reached the endpoint in 2 minutes, whereas it took 30 seconds longer for supine position with the back elevated 30° and 1 minute longer using 30° reverse Trendelenburg position. Use of 30° reverse Trendelenburg position in obese patients undergoing bariatric surgery was also shown to reduce the alveolar-to-arterial oxygen difference, as well as increase total ventilatory compliance and reduce peak and plateau airway pressures, when compared with supine position.[15] Vital capacity has also been shown to decrease to a greater extent under general anesthesia in obese patients compared with normal-weight patients.[16]

Intraoperative maneuvers to maintain lung volume and oxygenation have also been studied. Increasing tidal volume incrementally from 13 to 22 mL/kg in obese patients ventilated under general anesthesia did not improve the gas exchange defect but did increase airway pressures.[17] Use of 10 cm H_2O PEEP has been demonstrated to have a greater effect in obese patients compared with normal subjects on improving ventilatory mechanics, increasing PaO_2, and decreasing alveolar-to-arterial oxygen difference during general anesthesia with neuromuscular blockade.[18] It is especially important to consider obese patients undergoing laparoscopic procedures, because pneumoperitoneum negatively affects pulmonary mechanics by increasing pulmonary resistance and decreases dynamic lung compliance.[19] During pneumoperitoneum, alterations in body position, tidal volume, and respiratory rate did not alter the alveolar-to-arterial oxygen difference in obese patients.[20] During pneumoperitoneum for laparoscopic bariatric surgery, alveolar recruitment by repeated sustained lung inflation to 50 cm H_2O followed by mechanical ventilation with 12 cm H_2O PEEP was shown to increase PaO_2 intraoperatively while causing hypotension that required vasopressor use.[21] An attempt to optimize PEEP in obese patients undergoing laparoscopic gastric bypass surgery showed that a normal functional residual capacity was maintained with 15 ± 1 cm H_2O PEEP, but intravascular volume expanders had to be infused to prevent PEEP-induced hemodynamic embarrassment.[22]

AREAS OF UNCERTAINTY

There is no ideal preinduction examination or test that clearly identifies patients at risk for difficult laryngoscopy and difficult intubation. Although some evidence indicates that difficult laryngoscopy and difficult intubation are more frequently encountered in the obese population, studies conducted with obese patients positioned in the ramped state clearly indicate that a superior laryngoscopic view is observed compared with that found in obese patients placed in the sniffing position. No studies have been conducted to determine the ideal position for proper alignment of the airway to optimize the likelihood of success of laryngoscopy and intubation of obese patients.

The optimal patient position and use of PEEP during preoxygenation, during induction of anesthesia, and intraoperatively have not been clearly defined for care of the obese patient. Use of noninvasive modes of ventilation, including pressure support and bilevel delivered by mask for preoxygenation, induction, and maintenance of anesthesia to maintain oxygenation and ventilatory mechanics in obese patients, has not been explored sufficiently. Ideal patient positioning, use of PEEP, and special modes of ventilation just before emergence and extubation to maintain pulmonary function and gas exchange after extubation have not been identified.

GUIDELINES

There are currently no guidelines published by national societies to address the issue of airway management of obese patients. As in any anesthetic induction, practitioners should be prepared to encounter difficulty. Therefore emergency methods of establishing and maintaining an airway should be readily available, as set forth in the American Society of Anesthesiologists algorithm for difficult airway management. Careful patient positioning in the ramped position should be accomplished before induction of general anesthesia. As to maintenance of oxygenation and ventilatory mechanics in obese patients undergoing general anesthesia, no guidelines have been published by national societies to address the issues. Considering both the airway management issues detailed previously and the oxygenation, lung volume, and ventilatory mechanics issues described as well for obese individuals, practitioners must aim to position patients to achieve the combined goals of providing a superior laryngoscopic view for ease of endotracheal intubation while establishing optimal conditions for oxygenation and preservation of pulmonary mechanical function.

AUTHOR'S RECOMMENDATIONS

AIRWAY MANAGEMENT, OXYGENATION, AND INTRAOPERATIVE MANAGEMENT

- Based on the evidence from randomized controlled trials and the body of literature for airway management of obese patients, patients should be readily intubated by direct laryngoscopy if placed carefully in ramped position.
- Obese patients should be thoroughly examined for the usual objective signs of potential difficult intubation such as small mouth opening, large protuberant teeth, limited neck mobility, and retrognathia.
- Techniques such as awake, topicalized direct laryngoscopy with modest sedation can be used to assess laryngoscopic view in deciding whether to proceed with induction of general anesthesia or awake, sedated fiber-optic intubation.
- Equipment for emergency airway management including laryngeal masks and a fiber-optic bronchoscope should be kept available.
- Put patients in ramped position and then use reverse Trendelenburg, if needed, to achieve a 25° to 30° incline of the thorax before preoxygenation.
- Preoxygenate patients for 3 to 5 minutes with 100% oxygen using some positive pressure. For a patient on CPAP for obstructive sleep apnea, use CPAP or pressure support ventilation by mask identical to the patient's home CPAP setting. Otherwise CPAP of 10 cm H_2O should be used.
- Maintain 10 to 12 cm H_2O PEEP intraoperatively, but be careful to treat hypotension that may occur.
- If patient position changes intraoperatively, return the patient to head-up position before emergence and extubation.

REFERENCES

1. Hensrud DD, Klein S: Extreme obesity: A new medical crisis in the United States. *Mayo Clinic Proc* 2006;81:S5-10.
2. Jense HG, Dubin SA, Silverstein PI, O'Leary-Escolas U: Effect of obesity on safe duration of apnea in anesthetized humans. *Anesth Analg* 1991;72:89-93.
3. Voyagis GS, Kyriakis KP, Dimitriou V, Vrettou I: Value of oropharyngeal Mallampati classification in predicting difficult laryngoscopy among obese patients. *Eur J Anaesthesiol* 1998;15:330-334.
4. Brodsky JB, Lemmens HJM, Brock-Utne JG, et al: Morbid obesity and tracheal intubation. *Anesth Analg* 2002;94:732-736.
5. Juvin P, Lavaut E, Dupont H, et al: Difficult tracheal intubation is more common in obese than in lean patients. *Anesth Analg* 2003;97:595-600.
6. Ezri T, Gewurtz G, Sessler DI, et al: Prediction of difficult laryngoscopy in obese patients by ultrasound quantification of anterior neck soft tissue. *Anaesthesia* 2003;58:1111-1114.
7. Shiga T, Wajima Z, Inoue T, Sakamoto A. Predicting difficult intubation in apparently normal patients—a meta-analysis of bedside screening test performance. *Anesthesiology* 2005;103:429-437.
8. Collins JS, Lemmens HJM, Brodsky JB, et al: Laryngoscopy and morbid obesity: A comparison of the "sniff" and "ramped" positions. *Obesity Surgery* 2004;14:1171-1175.
9. Coussa M, Proietti S, Schnyder P, et al: Prevention of atelectasis formation during the induction of general anesthesia in morbidly obese patients. *Anesth Analg* 2004;98:1419-1495.
10. Cressey DM, Berthoud MC, Reilly CS: Effectiveness of continuous positive airway pressure to enhance pre-oxygenation in morbidly obese women. *Anaesthesia* 2001;56:680-684.
11. Gander S, Frascarolo P, Suter M, et al: Positive end-expiratory pressure during induction of general anesthesia increases duration of nonhypoxic apnea in morbidly obese patients. *Anesth Analg* 2005;100:580-584.
12. Dixon BJ, Dixon JB, Carden JR, et al: Preoxygenation is more effective in the 25 degrees head-up position than in the supine position in severely obese patients: A randomized controlled study. *Anesthesiology* 2005;102:1110-1115.
13. Zavorsky GS, Murias JM, Kim dJ, et al: Waist-to-hip ratio is associated with pulmonary gas exchange in the morbidly obese. *Chest* 2007;131:362-367.
14. Boyce JR, Ness T, Castroman P, Gleysteen JJ: A preliminary study of the optimal anesthesia positioning for the morbidly obese patient. *Obesity Surgery* 2003;13:4-9.
15. Perilli V, Sollazzi L, Bozza P, et al: The effects of the reverse Trendelenburg position on respiratory mechanics and blood gases in morbidly obese patients during bariatric surgery. *Anesth Analg* 2000;91:1520-1525.
16. von Ungern-Sternberg BS, Regli A, Schneider MC, et al: Effect of obesity and site of surgery on perioperative lung volumes. *Br J Anaesth* 2004;92:202-207.
17. Bardoczky GI, Yernault JC, Houben JJ, d'Hollander AA: Large tidal volume ventilation does not improve oxygenation in morbidly obese patients during anesthesia. *Anesth Analg* 1995;81:385-388.
18. Pelosi P, Ravagnan I, Giurati G, et al: Positive end-expiratory pressure improves respiratory function in obese but not in normal subjects during anesthesia and paralysis. *Anesthesiology* 1999;91:1221-1231.
19. El Dawlatly AA, Al Dohayan A, Abdel-Meguid ME, et al: The effects of pneumoperitoneum on respiratory mechanics during general anesthesia for bariatric surgery. *Obesity Surgery* 2004;14:212-215.
20. Sprung J, Whalley DG, Falcone T, et al: The effects of tidal volume and respiratory rate on oxygenation and respiratory mechanics during laparoscopy in morbidly obese patients. *Anesth Analg* 2003;97:268-274.
21. Whalen FX, Gajic O, Thompson GB, et al: The effects of the alveolar recruitment maneuver and positive end-expiratory pressure on arterial oxygenation during laparoscopic bariatric surgery. *Anesth Analg* 2006;102:298-305.
22. Erlandsson K, Odenstedt H, Lundin S, Stenqvist O: Positive end-expiratory pressure optimization using electric impedance tomography in morbidly obese patients during laparoscopic gastric bypass surgery. *Acta Anaesthesiol Scand* 2006;50:833-839.

39 Is There an Ideal Approach to the Malignant Hyperthermia–Susceptible Patient?

Charles B. Watson, MD, FCCM

INTRODUCTION

Malignant hyperthermia crisis (MHC) is a potentially lethal inherited syndrome triggered by exposure to anesthetic agents. The anesthesia community is best prepared to deal with the MHC and patients who have a diagnosis of malignant hyperthermia susceptibility (MHS), because MH is triggered by anesthesia and stress and early identification of the MHC and treatment is most common in the perioperative setting.[1] The outcome of MHC has improved, and alternative methods of identifying other family members at risk (2) have supplemented the expensive in vivo caffeine halothane contracture test (CHCT) and positive family history as a basis for establishing risk. There is an increasing population of MHS individuals who may require elective or emergent surgery. Anesthesia for MHS is high risk because anesthetic drugs or stress may induce an MHC with resultant death or major morbidity.

Malignant Hyperthermia Update

The incidence of unexpected MHC reported in surgical populations ranges from 1:5,000 to 1:50,000 patients.[3] MHC can follow anesthetic exposure to succinylcholine and all of the potent volatile anesthetic agents. It is characterized by accelerating hypermetabolism with mounting fever and evolving multiple organ failure. Clinical signs of MHC are progressive and nonspecific: tachydysrhythmias, tachypnea with hypercapnia, unstable blood pressure, and fever. Laboratory findings of progressive mixed metabolic and respiratory acidosis, hyperkalemia, and rising creatine phosphokinase presage arrhythmias, rhabdomyolysis, disseminated intravascular coagulation, hepatic injury, renal dysfunction, encephalopathy, and death unless recognized promptly and treated. Treatment requires withdrawal of inhalational agents, hyperventilation, treatment of acidosis and hyperkalemia, control of fever, administration of dantrolene sodium, and preventive critical care.[1,4,5] Malignant hyperthermia susceptibility is genetically determined.[6]

Before the introduction of early recognition and treatment protocols, MHC was largely fatal. After widespread educational efforts in the 1970s that highlighted early

suspicion of MHC and expectant management, the fatality rate fell to 60% to 80%. With the introduction of dantrolene sodium and increased awareness of the syndrome in the late 1970s to 1980s, mortality rates fell to very low levels,[3,7,8] but there continue to be perioperative deaths attributed to MHC.[9,10] Since the 1990s, genetics has been an important focus of MH research.[11] A number of genetic variations have been identified in patients who have exhibited MHC in response to anesthetic triggers or demonstrated a phenotypic, positive reaction to the CHCT. Most genotypes are associated with abnormalities in the skeletal muscle ryanodine recepter. Although genetic testing offered the hope for a simple means of establishing which patients are MHS, the genetic background of individuals with phenotypic MH is increasingly complex.[12-17] Indeed, genetic variability, together with the development of isolated mutations, may account for observed variation in clinical presentations and severity of MHC.[18]

Who Is Malignant Hyperthermia Susceptible?

MHC has been observed in very young and elderly patients of both sexes. It is common in patients who have negative histories and uneventful anesthetics.[19] In one report, only 35% to 50% of patients who were MHS developed MHC when exposed to triggering anesthetic agents.[20] Anesthetic agents that trigger MHC are widely used because they are convenient and effective, there is no simple means of establishing MH risk, and MHC is relatively uncommon. Consequently, clinicians must assume that all patients may be MHS. MHC and other hypermetabolic perioperative crises provide a strong rationale for monitoring all anesthesia patients for signs of unexpected hypermetabolism, rigidity, and fever.

Although there is an association between MH and several neuromuscular syndromes,[21-23] there are no physical findings that identify MHS patients.[24] Individuals who have had family members die in the perioperative period of MHC or who, themselves, have had MH-like events often give a suggestive history or identify a family relationship with an MHS patient. When patients report an obvious, well-documented MHC, positive genetic screening, or a strong family history of the MHC, the clinician must be alert to a heightened risk of MHC in the perioperative period and treat the patient as MHS. When a patient provides a history of a suggestive perianesthetic episode without having had a CHCT, most clinicians would assume that the patient is MHS. Some recommend that any patient with a neuromuscular disease be treated as MHS because of a high correlation between CHCT MH and specific neuromuscular diseases such as central core and multi-mini central core disease.[25] Both retrospective and prospective outcome data show that outcome will be optimal for patients who are thought to be MHS when they have anesthesia that is designed to prevent triggering the MHC.

TREATMENT OPTIONS FOR MHS PATIENTS

Anesthesia plans for MHS patients should avoid known triggering agents. These include all the potent, volatile, inhalational anesthetics and the nondepolarizing muscle relaxant succinylcholine. General anesthesia with a "balanced" technique that uses nitrous oxide and intravenous (IV) agents and total intravenous anesthesia (TIVA) with or without nondepolarizing muscle relaxants is considered safe. Regional anesthesia with any technique and any local anesthetic agent is safe. Nitrous oxide analgesia, regional analgesia, and all levels of sedation with any narcotic/sedative/hypnotic combination are acceptable. Nontriggering anesthetics are less likely to evoke MHC, but close monitoring is required because the anesthetic and procedural experience may trigger MHC even when specific triggering agents are not used.

Pretreatment of MHS patients with oral or intravenous dantrolene may prevent or abort the MHC but is no longer recommended.

The ideal anesthetic approach should meet the needs of the patient, surgeon, and anesthesiologist. Unusual techniques that involve rarely used drugs, skills, or equipment are ill advised. Whatever the specific anesthetic chosen, MHC treatment protocols, equipment, and drugs must be available for management of the patient who develops MHC or MH-like reactions during anesthesia and surgery. Procedural facilities or offices that provide anesthesia but do not employ known triggering agents should carefully screen MHS individuals. Rarely, MHS patients may develop MH when stressed, even though triggering agents are not used.[26-28] Evidence for the idea that MHC is a "stress syndrome" is tenuous and the issue is controversial. If a patient presents a history of unstable myopathic syndromes and is MHS, anesthesia care should not be undertaken without preparation because of phenotypic variability and an unknown risk of MH-like symptoms. If the anesthesia provider at an institution does not have access to MH support protocols, trained staff, rapidly available laboratory tests, and resuscitation equipment, the MHS patient should be referred to another institution (Table 39-1).

EVIDENCE

Both experiential and prospective data support these approaches to the MHS patient. Data regarding management of MHS are most often evidentiary or experiential. Important ethical questions limit prospective exposure of

Table 39-1	
Safe Anesthesia for the MHS Patient	**Drug Choices**
Local anesthesia with or without sedation	All local anesthetics
	All sedative/narcotic drugs
General "balanced" anesthesia	Nitrous oxide, nondepolarizing muscle relaxants, opiates, all induction agents, sedatives, TIVA
Regional anesthesia and analgesia with or without sedation	All local anesthetic agents
	All IV/IM sedative, opiate, hypnotic agents

individuals to experimental anesthetic protocols who are thought to be at risk for life-threatening MHC.

Experiential data demonstrate improving outcome following MHC over the past four decades. A historic decrease in death and other morbidity following MHC is likely multifactorial. Improved outcome is attributed to earlier recognition, withdrawal of triggering agents, early use of dantrolene, and supportive care designed to minimize secondary insults associated with MHC, together with attempts to identify MHS patients for receipt of trigger-free anesthetics.[21,29] One retrospective review of outcome from New Zealand reported no deaths associated with MHC over two decades from 1981 to 2001.[8]

In contrast with recent findings reported by Pollock and colleagues,[8] sporadic case reports, court cases, and deaths reported in the press[10] or known to volunteer physician MH Hotline Consultants (MHHLC) in the United States (https://about.mhaus.org/index.cfm/FUSEACTION/Hotline.Home.cfm, Malignant Hyperthermia Association of the United States, Sherbourne, NY) and abroad,[30] confirm the impression of continued perioperative mortality from catastrophic MHC. Legal issues likely prevent or delay scientific reporting of MH deaths. Secondary complications of MHC also may be underreported as demonstrated by sporadic case publications[31] and MHHLC reports.

In the pre-dantrolene era, clinicians were unwilling to provide elective anesthesia for MHS patients, judging the risk of MHC to be too great. No one would undertake a comparison of management approaches involving triggering agents in humans known to be MHS for ethical reasons. Experience with animal models of MHC showed that anesthesia performed without triggering agents was safe. A specific in vivo test for MHS that required muscle biopsy, the CHCT, was developed. Muscle biopsy could be performed in adults with local anesthesia or nerve block. In small children where muscle biopsy for CHCT is not feasible without anesthesia, prospective controlled studies of the best elective anesthetic for the MHS patient were undertaken as the only recourse. Experience with children using nontriggering agents for CHCT muscle biopsy was reported to be safe.[32] These experiences, together with sporadic case reports of successful avoidance of MHC in MHS patients who required urgent anesthesia, provided evidence for a cautious approach to elective surgery for the MHS patient.[26,33,34] Consequently, anesthesia and surgical staff are more willing to undertake both emergency and elective surgery for MHS patients.[35-38]

Additional experiential evidence includes the content of approximately 650 phone calls a year[39] made to volunteer advisory physicians serving as MHHLC, sponsored by the Malignant Hyperthermia Association of the United States (MHAUS, Sherborne, NY, www.mhaus.org), a lay advocacy organization established in 1981, summarized and published quarterly in *The Communicator*, published by MHAUS. MHAUS also provides information on its website and produces a "case of the month" that discusses management of MHC or MH-like events. MHC and MH-like experiences collected as voluntary "Adverse Metabolic Reaction to Anesthesia" reports form the basis of a privacy-protected database, the MH Registry, that was established in 1987 (www.mhreg.org). These growing databases provide retrospective information, but no denominator of MHC and MH-like events experienced by the general population. Nor is there information establishing the frequency of MHS in the general population. Retrospective data provide invaluable insight into MHC management and MH-like episodes that take place in the anesthesia setting.[9,40,41] It has also highlighted key aspects of MHC management. For example, although the average effective dose of dantrolene was approximately 2.5 mg/kg, with MH registry reports of patients requiring as much as 10 mg/kg for control of MHC, occasional case reports illustrated the value of increasing dantrolene doses when the typical ceiling dose of 10 mg/kg has been exceeded.[30] Similarly, case reports of delayed-onset MHC[42] and recurrent MHC have led to evidence-based recommendations by MH hotline consultants for continued therapy of the MHC and at least an hour's observation postoperatively.

Only a small number of prospective studies of management of MHS/MHC patients have been published. These, together with subsequent experience, add a higher level of evidence-based support for current management strategies. The multicenter, U.S. Food and Drug Administration (FDA)–approved, dantrolene trial, published in 1982,[43,44] demonstrated that dantrolene sodium was effective in treating MHC, provided it was recognized and treated before sudden death or outcome-limiting organ system injury. In fact, the FDA approved the drug for this purpose in 1979, before formal peer-reviewed publication of outcome data. Subsequent experience with dantrolene after its acceptance as a treatment for MHC[45] allowed prospective studies of muscle biopsy patients using sedation, as well as "trigger-free" general and regional anesthetics, of which the majority were general anesthetics.[19,32]

This prospective evidence, together with published case reports,[46,47] and the accumulated encounters reported to the MH Registry and voluntary physician MHHLC, has changed the anesthetic approach to MHS patients by demonstrating that trigger-free anesthetics are safe. Not only is the frequency of MHC low when patients are given anesthetics that avoid triggering agents, but the outcome of MHC in this population, when it occurs and is managed in a prepared setting, is better than that following unexpected MHC in other environments.

AREAS OF UNCERTAINTY

Dantrolene Pretreatment

Initial recommendations included preoperative pretreatment with dantrolene.[26] Subsequently, clinical experience with MHS patients,[32] side effects of dantrolene,[48] a small number of complications after oral dantrolene therapy,[49] and the ability to measure serum dantrolene levels,[50] with Flewellen's demonstration that effective serum dantrolene levels can be achieved after acute IV loading,[51] supported a rationale for eliminating routine pretreatment of MHS patients by loading oral dantrolene before anesthesia.[52] IV dantrolene treatment was extended to children after demonstration of dantrolene pharmacokinetics in that population.[53] Also, intermittent IV dantrolene injections and/or maintenance IV infusions for continuing MH suppression after the crisis have been based on necessity during case experience. Evolving practice has been tested by experience, although not in controlled, prospectively blinded trials. Dantrolene pretreatment is no longer recommended for MHS patients having elective surgery with trigger-free anesthetics.

There are unusual patients whose underlying muscle disease is so symptomatic that they take oral dantrolene when stressed in daily life outside of the anesthesia setting.[27,54] This, together with pathologic similarity between MHC and heat stroke fatality, has raised the question of whether heat stroke is a variant, or more common, in MHS.[55-58] Stress-induced MHC may be associated with unknown myopathy or may occur only in a unique genetic subset of MHS patients. Data repositories are inadequate to guide the practitioner, but it would seem prudent to give dantrolene preoperatively and for some time postoperatively to very symptomatic patients who have myopathic, MH-like symptoms with stress and exercise.

Masseter Muscle Rigidity Is MHC Until Proven Otherwise?

Masseter muscle spasm or rigidity (MMR) in response to depolarizing muscle relaxants[59] and/or MH triggering agents has been identified as an early clinical sign of MHC[60,61] and/or a myotonic reaction[62,63] commonly followed by elevated muscle enzymes, hyperkalemia, dysrhythmias, and metabolic acidosis. The relationship between MMR and both acute myopathic response and MHC argued for a conservative approach to MMR.[64] It is recommended that triggering agents and anesthesia be discontinued after observation of MMR while possible causes for MMR are evaluated.[65] CHCT examination of adults who had various myopathies subsequently demonstrated a high incidence of MH-positive and MH-equivocal contracture responses.[66] The extent to which the myopathic response to anesthetic agents resembles the MHC is further confused by the fact that MH CHCT is probably less specific in these patients.[25] This supported a clinical impression that various myopathies, in addition to MH, may manifest with MMR or muscle injury following anesthetic induction with MH-triggering agents.

The recognition of sudden cardiac arrest and rhabdomyolysis following succinylcholine administration to male infants and children amplified recognition of the risk, whether the etiology was the same or not.[67] Cardiac arrest and dysrhythmias following triggering agents that are seen during myotonic reactions are caused by acute hyperkalemia, myopathic muscle responses, or both.[68] Subsequently, case reports[69] and retrospective reviews[70,71] of MMR following succinylcholine in children without either severe myotonic reactions or MHC generated controversy. Is MMR observed during anesthesia in children or adults a normal variant of the succinylcholine response, or is it a high-probability sign of significant muscle injury associated with potentially lethal MHC or myotonic crisis?

It has long been known that adults and children who receive succinylcholine develop creatine phosphokinase (CK) elevation and myoglobinuria.[72,73] One prospective study of 500 children has shown a low incidence of MMR and, more commonly, incomplete jaw relaxation following halothane anesthesia and succinylcholine.[74] In a prospective study of more than 5000 children who had succinylcholine or a nondepolarizing relaxant following an induction and intubation technique with or without inhalational halothane,[75] it was evident that the inhalational agent was associated with MMR. Of note, although the MHC did not occur, 3 of 600 (0.5%) patients developed MMR after paralysis for intubation following a technique that used halothane before intubation. Two of these had MMR with large CK enzyme increases following halothane and thiopental with nondepolarizing relaxants. Therefore MMR is not simply a normal variant of the succinylcholine response in children, and also is seen during administration of inhalational agents and nondepolarizing muscle relaxants.

The incidence of MH and sudden death following MMR is not as high as initially thought, but the implications of MMR are clear—a significant percentage of those who demonstrate MMR have rhabdomyolysis associated with an unknown myopathy that should be evaluated. Young boys with unrecognized muscular dystrophy, in particular, are at risk for hyperkalemia that could cause death or significantly complicate anesthesia and surgical care. Whether unrecognized myopathy or dystrophinopathy is the cause or not, MMR is often associated with significant muscle injury and the risk of concomitant secondary insults associated with rhabdomyolysis—hyperkalemic dysrhythmia, myalgias, peripheral compartment syndrome and limb compromise, renal failure, and sudden death.

Although the subsequent anesthetic course may appear benign, MMR may be associated with rhabdomyolysis and the aforementioned associated insults. The incidence may vary with population, but MMR is abnormal. MMR signals a need for careful monitoring of cardiorespiratory and metabolic parameters, urine testing for myoglobin, blood testing for electrolytes, CK measurement, and, possibly, arterial blood gases. MMR associated with MHC or a severe myopathic response may require withdrawal of triggering anesthetic agents, together with aggressive critical care management. It may be necessary to abort surgery. Clinical MMR should be investigated whenever it is observed.

The Pregnant MHS Patient

Aside from the recommendation that pregnant patients who are MHS should have a trigger-free anesthetic, whether regional or general, no one has specific data on risk to the fetus. Nor is there any evidence regarding safe maternal anesthesia when the infant in utero is MHS and the mother is not. The topic of infant exposure to maternally administered dantrolene has been raised,[76] but withholding dantrolene treatment of the MHC during cesarean section or other maternal surgery has not been recommended.[77] No dantrolene side effect other than uterine atony following cesarean section has been reported.[78,79] Collected case reports and inferential reasoning provide our only source of guidance.[77,80-83] Newborn MHC has been suspected but not definitively confirmed,[84] although MH has been sporadically reported in infants from 7 days to 6 months old.[85-89]

The MHS parturient should be given appropriate regional analgesia when needed. She should have operative procedures under trigger-free anesthetic techiques. Dantrolene prophylaxis is not indicated, but it should not be witheld in acute MHC for fear of fetal compromise or maternal complications.

AUTHOR'S RECOMMENDATIONS

- Elicit a patient history of neuromuscular disease, MHS, MH-like family or personal events, or hyperthermic demise associated with anesthesia.
- Assume patients with suggestive history to be MHS.
- Inform patient of MHS concerns.
- Plan anesthesia with nontriggering agents.
- Preoperative dantrolene prophylaxis is generally not necessary.
- Avoid unfamiliar drugs or techniques.
- Have recommended supply of dantrolene and MH kit available.
- Ensure facility and clinical support sufficient to treat the MHC.
- Monitor MHS or suspect MHS patients more closely for signs of MHC.
- Treat suspicious episodes promptly with dantrolene and supportive care.
- Assume that MMR is associated with MH, dystrorhinopathy, or other cause of critical rhabdomyolysis and monitor carefully.

REFERENCES

1. Denborough MA: Malignant hyperpyrexia. *Compr Ther* 1975;1 (8):51-56.
2. Girard T, Treves S, et al: Molecular genetic testing for malignant hyperthermia susceptibility. *Anesthesiology* 2004;100(5):1076-1080.
3. Rosenberg H, Davis M, et al: Malignant hyperthermia. *Orphanet J Rare Dis* 2007;2:21.
4. King JO, Denborough MA: Malignant hyperpyrexia in Australia and New Zealand. *Med J Aust* 1973;1(11):525-528.
5. Strazis KP, Fox AW: Malignant hyperthermia: A review of published cases. *Anesth Analg* 1993;77(2):297-304.
6. Barlow MB, Isaacs H: Malignant hyperpyrexial deaths in a family. Reports of three cases. *Br J Anaesth* 1970;42(12):1072-1076.
7. Rosenberg H, Fletcher JE: An update on the malignant hyperthermia syndrome. *Ann Acad Med Singapore* 1994;23(6 suppl):84-97.
8. Pollock AN, Langton EE, et al: Suspected malignant hyperthermia reactions in New Zealand. *Anesth Intensive Care* 2002;30(4): 453-461.

9. Larach MG, Brandom BW, et al: Cardiac arrests and deaths associated with malignant hyperthermia in North America from 1987 to 2006—a report from the North American malignant hyperthermia registry of the malignant hyperthermia association of the United States. *Anesthesiology* 2008;108(4):603-611.
10. Sarmiento G: Autopsy confirms Boca Raton cheerleader died of rare genetic ailment. *Palm Beach Post*, May 30, 2008.
11. MacLennan DH: The genetic basis of malignant hyperthermia. *Trends Pharmacol Sci* 1992;13(8):330-334.
12. Allen GC: Malignant hyperthermia and associated disorders. *Curr Opin Rheumatol* 1993;5(6):719-724.
13. Hopkins PM: Malignant hyperthermia: Advances in clinical management and diagnosis. *Br J Anaesth* 2000;85(1):118-128.
14. Girard T, Treves S, et al: Phenotype/genotype presentation of malignant hyperthermia. *Anesthesiology* 2001;95(10S):A-1175.
15. Robinson RL, Anetseder MJ, et al: Recent advances in the diagnosis of malignant hyperthermia susceptibility: How confident can we be of genetic testing? *Eur J Hum Genet* 2003;11(4):342-348.
16. Monnier N, Kozak-Ribbens G, et al: Correlations between genotype and pharmacological, histological, functional, and clinical phenotypes in malignant hyperthermia susceptibility. *Human Mutation* 2005;26(5):413-425.
17. Anderson AA, Brown RL, et al: Identification and biochemical characterization of a novel ryanodine receptor gene mutation associated with malignant hyperthermia. *Anesthesiology* 2008;108(2):208-215.
18. Fiege M, Wappler F, et al: Results of contracture tests with halothane, caffeine, and ryanodine depend on different malignant hyperthermia-associated ryanodine receptor gene mutations. *Anesthesiology* 2002;97(2):345-350.
19. Carr AS, Cunliffe M, et al: Incidence of malignant hyperthermia reactions in 2,214 patients undergoing muscle biopsy. *Can J Anaesth* 1995;42(4):281-286.
20. Bendixen D, Skovgaard LT, et al: Analysis of anaesthesia in patients suspected to be susceptible to malignant hyperthermia before diagnostic in vitro contracture test. *Acta Anaesthesiol Scand* 1997;41(4):480-484.
21. Britt BA: Preanesthetic diagnosis of malignant hyperthermia. *Int Anesthesiol Clin* 1979;17(4):63-96.
22. Deufel T, Muller-Felber W, et al: Chronic myopathy in a patient suspected of carrying two malignant hyperthermia susceptibility (MHS) mutations. *Neuromuscul Disord* 1992;2(5-6):389-396.
23. Brandt A, Schleithoff L, et al: Screening of the ryanodine receptor gene in 105 malignant hyperthermia families: Novel mutations and concordance with the in vitro contracture test. *Hum Mol Genet* 1999;8(11):2055-2062.
24. Ranklev E, Henriksson KG, et al: Clinical and muscle biopsy findings in malignant hyperthermia susceptibility. *Acta Neurol Scand* 1986;74(4):452-459.
25. Wappler F, Scholz J, et al: [Incidence of disposition for malignant hyperthermia in patients with neuromuscular diseases]. *Anasthesiol Intensivmed Notfallmed Schmerzther* 1998;33(6):373-380.
26. Gronert GA: Malignant hyperthermia. *Anesthesiology* 1980;53(5):395-423.
27. Gronert GA: Dantrolene in malignant hyperthermia (MH)-susceptible patients with exaggerated exercise stress. *Anesthesiology* 2000;93(3):905.
28. Wappler F, Fiege M, et al: Evidence for susceptibility to malignant hyperthermia in patients with exercise-induced rhabdomyolysis. *Anesthesiology* 2001;94(1):95-100.
29. Britt B: Management of malignant hyperthermia susceptible patients—a review. In *Malignant hyperthermia current concepts*. New York, Appleton-Century-Crofts, 1977, pp 63-76.
30. Blank JW, Boggs SD: Successful treatment of an episode of malignant hyperthermia using a large dose of dantrolene. *J Clin Anesth* 1993;5(1):69-72.
31. Burns AP, Hopkins PM, et al: Rhabdomyolysis and acute renal failure in unsuspected malignant hyperpyrexia. *Q J Med* 1993;86(7):431-434.
32. Dubrow TJ, Wackym PA, et al: Malignant hyperthermia: Experience in the prospective management of eight children. *J Pediatr Surg* 1989;24(2):163-166.
33. Byrick RJ, Rose DK, et al: Management of a malignant hyperthermia patient during cardiopulmonary bypass. *Can Anaesth Soc J* 1982;29(1):50-54.
34. Ording H, Hedengran AM, et al: Evaluation of 119 anaesthetics received after investigation for susceptibility to malignant hyperthermia. *Acta Anaesthesiol Scand* 1991;35(8):711-716.
35. Relton JE: Anesthesia for elective surgery in patients susceptible to malignant hyperthermia. *Int Anesthesiol Clin* 1979;17(4):141-151.
36. Jantzen JP, Erdmann K, et al: Malignant hyperthermia susceptibility—successful management with a stressfree technique. *Acta Anaesthesiol Belg* 1987;38(1):107-113.
37. Dershwitz M, Ryan JF, et al: Safety of amide local anesthetics in patients susceptible to malignant hyperthermia. *J Am Dent Assoc* 1989;118(3):276-278, 280.
38. Derkay CS, Grundfast KM: Management of otolaryngic patients susceptible to malignant hyperthermia without dantrolene. *Otolaryngol Head Neck Surg* 1991;105(5):680-686.
39. O'Flynn RP, Shutack JG, et al: Masseter muscle rigidity and malignant hyperthermia susceptibility in pediatric patients: An update on management and diagnosis. *Anesthesiology* 1994;80(6):1228-1229.
40. Landro L: A fresh focus on a rare risk of anesthesia. *Wall Street Journal*, April 30, 2008, p D1.
41. Allen GC, Larach MG, et al: The sensitivity and specificity of the caffeine-halothane contracture test: A report from the North American Malignant Hyperthermia Registry. The North American Malignant Hyperthermia Registry of MHAUS. *Anesthesiology* 1998;88(3):579-588.
42. Souliere CR Jr, Weintraub SJ, et al: Markedly delayed postoperative malignant hyperthermia. *Arch Otolaryngol Head Neck Surg* 1986;112(5):564-566.
43. Forrest WH, Jr: A collaborative clinical trial on trial. *Anesthesiology* 1982;56(4):249-250.
44. Kolb ME, Horn ML, et al: Dantrolene in human malignant hyperthermia, a multicenter study. *Anesthesiology* 1982;56:254-262.
45. Bronstein SL, Ryan DE, et al: Dantrolene sodium in the management of patients at risk from malignant hyperthermia. *J Oral Surg* 1979;37(10):719-724.
46. Bracali AM, Sette MP, et al: Risk and choice of anesthetics for patients with previous malignant hyperthermia syndrome. *Minerva Anestesiol* 1979;45(10):749-753.
47. Wagner W, Feldmann E: Malignant hyperthermia—therapy results with dantrolene. A case report. *Anasth Intensivther Notfallmed* 1983;18(5):270-271.
48. Wedel DJ, Quinlan JG, et al: Clinical effects of intravenously administered dantrolene. *Mayo Clin Proc* 1995;70(3):241-246.
49. Watson CB, Reierson N, et al: Clinically significant muscle weakness induced by dantrolene sodium prophylaxis for malignant hyperthermia. *Anesthesiology* 1986;65:312-314.
50. Wuis EW, Driessen JJ, et al: Dantrolene plasma and urine concentrations after oral pretreatment for malignant hyperthermia: Report of a case. *Eur J Anaesthesiol* 1986;3(3):219-223.
51. Flewellen EH, Nelson TE, et al: Dantrolene dose response in awake man: Implications for management of malignant hyperthermia. *Anesthesiology* 1983;59(4):275-280.
52. Mauritz W, Hackl W, et al: Malignant hyperthermia in Austria. III. Anesthesia in susceptible patients. *Anaesthesist* 1988;37(8):522-528.
53. Lerman J, McLeod ME, et al: Pharmacokinetics of intravenous dantrolene in children. *Anesthesiology* 1989;70(4):625-629.
54. Gronert GA, Thompson RL, et al: Human malignant hyperthermia: Awake episodes and correction by dantrolene. *Anesth Analg* 1980;59(5):377-378.
55. Denborough MA: Heat stroke and malignant hyperpyrexia. *Med J Aust* 1982;1(5):204-205.
56. Figarella-Branger D, Kozak-Ribbens G, et al: Pathological findings in 165 patients explored for malignant hyperthermia susceptibility. *Neuromuscul Disord* 1993;3(5-6):553-556.
57. Ali SZ, Taguchi A, et al: Malignant hyperthermia. *Best Pract Res Clin Anaesthesiol* 2003;17(4):519-533.
58. Wappler F: Is there a link between malignant hyperthermia and exertional heat illness? Commentary. *Br J Sports Med* 2007;41(5):284.
59. Cornet C, Moeller R, et al: Clinical features of malignant hyperthermia crisis. *Ann Fr Anesth Reanim* 1989;8(5):435-443.
60. Flewellen EH, Nelson TE: Halothane-succinylcholine induced masseter spasm: Indicative of malignant hyperthermia susceptibility? *Anesth Analg* 1984;63(7):693-697.

61. Ramirez JA, Cheetham ED, et al: Suxamethonium, masseter spasm and later malignant hyperthermia. *Anaesthesia* 1998;53(11):1111-1116.
62. Gronert GA: Myotonias and masseter spasm: Not malignant hyperthermia? *Anesthesiology* 1995;83(6):1382-1383.
63. Habre W, Sims C: Masseter spasm and elevated creatine kinase after intravenous induction in a child. *Anaesth Intensive Care* 1996;24(4):496-499.
64. Rosenberg H: Trismus is not trivial. *Anesthesiology* 1987;67(4):453-455.
65. Rosenbaum HK, Miller JD: Malignant hyperthermia and myotonic disorders. *Anesthesiol Clin North Am* 2002;20(3):623-664.
66. Heytens L, Martin JJ, et al: In vitro contracture tests in patients with various neuromuscular diseases. *Br J Anaesth* 1992;68(1):72-75.
67. Larach MG, Rosenberg H, et al: Hyperkalemic cardiac arrest during anesthesia in infants and children with occult myopathies. *Clin Pediatr (Phila)* 1997;36(1):9-16.
68. Sullivan M, Thompson WK, et al: Succinylcholine-induced cardiac arrest in children with undiagnosed myopathy. *Can J Anaesth* 1994;41(6):497-501.
69. Kaplan RF, Rushing E: Isolated masseter muscle spasm and increased creatine kinase without malignant hyperthermia susceptibility or other myopathies. *Anesthesiology* 1992;77(4):820-822.
70. Littleford JA, Patel LR, et al: Masseter muscle spasm in children: Implications of continuing the triggering anesthetic. *Anesth Analg* 1991;72(2):151-160.
71. Kosko JR, Brandom BW, et al: Masseter spasm and malignant hyperthermia: A retrospective review of a hospital-based pediatric otolaryngology practice. *Int J Pediatr Otorhinolaryngol* 1992;23(1):45-50.
72. Airaksinen MM, Tammisto T: Myoglobinuria after intermittent admistration of succinylcholine during halothane anesthesia. *Clin Pharmacol Ther* 1966;7(5):583-587.
73. Thomas ET, Dobkin AB: Untoward effects of muscle relaxant drugs. *Int Anesthesiol Clin* 1972;10(1):207-225.
74. Hannallah RS, Kaplan RF: Jaw relaxation after a halothane/succinylcholine sequence in children. *Anesthesiology* 1994;81(1):99-103, discussion 28A.
75. Lazzell VA, Carr AS, et al: The incidence of masseter muscle rigidity after succinylcholine in infants and children. *Can J Anaesth* 1994;41(6):475-479.
76. Fricker RM, Hoerauf KH, et al: Secretion of dantrolene into breast milk after acute therapy of a suspected malignant hyperthermia crisis during cesarean section. *Anesthesiology* 1998;89(4):1023-1025.
77. Douglas MJ, McMorland GH: The anaesthetic management of the malignant hyperthermia susceptible parturient. *Can Anaesth Soc J* 1986;33(3 pt 1):371-378.
78. Weingarten AE, Korsh JI, et al: Postpartum uterine atony after intravenous dantrolene. *Anesth Analg* 1987;66(3):269-270.
79. Houvenaeghel M, Achilli-Cornesse E, et al: [Oral dantrolene in a parturient with myotonic dystrophy and susceptibility to malignant hyperthermia]. *Ann Fr Anesth Reanim* 1988;7(5):408-411.
80. Kaplan RF, Kellner KR: More on malignant hyperthermia during delivery. *Am J Obstet Gynecol* 1985;152(5):608-609.
81. Sorosky JI, Ingardia CJ, et al: Diagnosis and management of susceptibility to malignant hyperthermia in pregnancy. *Am J Perinatol* 1989;6(1):46-48.
82. Lucy SJ: Anaesthesia for caesarean delivery of a malignant hyperthermia susceptible parturient. *Can J Anaesth* 1994;41(12):1220-1226.
83. Foster RN, Boothroyd KP: Caesarean section in a complicated case of central core disease. *Anaesthesia* 2008;63(5):544-547.
84. Sewall K, Flowerdew RM, et al: Severe muscular rigidity at birth: Malignant hyperthermia syndrome? *Can Anaesth Soc J* 1980;27(3):279-282.
85. Mayhew JF, Rudolph J, et al: Malignant hyperthermia in a six-month old infant: A case report. *Anesth Analg* 1978;57(2):262-264.
86. Bailey AG, Bloch EC: Malignant hyperthermia in a three-month-old American Indian infant. *Anesth Analg* 1987;66(10):1043-1045.
87. Puschel K, Koops E, et al: [Postoperative malignant hyperthermia in a 7-day-old infant?] *Anaesthesist* 1989;38(2):81-84.
88. Wilhoit RD, Brown RE Jr, et al: Possible malignant hyperthermia in a 7-week-old infant. *Anesth Analg* 1989;68(5):688-691.
89. Chamley D, Pollock NA, et al: Malignant hyperthermia in infancy and identification of novel RYR1 mutation. *Br J Anaesth* 2000;84(4):500-504.

40 What Is the Best Strategy to Prevent Postoperative Nausea and Vomiting?

Ashraf S. Habib, MBBCh, MSc, FRCA, and Tong J. Gan, MBBS, FRCA, FFARCSI

INTRODUCTION

Postoperative nausea and vomiting (PONV) are among the most common side effects associated with anesthesia and surgery. Currently, the overall incidence of PONV for all surgeries and patient populations is estimated to be 25% to 30%.[1] Furthermore, it is estimated that approximately 0.18% of all patients may experience intractable PONV, leading to a delay in postanesthesia care unit (PACU) discharge or unanticipated hospital admission, thereby increasing medical costs.[2] Symptoms of PONV are also among the most unpleasant experiences associated with surgery and one of the most common reasons for poor patient satisfaction rating in the postoperative period.[3] In one survey, surgical patients were willing to pay up to $100 to avoid PONV.[4]

Because, overall, only 25% to 30% of the surgical patient population will experience PONV, not all patients will require antiemetic prophylaxis. Identification of patients at high risk for PONV is therefore important. Anesthesia-, patient-, and surgery-related risk factors have been identified (Table 40-1).[5] Apfel and colleagues[6] developed a simplified risk score consisting of four predictors: female gender, history of motion sickness or PONV, nonsmoking status, and the use of opioids for postoperative analgesia. If none, one, two, three, or four of these risk factors were present, the incidences of PONV were 10%, 21%, 39%, 61%, and 79%, respectively.[6]

THERAPIES

Pharmacologic Agents

Pharmacologic agents available for the prevention of PONV can be summarized as follows:

- Conventional antiemetics:
  - Dopamine (D_2) receptor antagonists: phenothiazines (e.g., promethazine, prochlorperazine), butyrophenones (e.g., droperidol, haloperidol), benzamides (e.g., metoclopramide)
  - Antihistamines (e.g., dimenhydrinate, cyclizine)
  - Anticholinergics (e.g., scopolamine)
  - Serotonin receptor antagonists (e.g., ondansetron, dolasetron, granisetron)
  - Neurokinin-1 receptor antagonists (e.g., Aprepitant)
- Nonconventional antiemetics:
  - Steroids, propofol
- Other therapies shown to be of benefit:
  - Benzodiazepines,[7,8] ephedrine,[9,10] aggressive intravenous hydration[11]

Nonpharmacologic Techniques

Nonpharmacologic techniques include acupuncture, acupressure, electroacupuncture, transcutaneous acupoint electrical stimulation, laser to the P6 pressure point, and hypnosis.[12]

EVIDENCE

There are hundreds of published randomized controlled trials investigating the efficacy of different antiemetic interventions. This plethora of data has resulted in a number of systematic reviews being published in this area. Although systematic reviews are a powerful tool to further our understanding of the efficacy of interventions and likelihood for harm when there are data from many small trials,[13] they are not a substitute for a well-conducted, large, randomized controlled trial. In this chapter, we will base the evidence reported on the results of randomized controlled trials and systematic reviews. Four issues will be addressed in providing evidence for the best strategy to prevent PONV:

1. Evidence for selecting a single antiemetic.
2. Is combination antiemetic therapy better than monotherapy?
3. What is the best available combination of antiemetics?
4. Evidence for using a multimodal approach to prevent PONV.

Evidence for Selecting a Single Antiemetic

There are at least five major receptor systems involved in the etiology of PONV: dopaminergic (D_2), cholinergic (muscarinic), histaminergic (H_1), serotonergic ($5\text{-}HT_3$),

269

Table 40-1	**Risk Factors for PONV**	
Anesthetic Factors	**Patient Factors**	**Surgical Factors**
1. Volatile agents 2. Nitrous oxide 3. Opioids 4. High doses of neostigmine	1. Female gender 2. History of PONV or motion sickness 3. Pain 4. High levels of anxiety	1. Long surgical procedures 2. Certain types of surgery (e.g., intra-abdominal, major gynecologic, laparoscopic, breast, ears/nose/throat, strabismus

and the neurokinin-1 (NK-1) receptors. Traditionally, antagonists at these receptors have been the mainstay of PONV management. Metoclopramide and droperidol are the most commonly studied dopamine receptor antagonists. Although metoclopramide has prokinetic effects, its antiemetic efficacy is uncertain, with approximately 50% of studies showing it to be no more effective than placebo when used in a dose of 10 mg.[14] Two recent studies, however, suggested that higher doses of metoclopramide (20 to 50 mg) might be efficacious.[15,16] Droperidol, on the other hand, has been shown to be an effective antiemetic and was widely used. In a meta-analysis of randomized controlled trials involving droperidol, the number needed to treat (NNT) was found to be 5 to 7.[17] However, following the Food and Drug Administration (FDA) black box warning on droperidol, there has been a significant decline in the use of this cost-effective agent.[18] Recently, some studies suggested that haloperidol 1 to 2 mg IV might be a suitable alternative.[19,20]

The 5-HT$_3$ receptor antagonists are highly specific and selective for nausea and vomiting. Their antivomiting efficacy is better than their antinausea efficacy.[21] Members of this group exert their effects by binding to the 5-HT$_3$ receptor in the chemoreceptor trigger zone and at vagal afferents in the gastrointestinal tract. Their favorable side-effect profile, particularly the lack of sedation, makes them particularly popular and suitable for ambulatory surgery. Currently available 5HT$_3$ receptor antagonists include ondansetron, granisetron, and dolasetron. There is no evidence that there is any difference in efficacy or side-effect profile between the various 5-HT$_3$ receptor antagonists, when appropriate doses are used for the management of PONV. Therefore acquisition cost is the main factor that differentiates the 5-HT$_3$ compounds from one another.[22] It is of note that ondansetron, the most commonly studied agent in this group, has recently become generic. The NNT for the prevention of PONV with ondansetron is 5 to 6.[21] Palonosetron is a new 5-HT$_3$ receptor antagonist that is currently being investigated for the prophylaxis of PONV. It has a unique pharmacokinetic profile with a duration of action of up to 72 hours. In two recent multicenter studies, a dose of 0.075 mg IV reduced the incidence of nausea and vomiting for up to 3 days after surgery.[23,24]

Dexamethasone has also proved to be an effective antiemetic. In a meta-analysis of 17 studies (1946 patients), dexamethasone was reported to be especially effective against late PONV. Using 8 or 10 mg IV in adults (1 or 1.5 mg/kg IV in children), the NNT to prevent early and

late vomiting compared with placebo was 7.1 and 3.8, respectively. In adults, the NNT to prevent late nausea was 4.3. There were no reports of dexamethasone-related side effects when used as a single dose for PONV prophylaxis.[25] More recently, smaller doses (4 mg) of dexamethasone also proved to be effective for PONV prophylaxis.[26]

In a large multicenter study involving patients having at least a 40% risk of PONV, ondansetron 4 mg, droperidol 1.25 mg, and dexamethasone 4 mg were reported to produce a similar reduction in the incidence of PONV of about 26%.[26] Any of these antiemetics could therefore be recommended for use as a first-line agent.

Scopolamine (hyoscine) is an anticholinergic agent that was widely used with opioid premedication.[27,28] Transdermal scopolamine was shown to be effective in controlling PONV following outpatient laparoscopy[29] and following neuraxial morphine administration.[30-32] There has recently been a renewed interest in this transdermal preparation, with one study reporting similar efficacy to ondansetron 4 mg and droperidol 1.25 mg.[33] The number needed to harm (NNH) for the most commonly reported side effects with scopolamine was 5.6 for dry mouth, 12.5 for visual disturbances, 50 for dizziness, and 100 for agitation.[34]

The antihistamines include the ethanolamines (dimenhydrinate, diphenhydramine) and the piperazines (cyclizine, hydroxyzine, meclizine). Their major disadvantages are sedation, dry mouth, blurred vision, urinary retention, and delayed recovery room discharge.[35] Promethazine is an effective antiemetic with a long duration of action. In a dose of 12.5 to 25 mg given toward the end of surgery, it has been shown to be effective for PONV management.[36] Its use, however, is limited by sedation and prolonged recovery from anesthesia.[5] One study did not show increased awakening time or duration of PACU stay when compared with ondansetron and placebo in patients undergoing middle ear surgery.[36] Recently, the use of low-dose promethazine (6.25 mg) was shown to be as effective as higher doses and might be associated with less sedation.[37-39] Another antihistamine, dimenhydrinate, appears to be effective in a recent meta-analysis.[40]

The neurokinin-1 (NK-1) receptor antagonists belong to a new class of antiemetics that may act on the final common pathway from the emetic center. In a recent multicenter study, oral aprepitant was compared with IV ondansetron in females undergoing abdominal surgery. The incidence of no vomiting (0 to 24 hours) was significantly higher with aprepitant 40 mg (90%) and aprepitant 125 mg (95%) versus ondansetron (74%) ($p < 0.001$ for both comparisons). Both aprepitant doses also had higher incidences of no vomiting over 0 to 48 hours ($p < 0.001$). Nausea incidence and severity and the need for rescue antiemetics were not different, however, across the three groups.[41] The results were reproduced in another large study. The severity of nausea was also lower with aprepitant in this second study.[42] The 40-mg dose of aprepitant was approved for the prophylaxis of PONV.

Total intravenous anesthesia (TIVA) using propofol has also been shown to reduce the incidence of PONV and to be as efficacious as ondansetron 4 mg in reducing postoperative nausea.[43,44] The protective effect of propofol against PONV was not evident when it was used as an induction agent only.[45] A dose-response relationship of propofol for improvement of nausea has also been established.[46]

In 1999, Lee and Done[47] performed a meta-analysis to assess the efficacy of nonpharmacologic techniques (acupuncture) for the prevention of PONV. There was a significant reduction in early PONV in adults using nonpharmacologic methods compared with placebo, and these were comparable to conventional antiemetics (metoclopramide, cyclizine, droperidol, prochlorperazine) in preventing early or late PONV in adults.[47] Transcutaneous acupoint electrical stimulation was also comparable with ondansetron for the prophylaxis and treatment of PONV in a number of more recent studies.[48-50] This modality was particularly effective for the prophylaxis against nausea.[48,51] The benefits and side effects of the main classes of agents used for the prophylaxis of PONV are summarized in Table 40-2.

Is Combination Antiemetic Therapy Better Than Monotherapy?

Because PONV is multifactorial, and there are a number of receptors involved in the pathogenesis of PONV, there has been a growing interest in investigating the efficacy of combining antiemetics targeting different receptors in the emetic pathway. Numerous randomized controlled trials compared combination versus single-agent antiemetic prophylaxis.[52] The combinations of one of the 5-HT$_3$ receptor antagonists with droperidol, dexamethasone, or metoclopramide were

Table 40-2   Benefits and Side Effects of the Main Classes of Agents Used for PONV Prophylaxis

Class of Antiemetics	Benefits	Side Effects
Dopamine receptor antagonists:		
• Phenothiazines (e.g., promethazine, prochlorperazine)	Long duration of action	Sedation, extrapyramidal side effects, hypotension, restlessness, anticholinergic syndrome
• Buterophenones (e.g., droperidol, haloperidol)	Improved prophylaxis against nausea	Sedation with high doses, hypotension, extrapyramidal side effects, neuroleptic malignant syndrome, droperidol has an FDA black box warning regarding prolongation of QTc, although the risk is considered minimal with antiemetic doses
• Benzamides (e.g., metoclopramide)	Have prokinetic effects	Sedation, restlessness, extrapyramidal side effects
Anticholinergics (e.g., scopolamine)	Effective against motion sickness Transdermal preparation with a long duration of action available	Sedation, blurred vision, dry mouth, restlessness, central cholinergic syndrome
Antihistamines (e.g., dimenhydrinate, cyclizine)	Effective against motion sickness Effective for PONV following middle ear surgery	Sedation, dry mouth, restlessness
5-HT$_3$ receptor antagonists (e.g., ondansetron, dolasetron, granisetron)	Specific for PONV Do not have sedative side effects	Headache, constipation, elevated liver enzymes
NK-1 receptor antagonists (e.g., aprepitant)	Long duration of action Improved efficacy against vomiting Do not have sedative side effects	Headache, constipation
Corticosteroids (e.g., dexamethasone)	Do not have sedative side effects Long duration of action	No data available regarding side effects following single dose for PONV prophylaxis
Acupuncture (P6 stimulation)	Improved efficacy against nausea	None reported when used for PONV prophylaxis

the most commonly studied. With the exception of combinations involving metoclopramide, the majority of these studies have reported improved antiemetic prophylaxis with combination compared with monotherapy.[53] Meta-analyses and a large multicenter study involving over 5000 patients confirmed the superiority of combination antiemetic prophylaxis compared with monotherapy.[25,26,54] Because the efficacy of antiemetics depends on the patients' underlying baseline risk, patients with moderate to high risk for PONV derive most benefit from receiving a combination of antiemetics.[26]

What Is the Best Available Antiemetic Combination?

There are few data directly comparing the efficacy of different antiemetic combinations. A meta-analysis suggested that there was no difference in antiemetic efficacy or side-effect profile between the combination of the 5-HT_3 receptor antagonists with droperidol, and their combination with dexamethasone.[54] These findings were subsequently confirmed in a large multicenter study that reported that there were no differences in antiemetic efficacy between the combination of ondansetron with droperidol, ondansetron with dexamethasone, and droperidol with dexamethasone.[26]

Evidence for Using a Multimodal Approach to Prevent PONV

Because the etiology of PONV is multifactorial, a multimodal approach may be the best strategy to successfully reduce the incidence, particularly in high-risk patients. Scuderi and colleagues[55] investigated a multimodal approach to the management of PONV in female patients undergoing outpatient laparoscopy. Their multimodal algorithm consisted of total intravenous anesthesia with propofol and remifentanil, no nitrous oxide, no neuromuscular blockade, aggressive intravenous hydration, triple prophylactic antiemetics (ondansetron 1 mg, droperidol 0.625 mg, and dexamethasone 10 mg), and ketorolac 30 mg. Control groups included standard balanced outpatient anesthetic with or without 4 mg ondansetron prophylaxis. Multimodal management resulted in a 98% complete response rate (no vomiting and no antiemetic rescue) in PACU. No patient in the multimodal group vomited before discharge, compared with 7% of patients in the ondansetron group ($p = 0.07$) and 22% of patients in the placebo group ($p = 0.0003$).[55]

Habib and colleagues[56] also found that a triple antiemetic combination with ondansetron and droperidol in the presence of propofol maintained anesthetic, was associated with a lower incidence of PONV, and was associated with greater patient satisfaction compared with a similar antiemetic combination with an isoflurane-based anesthetic.

In a large prospective study, Apfel and colleagues[26] evaluated three antiemetic interventions (ondansetron 4 mg, droperidol 1.25 mg, and dexamethasone 4 mg) and three anesthetic interventions (TIVA with propofol, omitting nitrous oxide, and substituting remifentanil for fentanyl) for the prophylaxis of PONV. The authors employed a multifactorial design allowing them to evaluate the effectiveness of each of the interventions plus all possible combinations of two or three interventions. The resulting data

suggest that antiemetics with different mechanisms of action have additive rather than synergistic effects on the incidence of PONV. Each antiemetic reduced the risk of PONV by about 26%. Using TIVA with propofol rather than a volatile-based anesthetic reduced the risk of PONV by about 19%, whereas avoiding nitrous oxide reduced the risk by about 12%. Substituting remifentanil for fentanyl was of no benefit. When combinations of interventions were used, the benefit of each subsequent intervention was always less than that of the first intervention. They also reported that the efficacy of the interventions depends on the patient's baseline risk; the greatest absolute risk reduction from the antiemetic interventions was achieved in patients with high risk for PONV.[26]

AREAS OF UNCERTAINTY

Droperidol has been used for the management of PONV for over 30 years with an acceptable side-effect profile. In December 2001, the FDA issued a new "black box" warning on droperidol, noting that its use has been associated with QTc-segment prolongation and torsades de pointes, and in some cases resulted in fatal cardiac arrhythmias. Although the package insert of droperidol included a warning about cases of sudden death at high doses greater than 25 mg in patients at risk for cardiac arrhythmias, the FDA noted that there have been cases of serious cardiac arrhythmias and death when droperidol is given at or below the currently labeled dose range and cautioned that droperidol should only be used when other first-line drugs fail. The FDA also recommended that all surgical patients should undergo a 12-lead electrocardiogram (ECG) before administration of droperidol to determine if a prolonged QTc interval is present, and to continue ECG monitoring for 3 hours after its administration.[57] A review of the cases based on which the FDA issued its warning revealed 10 cases where droperidol 1.25 mg or less was used. It was difficult to draw any definitive evidence of a cause-and-effect relationship because of the presence of several confounding factors.[18] Experts in the field, as well as practicing anesthesiologists, believe that this warning is not justified.[58,59]

There have been no reported serious side effects related to the use of a single dose of dexamethasone for PONV prophylaxis. There are, however, some potential concerns. Avascular necrosis of the femoral head (AVN) is a recognized complication of glucocorticoid therapy.[60] There are case reports in which AVN developed following relatively brief courses (7 days) of orally administered steroids.[61-63] It has also been described when dexamethasone was used for antiemetic prophylaxis in chemotherapy.[64] It is not known if a single dose of dexamethasone given for PONV prophylaxis might lead to AVN in a high-risk patient. Other potential side effects of steroids, such as immunosuppression and dysfunction of the hypothalamic-pituitary-adrenal axis, were not tested or reported when used for PONV management. Other groups of patients who might be at risk from the administration of dexamethasone include diabetics, patients with peptic ulcer disease, and immunocompromised patients. The effect of giving a single dose of dexamethasone for PONV prophylaxis in such patients is unknown.

AUTHORS' RECOMMENDATIONS

Because the etiology of PONV is multifactorial, and there is evidence that combination antiemetic therapy appears to be more effective than single agents, a multimodal approach for the management of PONV should be adopted (Table 40-3). First, high-risk patients should be identified (Figure 40-1); second, steps should be taken to reduce the avoidable risk factors; and third, the use of combination antiemetics should be considered.[65] These recommendations follow the recently published guidelines for the management of PONV.[22]

Table 40-3   Recommended Strategies for Minimizing the Incidence of PONV

A. Identify high-risk patients (see Figure 40-1)
B. Avoid emetogenic stimuli

- Etomidate
- Nitrous oxide/inhalational agents
- Opioids (optimal analgesia should, however, be achieved by incorporating local anesthetics, nonsteroidal antiinflammatory drugs, and opioids as required)

C. Multimodal therapy

- Antiemetics (consider combination therapy)
- Total intravenous anesthesia with propofol
- Adequate hydration
- Effective analgesia
- Anxiolytics (e.g., benzodiazpines)
- Nonpharmacologic techniques (e.g., acupuncture)

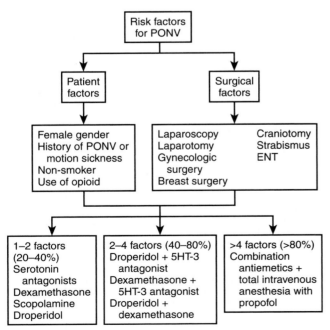

Figure 40-1. Risk Factors for PONV and Guidelines for Prophylactic Antiemetic Therapy. Number in brackets indicates risk of developing PONV. (Modified from references 6, 65, 66)

REFERENCES

1. Kovac AL: Prevention and treatment of postoperative nausea and vomiting. *Drugs* 2000;59:213-243.
2. Gold BS, Kitz DS, Lecky JH, Neuhaus JM: Unanticipated admission to the hospital following ambulatory surgery. *JAMA* 1989; 262:3008-3010.
3. Myles PS, Williams DL, Hendrata M, Anderson H, Weeks AM: Patient satisfaction after anaesthesia and surgery: Results of a prospective survey of 10,811 patients. *Br J Anaesth* 2000;84: 6-10.
4. Gan T, Sloan F, Dear G, El-Moalem HE, Lubarsky DA: How much are patients willing to pay for a completely effective antiemetic? *Anesth Analg* 2001;92:393-400.
5. Rowbotham DJ: Current management of postoperative nausea and vomiting. *Br J Anaesth* 1992;69:46S-59S.
6. Apfel CC, Laara E, Koivuranta M, Greim CA, Roewer N: A simplified risk score for predicting postoperative nausea and vomiting: Conclusions from cross-validations between two centers. *Anesthesiology* 1999;91:693-700.
7. Splinter WM, MacNeill HB, Menard EA, Rhine EJ, Roberts DJ, Gould MH: Midazolam reduces vomiting after tonsillectomy in children. *Can J Anaesth* 1995;42:201-203.
8. Khalil SN, Berry JM, Howard G, Lawson K, Hanis C, Mazow ML, Stanley TH: The antiemetic effect of lorazepam after outpatient strabismus surgery in children. *Anesthesiology* 1992;77:915-919.
9. Rothenberg DM, Parnass SM, Litwack K, McCarthy RJ, Newman LM: Efficacy of ephedrine in the prevention of postoperative nausea and vomiting. *Anesth Analg* 1991;72:58-61.
10. Naguib K, Osman HA, Al-Khayat HC, Zikri AM: Prevention of post-operative nausea and vomiting following laparoscopic surgery—ephedrine vs propofol. *Middle East Journal of Anesthesiology* 1998;14:219-230.
11. Yogendran S, Asokumar B, Cheng DC, Chung F: A prospective randomized double-blinded study of the effect of intravenous fluid therapy on adverse outcomes on outpatient surgery. *Anesth Analg* 1995;80:682-686.
12. Enqvist B, Bjorklund C, Engman M, Jakobsson J: Preoperative hypnosis reduces postoperative vomiting after surgery of the breasts. A prospective, randomized and blinded study. *Acta Anaesthesiol Scand* 1997;41:1028-1032.
13. Tramer MR: A rational approach to the control of postoperative nausea and vomiting: Evidence from systematic reviews. Part I. Efficacy and harm of antiemetic interventions, and methodological issues. *Acta Anaesthesiol Scand* 2001;45:4-13.
14. Rowbotham DJ: Current management of postoperative nausea and vomiting. *Br J Anaesth* 1992;69:46S-59S.
15. Quaynor H, Raeder JC: Incidence and severity of postoperative nausea and vomiting are similar after metoclopramide 20 mg and ondansetron 8 mg given by the end of laparoscopic cholecystectomies. *Acta Anaesthesiol Scand* 2002;46:109-113.
16. Wallenborn J, Gelbrich G, Bulst D, Behrends K, Wallenborn H, Rohrbach A, et al: Prevention of postoperative nausea and vomiting by metoclopramide combined with dexamethasone: Randomised double blind multicentre trial. *BMJ* 2006;333:324.
17. Henzi I, Sonderegger J, Tramer MR: Efficacy, dose-response, and adverse effects of droperidol for prevention of postoperative nausea and vomiting. *Can J Anaesth* 2000;47:537-551.
18. Habib AS, Gan TJ: Food and drug administration black box warning on the perioperative use of droperidol: A review of the cases. *Anesth Analg* 2003;96:1377-1379.
19. Lee Y, Wang PK, Lai HY, Yang YL, Chu CC, Wang JJ: Haloperidol is as effective as ondansetron for preventing postoperative nausea and vomiting. *Can J Anaesth* 2007;54:349-354.
20. Buttner M, Walder B, von Elm E, Tramer MR: Is low-dose haloperidol a useful antiemetic? A meta-analysis of published and unpublished randomized trials. *Anesthesiology* 2004;101: 1454-1463.
21. Tramer MR, Reynolds DJ, Moore RA, McQuay HJ: Efficacy, dose-response, and safety of ondansetron in prevention of postoperative nausea and vomiting: A quantitative systematic review of randomized placebo-controlled trials. *Anesthesiology* 1997;87: 1277-1289.
22. Gan TJ, Meyer T, Apfel CC, Chung F, Davis PJ, Habib AS, et al: Society for Ambulatory Anesthesia guidelines for the management of postoperative nausea and vomiting. *Anesth Analg* 2007;105:1615-1628.

23. Candiotti KA, Kovac AL, Melson TI, Clerici G, Gan TJ: A randomized, double-blind study to evaluate the efficacy and safety of three different doses of palonosetron versus placebo for preventing postoperative nausea and vomiting. *Anesth Analog* 2008;107:445-451.

24. Kovac AL, Eberhart L, Kotarski J, Clerici G, Apfel C. A randomized, double-blind study to evaluate the efficacy and safety of three different doses of palonosetron versus placebo in preventing postoperative nausea and vomiting over a 72-hour period. *Anesth Analog* 2008;107:439-444.

25. Henzi I, Walder B, Tramer MR: Dexamethasone for the prevention of postoperative nausea and vomiting: A quantitative systematic review. *Anesth Analg* 2000;90:186-194.

26. Apfel CC, Korttila K, Abdalla M, Kerger H, Turan A, Vedder I, et al: A factorial trial of six interventions for the prevention of postoperative nausea and vomiting. *N Engl J Med* 2004;350:2441-2451.

27. Dundee JW, Moore J, Clarke RSJ: Studies of drugs given before anaesthesia V: Pethidine 100 mg alone and with atropine or hyoscine. *Br J Anaesth* 1964;36:703-710.

28. Dundee JW, Kirwan MJ, Clarke RS: Anaesthesia and premedication as factors in postoperative vomiting. *Acta Anaesthesiol Scand* 1965;9:223-231.

29. Bailey PL, Streisand JB, Pace NL, Bubbers SJ, East KA, Mulder S, Stanley TH: Transdermal scopolamine reduces nausea and vomiting after outpatient laparoscopy. *Anesthesiology* 1990;72:977-980.

30. Loper KA, Ready LB, Dorman BH: Prophylactic transdermal scopolamine patches reduce nausea in postoperative patients receiving epidural morphine. *Anesth Analg* 1989;68:144-146.

31. Kotelko DM, Rottman RL, Wright WC, Stone JJ, Yamashiro AY, Rosenblatt RM: Transdermal scopolamine decreases nausea and vomiting following cesarean section in patients receiving epidural morphine. *Anesthesiology* 1989;71:675-678.

32. Harnett MJ, O'Rourke N, Walsh M, Carabuena JM, Segal S: Transdermal scopolamine for prevention of intrathecal morphine-induced nausea and vomiting after cesarean delivery. *Anesth Analg* 2007;105:764-769.

33. White PF, Tang J, Song D, Coleman JE, Wender RH, Ogunnaike B, et al: Transdermal scopolamine: An alternative to ondansetron and droperidol for the prevention of postoperative and postdischarge emetic symptoms. *Anesth Analg* 2007;104:92-96.

34. Kranke P, Morin AM, Roewer N, Wulf H, Eberhart LH: The efficacy and safety of transdermal scopolamine for the prevention of postoperative nausea and vomiting: A quantitative systematic review. *Anesth Analg* 2002;95:133-143.

35. Dundee JW, Loan WB, Morrison JD: A comparison of the efficacy of cyclizine and perhenazine in reducing the emetic effects of morphine and pethidine. *Br J Clin Pharmacol* 1975;2:81-85.

36. Khalil S, Philbrook L, Rabb M, Wells L, Aves T, Villanueva G, et al: Ondansetron/promethazine combination or promethazine alone reduces nausea and vomiting after middle ear surgery. *J Clin Anesth* 1999;11:596-600.

37. Chia YY, Lo Y, Liu K, Tan PH, Chung NC, Ko NH: The effect of promethazine on postoperative pain: A comparison of preoperative, postoperative, and placebo administration in patients following total abdominal hysterectomy. *Acta Anaesthesiol Scand* 2004;48:625-630.

38. Habib AS, Reuveni J, Taguchi A, White WD, Gan TJ: A comparison of ondansetron with promethazine for treating postoperative nausea and vomiting in patients who received prophylaxis with ondansetron: A retrospective database analysis. *Anesth Analg* 2007;104:548-551.

39. Habib AS, Breen TW, Gan TJ: Comment: Promethazine adverse events after implementation of a medication shortage interchange. *Ann Pharmacother* 2005;39:1370.

40. Kranke P, Morin AM, Roewer N, Eberhart LHJ: Dimenhydrinate for prophylaxis of postoperative nausea and vomiting: A meta-analysis of randomized controlled trials. *Acta Anaesthesiol Scand* 2002;46:238-244.

41. Gan TJ, Apfel CC, Kovac A, Philip BK, Singla N, Minkowitz H, et al: A randomized, double-blind comparison of the NK1 antagonist, aprepitant, versus ondansetron for the prevention of postoperative nausea and vomiting. *Anesth Analg* 2007;104:1082-1089.

42. Diemunsch P, Gan TJ, Philip BK, Girao MJ, Eberhart L, Irwin MG, et al: Single-dose aprepitant vs ondansetron for the prevention of postoperative nausea and vomiting: A randomized, double-blind phase III trial in patients undergoing open abdominal surgery. *Br J Anaesth* 2007;99:202-211.

43. Tramer M, Moore A, McQuay H: Meta-analytic comparison of prophylactic antiemetic efficacy for postoperative nausea and vomiting: Propofol anaesthesia vs omitting nitrous oxide vs total I.V. anaesthesia with propofol. *Br J Anaesth* 1997;78:256-259.

44. Gan TJ, Ginsberg B, Grant AP, Glass PS: Double-blind, randomized comparison of ondansetron and intraoperative propofol to prevent postoperative nausea and vomiting. *Anesthesiology* 1996;85:1036-1042.

45. Tramer M, Moore A, McQuay H: Propofol anaesthesia and postoperative nausea and vomiting: Quantitative systematic review of randomized controlled studies. *Br J Anaesth* 1997;78:247-255.

46. Gan TJ, Glass PS, Howell ST, Canada AT, Grant AP, Ginsberg B: Determination of plasma concentrations of propofol associated with 50% reduction in postoperative nausea. *Anesthesiology* 1997;87:779-784.

47. Lee A, Done ML: The use of nonpharmacologic techniques to prevent postoperative nausea and vomiting: A meta-analysis. *Anesth Analg* 1999;88:1362-1369.

48. Gan TJ, Jiao KR, Zenn M, Georgiade G: A randomized controlled comparison of electro-acupoint stimulation or ondansetron versus placebo for the prevention of postoperative nausea and vomiting. *Anesth Analg* 2004;99:1070-1075.

49. White PF, Issioui T, Hu J, Jones SB, Coleman JE, Waddle JP, et al: Comparative efficacy of acustimulation (ReliefBand) versus ondansetron (Zofran) in combination with droperidol for preventing nausea and vomiting. *Anesthesiology* 2002;97:1075-1081.

50. Coloma M, White PF, Ogunnaike BO, Markowitz SD, Brown PM, Lee AQ, et al: Comparison of acustimulation and ondansetron for the treatment of established postoperative nausea and vomiting. *Anesthesiology* 2002;97:1387-1392.

51. Zarate E, Mingus M, White PF, Chiu JW, Scuderi P, Loskota W, Daneshgari V: The use of transcutaneous acupoint electrical stimulation for preventing nausea and vomiting after laparoscopic surgery. *Anesth Analg* 2001;92:629-635.

52. Habib AS, Gan TJ: Combination therapy for postoperative nausea and vomiting—a more effective prophylaxis? *Ambulatory Surgery* 2001;9:59-71.

53. Habib AS, Gan TJ: Combination antiemetics: What is the evidence? *Int Anesthesiol Clin* 2003;41:119-144.

54. Habib AS, El-Moalem HE, Gan TJ: The efficacy of the 5-HT(3) receptor antagonists combined with droperidol for PONV prophylaxis is similar to their combination with dexamethasone. A meta-analysis of randomized controlled trials. *Can J Anaesth* 2004;51:311-319.

55. Scuderi PE, James RL, Harris L, Mims GR 3rd: Multimodal antiemetic management prevents early postoperative vomiting after outpatient laparoscopy. *Anesth Analg* 2000;91:1408-1414.

56. Habib AS, White WD, Eubanks S, Pappas TN, Gan TJ: A randomized comparison of a multimodal management strategy versus combination antiemetics for the prevention of postoperative nausea and vomiting. *Anesth Analg* 2004;99:77-81.

57. U.S. Food and Drug Administration: FDA strengthens warnings for droperidol. Available at www.fda.gov/bbs/topics/ANSWERS/2001/ANS01123.html.

58. Gan TJ, White PF, Scuderi PE, Watcha MF, Kovac A: FDA "black box" warning regarding use of droperidol for postoperative nausea and vomiting: Is it justified? *Anesthesiology* 2002;97:287.

59. Habib AS, Gan TJ: The use of droperidol before and after the FDA black box warning: A survey of the members of the Society of Ambulatory Anesthesia (SAMBA). *J Clin Anesth* 2008;20:35-39.

60. Felson DT, Anderson JJ: A cross study evaluation of association between steroid dose and bolus steroids and avascular necrosis of bone. *Lancet* 1987;1:902-906.

61. Fast A, Alon M, Weiss S, Zer-Aviv FR: Avascular necrosis of bone following short-term dexamethasone therapy for brain edema. Case report. *J Neurosurg* 1984;61:983-985.

62. Cameron HA, Reyntjens AJ, Lake-Bakaar G: Cardiac arrest after treatment with intravenous domperidone. *Br Med J Clin Res Ed* 1985;290:160.
63. Taylor LJ: Multifocal avascular necrosis after short-term high-dose steroid therapy. A report of three cases. *J Bone Joint Surg Br* 1984;66:431-433.
64. Virik K, Karapetis C, Droufakou S, Harper P: Avascular necrosis of bone: The hidden risk of glucocorticoids used as antiemetics in cancer chemotherapy. *Int J Clin Pract* 2001;55:344-345.
65. Gan TJ: Postoperative nausea and vomiting—can it be eliminated? *JAMA* 2002;287:1233-1236.
66. Watcha MF: The cost-effective management of postoperative nausea and vomiting. *Anesthesiology* 2000;92:931-933.

How Can We Prevent Postoperative Cognitive Dysfunction?

Terri G. Monk, MD, MS, and Catherine C. Price, PhD

INTRODUCTION/BACKGROUND

Postoperative cognitive changes have been reported in elderly patients for over a century, and anesthesia has often been mentioned as a possible cause of this problem.[1] In 1955, Bedford published a retrospective review of 1193 elderly patients who had surgery under general anesthesia during a 5-year period.[1] He found that cognitive problems occurred in approximately 10% of older patients after surgery and described 18 cases in which patients developed extreme dementia and remained confused until their death.

Postoperative cognitive problems can be classified as delirium, postoperative cognitive dysfunction (POCD), or dementia. Although POCD is not a formal psychiatric diagnosis, the term is commonly used in current literature and is considered to be a mild neurocognitive disorder.[2-4] The *Diagnostic and Statistical Manual of Mental Disorders, Fourth Edition* (DSM-IV) states that a mild neurocognitive disorder can only be diagnosed if the cognitive disturbance does not meet the criteria for three other conditions (delirium, dementia, or amnestic disorder).[5] The diagnosis of mild neurocognitive disorder must be corroborated by the results of neuropsychologic testing showing that an individual has a new onset of deficits in at least two areas of cognitive functioning lasting for a period of at least 2 weeks.[5] These diagnostic criteria make it nearly impossible to make a clinical diagnosis of POCD during the hospital stay.

Cognitive problems are common at hospital discharge, but the majority of these problems resolve soon after surgery.[2,3] It is likely that the lingering effects of anesthetic agents, pain medications, sleep deprivation, and the stress response to surgery may interfere with patients' ability to take the sensitive neurocognitive tests in the early postoperative period.[3] Thus early cognitive decline may reflect recovery from major surgery and not true cognitive impairment. As such, this review will only focus on POCD occurring at least 4 weeks after surgery.

Recently, several prospective longitudinal studies have presented evidence that postoperative cognitive dysfunction is indeed a reality.[2,3,6] A prospective longitudinal study of 261 patients who underwent coronary artery bypass graft (CABG) surgery found that 53% of the patients had cognitive decline at hospital discharge, 36% at 6 weeks, 24% at 6 months, and 42% at 5 years after surgery.[6] These investigators evaluated predictors of cognitive decline at 5 years after surgery and found that cognitive impairment at hospital discharge was a significant predictor of long-term cognitive impairment. A second multinational, prospective study reported on postoperative cognitive decline following noncardiac surgery. In this study, Moller and colleagues[2] evaluated cognitive function in patients ages 60 years or older after major abdominal and orthopedic surgery. These patients completed a battery of psychometric tests before surgery and at 1 week and 3 months after surgery. In this study, 25% of the patients had measurable cognitive dysfunction 1 week after the operation and 10% had cognitive changes 3 months after surgery. Advancing age was the only significant predictor for POCD at 3 months after surgery. Using the same study design, Monk and colleagues[3] evaluated adults of all ages undergoing major noncardiac surgery and diagnosed POCD in 30% to 40% of adult patients at hospital discharge with only the elderly at significant risk for POCD at 3 months after surgery. This study demonstrated that approximately 13% of patients, age 60 or over, exhibited late POCD (3 months after surgery). The independent risk factors for POCD at this time point were increasing age, lower educational level, a history of a previous cerebral vascular accident (CVA) with no residual impairment, and POCD at hospital discharge. These investigators also found that the occurrence of POCD increased the risk of death in the first year after surgery.[3]

POTENTIAL MECHANISMS FOR POCD

The mechanisms responsible for POCD after noncardiac surgery are unknown, but potential risk factors can be classified into patient, surgical, and anesthetic categories. It is likely that the etiology of POCD in the elderly patient is multifactorial and may include the preoperative health status of the patient, the patient's preoperative level of cognition, intraoperative events related to the surgery itself, and neurotoxic effects of anesthetic agents.

POTENTIAL INTERVENTIONS TO REDUCE POCD

To date, research has attempted to prevent or minimize POCD by focusing on surgical or anesthetic alternatives such as the following:

1. *General versus regional anesthesia:* The hypothesis for these studies is that postoperative cognitive outcome will be better after regional than after general anesthesia (Table 41-1).
2. *Alterations in surgical techniques during CABG:* The hypothesis for these studies is that postoperative cognitive outcome will be better if cardiopulmonary bypass and cerebral embolic events can be avoided during CABG (Table 41-2).
3. *Alterations in anesthetic management:* These studies have multiple hypotheses investigating hypothermia and specific pharmacologic agents (vitamins, fentanyl, inhalational agents; Table 41-3).

RESULTS OF RANDOMIZED CLINICAL TRIALS EVALUATING COGNITIVE OUTCOMES

Methodologic Issues

The methodologic issues associated with identifying POCD have been a major concern for investigators. Problems with the methodology include differences in neurocognitive test batteries, intervals between sessions, the definitions of cognitive decline, and statistical analysis methods.[4,7] It is only within the last several years that some uniformity has developed regarding methodologic approaches and statistical issues. This is in large part due to consensus statements[8,9] and definition papers[4,10] bringing attention to issues such as practice effects, the value of an age-matched control group, group versus individual change scores, and ceiling and floor effects. Tables 41-1 through 41-3 compare randomized clinical trials (RCTs) evaluating interventions to minimize POCD, but the methodology is not consistent across these trials, making it difficult to compare results.

EVIDENCE

Trials Comparing the Effects of General Versus Regional Anesthesia on POCD

Within the last 30 years, there have been numerous investigations examining Bedford's original claim regarding general anesthesia.[1] The 10 RCTs included in Table 41-1 varied in the type of surgery, the time of postoperative testing, the type of neuropsychologic tests administered, and the definition of POCD.[11-20] When one evaluates these studies, which all used prospective randomization and objective cognitive measures, there is little evidence that *long-term* (30 days or greater) postoperative cognitive dysfunction occurs more often following general relative to regional anesthesia. At most, there is some evidence that general anesthesia is associated with reduced global cognitive functioning in the early postoperative recovery hours and days. The two most recent studies by Rasmussen and colleagues[19] and

Table 41-1	**Prospective Randomized Trials Evaluating Cognitive Outcomes after General versus Regional Anesthesia**						
Author	**Year**	**Age (Years)**	**Surgical Procedure**	**Anesthetic Technique**	**Sample Size**	**Time of Testing (Days Postop)**	**Cognitive Differences**
Chung[11]	1987	Mean = 72	TURP or pelvic floor repair	GA vs. spinal	44	30	NS
Chung[12]	1989	Mean = 72	TURP	GA vs. spinal	44	30	NS
Riis[13]	1983	Mean = 70	THA	GA vs. epidural vs. GA + epidural	30	90	NS
Bigler[14]	1985	Mean = 79	Hip Fx	GA vs. spinal	40	90	NS
Ghoneim[15]	1988	Mean = 61	TURP, THA, TKA, Vag Hyst	GA vs. regional	105	90	NS
Jones[16]	1990	≥60	TKA, THA	GA vs. spinal	146	90	NS
Nielson[17]	1990	Mean = 69	TKA	GA vs. spinal	64	90	NS
Haan[18]	1990	Mean = 72	TURP	GA vs. spinal	53	90	NS
Rasmussen[19]	2003	Mean = 71 years	Major noncardiac	GA vs. regional	428	90	NS
Williams-Russo[20]	1995	Median = 69	TKA	GA vs. epidural	262	180	NS

GA, general anesthesia, *Hip FX,* hip fracture; *NS,* no significant differences in cognitive outcomes between the groups at the time of testing indicated in this table; *THA,* total hip arthroplasty; *TKA,* total knee arthroplasty; *TURP,* transurethral resection of the prostate; *Vag Hyst,* vaginal hysterectomy.

Table 41-2 Prospective Randomized Trials Evaluating Cognitive Outcomes after Alterations in Operative Techniques for Coronary Artery Bypass Graft Surgery

Author	Year	Age (Years)	Intervention	Sample Size	Time of Testing (Postop)	Cognitive Differences
Lloyd[21]	2000	Median = 61	Off vs. on pump	60	12 weeks	NS
Van Dijk[22]	2002	Mean = 61	Off vs. on pump	281	90 days and 1 year	Off pump: better cognitive outcome at 3 months NS at 1 year
Zamvar[23]	2002	Mean = 63	Off vs. on pump	60	10 weeks	Off pump: better cognitive outcome
Rankin[24]	2003	Mean = 61	Off vs. on pump	43	60-90 days	NS
Lee[25]	2003	Mean = 66	Off vs. on pump	60	1 year	Off pump: better cognitive outcome
Lund[26]	2005	40-80	Off vs. on pump	120	90 days	NS
Jensen[27]	2006	≥55	Off vs. on pump	120	103 days	NS
Ernest[28]	2006	Mean = 63	Off vs. on pump	107	60 and 180 days	NS
Vedin[29]	2006	Mean = 65	Off vs. on pump	70	1 and 6 months	NS
Van Dijk[30]	2007	Mean = 61	Off vs. on pump	281	5 years	NS
Boodhwani[32]	2007	≥60	Hypothermia 34°C vs. 36°C	267	90 days	NS
Rubens[33]	2007	Mean = 59	Processed vs. unprocessed shed blood	269	90 days	NS
Hammon[34]	2007	≥60	Single vs. multiple cross-clamp	107	180 days	Cognitive outcomes significantly better with single cross-clamp
Mathew[35]	2007	Mean = 69	Moderate hemodilution to Hct = 27% vs. Profound hemodilution to Hct = 15%-18% during CPB	108	6 weeks	Profound hemodilution in elderly patients associated with cognitive decline

CPB, cardiopulmonary bypass; Hct, hematocrit; NS, no significant differences in cognitive outcomes between the groups at the time of testing indicated in this table.

Table 41-3 Prospective Randomized Trials Evaluating the Effect of Anesthetic Management on Postoperative Cognitive Outcome Techniques

Author	Year	Age (Years)	Surgical Procedure	Intervention	Sample Size	Time of Testing (Postop)	Cognitive Differences
Day[37]	1988	Mean = 79	Femur Fx	Vitamins B and C	60	3 months	NS
Jhaveri[38]	1989	≥65	Cataract surgery	Hypocapnic ventilation to $PaCO_2$ of 4.9 vs. 2.9 kPa vs. local block	83	4 weeks	NS
Enlund[39]	1998	Mean = 36	Orthognathic surgery	Isoflurane vs. propofol anesthesia	29	28-56 days	NS
Williams-Russo[40]	1999	Mean = 72	THA	Hypotensive (MAP = 45-55) vs. less hypotensive (MAP = 55-70) BP	235	4 months	NS
Faraq[41]	2006	Mean = 64	Elective surgery >2 hours	Low BIS (median = 39) vs. High BIS (median = 51)	74	4-6 weeks	Low BIS had better information-processing speed
Silbert[42]	2006	Mean = 68	CABG	High (50 mcg/kg) vs. low (10 mcg/kg) dose fentanyl	350	3 months and 1 year	NS

BIS, bispectral index; CABG, coronary artery bypass graft surgery; Fx, fracture; NS, no significant differences in cognitive outcomes between the groups at the time of testing indicated in this table; THA, total hip arthroplasty.

Williams-Russo and colleagues[20] best exemplify this finding. Both studies included a large participant pool and applied rigorous methodologic approaches to assess the effects of general versus regional anesthesia for up to 6 months following surgery.[19,20] They both clearly demonstrate that the type of anesthesia (general versus regional) made no difference in long-term cognitive outcome. However, all the patients receiving regional anesthesia also received intravenous opioids and sedatives during the surgical procedure, so it is not known if regional anesthesia with no additional intravenous agents would improve postoperative cognitive outcome.

Trials Evaluating the Effects of Surgical Techniques on POCD

There is increasing evidence that CABG can produce long-term cognitive decline.[6] The use of cardiopulmonary bypass has long been regarded as one of the potential causes of neurocognitive impairment following CABG. It has been suggested that off-pump CABG, in which surgery is performed on a beating heart without cardiopulmonary bypass, should result in improved neurocognitive outcomes. Table 41-2 illustrates 10 RCTs that have evaluated neurocognitive function after on-pump versus off-pump CABG.[21-30] Only three trials were able to demonstrate that off-pump surgery improved postoperative cognitive function.[22,23,25] The remainder of these trials were unable to find significant differences in late cognitive outcome (greater than 1 month after surgery) after CABG regardless of whether the procedure used cardiopulmonary bypass or not.[21,24,26-30] Van Dijk and colleagues[22,30] performed the longest postoperative follow-up and found that avoidance of cardiopulmonary bypass in low-risk patients undergoing CABG improved cognitive outcomes at 3 months after the procedure but had no beneficial effect on cognitive outcomes at either 1 or 5 years after surgery. A recent meta-analysis analyzing prospective RCTs evaluating off- versus on-pump CABG concluded that the findings of these studies "suggest that factors other than cardiopulmonary bypass may be responsible for cognitive decline, such as anesthesia and the generalized inflammatory response that is associated with major surgical procedures."[31]

Other variations in operative technique during CABG with cardiopulmonary bypass are outlined in Table 41-2. Boodhwani and colleagues[32] randomized patients undergoing CABG to either an intraoperative nasopharyngeal temperature of 34°C (hypothermia) or 37°C (normothermia) to determine if mild hypothermia would have a neuroprotective effect. Although mild hypothermia had no major adverse effects on outcome, it did not improve neurocognitive outcome at 3 months after surgery.[32]

Cerebral emboli are common during CABG and are also considered to be one of the primary mechanisms for POCD. Several recent studies have investigated techniques to minimize cerebral emboli during cardiac surgery.[33,34] Cardiotomy blood that is aspirated from the pericardial cavity during cardiopulmonary bypass may contain cellular debris and fat particles, and it is possible

that these microemboli may cause cerebral damage. However, a study randomizing patients to receive either nonprocessed or processed blood (blood that is centrifuged to remove debris from the blood before return to the patient) failed to demonstrate improved postoperative neurocognitive outcomes.[33] A reanalysis of data from a large group of patients undergoing CABG suggests that cardiopulmonary bypass performed with the use of a single cross-clamp may reduce cerebral emboli and improve postoperative cognitive outcome, but additional research is needed to confirm this finding.[34] Extreme hemodilution to hematocrit (Hct) values less than 18% during cardiopulmonary bypass is common during CABG.[35] Mathew and colleagues[35] randomized patients undergoing CABG to either moderate hemodilution (Hct $\geq$27%) or profound hemodilution (Hct = 15% to 18%) on cardiopulmonary bypass and found that older patients in the profound hemodilution group experienced greater postoperative neurocognitive decline.

Trials Evaluating the Effects of Various Anesthesia Techniques on POCD

Exposure to anesthetic agents has been suggested as a possible cause of postoperative cognitive dysfunction in elderly patients. Anesthetic agents affecting the release of central nervous system neurotransmitters such as acetylcholine, dopamine, and norepinephrine could potentially impair memory, especially in elderly patients. A systematic review of the literature concerning the impact of anesthesia on memory revealed that the majority of the studies have serious shortcomings in the psychometric test measures used, the selection of study populations, and interpretation of the results.[36] At this time there are no definitive conclusions on the effects of anesthesia on learning and memory, and additional research is needed to clarify the relationship between anesthetic agents and postoperative cognitive changes.

Table 41-3 contains RCTs evaluating the effect of perioperative anesthetic management on POCD.[37-42] The perioperative use of intravenous vitamins did not decrease the risk of postoperative confusion in patients with femur fractures.[37] Likewise, varying the type of anesthesia (propofol or isoflurane) or the intraoperative dose of fentanyl administered did not affect postoperative cognitive outcome.[39,42] In one study, patients anesthetized with deeper (both groups were still within the recommended range for depth of anesthesia) levels of anesthesia were able to process information more quickly at 4 to 6 weeks after surgery, but did not perform differently on working or verbal memory tests.[41]

Although it may seem obvious that intraoperative hypotension would be associated with increased postoperative cognitive problems, the literature does not support this theory. Williams-Russo and colleagues[40] randomized older adults undergoing total hip replacement to either mild hypotension (mean blood pressure of 55 to 70) or marked hypotension (mean blood pressure of 45 to 55). At 4 months after surgery, there were no significant differences in the rates of POCD between the groups, as well as no significant differences in other complications, including cardiac, renal, and thromboembolic events.[40] These findings are in agreement with an earlier longitudinal study that found no relationship between intraoperative hypotension or hypoxemia and POCD in elderly patients.[2] It has also been hypothesized that hyperventilation and the resultant decrease in cerebral blood flow might result in insufficient cerebral oxygenation and cause POCD. In a study of patients undergoing cataract surgery, patients were randomized to three groups: general anesthesia and ventilation to 4.9 kPa (37 torr) versus general anesthesia and hyperventilation to 2.9 kPa (22 torr) versus local anesthesia with spontaneous ventilation.[38] There were no significant differences in cognitive outcome among the groups at 4 days and 4 weeks after surgery.

AREAS OF UNCERTAINTY

It is now accepted that POCD occurs in a significant number of elderly patients, but the mechanisms responsible for this problem are unknown. Likewise, there are no known interventions to minimize or prevent this complication.

Because advancing age, lower educational level, and previous CVA with no residual deficit have been found to be independent predictors of POCD, it is likely that a patient's preoperative cognition may be the most important determinant of postoperative cognitive problems.[2,3,6] The brain reserve hypothesis argues that individuals with larger cognitive reserve have greater capacity to replace compromised brain areas and maintain high functioning.[43] This theory suggests that elders who are cognitively impaired before surgery might be at higher risk for postoperative cognitive problems. Thus, even mild perioperative neurologic trauma may be a sufficient proximal cause to move people over that functional cliff and into the range of cognitive functioning that might be classified as impaired.[44] It is, therefore, possible that patients with borderline cognition before surgery may be predisposed to POCD when exposed to anesthetic agents, surgical trauma, the perioperative inflammatory response, or other perioperative events. One reason that the RCTs (see Tables 41-1, 41-2, and 41-3) evaluating interventions to improve cognitive outcome have had limited success may be that the subject groups may not include enough high-risk patients to detect differences in treatments.

Extensive data support the use of cholinesterase inhibitors, including tacrine, donepezil, rivastigmine, and galantamine, for the treatment of mild to moderate Alzheimer's disease. A small pilot study evaluated the efficacy of donepezil in treating patients with cognitive decline at 1 year after CABG and found cognitive improvement on delayed and immediate recall tests at 12 weeks after surgery but no changes on tests of executive function or word association.[45] Although the findings in this study are preliminary, they provide hope that pharmacologic interventions to treat POCD will be developed in the future.

GUIDELINES

There are no formal guidelines regarding avoidance and treatment of POCD.

AUTHORS' RECOMMENDATIONS

The authors have the following suggestions:

- Anesthesiologists should be aware that POCD occurs in a significant number of elderly patients.
- Anesthesiologists should also be informed about postoperative cognitive problems so that they can discuss these issues with concerned patients and their families.
- The preoperative cognitive status of the patient should be assessed during the preoperative interview. The Mini-Mental State Examination is a valid screening instrument for cognitive status.[46]
- Until further studies are done, it is impossible to recommend an anesthetic technique that will change cognitive outcomes; however, it makes sense to avoid drugs with long-acting central nervous system effects such as benzodiazepines in the elderly.
- Despite the lack of evidence, it is likely that the maintenance of adequate tissue oxygenation, hemodynamic stability, and appropriate anesthetic depth will be associated with the best cognitive outcomes in elderly patients.

REFERENCES

1. Bedford PD: Adverse cerebral effects of anaesthesia on old people. *Lancet* 1955;2:857-861.
2. Moller JT, Cluitmans P, Rasmussen LS, et al: Long-term postoperative cognitive dysfunction in the elderly, ISPOCD 1 Study. *Lancet* 1998;351:857-861.
3. Monk TG, Weldon BC, Garvan CW, Dede DE, van der Aa MT, Heilman KM, Gravenstein JS: Predictors of cognitive dysfunction after major noncardiac surgery. *Anesthesiology* 2008;108:18-30.
4. Rasmussen LS, Larssen K, Houx P, et al: The assessment of postoperative cognitive function. *Acta Anaesthesiol Scand* 2001;45:275-289.
5. *Diagnostic and statistical manual of mental disorders, fourth edition.* Washington, DC, American Psychiatric Association, 1994.
6. Newman MF, Kirchner JL, Phillips-Bute B, et al: Longitudinal assessment of neurocognitive function after coronary-artery bypass surgery. *N Engl J Med* 2001;344:395-402.
7. Newman S, Stygall J, Hirani S, et al: Postoperative cognitive dysfunction after noncardiac surgery. *Anesthesiology* 2007;106:572-590.
8. Murkin JM et al: Statement of consensus on assessment of neurobehavioral outcomes after cardiac surgery. *Ann Thorac Surg* 1995;59:1289-1295.
9. Murkin JM et al: Defining dysfunction: Group means versus incidence analysis—a statement of consensus. *Ann Thorac Surg* 1997;64:904-905.
10. Rasmussen LS: Defining postoperative cognitive dysfunction. *Eur J Anaesthesiol* 1998;15:761-764.
11. Chung F, Meier R, Lautenschlager E, et al: General or spinal anesthesia: Which is better in the elderly? *Anesthesiology* 1987;67:422-427.
12. Chung F, Meier RH, Lautenschlaeger E: Comparison of perioperative mental function after general anaesthesia and spinal anaesthesia with intravenous sedation. *Can J Anaesth* 1989;36:382-387.
13. Riis J, Lombolt B, Haxholdt O, et al: Immediate and long-term recovery from general versus epidural anesthesia in elderly patients. *Acta Anaesthesiol Scand* 1983;27:44-49.

14. Bigler D, Adelhøj B, Petring OU, et al: Mental function and morbidity after acute hip surgery during spinal and general anaesthesia. *Anaesthesia* 1985;40:672-676.
15. Ghoneim MM, Hinrichs JV, O'Hara MW, et al: Comparison of psychologic and cognitive functions after general or regional anesthesia. *Anesthesiology* 1988;69:507-515.
16. Jones MJT, Piggott SE, Vaughan RS, et al: Cognitive and functional competence after anaesthesia in patients aged over 60: Controlled trial of general and regional anaesthesia for elective hip or knee replacement. *BMJ* 1990;300:1683-1687.
17. Nielson WR, Gelb AW, Casey JE, et al: Long-term cognitive and social sequelae of general versus regional anesthesia during arthroplasty in the elderly. *Anesthesiology* 1990;73:1103-1109.
18. Haan J, van Kleef JW, Bloem BR, et al: Cognitive function after spinal or general anesthesia for transurethral prostatectomy in elderly men. *J Am Geriatr Soc* 1991;39:596-600.
19. Rasmussen LS, Johnson T, Kuipers HM, et al: Does anaesthesia cause postoperative cognitive dysfunction? A randomised study of regional versus general anaesthesia in 438 elderly patients. *Acta Anaesthesiol Scand* 2003;47:260-266.
20. Williams-Russo P, Sharrock NE, Mattis S, et al: Cognitive effects after epidural vs. general anesthesia in older adults. A randomized trial. *JAMA* 1995;274:44-50.
21. Lloyd CT, Ascione R, Underwood MJ, et al: Serum S-100 protein release and neuropsychologic outcome during coronary revascularization on the beating heart: A prospective randomized study. *J Thorac Cardiovasc Surg* 2000;119:148-154.
22. Van Dijk D, Jansen EW, Hijman R, et al: Cognitive outcome after off-pump and on-pump coronary artery bypass graft surgery. *JAMA* 2002;287:1405-1412.
23. Zamvar V, William D, Hall J, et al: Assessment of neurocognitive impairment after off-pump and on-pump techniques for coronary artery bypass graft surgery: Prospective randomized controlled trial. *BMJ* 2002;325:1268.
24. Rankin KP, Kochamba GS, Boone KB, et al: Presurgical cognitive deficits in patients receiving coronary artery bypass surgery. *JINS* 2003;9:913-924.
25. Lee JD, Lee SJ, Tsushima WT, et al: Benefits of off-pump bypass on neurologic and clinical morbidity: A prospective randomized trial. *Ann Thorac Surg* 2003;76:18-26.
26. Lund C, Sundet K, Tennøe B, et al: Cerebral ischemic injury and cognitive impairment after off-pump and on-pump coronary artery bypass grafting surgery. *Ann Thorac Surg* 2005;80:2126-231.
27. Jensen BO, Hughes P, Rasmussen LS, et al: Cognitive outcomes in elderly high-risk patients after off-pump versus conventional coronary artery bypass grafting: A randomized trial. *Circulation* 2006;113:2790-2795.
28. Ernest CS, Worcester MUC, Tatoulis J, et al: Neurocognitive outcomes in off-pump versus on-pump bypass surgery: A randomized controlled trial. *Ann Thorac Surg* 2006;81:2105-2114.
29. Vedin J, Nyman H, Ericsson A, et al: Cognitive function after on or off pump coronary artery bypass grafting. *Eur J Cardiothorac Surg* 2006;30:305-310.
30. Van Dijk D, Spoor M, Hijman R, et al: Cognitive and cardiac outcomes 5 years after off-pump vs on-pump coronary artery bypass graft surgery. *JAMA* 2007;297:701-708.
31. Takagi H, Tanabashi T, Kawai N, Umemoto T: Cognitive decline after off-pump versus on-pump coronary artery bypass graft surgery: Meta-analysis of randomized controlled trials. *J Thorac Cardiovasc Surg* 2007;134:512-513.
32. Boodhwani M, Rubens F, Wozny D, et al: Effects of sustained mild hypothermia on neurocognitive function after coronary artery bypass surgery: A randomized, double-blind study. *J Thorac Cardiovasc Surg* 2007;134:1443-1452.
33. Rubens FD, Boodhwani M, Mesana T, et al: The cardiotomy trial: A randomized, double-blind study to assess the effect of processing of shed blood during cardiopulmonary bypass on transfusion and neurocognitive function. *Circulation* 2007;116(suppl I):I89-I97.
34. Hammon JW, Stump DA, Butterworth, et al: Coronary artery bypass grafting with single cross-clamp results in fewer persistent neuropsychological deficits than multiple clamp or off-pump coronary artery bypass grafting. *Ann Thorac Surg* 2007;84:1174-1179.
35. Mathew JP, Mackensen GB, Phillips-Bute B, et al: Effects of extreme hemodilution during cardiac surgery on cognitive function in the elderly. *Anesthesiology* 2007;107:577-584.
36. Ritchie K, Polge C, de Roquefeuil G, et al: Impact of anesthesia on the cognitive functioning of the elderly. *Int Psychogeriat* 1997;9:309-326.
37. Day JJ, Bayer AJ, McMahon M, et al: Thiamine status, vitamin supplements, and postoperative confusion. *Age Ageing* 1988;17:29-34.
38. Jhaveri RM: The effects of hypocapnic ventilation on mental function in elderly patients undergoing cataract surgery. *Anaesthesia* 1989;44:635-640.
39. Enlund M, Mentell O, Flenninger A, et al: Evidence of cerebral dysfunction associated with isoflurane or propofol based anaesthesia for orthognathic surgery, as assessed by biochemical and neuropsychological methods. *Ups J Med Sci* 1998;103:43-59.
40. Williams-Russo P, Sharrock NE, Mattis S, et al: Randomized trial of hypotensive epidural anesthesia in older adults. *Anesthesiology* 1999;91:926-935.
41. Faraq E, Chelune GJ, Schubert A, Mascha EJ: Is depth of anesthesia, as assessed by the bispectral index, related to postoperative cognitive dysfunction and recovery? *Anesth Analg* 2006;103:633-640.
42. Silbert BS, Scott DA, Evered LA, et al: A comparison of the effect of high- and low-dose fentanyl on the incidence of postoperative cognitive dysfunction after coronary artery bypass surgery in the elderly. *Anesthesiology* 2006;104:1137-1145.
43. Christensen H, Anstey K, Leach LS, Mackinnon AJ: Intelligence, education and the brain reserve hypothesis. In Craik FI, Salthouse TA, editors: *The handbook of aging and cognition*, ed 3. New York, Psychology Press, 2008.
44. Valenzuela MJ, Sachdev P: Brain reserve and cognitive decline: A nonparametric systematic review. *Psychol Med* 2006;36:1065-1073.
45. Doraiswamy PM, Babyak MA, Hennig T, et al: Donepezil for cognitive decline following coronary artery bypass surgery: A pilot randomized controlled trial. *Psychopharmacol Bull* 2007;40:54-62.
46. Folstein MF, Folstein SE, McHugh PR: "Mini-Mental State": A practical method for grading the cognitive state of patients for the clinician. *J Psychiatr Res* 1975;12:189-198.

42 Do Intensive Care Specialists Improve Patient Outcomes?

Patrick Neligan, MA, MB, FCARCSI, and Clifford S. Deutschman, MD, MS, FCCM

INTRODUCTION

Intensive (critical) care units (ICUs) first appeared in the 1950s as specialized wards to care for patients with acute respiratory failure. Subsequent technical and pharmacologic advances led to the provision of life-sustaining care for a medley of medical and surgical problems. Admission to intensive care is determined by a requirement for ventilatory or cardiovascular support, invasive monitoring or correction of life-threatening fluid and electrolyte abnormalities, or the expectation that severe, life-threatening abnormalities may arise without warning. Although ICUs are characterized by a high ratio of nurses to patients (usually 1:2 or less), physician staffing is variable. Based on the size of the hospital, ICUs may be generalized ("mixed") or specialized. Subtypes include coronary care units (CCUs), burn units, medical ICUs (MICUs), surgical and trauma ICUs (SICUs), and cardiac surgical and neurosurgical units.

The use and availability of critical care beds have increased dramatically over the past 50 years. There are more than 6000 ICUs in the United States.[1,2] Since its inception, intensive care has cost the United States approximately $1 trillion.[3] Overall health care costs in the United States are now over $2 trillion annually, 16% of gross domestic product (GDP), and this is rising.[4] Currently, more than 1% of GDP[5] is spent on critical care. The number of critical care beds in hospitals in increasing, while the number of non–critical care beds is diminishing.[6] Consequently, the cost of providing critical care services will continue to escalate. Inevitably, rationing of resources will result.[7] Only recently has utility of critical care been rigorously validated. Consequently, it is essential that critical care services are efficient, effective, and economic.

THE ARGUMENT FOR INTEGRATED CRITICAL CARE SERVICES

There has been significant historic diversity in the operation and organization of intensive care units. An early consultant-based model is being supplanted by one featuring an intensive care specialist ("intensivist"). In the consultant model one physician typically manages mechanical ventilation while dysfunction of other organs is directed by a combination of the primary care team and a series of specialist consultants. Responsibility for orders, consultations, and decision making may lie with the primary physician, but this often is unclear. Faults with this system include diffusion of responsibility, expertise imbalance between the decision maker and consultant, high cost, competing and conflicting orders, duplication of services, lack of cohesive planning, inconsistent coverage (particularly nights and weekends), and potentially worse patient outcomes.[8]

Specialized critical care training has been introduced over the past 30 years to deal with the shortcomings of this system. This has led to an integrated model whereby the intensivist coordinates the care of the patient, taking primary responsibility for the patient while in the ICU, and requests consultations if necessary. At the extreme is a "closed" model in which the full-time intensive care physician controls all admissions, discharges, orders, clinical management, and consultations for all patients admitted to the ICU. Advantages of this system include consistency of care, cost control, communication, availability, a clear hierarchy of responsibility, facilitation of standards, and improved nurse-physician relations. Faults with this system include the capacity to "lock out" the primary physician, loss of continuity of care, and the potential for conflict.

Unlike other specialties, critical care medicine has not been accepted universally. In several countries specific vocational training is available.[9] In the United States critical care is a subspecialty of anesthesiology, surgery, internal medicine, and pediatrics. Wide variations in the duration and nature of training exist.[9] It has been necessary for intensivists to justify their existence, using the evidence-based platform, a situation that distinguishes critical care from other specialties such as cardiology, trauma surgery, and emergency medicine, which share common features. At its core critical care requires an integrationist approach: the 1970s and 1980s were characterized by the hyperspecialization of the medical profession along system lines—the cardiovascular system, the renal system, the gastrointestinal tract, and even systems within systems. Intensive care specialists provide general holistic medical care according to severity of illness.

Conceptually, critical care may be both horizontally and vertically integrated, with its own specialists, its own team, and its own management structure. This includes an intensive care director and a multidisciplinary critical care team.

Thus, evaluation of outcomes relating to the appointment of an intensive care specialist mandates appraisal of all literature relating to critical care organization. Three questions are asked: (1) Do intensive care specialists improve outcomes—mortality, morbidity, cost reduction, length of stay? (2) What impact does the appointment of a critical care director have on ICU performance and outcomes? and (3) Does the conversion of an ICU from open to closed format, with concomitant introduction of an intensive care team, confer additional benefit?

EVIDENCE

The Intensive Care Specialist

Physician staffing in intensive care has not been rigorously studied. The literature is largely anecdotal or observational, usually detailing changes in costs and outcomes following planned changes in critical care staffing or configuration. Changes in physician staffing were usually accompanied by other alterations—the introduction of a critical care team or an ICU director, for example. Simultaneous changes in case-mix or severity of illness require adjustment in statistical results. The definition of physician staffing varies from an intensivist doing daily rounds (often in collaboration with the primary care team) to a "closed" 24-hour critical care service. Different styles of critical care service that involve the intensivist may or may not use external physician consultants, or may envelop consultation services such as nutrition or pharmacy, and may operate quite differently but carry the same "intensivist" label.[10-12] Attention should also be paid to specialist nurse training, nurse-to-patient ratios, and the presence or absence of certified nurse practitioners.[13]

Li and colleagues[14] looked at outcomes and interventions in a community hospital ICU before ($n = 463$) and after ($n = 491$) the introduction of an ICU physician. There was a significant reduction in adjusted (reason for admission, age, mental status) hospital mortality rate following the change, with a concomitant increase in the use of invasive monitors.

Pollack and colleagues[11] studied ICU mortality rates, the use of monitoring and therapeutic modalities, and efficiency of ICU bed utilization in the 3 months before ($n = 149$) and after ($n = 113$) the appointment of a pediatric intensivist and daytime ICU team. There was a clear improvement in the efficiency of bed utilization following the arrival of the intensivist. There was a reduction in the number of admissions of patients with low severity of illness and for monitoring, with a parallel increase in therapeutic and monitoring interventions in the post intensivist period. Mortality rate, adjusted for case mix, reduced in the intensivist period by 5.3% (number needed to treat to prevent one death [NNT] 19, odds ratio [OR] 0.51 [0.16 to 1.67, 95% confidence interval (CI)]).

Reynolds and colleagues[15] studied outcomes in patients with septic shock in the year before ($n = 100$) and after ($n = 112$) the introduction of a critical care service, staffed by intensivists. There was a significant reduction in hospital mortality rate from 74% to 64% (absolute risk reduction [ARR] 10%, NNT 10, OR 0.46 [0.26 to 0.83, 95% CI]), following introduction of the critical care service. There was also a significant increase in the use of invasive monitors, but no change in the number of external consultations.

Brown and colleagues[16] performed a cohort analysis of 223 patients admitted to ICU before, and 216 patients after, the introduction of an intensivist operating in an open model. Intensive care mortality rate decreased from 28% to 13% (ARR 15%, NNT 6.6, OR 0.40 [0.25 to 0.66, 95% CI]). Hospital mortality rate decreased from 36% to 25% (ARR 11%, NNT 9, OR 0.59 [0.39 to 0.90, 95% CI]). This effect was consistent irrespective of severity of illness.

Hanson and colleagues[17] undertook a cohort study comparing two parallel models of critical care. One group of patients was looked after by an on-site critical care team, supervised by an intensivist. The other was managed by a surgical team supervised by a general surgeon, with multiple commitments. Despite having higher Acute Physiology and Chronic Health Evaluation II scores, patients cared for by the critical care team spent less time in the surgical intensive care unit, had fewer complications, used fewer resources, and had lower total hospital charges. There was no significant difference in hospital or ICU mortality rates. Selection bias may have been an issue with this study.

Blunt and colleagues[18] compared outcomes in intensive care units covered by intensivist versus nonspecialist consultants (anesthesiologists) covering multiple sites using standardized mortality ratios. The case-mix-adjusted hospital mortality rate of intensive care patients improved significantly in the intensivist group compared with the nonspecialist group (standardized mortality ratios 0.81 versus 1.11, OR 0.73 [0.55 to 0.97, 95% CI]).

Dimick and colleagues[19] and Pronovost and colleagues,[20] using similar methodology, studied outcomes following high-risk surgery in the state of Maryland via a large database.[21] Following esophageal resection, lack of daily rounds by an ICU physician was associated with longer lengths of stay (7 days; 1 to 15, 95% CI; $p = .012$), higher hospital costs (61% increase or $8,839; 95% CI, $1,674 to $19,192; $p = .013$), and increased frequency of postoperative complications.[22] Following aortic repair surgery, not having daily rounds by an ICU physician was associated with a threefold increase in in-hospital mortality rate (OR, 3.0; 95% CI, 1.9 to 4.9), and in major postoperative complications such as cardiac arrest (OR, 2.9; 1.2 to 7.0, 95% CI), acute renal failure (OR, 2.2; 1.3 to 3.9, 95% CI), and sepsis (OR, 1.8; 1.2 to 2.6, 95% CI). Thus daily rounds by an intensive care physician are efficient, effective, and economical.

Numerous other studies have haphazardly appeared in the literature in abstract form. Pronovost and colleagues[23] have completed a systematic review to include these data. ICU physician staffing was divided into low intensity (no intensivist or elective intensivist consultation) or high intensity (mandatory intensivist consultation). High-intensity staffing reduced the risk of ICU mortality (pooled relative risk [RR] 0.61, 0.50 to 0.75, 95% CI), hospital mortality (RR 0.71, 0.62 to 0.82, 95% CI), and ICU and hospital length of stay, whether adjusted for case mix or not.

Levy and colleagues[24] studied the impact of intensive care specialists on hospital mortality rate using a large database (Project IMPACT) that had been designed to address resource use in 123 ICUs across the United States.

The study was performed by intensivists using a database constructed by intensivists. Patients who were managed by intensive care specialists had greater severity of illness than those managed by the primary physician and they underwent more procedures. When outcomes were adjusted for illness severity and a propensity score was used, patients cared for by intensive care specialists had greater in-hospital mortality rates than those who were not. Critical care predicted hospital mortality rate with a crude odds ratio (OR) of 2.13 (p <0.001). The addition of SAPS II (a severity of illness scoring system) to this model reduced this OR to 1.42 (p <0.001). Further inclusion of the propensity score decreased the OR to 1.40 (p <0.001). Several potential limitations to this study should be noted. The study tests two different hypotheses. The first looked at outcomes depending on whether an intensivist was chosen or not by the primary physician. This likely resulted in selection bias, because choice patients were likely to be less severely ill, and intensivists presumably consulted due to clinical concerns. The second study involved more robust groups—critical care for the entire stay (18,618 patients, critical care medicine [CCM] group) versus no critical care (22,870 patients, no CCM group), presumably due to lack of availability. The CCM group were more likely to be academic medical centers in urban locations, indicating that selection bias, which included racial background, chronic health problems, and socioeconomic status, may have had an impact. Another form of selection bias may have been evident—that of the units themselves.[25] It is likely that there is a cohort of nursing-led ICUs that may function at a very high level of care. This may result from strict adherence to protocols and guidelines, with meticulous attention to infection control and involvement in, and submission to, national benchmarking databases (such as Project IMPACT).[26] Thus, this study may illuminate the effectiveness of an elite group of ICUs, absent an intensive care specialist, that through tight organizational controls may have better outcomes.

In conclusion, the majority of studies have demonstrated that availability of an intensive care specialist may reduce mortality rate, length of stay, and costs in intensive care. Interestingly, there are impressive epidemiologic data that intensive care outcomes for many diagnoses are improving.[27-32] This may reflect the overall increase in awareness of critical illness; improved vertical integration between emergency medicine, medicine, surgery, and anesthesia; and a problem-oriented, systems-based approach to medical education and practice. Young and Birkmeyer[33] have estimated that full implementation of intensivist-model ICUs would save approximately 53,850 lives each year in the United States. Conversely, Levy and colleagues[24] have suggested that management of patients in "choice" ICUs by intensivists and in units with full critical care management of patients, compared with a no-intensivists model, may be associated with worse outcomes. No clear explanation for the adverse outcomes in this patient subgroup has emerged. However, it is worth noting that the presence of an intensive care specialist alone is not a "critical care service" and that improved outcomes may result from an integrated model of specialist and multidisciplinary team care, strategic management, and tight organizational structure.

Intensive Care Organization

As previously noted, the introduction of intensive care specialists is one part of a system, usually referred to as a "critical care service." A critical care team, led by an intensivist and including residents, fellows, nurse practitioners, respiratory therapists, and a pharmacist, provide 24-hour care to the patient. This may be in full collaboration with the primary care team (the "open" model), or to replace that team as primary caregivers (the "closed" model).

Baldock and colleagues[34] prospectively studied 1140 patients admitted into a mixed medical-surgical ICU over a 3-year period, during which time resident medical staff and a closed configuration were introduced. ICU mortality rate was reduced from 28% to 19% (ARR 9%, NNT 11), OR 0.61 (0.42 to 0.89, 95% CI). Hospital mortality rate was reduced from 36% to 24% (ARR 12%, NNT 8), OR 0.54 (0.38 to 0.77, 95% CI).

Carson and colleagues[35] studied change from an open ($n = 121$) to a closed ($n = 124$) format in a medical ICU. Apache II scores indicated that patients admitted following closure of the unit were significantly sicker. Mortality rates increased following unit closure. However, the ratio of actual mortality to predicted mortality rate was lower in this system. Resource utilization remained similar, which is surprising in view of the increase in severity of illness. Consequently this paper suggests the cost-effectiveness and probable clinical effectiveness of the closed unit format.

Ghorra and colleagues[36] retrospectively studied the conversion of a surgical ICU from open ($n = 125$) to closed ($n = 149$) format. Again, primary care was provided by an intensive care team. There was a significant reduction in mortality rate, from 14% to 6% (ARR 8, NNT 12, OR 0.38 [0.17 to 0.88, 95% CI]), and in complications from 56% to 44% (ARR 12, NNT 8). This was accompanied by a reduction in the number of consultations (from 0.6 to 0.4 per patient). The incidence of renal failure and the use of low-dose dopamine were higher in the open format, reflecting outdated approaches to critical illness.[37]

Multz and colleagues[38] retrospectively looked at outcomes in a community hospital before and after conversion to a closed ICU model, and prospectively compared outcomes with a nearby hospital's open ICU. Although no significant differences in mortality rate were found in either arm of this underpowered study, there was a significant reduction in ICU length of stay (retrospective 6.1 versus 9.3 days, p <0.05; prospective 6.1 versus 12.6 days, p <0.0001), hospital length of stay (retrospective 22.2 versus 31.2 days, p <0.02; prospective 19.2 versus 33.2 days, p <0.008) and days of mechanical ventilation (retrospective 3.3 versus 6.4 days, p <0.05; prospective 2.3 versus 8.5 days, p <0.0005).

Treggiari and colleagues[39] studied outcomes for patients with acute lung injury in open versus closed ICUs. A total of 24 intensive care units were evaluated, with complete data for 23; 13 units were closed and 11 were open. Hospital mortality rate was improved significantly in the closed versus open units (adjusted OR, 0.68; 95% CI, 0.53, 0.89; $p = 0.004$). The presence of a consulting pulmonologist, presumably with critical care training, and thus an "intensivist," did not appear to confer benefit in open ICUs.

Using data from a prospective cohort study, Nathens and colleagues[40] looked at mortality rates in trauma patients across 68 intensive care units. After adjusting for differences in baseline characteristics, the relative risk of death in intensivist-model ICUs was 0.78 (0.58 to 1.04) compared with an open ICU model. The effect was greatest in the elderly (RR, 0.55 [0.39 to 0.77]), in units led by surgical intensivists (RR, 0.67 [0.50 to 0.90]), and in designated trauma centers 0.64 (0.46 to 0.88). It is worth noting that in this study, as in other studies of surgical ICUs, high-volume surgical centers are more likely to have intensivists, and these factors may reinforce one another.[41-43]

Tai and colleagues[44] retrospectively studied quality of patient care and procedure use in a medical ICU over two 3-month periods before ($n = 112$) and after ($n = 127$) change in unit organization. In the first period, an open model prevailed. In the second, an intensivist provided daytime care, acting as primary physician and gatekeeper, with rotational medical cover at night. There was a reduction in median length of stay. Interestingly, the use of invasive monitors increased from 0% to 24% for arterial lines, and from 0% to 5.5% for pulmonary artery catheters, without evidence of improvements in outcomes.

The introduction of a physician-manager for intensive care services (ICU director) has become universal. However, there is significant variability in the director's day-to-day involvement in medical care, protocols, bed management, and audit.

Manthous and colleagues[45] studied outcomes and educational standards in a medium-sized community hospital in the year before ($n = 459$) and after ($n = 471$) the appointment of a director of critical care. ICU mortality rate was reduced from 21% to 15% (ARR 6%, NNT 16, OR 0.66 [0.47 to 0.93, 95% CI]). This reduction in mortality rate was consistent for most disease processes and severity of illness. In addition, there was a significant reduction in hospital mortality rate from 34% to 25% (ARR 9%, NNT 11, OR 0.63 [0.48 to 0.84, 95% CI]). There was a concomitant reduction in mean stays in the ICU (from 5.0 ± 0.3 days to 3.9 ± 0.3 days [$p <0.05$]) and in the hospital (from 22.6 ± 1.4 days to 17.7 ± 1.0 days), along with an improvement in standard of knowledge of residents.

Mallick and colleagues[46] examined a 1991 survey by the Society of Critical Care Medicine (SCCM) of nearly 3000 ICUs to determine the effectiveness of the role of the ICU director. They concluded that significant involvement of the ICU director in the day-to-day operation of the unit reduced inappropriate bed occupancy, thus improving efficiency. Strosberg and colleagues[47] questioned nurse managers from 137 ICUs on the involvement of ICU directors in bed management at their hospitals. This revealed that although many hospitals had ICU directors, there was a perception of limited nocturnal availability.

Zimmerman and colleagues[48] looked at organizational issues in nine ICUs and determined that superior organization was characterized by a patient-centered culture, strong medical and nursing leadership, effective communication and coordination, and open, collaborative approaches to solving problems and managing conflict.

They failed to equate superior organization to improved risk-adjusted survival.

Shortell and colleagues[49] examined risk-adjusted mortality rates in 42 ICUs involving 17,440 patients using Apache III. They found that high-quality organization was associated with lower risk-associated mortality rate, lower risk-adjusted length of stay, lower nurse turnover, and higher patient and family member satisfaction. Examples of organizational excellence included technologic availability, lack of diagnostic diversity, and caregiver interaction comprising the culture, leadership, coordination, communication, and conflict management abilities of the unit.

A large European study of ICU organization, EURICUS-1,[50] published in 1998, looked at the organizational characteristics of 89 ICUs in 12 European countries. It was determined that the optimal model of ICU organization—where the strategic apex of shared medical-nursing administration lies within the ICU—exists in only 12% of ICUs studied. Further, there was no clear concept of "intensive care," little planning or purposeful organization, and few defined objectives.[30]

The Leapfrog group has proposed that intensive care services provided by telemedicine, involving an intensive care specialist covering several ICUs from a remote location,[51] would be a reasonable surrogate for a full-time intensivist.[52] This has been a widely embraced system of alternative intensivist staffing,[53] and it has demonstrated some outcome benefit.[54] Breslow and colleagues[55] have shown that tele-ICU services improve outcomes (reduced hospital mortality rate, 9.4% versus 12.9%; relative risk, 0.73; 95% CI, 0.55 to 0.95) and reduce length of stay (3.63 days [95% CI, 3.21 to 4.04] versus 4.35 days [95% CI, 3.93 to 4.78]). This approach should be envisioned as complementing and extending organized ICU services rather than manifesting an alternative model for critical care service delivery.

In conclusion, the conversion of intensive care units from open to closed formats and the appointment of an ICU medical director appears to confer modest benefits in terms of mortality rate, morbidity, resource utilization, and length of stay. At least in part, these outcome benefits relate to more advanced critical care built on the intensivist model.

AREAS OF UNCERTAINTY

The limited literature published in this field supports the appointment of intensive care specialists alongside the development of multidisciplinary critical care teams, standards-based care, and an integrated organizational structure. There are a number of significant limitations. The majority were cohort studies using historical controls. Hawthorne effects cannot be discounted. Only one group, Hanson and colleagues,[56] concurrently studied patients in the same ICU. This study was limited by lack of randomization and multiple potentially confounding variables because significant selection bias may have been present. Similarly, the large cross-sectional studies by Pronovost and colleagues,[57] Dimick and colleagues,[58] and Nathens and colleagues[40] were limited by single diagnoses and the possibility that poorer outcomes related not to critical care but to hospital volume and expertise.[59] However, Pronovost and colleagues,[60] having corrected for these factors, demonstrated a threefold increase in mortality rate in hospitals without daily intensivist rounds. A number of the studies required statistical adjustments to demonstrate mortality rate differences.[11,36,40,61,62] This is consistent with validated prediction models.[63]

Another potential limitation is publication bias. Studies of this nature are performed by intensivists to promote their specialty. Thus, it is unlikely that studies will be published demonstrating worse outcomes. Conversely, a number of studies have been published in abstract form alone. When systematically reviewed with published data,

support for the intensivist model persists.[64] Moreover, Pronovost and colleagues[64] have been unable to demonstrate publication bias in the literature.

Many authors have questioned whether the intensivist model improves outcomes only during the daytime when intensivists are physically present in the ICU. Although a 24-hour intensivist may be associated with improved outcomes,[65] there is no compelling evidence that patient outcomes are worse when admitted at night, on weekends, or during the month of July[66-70] (Table 42-1).

Finally, the study by Levy and colleagues[24] may lead to a reassessment of the entire intensivist paradigm. Although it was a data-mining exercise of a database that was designed to examine workload, not outcomes, the results

Table 42-1 Summary of Published Studies on Intensive Care Specialists

Study	Intervention	Design	Unit Type	Number Study group	Number Control group	Mortality Benefit (OR)	Hospital LOS reduced	Cost Benefit	Morbidity Benefit
Li[91]	Intensivist	Cohort Retrospective observational	Mixed	463	491	0.91* Hosp	—	Yes	—
Pollack[92]	Intensivist plus daytime ICU team	Cohort Prospective observational	Pediatric	149	113	0.51*	—	—	—
Reynolds[93]	Intensivist plus team	Cohort Prospective HC	MICU	100	112	0.46	—	—	—
Brown[94]	Intensivist	Cohort Prospective HC	Mixed	223	216	0.40 ICU 0.59 Hosp	—	—	—
Hanson[95]	Intensivist plus team	Cohort Retrospective Concurrent	SICU	100	100	—	Yes	Yes	Yes
Blunt[96]	Intensivist	Cohort HC	MICU	393	328	0.59*	—	—	—
Dimick[97]	Intensivist daily rounds	Cross-sectional	SICU	182	169	—	Yes	Yes	Yes
Pronovost[98]	Intensivist daily rounds	Cross-sectional	SICU	2036	472	0.56	Yes	Yes	Yes
Baldock[99]	Intensivist Closed	Cohort HC	Mixed	330	395	0.61 ICU 0.54 Hosp	—	—	—
Carson[100]	Intensivist Closed	Cohort HC	MICU	121	124	0.89‡ predicted	No	Yes	—
Ghorra[101]	Intensivist Closed	Cohort HC	SICU	125	149	0.36* ICU	—	Yes	Yes
Multz[102]	Intensivist Closed	Cohort HC	MICU	154	152	—	Yes	Yes	Yes
Multz[102]	Intensivist Closed	Prospective Cohort HC	MICU	185	95	—	Yes	Yes	Yes
Tai[103]	Intensivist During day	Cohort HC	MICU	127	112	—	—	Yes	—
Manthous[104]	ICU director	Cohort HC	MICU	930	459	0.63 ICU 0.66 Hosp	Yes	Yes	—

(Continued)

Study	**Intervention**	**Design**	**Unit Type**	**Number Study group**	**Number Control group**	**Mortality Benefit (OR)**	**Hospital LOS reduced**	**Cost Benefit**	**Morbidity Benefit**
Nathens[40]	Intensivist Intensive care team	Prospective Cohort	Trauma SICU			0.78 ICU 0.64 trauma centers	—	—	—
Treggiari[39]	Intensive care team Closed	Cohort	MICU (ARDS)	684	391	0.68 Hosp	—	—	—
Levy[24]	Intensivist	Cohort	All types	18,618	22,870	1.40[†]Hosp	—	—	—

Table 42-1 Summary of Published Studies on Intensive Care Specialists—Cont'd

HC, historic control; *MICU*, medical intensive care unit; *SICU*, surgical intensive care unit.
*Adjusted for severity of illness.
[†]Indicates unfavorable outcome with intensive care specialist.
[‡]Adjusted for standardized mortality ratios.

appear to be robust. However, the self-selection of highly functioning ICUs to the Project IMPACT database is problematic when applied to the population as a whole ("we measure what we value"), and this may represent an alternative model of ICU organization, rather than a repudiation of the critical care concept.[25] Guidelines and standards used in these units were developed by intensivists in academic medical centers and adopted by community hospitals, and this may represent the ultimate example of the effectiveness of evidence-based medicine.

AUTHORS' RECOMMENDATIONS

Most data support the contention that patient outcomes improve with the provision of an intensivist as part of an intensive care team. However, it is important to note that the data are heterogeneous—varying from daytime availability of an intensivist,[71] to "not consulted but available,"[72] to 24-hour cover,[73] to complete service closure.[74] It is tempting to suggest that outcome improvement is related to the degree of involvement and responsibility of the critical care team, and indeed a dose-response relationship has been described,[75,76] but more proof is required.

Although the intensivist model is ubiquitous outside the United States, there is significant geographic variability in outcomes.[77-79] Identifying why this is so is difficult. Some factors worth considering are bed availability,[78] nurse and physician workload,[80,81] and practice patterns and resource availability.[82] There is emerging evidence that subspecialist ICUs further improve outcomes.[83] Conversely, there is evidence that in certain circumstances, intensivists may be associated with worse outcomes.[24] Perhaps this illustrates the paradox of intensive care: hospital mortality rates of intensive care patients can be manipulated by admission and transfer criteria and end-of-life decision making. By "cherry picking" admissions with likely more favorable outcomes, by transferring to alternative (specialist) units the sickest patients, and by delaying end-of-life decision making (for example, by using long-stay ventilator facilities), more favorable outcomes may be presented without better health care delivered.

Intensivists, then, appear to be valuable, but are they available? In 1997 intensivists cared for only 37% of critically ill patients.[84] This is expected to fall significantly over the next 20 years. Currently, 78.9% of intensivists are pulmonologists, 11.9% are internists, 6.1% are anesthesiologists, and 3.2% are surgeons. The percentage of intensivists who are anesthesiologists is declining.[85] In spite of this the Committee on Manpower for Pulmonary and Critical Care Services has determined that surgical ICUs are particularly underserved by intensivists compared with medical units.[86] In 1996 there were 130 graduates from surgically oriented (50% were anesthesiologists) critical care training programs, compared with 464 from internal medicine–based programs.[86] This reflects the high opportunity cost of practicing critical care versus operating room activity.[85] Nevertheless, economically powerful patient advocate organizations[87] are demanding intensivist involvement in patient care. Increased remuneration or income redistribution may result. It is unlikely that this demand can be met[86,88] for the foreseeable future. Novel concepts such as telemedicine[89] may provide a bridge.

In summary, focused, standardized care with clear leadership, rapid specialist availability, and a well-developed team approach appears to be the optimal model for critical care organization.[26] Unquestionably, there will be an increased demand for intensivists trained in anesthesiology; the question is—are you in or are you out?[90]

REFERENCES

1. Groeger JS, Strosberg MA, Halpern NA, Raphaely RC, Kaye WE, Guntupalli KK, et al: Descriptive analysis of critical care units in the United States. *Crit Care Med* 1992;20:846-863.
2. Angus DC, Kelley MA, Schmitz RJ, White A, Popovich J Jr: Caring for the critically ill patient. Current and projected workforce requirements for care of the critically ill and patients with pulmonary disease: Can we meet the requirements of an aging population? *JAMA* 2000;284:2762-2770.
3. Angus DC, Ramakrishnan N: National intensive care unit datasets: Lost at sea without a compass? *Crit Care Med* 1999;27:1659-1661.
4. Catlin A, Cowan C, Hartman M, Heffler S: National health spending in 2006: A year of change for prescription drugs. *Health Aff* 2008;27:14-29.

5. Jacobs P, Noseworthy TW: National estimates of intensive care utilization and costs: Canada and the United States. *Crit Care Med* 1990;18:1282-1286.

6. Halpern NA, Pastores SM, Thaler HT, Greenstein RJ: Changes in critical care beds and occupancy in the United States 1985-2000: Differences attributable to hospital size. *Crit Care Med* 2006;34: 2105-2112.

7. Ward NS, Teno JM, Curtis JR, Rubenfeld GD, Levy MM: Perceptions of cost constraints, resource limitations, and rationing in United States intensive care units: Results of a national survey. *Crit Care Med* 2008;36:471-476.

8. Carlson RW, Weiland DE, Srivathsan K: Does a full-time, 24-hour intensivist improve care and efficiency? *Crit Care Clin* 1996;12:525-551.

9. Hanson CW III, Durbin CG Jr, Maccioli GA, Deutschman CS, Sladen RN, Pronovost PJ, Gattinoni L: The anesthesiologist in critical care medicine: Past, present, and future. *Anesthesiology* 2001;95:781-788.

10. Leape LL, Cullen DJ, Clapp MD, Burdick E, Demonaco HJ, Erickson JI, Bates DW: Pharmacist participation on physician rounds and adverse drug events in the intensive care unit. *JAMA* 1999;282:267-270.

11. Pollack MM, Katz RW, Ruttimann UE, Getson PR: Improving the outcome and efficiency of intensive care: The impact of an intensivist. *Crit Care Med* 1988;16:11-17.

12. Groeger JS, Guntupalli KK, Strosberg M, Halpern N, Raphaely RC, Cerra F, Kaye W: Descriptive analysis of critical care units in the United States: Patient characteristics and intensive care unit utilization. *Crit Care Med* 1993;21:279-291.

13. Amaravadi RK, Dimick JB, Pronovost PJ, Lipsett PA: ICU nurse-to-patient ratio is associated with complications and resource use after esophagectomy. *Intensive Care Med* 2000;26: 1857-1862.

14. Li TC, Phillips MC, Shaw L, Cook EF, Natanson C, Goldman L: On-site physician staffing in a community hospital intensive care unit. Impact on test and procedure use and on patient outcome. *JAMA* 1984;252:2023-2027.

15. Reynolds HN, Haupt MT, Thill-Baharozian MC, Carlson RW: Impact of critical care physician staffing on patients with septic shock in a university hospital medical intensive care unit. *JAMA* 1988;260:3446-3450.

16. Brown JJ, Sullivan G: Effect on ICU mortality of a full-time critical care specialist. *Chest* 1989;96:127-129.

17. Hanson CW III, Deutschman CS, Anderson HL III, Reilly PM, Behringer EC, Schwab CW, Price J: Effects of an organized critical care service on outcomes and resource utilization: A cohort study. *Crit Care Med* 1999;27:270-274.

18. Blunt MC, Burchett KR: Out-of-hours consultant cover and case-mix-adjusted mortality in intensive care. *Lancet* 2000;356: 735-736.

19. Dimick JB, Pronovost PJ, Heitmiller RF, Lipsett PA: Intensive care unit physician staffing is associated with decreased length of stay, hospital cost, and complications after esophageal resection. *Crit Care Med* 2001;29:753-758.

20. Pronovost PJ, Jenckes MW, Dorman T, Garrett E, Breslow MJ, Rosenfeld BA, et al: Organizational characteristics of intensive care units related to outcomes of abdominal aortic surgery. *JAMA* 1999;281:1310-1317.

21. Pronovost P, Angus DC: Using large-scale databases to measure outcomes in critical care. *Crit Care Clin* 1999;15:615-viii.

22. Dimick JB, Pronovost PJ, Heitmiller RF, Lipsett PA: Intensive care unit physician staffing is associated with decreased length of stay, hospital cost, and complications after esophageal resection. *Crit Care Med* 2001;29:753-758.

23. Pronovost PJ, Angus DC, Dorman T, Robinson KA, Dremsizov TT, Young TL: Physician staffing patterns and clinical outcomes in critically ill patients: A systematic review. *JAMA* 2002;288:2151-2162.

24. Levy MM, Rapoport J, Lemeshow S, Chalfin DB, Phillips G, Danis M: Association between critical care physician management and patient mortality in the intensive care unit. *Ann Intern Med* 2008;148:801-809.

25. Rubenfeld GD, Angus DC: Are intensivists safe? *Ann Intern Med* 2008;148:877-879.

26. Zimmerman JE, Alzola C, Von Rueden KT: The use of benchmarking to identify top performing critical care units: A preliminary assessment of their policies and practices. *J Crit Care* 2003;18:76-86.

27. Moran JL, Bristow P, Solomon PJ, George C, Hart GK: Mortality and length-of-stay outcomes, 1993-2003, in the binational Australian and New Zealand intensive care adult patient database. *Crit Care Med* 2008;36:46-61.

28. Halpern NA, Bettes L, Greenstein R: Federal and nationwide intensive care units and healthcare costs: 1986-1992. *Crit Care Med* 1994;22:2001-2007.

29. Zimmerman JE, Shortell SM, Rousseau DM, Duffy J, Gillies RR, Knaus WA, et al: Improving intensive care: Observations based on organizational case studies in nine intensive care units: A prospective, multicenter study. *Crit Care Med* 1993;21: 1443-1451.

30. Miranda DR, Rivera-Fernandez R, Nap RE: Critical care medicine in the hospital: Lessons from the EURICUS-studies. *Med Intensiva* 2007;31:194-203.

31. Deans KJ, Minneci PC, Cui X, Banks SM, Natanson C, Eichacker PQ: Mechanical ventilation in ARDS: One size does not fit all. *Crit Care Med* 2005;33:1141-1143.

32. Milberg JA, Davis DR, Steinberg KP, Hudson LD: Improved survival of patients with acute respiratory distress syndrome (ARDS): 1983-1993. *JAMA* 1995;273:306-309.

33. Young MP, Birkmeyer JD: Potential reduction in mortality rates using an intensivist model to manage intensive care units. *Eff Clin Pract* 2000;3:284-289.

34. Baldock G, Foley P, Brett S: The impact of organisational change on outcome in an intensive care unit in the United Kingdom. *Intensive Care Med* 2001;27:865-872.

35. Carson SS, Stocking C, Podsadecki T, Christenson J, Pohlman A, MacRae S, et al: Effects of organizational change in the medical intensive care unit of a teaching hospital: A comparison of "open" and "closed" formats. *JAMA* 1996;276:322-328.

36. Ghorra S, Reinert SE, Cioffi W, Buczko G, Simms HH: Analysis of the effect of conversion from open to closed surgical intensive care unit. *Ann Surg* 1999;229:163-171.

37. O'Leary MJ, Bihari DJ: Preventing renal failure in the critically ill. There are no magic bullets—just high quality intensive care. *BMJ* 2001;322:1437-1439.

38. Multz AS, Chalfin DB, Samson IM, Dantzker DR, Fein AM, Steinberg HN, et al: A "closed" medical intensive care unit (MICU) improves resource utilization when compared with an "open" MICU. *Am J Respir Crit Care Med* 1998;157:1468-1473.

39. Treggiari MM, Martin DP, Yanez ND, Caldwell E, Hudson LD, Rubenfeld GD: Effect of intensive care unit organizational model and structure on outcomes in patients with acute lung injury. *Am J Respir Crit Care Med* 2007;176:685-690.

40. Nathens AB, Rivara FP, Mackenzie EJ, Maier RV, Wang J, Egleston B, et al: The impact of an intensivist-model ICU on trauma-related mortality. *Ann Surg* 2006;244:545-554.

41. Volkert T, Hinder F, Ellger B, Van AH: Changing from a specialized surgical observation unit to an interdisciplinary surgical intensive care unit can reduce costs and increase the quality of treatment. *Eur J Anaesthesiol* 2008;1-6.

42. Halpern NA, Pastores SM, Thaler HT, Greenstein RJ: Changes in critical care beds and occupancy in the United States 1985-2000: Differences attributable to hospital size. *Crit Care Med* 2006;34: 2105-2112.

43. Birkmeyer JD, Siewers AE, Finlayson EV, Stukel TA, Lucas FL, Batista I, et al: Hospital volume and surgical mortality in the United States. *N Engl J Med* 2002;346:1128-1137.

44. Tai DY, Goh SK, Eng PC, Wang YT: Impact on quality of patient care and procedure use in the medical intensive care unit (MICU) following reorganisation. *Ann Acad Med Singapore* 1998;27:309-313.

45. Manthous CA, Amoateng-Adjepong Y, al Kharrat T, Jacob B, Alnuaimat HM, Chatila W, Hall JB: Effects of a medical intensivist on patient care in a community teaching hospital. *Mayo Clin Proc* 1997;72:391-399.

46. Mallick R, Strosberg M, Lambrinos J, Groeger JS: The intensive care unit medical director as manager. Impact on performance. *Med Care* 1995;33:611-624.

47. Strosberg MA, Teres D, Fein IA, Linsider R: Nursing perception of the availability of the intensive care unit medical director for triage and conflict resolution. *Heart Lung* 1990;19:452-455.

48. Zimmerman JE, Shortell SM, Rousseau DM, Duffy J, Gillies RR, Knaus WA, et al: Improving intensive care: Observations based on organizational case studies in nine intensive care units: A prospective, multicenter study. *Crit Care Med* 1993;21: 1443-1451.

49. Shortell SM, Zimmerman JE, Rousseau DM, Gillies RR, Wagner DP, Draper EA, et al: The performance of intensive care units: Does good management make a difference? *Med Care* 1994;32: 508-525.

50. Reis Miranda D, editor: *Organisation and management of intensive care. The EURICUS-1 study.* Berlin, Springer, 1998, pp 81-86.

51. Breslow MJ, Rosenfeld BA, Doerfler M, Burke G, Yates G, Stone DJ, et al: Effect of a multiple-site intensive care unit telemedicine program on clinical and economic outcomes: An alternative paradigm for intensivist staffing. *Crit Care Med* 2004;32:31-38.

52. Milstein A, Galvin RS, Delbanco SF, Salber P, Buck CR Jr: Improving the safety of health care: The leapfrog initiative. *Eff Clin Pract* 2000;3:313-316.

53. Breslow MJ: Remote ICU care programs: Current status. *J Crit Care* 2007;22:66-76.

54. Rosenfeld BA, Dorman T, Breslow MJ, Pronovost P, Jenckes M, Zhang N, et al: Intensive care unit telemedicine: Alternate paradigm for providing continuous intensivist care. *Crit Care Med* 2000;28:3925-3931.

55. Breslow MJ, Rosenfeld BA, Doerfler M, Burke G, Yates G, Stone DJ, et al: Effect of a multiple-site intensive care unit telemedicine program on clinical and economic outcomes: An alternative paradigm for intensivist staffing. *Crit Care Med* 2004;32:31-38.

56. Hanson CW III, Deutschman CS, Anderson HL III, Reilly PM, Behringer EC, Schwab CW, Price J: Effects of an organized critical care service on outcomes and resource utilization: A cohort study. *Crit Care Med* 1999;27:270-274.

57. Pronovost PJ, Jenckes MW, Dorman T, Garrett E, Breslow MJ, Rosenfeld BA, et al: Organizational characteristics of intensive care units related to outcomes of abdominal aortic surgery. *JAMA* 1999;281:1310-1317.

58. Dimick JB, Pronovost PJ, Heitmiller RF, Lipsett PA: Intensive care unit physician staffing is associated with decreased length of stay, hospital cost, and complications after esophageal resection. *Crit Care Med* 2001;29:753-758.

59. Birkmeyer JD, Siewers AE, Finlayson EV, Stukel TA, Lucas FL, Batista I, et al: Hospital volume and surgical mortality in the United States. *N Engl J Med* 2002;346:1128-1137.

60. Pronovost PJ, Jenckes MW, Dorman T, Garrett E, Breslow MJ, Rosenfeld BA, et al: Organizational characteristics of intensive care units related to outcomes of abdominal aortic surgery. *JAMA* 1999;281:1310-1317.

61. Blunt MC, Burchett KR: Out-of-hours consultant cover and case-mix-adjusted mortality in intensive care. *Lancet* 2000;356:735-736.

62. Li TC, Phillips MC, Shaw L, Cook EF, Natanson C, Goldman L: On-site physician staffing in a community hospital intensive care unit. Impact on test and procedure use and on patient outcome. *JAMA* 1984;252:2023-2027.

63. Knaus WA, Wagner DP, Zimmerman JE, Draper EA: Variations in mortality and length of stay in intensive care units. *Ann Intern Med* 1993;118:753-761.

64. Pronovost PJ, Angus DC, Dorman T, Robinson KA, Dremsizov TT, Young TL: Physician staffing patterns and clinical outcomes in critically ill patients: A systematic review. *JAMA* 2002;288: 2151-2162.

65. Gajic O, Afessa B, Hanson AC, Krpata T, Yilmaz M, Mohamed SF, et al: Effect of 24-hour mandatory versus on-demand critical care specialist presence on quality of care and family and provider satisfaction in the intensive care unit of a teaching hospital. *Crit Care Med* 2008;36:36-44.

66. Arabi Y, Alshimemeri A, Taher S: Weekend and weeknight admissions have the same outcome of weekday admissions to an intensive care unit with onsite intensivist coverage. *Crit Care Med* 2006;34:605-611.

67. Finkielman JD, Morales J, Peters SG, Keegan MT, Ensminger SA, Lymp JF, Afessa B: Mortality rate and length of stay of patients admitted to the intensive care unit in July. *Crit Care Med* 2004;32:1161-1165.

68. Morales IJ, Peters SG, Afessa B: Hospital mortality rate and length of stay in patients admitted at night to the intensive care unit. *Crit Care Med* 2003;31:858-863.

69. Ensminger SA, Morales IJ, Peters SG, Keegan MT, Finkielman JD, Lymp JF, Afessa B: The hospital mortality of patients admitted to the ICU on weekends. *Chest* 2004;126:1292-1298.

70. Luyt CE, Combes A, Aegerter P, Guidet B, Trouillet JL, Gibert C, Chastre J: Mortality among patients admitted to intensive care units during weekday day shifts compared with "off" hours. *Crit Care Med* 2007;35:3-11.

71. Tai DY, Goh SK, Eng PC, Wang YT: Impact on quality of patient care and procedure use in the medical intensive care unit (MICU) following reorganisation. *Ann Acad Med Singapore* 1998;27:309-313.

72. Hanson CW III, Deutschman CS, Anderson HL III, Reilly PM, Behringer EC, Schwab CW, Price J: Effects of an organized critical care service on outcomes and resource utilization: A cohort study. *Crit Care Med* 1999;27:270-274.

73. Baldock G, Foley P, Brett S: The impact of organisational change on outcome in an intensive care unit in the United Kingdom. *Intensive Care Med* 2001;27:865-872.

74. Ghorra S, Reinert SE, Cioffi W, Buczko G, Simms HH: Analysis of the effect of conversion from open to closed surgical intensive care unit. *Ann Surg* 1999;229:163-171.

75. Dara SI, Afessa B: Intensivist-to-bed ratio: Association with outcomes in the medical ICU. *Chest* 2005;128:567-572.

76. Parshuram CS, Kirpalani H, Mehta S, Granton J, Cook D: In-house, overnight physician staffing: A cross-sectional survey of Canadian adult and pediatric intensive care units. *Crit Care Med* 2006;34:1674-1678.

77. Knaus WA, Wagner DP, Zimmerman JE, Draper EA: Variations in mortality and length of stay in intensive care units. *Ann Intern Med* 1993;118:753-761.

78. Beck DH, Taylor BL, Millar B, Smith GB: Prediction of outcome from intensive care: A prospective cohort study comparing Acute Physiology and Chronic Health Evaluation II and III prognostic systems in a United Kingdom intensive care unit. *Crit Care Med* 1997;25:9-15.

79. Angus DC, Sirio CA, Clermont G, Bion J: International comparisons of critical care outcome and resource consumption. *Crit Care Clin* 1997;13:389-407.

80. Amaravadi RK, Dimick JB, Pronovost PJ, Lipsett PA: ICU nurse-to-patient ratio is associated with complications and resource use after esophagectomy. *Intensive Care Med* 2000;26:1857-1862.

81. Tarnow-Mordi WO, Hau C, Warden A, Shearer AJ: Hospital mortality in relation to staff workload: A 4-year study in an adult intensive-care unit. *Lancet* 2000;356:185-189.

82. Bell CM, Redelmeier DA: Mortality among patients admitted to hospitals on weekends as compared with weekdays. *N Engl J Med* 2001;345:663-668.

83. Diringer MN, Edwards DF: Admission to a neurologic/neurosurgical intensive care unit is associated with reduced mortality rate after intracerebral hemorrhage. *Crit Care Med* 2001;29:635-640.

84. Angus DC, Kelley MA, Schmitz RJ, White A, Popovich J Jr: Caring for the critically ill patient. Current and projected workforce requirements for care of the critically ill and patients with pulmonary disease: Can we meet the requirements of an aging population? *JAMA* 2000;284:2762-2770.

85. Hanson CW III, Durbin CG Jr, Maccioli GA, Deutschman CS, Sladen RN, Pronovost PJ, Gattinoni L: The anesthesiologist in critical care medicine: Past, present, and future. *Anesthesiology* 2001;95:781-788.

86. Angus DC, Kelley MA, Schmitz RJ, White A, Popovich J Jr: Caring for the critically ill patient. Current and projected workforce requirements for care of the critically ill and patients with pulmonary disease: Can we meet the requirements of an aging population? *JAMA* 2000;284:2762-2770.

87. Milstein A, Galvin RS, Delbanco SF, Salber P, Buck CR Jr: Improving the safety of health care: The leapfrog initiative. *Eff Clin Pract* 2000;3:313-316.

88. Carlson RW, Weiland DE, Srivathsan K: Does a full-time, 24-hour intensivist improve care and efficiency? *Crit Care Clin* 1996;12:525-551.

89. Rosenfeld BA, Dorman T, Breslow MJ, Pronovost P, Jenckes M, Zhang N, et al: Intensive care unit telemedicine: Alternate paradigm for providing continuous intensivist care. *Crit Care Med* 2000;28:3925-3931.

90. Hanson CW III, Durbin CG Jr, Maccioli GA, Deutschman CS, Sladen RN, Pronovost PJ, Gattinoni L: The anesthesiologist in critical care medicine: Past, present, and future. *Anesthesiology* 2001;95:781-788.

91. Li TC, Phillips MC, Shaw L, Cook EF, Natanson C, Goldman L: On-site physician staffing in a community hospital intensive care unit. Impact on test and procedure use and on patient outcome. *JAMA* 1984;252:2023-2027.

92. Pollack MM, Katz RW, Ruttimann UE, Getson PR: Improving the outcome and efficiency of intensive care: The impact of an intensivist. *Crit Care Med* 1988;16:11-17.

93. Reynolds HN, Haupt MT, Thill-Baharozian MC, Carlson RW: Impact of critical care physician staffing on patients with septic shock in a university hospital medical intensive care unit. *JAMA* 1988;260:3446-3450.

94. Brown JJ, Sullivan G: Effect on ICU mortality of a full-time critical care specialist. *Chest* 1989;96:127-129.

95. Hanson CW III, Deutschman CS, Anderson HL, III, Reilly PM, Behringer EC, Schwab CW, Price J: Effects of an organized critical care service on outcomes and resource utilization: A cohort study. *Crit Care Med* 1999;27:270-274.

96. Blunt MC, Burchett KR: Out-of-hours consultant cover and case-mix-adjusted mortality in intensive care. *Lancet* 2000;356:735-736.

97. Dimick JB, Pronovost PJ, Heitmiller RF, Lipsett PA: Intensive care unit physician staffing is associated with decreased length of stay, hospital cost, and complications after esophageal resection. *Crit Care Med* 2001;29:753-758.

98. Pronovost PJ, Jenckes MW, Dorman T, Garrett E, Breslow MJ, Rosenfeld BA, et al: Organizational characteristics of intensive care units related to outcomes of abdominal aortic surgery. *JAMA* 1999;281:1310-1317.

99. Baldock G, Foley P, Brett S: The impact of organisational change on outcome in an intensive care unit in the United Kingdom. *Intensive Care Med* 2001;27:865-872.

100. Carson SS, Stocking C, Podsadecki T, Christenson J, Pohlman A, MacRae S, et al: Effects of organizational change in the medical intensive care unit of a teaching hospital: A comparison of "open" and "closed" formats. *JAMA* 1996;276:322-328.

101. Ghorra S, Reinert SE, Cioffi W, Buczko G, Simms HH: Analysis of the effect of conversion from open to closed surgical intensive care unit. *Ann Surg* 1999;229:163-171.

102. Multz AS, Chalfin DB, Samson IM, Dantzker DR, Fein AM, Steinberg HN, et al: A "closed" medical intensive care unit (MICU) improves resource utilization when compared with an "open" MICU. *Am J Respir Crit Care Med* 1998;157:1468-1473.

103. Tai DY, Goh SK, Eng PC, Wang YT: Impact on quality of patient care and procedure use in the medical intensive care unit (MICU) following reorganisation. *Ann Acad Med Singapore* 1998;27:309-313.

104. Manthous CA, Amoateng-Adjepong Y, al Kharrat T, Jacob B, Alnuaimat HM, Chatila W, Hall JB: Effects of a medical intensivist on patient care in a community teaching hospital. *Mayo Clin Proc* 1997;72:391-399.

43 Can We Prevent Recall during Anesthesia?

T. Andrew Bowdle, MD, PhD

INTRODUCTION

Three large prospective studies of the incidence of intraoperative awareness from Australia, Europe, and North America suggest that the overall rate is in the range of 0.1% to 0.2% or 1 to 2 per thousand patients.[1-3] Intraoperative awareness can be a minor or a major complication depending on the severity and the response of the individual patient; in severe cases posttraumatic stress disorder may occur.[4-6] In select patient populations the rate of intraoperative awareness may be substantially higher, such as in cardiac surgery patients where the rate has been reported to be in the range of 0.4% to 1%.[3,7-12] Recent prospective studies of intraoperative awareness in children found a rate of 0.8% to 1.1%.[13, 14] Conversely, the rate of intraoperative awareness may be lower in a particular setting. A recent retrospective analysis of quality assurance data from a single medical center suggested that the incidence of intraoperative awareness was 0.0068% or 1 per 14,560 patients.[15] Methodologic criticisms can be made of all of these studies of the incidence of intraoperative awareness.[16] However, as a whole the literature suggests that intraoperative awareness is a significant problem. Many anesthesiologists find a rate of intraoperative awareness in the vicinity of 0.1% to be unacceptably high. Most patients affected by intraoperative awareness find the experience to be unacceptable, especially if they experience pain and anxiety.[1] Can we prevent recall during anesthesia, or at least lower the rate substantially?

OPTIONS

Some episodes of intraoperative awareness are caused by specific, identifiable errors in anesthetic drug administration. Examples of these errors include the following:

1. Administration of a muscle relaxant instead of a hypnotic during induction of anesthesia resulting in an awake, paralyzed patient.
2. Unrecognized failure of a pump to deliver an intravenous hypnotic drug such as propofol. See Rowan[17] for a particularly vivid example.
3. An unrecognized empty vaporizer.

Thus, prevention of drug administration errors could be useful for reducing intraoperative awareness. Discussion of drug administration errors and strategies for prevention are beyond the scope of this chapter, and readers are referred to previous publications.[18-23]

Many, if not most, cases of intraoperative awareness occur without the occurrence of a specific error in drug administration and are probably related to an unusually large anesthetic dose requirement, due either to lower than average sensitivity to one or more drugs or faster than average clearance of one or more drugs. Large variation between individuals in anesthetic drug effect or anesthetic drug clearance is well documented for a variety of anesthetic drugs.[24] Identification of higher-risk individuals in advance and administration of larger doses of anesthetic to these individuals might reduce the rate of intraoperative awareness. Unfortunately, there is not currently a practical clinical method for identifying such individuals.

Patients receiving nondepolarizing muscle relaxants during the maintenance phase of anesthesia may be at greater risk of intraoperative awareness, presumably because they may not be able to move as readily and thereby give a clue to the anesthesiologist that the anesthetic depth is inadequate.[2] Some anesthesiologists take the approach of using as small a dose of muscle relaxant as possible to provide surgical exposure, with the idea that if the patient is too lightly anesthetized he or she will still be able to move. This practice probably makes sense, although it is clear from case reports that patients may not move during an episode of intraoperative awareness even in the absence of neuromuscular blocking drugs.[25]

Another option could be to give all patients very large doses of anesthetic drugs that would be adequate for even the least sensitive patient. There are numerous drawbacks to this approach, including cost, the potential for slow wakeup, and cardiovascular side effects, not to mention that there are no data that show what dose of anesthetic drug would be large enough to prevent intraoperative awareness under every circumstance in every patient.

Likewise, no particular drug has ever been shown to be uniquely reliable for preventing awareness in every circumstance in every patient; intraoperative awareness has been reported in patients receiving apparently adequate doses of just about every possible anesthetic agent. The available evidence suggests that total intravenous anesthesia has the same risk of intraoperative awareness as inhalational anesthesia.[2,26-28]

Finally, there is the option to somehow monitor the depth of anesthesia and titrate anesthetic drugs accordingly. Hypothetically, such an approach might prevent intraoperative awareness by identifying the patients who require larger doses of anesthetic drugs. The rest of this chapter will focus on this last approach.

EVIDENCE

Electroencephalography (EEG) has been the most widely applied technology for measuring anesthetic depth. Auditory evoked potentials have also been used either alone or in combination with EEG. For a comprehensive review of the methodology of using EEG and/or auditory evoked potentials to measure anesthetic depth, the reader is referred to previous publications.[29,30]

Although it may seem reasonable that depth of anesthesia monitoring would reduce the incidence of intraoperative awareness, that outcome was certainly not assured. The opposite hypothesis was entertained by some—that depth of anesthesia monitoring would actually increase the incidence of intraoperative awareness, because numerous studies had previously shown that on average patients received less anesthetic drug when monitored with an EEG depth of anesthesia monitor.[31]

Three clinical trials have suggested that intraoperative monitoring with EEG (specifically the Bispectral Index [BIS] monitor) can significantly reduce the incidence of intraoperative awareness (Table 43-1). The first was a retrospective case-comparison study of 5057 consecutive BIS-monitored patients from two hospitals in Sweden, compared with 7826 non–BIS-monitored patients from the same institutions.[32] There were 2 cases of intraoperative awareness in the BIS-monitored series compared with 14 in the non–BIS-monitored case-matched controls. This difference was statistically significant ($p < 0.039$).

The second study was a prospective, randomized, international multicenter trial of 2463 patients at high risk for intraoperative awareness (e.g., cardiac, trauma, obstetrics) assigned randomly to BIS or non-BIS groups (the so-called B-AWARE trial).[9] High-risk patients were chosen for this trial in order to increase the statistical power of the study. There were 2 cases of intraoperative awareness in the BIS-monitored group and 11 in the non–BIS-monitored group. Again, the difference was statistically significant ($p = 0.022$).

The most recent trial, published by Avidan and colleagues,[33] was a single-center, randomized trial of BIS monitoring (target BIS range 40 to 60) compared to *targeted end-tidal anesthetic gas analysis* (target range 0.7 to 1.3 MAC) with nearly 2000 total patients. The patients were required to be at "high risk" for intraoperative awareness based on a specific set of criteria. Approximately 25% of the patients had cardiac surgery. BIS and end-tidal anesthetic gas data were collected for both groups, but BIS values were not visible in the operating room for the targeted end-tidal anesthetic gas analysis group. Patients were assessed for intraoperative awareness three times, at 0 to 24 hours, 24 to 72 hours, and 30 days after extubation. Classification of no awareness, possible awareness, or definite awareness was made by a panel of blinded reviewers.

There were two cases of definite awareness in each group. There were BIS values greater than 60 in one of the patients with awareness (in the BIS-monitored group), and end-tidal anesthetic gas concentration less than 0.7 MAC in three patients with awareness (including both patients in the targeted end-tidal anesthetic gas group). The incidence of awareness was approximately 0.2%. The authors concluded that their findings "do not support routine BIS monitoring as part of standard practice," a conclusion that may not be warranted by the data.

The other randomized trial of BIS monitoring (the so-called B-AWARE trial by Myles and colleagues[9]) was a comparison of BIS monitoring to "standard practice" in high-risk patients. The "standard practice" group had an incidence of awareness of approximately 1%, which was the expected incidence, compared with approximately 0.2% in the BIS-monitored group, a statistically significant difference in favor of BIS monitoring. The study by Avidan and colleagues[33] was not a comparison of BIS monitoring with "standard practice"; rather, it was a comparison of BIS monitoring with another intervention in which practitioners were instructed to keep end-tidal anesthetic gas concentrations within a particular range, and the gas monitor audible alarms were set to activate when the concentrations were outside the prescribed range. Given that the expected incidence of awareness in the study by Avidan and colleagues[33] was approximately 1% (as estimated by the authors), and the observed incidence of awareness was 0.2% with BIS monitoring or targeted end-tidal anesthetic gas analysis, one could conclude that either BIS monitoring or targeted end-tidal anesthetic gas analysis were similarly effective in

Table 43-1	Summary of Clinical Trials of Bispectral Index (BIS) Monitoring for Reduction of Intraoperative Awareness		
Ekman et al., 2004[32]	5057 consecutive BIS-monitored patients compared with 7826 non–BIS-monitored case-control patients	Two hospitals in Sweden	Two cases of intraoperative awareness in BIS-monitored group versus 14 in non–BIS-monitored group ($p < 0.039$)
Myles et al., 2004, "B-AWARE" trial[9]	Randomized, prospective; patients at high risk for awareness, 1225 BIS-monitored, 1238 non–BIS-monitored standard practice	International, 21 hospitals, most in Australia	Two cases of intraoperative awareness in BIS-monitored group versus 11 in non–BIS-monitored group ($p = 0.022$)
Avidan et al., 2008[33]	Randomized, prospective; patients at high risk for awareness, 967 BIS-guided, 974 target end-tidal anesthetic gas guided	Single center	Two cases of intraoperative awareness in BIS group, two cases in targeted end-tidal anesthetic group

reducing the expected incidence of intraoperative awareness. Unfortunately, Avidan and colleagues[33] did not have a true "standard practice" control group for comparison, so we cannot know with certainty what the incidence of intraoperative awareness would have been in their patients without either BIS monitoring or targeted end-tidal anesthetic gas analysis.

Another problem with the study by Avidan and colleagues[33] concerns missing data. Three of the four patients with intraoperative awareness, including both patients in the BIS group, had epochs of missing BIS data lasting approximately 20 to 30 minutes. No explanation for the missing data was provided. One cannot help but wonder whether intraoperative awareness may have occurred during an epoch of missing BIS data in the BIS-monitored patients, and whether the availability of BIS data would have enabled the anesthesia providers to prevent awareness in these patients. The argument can be made that no monitoring device is able to provide usable data under all circumstances, and the prevalence of missing data contributes (negatively) to the overall performance and usefulness of any monitor. Nevertheless, it would be very valuable to distinguish intraoperative awareness that occurs with BIS values in the target range (less than 60) from intraoperative awareness that occurs in the absence of usable BIS data. Unfortunately, it is not possible to make that distinction for three of the four patients with intraoperative awareness in the study by Avidan and colleagues[33] because of significant amounts of missing BIS data.

It may be instructive to look more closely at patients who have had intraoperative awareness despite the use of a BIS monitor. In the Swedish case-control study there were two BIS-monitored patients with intraoperative awareness, both of which occurred during intubation, with a BIS value greater than 60 (BIS values less than 60 are generally considered to be desirable for the purpose of avoiding intraoperative awareness).[32] In the multicenter randomized prospective trial (B-AWARE) there were two BIS-monitored patients with intraoperative awareness, one during laryngoscopy with a BIS value of 79 to 82 and one during cardiac surgery with a BIS value of 55 to 59.[9] In this later case, intraoperative awareness occurred despite BIS values in the recommended range. In the study by Avidan and colleagues,[33] one patient with intraoperative awareness had a complete record of BIS and end-tidal anesthetic gas data, except for a few minutes following induction of anesthesia. This patient appears to have had intraoperative awareness with a BIS less than 60. Despite the possibility that intraoperative awareness can occur with a BIS less than 60, the use of BIS resulted in reduction of the incidence of intraoperative awareness from about 1% (either an actual measured incidence with Myles and colleagues[9] or an expected incidence with Avidan and colleagues[33]) to about 0.2% in both the Myles and Avidan studies, suggesting that BIS is useful.

Although intraoperative awareness appears to be less likely at depth of anesthesia monitoring index values in the recommended range (e.g., less than 60 for BIS), clearly it is possible for index values to exceed the recommended range without the occurrence of intraoperative awareness, and the sufficient conditions to produce intraoperative awareness

are not known. The Swedish case-control study[32] reported the distribution of BIS index values greater than 60 found in 5057 consecutive BIS-monitored patients. They found an average time with BIS index greater than 60 of 1.9 minutes during induction of anesthesia (range 0 to 10 minutes) and 2.0 minutes during maintenance (range 0 to 178 minutes). As noted previously, only two of these patients had intraoperative awareness.

Given that intraoperative awareness can occur at BIS less than 60, it is important to use the traditional methods of detecting light anesthesia (movement, vital signs, etc.) and give reasonable doses of anesthetic drugs regardless of the BIS—those who understand the BIS technology have never seriously suggested otherwise. As a general principle, the wise practitioner realizes that no monitoring device, single "number," or data point should be used as the sole guide to patient care.

There have been very few individual case reports of intraoperative awareness in the presence of BIS values in the recommended range, that is, less than 60. In two published case reports of purported intraoperative awareness with BIS values less than 60, the BIS data were taken retrospectively from an anesthesia record, not from the continuous record stored in the memory of the monitor.[34,35] Because the BIS values are recorded intermittently on a handmade anesthesia record, it is possible that the BIS values pertinent to the episode of intraoperative awareness may not appear on the anesthesia record. In the instance of one of the case reports,[34] when the complete record was obtained at a later time from the flash memory of the monitor, there were substantial time periods with BIS greater than 60 that were not recorded on the anesthesia record.[36]

AREAS OF UNCERTAINTY

Whether the clinical trials discussed previously constitute a convincing argument that BIS monitoring reduces the incidence of intraoperative awareness depends perhaps on whether you think the glass is half empty or half full. It would be desirable to have additional trials of depth of anesthesia monitoring for the prevention of intraoperative awareness. However, by historical standards, that three studies suggest better outcomes for patients monitored with a particular device is significant. By comparison, it has not been possible to demonstrate that pulse oximetry affects outcome,[37-39] and most studies suggest that the use of pulmonary artery catheters produces worse outcomes or outcomes that are no better than when pulmonary artery catheters are not used.[40-42] The BIS monitor is probably the only monitoring device used in anesthesiology that has been shown by a clinical trial to improve outcome.

The BIS monitor is not the only depth of anesthesia monitor available today. Several other monitors use EEG and/or auditory evoked potential monitoring to assess anesthetic depth.[30] Although similar in principle to BIS, each of these monitors uses different hardware and software. Whether the use of non-BIS depth of anesthesia monitors will result in a reduction in the rate of intraoperative awareness is unknown.

As noted previously, intraoperative awareness can occur during the use of a BIS monitor. There are limitations to the monitor that have to be taken into account.[30] An evaluable, suitably artifact-free EEG signal is not available under all circumstances. There is a time lag of around 15 to 30 seconds related to EEG processing so that the BIS number slightly lags behind the current anesthetic state. This may be especially important during induction and intubation, when events occur relatively quickly and BIS processing may lag significantly behind. Interestingly, in the three clinical trials of BIS for the prevention of intraoperative awareness there were three cases of intraoperative awareness during laryngoscopy or intubation in patients monitored with BIS, associated with BIS greater than 60. The circumstances under which intraoperative awareness occurs at BIS values greater than 60 are not understood; clearly, not all patients having values greater than 60 experience intraoperative awareness. Some patients with BIS values less than 60 may experience intraoperative awareness.

One wonders whether the combined, simultaneous application of BIS monitoring and targeted end-tidal anesthetic gas analysis (as described by Avidan and colleagues[33]) or target-controlled infusion (TCI) for intravenous anesthetics would result in a lower incidence of intraoperative awareness than either modality alone.

GUIDELINES

The American Society of Anesthesiologists published a practice advisory on intraoperative awareness and monitoring in 2006 (available at www.asahq.org/publications AndServices/AwareAdvisoryFinalOct05.pdf). It is important to note that an advisory does not have the force of a practice guideline or standard of care. As noted in the publication, "Practice advisories are not supported by scientific literature to the same degree as are standards or guidelines because sufficient numbers of adequately controlled studies are lacking." The reader is urged to read the complete text of the advisory, but the "bottom line" recommendation follows: "It is the consensus of the Task Force that the decision to use a brain function monitor should be made on a case-by-case basis by the individual practitioner for selected patients. . . . It is the opinion of the Task Force that brain function monitors currently have the status of the many other monitoring modalities that are currently used in selected situations at the discretion of individual clinicians."

The Joint Commission on Accreditation of Healthcare Organizations has published a "sentinel event alert" concerning intraoperative awareness (available at www.jointcommission.org/SentinelEvents/SentinelEventAlert/sea_32.htm). The reader is urged to read the complete text of the sentinel event alert. The portion relevant to depth of anesthesia monitoring follows:

To overcome the limitations of current methods to detect anesthesia awareness, new methods are being developed that are less affected by the drugs typically used during general anesthesia. These devices measure brain activity rather than physiological responses. These electroencephalography (EEG) devices (also called level-of-consciousness, sedation-level and anesthesia-depth monitors) include the Bispectral Index (BIS)®, spectral edge frequency (SEF) and median frequency (MF) monitors. These devices may have a role in preventing and detecting anesthesia awareness in patients with the highest risk, thereby ameliorating the impact of anesthesia awareness. A body of evidence has not yet accumulated to definitely define the role of these devices in detecting and preventing anesthesia awareness; the Joint Commission expects additional studies on these subjects to emerge.

SUMMARY

Intraoperative awareness is a significant clinical problem. Several large studies suggest that the incidence is around 0.1% overall, with higher and lower rates possible for specific circumstances. There is no simple, completely reliable way to prevent intraoperative awareness. Prevention of intraoperative awareness requires a comprehensive approach, including meticulous attention to correct drug administration, careful clinical observation of the patient for movement or autonomic responses to surgical stimulation, avoidance of muscle relaxant overuse, and appropriate use of monitors of anesthetic depth. Two clinical trials have indicated that BIS monitoring may significantly reduce the incidence of intraoperative awareness.

AUTHOR'S RECOMMENDATIONS

1. Because some cases of intraoperative awareness are related to errors in drug administration, do everything possible to avoid these errors. See previous publications for suggestions of methodology for avoiding drug administration errors.[18-23]
2. Use only the smallest dose of neuromuscular blocking drugs necessary to achieve adequate surgical exposure.
3. If available, BIS monitoring may help reduce the incidence of intraoperative awareness, as suggested by three clinical trials.[9,32,33] As with any monitor, BIS monitors have limitations. Users of BIS monitors (or other depth of anesthesia monitors) are encouraged to be very familiar with the correct operation of the monitor, interpretation of the data, and inherent limitations. Whether the use of non-BIS monitors of anesthetic depth can result in reduced incidence of intraoperative awareness is currently unknown.
4. Awareness during intubation appears to be relatively common. Therefore if depth of anesthesia monitoring is available, it may be valuable to initiate monitoring before induction of anesthesia. Nevertheless, it is important to note that monitors typically lag behind the current anesthetic state by at least 15 to 30 seconds because of the time required for processing the raw EEG signal, which may limit the usefulness of monitoring during induction or at other times when rapid changes in the EEG are taking place.
5. Prevention of intraoperative awareness requires a comprehensive approach, including meticulous attention to correct drug administration, careful clinical observation of the patient for movement or autonomic responses to surgical stimulation, avoidance of muscle relaxant overuse, and appropriate use of monitors of anesthetic depth.

REFERENCES

1. Myles PS, Williams DL, Hendrata M, Anderson H, Weeks AM: Patient satisfaction after anaesthesia and surgery: Results of a prospective survey of 10,811 patients. *Br J Anaesth* 2000;84:6-10.
2. Sandin RH, Enlund G, Samuelsson P, Lennmarken C: Awareness during anaesthesia: A prospective case study. *Lancet* 2000;355: 707-711.
3. Sebel PS, Lang E, Rampil IJ, White PJ, Cork R, Jopling M, et al: A multicenter study of bispectral electroencephalogram analysis for monitoring anesthetic effect. *Anesth Analg* 1997;84:891-899.
4. Lennmarken C, Bildfors K, Enlund G, Samuelsson P, Sandin R: Victims of awareness. *Acta Anaesthesiol Scand* 2002;46:229-231.
5. Osterman JE, Hopper J, Heran WJ, Keane TM, van der Kolk BA: Awareness under anesthesia and the development of posttraumatic stress disorder. *Gen Hosp Psychiatry* 2001;23:198-204.
6. Osterman JE, van der Kolk BA: Awareness during anesthesia and posttraumatic stress disorder. *Gen Hosp Psychiatry* 1998; 20:274-281.
7. Domino KB, Posner KL, Caplan RA, Cheney FW: Awareness during anesthesia: A closed claims analysis. *Anesthesiology* 1999; 90:1053-1061.
8. Dowd NP, Cheng DCH, Karski JM, Wong DT, Munro JA, Sandler A: Intraoperative awareness in fast-track cardiac anesthesia. *Anesthesiology* 1998;89:1068-1073.
9. Myles PS, Leslie K, McNeil J, Forbes A, Chan MTV: Bispectral Index monitoring to prevent awareness during anaesthesia: The B-AWARE randomized controlled trial. *Lancet* 2004:1757-1763.
10. Phillips AA, McLean RF, Devitt JH, Harrington EM: Recall of intraoperative events after general anaesthesia and cardiopulmonary bypass. *Can J Anaesth* 1993;40:922-966.
11. Ranta S, Jussila J, Hynynen M: Recall of awareness during cardiac anesthesia: Influence of feedback information to the anesthesiologist. *Acta Anaesthesiol Scand* 1996;40:554-560.
12. Ranta SO-V, Hernanen P, Hynynen M: Patient's conscious recollections from cardiac anesthesia. *J Cardiothorac Vasc Anesth* 2002;16:426-430.
13. Davidson AJ, Huang GH, Czarnecki C, Gibson MA, Stewart SA, Jamsen K, Stargatt R: Awareness during anesthesia in children: A prospective cohort study. *Anesth Analg* 2005;100:653-661.
14. Lopez U, Habre W, Laurencon M, Haller G, Van der Linden M, Iselin-Chaves IA: Intra-operative awareness in children: The value of an interview adapted to their cognitive abilities. *Anaesthesia* 2007;62:778-789.
15. Pollard RJ, Coyle JP, Gilbert RL, Beck JE: Intraoperative awareness in a regional medical system: A review of 3 years' data. *Anesthesiology* 2007;106:269-274.
16. Bowdle TA, Sebel PS, Ghoneim MM, Rampil IJ, Padilla RE, Gan TJ, Domino KB: How likely is awareness during anesthesia? *Anesth Analg* 2005;100:1545.
17. Rowan KJ: Awareness under TIVA: A doctor's personal experience. *Anaesth Intensive Care* 2002;30:505-506.
18. Bowdle A, Kruger C, Grieve R, Emmens D, Merry A: Anesthesia drug administration errors in a university hospital. *Anesthesiology* 2003;99:A1358.
19. Bowdle TA: Drug administration errors from the ASA closed claims project. *American Society of Anesthesiologists Newsletter* 2003;67:11-13.
20. Merry AF, Webster CS, Mathew DJ: A new, safety-oriented, integrated drug administration and automated anesthesia record system. *Anesth Analg* 2001;93:385-390.
21. Webster CS, Merry AF, Gander PH, Mann NK: A prospective, randomized clinical evaluation of a new safety-oriented injectable drug administration system in comparison with conventional methods. *Anaesthesia* 2004;59:80-87.
22. Webster CS, Merry AF, Larsson L, McGrath KA, Weller J: The frequency and nature of drug administration error during anaesthesia. *Anaesth Intensive Care* 2001;29:494-500.
23. Bowdle TA, Edwards M, Domino KB: Reducing errors in cardiac anesthesiology. In Kaplan JA, editor: *Kaplan's cardiac anesthesia*, ed 5 Philadelphia, Saunders Elsevier, 2006, pp 1217-1234.
24. Iohom G, Fitzgerald D, Cunningham AJ: Principles of pharmacogenetics—implication for the anaesthetist. *Br J Anaesth* 2004; 93:440-450.
25. Saucier N, Walts LF, Moreland JR: Patient awareness during nitrous oxide, oxygen, and halothane anesthesia. *Anesth Analg* 1983;62:239-240.
26. Enlund M: TIVA, awareness, and the Brice interview. *Anesth Analg* 2006;102:967, author reply 967.
27. Enlund M, Hassan HG: Intraoperative awareness: Detected by the structured Brice interview? *Acta Anaesthesiol Scand* 2002; 46:345-349.
28. Nordstrom O, Engstrom AM, Persson S, Sandin R: Incidence of awareness in total I.V. anaesthesia based on propofol, alfentanil and neuromuscular blockade. *Acta Anaesthesiol Scand* 1997;41:978-984.
29. Bowdle TA: The Bispectral Index (BIS): An update. *Curr Rev Clin Anesth* 2004;25:17-28.
30. Bowdle TA: Depth of anesthesia monitoring. *Anesthesiol Clin* 2006;24:793-822.
31. Kalkman CJ, Drummond JC: Monitors of depth of anesthesia, quo vadis? *Anesthesiology* 2002;96:784-787.
32. Ekman A, Lindholm M-L, Lennmarken C, Sandin RH: Reduction in the incidence of awareness using BIS monitoring. *Acta Anaesthesiol Scand* 2004;48:20-26.
33. Avidan MS, Zhang L, Burnside BA, Finkel KJ, Searleman AC, Selvidge JA, et al: Anesthesia awareness and the Bispectral Index. *N Engl J Med* 2008;358:1097-1108.
34. Mychaskiw G 2nd, Horowitz M, Sachdev V, Heath BJ: Explicit intraoperative recall at a Bispectral Index of 47. *Anesth Analg* 2001;92:808-809.
35. Rampersad SE, Mulroy MF: A case of awareness despite an "adequate depth of anesthesia" as indicated by a Bispectral Index monitor. *Anesth Analg* 2005;100:1363-1364, table of contents.
36. Rampil I: False negative BIS? Maybe, maybe not! *Anesth Analg* 2001;93:798-799.
37. Moller JT, Johannessen NW, Espersen K, Ravlo O, Pedersen BD, Jensen PF, et al: Randomized evaluation of pulse oximetry in 20,802 patients: II. Perioperative events and postoperative complications. *Anesthesiology* 1993;78:445-453.
38. Moller JT, Pedersen T, Rasmussen LS, Jensen PF, Pedersen BD, Ravlo O, et al: Randomized evaluation of pulse oximetry in 20,802 patients: I. Design, demography, pulse oximetry failure rate, and overall complication rate. *Anesthesiology* 1993;78: 436-444.
39. Pedersen T, Moller AM, Pedersen BD: Pulse oximetry for perioperative monitoring: Systematic review of randomized, controlled trials. *Anesth Analg* 2003;96:426-431, table of contents.
40. Connors AF Jr, Speroff T, Dawson NV, Thomas C, Harrell FE Jr, Wagner D, et al: The effectiveness of right heart catheterization in the initial care of critically ill patients. SUPPORT Investigators. *JAMA* 1996;276:889-897.
41. Dalen JE, Bone RC: Is it time to pull the pulmonary artery catheter? *JAMA* 1996;276:916-918.
42. Shah MR, Hasselblad V, Stevenson LW, Binanay C, O'Connor CM, Sopko G, Califf RM: Impact of the pulmonary artery catheter in critically ill patients: Meta-analysis of randomized clinical trials. *JAMA* 2005;294:1664-1670.

44 What Is the Best Technique in the Patient with an Open Globe and Full Stomach?

Kathryn E. McGoldrick, MD

INTRODUCTION

The anesthesiologist who cares for a patient with a penetrating eye injury and a full stomach must confront special challenges. The risk of blindness in the injured eye that could result from increased intraocular pressure (IOP) producing extrusion of intraocular contents must be weighed against the risk of aspiration associated with suboptimal airway management. Although succinylcholine is commonly used as part of a rapid-sequence induction technique for the patient with a full stomach having nonocular emergency surgery, the use of succinylcholine in ocular trauma is controversial. Clearly, succinylcholine causes a small, transient increase in IOP that dissipates within 7 minutes of administration.[1] The precise mechanism of this increase has not been established. In the past, it was postulated that tonic contractions of the extraocular muscles were responsible for the IOP increase. However, in a feline model of anterior and posterior ocular trauma, the only apparent effect of succinylcholine was forward displacement the lens and iris, unaccompanied by any extrusion of ocular contents.[2] Moreover, in a study of 15 patients having elective enucleation, succinylcholine was administered after all the extraocular muscles to the diseased eye had been detached. There was no difference in IOP increase between the intact and the detached eyes.[3] It is now generally hypothesized that the succinylcholine-induced increase in IOP is associated with choroidal vascular dilation or a reduction in drainage resulting from increased central venous pressure, transiently reducing the flow of aqueous humor through the canal of Schlemm.[4] Nonetheless, assorted methods may be selected to attenuate the effect of succinylcholine on IOP, if it is administered.

Alternatives to succinylcholine are available, and the advantages and disadvantages of these approaches are numerous, and will be discussed. As in all cases of trauma, it is axiomatic that other injuries, such as skull and orbital fractures, intracranial trauma associated with subdural hematoma formation, and the possibility of thoracic or abdominal injury, must be excluded before surgically addressing the penetrating eye injury.

OPTIONS/THERAPIES

Although regional anesthesia is often a valuable option for the management of trauma patients who have recently eaten, this alternative traditionally had been considered contraindicated in patients with penetrating eye injuries owing to concerns about potential extrusion of intraocular contents from the pressure generated by administration of local anesthetics, from the force associated with instrumentation of the orbit, from squeezing of the eyelids associated with pain on injection, or from potential bleeding subsequent to injection. Nevertheless, there are case reports of successful use of ophthalmic blocks in this setting. Several techniques are available that may be selected in appropriate patients. These include cannula-based sub-Tenon block techniques, intracameral injection, topical anesthesia,[5] and peribulbar and/or retrobulbar anesthesia. Because there are many distinct permutations of eye injuries, Scott and colleagues[6] developed techniques to safely block patients with *selective* open-globe injuries. During a 4-year interval, 220 open eyes were repaired with regional anesthesia at Bascom Palmer Eye Institute. Many of the injuries were the result of either intraocular foreign bodies or dehiscence of cataract or corneal transplant incisions. Eyes in which regional techniques were selected tended to have more anterior, smaller wounds than those repaired with general anesthesia, and were less likely to have a pupillary defect. Indeed, in some cases the wounds may have been self-sealing. No outcome difference—that is, change of visual acuity from presenting evaluation until final examination—between eyes repaired under regional compared with general anesthesia was detected. Given the relevant caveats and surgical issues involved, the decision to administer regional anesthesia to a traumatized eye is best left to the ophthalmic surgeon.

It is not always possible, however, to determine the precise extent of ocular disruption preoperatively. Therefore general anesthesia is typically considered a prudent choice in this setting. Preoperative prophylaxis against aspiration may include administration of H_2 receptor antagonists to increase gastric fluid pH and to decrease gastric acid production. Additionally, metoclopramide may be given in an attempt to stimulate peristalsis and promote gastric emptying.

Once the decision has been made to administer general endotracheal anesthesia, the patient's airway can be secured using either succinylcholine after pretreatment to blunt its effect on IOP or by administering a nondepolarizing muscle relaxant with the appropriate dose adjustment to facilitate rapid-sequence induction. On rare occasions, it may be deemed advisable to perform an awake fiber-optic intubation to secure the airway. This latter approach may be the safest alternative in a patient, for example, whose airway assessment suggests a difficult intubation and whose eye has been seriously injured and may not be salvageable. This approach, however, may dramatically increase IOP if the patient gags or retches from the local anesthetic spray or coughs when the transtracheal injection is performed.

EVIDENCE AND CONTROVERSIES

Nondepolarizing Muscle Relaxants

One of several nondepolarizing muscle relaxants can be administered to facilitate rapid-sequence induction for open eye injuries. In general, however, onset time is slower and somewhat less predictable than with succinylcholine. To overcome this disadvantage, various methods have been proposed to accelerate the onset of nondepolarizing agents. These approaches include priming[7,8] and using high-dose regimens.

The priming principle involves using approximately one tenth of an intubating dose of nondepolarizing drug, followed 3 or 4 minutes later by an intubating dose. Then, after waiting an additional 90 seconds, intubation of the trachea may be performed. Priming, however, is not devoid of risk; partial paralysis may occur from the priming dose itself, and a case of pulmonary aspiration after a priming dose of vecuronium has been reported.[9]

Several studies have explored the use of large doses of nondepolarizing neuromuscular blockers to accelerate the onset of adequate relaxation for endotracheal intubation. Using vecuronium doses of 0.2 and 0.4 mg/kg, Casson and Jones[10] found mean onset times of 95 and 87 seconds, respectively. Ginsberg and colleagues[11] found comparable, albeit slightly longer, onset times.

Some have proposed rocuronium 0.6 mg/kg as a satisfactory substitute for succinylcholine in rapid-sequence induction and intubation.[12,13] Others, however, indicate that as much as 0.9 to 1.2 mg/kg of rocuronium is necessary to produce equivalent intubating conditions to succinylcholine.[14-16] These high doses have the disadvantage of protracted duration of action, a factor that could prove hazardous in a patient with an unrecognized difficult airway. Nonetheless, when the promising new selective relaxant binding agent sugammadex (Org 25969) becomes commercially available, this risk could be minimized, if not eliminated. Initial studies with sugammadex to antagonize rocuronium- and vecuronium-induced neuromuscular blockade have been encouraging.[17-19]

Less than a decade ago, it was hoped that rapacuronium (Org 9487), with its swift onset, would offer a reliable, nondepolarizing alternative to succinylcholine. However, rapacuronium is no longer available because it produced intractable bronchospasm in some patients. A new ultra-short-acting nondepolarizing agent (GW280430A) is currently undergoing investigation as a possible substitute for succinylcholine.

Regardless of the particular nondepolarizing agent administered, it is mandatory to appreciate that a premature attempt at endotracheal intubation produces coughing, straining, and a dramatic increase in IOP of as much as 40 mm Hg, underscoring the necessity of confirming the onset of paralysis with a peripheral nerve stimulator. One must keep in mind, however, that muscle groups vary in their response to muscle relaxants; abolition of twitch responses in the thumb does not necessarily indicate that the larynx is fully relaxed. Despite the panoply of methods to optimize their efficacy, nondepolarizing muscle relaxants often produce imperfect intubating conditions at 60 seconds, a protracted period of paralysis, and a longer time when the patient has an unprotected airway when compared with succinylcholine.

Attenuating the Effect of Succinylcholine on IOP

To maintain appropriate perspective, it is important to remember that the small, transient increase in IOP induced by succinylcholine pales in comparison with the dramatic intraocular hypertension that occurs with such maneuvers as coughing, straining, vomiting, or attempting to intubate an inadequately anesthetized patient. These occurrences can produce devastating consequences in the setting of an open eye injury.

Moreover, in 1993, McGoldrick[20] pointed out that Lincoff's 1957 watershed article states: "Various communications have been received from ophthalmologists who have used succinylcholine in surgery. This includes several reports of cases in which succinylcholine was given *to forestall impending vitreous prolapse* only to have a prompt expulsion of vitreous occur" (emphasis added).[21] Under such desperate circumstances, it seems inappropriate to attribute the expulsion of vitreous directly to succinylcholine.[20]

Nonetheless, numerous methods have been devised to blunt the effect that succinylcholine has on IOP. These include self-taming, and pretreatment with acetazolamide,[22] narcotics,[23-26] nifedipine,[27] nitroglycerin,[28] propranolol,[29] lidocaine,[30,31] and nondepolarizing muscle relaxants. In reality, although some attenuation of the succinylcholine-induced increase in IOP results, none of these drugs consistently and completely blocks the ocular hypertensive response associated with administration of this rapid-onset, short-acting, depolarizing muscle relaxant.

Self-taming[32,33] is a technique whereby a small amount of succinylcholine is given before proceeding to administer the full intubating dose for rapid-sequence induction. Although Verma,[32] in 1979, claimed that a self-taming dose was protective, Meyers[33] found this approach to be ineffective.

Pretreatment with a small defasciculating dose of nondepolarizing agent has yielded conflicting results. In 1968, Miller and colleagues,[34] using indentation tonometry, reported that pretreatment with small amounts of gallamine or d-tubocurarine prevented succinylcholine-associated increases in IOP. Ten years later, however, Meyers and colleagues,[35] using the more sensitive applanation tonometer, were unable to consistently block the ocular hypertensive response after similar pretreatment therapy. More recently, it has been suggested that mivacurium obtunds the IOP increase from succinylcholine.[36]

AREAS OF UNCERTAINTY

There are no prospective, randomized, controlled trials currently available to compare the safety and efficacy of the various approaches to management of the patient with an open eye and full stomach. The decision to administer or avoid succinylcholine is a matter of assessing and balancing risks for the individual patient. The critical factors to be considered in this individual calculus are the airway assessment, the extent of ocular damage, and any potential medical contraindications to a particular approach.

Although succinylcholine increases IOP, it allows intubation reliably within 45 to 60 seconds after administration. Its brief half-life enables swift recovery of muscle power if intubation or ventilation becomes difficult. No currently available shorter-acting nondepolarizing muscle relaxant can compete with the pharmacokinetic profile of succinylcholine in terms of quick onset and offset. Perhaps in the future, an ideal replacement that has an onset as rapid as succinylcholine, dissipates as quickly as succinylcholine, and causes no hemodynamic perturbation or increase in IOP will be developed. Currently, we have no such holy grail. We do know, however, that the small increase in IOP produced by succinylcholine can be attenuated with various pretreatments, and is notably less than the elevation in IOP encountered if paralysis is inadequate at the time of attempted laryngoscopy and intubation after an augmented dose of nondepolarizing agent was given in hope of accelerating its onset. Moreover, retrospective reports from such eminent institutions as the Wills Eye Hospital in Philadelphia[37] and the Massachusetts Eye and Ear Infirmary in Boston[38] indicated no instances of vitreous extrusion or expulsion associated with succinylcholine administration to patients with open eye injuries during more than one decade of tracking.

GUIDELINES

There are no guidelines that address the best agent to use in a patient with an open globe and full stomach.

AUTHOR'S RECOMMENDATIONS

Recognizing that the use of succinylcholine may decline with the development of new and improved drugs, the author believes that succinylcholine, except when contraindicated (malignant hyperthermia susceptibility, for example), is the preferred neuromuscular blocking drug in patients with an open globe and full stomach. Its rapid, reliable onset permits swift, smooth intubation and airway protection without coughing, straining, or other highly detrimental responses. Our currently available nondepolarizing agents do not provide such excellent intubating conditions quite so rapidly or predictably. Furthermore, it is not always possible to foretell which patients may be difficult to intubate or ventilate.[39-41] The quick return of spontaneous respiration is often invaluable in the management of a difficult airway. Clearly, the use of appropriate intubating doses for rapid-sequence induction with nondepolarizing drugs eliminates this helpful option, although the addition of sugammadex to our armamentarium may nullify, or at least mitigate, this potentially dangerous obstacle.

Patients requiring general anesthesia whose airway assessment is reassuring may occasionally have a contraindication, such as malignant hyperthermia susceptibility, Duchenne muscular dystrophy, or certain types of myotonia, to the administration of succinylcholine. These patients may be managed using sufficiently large doses of a nondepolarizing neuromuscular blocker to enable accelerated onset of paralysis and satisfactory intubating conditions. Maintenance could then be accomplished with a total intravenous anesthetic technique.

When confronted with a patient whose airway anatomy suggests potential difficulties, the anesthesiologist should consult with the ophthalmologist regarding the likelihood of salvaging the injured eye. In selective instances outlined previously in which ocular injury is less devastating, general anesthesia may be avoided by proceeding under topical or regional anesthesia. If this approach is not feasible because the eye is severely damaged and probably not salvageable, awake fiber-optic laryngoscopy and intubation may be the safest management choice, realizing that substantial increases in IOP may be associated with gagging, retching, and coughing. These hazards, however, become relatively unimportant when balanced against the risk of losing the airway.

REFERENCES

1. Pandey K, Badolas RP, Kumar S: Time course of intraocular hypertension produced by suxamethonium. *Br J Anaesth* 1972;44:191-195.
2. Moreno RJ, Kloess P, Carlson DW: Effect of succinylcholine on the intraocular contents of open globes. *Ophthalmology* 1991;98:636-638.
3. Kelly RE, Dinner M, Turner LS, et al: Succinylcholine increases intraocular pressure in the human eye with the extraocular muscles detached. *Anesthesiology* 1993;79:948-952.
4. Metz HS, Venkatesh B: Succinylcholine and intraocular pressure. *J Pediatr Ophthalmol Strabismus* 1981;18:12-14.
5. Boscia F, LaTegola MG, Columbo G, et al: Combined topical anesthesia and sedation for open-globe injuries in selected patients. *Ophthalmology* 2003;110:1555-1559.
6. Scott IU, McCabe CM, Flynn HW Jr, et al: Local anesthesia with intravenous sedation for surgical repair of selected open globe injuries. *Am J Ophthalmol* 2002;134:707-711.
7. Foldes FF: Rapid tracheal intubation with nondepolarizing neuromuscular blocking drugs: The priming principle (correspondence). *Br J Anaesth* 1984;56:663.
8. Jones RM. The priming principle: How does it work and should we be using it? *Br J Anaesth* 1989;63:1-3.
9. Musich J, Walts LF: Pulmonary aspiration after a priming dose of vecuronium. *Anesthesiology* 1986;64:517-519.
10. Casson WR, Jones RM: Vecuronium-induced neuromuscular blockade: The effect of increasing dose on speed of onset. *Anaesthesia* 1986;41:354-357.
11. Ginsberg B, Glass PS, Quill TS, et al: Onset and duration of neuromuscular blockade following high-dose vecuronium administration. *Anesthesiology* 1989;71:201-205.
12. Puhringer FK, Khuenl-Brady KS, Koller J, et al: Evaluation of the endotracheal intubating conditions of rocuronium and succinylcholine in outpatient surgery. *Anesth Analg* 1992;75: 37-40.
13. Vinik HR: Intraocular pressure changes during rapid-sequence induction and intubation: A comparison of rocuronium, atracurium, and succinylcholine. *J Clin Anesth* 1999;11:95-100.

14. Weiss JH, Gratz I, Goldberg ME: Double-blind comparison of two doses of rocuronium and succinylcholine for rapid-sequence intubation. *J Clin Anesth* 1997;9:379-382.
15. Magorian T, Flannery KB, Miller RD: Comparison of rocuronium, succinylcholine, and vecuronium for rapid-sequence induction of anesthesia in adult patients. *Anesthesiology* 1993;79:913-918.
16. Heier T, Caldwell JE: Rapid tracheal intubation with large-dose rocuronium: A probability-based approach. *Anesth Analg* 2000;90:175-179.
17. Sorgenfrei IF, Norrild K, Larsen PO, et al: Reversal of rocuronium-induced neuromuscular block by the selective relaxant binding agent sugammadex: A dose-finding and safety study. *Anesthesiology* 2006;104:667-674.
18. Shields M, Biovanelli M, Mirakur RK, et al: Org 25969 (sugammadex), a selective relaxant binding agent for antagonism of prolonged rocuronium-induced neuromuscular block. *Br J Anaesth* 2006;96:36-43.
19. Suy K, Morias K, Cammu G, et al: Effective reversal of moderate rocuronium- or vecuronium-induced neuromuscular block with sugammadex, a selective relaxant binding agent. *Anesthesiology* 2007;106:283-288.
20. McGoldrick KE: The open globe: Is an alternative to succinylcholine necessary? *J Clin Anesth* 1993;5:1-4 (editorial).
21. Lincoff HA, Breinin GM, DeVoe AG: Effect of succinylcholine on the extraocular muscles. *Am J Ophthalmol* 1957;44:440-444.
22. Carballo AS: Succinylcholine and acetazolamide in anesthesia for ocular surgery. *Can Anaesth Soc J* 1965;12:486-498.
23. Sweeney J, Underhill S, Dowd T, et al: Modification by fentanyl and alfentanil of intraocular pressure response to suxamethonium and tracheal intubation. *Br J Anaesth* 1989;63:688-691.
24. Ng HP, Chen FG, Yeong SM, et al: Effect of remifentanil compared with fentanyl on intraocular pressure after succinylcholine and tracheal intubation. *Br J Anaesth* 2000;85:785-787.
25. Alexander R, Hill R, Lipham WJ, et al: Remifentanil prevents an increase in IOP after succinylcholine and tracheal intubation. *Br J Anaesth* 1998;81:606-607.
26. Georgiou M, Parlapani A, Argiriadou H, et al: Sufentanil or clonidine for blunting the increase in intraocular pressure during rapid-sequence induction. *Eur J Anaesthesiol* 2002;19:819-822.
27. Indu B, Batra YK, Puri GD, et al: Nifedipine attenuates the intraocular pressure response to intubation following succinylcholine. *Can J Anaesth* 1989;36:269-272.
28. Mahajan RP, Grover VK, Sharma SL, et al: Intranasal nitroglycerin and intraocular pressure during general anesthesia. *Anesth Analg* 1988;67:631-636.
29. Cook JH, Feneck RO, Smith MB: Effect of pretreatment with propranolol on intraocular pressure changes during induction of anaesthesia. *Eur J Anaesthesiol* 1986;3:449-457.
30. Mahajan RP, Grover VK, Munjal VP, et al: Double-blind comparison of lidocaine, tubocurarine and diazepam pretreatment in modifying intraocular pressure increases. *Can J Anaesth* 1987;34:41-45.
31. Grover VK, Lata K, Sharma S, et al: Efficacy of lignocaine in the suppression of the intraocular pressure response to suxamethonium and tracheal intubation. *Anaesthesia* 1989;44:22-25.
32. Verma RS: "Self-taming" of succinylcholine-induced fasciculations and intraocular pressure. *Anesthesiology* 1979;50:245-247.
33. Meyers EF, Singer P, Otto A: A controlled study of the effect of succinylcholine self-taming on intraocular pressure. *Anesthesiology* 1980;53:72-74.
34. Miller RD, Way WL, Hickey RF: Inhibition of succinylcholine-induced increased intraocular pressure by nondepolarizing muscle relaxants. *Anesthesiology* 1968;29:123-126.
35. Meyers EF, Krupin T, Johnson M, et al: Failure of nondepolarizing neuromuscular blockers to inhibit succinylcholine-induced increased intraocular pressure: A controlled study. *Anesthesiology* 1978;48:149-151.
36. Chiu CL, Lang CC, Wong PK, et al: The effect of mivacurium pretreatment on intraocular pressure changes induced by suxamethonium. *Anaesthesia* 1998;53:501-505.
37. Libonati MM, Leahy JJ, Ellison N: The use of succinylcholine in open eye surgery. *Anesthesiology* 1986;62:637-640.
38. Donlon JV: Succinylcholine and open eye injuries (letter to the editor). *Anesthesiology* 1986;65:526-527.
39. Wilson ME, Spiegelhalter D, Robertson JA, Lesser P: Predicting difficult intubation. *Br J Anaesth* 1988;61:211-216.
40. Frerk CM: Predicting difficult intubation. *Anaesthesia* 1991;46:1005-1008.
41. Rocke DA, Murray WB, Rout CC, Gouws E: Relative risk analysis of factors associated with difficult intubation in obstetric anesthesia. *Anesthesiology* 1992;77:67-73.

45 Are Patients with Sleep Apnea Appropriate for Ambulatory Surgery?

Tracey L. Stierer, MD, and Nancy Collop, MD

INTRODUCTION/BACKGROUND

Obstructive sleep apnea (OSA) is a chronic condition that is characterized by recurrent episodes of partial or complete collapse of the upper airway during sleep. The reduction or cessation of airflow during these obstructive episodes may result in significant decreases in oxyhemoglobin saturation and hypercarbia, and eventual arousal from sleep. Patients with sleep apnea may have a variety of nocturnal symptoms, such as loud disruptive snoring, choking, and gasping, and they may have observed pauses in breathing. Because sleep is fragmented, daytime symptoms include excessive daytime sleepiness, mood disorders, and neurocognitive impairment, which lead to an increased likelihood of accidental injury or death.[1] Additionally, it is well accepted that the abnormalities in gas exchange that result from OSA are associated with adverse cardiovascular, endocrine, and cerebrovascular consequences.[2-6]

There is increasing public awareness of OSA and its health consequences, and a growing concern among health care providers that patients with sleep apnea may be at risk for adverse perioperative outcomes, including death. General population studies suggest that 5% of middle-aged women and 9% of middle-aged men suffer from OSA, and there are data to suggest that the prevalence of OSA is even higher in the elderly population.[7,8] Unfortunately, the prevalence OSA in adult patients undergoing outpatient surgery is still unknown. Furthermore, it has been estimated that up to 90% of those with the disease carry no formal diagnosis.[7,9] With 15 million patients undergoing outpatient surgeries in free-standing ambulatory surgical centers each year, statistically, more than 1 million of them may suffer from disordered breathing.

The presence of OSA in the surgical patient is thought to lead to potential problems with mask ventilation, tracheal intubation, extubation, and the ability to provide adequate analgesia without respiratory compromise.[10] When the diagnosis of OSA is known, there is an opportunity to arrange for additional resources to deal with anticipated potential airway complications and the need for possible prolonged postoperative monitoring. However, the patient who has signs and symptoms of OSA, but does not have a formal diagnosis, poses a particular problem for the ambulatory anesthesiologist who must decide whether to proceed with surgery or delay the case until the patient undergoes a formal evaluation. Additionally, the anesthesiologist must decide if the patient is a candidate for a free-standing ambulatory surgical center.

The gold standard test used to determine the presence of OSA is the polysomnogram (PSG). Polysomnography is a relatively expensive, time-consuming, and labor-intensive test, and cannot be performed on the day of the surgical procedure. The patient who undergoes PSG is brought to a sleep laboratory in the evening, monitors are applied, and simultaneous recordings of several physiologic signals are acquired over an 8-hour period while the patient sleeps. Most sleep laboratories define an abnormal breathing episode of obstructive apnea as the complete cessation of airflow for a minimum of 10 seconds during sleep while the patient makes persistent efforts to breathe. Although the definition of hypopnea is less uniform, the most common description is a decrease in airflow of greater than 30% associated with a decrease in oxyhemoglobin saturation of 4% or more. The apnea hypopnea index (AHI) is the total number of all recorded episodes of apneas and hypopneas per hour of total sleep time, and if sleep-disordered breathing is detected, it is reported as mild, moderate, or severe, based on the AHI. It is important to note that the criteria for diagnosis and the presentation of OSA differ between the adult and pediatric populations, and what is discussed in this review applies only to the management of adults.

OPTIONS

At present, there is no consensus to define the specific additional risk, if any, that the presence of OSA poses to the ambulatory surgical patient. Because the risk of potential OSA during outpatient surgery is poorly defined, postponement of a surgical procedure to define the patient's risk may seem unreasonable to the patient and the surgeon. There are both financial and social pressures to proceed as the patient may have made arrangements for time away from work, as well as provisions for family members to help during the recovery period. Additionally, even though the procedure may have been scheduled as an elective outpatient procedure, the nature of the surgery may still be considered relatively urgent as in the case of a breast biopsy to rule out cancer. Delay of this type of procedure can have tremendous psychologic consequences for the patient, and may result in delay of treatment. Although there are no large-scale, randomized trials that compare perioperative adverse outcomes of patients with OSA with normal patients, several observational studies have examined this question. Therefore current perioperative care is based on clinical judgment and an understanding of the pathophysiologic mechanism and consequences of OSA.

PATHOPHYSIOLOGY/MECHANISM OF ACTION

The occurrence of pharyngeal collapse during sleep suggests that sleep onset is associated with functional alterations in airflow in the upper airway that reduce patency and increase resistance to airflow. The point of obstruction can occur anywhere in the upper airway, from the soft palate and nasopharynx to the base of the tongue and epiglottis, and frequently occurs at different sites during the various stages of sleep.[11] Bachar and colleagues[12] demonstrated sites and patterns of obstruction with the use of sleep endoscopy in 55 surgical patients. They found that the most common site of obstruction was uvulopalatine, and also noted that many patients (72%) had multiple sites of obstruction.[12] Regardless of where the obstruction occurs, two subsequent effects are thought to follow. First, with repetitive episodes of hypoxia and hypercapnia, and the reoxygenation that occurs during arousal, oxidative stress ensues and systemic inflammation follows.[13] Reactive oxygen species are formed and cause injury to the surrounding tissue. Although these molecules trigger pathways that are adaptive to hypoxia, they have also been found to have an association with harmful inflammatory and immune responses. Among the changes are activation of endothelial cells, leukocytes, and platelets.[14,15] There is increased sympathetic activity, which, after repetitive cycles of hypoxia and hypercarbia, results in upregulation of both alpha and beta receptors. This may have a role in the pathogenesis of coronary and cerebrovascular disorders.

One of the most commonly recognized cardiac sequelae of OSA is right-sided heart dysfunction. The increased sympathetic activity associated with the hypoxia and hypercarbia leads to an increase in pulmonary vascular resistance. The endothelial wall thickens and pulmonary hypertension can ensue. The right ventricle hypertrophies to meet the demand, and if unremedied can eventually dilate and enlarge. However, while historically most attention has been directed toward the status of the right side of the heart during a preoperative assessment in the patient suspected of having OSA, there is a far greater association with systemic hypertension and, more specifically, uncontrolled hypertension.[16] Sixty percent to 70% of patients with documented OSA have a concomitant diagnosis of systemic hypertension, whereas only about 20% of those with OSA have progression of the disease resulting in pulmonary hypertension severe enough to cause right ventricular dysfunction.

OSA has been implicated in the pathogenesis of various other comorbidities, including coronary artery disease, congestive heart failure, cardiac arrhythmias, sudden death, stroke, and impaired glucose metabolism.[14,15,17]

EVIDENCE

To date, there is a paucity of outcome data on surgical patients with diagnosed, or undiagnosed, OSA, and even less that addresses outcomes in the ambulatory surgical population. Recent studies suggest that 24-hour observation in a monitored environment confers minimal, if any, advantage in risk reduction for ambulatory surgical patients with uncomplicated obstructive sleep apnea.

Most available data arise from otolaryngologic studies, specifically patients undergoing uvulopalatopharyngoplasty (UPPP). Several studies have addressed the question of whether patients with OSA undergoing upper airway procedures should be monitored in an intensive care unit postoperatively, but the data are retrospective and inconclusive. Mickelson and Hakim[18] retrospectively analyzed 347 consecutive patients who underwent UPPP. Of the 14 patients who suffered complications, 5 involved airway and the episodes occurred in the immediate perioperative period. Additionally, there was no correlation between the rate of complication and the severity of OSA. Of the five patients with airway complications, three required reintubation. One patient suffered bronchospasm immediately postextubation, one patient was thought to have been prematurely extubated in the operating room and experienced subsequent respiratory arrest, and one patient was reported to have respiratory distress in the recovery room of unknown etiology. Respiratory complications developed in two of the five patients after admission to the ward; however, neither required reintubation. The authors concluded that intensive care unit (ICU) care postoperatively was not required for most patients undergoing UPPP, and that the rate of complication was substantially higher in patients who had undergone simultaneous otolaryngologic procedures in addition to UPPP. Hathaway and Johnson[19] examined the outcomes of 110 patients scheduled for outpatient UPPP. Twenty of the 110 patients required admission (18%); however, no patient required transfer to an ICU. Although three patients were admitted for postoperative oxygen desaturation, this did not correlate with severity of AHI. Additionally, the majority of admissions were for control of pain and nausea. The authors emphasized that appropriate patient selection is essential in minimizing the risk of perioperative complications in patients undergoing UPPP, and in their study, any patient with severe cardiopulmonary comorbidities was eliminated as a candidate for UPPP. Terris and colleagues[20] found similar results when they performed a retrospective analysis of 109 patients with OSA who were scheduled for 125 upper airway procedures. The rate of airway complications was 0.8% (1 of 109), and the one patient who experienced airway obstruction did so in the immediate postoperative period. Again, the authors concluded that ICU monitoring for all patients undergoing UPPP was unnecessary, and that the decision for discharge to the floor or home could be made based on the patient's status in the recovery room within 2 hours of the surgical procedure. In another retrospective analysis of OSA patients undergoing airway procedures, Spiegel and Tejas[20a] found that if airway complications were to occur, they could be identified within 2 to 3 hours postoperatively, and also concluded that same-day discharge was an option for some patients. Although it appears that selected patients with OSA can be safely discharged to home after UPPP, it seems prudent that this be done in a facility with provisions for transfer to an overnight ward for observation.

Literature examining nonotorhinolaryngologic surgeries in patients with OSA is scant. However, studies that retrospectively analyze outcome of inpatient surgical procedures have suggested that OSA is an independent risk factor for adverse outcome. Gupta and colleagues[21] studied 110 patients with OSA diagnosed either before or after total hip or knee replacement, and matched the population with controls. OSA was associated with an increased incidence of "serious" adverse perioperative events requiring transfer to an ICU.[21] Although severity of OSA or AHI was not related to the incidence of complications, OSA patients who were compliant with continuous positive airway pressure (CPAP) preoperatively were noted to have a decreased incidence of complications when compared with patients with OSA who did not use CPAP.

Sabers and colleagues[22] at the Mayo Clinic in Rochester, Minnesota, designed a retrospective study to determine whether the preoperative diagnosis of OSA was an independent risk factor for perioperative complications after outpatient surgery. Two hundred thirty-four patients who had been previously diagnosed with OSA by polysomnography were scheduled for ambulatory surgical procedures and were matched with controls. All types of surgery were included with the exception of otorhinolaryngologic procedures. The primary outcome measured was unplanned hospital admission or readmission; however, recorded data included episodes of bronchospasm, airway obstruction, and reintubation during the recovery period. Previously diagnosed OSA was not found to be an independent risk factor for unplanned admissions or for other adverse perioperative events.

The authors have examined the prevalence of OSA and propensity to OSA in our own outpatient surgical population at Johns Hopkins Hospital. A previously validated prediction model was used to determine the pretest probability for OSA in 3557 consecutive adult patient undergoing ambulatory surgical procedures of all types except ophthalmologic.[23] Propensity to OSA was determined by logistic regression analysis. Relevant perioperative data such as anesthetic technique, difficulty with endotracheal intubation, need for supplemental oxygen and need for assisted ventilation, reintubation, unplanned admission, and death were recorded; 2.6% of the patients had a greater than 70% propensity for OSA but had not yet been diagnosed. Of these high-risk patients, only 28.2% (31 of 110) of males and 21.6% (11 of 51) of female patients had a previous self-reported diagnosis of possible OSA. The results of the study suggested that OSA is relatively common in an ambulatory surgical population and that a majority of patients with a propensity for OSA

who undergo ambulatory surgery remain undiagnosed. There was a positive correlation of patients with a higher propensity to OSA (versus non-OSA) and increased difficulty of intubation, administration of intraoperative ephedrine, metoprolol, and labetolol, and need for prolonged supplemental oxygen. However, we found no relationship between unplanned admission or readmission, life-threatening events such as reintubation, cardiac arrhythmia, or death in patients with either a diagnosis or higher propensity for OSA. Therefore our data suggest that patients with OSA may require additional perioperative interventions; however, they can be treated safely in an ambulatory care center.[24]

Acknowledging the weakness of the data available to guide the perioperative management of patients with uncomplicated OSA, it appears that these patients can be safely managed as outpatients. However, those patients with comorbid illnesses may need to be managed differently. Moreover, as the complexity and invasiveness of ambulatory surgical procedures increase with advances in technique and technology, the appropriateness of care of patients with OSA in an ambulatory surgical center may need further exploration.

CONTROVERSIES

The greatest controversy in the management of surgical patients with known or suspected sleep apnea involves the postoperative disposition of the patient. Although there are current recommendations for prolonged postoperative monitoring, there are no data to show what type of monitoring, or duration, is necessary to decrease risk.

GUIDELINES

The American Society of Anesthesiologists task force approved practice parameters for the perioperative management of patients with obstructive sleep apnea in October 2005.[25] The systematically developed guidelines were intended as recommendations aimed at reducing adverse outcomes, and although based on review of current literature, have not been validated and are not intended to replace the judgment of the practitioner. The recommendations are consensus based.

The ASA practice parameters include a scoring system based on the documented severity of the patient's sleep apnea and the invasiveness of the surgical procedure, combined with the perioperative opioid requirements.

The task force recognized that the majority of patients with OSA may not carry a formal diagnosis, and therefore provided recommendations for the preoperative identification of patients who may be at risk of OSA. Determination of risk for OSA is ascertained by assessment of predisposing physical characteristics, history of apparent airway obstruction during sleep, and presence of daytime somnolence. If the patient is found to have signs and symptoms from two or more of these categories, the guidelines state that the patient should be treated as though he or she has moderate sleep apnea. If any of the signs and symptoms are extraordinarily severe, the patient should be treated as though he or she has severe OSA. Although the literature was insufficient to construct guidelines for recommended criteria for discharge to home for patients with OSA, the consensus opinion was that outpatient procedures could be safely performed if regional or local anesthesia was administered. The consultants were equivocal regarding whether minor-risk procedures could be safely performed under general anesthesia in patients at risk for OSA in an ambulatory setting. Furthermore, they stated that otorhinolaryngologic surgery such as UPPP should not be performed in patients with OSA on an ambulatory basis. Moreover, the consultants acknowledge that the literature is insufficient to determine the efficacy of postoperative monitoring in reducing perioperative risk in patients with OSA. The consultants did agree that intermittent pulse oximetry was of little use in reducing patient risk. Although the guidelines recommend monitoring a patient with OSA for 3 hours longer than their non-OSA counterparts before discharge from a facility, they also indicate that monitoring of patients with OSA should be continuous for a median of 7 hours after the last episode of obstruction of the airway or documented hypoxemia while the patient is breathing room air. Again, we want to emphasize that this is a consensus of expert opinion based on a relative paucity of published literature.

AUTHORS' RECOMMENDATIONS

Ambulatory patients with known or suspected OSA should be scheduled early in the day to allow for potential prolonged postoperative observation. Additionally, those who have been prescribed CPAP should be instructed to bring the device with them to the facility on the day of surgery for postoperative use. Provisions should be made to deal with a potential difficult airway, and there should be a plan in place for transfer to a monitored care environment if necessary. There is no validated optimal anesthetic technique for patients with diagnosed or suspected OSA. Local and regional anesthesia seem to be logical choices because they may decrease the amount of postoperative systemic narcotic required for adequate analgesia. Neuraxial blockade with local anesthetic may also confer the advantage of avoidance of further airway compromise; however, it must be recognized that a high block may exacerbate cardiopulmonary dysfunction. Additionally, epidural narcotics have been implicated in postoperative respiratory arrest.[26,27]

If general anesthesia is required, consideration should be given to securing the airway with the patient awake and spontaneously ventilating. Obese patients should be placed in the semiupright position during induction, and consideration should be given to aspiration prophylaxis. On tracheal extubation there should be unequivocal confirmation of reversal of neuromuscular blockade, and extubation should occur with the patient returned to the semiupright position, breathing 100% oxygen, and fully awake.

On arrival to the postanesthesia care unit, the patient with OSA requires constant surveillance for airway obstruction, hypoxemia, dysrhythmias, and hypertension. During the immediate postoperative period, the patient is particularly at risk for the residual effects of anesthetics in the absence of a secured airway. Supplemental oxygen therapy should be continued and weaned cautiously. However, because respiratory status is frequently based on pulse oximetry readings, the patient may suffer from hypercarbia due to unrecognized hypoventilation. Hypercarbia should be suspected

if the patient exhibits persistent hypertension or dysrhythmia, and arterial blood gas analysis should be considered.

In addition to narcotics, other sedating drugs such as benzodiazepines, antihistamines, and phenothiazines should be administered only if required, and then only judiciously to the patient with OSA. Before discharge, the authors recommend administration of the patient's first dose of prescribed narcotic analgesic while the patient is still in the recovery room, followed by a period of observation for hypersomnolence and airway compromise, which might necessitate overnight observation. Additionally, the patient should be counseled about the potentiated respiratory depressant effects of alcohol consumption or other over-the-counter sedating medications in conjunction with narcotic analgesics.[28]

REFERENCES

1. Malhotra A, White DP: Obstructive sleep apnoea. *Lancet* 2002;360:237-245.
2. Alonso-Fernandez A, Garcia-Rio F, Racionero MA Pino JM, Ortuno F, Martinez I, Villamor J: Cardiac rhythm disturbances and ST-segment depression episodes in patients with obstructive sleep apnea-hypopnea syndrome and its mechanisms. *Chest* 2005; 127:15-22.
3. Bassetti CL, Milanova M, Gugger M: Sleep-disordered breathing and acute ischemic stroke: Diagnosis, risk factors, treatment, evolution, and long-term clinical outcome. *Stroke* 2006;37:967-972.
4. Nieto FJ, Young TB, Lind BK, Shahar E, Samet JM, Redline S, et al: Association of sleep-disordered breathing, sleep apnea, and hypertension in a large community-based study: Sleep Heart Health Study. *JAMA* 2000;283:1829-1836.
5. Punjabi NM, Ahmed NM, Polotsky VY, Beamer BA, O'Donnell CP: Sleep-disordered breathing, glucose intolerance, and insulin resistance. *Respir Physiol Neurobiol* 2003;136:167-178.
6. Shepard JW Jr: Hypertension, cardiac arrhythmias, myocardial infarction, and stroke in relation to obstructive sleep apnea. *Clin Chest Med* 1992;13:437-458.
7. Young T, Palta M, Dempsey J, et al: The occurrence of sleep-disordered breathing among middle-aged adults. *N Eng J Med* 1993;328:130-135.
8. Ancoli-Israel S, Ayalon L: Diagnosis and treatment of sleep disorders in older adults. *Am J Geriatr Psychiatry* 2006;14(2):95-103.
9. Strollo PJ Jr, Rogers RM: Obstructive sleep apnea. *N Engl J Med* 1996;334:99-104.
10. Hiremath AS, Hillman DR, James AL, et al: Relationship between difficult tracheal intubation and obstructive sleep apnoea. *Br J Anaesth* 1998;80:606-611.
11. Boudewyns AN, Van de Heyning PH, De Backer WA: Site of upper airway obstruction in obstructive apnoea and influence of sleep stage. *Eur Respir J* 1997;10(11):2566-2572.
12. Bachar G, Feinmesser R, Shpitzer T, Yaniv E, Nageris B, Eldelman L: Laryngeal and hypopharyngeal obstruction in sleep disordered breathing patients, evaluated by sleep endoscopy. *Eur Arch Otorhinolaryngol*, Mar 8, 2008 [Epub ahead of print].
13. Lavie L: Obstructive sleep apnoea syndrome and oxidative stress disorder. *Sleep Med Rev* 2003;7:35-51.
14. Davignon J, Ganz P: Role of endothelial dysfunction in atherosclerosis. *Circulation* 2004;109:1127-1132.
15. Dyugovskaya L, Lavie P, Lavie L: Increased adhesion molecules expression and production of reactive species in leukocytes of sleep apnea patients. *Am J Respir Crit Care Med* 2002;165:934-939.
16. Haas DC, Foster GL, Nieto FJ, Redline S, Resnick HE, Robbins JA, et al: Age-dependent associations between sleep-disordered breathing and hypertension. *Circulation* 2005;111:614-621.
17. Coughlin SR, Mawdsley L, Mugarza JA, Calverley PMA, Wilding JPH: Obstructive sleep apnea is independently associated with an increased prevalence of metabolic syndrome. *Eur Heart* 2004; 25:735-741.
18. Mickelson SA, Hakim I: Is postoperative intensive care monitoring necessary after uvulopalatopharyngoplasty? *Otolaryngol Head Neck Surg* 1998;119:352-356.

19. Hathaway B, Johnson JT: Safety of uvulopalatopharyngoplasty as outpatient surgery. *Otolaryngol Head Neck Surg* 2006;134(4):542-544.

20. Terris DJ, Fincher EF, Hanasono MM, et al: Conservation of resources: Indications for intensive care monitoring after upper airway surgery on patients with obstructive sleep apnea. *Laryngoscope* 1998;108:784-788.

20a.Spiegel JH, Tejas RH: Overnight stay is not always necessary after uvulopalatopharyngoplasty. *Laryngoscope* 2005;115: 167-171.

21. Gupta RM, Parvizi J, Hanssen AD, Gay PC: Postoperative complications in patients with obstructive sleep apnea syndrome undergoing hip or knee replacement: A case-control study. *Mayo Clin Proc* 2001;76:897-905.

22. Sabers C, Plevak DJ, Schroeder D, Warner DO: The diagnosis of obstructive sleep apnea as a risk factor for unanticipated admissions in outpatient surgery. *Anesth Analg* 2003;96:1328-1335.

23. Maislin G, Pack AI, Kribbs NB, Smith PL, Schwartz AR, Kline LR, et al: A survey screen. *Sleep* 1995;18(3):158-166.

24. Stierer TL, Cohen D, Wright C, George A, Wu C, Brown RH: Propensity for obstructive sleep apnea and perioperative outcome in an ambulatory surgical population. Abstract/poster, IARS, March 2007, Orlando, Florida.

25. Gross J, Bachenberg K, Bellingham WA, Benumof J, Caplan R, Connis R, et al: Practice guidelines for the perioperative management of patients with obstructive sleep apnea. *Anesthesiology* 2006;104:1081-1093.

26. Lamarche Y, Martin R, Reiher J, Blaise G: The sleep apnea syndrome and epidural morphine. *Can Anaesth Soc J* 1986:33:231-233.

27. Ostermeier AM, Roizen MF, Hautkappe M, et al: Three sudden postoperative respiratory arrests associated with epidural opioids in patients with sleep apnea. *Anesth Analg* 1997;85: 452-460.

28. Mitler MM, Dawson A. Henriksen SJ, Sobers M, Bloom FE: Bedtime ethanol increases resistance of upper airways and produces sleep apneas in asymptomatic snorers. *Alcohol Clin Exp Res* 1988; 12:801-805.

46 What Criteria Should Be Used for Discharge after Outpatient Surgery?

Vinod Chinnappa, MBBS, MD, FCARCSI, and Frances Chung, FRCPC

INTRODUCTION

The concept of ambulatory procedure with admission, operation, and discharge on the same day has evolved considerably over the last two decades. The number of ambulatory surgical procedures has grown tremendously throughout the world. The rapid growth of ambulatory surgical care worldwide is attributed to its multiple advantages, such as early return to preoperative physiologic state, fewer complications, reduced physical and mental disturbance, early resumption of normal activities, and reduced hospital costs. The major advance in anesthetic techniques includes the use of rapidly dissipated anesthetic agents and the increasing use of regional anesthetic techniques. It is expected that the number, diversity, and complexity of operations performed in the outpatient setting will continue to increase.

Time to discharge from an ambulatory surgical unit is considered to be a measure of the efficiency of the unit. Counterbalancing efficiency, patient safety is also an important issue in terms of a good practice. Hence, for a successful ambulatory surgical unit, emphasis is not only on patient selection but also on scientifically sound and safe discharge criteria. This chapter outlines the current literature available on discharge criteria and reviews the factors affecting the discharge.

EVIDENCE

The knowledge regarding the process of recovery and the concept of fast-tracking are essential in understanding the application of the appropriate discharge criteria that are presently available. Recovery is an ongoing process that begins from the end of intraoperative care until the patient returns to his or her preoperative physiologic state. This process is divided into three distinct phases: early, intermediate, and late recovery. Early recovery (phase 1) is from the discontinuation of anesthetic agents to the recovery of the protective reflexes and motor function. At most institutions, the phase 1 recovery occurs in the post-anesthesia care unit (PACU).

Intermediate recovery (phase 2) occurs when the patient achieves criteria for discharge from the PACU and occurs mostly in the step-down or ambulatory surgical unit (ASU). Late recovery (phase 3) continues at home under the supervision of a responsible adult and continues until the patient returns to his or her preoperative physiologic state.[1]

Traditionally, most patients are transferred from the operating room to the PACU and then to the ASU before they are discharged home. However, the recovery care after ambulatory surgery is now in a state of change with advances in surgical and anesthetic techniques. This has facilitated an early recovery process. It is now possible to have patients who are awake, alert, and comfortable in the operating room to bypass the labor-intensive PACU directly into the step 2 recovery area. This new concept is referred as *fast-tracking* in ambulatory surgery.[2]

DISCHARGE CRITERIA

The many discharge criteria commonly employed are identified in Table 46-1. There are discharge criteria for the PACU, the ASU, and fast-tracking.

Discharge Criteria for the PACU

The Aldrete score has been successful in addressing the early phase 1 recovery. This score, created in 1970, is a modification of the Apgar score used in neonates.[3] This score assesses five parameters: respiration, circulation, consciousness, color, and level of activity. Each parameter is scored 0, 1, or 2, and patients scoring 9 or greater are eligible to be transferred from the high-dependency PACU to the ASU. However, with the advent of pulse oximetry, the Aldrete score was modified in 1995 to include this technologic improvement[4] (Table 46-2).

Although the Aldrete score is an effective screening tool, it has a few limitations.[5] It does not provide an assessment for home-readiness, and it does not address some of the common side effects seen in the PACU, such as pain, nausea and vomiting, and bleeding at the incision site.

Discharge Criteria for the ASU

Discharge criteria applied in the ASU are designed to assess home-readiness of patients, and hence strict adherence to the criteria to ensure patient safety is important. There are a number of available criteria, but the most

Table 46-1 Common Discharge Criteria

Discharge Scoring Criteria

DISCHARGE CRITERIA APPLIED AT DIFFERENT PHASES OF RECOVERY

Discharge criteria at PACU (phase 1 recovery)
   Aldrete score
Discharge criteria at ASU (phase 2 recovery)
   Postanesthesia discharge score (PADS)
   Outcome-based discharge criteria
Discharge criteria for fast-tracking
   White fast-tracking score

DISCHARGE CRITERIA USED FOR RESEARCH PURPOSES

Psychomotor test of recovery (phase 3 recovery)

DISCHARGE CRITERIA USED UNDER SPECIFIC CIRCUMSTANCES

Discharge home criteria after neuraxial blockade
Discharge home criteria after peripheral nerve block
Discharge home criteria for suspected MH

Table 46-2 The Modified Aldrete Scoring System*

	Discharge Criteria from PACU	Score
Activity	Able to move voluntarily or on command	
	Four extremity	2
	Two extremity	1
	Zero extremity	0
Respiration		
	Able to breathe and cough freely	2
	Dyspnea, shallow or limited breathing	1
	Apneic	0
Circulation		
	Blood pressure 20 mm of preanesthetic level	2
	Blood pressure 20 to 50 mm of preanesthesia level	1
	Blood pressure - 50 mm of preanesthesia level	0
Consciousness		
	Fully awake	2
	Arousable on calling	1
	Not responding	0
O_2 saturation		
	O_2 saturation able to maintain O_2 saturation >92% on room air	2
	Needs O_2 inhalation to maintain O_2 saturation >90%	1
	O_2 saturation <90% even with O_2 supplementation room	0

*To determine readiness for discharge from postanesthesia care unit. A score >9 is required for discharge. Aldrete JA: *J Clin Anesth* 1995;7:89-91.

common criteria that are applied at the ASU are the safe discharge criteria proposed by Korttila[6] and the postanesthesia discharge score (PADS) devised by Chung and colleagues.[7]

The safe discharge criteria use outcome-based clinical observations and all parameters have to be met before discharge. It is important to note that clinical observations such as the need to drink and void before discharge, which were initial prerequisites in "safe discharge criteria," are no longer applicable. Current outcome-based discharge criteria are listed in Table 46-3.[1]

Chung and colleagues[7] devised the PADS in 1993. The PADS was later modified to eliminate the requirements for oral fluid intake and urinary output before discharge.[8] It has been demonstrated that the implementation of PADS as a criterion for discharge from the ASU facilitates expeditious discharge, with 80% of patients able to be discharged within 1 to 2 hours.[9] PADS is a cumulative index that measures the home-readiness of patients based on five major criteria: (1) vital signs, (2) ambulation, (3) pain, (4) postoperative nausea and vomiting, and (5) surgical bleeding.[1] The pain criteria have been further refined to score pain with a visual analog scale ranging from 1 to 10 (Table 46-4). Patients who achieve a score of 9 or greater are considered fit for discharge with an adult escort. PADS also provides for an objective determination of the optimal length of patient stay following ambulatory surgery (see Table 46-4).

Discharge Criteria for Fast-tracking

The success of fast-tracking depends on the appropriate modification of anesthetic technique, which would allow rapid emergence from anesthesia and the prevention of common postoperative complications such as pain, nausea, and vomiting using a multimodal approach. White and Song[2] devised a fast-tracking score, which incorporated assessment of pain and emetic symptoms, to the original Aldrete score. The maximum possible score is 14. A score of 12 (with no score less than 1 in any category) is considered sufficient for discharge from the operating room to the ASU (Table 46-5).

Studies have shown that outpatients who are fast-tracked can be discharged earlier without any increase in

Table 46-3 "Safe Discharge" Criteria*

Patient alert and oriented to time, place, and person
- Stable vital signs
- Pain controlled by oral analgesics
- Nausea and emesis controlled
- Able to walk without dizziness
- No unexpected bleeding from the operating sites
- Discharge instruction and prescription received
- Patient accepts readiness for discharge
- Responsible escort

*A set of typical discharge criteria to determine readiness for discharge from postanesthesia care unit. All parameters of safe discharge criteria need to be met before discharge. Awad IT, Chung F: Factors affecting recovery and discharge following ambulatory surgery. *Can J Anaesth* 2006;53:858-872.

Table 46-4	Postanesthetic Discharge Scoring System (PADS)	

VITAL SIGNS

Within 20% of preoperative baseline	2
20%-40% of preoperative baseline	1
40% of preoperative baseline	0

ACTIVITY LEVEL

Steady gait, no dizziness, consistent with preoperative level	2
Requires assistance	1
Unable to ambulate/assess	0

NAUSEA AND VOMITING

Minimal: mild, no treatment required	2
Moderate: treatment effective	1
Severe: treatment not effective	0

PAIN

VAS = 0-3: the patient has minimal or no pain before discharge	2
VAS = 4-6: the patient has moderate pain	1
VAS = 7-10: the patient has severe pain	0

SURGICAL BLEEDING

Minimal: does not require dressing change	2
Moderate: required up to two dressing changes with no further bleeding	1
Severe: required three or more dressing changes and continues to bleed	0

VAS, visual analog scale; maximum score = 10: patients scoring >9 are fit for discharge. Awad IT, Chung F: Factors affecting recovery and discharge following ambulatory surgery. *Can J Anaesth* 2006;53:858-872.

Table 46-5	White Fast-tracking Score

Discharge Criteria	Score
LEVEL OF CONSCIOUSNESS	
Awake and oriented	2
Arousable with minimal stimulation	1
Responsive to tactile stimulation	0
PHYSICAL ACTIVITY	
Able to move all extremities on command	2
Some weakness in movement of extremities	1
Unable to voluntarily move extremities	0
HEMODYNAMIC STABILITY	
Blood pressure <15% of baseline MAP value	2
Blood pressure 15%-30% of baseline MAP value	1
Blood pressure >30% below the baseline MAP value	0
RESPIRATORY STABILITY	
Able to breathe deeply	2
Tachypnea with good cough	1
Dyspneic with good cough	0
OXYGEN SATURATION STATUS	
Maintains value >90% on room air	2
Requires supplemental oxygen	1
Saturation <90% with supplemental oxygen	0
POSTOPERATIVE PAIN ASSESSMENT	
None, or mild discomfort	2
Moderate to severe pain controlled with IV analgesics	1
Persistent severe pain	0
POSTOPERATIVE EMETIC SYMPTOMS	
None, or mild nausea with no active vomiting	2
Transient vomiting	1
Persistent moderate to severe nausea and vomiting	0
Total possible score	**14**

Scoring system to determine whether outpatients can be transferred directly from the operating room to the step-down unit. A minimum score of 12 (with no score <1 in any individual category) would be required for patients to be fast-tracked after general anesthesia. White et al: *Anesth Analg* 1999;88:1069-1072.

complications or side effects.[10-12] Apfelbaum and colleagues[12] undertook a multicenter prospective study to determine the safe bypass of PACU of patients after ambulatory surgery. After education of the health personnel, the PACU bypass rate of patients having general anesthesia increased from baseline 15.9% to 58%. These patients had a significantly shorter duration of recovery when compared with patients who had a standard recovery at the PACU.

However, the advantages of a faster recovery and saving time may not reflect the true nursing workload and real cost savings. A recent randomized control trial compared fast-tracking of bypassing PACU with no bypassing of PACU.[13] In this study, patients were randomly assigned to either a routine or a fast-tracking group. Patients in the fast-tracking group were transferred from the operating room directly to the ASU (i.e., bypassing the PACU) if they achieved the fast-tracking criteria. All other patients were transferred to the PACU and then to the ASU. The mean time to discharge was 17 minutes less in the fast-tracking group, but the overall nursing workload and the associated cost were not significantly different between the two groups.[13]

A number of psychomotor tests are available[14-21] (Table 46-6) to determine recovery of patients; however, the tests have a number of disadvantages. They require equipment and trained personnel to use and interpret the equipment. The tests are time consuming, and usually only assess one area of brain function. Therefore they are mostly used for research purposes rather than for clinical use.

Evaluation of the Scores

Various scores have been devised to guide the process of discharge and home-readiness to ensure patient safety, but none have been formally evaluated. An ideal discharge score should be practical, simple, and easy to remember and should be applicable to all postanesthesia settings.[22] Use of common physical signs with scores assigned to each parameter makes the assessment more objective. The presently available discharge criteria in literature have been successful to a very large extent, but have some limitations. The Aldrete scoring system and the PADS are widely used.

Table 46-6	Common Psychomotor Tests*
Simple reaction time[14]	Time to press a keyboard in response to a stimulus (e.g., buzzer)
Choice reaction time[14]	Involves choice of optical stimulus (e.g., green/red)
Critical flicker fusion time[15]	Involves the time it takes for the patient to notice a flickering light at a particular frequency that appears and becomes continuous
Digital symbol substitution test[16]	
Perceptive accuracy test[17]	
Digital span	The ability to recall strings of numbers
California verbal test[18]	Ability to remember a list of words from a previously presented list
Treiger dot test (gestalt test)[19]	Ability to connect a series of dots on paper to form a pattern; the more dots the patient misses, the lower the recovery score
Driving simulation test[20]	
Maddox wing test[21]	A device to test extraocular muscle balance

*Used as discharge criteria for research purposes.

Table 46-7	Risk Factors for Postoperative Urinary Retention

LOW RISK FOR URINARY RETENTION

Low-risk patients can be defined as having the following characteristics:
- General anesthesia, peripheral nerve block, monitored anesthesia care
- Nonpelvic and nonurologic surgery
- Most outpatient gynecologic surgeries (transvaginal, or pelvic laparoscopy who undergo intraoperative bladder drainage)
- Most patients having spinal or epidural anesthesia with short-acting local anesthetic such as lidocaine, procaine, or 2-chloroprocaine

HIGH RISK FOR URINARY RETENTION

High risk of urinary retention can be defined as having
- Pelvic surgery (hernia, rectal, penile, urologic)
- Positive family history of retention or spinal cord disease
- Spinal or epidural anesthesia with agents of long-acting duration such as bupivacaine, tetracaine, and ropivicaine
- The use of neuraxial opioids combined with local anesthetics

Souter KJ, Pavlin DJ: Bladder function after ambulatory surgery. *Journal of Ambulatory Surgery* 2005;12:89-97.

Shift from the Traditional Discharge Criteria

Traditionally, clinical parameters such as oral intake and urinary output were considered a prerequisite for discharge criteria from the ASU. However, this practice is increasingly being questioned.

Urinary retention is defined by the inability to void at a bladder volume of 600 mL, a volume at which there is a strong desire to void.[23] The risk for postoperative urinary retention can be classified as high and low risk.[24] The identified risk factors for postoperative urinary retention are presented in Table 46-7.

The incidence of urinary retention is 1% in low-risk ambulatory surgical procedures and ranges from 3% to 20% in high-risk patients.[24] Prolonged urinary retention can cause bladder atony and may also cause impaired voiding after return of function.[24] Prolonged urinary retention can also cause delay in discharge in 5% to 11% of ambulatory care patients.[25] Mulroy and colleagues[26] undertook a prospective study to determine the risk of developing postoperative urinary retention in the low-risk group. In this study standard patients were required to void before discharge. Accelerated-pathway patients were discharged home if the bladder volume was less than 400 mL as evidenced by ultrasound. Patients who had bladder volume greater than 400 mL were reassessed after 1 hour and catheterized if they did not void. All patients were advised to return to the emergency department if they were not able to void after 8 hours. Mean discharge time in patients with the accelerated pathway was 22 minutes shorter than the standard pathway. No patients reported urinary retention after they were discharged home.[26]

In summary, low-risk patients can be discharged home without voiding. They should be instructed to return to the hospital if they are unable to void within 6 to 8 hours. Patients at high risk of urinary retention should be required to void before discharge and display a residual volume of less than 400 mL. If the bladder volume is greater than 500 to 600 mL, catheterization should be performed before discharge. It is important to note that the use of ultrasound in detecting bladder volume is better than clinical judgment.[27]

Patients are no longer required to drink fluids before discharge. The studies that questioned mandatory oral fluids before discharge were Schreiner and colleagues[28] and Kearney and colleagues[29] in the pediatric population and Jin and colleagues[30] in the adult population. Schreiner assigned children undergoing ambulatory surgery into either mandatory drinker or elective drinker.[28] Children in the mandatory drinker group experienced a higher incidence of vomiting and prolonged hospital stay. Kearney evaluated the incidence of vomiting in 317 children undergoing day surgery.[29] Children were randomized into two groups: either drinking oral fluids or having oral fluids withheld for 4 to 6 hours. Vomiting was assessed in the hospital and throughout the first postoperative day. The incidence of vomiting in the group with fluids withheld was significantly less than that of the group that drank (38% versus 56%, $p < 0.004$). The greatest effect of withholding fluids was seen in patients receiving opioids ($p < 0.004$), where vomiting was reduced from 76% to 36%.

To answer the question of whether adult outpatients should drink before discharge after minor surgical procedures, 726 patients were randomized to either drinking oral fluids or not drinking after surgery.[30] Neither drinking nor nondrinking worsened postoperative nausea or vomiting or prolonged hospital stay. Therefore drinking oral fluids is not a requirement before discharge. These changes have been incorporated in the American Society of Anesthesiologists' practice guidelines for postanesthetic care. Mandating oral fluid intake before discharge should be done only for selected patients on a case-by-case basis.

Discharge Criteria after Regional Anesthesia

The role of regional anesthesia in ambulatory surgery is very promising and has demonstrated benefits of better pain control, lower incidence of nausea and vomiting,[31] and potentially faster discharge and reduction in the incidence of chronic pain syndrome.[32]

Spinal anesthesia is a simple and reliable technique, widely used in ambulatory surgical care. There has been ongoing effort to refine anesthetic technique to tailor faster recovery with minimal side effects. Two specific low-dose techniques, unilateral[33,34] and selective spinal anesthesia,[35] have been described, although there is an overlap between the two. With adequate doses of local anesthetic agents, the time to home-readiness after unilateral spinal anesthesia,[36] or selective spinal anesthesia[37-40] with bupivacaine, or low-dose spinal anesthetic with lidocaine and fentanyl,[41] or sufentanil,[42] has been equal to that for general anesthesia maintained with propofol or desflurane.[40,41]

Lidocaine was previously the agent used for short-acting spinal anesthesia until it was reported to cause transient neurologic symptoms.[43-45] These neurologic problems have made anesthesiologists seek alternative suitable local aesthetic agents. The incidence of transient neurologic symptoms has been highest after lidocaine spinal anesthesia (37%) and in patients undergoing knee arthroscopy (22%) or surgery in the lithotomy position (0% to 3%),[46] whereas after bupivacaine or ropivacine it has been as low as 0% to 3%.[38,39,47,48] Recently the use of 2-chloroprocaine as an alternative to lidocaine in ambulatory anesthesia has been revisited.[49] In this study, volunteers received either 40 mg of 2% lidocaine or 40 mg of 3% 2-chloroprocaine intrathecally. The quality of surgical anesthesia and motor block was similar in the two groups. No patient developed transient neurologic symptoms in the 2-chloroprocaine groups. Patients in this group also experienced faster resolution of sensory block, and achieved discharge criteria earlier. In another study, 40 mg of 3% 2-chloroprocaine produced similar motor block compared with bupivicaine 7.5 mg. Low-dose 2-chloroprocaine may be the local anesthetic for short-acting bilateral procedures in the future, but its safety has not been proven.[50]

The main factor restricting the popularity of spinal anesthesia is postdural puncture headache (PDPH). The incidence of PDPH is less than 1% with the use of a standard 25 G Whitacre spinal needle.[51] This complication is reduced to a large extent by choosing an appropriate needle, decreasing to 0.4% with a 27 G Whitacare needle versus 1.5% with a 27 G Quinke needle (1.5%).[52]

There are limited reports in the literature on epidural anesthesia for ambulatory care, as it is generally regarded as a time-consuming technique when compared with other techniques. Milroy and colleagues[26] showed a faster discharge after epidural with either lidocaine or 2-chloroprocaine versus spinal lidocaine or low-dose bupivicaine. Other studies have used epidural successfully for hemorrhoidectomy and lower abdominal surgery,[53,54] with observation time in hospital ranging from 5 to 6 hours, respectively. However, there is an isolated case report of epidural hematoma in a patient receiving nonsteroidal antiinflammatory drugs (NSAIDs) after discharge from an ambulatory arthroscopy after epidural anesthesia.[55]

Patients undergoing regional anesthesia should expect the same discharge criteria and standard postoperative care as those who have undergone general anesthesia. It is important to ensure that motor, sensory, and sympathetic blocks have regressed; suitable criteria to judge block regression include normal perianal (S4–S5) sensation, plantar flexion of the foot, and proprioception in the big toe.[56]

Discharge after Single Shot Peripheral Block

For peripheral nerve block, it is safe to discharge patients home before full regression of motor and sensory block. Although the risk of accidental injury is very low,[57] patients should be given written instructions advising them (1) to avoid driving while the leg is insensate, (2) to avoid placing hot pads on the numb limb, (3) to keep the limb elevated as much as possible in the first 24 hours to avoid swelling, (4) to use walkers or crutches when the leg is numb, and (5) to take analgesic medication as soon as the numbness starts to subside and is replaced by a tingling sensation.[1,58]

Discharge after Continuous Peripheral Block

The ability to provide continuous peripheral nerve block to patients safely on an outpatient basis has been a major advance in ambulatory surgery over the past several years. There are more studies showing the efficacy and safety of ambulatory continuous interscalene blocks,[59,60] infraclavicular blocks,[61] axillary block,[62] sciatic nerve blocks,[63-65] femoral nerve block,[66] psoas compartment blocks,[67] and paravertebral block.[68] However, these techniques have the potential for significant complications such as nerve injury, catheter migration leading to local anesthetic toxicity, and unintentional spread of blockade epidurally or intrathecally.[69-71] Discharge in patients with regional anesthesia should include clear instructions with a written copy regarding cautions and limitation of continuous regional blocks.[72] Telephone communication must be available to the patient at all times. The instructions should also vary depending on the site of catheter placement. Patients with an upper-extremity catheter should be instructed to protect their arm in a sling. Patients with a lower-extremity catheter must be instructed to have aid for ambulation and to avoid weight bearing on the surgical extremity. These precautions, along with standard discharge criteria, are an essential part of good practice.

Discharge for Patients with Suspected Malignant Hyperthermia

Malignant hyperthermia (MH) is a rare condition and does not lend itself to large prospective studies. Knowledge of this condition and its management in the ambulatory setting is largely derived from case reports, audits, and retrospective cases and hence the level of evidence is poor. Traditionally, overnight hospitalization of the patient with suspected or confirmed MH was a common practice. To determine whether hospitalization for MH-susceptible (MHS) patients is required, the charts of 303 children labeled MHS who underwent surgery with trigger-free anesthesia on 431 occasions were reviewed.[73] Ten cases developed fever, but none were considered to be MH. The authors recommend that MHS is not an indication for postoperative hospital admission. These findings are again confirmed in a large prospective audit investigating possible adverse reactions in patients suspected of MH.[74] The incidence of MH after a trigger-free anesthetic has been estimated to be less than 1%.[75,76] In a large population of MHS patients, the charts of 2124 who underwent elective muscle biopsy for MH were reviewed.[75] Five patients (0.46%) had MH-like reactions, and all the reactions were seen in the immediate recovery room; four of these patients received intravenous dantrolene as a part of therapy. Current available literature suggests that overnight hospitalizations may not be required as long as a trigger-free anesthetic is provided and body temperature is monitored and remains normal for at least 4 hours postoperatively. These are recommendations in keeping with the guidelines of the Malignant Hyperthermia Association of the United States. It is important to give written instructions regarding how to monitor temperature of the patient at home and how to recognize signs of malignant hyperthermia with contact details to seek medical attention if necessary before discharge of patients.

Reliable Escort

Meeting a set of standard discharge criteria before discharge is not the end of quality ambulatory surgical care. The presence of an escort, clear verbal instructions, and written postoperative instructions are crucial for safety of patients before discharge. A recent study reported that 0.2% of ambulatory surgical patients did not have an escort.[77] Another survey indicated that 11% of anesthesiologists would be willing to anesthetize patients for ambulatory surgery without the availability of an escort to take patients home.[78] This is in contrast to the guidelines issued by professional associations such as the American Society of Anesthesiologists (ASA), Canadian Anesthesiologists Society (CAS), Association of Anaesthetists of Great Britain and Ireland (AAGBI), and Australian Day Surgery Council.[79-82] The major concern with an absence of an escort is that the patient may drive, operate machinery, or become involved in unsafe activities that are not intended. These may lead to serious consequences such as car accidents and may have medicolegal implications for the anesthesiolgist. A number of factors can impair performance of patients[83-87] (Table 46-8).

Table 46-8 Common Factors Impairing Driving
• Lack of sleep
• Stress of surgery
• Residual effects of anesthetic[87-90]
• Type of surgery[91]
• Residual motor block after local or regional anesthesia

Chung and colleagues[88] compared the driving performance in a simulator in patients who had their surgery performed under general anesthesia with healthy, nonanesthetized controls. In this study, simulated driving in patients was impaired both preoperatively and postoperatively. Performance was worst 2 hours postoperatively, a crucial time, as many patients met discharge criteria within 2 to 3 hours. Within 24 hours, driving simulation performance had returned to normal. The results of this trial support the current recommendations not to drive for 24 hours after ambulatory surgery.[88]

In another study the brake response time for driving returned to normal at 3 weeks in patients who underwent total knee arthroplasty for osteoarthritis.[89] These studies denote that the degree of functional recovery may vary depending on the type of anesthetic and the type of surgery. In the context of the available literature, if no escort is available before surgery, the elective procedure should be canceled or the patient should be admitted overnight. If an escort is not available after anesthesia is given, elective hospital admission should be arranged.

Most ambulatory surgical units verify the presence of an escort, but it may be difficult to ensure the compliance of postoperative instruction. Correa and colleagues[90] reported that 4% of patient drove within 24 hours and 4% of patients were alone despite a clear postoperative instruction.[90] These results were confirmed by another survey where 1.3% of patients spent the night alone and 4.1% drove home within 24 hours after ambulatory surgery.[91] Although it is impossible to ensure the compliance of postoperative instructions, it is essential to educate patients, and their caregivers, regarding the potential hazards of not complying with the recommendation.

POSTANESTHESIA CARE

The safe transition of patients through the three phases of recovery requires standard patient care in the PACU and ASU. Postanesthesia care refers to those activities undertaken to manage patients following the completion of surgical procedures and the concomitant primary anesthetic.[92] The American Society of Anesthesiologists Task Force provides a practice guideline for standard postanesthesia care.[92] The guideline emphasizes the need for periodic perioperative patient assessment and monitoring and recommends treatment during emergence and recovery in the PACU. Perioperative patient assessment includes monitoring of respiratory and cardiovascular function, neuromuscular function, mental status, temperature, pain, nausea and vomiting, drainage and bleeding, and urine output. Treatment recommendations during emergence and recovery in the PACU include prophylaxis and treatment of nausea and vomiting, administration of supplemental oxygen, fluid administration and management, normalizing patient temperature, and pharmacologic agents for reduction of shivering and antagonism of the effects of sedatives, analgesics, and neuromuscular blocks.

The guidelines do not recommend any specific discharge criteria, but focus on the need to adopt discharge criteria that are suitable to the local ambulatory surgical setting. The guidelines also suggest that a discharge scoring system may be helpful in documentation of fitness for discharge.

AREAS OF UNCERTAINTIES

Anesthesiologists, to a large extent, have focused on patient care to the point of the patient's discharge. Unfortunately, postdischarge symptoms such as nausea and vomiting are aspects of ambulatory anesthesia that have been overlooked. Relatively little research to date has examined these unpleasant and distressing symptoms. The incidence of postdischarge nausea and vomiting (PDNV) can be as high as 30% to 50%.[93,94] This high incidence of PDNV is clinically important, especially when recognizing that 65% to 70% of surgeries are performed in the ambulatory surgical setting. The treatment of this complication should extend beyond discharge from the hospital because one third of patients continue to have PDNV after returning home. More research needs to be conducted in this area. The scope for further study includes identification of specific risk factors, antiemetic efficacy in postdischarge settings, the effectiveness of a detailed education program for patients, and the possible economic impact.

The presence of a reliable escort before the patient is discharged is emphasized by most anesthesia professional associations. However, the presence of a responsible caregiver at home, who can cater to the needs of the discharged patient in the postdischarge setting, is not clear. The functional status of these discharged patients may be reduced for up to 7 days, which is both unpleasant and disturbing.[95] More studies are needed to address the functional status of patients during the postdischarge period and the need for a responsible adult during those times.

GUIDELINES

The major concern for patients without an escort is that they may drive home after ambulatory surgery. Patients may be noncompliant with postoperative instructions, which can lead to potential hazards. The American Society of Anesthesiologists' guidelines do not comment on the issue of driving. The minimum duration required for patients to resume driving based on the type of surgery is still an area of uncertainty, which emphasizes the need for further focused research.

AUTHORS' RECOMMENDATIONS

- The success of safe ambulatory surgical care depends on appropriate patient selection and timely discharge.
- Discharge scoring systems such as the Aldrete score, the post-anesthesia discharge score (PADS), and fast-tracking can facilitate safe transition through the three phases of recovery.
- Shifting from previous traditional discharge criteria by excluding mandatory drinking and voiding will enhance the speedy discharge.
- Patients at low risk for urinary retention can be discharged home without voiding, and should be instructed to return to the hospital if they are unable to void within 6 to 8 hours. Patients at a high risk of urinary retention should be required to void before discharge and display a residual volume of less than 400 mL. If the bladder volume is more than 500 to 600 mL, catheterization should be performed before discharge.
- Patients are no longer required to drink fluids before discharge.
- Regional anesthetic techniques are well suited for ambulatory surgery, but discharging such patients requires specific considerations and patient education, apart from the standard discharge criteria.
- Inclusion of antiemetics in the postdischarge prescription, along with analgesics and other required medication, may improve the patient's overall comfort in postdischarge settings.
- Discharge criteria and discharge scores assess home-readiness but not street fitness as functional recovery may vary depending on the type of anesthetic and type of surgery.
- The presence of a reliable escort, clear written instructions, and clear verbal instructions are crucial for patient safety before discharge.
- If an escort is not available after anesthesia is given, elective admission should be arranged.
- Patients should not drive or operate machinery for 24 hours after ambulatory surgery.

REFERENCES

1. Awad IT, Chung F: Factors affecting recovery and discharge following ambulatory surgery. *Can J Anesth* 2006;53:858-872.
2. White PF, Song D: New criteria for fast-tracking after outpatient anesthesia: A comparison with the modified Aldrete's scoring system. *Anesth Analg* 1999;88:1069-1072.
3. Aldrete JA, Kroulik D: A postanesthetic recovery score. *Anesth Analg* 1970;49:924-934.
4. Aldrete JA: The post-anesthesia recovery score revisited. *J Clin Anesth* 1995;7:89-91.
5. Aldrete JA: Modifications to the postanesthesia score for use in ambulatory surgery. *J Perianesth Nurs* 1998;13:148-155.
6. Korttila KT: Post-anaesthetic psychomotor and cognitive function. *Eur J Anaesthesiol Suppl* 1995;10:43-46.
7. Chung F, Chan VW, Ong D: A post-anesthetic discharge scoring system for home readiness after ambulatory surgery. *J Clin Anesth* 1995;7:500-506.
8. Chung F: Recovery pattern and home-readiness after ambulatory surgery. *Anesth Analg* 1995;80:896-902.
9. Marshall S, Chung F: Assessment of "home readiness"—discharge criteria and post discharge complication. *Curr Opin Aanesthesiol* 1997;10:445-450.
10. Duncan PG, Shandro J, Bachand R, Ainsworth L. A pilot study of recovery room bypass (fast-track protocol) in a community hospital. *Can J Anaesth* 2001;48:630-636.
11. Williams BA, Kentor ML, Williams JP, et al: PACU bypass after outpatient knee surgery is associated with fewer unplanned hospital admissions but more phase II nursing interventions. *Anesthesiology* 2002;97:981-988.
12. Apfelbaum JL, Walawander CA, Grasela TH, et al: Eliminating intensive postoperative care in same-day surgery patients using short-acting anesthetics. *Anesthesiology* 2002;97:66-74.
13. Song D, Chung F, Ronayne M, Ward B, Yogendran S, Sibbick C: Fast-tracking (bypassing the PACU) does not reduce nursing workload after ambulatory surgery. *Br J Anaesth* 2004;93:768-774.
14. Nightingale JJ, Lewis IH: Recovery from day-case anaesthesia: Comparison of total IV anaesthesia using propofol with an inhalation technique. *Br J Anaesth* 1992;68:356-359.
15. Salib Y, Plourde G, Alloul K, Provost A, Moore A: Measuring recovery from general anaesthesia using critical flicker frequency: A comparison of two methods. *Can J Anaesth* 1992;39:1045-1050.
16. Tarazi EM, Philip BK: A comparison of recovery after sevoflurane or desflurane in ambulatory anesthesia. *J Clin Anesth* 1998; 10:272-277.

17. Larsen LE, Gupta A, Ledin T, Doolan M, Linder P, Lennmarken C: Psychomotor recovery following propofol or isoflurane anaesthesia for day-care surgery. *Acta Anaesthesiol Scand* 1992;36:276-282.
18. Schwender D, Müller A, Madler M, Faber-Züllig E, Ilmberger J: Recovery of psychomotor and cognitive functions following anesthesia. Propofol/alfentanil and thiopental/isoflurane/alfentanil. *Anaesthesist* 1993;42:583.
19. Newman MG, Trieger N, Miller JC: Measuring recovery from anesthesia—a simple test. *Anesth Analg* 1969;48:136-140.
20. Korttila K, Tammisto T, Ertama P, Pfäffli P, Blomgren E, Häkkinen S: Recovery, psychomotor skills, and simulated driving after brief inhalational anesthesia with halothane or enflurane combined with nitrous oxide and oxygen. *Anesthesiology* 1977;46:20-27.
21. Hannington-Kiff JG: Measurement of recovery from outpatient general anaesthesia with a simple ocular test. *BMJ* 1970;3:132-135.
22. Ead H: From Aldrete to PADSS: Reviewing discharge criteria after ambulatory surgery. *J Perianesth Nurs* 2006;21:259-267.
23. Pavlin DJ, Pavlin EG, Gunn HC, Taraday JK, Koerschgen ME: Voiding in patients managed with or without ultrasound monitoring of bladder volume after outpatient surgery. *Anesth Analg* 1999;89:90-97.
24. Souter KJ, Pavlin DJ: Bladder function after ambulatory surgery. *Journal of Ambulatory Surgery* 2005;12:89-97.
25. Pavlin DJ, Rapp SE, Polissar NL, Malmgren JA, Koerschgen M, Keyes H: Factors affecting discharge time in adult outpatients. *Anesth Analg* 1998;87:816-826.
26. Mulroy MF, Salinas FV, Larkin KL, Polissar NL: Ambulatory surgery patients may be discharged before voiding after short-acting spinal and epidural anesthesia. *Anesthesiology* 2002;97:315-319.
27. Rosseland LA, Stubhaug A, Breivik H: Detecting postoperative urinary retention with an ultrasound scanner. *Acta Anaesthesiol Scand* 2002;46:279-282.
28. Schreiner MS, Nicolson SC, Martin T, Whitney L: Should children drink before discharge from day surgery? *Anesthesiology* 1992;76:528-533.
29. Kearney R, Mack C, Entwistle L: Withholding oral fluids from children undergoing day surgery reduces vomiting. *Paediatr Anaesth* 1998;8:331-336.
30. Jin FL, Norris A, Chung F, Ganeshram T: Should adult patients drink fluids before discharge from ambulatory surgery? *Anesth Analg* 1998;87:306-311.
31. Liu SS, Strodtbeck WM, Richman JM, Wu CL: A comparison of regional versus general anesthesia for ambulatory anesthesia: A meta-analysis of randomized controlled trials. *Anesth Analg* 2005;101:1634-1642.
32. Reuben SS, Pristas R, Dixon D, Faruqi S, Madabhushi L, Wenner S: The incidence of complex regional pain syndrome after fasciectomy for Dupuytren's contracture: A prospective observational study of four anesthetic techniques. *Anesth Analg* 2006;102:499-503.
33. Enk D, Prien T, Van Aken H, Mertes N, Meyer J, Brussel T: Success rate of unilateral spinal anesthesia is dependent on injection flow. *Reg Anesth Pain Med* 2001;26:420-427.
34. Enk D: Unilateral spinal anaesthesia: Gadget or tool? *Curr Opin Anaesthesiol* 1998;11:511-515.
35. Vaghadia H, Viskari D, Mitchell GW, Berrill A: Selective spinal anesthesia for outpatient laparoscopy. I: Characteristics of three hypobaric solutions. *Can J Anaesth* 2001;48:256-260.
36. Jankowski CJ, Hebl JR, Stuart MJ, Rock MG, Pagnano MW, Beighley CM, et al: A comparison of psoas compartment block and spinal and general anesthesia for outpatient knee arthroscopy. *Anesth Analg* 2003;97:1003-1009.
37. Korhonen AM, Valanne JV, Jokela RM, Ravaska P, Volmanen P, Korttila K: Influence of the injection site (L2/3 or L3/4) and the posture of the vertebral column on selective spinal anesthesia for ambulatory knee arthroscopy. *Acta Anaesthesiol Scand* 2005;49:72-77.
38. Korhonen AM, Valanne JV, Jokela RM, Ravaska P, Korttila K: Intrathecal hyperbaric bupivacaine 3 mg + fentanyl 10 microg for outpatient knee arthroscopy with tourniquet. *Acta Anaesthesiol Scand* 2003;47:342-346.
39. Valanne JV, Korhonen AM, Jokela RM, Ravaska P, Korttila KK: Selective spinal anesthesia: A comparison of hyperbaric bupivacaine 4 mg versus 6 mg for outpatient knee arthroscopy. *Anesth Analg* 2001;93:1377-1379.
40. Korhonen AM, Valanne JV, Jokela RM, Ravaska P, Korttila KT: A comparison of selective spinal anesthesia with hyperbaric bupivacaine and general anesthesia with desflurane for outpatient knee arthroscopy. *Anesth Analg* 2004;99:1668-1673.
41. Ben-David B, DeMeo PJ, Lucyk C, Solosko D: A comparison of minidose lidocaine-fentanyl spinal anesthesia and local anesthesia/propofol infusion for outpatient knee arthroscopy. *Anesth Analg* 2001;93:319-325.
42. Lennox PH, Vaghadia H, Henderson C, Martin L, Mitchell GW: Small-dose selective spinal anesthesia for short-duration outpatient laparoscopy: Recovery characteristics compared with desflurane anesthesia. *Anesth Analg* 2002;94:346-350.
43. Tarkkila P, Huhtala J, Tuominen M, Lindgren L: Transient radicular irritation after bupivacaine spinal anesthesia. *Reg Anesth* 1996;21:26-29.
44. Schneider M, Ettlin T, Kaufmann M, Schumacher P, Urwyler A, Hampl K, von Hochstetter A: Transient neurologic toxicity after hyperbaric subarachnoid anesthesia with 5% lidocaine. *Anesth Analg* 1993;76:1154-1157.
45. Rodríguez-Chinchilla R, Rodríguez-Pont A, Pintanel T, Vidal-López F: Bilateral severe pain at L3-4 after spinal anaesthesia with hyperbaric 5% lignocaine. *Br J Anaesth* 1996;76:328-329.
46. Pollock JE: Neurotoxicity of intrathecal local anaesthetics and transient neurological symptoms. *Best Pract Res Clin Anaesthesiol* 2003;17:471-484.
47. Kuusniemi KS, Pihlajamaki KK, Pitkanen MT: A low dose of plain or hyperbaric bupivacaine for unilateral spinal anesthesia. *Reg Anesth Pain Med* 2000;25:605-610.
48. Buckenmaier CC 3rd, Nielsen KC, Pietrobon R, Klein SM, Martin AH, Greengrass RA, Steele SM: Small-dose intrathecal lidocaine versus ropivacaine for anorectal surgery in an ambulatory setting. *Anesth Analg* 2002;95:1253-1257.
49. Kouri ME, Kopacz DJ: Spinal 2-chloroprocaine: A comparison with lidocaine in volunteers. *Anesth Analg* 2004;98:75-80.
50. Yoos JR, Kopacz DJ: Spinal 2-chloroprocaine: A comparison with small-dose bupivacaine in volunteers. *Anesth Analg* 2005;100:566-572.
51. Pittoni G, Toffoletto F, Calcarella G, Zanette G, Giron GP: Spinal anesthesia in outpatient knee surgery: 22-gauge versus 25-gauge Sprotte needle. *Anesth Analg* 1995;81:73-79.
52. Santanen U, Rautoma P, Luurila H, Erkola O, Pere P: Comparison of 27-gauge (0.41-mm) Whitacre and Quincke spinal needles with respect to post-dural puncture headache and non-dural puncture headache. *Acta Anaesthesiol Scand* 2004;48:474-479.
53. Labas P, Ohradka B, Cambal M, Olejnik J, Fillo J: Haemorrhoidectomy in outpatient practice. *Eur J Surg* 2002;168:619-620.
54. Weinbroum AA, Lalayev G, Yashar T, Ben-Abraham R, Niv D, Flaishon R: Combined pre-incisional oral dextromethorphan and epidural lidocaine for postoperative pain reduction and morphine sparing: A randomised double-blind study on day-surgery patients. *Anaesthesia* 2001;56:616-622.
55. Gilbert A, Owens BD, Mulroy MF: Epidural hematoma after outpatient epidural anesthesia. *Anesth Analg* 2002;94:1:77-78.
56. Pflug AE, Aasheim GM, Foster C: Sequence of return of neurological function and criteria for safe ambulation following subarachnoid block (spinal anaesthetic). *Can Anaesth Soc J* 1978;25:133-139.
57. Klein SM, Nielsen KC, Greengrass RA, Warner DS, Martin A, Steele SM: Ambulatory discharge after long-acting peripheral nerve blockade: 2382 blocks with ropivacaine. *Anesth Analg* 2002;94:65-70.
58. Enneking FK, Chan V, Greger J, Hadzic A, Lang SA, Horlocker TT: Lower-extremity peripheral nerve blockade: Essentials of our current understanding. *Reg Anesth Pain Med* 2005;30:4-35.
59. Klein SM, Grant SA, Greengrass RA, Nielsen KC, Speer KP, White W, et al: Interscalene brachial plexus block with a continuous catheter insertion system and a disposable infusion pump. *Anesth Analg* 2000;91:1473-1478.
60. Ilfeld BM, Morey TE, Wright TW, Chidgey LK, Enneking FK: Continuous interscalene brachial plexus block for postoperative pain control at home: A randomized, double-blinded, placebo-controlled study. *Anesth Analg* 2003;96:1089-1095.

61. Ilfeld BM, Morey TE, Enneking FK: Continuous infraclavicular brachial plexus block for postoperative pain control at home: A randomized, double-blinded, placebo-controlled study. *Anesthesiology* 2002;96:1283-1285.
62. Rawal N, Allvin R, Axelsson K, Hallén J, Ekbäck G, Ohlsson T, Amilon A: Patient-controlled regional analgesia (PCRA) at home: Controlled comparison between bupivacaine and ropivacaine brachial plexus analgesia. *Anesthesiology* 2002;96: 1290-1296.
63. Ilfeld BM, Morey TE, Wang RD, Enneking FK: Continuous popliteal sciatic nerve block for postoperative pain control at home: A randomized, double-blinded, placebo-controlled study. *Anesthesiology* 2002;97:959-965.
64. Klein SM, Greengrass RA, Grant SA, Higgins LD, Nielsen KC, Steele SM: Ambulatory surgery for multi-ligament knee reconstruction with continuous dual catheter peripheral nerve blockade. *Can J Anaesth* 2001;48:375-378.
65. Zaric D, Boysen K, Christiansen J, Haastrup U, Kofoed H, Rawal N: Continuous popliteal sciatic nerve block for outpatient foot surgery—a randomized, controlled trial. *Acta Anaesthesiol Scand* 2004;48:337-341.
66. Chelly JE, Gebhard R, Coupe K, et al: Local anesthetic delivered via a femoral catheter by patient-controlled analgesia pump for pin relief after anterior cruciate ligament outpatient procedure. *Am J Anesthesiol* 2001;28:192-194.
67. Ilfeld BM, Gearen PF, Enneking FK, Berry LF, Spadoni EH, George SZ, Vandenborne K: Total hip arthroplasty as an overnight-stay procedure using an ambulatory continuous psoas compartment nerve block: A prospective feasibility study. *Reg Anesth Pain Med* 2006;3:113-118.
68. Buckenmaier CC 3rd, Klein SM, Nielsen KC, Steele SM: Continuous paravertebral catheter and outpatient infusion for breast surgery. *Anesth Analg* 2003;97:3:715-717.
69. Borgeat A, Ekatodramis G, Kalberer F, Benz C: Acute and nonacute complications associated with interscalene block and shoulder surgery: A prospective study. *Anesthesiology* 2001;95: 875-880.
70. Tuominen MK, Pere P, Rosenberg PH: Unintentional arterial catheterization and bupivacaine toxicity associated with continuous interscalene brachial plexus block. *Anesthesiology* 1991;75:356-358.
71. Cook LB: Unsuspected extradural catheterization in an interscalene block. *Br J Anaesth* 1991;67:473-475.
72. Enneking FK, Ilfeld BM: Major surgery in the ambulatory environment: Continuous catheters and home infusions. *Best Pract Res Clin Anaesthesiol* 2002;16:285-294.
73. Yentis SM, Levine MF, Hartley EJ: Should all children with suspected or confirmed malignant hyperthermia susceptibility be admitted after surgery? A 10-year review. *Anesth Analg* 1992;75:345-350.
74. Pollock N, Langton E, McDonnell N, Tiemessen J, Stowell K: Malignant hyperthermia and day stay surgery. *Anaesth Intensive Care* 2006;34:40-45.
75. Carr AS, Lerman J, Cunliffe M, McLeod ME, Britt BA: Incidence of malignant hyperthermia reactions in 2,214 patients undergoing muscle biopsy. *Can J Anaesth* 1995;42:281-286.
76. Hackl W, Mauritz W, Winkler M, Sporn P, Steinbereithner K: Anaesthesia in malignant hyperthermia-susceptible patients without dantrolene prophylaxis: A report of 30 cases. *Acta Anaesthesiol Scand* 1990;34:534-537.
77. Chung F, Imasogie N, Ho J, Ning X, Prabhu A, Curti B: Frequency and implications of ambulatory surgery without a patient escort. *Can J Anaesth* 2005;52:1022-1026.
78. Friedman Z, Chung F, Wong D: Ambulatory surgery adult patient selection criteria—a survey of Canadian anesthesiologists. *Can J Anesth* 2004;56:481-484.
79. Canadian Anesthesiologists' Society: Guidelines to the practice of anesthesia 2006. The Canadian Anesthesiologists' Society (CAS). Available at www.cas.ca/members/sign_in/guidelines.
80. Association of Anaesthetists of Great Britain and Ireland: *Day surgery—revised edition.* London: Association of Anaesthesiologists of Great Britain and Ireland, 2005, www.aagbi.org.
81. Australia Day Surgery Council: *Day surgery in Australia. Report and recommendations of the Australian Day Surgery Council, of Royal Australasian College of Surgeons, Australian and New Zealand College of Anaesthetists and the Australian Society of Anaesthetists. Revised edition.* Melbourne: Royal Australasian College of Surgeons, 2004, www.surgeons.org.
82. American Society of Anesthesiologists: Practice guidelines for postanesthetic care. A report by the American Society of Anesthesiologists Task Force on postanesthetic care. *Anesthesiology* 2002;96:742-752.
83. Lichtor JL, Alessi R, Lane BS: Sleep tendency as a measure of recovery after drugs used for ambulatory surgery. *Anesthesiology* 2002;96:878-883.
84. Fredman B, Lahav M, Zohar E, Golod M, Paruta I, Jedeikin R: The effect of midazolam premedication on mental and psychomotor recovery in geriatric patients undergoing brief surgical procedures. *Anesth Analg* 1999;89:1161-1166.
85. Grant SA, Murdoch J, Millar K, Kenny GN: Blood propofol concentration and psychomotor effects on driving skills. *Br J Anaesth* 2000;85:396-400.
86. Thapar P, Zacny JP, Choi M, Apfelbaum JL: Objective and subjective impairment from often-used sedative/analgesic combinations in ambulatory surgery, using alcohol as a benchmark. *Anesth Analg* 1995;80:1092-1098.
87. Myles PS, Hung JO, Nightingale CE, et al: Development and psychomotor testing of a quality of life recovery score after general anesthesia and surgery in adults. *Anesth Analg* 1999;88:83-89.
88. Chung F, Kayumov L, Sinclair DR, Moller HJ, Shapiro CM: What is the driving performance of ambulatory surgical patients after general anesthesia? *Anesthesiology* 2005;103:951-956.
89. Pierson JL, Earles DR, Wood K: Brake response time after total knee arthroplasty: When is it safe for patients to drive? *J Arthroplasty* 2003;18:840-843.
90. Correa R, Menezes RB, Wong J, Yogendran S, Jenkins K, Chung F: Compliance with postoperative instructions: A telephone survey of 750 day surgery patients. *Anaesthesia* 2001;56: 481-484.
91. Cheng CJC, Smith I, Watson BJ: A multicentre telephone survey of compliance with postoperative instructions. *Anaesthesia* 2002;57:778-817.
92. American Society of Anesthesiologists: Practice parameters. Available at www.asahq.org/publicationsAndServices/practice-param.htm.
93. Carroll NV, Miederhoff P, Cox FM, Hirsch JD: Postoperative nausea and vomiting after discharge from outpatient surgery centers. *Anesth Analg* 1995;80:5:903-909.
94. Gan TJ, Franiak R, Reeves J: Ondansetron orally disintegrating tablet versus placebo for the prevention of postdischarge nausea and vomiting after ambulatory surgery. *Anesth Analg* 2002;94:5: 1199-2000.
95. Swan BA, Maislin G, Traber KB: Symptom distress and functional status changes during the first seven days after ambulatory surgery. *Anesth Analg* 1998;86:4:739-745.

47 What Must I Consider to Safely Anesthetize Someone in the Office Setting?

Laurence M. Hausman, MD, and Meg A. Rosenblatt, MD

INTRODUCTION

Providing anesthetic care in a surgical office is often a significant component of the responsibilities of an anesthesiologist. It is estimated that 9.2 million cosmetic procedures were performed in plastic surgical offices in 2004.[1] This number does not take into account office-based procedures performed by dermatologists, dentists, general surgeons, gastroenterologists, otolaryngologists, and others. Office-based procedures offer many advantages over the traditional hospital or freestanding ambulatory surgery center–based ones, including cost containment, patient privacy, ease of scheduling, and decreased risk of nosocomial infection.

The lay press often claims that office-based surgery is not as safe as traditional hospital or ambulatory surgery center–based surgery.[2] However, contradictory data do exist.[3-6] A report by Hoefflin and colleagues[4] found no complications after 23,000 procedures that occurred in an office under general anesthesia. Sullivan and Tattini[7] retrospectively reviewed the outcomes of an office performing over 5000 surgical procedures by five independent surgeons, and no deaths occurred over the 5-year period. A retrospective study of adverse outcomes in 3615 consecutive patients undergoing 4778 procedures in offices between 1995 and 2000, employing monitored anesthesia care, reported no deaths.[8] Safety in the office-based setting is contingent on a number of factors, all of which must be ensured before embarking on an anesthetic.

COMPONENTS OF OFFICE SAFETY

Physical Considerations

The physical design of the office (i.e., ensuring adequate space for all operating room functions, consideration for anesthesia equipment, particularly the availability and placement of oxygen lines and venting opportunities, emergency egress for an anesthetized patient, etc.), perioperative monitoring capabilities, office staffing, governance, policies and procedures (including emergency admission planning, fire safety, and infection control), and accreditation status are important components of office safety. Presently, there are several nationally recognized agencies that

can accredit an office-based surgical site. These agencies include the Joint Commission, the American Association for Accreditation of Ambulatory Surgery Facilities, and the Accreditation Association for Ambulatory Health Care. Most states that regulate office-based surgery and anesthesia require that the office be accredited by one of these bodies or that the office be Medicare certified under Title XVIII. Additionally, the American Society of Plastic Surgeons (ASPS) requires that all of its members operate exclusively in an accredited office or forfeit their societal membership. It must be noted though that accreditation is on a cycle, and between site visits, it is imperative that practitioners be constantly vigilant in maintaining a safe anesthetizing location.[9]

Physician Qualifications

The qualifications of the surgeon/proceduralist, as well as the anesthesia provider, must be considered. The physician performing the office-based procedure should be certified by one of the boards recognized by the American Board of Medical Specialties or the American Osteopathic Association. It is also recommended that the surgeon/proceduralist have privileges to perform the proposed procedure at a local hospital. She or he should also have admitting privileges in a nearby hospital for an unplanned emergency admission.

For both the anesthesiologist and proceduralist, active license, registration, and Drug Enforcement Administration (DEA) certificate, as well as adequate malpractice coverage, must be maintained and continued medical education (CME) credit earned. Peer review/performance improvement must occur. Anesthesiologists must be held to these same high standards of certification and continuing education and should participate in peer review/performance improvement in each of their anesthetizing locations.

Patient and Procedure Selection

A determination of the procedures to be performed and appropriateness of individual patients to undergo that procedure in this venue must be clearly defined. Patients with significant comorbidities are not ideal candidates and should be excluded from this type of surgical environment. Specifically, only American Society of Anesthesiologists

(ASA) physical status (PS) 1 and 2 patients should undergo general anesthesia, although occasionally an ASA 3 patient may be acceptable.[10,11]

The patient with the anticipated difficult airway raises a potential problem for the office-based practice. One of the earliest steps in the difficult airway algorithm endorsed by the ASA is to call for help. In the office-based setting, there will, likely, be no other experienced individuals present. It is therefore intuitive that patients with anticipated difficult airways should be avoided in this venue. It would, however, be difficult to design a randomized prospective study to evaluate this issue.

All procedures cannot be safely performed in an office. Procedures that create significant physiologic derangements, including pain or large fluid shifts, are better suited for a hospital or an ambulatory surgery center. When deciding on the appropriateness of a particular procedure consideration must be given to the patient's comorbidities. For example, an obese, asthmatic ASA PS 3 patient may safely undergo a cataract extraction in an office, with local anesthesia, whereas this patient may not be suitable for a rhytidectomy under general anesthesia.

EVIDENCE

The ASA is a strong proponent of patient safety. Consequently, it has become a leader in advocating that all anesthetizing locations meet the same safety standards, and has published recommendations specifically for the office-based anesthesiologist.[10] The ASPS has likewise published guidelines for its members.[11,12] However, the field of office-based surgery and anesthesia is completely unregulated in many states; it thus becomes the joint responsibility of the individual surgeon/proceduralist and anesthesia provider to ensure that patient safety is a priority in each office and to follow all local, state, and society-mandated regulations.

Because the field of office-based anesthesia is primarily conducted outside of academic medical centers and the reporting of adverse outcomes is often voluntary, scientific data in the field of office-based anesthesia and surgery in the literature are sparse.[13] Therefore it is necessary to extrapolate data regarding procedure and patient selection from the specialty of ambulatory anesthesia and apply it to the office-based setting. Much of the available literature regarding office-based anesthesia comes from a retrospective analysis of the experience in Florida.[14,15] Most of these data look at perioperative deaths and what may have been done to prevent these occurrences. Vila and colleagues[16] determined that whereas adverse incidents occurred at a rate of 5.3 per 100,000 procedures in ambulatory surgery centers, it occurred at a rate of 66 per 100,000 in offices. Similarly, the death rate per 100,000 procedures was 0.78 in ambulatory surgery centers and 9.2 in offices.[16]

One certainty in office-based anesthesia is a direct relationship between a patient's preoperative health and the potential to develop a perioperative deep vein thrombosis. Pulmonary embolism has been shown to be a significant cause of death following office-based surgical procedures.[14,15] Reinish and colleagues[17] found that 0.39% (37

Table 47-1	**Risk Factors for the Development of Deep Vein Thrombosis (DVT)**

- Age greater than 40
- Antithrombin III deficiency
- Central nervous system disease
- Family history of DVT
- Heart failure
- History of a DVT
- Hypercoagulable states
- Lupus anticoagulant
- Malignancy
- Obesity
- Oral contraceptive use
- Polycythemia
- Previous miscarriage
- Radiation therapy for pelvic neoplasms
- Severe infection
- Trauma
- Venous insufficiency

of 9493) of patients who underwent rhytidectomy developed a deep vein thrombosis (DVT). Of these, 40.5% (15 of 37) progressed to have a pulmonary embolism. Further, it was noted that although general anesthesia had accounted for only 43% of the anesthetic techniques used for the rhytidectomy, 83.7% of the embolic events were associated with the patient having undergone a general anesthetic.[17] Risk factors for the development of DVT appear in Table 47-1.[18]

When unfavorable outcomes do occur, they are often secondary to inadequate perioperative patient monitoring, oversedation, and thromboembolitic events.[19,20]

GUIDELINES

The ASPS has published a practice advisory dealing with procedure and patient selection for the office-based practitioner.[11,12] It should be noted that although there are few data to support the exclusion of specific procedures or specific patient populations from an office-based surgical procedure, certain basic physiologic principles can be applied to this venue.

Acute blood loss will limit oxygen carrying capacity and may lead to hemodynamic instability. It is therefore recommended that procedures with anticipated blood loss exceeding 500 mL be done only in centers where blood products are readily available.[12]

Hypothermia is associated with marked physiologic impairment, including platelet dysfunction, altered drug metabolism, tissue hypoxia, and increased incidence of postoperative infection. General anesthesia will routinely cause some degree of hypothermia because of redistribution of body heat from the core to the periphery secondary to vasodilation. Additionally, there is direct inhibition of thermoregulation of the hypothalamus by most general anesthetic agents.[21] The ASPS recommends that active patient warming devices such as forced-air warming devices and fluid warmers be used. If these apparatuses are not available, it is recommended that the procedures be less than 2 hours in duration and be limited to 20% of body surface area.[12]

Large-volume liposuction (greater than 5 L of lipoaspirant) is associated with significant derangements of normal physiology.[22] Although the data to exclude specific volumes of aspirant from an office-based procedure are not available, the ASPS limits total aspirant to 5000 mL or less. It also cautions against performing large-volume liposuction when combined with another procedure.[23]

There is debate among clinicians about the suitability of a patient with obstructive sleep apnea syndrome (OSAS) for an ambulatory-based procedure. Recently, the ASA published "Practice Guidelines for the Perioperative Management of Patients with Obstructive Sleep Apnea."[24] The scientific data for the ASA recommendations regarding patient selection are considered insufficient (too few studies to investigate a relationship between intervention and outcome). However, the consultants had recommendations regarding patient and procedure suitability for an ambulatory anesthetic. Most agree that superficial surgery or minor orthopedic procedures under local or regional anesthesia and lithotripsy are acceptable ambulatory procedures. They also believe that airway surgery such as uvulopalatopharyringoplasty, tonsillectomy in patients younger than 3 years, and upper abdominal laparoscopy should not be performed on an outpatient basis. They were equivocal in their opinions about the suitability of superficial surgery under general anesthesia, tonsillectomy in patients older than 3 years, minor orthopedic procedures under general anesthesia, and pelvic laparoscopy. These recommendations were created for ambulatory procedures, and it is intuitive that they, at a minimum, should be adhered to in an office when considering the risks of treating patients with OSAS.

The ASPS recommends that patients be stratified according to risk and the prophylactic treatment be directed by risk (Table 47-2).

Duration of procedure has long been correlated with the need for hospital admission. Originally, procedures lasting more than 1 hour were found to be associated with a higher incidence of unplanned hospital admission.[25] More recent data suggest that procedure duration alone is not predictive of an unplanned admission. Rather, the patient's preexisting comorbidities and the procedure itself are more predictive.[26] It is also important to note that longer procedures are often associated with postoperative nausea and vomiting, postoperative pain, and bleeding.[27,28] These conditions may go on to warrant admission. For these reasons the ASPS has recommended that procedures be limited to 6 hours and be completed by 3 PM. Finishing the procedure by 3 PM will allow a full patient recovery with maximum office staffing.[12]

Table 47-3 Safety "Checklist" for OBA Providers

OFFICE

Accreditation status
Design and layout
   Adequate space for procedure
   Adequate space for recovery
   Safe emergency egress for an anesthetized patient
Policies and procedures manual
   Office governance
   Infection control
   Emergency preparedness
   Narcotic storage and maintenance
   Gas transport and storage
Perioperative monitoring capabilities and defibrillator
   Maintenance and servicing
Oxygen, suction, positive pressure ventilation (anesthesia machine)
"Crash cart"
Emergency/anesthetic drugs and supplies
Staffing

PROCEDURALIST/SURGEON/ANESTHESIA PROVIDER

Active license and registration
Current DEA number
Malpractice
Evidence of proficiency/board certification
Admitting privileges
Current curriculum vitae
CME
Peer review/performance improvement
Admitting privileges
Basic life support/advanced cardiac life support/pediatric advanced life support

PATIENT SELECTION

ASA PS status
Coexisting diseases
Difficult airway
DVT prophylaxis

PROCEDURE SELECTION

Duration
Risk of hypothermia
Risk of blood loss
Postoperative pain
Postoperative nausea and vomiting
Fluid shifts

Table 47-2 Stratification of the Risk for the Development of Thromboembolism

	Cohort	Treatment
Low risk	• No risk factors • Uncomplicated surgery • Short duration	• Comfortable position • Knees flexed at 5 degrees • Avoid constriction and external pressure
Moderate risk	• Age >40 with no other risks • Procedure >30 min • Oral contraceptive use	• Proper positioning • Intermittent pneumatic compression of calf or ankle (before sedation and continued until patient is awake and moving) • Frequent alterations of the operating room table
High risk	• Age >40 with concomitant risk factors • Procedure >30 min	• Treatment as per patients with moderate risk • Preoperative hematology consultation with consideration of perioperative antithrombotic therapy

AREAS OF UNCERTAINTY

Because there are few scientific data to exclude any particular patient from undergoing an office-based anesthetic, there are no hard and fast standards for patient selection. However, the ASA does recommend that the anesthesia provider specifically consider coexisting diseases, previous adverse reaction to anesthesia, current medications and allergies, nothing-by-mouth status, potential difficult airway, substance abuse, and the presence of an escort when considering a patient for an office-based surgical procedure.[10]

AUTHORS' RECOMMENDATIONS

Before undertaking an office-based anesthetic, many considerations must be discussed and agreed on by the anesthesiologist and surgeon/proceduralist, remembering that many of the safeguards inherent in a hospital system will not be present. The "checklist" provided in Table 47-3 should serve as template for the delivery of safe office-based anesthesia.

REFERENCES

1. American Society of Plastic Surgeons: National plastic surgery statistics 2002-2004. Available at www.plasticsurgery.org/public_education/loader.cfm?url=/commonspot/security/getfile.cfm&PageID=16158.
2. Fields H: Health hazards of office-based surgery. *U.S. News and World Report*, 2003. Available at http://health.usnews.com/usnews/health/articles/031006/6surgery.htm. Accessed November 17, 2008.
3. Morello DC, Colon GA, Fredericks S, et al: Patient safety in accredited office surgical facilities. *Plast Reconstr Surg* 1997;99:1496-1500.
4. Hoefflin SM, Bornstein JB, Gordon M: General anesthesia in an office-based plastic surgical facility: A report on more than 23,000 consecutive office-based procedures under general anesthesia with no significant anesthetic complications. *Plast Reconstr Surg* 2001;107:243-251.
5. Balkrishnan R, Hill A, Feldman SR, Graham GF: Efficacy, safety, and cost of office-based surgery: A multidisciplinary perspective. *Dermatol Surg* 2003;29:1-6.
6. Byrd HS, Barton FE, Orenstein HH, et al: Safety and efficacy in an accredited outpatient plastic surgery facility: A review of 5316 consecutive cases. *Plast Reconstr Surg* 2003;112:636-641.
7. Sullivan PK, Tattini CD: Office-based operatory experience: An overview of anesthetic technique, procedures and complications. *Med Health RI* 2001;84:392-394.
8. Bitar G, Mullis W, Jacobs W, et al: Safety and efficacy of office-based surgery with monitored anesthesia care/sedation in 4778 consecutive plastic surgery procedures. *Plast Reconstr Surg* 2003;111:150-156.
9. Rohrich RJ, White PF: Safety of outpatient surgery: Is mandatory accreditation of outpatient surgery centers enough? *Plast Reconstr Surg* 2001;107:189-192.
10. American Society of Anesthesiologists Committee on Ambulatory Surgical Care and the American Society of Anesthesiologists Task Force on Office-Based Anesthesia: Considerations for anesthesiologists in setting up and maintaining a safe office anesthesia environment. Park Ridge, IL: American Society of Anesthesiologists, 2000.
11. Iverson RE, Lynch DJ, ASPS Task Force on Patient Safety in Office-Based Surgery Facilities: Patient safety in office-based surgery facilities: II. Patient selection. *Plast Reconstr Surg* 2002;110:1785-1790.
12. Iverson RE, ASPS Task Force on Patient Safety in Office-based Surgery Facilities: Patient safety in office-based surgery facilities: I. Procedures in the office-based surgery setting. *Plast Reconstr Surg* 2002;1337-1342.
13. Hausman LM, Levine AI, Rosenblatt MA: A survey evaluating the training of anesthesiology residents in office-based anesthesia. *J Clin Anesth* 2006;18:499-503.
14. Coldiron B, Shreve E, Balkrishnan R: Patient injuries from surgical procedures performed in medical offices: Three years of Florida data. *Dermatol Surg* 2004;30:1435-1443.
15. Claymen MA, Seagle BM: Office surgery safety: The myths and truths behind the Florida moratoria—six years of Florida data. *Plast Reconstr Surg* 2006;118:777-785.
16. Vila H, Soto R, Cantor AB, Mackey D: Comparative outcomes analysis of procedures performed in physician offices and ambulatory surgery centers. *Arch Surg* 2003;138:991-995.
17. Reinish JF, Russo RF, Bresnick SD: Deep vein thrombosis and pulmonary embolus following face lift: A study of incidence and prophylaxis. *Plast Surg Forum* 1998;21:159.
18. Davison SP, Venturi ML, Attinger CE, et al: Prevention of venous thromboembolism in the plastic surgery patient. *Plast Reconstr Surg* 2004;114:43e-51e.
19. Clayman MA, Caffee HH: Office surgery safety and the Florida moratoria. *Ann Plast Surg* 2006;56:78-81.
20. McDevitt NB: Deep vein thrombosis prophylaxis. *Plast Reconstr Surg* 1999;104:1923-1928.
21. Sessler DI: Complications and treatment of mild hypothermia. *Anesthesiology* 2001;95:531-543.
22. Iverson RE, Lynch DJ, American Society of Plastic Surgeons Committee on Patient Safety: Practice advisory on liposuction. *Plast Reconstr Surg* 2004;113:1478-1490.
23. Hughes CE 3rd: Reduction of lipoplasty risks and mortality: An ASAPS survey. *Aesth Surg J* 2001;21:120-127.
24. Practice guidelines for the perioperative management of patients with obstructive sleep apnea: A report by the American Society of Anesthesiologists Task Force on Perioperative Management of Patients with Obstructive Sleep Apnea. *Anesthesiology* 2002;104:1081-1093.
25. Mingus ML, Bodian CA, Bradford CN, Eisenkraft JB: Prolonged surgery increases the likelihood of admission of scheduled ambulatory surgery patients. *J Clin Anesth* 1997;9:446-450.
26. Fogarty BJ, Khan K, Ashall G, Leonard AG: Complications of long operations: A prospective study of morbidity associated with long operative time (>6h). *Br J Plast Surg* 1999;52:33-36.
27. Fortier J, Chung F, Su J: Unanticipated admission after ambulatory surgery—a prospective study. *Can J Anaesth* 1997;45:612-619.
28. Gold BS, Kitz DS, Lecky JH, Neuhaus JM: Unanticipated admission to the hospital following ambulatory surgery. *JAMA* 1989;262:3008-3010.

48 Should Propofol Be Given by Nonanesthesia Providers?

McCallum R. Hoyt, MD, MBA, and Beverly K. Philip, MD

INTRODUCTION

Propofol is a sedative-hypnotic that was commercially introduced into U.S. anesthetic practice in 1989.[1] Released under the trade name of Diprivan, it rapidly gained acceptance in the anesthesia community as an induction agent because of its rapid onset of action and other favorable pharmacokinetic properties. Because propofol undergoes a two-phase distribution with the first phase lasting only 4 to 6 minutes, the sedative effects of a single bolus dissipate rapidly.[1] Thus it was soon recognized that the "rapid-on, rapid-off" profile of propofol also made it an ideal agent for sedation either as a continuous infusion or in small boluses.[2,3]

OPTIONS

Even before its commercial release in the United States, specialties outside anesthesiology began to report on the use of propofol for procedures requiring sedation.[4] Opioids and long-acting sedatives such as benzodiazepines were the standard agents for procedures occurring in the radiology and emergency departments, endoscopy suites, and dental offices. But recovery from the prolonged effects of these medications was problematic, and clinically significant side effects such as respiratory depression limited the amounts administered. The rapid redistribution properties of propofol and its minimal effects on most patients' hemodynamic parameters made it appear to be a much safer alternative.

Patients emerge more quickly after propofol administration and appear to be less sedated compared with other barbiturate or benzodiazepine combinations, even though complete elimination from the body can take hours or even days.[1] It also may produce amnesia and has a dose-dependent mood-altering effect that can be euphorogenic.[5] However, studies have shown that mood and psychomotor function as determined by specific tests return to baseline within an hour or less after the medication is stopped in healthy volunteers,[5,6] similar to other modern general anesthetics.[7] Propofol also has an antiemetic effect[1] that further supports its selection in the ambulatory setting.

Unfortunately, the ideal anesthetic agent does not exist, and propofol has its share of undesirable side effects. Most notable is the dose-dependent respiratory depression that can abruptly result in apnea or airway obstruction. This effect ends quickly when administration is stopped,[1] giving a false sense of safety to those providing or directing the sedation. Another commonly encountered effect is the decrease in mean arterial pressure that is similar[8,9] or somewhat more pronounced[6,10] when compared with other sedative-hypnotics. Again, these observed effects end quickly when dosing stops.

EVIDENCE

Investigators in three medical specialties and dentistry have compared propofol with other traditional options and currently recommend propofol as a safe addition to everyday practice, supporting its administration by practitioners who are not anesthesia professionals. In nearly every instance, the studies concluded that propofol has little postprocedural sedation, provides amnesia and comfort to the patient, provides better procedural conditions, and has a better safety profile than traditional medications.

Evaluation of the data on propofol use by nonanesthesia providers is complex because a direct comparison among the different specialties cannot be made. Procedural needs, patient presentation, and defined endpoints are quite different for each specialty. Gastroenterology has developed more invasive procedures, such as esophagogastroduodenoscopy (EGD) and endoscopic retrograde cholangiopancreatography/endoscopic ultrasound (ERCP/EUS), in addition to colonoscopy. The diagnostic and therapeutic value of these three procedures has led to a substantial increase in the numbers performed annually.[11] All are carried out with various levels of sedation and drugs, of which the traditional methods have been to combine a benzodiazepine with an opioid.[12] Gastrointestinal endoscopies vary in duration depending on the skill of the physician and the complexity of the procedure but rarely last longer than an hour. The specialty of radiology has supported the development of pediatric sedation units (PSUs) primarily for radiologic procedures. The sedation teams are led by pediatric intensivists[13] or emergency department physicians.[14] The cases can require hours of sedation.[13,14] Patients are seen in a sedation unit, the sedation plan is made, baseline vital signs are noted, and sedation is initiated. The child is then transported to the required area where the sedation is maintained under monitoring during the procedure. After the procedure, the child is returned to the sedation unit and allowed to recover. In one of the described formats, specially trained pediatric sedation nurses are described as a part of the team and may be the individual who provides the monitoring and sedation to the patient during transport and through the procedure.[13] Propofol is one of several options used. In the specialty of emergency medicine, physicians are often faced with the need for sedation and analgesia to perform short, painful procedures such as dislocation or closed fracture reductions.[15] Patients rarely meet surgical fasting requirements.[16] As with gastroenterology, the traditional methods have been a benzodiazepine or an opioid (or both). Finally, dentistry has long been associated with painful procedures. Although local infiltration or nerve blocks remain the techniques of choice, patients may receive supplemental sedation to accompany the procedure, especially at the time of the nerve block or infiltration.[17] Current studies report sedation being maintained throughout the entire procedure, albeit at a more responsive level.[18]

The American Society of Anesthesiologists (ASA) House of Delegates approved a document in 1999 describing the continuum of depth of sedation.[19] However, the aforementioned specialties had already begun to report on sedation with propofol against other traditional medications, and in so doing, used the definitions for sedation depth to which they were accustomed. This makes comparisons between fields difficult (Table 48-1). Basic monitors such as an electrocardiogram, pulse oximeter, and automated blood pressure cuff are typically used (except in dentistry), but supplemental oxygen and capnography are not standard. Although the use of propofol for sedation in the critical care unit is common, there is often input from the available anesthesiology service and the situation involves ventilated patients under a heightened monitored situation and will not be considered in this chapter.

Gastroenterology

Only one meta-analysis has been published on the use of propofol by nonanesthesia professionals and it is in the endoscopic literature.[23] It reported on 12 randomized controlled trials (RCTs) in which propofol was compared with traditional sedation protocols. In two studies it was not reported who administered the sedation, in two other studies an anesthesiologist did so, and in eight studies sedation was nurse or endoscopist administered. Although the number of studies is small, this meta-analysis is of interest because only 84 of the 1161 patients were documented to have anesthesiologist care involved. The complications reported were hypoxia with oximetry saturations below 90%, hypotension with systolic pressure less than 90 mm Hg, arrhythmias, apnea, and the overall number of complications. As hypoxia and hypotension were the most consistently recorded complications, these were further compared in a pooled odds ratio analysis. Propofol caused less hypoxia and so was favored in 5 out of 12 studies, and traditional methods were favored in 4 out of 12. A similar pooled odds ratio performed for hypotension summarized no difference among the eleven studies reporting that complication. The analysis concluded that propofol had a slightly lower risk profile than traditional methods but that further studies were needed to prove its superiority.

Table 48-1	**Sedation Scales**				
Ramsay Sedation Scale[20]		**ASA Continuum of Depth of Sedation (Responsiveness)**[19]	**Observer's Assessment of Alertness/ Sedation (OAA/S)**[21]		
6	No response	General anesthesia	0	No response to pain
5	Sluggish to light glabellar tap/noise	Deep sedation/ analgesia	1	No response to mild prodding/ shaking
4	Response to light glabellar tap/noise	Moderate sedation/ analgesia	2	Responds to mild prodding/ shaking
			3	Responds to loud noise or repeated name
3	Responds to commands only		4	Lethargic response to name called
2	Cooperative, oriented, calm	Minimal sedation to awake	5	Responds to name, alert
1	Anxious, agitated Restless	Not defined	6*	Anxious, agitated Restless

*The Modified Observer's Assessment of Alertness/Sedation (MOAA/S) includes level 6.[22]

The overall cardiopulmonary complication rate was 14.5% for propofol and 16.9% for traditional methods.

Outside of the studies reported in the meta-analysis, only nine RCTs published within the past decade compared propofol against a traditional sedation protocol and used a nonanesthesia professional to administer the sedation. Unfortunately, two did not report intraprocedural cardiopulmonary changes.[24,25] Of the remaining seven studies (Table 48-2), two were designed to demonstrate the safety of using registered nurses to administer the sedation while under the direction of the endoscopist,[26,27] one compared patient-controlled sedation against nurse-administered sedation (arguing that nurse administration was preferred),[28] and one other argued that the use of another endoscopist to administer the propofol was not cost-effective.[29] Trained nurses were identified as the most cost-effective providers of propofol.[29,30] Endoscopic procedures can be painful, but analgesics were not used with the propofol in five of the seven studies.[26,28,29,31,32] Supplemental oxygen was not given in one study,[29] only 2 L per minute was delivered in four,[27,28,31,32] and hypoxia was the most common complication. However, the incidence of hypoxia was similar with either sedation technique. Only one study compared deep sedation with propofol alone to moderate sedation with propofol in

Table 48-2 Randomized Clinical Trails of Endoscopic Literature

Author (Date)	Study	Responsible for Administration of Medications	Medications	Population (N)	Mean Dose (mg/kg)	Hypoxia <90% (%)	Hypotension <25% (%)	Heart Rate Changes (%)	Study Conclusions
Lee (2002)[27]	Colonoscopy in >65-year-olds	Patient-controlled	Pfl and A	50	0.79 NR	0	4	NR	Total Pfl dose was low and had a faster recovery. Patient satisfaction was high in both.
		Endoscopist-directed registered nurse (RN)	D and Mep	50	5.8 30.1	8	28	NR	
Vargo (2002)[29]	ERCP/EUS	Endoscopist	Pfl	38	4.67 0.12	37	16	0	Cost analysis study. End-expired CO_2 measured. No differences in cardiopulmonary parameters. Pfl had a shorter recovery. Author argued for RN delivery because of expense of second physician.
		Endoscopist	Mid and Mep	37	1.54	57	19	8	
Sipe (2002)[26]	Colonoscopy	RN	Pfl	40	2.61 0.06	0	0	0	Pfl had faster onset, greater sedation (unresponsive to pain vs. response to verbal), and faster recovery. Author claimed within the past decade safety in RN administration
		RN	Mid and Mep	40	1.09	0	5	5	
Heuss (2004)[28]	Colonoscopy	PCS	Pfl	36	1.78	2	23	NR	Similar cardiopulmonary changes regardless of technique, but 35% of patients refused PCS. Author concluded that patient preference makes NAPS the preferred method.
		NAPS	Pfl	40	1.53	2	25	NR	
Riphaus (2005)[31]	ERCP in >80-year-olds	Intensivists	Pfl	75	322 mg mean total	9	4	8	ASA III and IV elderly patients. No statistical difference in clinical parameters except desaturation during recovery was less and recovery faster with Pfl.
		Intensivists	Mid and Mep	75	6.3 mg and 50 mg mean totals	11	5	4	

Study	Procedure	Provider	Agent						Comments
Chen (2005)[32]	ERCP	Intensivists	Pfl	35	NR	6	20	6	43% with Pfl had significant changes in blood pressure vs. 60%. Heart rate and SpO$_2$ changes similar. Recovery time was faster with Pfl.
		Intensivists	Mid and Mep	35	NR	9	0	11	
VanNatta (2006)[33]	Colonoscopy	Endoscopist-directed RN	Pfl	50	215 mg median dose	0	Cannot interpret	Occurred but cannot interpret data as presented	The mean sedation score (MOAA/S) with Pfl was 0.9 but was >3.0 for the three combinations. The Pfl + F group had the lightest mean sedation score and never reached deep sedation. None desaturated below 90%. Shorter recovery times occurred with the mixtures vs. Pfl alone.
		Endoscopist-directed RN	Pfl + F	50	140 mg Pfl median dose F: NR	0	0		
		Endoscopist-directed RN	Pfl + Mid	50	125 mg Pfl median dose Mid: NR	0	0		
		Endoscopist-directed RN	Pfl + Mid + F	50	82.5 mg Pfl median dose F and Mid: NR	0	Cannot interpret		

A, alfentanil; *D*, diazepam; *EGD/US*, endoscopic retrograde cholangiopancreatography/endoscopic ultrasound; *ERCP*, esophagogastroduodenoscopy; *F*, fentanyl; *Mep*, meperidine; *Mid*, midazolam; *NAPS*, nurse-administered propofol sedation; *NR*, not recorded; *PCS*, patient-controlled sedation; *Pfl*, propofol.

combination with four different protocols using opioids and/or benzodiazepines.[33] The authors reported that intraprocedural doses of propofol were less when used with a benzodiazepine, an opioid, or both and that there were no cardiopulmonary complications that required intervention. Also, all patients stayed at or above 93% saturation except in the study group that had deep sedation with propofol as the sole agent. The lowest recorded saturation in this group was 91%. Finally, recovery was faster in the study groups that received combination therapy and were kept to a moderate level of sedation.

Among the 10 prospective, non–evidence-based studies reviewed, several trends were apparent. Within the endoscopy literature, depth of sedation was most often assessed using either the Observer's Assessment of Alertness/Sedation (OAA/S) scale or its modified version (MOAA/S) (see Table 48-1). The ASA sedation continuum scale was not used. The deepest sedation level on the OAA/S scale is 0, defined as no response to painful stimulation. This corresponds to the ASA definition of general anesthesia. In studies where sedation levels were reported, intraprocedural levels were often in the 0 to 2 range of the OAA/S scale,[22,34,35] except when patients controlled their own level of sedation.[36] Hypoxia as measured by the pulse oximeter and typically defined as SpO_2 less than 90% was the most frequent finding, yet some studies did not report the use of supplemental oxygen,[37,38] and the amount of supplemental oxygen used ranged from 1 to 6 L/min.[22,34-36,39] Additionally, only two studies monitored respiratory activity. One did so using a capnograph[38] to look for the presence of a waveform, but in the other, the sedating nurse only felt for a breath on the back of a hand.[37] None of the other studies monitored ventilations or respiratory effort.[22,34-36,39] Yet, compared with more traditional agents, the clinical and recovery profile of propofol was reported as consistently better, and there were no reports of death or significant morbidity. Although its usefulness is generally not supported in the gastroenterology literature, one study evaluated bispectral electroencephalogram analysis (Bispectral Index [BIS]) monitoring.[22] The nurses responsible for sedation were asked to use the BIS monitor as a dosing guide, but in practice this did not alter their behavior. Mean BIS scores remained in the 59 to 64 range whether or not the monitor was available, and the mean MOAA/S scores were less than 2.

A frequently studied and reported-on parameter in both the RCT literature and nonrandomized articles is the use of nurse-administered propofol sedation (NAPS).[22,25,26,28,37] The concept has evolved from that of a nurse solely devoted to the process of sedation and following endoscopist direction to the nurse following a set protocol with less input from the endoscopist.[22,37] Most recently, a published article reported on the success of NAPS for endoscopy where the nurse was no longer devoted to sedation with propofol but was performing the other nursing aspects of the endoscopic procedure as well.[40]

Emergency Medicine

In emergency medicine, five RCTs comparing the use of propofol against traditional techniques for sedation and analgesia have been published since 1999.[15,41-44] Three types of emergency department procedures were used to evaluate medication effectiveness: fracture reductions, dislocation reductions, and cardioversions. The common factors under study were suitability of conditions to do the necessary procedure, recovery time, and any clinically significant complications as defined by the particular study protocol.

One of the RCTs evaluated closed fracture reduction and casting in the pediatric population.[41] Of the 89 randomly assigned patients ranging in age from 2 to 18, 43 received propofol, 46 received midazolam, and all received morphine preprocedurally. No child received supplemental oxygen initially, and hypoxemia was defined as a pulse oximetry reading of less than 93%; 11.6% of those receiving propofol and 10.9% of those receiving midazolam met the criteria for hypoxemia in the study. Agitation was observed more frequently with midazolam (6.5% versus 4.7%, $p = 1.0$) and pain on injection was more frequent with the use of propofol (7.0% versus 4.3%, $p = 0.67$). Oversedation was the most common complication and was defined as a Ramsay score of 6 for two or more consecutive scoring intervals of 5 minutes (see Table 48-1); 32.6% of those receiving propofol and 34.8% of those receiving midazolam met this definition. Although the levels of sedation and oversedation were comparable during the procedures, propofol demonstrated a threefold faster recovery time.

The four other studies evaluated different sedation techniques in the adult population. Coll-Vinent and colleagues[42] looked at sedation for cardioversion and analyzed four different sedative regimens including propofol. Measured parameters were blood pressure, heart rate, respiratory rate, sedation level, oxygen saturation, and recovery. The group sizes were small, being nine for etomidate, nine for propofol, eight for midazolam, and six for midazolam followed by flumazenil. All patients were sedated to a Ramsay score of 5 or 6. Desaturation was defined as SpO_2 less than 90% and occurred in all protocols except when midazolam was used alone. Apnea was defined as a lack of spontaneous respirations for at least 20 seconds. Midazolam without flumazenil had the highest incidence of apnea at 37.5%, although none of the patients met criteria for desaturation. Propofol had the highest percentage of desaturated patients at 44%, but none required management of the airway beyond assisted ventilation for less than 2 minutes. Apnea and desaturation were considered outcome measures and not adverse events. Reported adverse events were myoclonus, bronchospasm, pain at the site of injection, cough, dizziness, and resedation. Among the nine patients receiving etomidate, 11 adverse events were reported. Of the six patients who received midazolam followed by flumazenil administered as a 0.5 mg bolus with another 0.5 mg in an intravenous infusion given over the next hour, five experienced resedation after the infusion was stopped. Propofol had the lowest incidence of adverse events at 11% (one with bronchospasm) and demonstrated the best recovery profile.

Miner (with different groups of colleagues)[15,43,44] performed the remaining three RCT studies using adults undergoing fracture and dislocation reductions. This author supplemented the traditional cardiopulmonary measurements of blood pressure, heart rate, and pulse oximetry recordings with end-tidal carbon dioxide ($ETCO_2$) and BIS.

In his earliest RCT study, he compared propofol against methohexital[43] and found no cardiac rhythm abnormalities or decrease in blood pressure as defined by a 20% drop from baseline. Respiratory depression, defined as either a loss of the capnographic waveform, an SpO_2 less than 90%, or a change from the recorded $ETCO_2$ of more than 10 torr, was 48% with methohexital and 49% with propofol. Of the total number of patients who experienced respiratory depression, 61.5% registered a BIS score of less than 70 at some point during the procedure. By comparison, the other 37.3% who developed respiratory depression remained above 70 at all times. Furthermore, the lowest mean BIS value for methohexital was 66.2 and for propofol it was 65.5. The author concluded that the BIS monitor was not helpful in detecting respiratory depression. The other parameters measured were patient satisfaction, return to baseline mental function, patient pain, and recall. For these parameters, the two drugs were comparable, leading the author to conclude that propofol was as safe as methohexital for sedation in the emergency department. Of note is that this paper defined sedation dosing regimens that have since gained wide acceptance within this specialty.

In 2007, Miner published another study that was similar in design but compared etomidate with propofol.[44] Measured outcome parameters were blood pressure, pulse, respiratory depression, oxygen saturation, BIS scores, MOAA/S scores (see Table 48-1), procedure success, and return to baseline status. The number of patients who met respiratory depression criteria as described in the previous study[43] was 36 of 105 (34.3%) receiving etomidate and 46 of 109 (42.2%) receiving propofol. Among etomidate patients with respiratory depression, 3.8% required bag-valve-mask assistance, 13.3% needed airway repositioning, and 11.4% were stimulated to induce breathing. Among propofol patients the incidences were 4.6%, 11.0%, and 11.9%, respectively. Sedation depth as measured by the BIS monitor and MOAA/S scale was similar. The mean BIS score nadir with etomidate was 63.6 with a range of 25 to 97, and for propofol it was 62.0 with a range of 5 to 94. The lowest MOAA/S was a median score of 1 for both sedation protocols, and no other information was provided. Myoclonus was reported as an adverse event with an incidence of 20% among those receiving etomidate and 1.8% of those receiving propofol. The study concluded that although the use of either medication was a safe option, etomidate produced more myoclonus and was associated with a lower procedural success (89.5% versus 97.2% with propofol).

The third Miner RCT study assessed whether assigning a preprocedural sedation level made a difference in outcome or complications.[15] As was done previously, heart rate, blood pressure, pulse oximetry, $ETCO_2$, and BIS levels were monitored. Patients were assigned to receive deep versus moderate sedation as defined by ASA sedation definitions,[19] and propofol was the only sedative used. The total dose of propofol administered was 1.69 mg/kg in the moderate group and 1.82 mg/kg in the deep group. Of the 75 patients enrolled, 39 were to receive moderate sedation and 36 were to receive deep sedation; 31% of the moderate sedation group reached deeper than intended levels and 46% of the deep sedation group reached only a moderate level of sedation. The mean minimum BIS score was 67.7 in the moderate group and 59.2 in the deep group. Respiratory depression as previously defined[43,44] was 49% in the moderate group and 50% in the deep sedation group. The incidence of hypotension, defined as a greater than 20% drop of the systolic pressure from baseline, was 11.4% in the moderate group and 9.3% in the deep. All other measured parameters were similar, and the authors' conclusion was that a preprocedural target sedation level did not influence outcomes or the occurrence of complications.

Radiology and Pediatric Sedation Units

The first report of a pediatric sedation unit (PSU) that provided services for primarily radiologic procedures and without anesthesia professionals directly involved occurred in 1998.[13] Since then, there have been no randomized controlled trials, but additional reports of primarily a retrospective[13,14] and an observational nature.[45] Most reports used propofol as a component of the sedation regimen along with opioids, benzodiazepines, and ketamine[13,14]; one used only propofol.[45] In all the reports, the physicians involved in drug selection and administration were pediatric intensivists or emergency department physicians. They did not consistently care for the child in transport or during the procedure, and maintenance monitoring was often performed by specially trained nurses who had variable levels of contact with the supervising physician. In two of the reports, the PSUs were established in consultation with the anesthesia department.[13,45] One study in which emergency department physicians were providing the sedation service did not state whether there was anesthesia involvement at any time.[14] Deep levels of sedation were intentionally achieved to prevent movement. One study did not report complications from the sedation medications used but concluded that the practice was safe.[14] Another reported a 4.4% incidence of hypotension, 2.6% incidence of hypoxia, 1.5% incidence of apnea, and 1.3% incidence of airway obstruction.[13] Most treatments for these complications were performed by the sedation nurse present acting under a protocol and with a radio communication device handy.[13] In the study in which propofol was the only medication used, desaturation occurred in 12.7%, and 0.8% required assisted ventilation for a short period.[45] The authors concluded that propofol for sedation in a PSU with rapid availability of anesthesia personnel as needed was safe.

Dentistry

The dentistry literature that reported RCT-style studies focused more on evaluating the effectiveness of different delivery modes for sedation with propofol rather than comparing propofol against other traditional medications. Patients having simple ambulatory surgical procedures such as extraction of third molar teeth comprised the study groups in all four papers, often with each patient serving as his or her own comparison in two separate sessions. In the studies reviewed, the goal was to achieve sedation that was satisfactory to the patient before the administration of the local infiltration or nerve block and then a level of sedation thereafter as determined by the individual controlling the sedation, be it the patient or the practitioner. Only one study compared propofol against another sedative using the same administration technique,[46] and another examined propofol against a different sedative and used different administration techniques as well.[47] The other two compared different modes of delivering propofol and no other sedative was used.[17,18]

When propofol was compared with methohexital[46] or midazolam,[47] propofol was found to have superior recovery and better patient acceptance without an increased complication rate,[47] or there was no difference between the two medications.[46] Parameters measured were heart rate, oxygen saturation, blood pressure, sedation level, patient cooperation, ease of procedure performance, patient satisfaction, and recovery.

The delivery systems evaluated in the two other studies using propofol were a continuous infusion, a patient-controlled bolus technique without an infusion, and a patient-maintained system (PMS). The PMS technique involved using a computerized pump set to infuse at a rate that would maintain a target plasma level of 1.4 mcg/mL. The computer set the rate based on the patient's age and weight. The patient could then increase the infusion to deliver a higher plasma level by pushing a button on a handset. Parameters measured were pulse, respiratory rate, blood pressure, oxygen saturation, sedation, recovery, and patient satisfaction. No cardiopulmonary complications were reported, and recovery times were similar, as were satisfaction rates. Only two patients were considered oversedated, defined as not arousable to mild stimulation, and this occurred with the PMS system only.[18] In another study, all patients who received the continuous infusion of propofol reached a sedation level where they were arousable to command,[17] and no patients in either study who received patient-controlled boluses reached a level of sedation where they were not arousable. In both studies, the patient-controlled groups used less propofol overall and satisfaction remained high.

AREAS OF UNCERTAINTY

It is evident from the literature that propofol use is growing among nonanesthesia professionals. However, areas of controversy revolve around acceptability of outcomes, adequate monitoring, consistent definitions of sedation depth, and whether the individual administering the medications and monitoring the patient has the necessary education and skills to identify developing problems and implement corrections.

The types and quantities of procedures requiring sedation and analgesia are increasing,[11] and there are mounting economic and social pressures for nonanesthesia specialties to provide procedural sedation without an anesthesia professional present.[48-51] Studies in the nonanesthesiology literature demonstrate that propofol, compared with traditional protocols, has a comparably safer recovery profile. Whether with sedation by propofol or by traditional medications, the studies report periods of apnea, hypotension, hypoxia, and the loss of response to stimulation as acceptable intraprocedural conditions. Unfortunately, there are no data showing whether such short-term events are insignificant and without morbidity over the long term, as assumed by the studies' authors.

Anesthesia professionals believe that monitoring the patient is the key to maintaining safety, and intraprocedural variations in cardiopulmonary parameters should be treated. Unfortunately, other specialties differ on which cardiopulmonary parameters are monitored, how changes are defined as significant, and whether they are treated. Although the basic heart rate, blood pressure, and oxygen saturation measurement, as well as simple observation, are commonly employed, other parameters such as adequate ventilation are not routinely assessed. Emergency medicine is one specialty that has actively defined monitoring requirements.[43] Researchers have identified that the routine use of supplemental oxygen may delay recognition of apnea or airway obstruction[50] because not all chest wall movement means air exchange. They advocate the measurement of end-expired CO_2 via nasal cannulae and have defined the parameters that signal the presence of subclinical respiratory depression. Aside from emergency medicine, other nonanesthesia fields do not routinely use more than basic monitoring. Finally, despite hopes that electroencephalographic monitoring such as the BIS would correlate with perceived sedation levels and perhaps reduce oversedation-related adverse events, studies have not shown a correlation.[21,22,43,44] This suggests that the technology as it now exists offers very little, and its use is not recommended by those practitioners.

Another area of concern is the many ways sedation depth is defined. Definitions are loosely similar among the scales used, but the numeric designations may cause confusion when comparing the literature (see Table 48-1). To avoid such confusion, it would be helpful if only one document describing the range of sedation, including the extremes of no sedation and general anesthesia, was universally accepted among the specialties. One-word descriptors such as "minimal," "moderate," or "deep" with an explicit, accepted description of the term would give a more comprehensive understanding of the level of sedation, as opposed to a numeric value. Furthermore, knowledge of the depth at which cardiopulmonary parameters may be affected or protective airway reflexes lost would provide better sedation endpoints and might reduce the incidence of adverse events. Unfortunately, the physician's desire to have an unresponsive patient during a procedure may concur with the patient's desire to be unaware and result in oversedation, even though several studies established that deep sedation is not a necessary endpoint for patient satisfaction or procedural success.[18,24,27,33,36,38,47,52,53]

Who is actually administering the medications and how they decide when and what dose is another area of concern to the professional anesthesia community. Endoscopy has been advocating the use of NAPS for some time as a cost-effective and efficient mode.[22,25-30,33] However, studies show that the depth of sedation achieved can slip beyond deep levels into what is commonly understood to be general anesthesia,[22,34,35] and it is sometimes unclear who is ordering the drug doses and their timing. Although in the United States the nurse involved in NAPS is separate from the nurse assisting with the procedure, in one European report this situation may be changing.[40] Also, patient-controlled computerized infusion systems to provide sedation such as the PMS system described in the dental literature[18,47] are in development. If these are the coming trends, the need for better monitoring standards, better sedation assessments, and education on the adverse effects of propofol and their treatment are underscored.

GUIDELINES

The ASA has published a number of well-defined guidelines on the use of propofol by nonanesthesia professionals. The most relevant here are "Continuum of Depth of Sedation,"[19] "Statement on the Safe Use of Propofol,"[54] and "Practice Guidelines for Sedation and Analgesia by Non-Anesthesiologists."[55] Although these documents have not yet gained universal acceptance outside anesthesiology, and there are competing documents promoted by other specialties,[56,57] the ASA classifications and guidelines are being acknowledged in the more recent nonanesthetic literature.[33,50,58]

AUTHORS' RECOMMENDATIONS

1. It is unlikely that the use of propofol by nonanesthesia professionals will cease. In many ways, propofol may be as safe as or safer than more traditional medications. However, education of nonanesthesia professionals, especially those responsible for the patient's safety, is needed to advance patient safety. Understanding the risks for nonfasted patients and providing the training to achieve only moderate levels of sedation are essential. The ASA provides documents to assist in many aspects of the educational and credentialing process, and these should be at the core of any training program.
2. Monitoring must be standardized and adequate. Given their training, experience, and everyday environment, we recommend that anesthesiologists should be at the forefront to determine protocols, initiate training, perform or oversee competency reviews, and set up the quality assurance programs. All data should undergo periodic review with appropriate responses to sentinel events.
3. All specialties using sedation should agree on a consistent set of definitions of sedation depth. This would help to advance research and develop evidence-based recommendations on patient safety. The ASA has published a document defining the continuum of depth of sedation that describes physiologic changes, as well as responsiveness at different depths, including general anesthesia. We recommend the universal use of such a document as it would open the discussion and comparison of data between fields.
4. Anesthesiologists did not anticipate such ready acceptance of a new anesthetic medication outside of the specialty. However, this is unlikely to be the last time such a scenario occurs. With a growing emphasis on ambulatory procedures and short-acting medications, a similar circumstance may occur again. Ideally, anesthesia professionals will be better prepared to address the use of such potent drugs by nonanesthesia professionals in a more proactive manner. The ASA has started to establish the necessary documentation to address future events.

REFERENCES

1. Smith I, White PF, Nathanson M, Gouldson R: Propofol: An update on its clinical use. *Anesthesiology* 1994;81(4):1005-1043.
2. MacKenzie N, Grant IS: Propofol for intravenous sedation. *Anaesthesia* 1987;42:3-6.
3. Smith I, Monk TG, White PF, Ding Y: Propofol infusion during regional anesthesia: Sedative, amnestic, and anxiolytic properties. *Anesth Analg* 1994;79:313-319.
4. Gepts E, Claeys MA, Camu F, Smekens L: Infusion of propofol ("Diprivan") as sedative technique for colonoscopies. *Postgrad Med J* 1985;61(suppl 3):120-126.
5. Zacny JP, Lichtor JL, Coalson DW, Finn RS, Uitvlugh AM, Glosten B, et al: Subjective and psychomotor effects of subanesthetic doses of propofol in healthy volunteers. *Anesthesiology* 1992;76:696-702.
6. MacKenzie N, Grant IS: Comparison of the new emulsion formulation of propofol with methohexitone and thiopentone for induction of anaesthesia in day cases. *Br J Anaesth* 1985;57:725-731.
7. Tarazi EM, Philip BK: A comparison of recovery after sevoflurane or desflurane in ambulatory anesthesia. *J Clin Anesth* 1998;10:272-277.
8. Rolly G, Versichelen L, Huyghe L, Mungroop H: Effect of speed of injection on induction of anaesthesia using propofol. *Br J Anaesth* 1985;57:743-746.
9. Chan VWS, Chung FF: Propofol infusion for induction and maintenance of anesthesia in elderly patients: Recovery and hemodynamic profiles. *J Clin Anesth* 1996;8:317-323.
10. Wells JKG: Comparison of IC 35868, etomidate and methohexitone for day-case anaesthesia. *Br J Anaesth* 1985;57:732-735.
11. Aisenberg J, Brill JV, Ladabaum U, Cohen LB: Sedation for gastrointestinal endoscopy: New practices, new economics. *Am J Gastroenterol* 2005;100:996-1000.
12. Arrowsmith JB, Gerstmann BB, Fleischer DE, Benjamin SB: Results from the American Society for Gastrointestinal Endoscopy/U.S. Food and Drug Administration collaborative study on complication rates and drug use during gastrointestinal endoscopy. *Gastrointest Endosc* 1991; 37:421-427.
13. Lowrie L, Weiss AH, Lacombe C: The pediatric sedation unit: A mechanism for pediatric sedation. *Pediatrics* 1998;102:e30-e39.
14. Pershad J, Gilmore B: Successful implementation of a radiology sedation service staffed exclusively by pediatric emergency physicians. *Pediatrics* 2006;117:e413-e422.
15. Miner JR, Huber D, Nichols S, Biros M: The effect of the assignment of a pre-sedation target level on procedural sedation using propofol. *J Emerg Med* 2007;32(3):249-255.
16. Green SM. Propofol for emergency department procedural sedation—not yet ready for prime time. *Acad Emerg Med* 1999;6: 975-978.
17. Osborne GA, Rudkin GE, Jarvis DA, Young IG, Barlow J, Leppard PI: Intra-operative patient-controlled sedation and patient attitude to control. *Anaesthesia* 1994;49:287-292.
18. Rodrigo MRC, Irwin MG, Tong CKA, Yan SY: A randomized crossover comparison of patient-controlled sedation and patient-maintained sedation using propofol. *Anaesthesia* 2003;58: 333-338.
19. American Society of Anesthesiologists: Continuum of depth of sedation definition of general anesthesia and levels of sedation/analgesia. Approved by the ASA House of Delegates on October 13, 1999, and amended on October 27, 2004.
20. Ramsay MAE, Savege TM, Simpson BRJ, Goodwin R: Controlled sedation with alphaxalone-alphadolone. *BMJ* 1974;2:656-659.
21. Bower AL, Ripepi A, Dilger J, Boparai N, Brody FJ, Ponsky JL: Bispectral Index monitoring of sedation during endoscopy. *Gastrointest Endosc* 2000;52:192-196.
22. Drake LM, Chen SC, Rex DK: Efficacy of bispectral monitoring as an adjunct to nurse-administered propofol sedation for colonoscopy: A randomized controlled trial. *Am J Gastroenterol* 2006; 101:2003-2007.
23. Qadeer MA, Vargo JJ, Khandwala F, Lopez R, Zuccaro G: Propofol versus traditional sedative agents for gastrointestinal endoscopy: A meta-analysis. *Clin Gastroent Hepatol* 2005;3:1049-1056.
24. Bright E, Roseveare C, Dalgleish D, Kimble J, Elliott J, Shepherd H: Patient-controlled sedation for colonoscopy: A randomized trial comparing patient-controlled administration of propofol and alfentanil with physician-administered midazolam and pethidine. *Endoscopy* 2003;35(8):683-687.
25. Weston BR, Chadalawada V, Chalasani N, Kwo P, Overly CA, Symms M, et al: Nurse-administered propofol versus midazolam

and meperidine for upper endoscopy in cirrhotic patients. *Am J Gastroenterol* 2003;98:2440-2447.

26. Sipe BW, Rex DK, Latinovich D, Oerley C, Kinser K, Bratcher L, Kareken D: Propofol versus midazolam/meperidine for outpatient colonoscopy: Administration by nurses supervised by endoscopists. *Gastrointest Endosc* 2002;55:815-825.

27. Lee DWH, Chan ACW, Sze TS, Ko CW, Poon CM, Chan KC, et al: Patient-controlled sedation versus intravenous sedation for colonoscopy in elderly patients: A prospective randomized controlled trial. *Gastrointest Endosc* 2002;56:629-632.

28. Heuss LT, Drewe J, Schnieper P, Tapparelli CB, Pflimlin E, Beglinger C: Patient-controlled versus nurse-administered sedation with propofol during colonoscopy. A prospective randomized trial. *Am J Gastroenterol* 2004;99:511-518.

29. Vargo JJ, Zuccaro G, Dumont JA, Shermock KM, Morrow JB, Conwell DL, et al: Gastroenterologist-administered propofol versus meperidine and midazolam for advanced upper endoscopy: A prospective, randomized trial. *Gastroenterology* 2002;123:8-16.

30. Vargo JJ: Big NAPS, little NAPS, mixed NAPS, computerized NAPS: What is your flavor of propofol? *Gastrointest Endosc* 2007;66:457-459.

31. Riphaus A, Stergiou N, Wehrmann T : Sedation with propofol for routine ERCP in high-risk octogenarians: A randomized controlled study. *Am J Gastroenterol* 2005;100:1957-1963.

32. Chen WX, Lin HJ, Zhang WF, Gu Q, Zhong XQ, Yu CH, et al: Sedation and safety of propofol for therapeutic endoscopic retrograde cholangiopancreatography. *Hepatobiliary Pancreat Dis Int* 2005;4(3):437-440.

33. VanNatta ME, Rex DK: Propofol alone titrated to deep sedation versus propofol in combination with opioids and/or benzodiazepines and titrated to moderate sedation for colonoscopy. *Am J Gastroenterol* 2006;101:2209-2217.

34. Khoshoo V, Thoppil D, Landry L, Brown S, Ross G: Propofol versus midazolam plus meperidine for sedation during ambulatory esophagogastroduodenoscopy. *J Pediatr Gastroenterol Nutr* 2003;37:146-149.

35. Koshy G, Nair S, Norkus EP, Hertan HI, Pitchumoni CS: Propofol versus midazolam and meperidine for conscious sedation in GI endoscopy. *Am J Gastroenterol* 2000;95:1476-1479.

36. Crepeau T, Poincloux L, Bonny C, Lighetto S, Jaffeux P, Artigue F, et al: Significance of patient-controlled sedation during colonoscopy. *Gastroenterol Clin Biol* 2005;29:1090-1096.

37. Walker JA, McIntyre RD, Schleinitz PF, Jacobson KN, Haulk AA, Adesman P, et al: Nurse-administered propofol sedation without anesthesia specialists in 9152 endoscopic cases in an ambulatory surgery center. *Am J Gastroenterol* 2003;98:1744-1750.

38. Cohen LB, Hightower CD, Wood DA, Miller KM, Aisenberg J: Moderate level sedation during endoscopy: A prospective study using low-dose propofol, meperidine/fentanyl, and midazolam. *Gastrointest Endosc* 2004;58:795-803.

39. Heuss LT, Schnieper P, Drewe J, Pflimlin E, Beglinger C: Safety of propofol for conscious sedation during endoscopic procedures in high-risk patients—a prospective, controlled study. *Am J Gastroenterol* 2003;98:1751-1757.

40. Kulling D, Orlandi M, Inauen W: Propofol sedation during endoscopic procedures: How much staff and monitoring are necessary? *Gastrointest Endosc* 2007;66:443-449.

41. Havel CJ, Strait RT, Hennes H: A clinical trial of propofol vs midazolam for procedural sedation in a pediatric emergency department. *Acad Emerg Med* 1999;6(10):989-997.

42. Coll-Vinent B, Sala X, Fernandez C, Bragulat E, Espinosa G, Miro O, et al: Sedation for cardioversion in the emergency department: Analysis of effectiveness in four protocols. *Ann Emerg Med* 2003;42:767-772.

43. Miner JR, Biros M, Krieg S, Johnson C, Heegaard W, Plummer D: Randomized clinical trial of propofol versus methohexital for procedural sedation during fracture and dislocation reduction in the emergency department. *Acad Emerg Med* 2003;10(9):931-937.

44. Miner JR, Danahy M, Moch A, Biros M: Randomized clinical trial of etomidate versus propofol for procedural sedation in the emergency department. *Ann Emerg Med* 2007;49:15-22.

45. Barbi E, Gerarduzzi T, Marchetti F, Neri E, Verucci E, Bruno I, et al: Deep sedation with propofol by non-anesthesiologists; a prospective pediatric experience. *Arch Pediatr Adolesc Med* 2003;157:1097-1103.

46. Johns FR, Snadler NA, Buckley MJ, Herlich A: Comparison of propofol and methohexital continuous infusion techniques for conscious sedation. *J Oral Maxillofac Surg* 1998;56:1124-1127.

47. Leitch JA, Anderson K, Gambhir S, Millar K, Robb ND, McHugh S, Kenny GNC: A partially blinded randomized controlled trial of patient-maintained propofol sedation and operator-controlled midazolam sedation in third molar extractions. *Anaesthesia* 2004;59:853-860.

48. Rex DK, Heuss LT, Walker JA, Qi R: Trained registered nurse/endoscopy teams can administer propofol safely for endoscopy. *Gastroenterology* 2005;129:1384-1391.

49. Yaster M, Cravero JP: The continuing conundrum of sedation for painful and nonpainful procedures. *J Pediatr* 2004;145:10-12.

50. Green SM: Research advances in procedural sedation and analgesia. *Ann Emerg Med* 2007;49:31-36.

51. Lazzaroni M, Bianchi Porro G: Preparation, premedication, and surveillance. *Endoscopy* 2005;37:101-109.

52. Fanti L, Agostoni M, Casati A, Guslandi M, Giollo P, Torri G, Testoni PA: Target-controlled propofol infusion during monitored anesthesia in patients undergoing ERCP. *Gastrointest Endosc* 2004;60:361-366.

53. Campbell L, Imrie G, Doherty P, Porteous C, Millar K, Kenny GNC, Fletcher G: Patient maintained sedation for colonoscopy using a target controlled infusion of propofol. *Anaesthesia* 2004;59:127-132.

54. American Society of Anesthesiologists: Statement on the safe use of propofol. Approved by the ASA House of Delegates on October 27, 2004.

55. ASA Task Force on Sedation and Analgesia by Non-Anesthesiologists: Practice guidelines for sedation and analgesia by non-anesthesiologists. *Anesthesiology* 2002;96:1004-1017.

56. Frank LR, Strote J, Hauff SR, Bigelow SK, Fay K: Propofol by infusion protocol for ED procedural sedation. *Am J Emerg Med* 2006;24:599-602.

57. Training guideline for use of propofol in gastrointestinal endoscopy. *Gastrointest Endosc* 2004;60:167-171.

58. Bailey PL, Zuccaro G: Sedation for endoscopic procedures: Not as simple as it seems. *Am J Gastroenterol* 2006;101:2008-2010.

49 Aspiration: Is There an Optimal Management Strategy?

Neal H. Cohen, MD, MPH, MS

INTRODUCTION

Aspiration is a known risk of anesthesia and surgery. When rendered unconscious, patients lose their normal airway protective reflexes. Other situations also increase the risk of aspiration during anesthesia and surgery. For example, the patient with known gastroesophageal reflux disease is at high risk for aspiration and its consequences, particularly in the perioperative period. Supine positioning increases the risk of regurgitation and subsequent aspiration. Aspiration can have significant physiologic and economic costs for the patient; there are also significant professional liability issues associated with aspiration. At the same time, aspiration is presumed to be avoidable with proper management strategies. Anesthesiologists therefore go to great lengths to identify patients at risk for aspiration, to reduce the risk, and to treat the complication when it is identified. A number of approaches are used to reduce the risk of aspiration and to treat it, although the evidence to support most therapies is limited.

To clarify the current state of knowledge regarding the risks, complications, and treatment for aspiration during anesthesia care, this chapter will review the available data regarding the diagnosis of aspiration, discuss its clinical significance, and address some of the controversial areas surrounding management of aspiration based on currently available data.

THERAPEUTIC OPTIONS

Minimizing the Risk

The key to reducing the complications associated with aspiration is to minimize the likelihood that it will occur at all. Even when aspiration is witnessed, the risk of complications associated with it varies considerably. As a result, the incidence of aspiration may be underestimated and its relationship to the patient's postoperative course underappreciated.[1]

A number of approaches have been recommended to reduce both the risk of aspiration and the physiologic consequences of aspiration should it occur. The primary method for reducing the risk of aspiration is to ensure that the patient has an empty stomach before induction of anesthesia, particularly for elective surgical procedures. Fasting is the recommended approach to reducing the quantity of gastric contents. Although there are no clear-cut data to define the exact duration of fasting that is required, a number of recommendations have been proposed related to the duration of fasting and the type of foods that should be avoided. Based on a review of the current guidelines and the data to support them, practice guidelines have been developed to define the most appropriate duration of fasting for adults and children based on the current state of knowledge. The guidelines suggest a minimum fasting period of 2 hours after ingesting clear liquids. Adult patients should fast for at least 6 hours after a light meal. Children taking breast milk should fast for 4 hours and those taking infant formulas should fast for 4 hours before elective surgical procedures for which anesthesia will be provided.[2,3]

To reduce the volume and acidity of gastric secretions, a number of pharmacologic agents have been recommended. Although many clinicians routinely recommend the use of a gastrointestinal stimulant, gastric acid secretion blockers, and antacids, there are few data to support their routine use. In general the routine use of any of these agents is not recommended except in patients with a high likelihood of delayed gastric emptying, such as an obese or diabetic patient.[4] For selected patients at high risk for aspiration, when antacids are used, they should be restricted to nonparticulate antacids. The routine use of other agents, such as antiemetics or anticholinergics, has not been demonstrated to reduce the risk of pulmonary aspiration, although they may be of value in selected patients at high risk for aspiration or in patients with known gastroesophageal reflux, including some elderly patients.[5,6]

Another strategy that is used to reduce regurgitation and possible aspiration is cricoid pressure. It is generally employed as part of the "rapid-sequence induction technique" to reduce the likelihood of regurgitation and aspiration (or at least minimize the quantity of aspirate),[7,8] thereby reducing the magnitude of sequelae even when silent aspiration does occur. Although commonly used, there are few objective data to support its value, perhaps because it is difficult to confirm proper application.[9]

Management Strategies

The primary treatment for aspiration is supportive. Supplemental oxygen should be provided to ensure adequate oxygenation. Routine bronchopulmonary hygiene and other supportive measures are the only additional approaches that have been demonstrated to be effective.[10] There are no data that support the empiric initiation of other therapies immediately after a witnessed or suspected aspiration.

In the event that an aspiration event is witnessed, the removal of debris from the oropharynx should be performed using a Yankauer suction catheter. If the patient continues to regurgitate or actively vomit, she or he should be placed in the head-down position on the side to prevent further aspiration into the airway. Placement of a nasogastric tube may be required to remove additional gastric contents and prevent ongoing aspiration. Bronchodilator therapy with beta-agonists is indicated, if bronchospasm is triggered by the aspiration. The bronchodilatory therapy will not only improve the wheezing, but might also improve mucociliary function and facilitate clearance of secretions in the postoperative period.

For some patients with large-volume aspiration or known to have aspirated particulate material or material with a low pH, additional interventions may be required. Bronchoalveolar lavage is not indicated, because it can cause the aspirate to move more distally into the smaller airways, rather than facilitate clearance of the aspirate.[10] Lavage does not reduce the likelihood of pneumonitis. Bronchoscopy can be used to facilitate removal of particulate aspirate, particularly if a foreign body is identified in the larger airways. Fluid resuscitation and vasopressors may be indicated if a systemic inflammatory process ensues.

For most patients who aspirate, antibiotic therapy is not required and may simply increase the risk of antibiotic-resistant infection. In general, antibiotics should be administered based on documented clinical infection with positive sputum Gram stain, positive cultures, or a focal-persistent infiltrate associated with fever and elevated white count. Later in the patient's postoperative course, if an infiltrate persists or the sputum culture becomes positive, antibiotic coverage directed toward the offending organism should be initiated. In selected clinical situations early administration of antibiotics may be appropriate. For example, if a patient has known bowel obstruction or the aspirated material is feculent, antibiotic therapy that provides adequate gram-negative bacterial coverage should be initiated.

EVIDENCE

Every anesthesiologist is concerned about aspiration in the perioperative period, although there are remarkably few data to support management strategies to reduce the risk of aspiration or treat it once it occurs. Although the risk of aspiration and its consequences, as well as clinical management strategies, have been evaluated in a wide variety of studies, there is little evidence to support our understanding of the risk factors, the actual incidence of aspiration, or the most effective ways to deal with it. Despite this lack of a large body of evidence to support clinical practice, some general principles have been defined and their use justified based on reasonably sound data.

Incidence of Clinically Significant Aspiration

Although aspiration is of concern to every anesthesiologist, the incidence of aspiration in patients receiving anesthesia is difficult to define. It has been found to occur in 1 per 2000 to 3000 adult patients undergoing elective surgery and 1 per 1200 to 2600 anesthetics in children. During emergency procedures, the incidence may be three to four times higher than it is during elective procedures.[9,11,12] One of the difficulties in evaluating information obtained from published studies of the risk of aspiration is that the diagnosis is difficult to make and the frequency varies considerably by patient population and approaches to airway management. In some cases the aspiration may be silent and unrecognized. In addition, most patients who aspirate demonstrate no evidence of complications from the aspiration. Even those patients who have a witnessed aspiration often have minimal, if any, sequelae. As a result the diagnosis may be missed because it is based primarily on the complications that result from the aspiration, rather than observation of aspiration itself.[1]

The incidence of aspiration reported in the literature is influenced by the method used to define aspiration. The clinical manifestations vary considerably, particularly based on the material aspirated. The patient who loses the normal cough reflex during induction of anesthesia may aspirate small amounts of oral secretions with no obvious clinical manifestations and no clinical consequence. On the other hand, the patient who regurgitates gastric contents, such as a recently completed large meal, and aspirates the material into the lung, may have significant clinical manifestations, including laryngospasm, bronchospasm, gas trapping, gas exchange abnormalities (both acute and extended), pneumonitis, pneumonia, or pulmonary abscess formation.

Differentiating Aspiration Pneumonitis from Aspiration Pneumonia

Because of the overlapping clinical findings, the differentiation of pneumonitis and pneumonia is challenging for every clinician. The definitive diagnosis of aspiration pneumonitis or pneumonia is difficult to confirm because there are no obvious markers. In general, the diagnosis is made based on the clinical presentation and clinical signs and symptoms. Aspiration pneumonitis often gives rise to an infiltrate, but it is usually fleeting, lasting only a few hours. In general it clears without therapy. On the other hand, the aspirate that is acidic can cause a chemical pneumonitis resulting in the exudation of fluid into the lung parenchyma. The risk of a chemical pneumonitis is greatest if the pH of the aspirate is less than 2.5 or if the quantity of aspirate is large or particulate.[13-15] If blood is aspirated, there may be an infiltrate immediately after the aspiration, but it usually clears rapidly with minimal consequences.

The greatest concern in the patient who aspirates is the risk of pneumonia. Although the clinical features of pneumonitis and pneumonia overlap, if the patient has persistent fevers that cannot be attributed to a wound infection or other surgical cause or develops other clinical evidence of infection or sepsis, a pulmonary infection must be considered. An elevated white blood cell count, purulent sputum, and worsening clinical status are most likely associated with pneumonia after aspiration rather than inflammation (pneumonitis) alone.[14]

Risk Factors for Aspiration

The largest body of evidence related to the diagnosis and management of aspiration has concentrated on identification of patients at increased risk, particularly in the setting of anesthesia and surgery. Unfortunately, these studies do not rigidly or consistently define pulmonary aspiration, making the estimation of risk and analysis of the natural history of aspiration difficult.

Despite the difficulty in identifying specific risk factors, a number of factors have been associated with an increased likelihood of aspiration. Trauma patients and any patient with impaired gastric emptying are at risk for aspiration when rendered unconscious. Many trauma patients have recently eaten, so their stomachs may be full; pain and discomfort will also delay gastric emptying. In addition, the trauma patient may have altered level of consciousness due to the injury, compromising the ability to protect the airway before tracheal intubation. The same is true for the patient experiencing severe pain and those who have recently received narcotic analgesics that reduce gastric emptying. Other patients at risk for aspiration include those with preexisting airway abnormalities, the patient with esophageal disease, motility disorders, and altered gastroesophageal sphincter tone.[5,6,13] The obese patient and the pregnant patient are also at increased risk for aspiration because of delayed gastric emptying and, in some cases, the lower pH of gastric contents.

In addition to the increased risk of aspiration in selected patient populations, the likelihood of developing aspiration pneumonitis also varies by patient population. The primary problem for the clinician is to understand which patients are vulnerable to the more serious sequelae of aspiration, such as pneumonitis and pneumonia, versus those who aspirate without physiologic consequences. For instance, aspiration pneumonitis is a well-known complication after drug overdose, seizure, and cerebrovascular accident, as well as associated with general anesthesia. Aspiration has long been considered as the most common cause of death for patients suffering from dysphagia and compromised cough reflex, as may occur in patients with neurologic disease. It has been estimated that 5% to 15% of community-acquired pneumonia is secondary to aspiration.[14] This complication is probably most common in elderly patients who reside in nursing homes.

In a study evaluating the significance of pulmonary aspiration during the perioperative period, pulmonary aspiration was defined based on the presence of bilious secretions or particulate matter in the tracheobronchial tree, or the presence of new pulmonary infiltrates on postoperative chest x-ray in patients without any clinical findings on preoperative examination.[12] Clearly, this definition may mistakenly include patients with postoperative pulmonary edema or patients with preexisting pneumonia that went undetected.

Some general conditions are associated with increased risk of aspiration. They include higher American Society of Anesthesiologists (ASA) physical status and patients undergoing emergency procedures. Many other conditions thought to be associated with aspiration were *not* found to be independent risk factors by these authors. Some of those include age, gender, obesity, ingestion of a meal within 3 hours, experience and type of anesthesia provider, and type of surgical procedure. And it is interesting that no pulmonary aspiration was detected in those patients undergoing cesarean sections under general anesthesia. The most common predisposing conditions associated with aspiration for patients undergoing elective procedures are gastrointestinal obstruction, lack of coordination of swallowing,[14] depressed level of consciousness,[14] and recent meal.[15]

Data from both animal and human studies suggest that a primary determinant in the development of aspiration pneumonitis is the pH of the aspirate. A pH of less than 2.5 in the aspirate is necessary to cause clinically significant aspiration pneumonitis.[15] The volume of aspirate also contributes to the likelihood of pneumonitis. A number of studies indicate that the critical volume is 25 mL, or 0.4 mL/kg, for causing pneumonitis.[16] Particulate antacids may increase the gastric pH, but may cause pulmonary problems due to the particulate matter if aspirated. Nonparticulate antacids, on the other hand, which are often administered to reduce the pH of the gastric contents, may contribute to the risk of pneumonitis, because they increase residual gastric volume.

The combined impact of the pH and volume on the risk of aspiration pneumonitis is not clearly defined. In at least one study evaluating the volume and pH implications, 80% of rats survived aspiration of volumes exceeding 2.0 mL/kg as long as the pH was greater than 2.5.[17] Other studies support this conclusion, suggesting that the administration of a nonparticulate antacid is appropriate for the patient at increased risk for aspiration in spite of its effect on intragastric volume.

Anesthetic Induction Strategies in Patients at Risk

For those patients at risk for aspiration, including those with a full stomach or delayed gastric emptying (e.g., the diabetic patient, the obese patient), the airway must be secured with extreme caution. Although the data on its value are limited, it is probably prudent to administer a nonparticulate antacid before induction of anesthesia. Cricoid pressure should be applied when the patient's normal protective reflexes are compromised or the patient is suspected of having a full stomach. These patients should also be placed in the head-up position, if clinically feasible, although positioning will be dictated by the overall clinical needs of the patient.

The specific airway to be used for the patient at risk for aspiration is not known. Although a cuffed endotracheal tube should be used for most patients at risk for aspiration, the presence of a cuff alone may not protect the patient from aspiration of fluids around the cuff, particularly if the patient has increased gastric pressure or volume of secretions and is in the supine position. Nonetheless, the cuffed endotracheal tube will protect against aspiration of larger particulate matter. There are now some case reports suggesting that endotracheal tubes with low-volume, low-pressure cuffs may reduce the risk of aspiration.[18] ProSeal laryngeal mask airways have also been shown to protect adult and pediatric patients from large-volume aspiration, although there are no studies that confirm that these airways are as effective as cuffed endotracheal tubes at reducing the risk of aspiration.[19-21]

Documentation of Aspiration

Aspiration of clear liquids of high pH and limited quantity is generally tolerated with minimal sequelae. However, it is difficult to predict whether an individual patient will develop clinically significant pneumonitis, pneumonia, or acute respiratory distress syndrome (ARDS) after aspiration. The underlying clinical condition of the patient, the physiologic status of the patient at the time of the aspiration, and other factors will influence the subsequent course. To ensure that the patient is being appropriately managed, if aspiration is suspected, the patient should be observed in a monitored setting for several hours after the aspiration. A chest x-ray should be obtained and reviewed for evidence of aspiration or pulmonary infiltrate.

TREATMENT

Antibiotics and steroids should not be given empirically to the patient. Antibiotics, however, should be given only if the patient's episode was associated with a high likelihood of gram-negative or anaerobic organisms, such as in the setting of known small bowel obstruction. Furthermore, if the patient's course continues to worsen or shows no sign of improvement after 2 to 3 days, broad-spectrum antibiotics are indicated at least until a positive diagnosis is established by culture and sensitivity studies. There are no data to support the administration of steroids in the setting of aspiration. Recent studies in animal models suggest that alveolar macrophages play an essential role in the inflammatory response to the aspiration, particularly in cases of acid-induced lung injury. In this situation, the administration of an agent that depleted macrophages was highly effective at reducing neutrophil recruitment and vascular permeability in the lung.[22] Whether this therapy has application in the treatment of aspiration in the human is unknown.

Sequelae of Aspiration Associated with Anesthesia

Most cases of aspiration resolve without specific treatment. However, in some specific situations aspiration can result in a number of clinically significant abnormalities. Aspiration can precipitate pneumonitis, give rise to pneumonia, or result in ARDS. Not only can aspiration lead to these serious sequelae, but it may also severely compromise oxygenation in the periprocedure period. Any aspirate in the upper airway, including particulate materials, can cause acute laryngospasm or bronchospasm. With supportive care, these consequences are generally easily managed. If the particulate material enters the smaller airways, however, the patient can develop either aspiration pneumonitis or aspiration pneumonia. The same sequelae can result from aspiration of feculent material or acidic aspirate. Aspiration of gastric contents high in fat can result in severe lipid pneumonia. Aspiration pneumonitis is an inflammatory response in the airways. It was initially described in obstetric patients by Mendelson and is often referred to as Mendelson's syndrome. Mendelson's syndrome occurs when gastric contents chemically injure the bronchopulmonary tree. In contrast to aspiration pneumonitis, aspiration pneumonia is an infectious process caused by the introduction and proliferation of bacteria in the lungs. Distinguishing these two diagnoses continues to be a clinical challenge, but it is important because the differentiation has both prognostic and therapeutic ramifications.

In addition to developing pneumonia after aspiration, patients are also at risk for pulmonary abscesses, most commonly in the setting of aspiration of anaerobic organisms. The patients at greatest risk for this complication are those with a depressed level of consciousness, swallowing dysfunction, or impaired cough and patients with a history of drug abuse. In these patients a cavity may be noted on chest x-ray. When a lung abscess is identified, antibiotics may or may not be effective. The patient may also require a surgical or interventional radiologic procedure to drain the abscess.

CONTROVERSIES

Antibiotic Therapy

The initiation of empiric antibiotic therapy after aspiration is discouraged, although many clinicians find it difficult to resist starting broad-spectrum antibiotics in the patient who has aspirated while under their care. In general, antibiotics should be administered cautiously and only when there is clinical evidence to confirm infection or the patient's underlying condition is deteriorating in spite of intensive supportive care. Most studies that have attempted to evaluate the optimal use of and timing for administration of antibiotics suggest that the initiation of antibiotics should only be considered when there have been persistent symptoms for about 3 days.[23] At that time, it becomes important to consider the clinical scenario, so that the proper antibacterial coverage is chosen. Patients who have been in the hospital for several days will be at increased risk for gram-negative pneumonia or, if already receiving antibiotics, antibiotic-resistant pneumonia, whereas most other patients are more likely at risk for anaerobic organisms found in healthy patients' oral flora.

Antibiotic therapy should be based on the results of blood and respiratory cultures and pleural fluid cultures when emphysema or abscess is suspected. If these results are unavailable or fail to isolate a specific species, a broad-spectrum agent should be chosen pending results of subsequent cultures.

There is one clinical situation in which early administration of antibiotics may be required. For the patient who aspirates feculent gastric contents, particularly in the setting of small bowel obstruction, the risk of pulmonary infection is high. These patients may benefit from immediate administration of broad-spectrum antibiotics to prevent the development of serious necrotizing pneumonia. If antibiotics are initiated in this situation, serial sputum cultures (mini-bronchoalveolar lavage) and sensitivities should be obtained and antibiotics adjusted based on the results of the studies.

Steroids

Although corticosteroids have often been administered in the setting of aspiration, there is no strong evidence that there is any benefit. Two studies from the early 1980s failed to show in animal models a benefit from corticosteroid therapy, particularly with regard to lung injury, pulmonary function, interstitial edema, and clinical outcome.[24,25] In a double-blind, placebo-controlled clinical trial, lung injury was found to resolve at a faster rate, as determined by chest radiograph, in patients who received corticosteroids.[26] Despite a more rapid resolution of infiltrates, no difference was noted in clinical outcome. Given the lack of convincing data to support the use of corticosteroids in the setting of aspiration, they do not have a role in the management of patients who have aspirated.

Bronchoscopy and Bronchoalveolar Lavage

The use of bronchoscopy or lavage after aspiration is limited.[10] For patients known to have aspirated a foreign body, such as a tooth, denture, or gum, bronchoscopy may be the only way to remove the foreign body. In most other situations, simple saline lavage and suctioning is sufficient. Selective segmental lavage is not indicated because the irrigation may force aspirated materials into smaller airways that are more difficult for the patient to mobilize. Because normal mucociliary clearance and cough are superior to selective suctioning, whenever possible, the patient's trachea should be extubated as soon as clinically appropriate to encourage normal bronchopulmonary hygiene. Only when the patient does not have a forceful cough or has a persistently depressed neurologic status is deep suctioning required.

GUIDELINES

Aspiration is a known complication of anesthesia and surgery. For most patients clinical management should be directed toward reducing the risk of aspiration. The risk reduction strategies include minimizing loss of airway-protective reflexes whenever possible, reducing the quantity and raising the pH of the gastric contents, and providing supplemental protective approaches such as cricoid pressure during airway manipulations. For patients at high risk for aspiration, the administration of nonparticulate antacids may be appropriate (obese patients, parturient). For patients with known delayed gastric emptying, such as a diabetic patient, preoperative administration of a gastric stimulant (e.g., metoclopramide) may be indicated.

When a patient has a witnessed aspiration or the clinical course is suggestive of aspiration, a thorough clinical examination and chest x-ray should be obtained. The patient should remain in a monitored setting until clinically stable without evidence of gas exchange or other physiologic complications. Based on the findings of the evaluation, further management strategies can be determined. If the patient

has wheezing or other evidence of increased airway resistance, bronchodilators should be administered. If the patient develops a pulmonary infiltrate, serial chest x-rays may be required for ongoing evaluation.

Routine administration of antibiotics or steroids should be avoided in the patient who aspirates. Care should be supportive, including administration of supplemental oxygen and monitoring of gas exchange and hemodynamics. Fluids should be administered to maintain normal intravascular volume. If the patient had known bowel obstruction or the aspirate was feculent, early administration of appropriate antibiotics may be required, although the antibiotic regimen should be guided by serial sputum cultures. Routine administration of antibiotics after aspiration is not indicated and may put the patient at risk for antibiotic-resistant infections. Steroid administration is not indicated.

AUTHOR'S RECOMMENDATIONS

- Minimize the risk of aspiration:
  - Elective patients should have nothing by mouth for at least 2 hours (clear liquids) or 6 hours (light meal) before initiation of anesthesia.
  - Administer nonparticulate antacid solution to high-risk patients.
  - Apply cricoid pressure and avoid positive pressure ventilation, whenever possible, during emergency airway management ("crash induction"), although neither approach has been documented to reduce the risk of aspiration.
- Diagnosing aspiration:
  - Obtain serial chest x-rays based on clinical course.
  - Obtain sputum for culture and sensitivity to diagnose pneumonia.
- Treating aspiration:
  - Therapy is supportive.
  - Provide supplemental oxygen.
  - Provide fluids to optimize intravascular volume.
  - Provide routine bronchopulmonary hygiene.
  - Routine antibiotics are not appropriate; treat known infections based on clinical evidence of pneumonia, cultures.
  - Avoid steroids.

REFERENCES

1. Shigemitsu H, Afshar K: Aspiration pneumonias: Under-diagnosed and under-treated. *Curr Opin Pulm Med* 2007;13: 192-198.
2. Practice guidelines for preoperative fasting and the use of pharmacologic agents to reduce the risk of pulmonary aspiration: Application to healthy patients undergoing elective procedures: A report by the American Society of Anesthesiologists Task Force on Preoperative Fasting. *Anesthesiology* 1999;90:896-905.
3. Soreide E, Ljungqvist O: Modern preoperative fasting guidelines: A summary of the present recommendations and remaining questions. *Best Pract Res Clin Anaesthesiol* 2006;20:483-491.
4. Tokumine J, Sugahara K, Fuchigami T, Teruya K, Nitta K, Satou K: Unanticipated full stomach at anesthesia induction in a type I diabetic patient with asymptomatic gastroparesis. *J Anesth* 2005;19:247-248.
5. Kikawada M, Iwamoto T, Takasaki M: Aspiration and infection in the elderly: Epidemiology, diagnosis and management. *Drugs Aging* 2005;22:115-130.
6. Ng A, Smith G: Gastroesophageal reflux and aspiration of gastric contents in anesthetic practice. *Anesth Analg* 2001;93:494-513.

7. Bell HE: Antacids and cricoid pressure in the prevention of fatal aspiration syndrome. *Lancet* 1979;2:354.
8. Lawes EG, Campbell I, Mercer D: Inflation pressure, gastric insufflation and rapid sequence induction. *Br J Anaesth* 1987;59: 315-318.
9. Janda M, Scheeren TW, Noldge-Schomburg GF: Management of pulmonary aspiration. *Best Pract Res Clin Anaesthesiol* 2006;20: 409-427.
10. Moore FA: Treatment of aspiration in intensive care unit patients. *J Parent Enteral Nutr* 2002;6:S569-574.
11. Olsson GL, Hallen B, Hambraeus-Jonzon K: Aspiration during anaesthesia: A computer-aided study of 185,358 anaesthetics. *Acta Anaesthesiol Scand* 1986;30:84-92.
12. Warner MA, Warner ME, Weber JG: Clinical significance of pulmonary aspiration during the perioperative period. *Anesthesiology* 1993;78:56-62.
13. Smith G, Ng A: Gastric reflux and pulmonary aspiration in anaesthesia. *Minerva Anestesiol* 2003;69:402-406.
14. Marik PE: Aspiration pneumonitis and aspiration pneumonia. *N Engl J Med* 2001;344:665-671.
15. Vandam LD: Aspiration of gastric contents in the operative period. *N Engl J Med* 1965;273:1206-1208.
16. Roberts RB, Shirley MA: Reducing the risk of acid aspiration during cesarean section. *Anesth Analg* 1974;53:859-868.
17. James CF, Modell JH, Gibbs CP, Kuck EJ, Ruiz BC: Pulmonary aspiration—effects of volume and pH in the rat. *Anesth Analg* 1984;63:665-668.
18. Young PJ, Pakeerathan S, Blunt MC, Subramanya S: A low-volume, low-pressure tracheal tube cuff reduces pulmonary aspiration. *Crit Care Med* 2006;34:900-902.
19. Evans NR, Llewellyn RL, Gardner SV, James MF: Aspiration prevented by the ProSeal laryngeal mask airway: A case report. *Can J Anaesth* 2002;49:413-416.
20. Wheeler M: ProSeal laryngeal mask airway in 120 pediatric surgical patients: A prospective evaluation of characteristics and performance. *Paediatr Anaesth* 2006;16:297-301.
21. Goldmann K, Jakob C: Prevention of aspiration under general anesthesia by use of the size 2 ProSeal laryngeal mask airway in a 6-year-old boy: A case report. *Paediatr Anaesth* 2005;886-889.
22. Beck-Schimmer B, Rosenberger DS, Neff SB, Jamnicki M, Suter D, Fuhrer T, et al: Pulmonary aspiration: New therapeutic approaches in the experimental model. *Anesthesiology* 2005;103: 556-566.
23. Marik PE, Brown WJ: A comparison of bronchoscopic vs blind protected specimen brush sampling in patients with suspected ventilator-associated pneumonia. *Chest* 1995;108:203-207.
24. Lowrey LD, Anderson M, Calhoun J, Edmonds H, Flint LM: Failure of corticosteroid therapy for experimental acid aspiration. *J Surg Res* 1982;32:168-172.
25. Wynne JW, DeMarco FJ, Hood CI: Physiological effects of corticosteroids in foodstuff aspiration. *Arch Surg* 1981;116:46-49.
26. Sukumaran M, Granada MJ, Berger HW, Lee M, Reilly TA: Evaluation of corticosteroid treatment in aspiration of gastric contents: A controlled clinical trial. *Mt Sinai J Med* 1980;47: 335–340.

REGIONAL ANESTHESIA

50 Nonsteroidal Antiinflammatory Drugs, Antiplatelet Medications, and Spinal Axis Anesthesia

Lynn M. Broadman, MD, and Edmund H. Jooste, MBChB

INTRODUCTION

Many individuals use cyclooxygenase-1 and cyclooxygenase-2 inhibitors (COX-1 and COX-2 nonsteroidal antiinflammatory drugs [NSAIDs]) on a regular basis. This is particularly true of the elderly, who are more prone to having osteoarthritis and rheumatoid diseases. The elderly are also more likely to have had cardiac stent placements or coronary angioplasties performed, and may be taking antiplatelet medications such as the thienopyridines (ticlopidine and clopidogrel) or the newer platelet antagonists, platelet glycoprotein (GP) IIb/IIIa agents (such as abciximab, eptifibatide, and tirofiban). All these agents alter platelet function and may increase the risk of spinal/epidural hematoma formation, if spinal axis anesthesia is used without following proper precautions. All anesthesiologists should be familiar with these agents and how they work. More important, they should be familiar with the established guidelines set forth by the American Society of Regional Anesthesia (ASRA),[1] the German Society of Anesthesiology and Intensive Care Medicine (DGAI),[2] and the Spanish Consensus Forum.[3] These guidelines will help one decide when these agents should be stopped before surgery/anesthesia and when it is safe to remove spinal/epidural catheters in order to provide all patients with the widest possible margin of safety.

OPTIONS

It would appear that we have come full circle in the use of aspirin (ASA) as the primary chemoprophylactic agent for the prevention of pulmonary embolism (PE) following hip pinning, total hip replacement surgery, and total knee replacement surgery. The material presented at the Third ASRA Consensus Conference (Vancouver, British Columbia, Canada, in April 2007) would suggest that there is a growing body of literature that shows that deep venous thrombosis (DVT) is not an accurate marker for the risk of embolic disease following total joint surgery, as the incidence of PE has not declined proportionally with the decrease in the incidence of DVT that results from the current use of the low-molecular-weight heparin (LMWH) regimens.[4] Furthermore, when LMWH is used as the primary DVT prophylactic agent, there is an increased risk that patients may develop a deep periprosthetic hematoma[4,5] or other surgical bleeding.[6] Should one's patient develop a deep periprosthetic hematoma there is a substantial risk that the patient will develop a prosthetic infection and need additional surgery. More important, the patient might require an amputation of the involved extremity. On the other hand, the use of ASA in conjunction with pneumatic compression devices allows one to provide epidural analgesia in the postoperative period. This in turn allows patients to ambulate with minimal discomfort in the immediate postoperative period and actively participate in physical therapy.[4,5] As a result of the aforementioned protocol the incidence of PE is the same as that seen with LMWH therapy following total joint arthroplasty.[4,5] In addition, an exhaustive literature survey and meta-analysis on spinal hematoma formations done by Kreppel and colleagues[7] showed that only 10% of all spinal hematomas were associated with the use of a spinal anesthetic procedure and that 60% of these epidural hematoma formations were either associated with the presence of a coagulopathy or an anticoagulant had been administered to the patient. More important, none of these hematoma formations occurred in the presence of ASA or NSAID therapy alone.[7] It would therefore appear that there is no increased risk of spinal hematoma formation with the timing of single shot or catheter techniques in relation to the dosing of NSAIDs or ASA. But what is the evidence that aspirin chemoprophylaxis reduces the risks of thromboembolic disease to an acceptable level following joint replacement surgery? A recent prospective study by Lotke and Lonner[4] used ASA chemoprophylaxis, early ambulation, an increased use of regional anesthesia and intermittent pneumatic compression to prevent fatal PE in 3473 consecutive patients undergoing a total knee arthroplasty. Again, the authors used a reduction in the incidence of fatal PE, not DVT, to determine the effectiveness of their study protocol and compared their results against those of multiple other studies in which more conventional chemoprophylactic agents, such as warfarin, fondaparinux, or LMWH, were used following total knee arthroplasty. The study period ran for a minimum of 6 weeks following each joint replacement. Lotke and Lonner[4] had a total of nine deaths during their study: two from PE, five from cardiac events, one from stroke, one from fat embolism, and three cardiac-related events for which PE could not be ruled out as the primary cause of death. Therefore the best- and worst-case scenarios for PE were 0.06% and 0.14%, respectively. Thirteen patients required reoperation to evacuate a deep wound hematoma (0.4%). The results of this study compare quite favorably with regard to the incidence of fatal PE when compared with multiple studies in which more conventional chemoprophylactic agents were used to prevent PE in patients having a total knee replacement. However, the incidence of fatal PE was found to be about 0.1% in the other studies, irrespective of the chemoprophylactic used. Finally, the incidence of adverse postoperative bleeding events in the Lotke and Lonner[4] study was only 0.3%. This incidence is substantially lower than the rate of 2% to 5% reported in the literature with the more conventional chemoprophylactic regimens.

EVIDENCE

Cyclooxygenase-1 Nonsteroidal Antiinflammatory Drugs (COX-1 and NSAIDs)

Aspirin causes inhibition of platelet function through inhibition of platelet cyclooxygenase, an enzyme that is instrumental in the biosynthesis of thromboxane A_2 from arachidonic acid. Thromboxane A_2 is necessary for the formation of thromboxane, a prostaglandin that is a potent stimulator of platelet aggregation and adhesion.[8] Because the reaction between aspirin and platelet membrane cyclooxygenase is irreversible, inhibition of platelet function lasts for the life of the platelet (7 to 10 days).

The remaining COX-1 NSAIDs such as naproxyn, ketorolac, diclofenac, piroxicam, ibuprofen, and others also act as prostaglandin synthesis inhibitors. All of them cause reversible competitive platelet inhibition, and platelet function usually returns to normal within 1 to 3 days after stopping the drug.[9]

Horlocker and colleagues[10-12] and Urmey and Rowlingson[9] all believe that there is a minimal risk of spinal hematoma formation when preoperative antiplatelet therapy has been administered with either aspirin or another COX-1 NSAID. All these authorities believe that it is *not* necessary to stop these agents before surgery or to avoid spinal or epidural anesthesia in patients who have been using these medications in the preoperative period.

They also believe that it is safe to remove epidural catheters from patients who have been administered aspirin or NSAIDs in the postoperative period.

Tryba[13] published an extensive review on spinal hematoma associated with regional anesthesia. Thirteen cases of hematoma were identified from the review of approximately 850,000 epidural anesthetics. Seven cases of spinal hematoma were identified from 650,000 spinal anesthetics. Statistical analysis of these data resulted in an estimated incidence of spinal hematoma of 1:150,000 with epidural anesthesia and 1:220,000 spinal blocks. These estimates represent the baseline risk of spinal hematoma formation with neuraxial anesthesia in the absence of antiplatelet agents.

Horlocker and colleagues[11] retrospectively reviewed 805 charts of patients who were receiving NSAIDs and who also were administered a spinal axis anesthetic. None of the patients developed a spinal hematoma in the postoperative period. In a more recent prospective study, Horlocker and colleagues[12] studied 924 patients who received 1000 spinal or epidural anesthetics. Three hundred eighty-six (39%) of these patients were either taking aspirin ($n = 193$) or another COX-1 NSAID ($n = 293$) in the preoperative period. Blood was noted during needle or catheter placement (minor hemorrhagic complications) in 223 of patients (22%), including 73 who had frank blood in either their needle or catheter. None of the patients developed a spinal hematoma in the postoperative period. The authors concluded that preoperative antiplatelet therapy was not a significant risk factor for the development of neurologic dysfunction from spinal hematoma in patients who undergo spinal or epidural anesthesia while receiving these medications.[12]

In another study by Horlocker and colleagues,[10] which involved 1035 patients who received 1214 epidural steroid injections, 383 of the 1035 patients (32%) were concurrently taking an NSAID. More specifically, 158 of these 383 patients were consuming ASA and 104 of the 158 were using low-dose aspirin (325 mg/day or less). The authors conclude that epidural steroid injection is safe in patients receiving either ASA or NSAIDs. Table 50-1 shows the combined results of the three Horlocker studies.[10-12]

Vandermeulen and colleagues,[14] in their review of the literature from 1906 to 1993, were able to find only three cases in which an NSAID was implicated in the formation of a postspinal/postepidural hematoma. One of the cases

Date of Study	Type of Study	Number of Epidurals/ Spinals	Number Taking NSAIDs	Number Taking Aspirin	Results
1990	Retrospective	924	301	N/A	No hematoma formations
1995	Prospective	1000	386	193	No hematoma formations
2002	Prospective	1214	383	158	No hematoma formations

Table 50-1 Horlocker Studies*

*Presents the results of three studies by Horlocker and colleagues[10-12] that demonstrate that there were no epidural hematoma formations in 3138 patients who received either a spinal or an epidural needle placement and who were also receiving aspirin therapy or another NSAID.

involved indomethacin; in the two other cases aspirin was implicated. One of these later two cases also involved the concurrent use of heparin. Two of the patients had epidural anesthesia and the third had a spinal anesthetic. The authors conclude that the incidence of spinal hematoma after the placement of either spinal or epidural blockade in patients taking aspirin or other NSAIDs is very low. However, Vandermeulen is also an author on the German Society of Anesthesiology and Intensive Care Medicine consensus statement that suggests that there is a risk of hematoma when aspirin and NSAIDs are not stopped several days before the placement of a spinal or an epidural block.[2]

The evidence that there is a risk of hematoma formation if aspirin and other COX-1 NSAIDs are not stopped several days before the placement of spinal or epidural blockade is quite sparse and is limited to single-incident case reports. A report by Litz and colleagues[15] implicates the perioperative administration of ibuprofen as the offending agent that led to the formation of a spinal-epidural hematoma following epidural catheter removal on the second postoperative day in a patient who had undergone a total knee replacement. However, the patient was also receiving LMWH.

The most alarming report is by Gerancher and colleagues.[16] Their patient was not anticoagulated and only received a single dose of ketorolac during surgery (30 mg intravenously [IV]) and then three doses in the postoperative period (15 mg intramuscularly [IM] every 6 hours). The patient's lumbar hematoma developed during the afternoon of the first postoperative day and its presence was confirmed by a magnetic resonance imaging [MRI] study. Even more alarming was the fact that it occurred as the result of a lumbar puncture with a small-gauge spinal needle. She had required three needle passes in order to place her block. The first two were performed with a 27-gauge Quincke needle and bone was encountered each time. The final pass was undertaken with a 25-gauge Quincke needle. No blood was aspirated or detected during any of the needle placements. Fortunately, the woman made a full recovery from her paraparesis without surgical decompression. Moreover, the concurrent use of ketorolac and LMWH has been implicated in three reports of spinal/epidural hematoma formations in conjunction with an axis anesthesia.[9] Two of these hematomas occurred immediately after the removal of an epidural catheter; therefore Litz and colleagues[15] warn that epidural catheter removal may be just as risky as catheter placement in regard to epidural hematoma formation in patients receiving anticoagulation or antiplatelet therapy.

A 1995 case report by Heye[17] presents a patient who was taking ASA 250 mg/day and who developed an epidural hematoma following spinal trauma. It was suggested by Heye[17] that while ASA did not cause the bleed, it did have a major impact on the extent of the epidural bleed. Finally, a more recent case report by Hyderally[18] describes a patient with ankylosing spondylitis who was undergoing total hip replacement and who was started on ASA for postoperative thromboprophylaxis. This patient subsequently developed a thoracic epidural hematoma 36 hours postoperatively. More important, this thoracic-level epidural hematoma extended from T-5 to T-10, which was quite distant from the lumbar epidural

catheter tip, which was confirmed by an MRI study to lie at L-2/L-3. Hyderally[18] concluded that the hematoma was not caused by the lumbar epidural catheter placement, but that it occurred spontaneously, possibly as the result of concurrent ASA therapy and the patient's primary disease of ankylosing spondylitis.

Areas of Uncertainty about Continuing COX-1 NSAIDs before the Placement of an Axis Anesthetic

Although Urmey and Rowlingson[9] believe that there is a minimal risk of spinal hematoma formation when preoperative antiplatelet therapy has been administered with either aspirin or another COX-1 NSAID, they question the conclusions reached by the Horlocker study[12] because it was their belief that the study lacked adequate statistical power to conclude that there was no increased risk of spinal/epidural hematoma formation in patients taking a COX-1 NSAID. This may be particularly true for aspirin administration before the placement of an axis anesthetic.[9] They point out that while no hematomas were detected in the study, fewer than 500 patients received both a spinal axis anesthetic and either aspirin or a COX-1 NSAID. Using Tryba's estimated incidence of spinal hematoma formation of 1:150,000 to 1:220,000,[13] one would need a study involving almost 200,000 patients to achieve adequate power, and then there would only be an 80% probability of detecting a tenfold increase in the frequency of hematoma formations in patients receiving both a neuraxial block and antiplatelet therapy.[9] Moreover, none of the patients in the Horlocker study[12] had received either the thienopyridines (ticlopidine and clopidogrel) or the newer platelet antagonists, platelet GP IIb/IIIa agents such as abciximab, eptifibatide, and tirofiban, in the preoperative period. Finally, the most recent Horlocker study[10] probably also lacks the statistical power to reach the conclusion that epidural steroid injections are probably safe in patients receiving aspirin and other COX-1 NSAIDs. Horlocker and colleagues[10] acknowledge that the rarity of spinal hematoma makes it impossible to make definitive conclusions on the safety of epidural steroid injection in patients who are also receiving NSAID therapy.

Another area of controversy is the use of bleeding time for determining if it is safe to place a spinal or an epidural anesthetic in a patient who has been taking ASA in the preoperative period. Hindman and Koka[19] do not believe that bleeding time is a reliable indicator of platelet function. Although the bleeding time may quickly normalize after aspirin ingestion, platelet function as measured by platelet response to adenosine diphosphate (ADP) or epinephrine may take up to a week to return to normal. Measurement of Ivy bleeding time before the placement of a spinal or an epidural anesthetic is not indicated and is of little value.[12]

Cyclooxygenase-2 Nonsteroidal Antiinflammatory Drugs (COX-2 NSAIDs)

The cyclooxygenase-2 specific inhibitors (COX-2 NSAIDs) are essentially devoid of platelet-altering activity. The COX-2 inhibitor valdecoxib (Bextra) is 28,000-fold more selective against COX-2 than COX-1.[20] In early clinical trials valdecoxib did not affect platelet function.[21] The same is true for the older COX-2 agents celecoxib (Celebrex)[22] and rofecoxib (Vioxx).[23] However, the aforementioned information is now a moot point because celecoxib is the only remaining COX-2 inhibitor on the market today in North America.

Antiplatelet Drugs

Thienopyridines (Ticlopidine and Clopidogrel) Inhibit Platelet Function

Ticlopidine (Ticlid) is a long-lasting inhibitor of both primary and secondary phases of platelet aggregation induced by ADP, collagen, thrombin, arachidonic acid, prostaglandin endoperoxidase, and thromboxane A_2–like substances.[24,25] Ticlopidine's effect on platelet function is irreversible, and the drug's action lasts for the lifetime of the platelet.[26] However, prolonged bleeding time is normalized within 2 hours following the intravenous administration of methylprednisolone (20 mg) or the transfusion of platelets.[26] The drug is indicated for reducing the risk of thrombotic events in patients who have experienced stroke precursors and who are also intolerant to aspirin.[26]

Clopidogrel (Plavix) irreversibly inhibits platelet aggregation by selectively binding to adenylate cyclase–coupled ADP receptors on the platelet surface.[27] Furthermore, by blocking the ADP receptor clopidogrel inhibits the binding of fibrinogen to the glycoprotein GP IIb/IIIa receptor.[27] Clopidogrel has almost completely replaced ticlopidine because it has a wider therapeutic index, has a reduced side-effect profile, and is more efficacious than ticlopidine at accepted clinical dosing parameters.

Ticlopidine prolongs template bleeding time.[26] It also displays nonlinear pharmacokinetics and its clearance decreases markedly with repeated dosing. The half-life after a single 250 mg oral dose is 12.6 hours, but with repeated dosing at 250 mg bid the elimination half-life rises to 4 to 5 days.[26]

Ticlopidine has been implicated as the medication that caused a spinal hematoma in a 70-year-old woman who was having her toe amputated.[28] Ticlopidine was administered for 10 days before surgery, but it was stopped just before the surgery. She had several unsuccessful attempts at placing a spinal block with a 23-gauge needle in the lumbar region, and she ultimately received a general anesthetic. On the sixth postoperative day the patient developed muscle weakness in both legs. On postoperative day 8 she received a cervical myelogram that showed an extramedullary block below the level of T-10. She underwent an emergency laminectomy and a hematoma was evacuated from the subarachnoid space. The clot extended from T-10 to L-5. She remained paralyzed following the laminectomy and expired the next day. This is the only case report that implicates ticlopidine as the offending agent in a patient who developed a spinal hematoma following spinal axis blockade.[28]

The elimination half-life of orally administered clopidogrel is only 7.7 hours following a single 75 mg dose,[27] but the irreversible platelet inhibition persists for several days after withdrawal of the drug and diminishes in proportion to platelet renewal.[29] Clopidogrel is 40 to 100 times more potent than ticlopidine,[30] and bleeding times

are significantly prolonged at 1 hour following the administration of a single oral loading dose of 375 mg.[27]

Clopidogrel was implicated as one of the agents that may have led to the development of a cervical epidural hematoma in a patient who had received a cervical epidural steroid injection.[31] He was taking several antiplatelet medications just before block placement (diclofenac, clopidogrel, and aspirin). Quadriparesis developed 30 minutes after the performance of a cervical epidural steroid injection, and he did not regain lower extremity function after his C-3/T-3 hematoma was surgically evacuated. There is no case report in the literature that implicates clopidogrel alone as the causative agent in the production of a post–neuraxial block spinal hematoma. The aforementioned epidural case report[31] highlights the fact that the effects of clopidogrel plus aspirin are additive and they may even be synergistic depending on the method one uses to ascertain platelet function. This may explain why cardiac surgical patients who have received this drug combination appear to have excessive bleeding[32-34] and why it would seem prudent to refrain from placing neuraxial blocks on patients who have received this drug combination without waiting the 7-day drug-free period of time suggested by the ASRA guidelines.[1]

Platelet Glycoprotein IIb/IIIa Antagonists

The identification of the platelet glycoprotein IIb/IIIa receptor, a fibrinogen receptor important for platelet aggregation, has led to the development of platelet receptor antagonists.[35] Activated glycoprotein IIb/IIIa receptors become receptive to fibrinogen, and when fibrinogen binds to the glycoprotein IIb/IIIa receptors located on two different platelets it builds the cross-links for platelet-to-platelet aggregation.[36] The glycoprotein IIb/IIIa also mediates platelet adhesion and spreading.[35]

Abciximab is a monoclonal antibody that binds nonspecifically to the glycoprotein IIb/IIIa receptor.[35] The binding of abciximab to the platelet IIb/IIIa receptor is a rapid high-affinity interaction, and all the receptors are blocked within 15 minutes following the parenteral administration of a bolus dose of 0.25 mg. The biologic half-life of abciximab is approximately 12 to 24 hours, but 24 hours after administration 50% to 60% of the platelet receptors are still blocked.[37] Abciximab can be detected on circulating platelets for more than 15 days, indicating platelet-to-platelet transfer.[35] Abciximab cannot be effectively reversed with the transfusion of platelets because the new platelets are inactivated by the free-circulating monoclonal antibody or platelet-to-platelet transfer of the drug. Platelet function recovers over the course of 48 hours due to platelet turnover.[35] Abciximab prolongs activated clotting time (ACT) by 30 to 80 seconds, and the activated partial thromboplastin time (aPTT) is also prolonged.[35] Comparative studies have shown that abciximab is superior to the other agents in preventing ischemic complications following percutaneous coronary interventions.[38] However, its potent inhibition of platelets also renders it likely to cause increased episodes of major bleeding.[39]

Eptifibatide is a small cyclic heptapetide.[35] The drug sits in the binding pocket between the IIb and IIIa arms of glycoprotein IIb/IIIa and prevents the binding of fibrinogen and thrombus formation.[40] Eptifibatide has a plasma half-life of 2.5 hours, with a rapid onset of action and a rapid reversibility of platelet inhibition.[35] Four hours after the termination of an eptifibatide infusion platelet aggregation recovers to approximately 70% of normal and there is normal hemostasis.[41] The majority of the drug is eliminated by renal clearance.[35] Eptifibatide prolongs ACT by 40 to 50 seconds, but it has no effect on prothrombin time (PT) or aPTT.[35]

Tirofiban is a tyrosine derivative.[35] Tirofiban occupies the binding pocket on the glycoprotein IIb/IIIa receptor and competitively inhibits platelet aggregation mediated by fibrinogen and von Willebrand factor.[41] It is given via an intravenous infusion and the plasma half-life is approximately 1.5 to 2.5 hours.[35] Greater than 70% of tirofiban is cleared by biliary elimination.[35] The remainder is eliminated by renal excretion and the drug may be removed by hemodialysis.[35] The ACT is prolonged by 40 to 50 seconds.[41]

There are no known case reports of a spinal/epidural hematoma forming as the result of spinal axis blockade being performed in a patient who was simultaneously being treated with a glycoprotein IIb/IIIa antagonist. However, two studies show that patients who were using glycoprotein IIb/IIIa medications and required emergency cardiac surgery were at increased risk of having major bleeding compared with patients having elective surgery.[42,43] Eleven consecutive patients who were taking abciximab and required emergency cardiac surgery after failed angioplasty or stent placement were randomized into two groups.[43] Group-1 patients ($n = 6$) had taken the last dose of abciximab 12 or less hours before surgery, and group-2 patients ($n = 5$) had taken it more than 12 hours before their surgery. Group-1 patients required 20 packs of platelets to control bleeding, whereas group-2 patients did not require any platelets ($p < 0.02$). Group-1 patients also required more packed erythrocyte transfusions (6 versus 0, $p < 0.02$). The results of the Gammie study[43] are outlined in Table 50-2.

Table 50-2	**Abciximab and Emergency Cardiac Surgery***		
$p < 0.02$, Group 1 vs. Group 2	**N**	**Number Packs Platelets**	**Number Packs Packed Cells**
Group 1: Last dose abciximab <12 hours before surgery	6	20	6
Group 2: Last dose abciximab >12 hours before surgery	5	0	0

*Results from a study by Gammie and colleagues[43] showing it is imperative that one attempt to delay emergent surgery for at least 12 hours following the administration of abciximab. The Gammie study does not attempt to ascertain the safety of placing a spinal or an epidural block in a patient who has received abciximab.

GUIDELINES FOR PERFORMING A SPINAL AXIS ANESTHETIC IN PATIENTS WHO ARE RECEIVING ASPIRIN OR A COX-1 NSAID

The American Society of Regional Anesthesiology and Pain Medicine (ASRA) provides the following guidelines for the anesthetic management of patients who are receiving aspirin or a COX-1 NSAID and in whom a spinal axis block is planned.[1]

The ASRA Guidelines[1]

1. NSAIDs appear to represent no added significant risk for the development of spinal hematoma in patients having epidural or spinal anesthesia. The use of NSAIDs alone does not create a level of risk that will interfere with the performance of neuraxial blocks.
2. At this time, there do not seem to be specific concerns as to the timing of single-shot or catheter techniques in relationship to the dosing of NSAIDs, postoperative monitoring, or the timing of neuraxial catheter removal.

The guidelines promulgated by both the German Society of Anesthesiology and Intensive Care Medicine and the Spanish Consensus Forum are quite different.[2,3] Both of these societies believe that there is a risk of hematoma formation when these agents are used in the perioperative period and they mandate a free interval of 1 to 2 days after the last administration of COX-1 NSAIDs and at least a 3-day interval without aspirin or aspirin-containing medications before neuraxial blocks are performed or epidural catheters are removed.[2,3]

The European Society of Regional Anesthesia (ESRA) is in the process of developing a set of guidelines for the performance of neuraxial anesthesia in patients who are receiving aspirin or another COX-1 NSAID. The ESRA guidelines will likely replace the older German Society of Anesthesiology and Intensive Care Medicine and the Spanish Consensus Forum guidelines.

The Spanish guidelines are quite rigid and they are the ones that express an emphasized concern about the long-term antiplatelet effects of aspirin.[3] These guidelines provide the following information about aspirin and other NSAIDs: acetylsalicylic acid is the best-studied NSAID and its antiaggregation effect is by COX-1 inhibition. This platelet inhibition is irreversible and its action lasts the entire life of the platelet (7 to 10 days), although by the third to fourth day there are sufficient new platelets to ensure adequate hemostasis.[3] Other NSAIDs such as meloxicam, sulindac, and nabumetone have a prolonged half-life; however, due to their mild or limited antiplatelet effect they can be continued up to 12 hours before the procedure.

The Spanish Consensus Forum Guidelines[3]

1. Regional anesthesia should be avoided in patients on multiple antiplatelet drugs.
2. Rule out the presence of any drug-related coagulopathy. Neuraxial anesthesia is not recommended when

there is a platelet count below 50,000 or when there is platelet dysfunction.

3. *Elective surgery should be delayed* if the patient is taking a potent NSAID. In such cases one should switch the patient to a different class of NSAID with a more moderate or mild antiplatelet effect (these more moderate platelet-inhibiting medications are not named in the guidelines but are construed to mean ibuprofen, naproxyn, or a COX-2 agent) several days before surgery.

One of the authors on the German Society of Anesthesiology and Intensive Care Medicine guideline project is Vandermeulen. In his extensive review of the literature on the effects of anticoagulants on the risk of spinal-epidural hematoma formation,[14] he suggests that aspirin or NSAID therapy should be restarted only after epidural (or subarachnoidal) catheter removal. Furthermore, the bleeding time may give some supplemental information if aspirin or nonaspirin NSAIDs have been taken in the days (aspirin, 7 to 8 days; nonaspirin NSAID, 1 to 3 days) before surgery.[14] This position is reflected in the German Society of Anesthesiology and Intensive Care Medicine guidelines.[2] Hindman and Koka[19] do not believe that bleeding time is a reliable indicator of platelet function, and Horlocker and colleagues[12] do not believe that there is any indication for the measurement of Ivy bleeding time before the placement of a spinal or an epidural anesthetic.

The German Society of Anesthesiology and Intensive Care Medicine Guidelines[2]

1. An interval of at least 3 days without the ingestion of aspirin-containing medications must be maintained before central neuraxial blocks should be performed or epidural catheters should be removed.
2. An interval of 1 to 2 days should be maintained after the administration of all other NSAIDs.

Readers will need to decide for themselves which guidelines, ASRA[1] or those of the German Society of Anesthesiology and Intensive Care Medicine,[2] they wish to follow and which information from the literature they may want to use to help guide their assessment of the risks involved in placing a spinal or an epidural block in a patient who is simultaneously receiving or who has only recently stopped receiving (the night before surgery) aspirin or a COX-1 NSAID. However, it must be pointed out that there is little evidence to support the conclusions and guidelines that have been reached by the two aforementioned societies.[2,3]

However, the concerns raised by both the German Society of Anesthesiology and Intensive Care Medicine[2] and the Spanish Consensus Forum[3] should heighten one's awareness that there may be potential risks associated with the concurrent administration of aspirin and other NSAIDs in patients who are about to receive a neuraxial block or who will have an epidural/spinal catheter removed. Unfortunately, the exact nature of these risks is unknown at this time. These concerns are also indirectly reflected by the ASRA Consensus Panel experts.[1,9] These experts are not concerned about the risks of spinal/epidural hematoma formation when aspirin is used before the placement of a spinal axis anesthetic.

Finally, a complete patient history and physical examination may be the most useful tools in guiding one's

decision regarding the risk/benefit ratio for the placement of a neuraxial block in a patient who has not curtailed aspirin or other NSAID therapy before surgery. The identification of alterations in health that might contribute to bleeding is crucial. These conditions include a history of easy bruisability/excessive bleeding, female gender, and increased age.[1]

GUIDELINES FOR PERFORMING A SPINAL AXIS ANESTHETIC IN PATIENTS WHO ARE RECEIVING A COX-2 NSAID

The American Society of Regional Anesthesia and Pain Medicine is the only group that provides guidelines for the anesthetic management of patients who are receiving a COX-2 NSAID.[1]

The ASRA Guidelines[1]

1. Cyclooxygenase-2 inhibitors have minimal effect on platelet function and should be considered in patients who require antiinflammatory therapy in the presence of antithrombotic therapy.

GUIDELINES FOR PERFORMING A SPINAL AXIS ANESTHETIC IN PATIENTS WHO ARE RECEIVING A THEINOPYRIDINE

The American Society of Regional Anesthesia and Pain Medicine is the only group that provides any guidance for the placement of spinal/epidural neuroblockade in patients who are receiving a theinopyridine.[1]

The ASRA Guidelines[1]

1. Ticlopidine should be discontinued 14 days before surgery.
2. It is recommended that clopidogrel be stopped 7 days before surgery.

Benzon and colleagues[31] recommend that neuraxial blocks be postponed for 5 to 7 days in patients who are receiving several antiplatelet drugs. The manufacturer of ticlopidine suggests that ticlopidine be stopped 10 to 14 days before elective surgery.[26] The general recommendation is that clopidogrel should be stopped 7 days before surgery.[1]

GUIDELINES FOR PERFORMING A SPINAL AXIS ANESTHETIC IN PATIENTS WHO ARE RECEIVING A GLYCOPROTEIN IIB/IIIA ANTAGONIST

The American Society of Regional Anesthesia and Pain Medicine is the only society that provides any guidelines for the anesthetic management of patients who are receiving a glycoprotein IIb/IIIa antagonist.[1]

The ASRA Guidelines[1]

1. Abciximab should be discontinued 48 hours before surgery.

2. It is recommended that eptifibatide and tirofiban be stopped 8 hours before surgery.

The guidelines also warn that the increase in perioperative bleeding noted in patients undergoing cardiac and vascular surgery after having received a glycoprotein IIb/IIIa antagonist warrants concern about the risks of spinal hematoma formations, should one believe that either spinal or epidural anesthesia is strongly indicated. Furthermore, Kam and Egan[35] indicate that literature concerning the safety of performing central neuraxial regional blockade (spinal or epidural anesthesia) in patients who have recently received a glycoprotein IIb/IIIa inhibitor is not available. Avoiding spinal or epidural anesthesia in these patients would appear to be wise.

Finally, assessing platelet function using platelet turbidometric aggregometry or platelet function analyzer PEA-100 may be useful in patients who have received a glycoprotein IIb/IIIa antagonist before anesthesia and surgery.[35] Unfortunately, neither of these tests is readily available.

Anesthesia offers guidelines for the management of this group of patients.[1] In brief, ticlopidine should be stopped 14 days before surgery and there should be a 7-day drug-free window following the last ingestion of clopidogrel.[1]

Finally, there is also a substantial risk of hematoma formation in patients who have used a platelet glycoprotein IIb/IIIa agent before placement of a spinal/epidural block or catheter removal. Although there are no direct reports of this having occurred in any patient, this position was derived from the cardiac surgery literature.[42,43] In brief, abciximab should be discontinued 48 hours before surgery, and eptifibatide and tirofiban should be stopped 8 hours before surgery.[1]

AUTHORS' RECOMMENDATIONS

The authors agree that cyclooxygenase-2 inhibitors have minimal effect on platelet function and the available evidence in the literature supports the contention that there is no reason to withhold COX-2 therapy before placing a neuraxial block or before the removal of either a spinal or an epidural catheter.

The development of a spinal/epidural hematoma is a rare event. Tryba[13] identified 13 cases of spinal hematoma following 850,000 epidural anesthetics and 7 cases involving 650,000 spinal blocks. Based on these observations he calculated the incidence of hematoma formation to be about 1 in 150,000 epidural blocks and 1 in 220,000 spinal anesthetics.[13] As such, none of the studies to date has a large enough patient population to predict with any degree of certainty that there is *no risk* of hematoma formation when one continues to use COX-1 NSAIDs before surgery, and there are divergent opinions on this topic. The German Society of Anesthesiology and Intensive Care Medicine and the Spanish Consensus Forum both believe that there is a risk of hematoma formation when these agents are used in the perioperative period. Both these groups mandate a free interval of 1 to 2 days after the last administration of COX-1 NSAIDs and at least a 3-day interval without aspirin or aspirin-containing medications before neuraxial blocks are performed or epidural catheters are removed.[2,3] On the other hand, the American Society of Regional Anesthesia does not believe that there is any risk and that cases should proceed as scheduled if patients without other risk factors are to undergo surgery and they have continued to take aspirin or another COX-1 NSAID in the perioperative period.[1] The ASRA position is supported by intuitive logic. Annually, millions of people worldwide undergo elective surgery who have continued to consume aspirin and other COX-1 NSAIDs, and the incidence of hematoma formation is almost nonexistent in this patient population.[12] More important, it would appear that we have come "full circle" in that many orthopedic surgeons now believe that the combination of ASA, epidural anesthesia, and early ambulation may be the anticoagulation protocol of choice for total joint arthroplasty.[4,5]

There appears to be no risk of hematoma formation in patients who continue to ingest COX-2 NSAIDs in the perioperative period, and surgery in such patients should proceed as scheduled.[1]

There is a substantial risk of hematoma formation in patients who have consumed either ticlopidine or clopidogrel in the preoperative period. Only the American Society of Regional

REFERENCES

1. Horlocker TT, Wedel DJ, Benzon H, et al: Regional anesthesia in the anticoagulated patient: Defining the risks (the second ASRA Consensus Conference on Neuraxial Anesthesia and Anticoagulation). *Reg Anesth Pain Med* 2003;28:172-197.
2. Gogarten W, Van Aken H, Wulf H, et al: Regional anaesthesia and thromboembolism prophylaxis/anticoagulation: Guidelines of the German Society of Anaesthesiology and Intensive Care Medicine (DGAI). *Anaesthesiol Intensivmed* 1997;38:623-628.
3. Llau JV, de Andres J, Gomar C, et al: [Drugs that alter hemostasis and regional anesthetic techniques: Safety guidelines. Consensus conference]. *Rev Esp Anestesiol Reanim* 2001;48:270-278.
4. Lotke PA, Lonner JH: The benefit of aspirin chemoprophylaxis for thromboembolism after total knee arthroplasty. *Clin Orthop Relat Res* 2006;452:175-180.
5. Hanssen AD, Lachiewicz PF, Soileau ES: Mechanical calf compression and aspirin prophylaxis for total knee arthroplasty. *Clin Orthop Relat Res* 2007;464:61-64.
6. Callaghan JJ, Dorr LD, Engh GA, et al: Prophylaxis for thromboembolic disease: Recommendations from the American College of Chest Physicians—are they appropriate for orthopaedic surgery? *J Arthroplasty* 2005;20:273-274.
7. Kreppel D, Antoniadis G, Seeling W: Spinal hematoma: A literature survey with meta-analysis of 613 patients. *Neurosurg Rev* 2003;26:1-49.
8. Schror K: Antiplatelet drugs. A comparative review. *Drugs* 1995;50:7-28.
9. Urmey WF, Rowlingson J: Do antiplatelet agents contribute to the development of perioperative spinal hematoma? *Reg Anesth Pain Med* 1998;23:146-151.
10. Horlocker TT, Bajwa ZH, Ashraf Z, et al: Risk assessment of hemorrhagic complications associated with nonsteroidal antiinflammatory medications in ambulatory pain clinic patients undergoing epidural steroid injection. *Anesth Analg* 2002;95: 1691-1697, table of contents.
11. Horlocker TT, Wedel DJ, Offord KP: Does preoperative antiplatelet therapy increase the risk of hemorrhagic complications associated with regional anesthesia? *Anesth Analg* 1990;70: 631-634.
12. Horlocker TT, Wedel DJ, Schroeder DR, et al: Preoperative antiplatelet therapy does not increase the risk of spinal hematoma associated with regional anesthesia. *Anesth Analg* 1995;80:303-309.
13. Tryba M: [Epidural regional anesthesia and low molecular heparin: Pro]. *Anasthesiol Intensivmed Notfallmed Schmerzther* 1993;28:179-181.
14. Vandermeulen EP, Van Aken H, Vermylen J: Anticoagulants and spinal-epidural anesthesia. *Anesth Analg* 1994;79:1165-1177.
15. Litz RJ, Hubler M, Koch T, Albrecht DM: Spinal-epidural hematoma following epidural anesthesia in the presence of antiplatelet and heparin therapy. *Anesthesiology* 2001;95:1031-1033.
16. Gerancher JC, Waterer R, Middleton J: Transient paraparesis after postdural puncture spinal hematoma in a patient receiving ketorolac. *Anesthesiology* 1997;86:490-494.
17. Heye N: Is there a link between acute spinal epidural hematoma and aspirin? *Spine* 1995;20:1931-1932.
18. Hyderally HA: Epidural hematoma unrelated to combined spinal-epidural anesthesia in a patient with ankylosing spondylitis

receiving aspirin after total hip replacement. *Anesth Analg* 2005;100:882-883.

19. Hindman BJ, Koka BV: Usefulness of the post-aspirin bleeding time. *Anesthesiology* 1986;64:368-370.

20. Camu F, Beecher T, Recker DP, Verburg KM: Valdecoxib, a COX-2-specific inhibitor, is an efficacious, opioid-sparing analgesic in patients undergoing hip arthroplasty. *Am J Ther* 2002;9:43-51.

21. Leese PT, Recker DP, Kent JD: The COX-2 selective inhibitor, valdecoxib, does not impair platelet function in the elderly: Results of a randomized controlled trial. *J Clin Pharmacol* 2003;43:504-513.

22. Leese PT, Hubbard RC, Karim A, et al: Effects of celecoxib, a novel cyclooxygenase-2 inhibitor, on platelet function in healthy adults: A randomized, controlled trial. *J Clin Pharmacol* 2000;40:124-132.

23. Cannon GW, Caldwell JR, Holt P, et al: Rofecoxib, a specific inhibitor of cyclooxygenase 2, with clinical efficacy comparable with that of diclofenac sodium: Results of a one-year, randomized, clinical trial in patients with osteoarthritis of the knee and hip. Rofecoxib Phase III Protocol 035 Study Group. *Arthritis Rheum* 2000;43:978-987.

24. Thebault JJ, Blatrix CE, Blanchard JF, Panak EA: Effects of ticlopidine, a new platelet aggregation inhibitor in man. *Clin Pharmacol Ther* 1975;18:485-490.

25. Ashida SI, Abiko Y: Inhibition of platelet aggregation by a new agent, ticlopidine. *Thromb Haemost* 1979;40:542-550.

26. *Physicians' desk reference*, ed 56. Montvale, NJ, Medical Economics, 2002, pp 3015-3018.

27. Coukell AJ, Markham A: Clopidogrel. *Drugs* 1997;54:745-750, discussion 751.

28. Mayumi T, Dohi S: Spinal subarachnoid hematoma after lumbar puncture in a patient receiving antiplatelet therapy. *Anesth Analg* 1983;62:777-779.

29. Savi P, Herbert JM, Pflieger AM, et al: Importance of hepatic metabolism in the antiaggregating activity of the thienopyridine clopidogrel. *Biochem Pharmacol* 1992;44:527-532.

30. Boneu B, Destelle G: Platelet anti-aggregating activity and tolerance of clopidogrel in atherosclerotic patients. *Thromb Haemost* 1996;76:939-943.

31. Benzon HT, Wong HY, Siddiqui T, Ondra S: Caution in performing epidural injections in patients on several antiplatelet drugs. *Anesthesiology* 1999;91:1558-1559.

32. Merritt JC, Bhatt DL: The efficacy and safety of perioperative antiplatelet therapy. *J Thromb Thrombolysis* 2004;17:21-27.

33. Hongo RH, Ley J, Dick SE, Yee RR: The effect of clopidogrel in combination with aspirin when given before coronary artery bypass grafting. *J Am Coll Cardiol* 2002;40:231-237.

34. Herbert JM, Dol F, Bernat A, et al: The antiaggregating and antithrombotic activity of clopidogrel is potentiated by aspirin in several experimental models in the rabbit. *Thromb Haemost* 1998;80:512-518.

35. Kam PC, Egan MK: Platelet glycoprotein IIb/IIIa antagonists: Pharmacology and clinical developments. *Anesthesiology* 2002;96:1237-1249.

36. Farrell DH, Thiagarajan P, Chung DW, Davie EW: Role of fibrinogen alpha and gamma chain sites in platelet aggregation. *Proc Natl Acad Sci U S A* 1992;89:10729-10732.

37. Tcheng JE, Ellis SG, George BS, et al: Pharmacodynamics of chimeric glycoprotein IIb/IIIa integrin antiplatelet antibody Fab 7E3 in high-risk coronary angioplasty. *Circulation* 1994;90: 1757-1764.

38. Brown DL, Fann CS, Chang CJ: Meta-analysis of effectiveness and safety of abciximab versus eptifibatide or tirofiban in percutaneous coronary intervention. *Am J Cardiol* 2001;87:537-541.

39. Lemmer JH Jr: Clinical experience in coronary bypass surgery for abciximab-treated patients. *Ann Thorac Surg* 2000;70:S33-S37.

40. Phillips DR, Scarborough RM: Clinical pharmacology of eptifibatide. *Am J Cardiol* 1997;80:11B-20B.

41. Tcheng JE: Clinical challenges of platelet glycoprotein IIb/IIIa receptor inhibitor therapy: Bleeding, reversal, thrombocytopenia, and retreatment. *Am Heart J* 2000;139:S38-S45.

42. Dyke C, Bhatia D: Inhibitors of the platelet receptor glycoprotein IIb-IIIa and complications during percutaneous coronary revascularization. Management strategies for the cardiac surgeon. *J Cardiovasc Surg (Torino)* 1999;40:505-516.

43. Gammie JS, Zenati M, Kormos RL, et al: Abciximab and excessive bleeding in patients undergoing emergency cardiac operations. *Ann Thorac Surg* 1998;65:465-469.

51

The Best Approaches to Prophylaxis against DVT Formation When Using a Combination of Neuraxial Anesthesia and One of the Heparins

Lynn M. Broadman, MD

INTRODUCTION

Many patients undergoing surgery benefit from spinal axis anesthesia and analgesia. To this end postoperative epidural analgesia provides many advantages over parenteral opioids, especially for patients undergoing lower-extremity orthopedic procedures; vascular, urologic, and gynecologic surgeries; and many cardiac and thoracic surgical procedures.[1-4] These benefits include improved pain relief, a decreased incidence of cardiopulmonary complications,[3] and reduced blood loss and the need for perioperative transfusions.[5,6] Numerous studies have documented the safety of spinal axis anesthesia and analgesia in the anticoagulated patient.[3,7-13] Spinal and continuous epidural infusion techniques provide effective operative and postoperative pain control, and frequently eliminate problems associated with general anesthesia.[1] However, there are some caveats to the use of neuraxial anesthesia. Many surgical patients require preoperative deep vein thrombosis (DVT) prophylaxis, or they will receive DVT prophylaxis in the postoperative period. More importantly, some cardiac and vascular procedures may even require that the patient receive significant intraoperative anticoagulation.

There are valid concerns surrounding the placement of a spinal axis anesthetic in an anticoagulated patient.[14-17] The placement of spinal access blocks can lead to the formation of spinal and epidural hematomas, and the incidence of this catastrophic complication is increased if the patient is anticoagulated.[14,18] The safe management of patients who will be receiving a neuraxial block and perioperative anticoagulation therapy can be improved by coordinating the timing of needle placement and catheter removal with the administration of the anticoagulant.[19]

Familiarity with the pharmacology of the heparins, as well as other hemostasis-altering drugs; knowledge of the literature pertaining to patients receiving spinal axis anesthesia while using these drugs; and the use of pertinent case reports can help guide the clinician in the management of these very special patients. The reasons for anticoagulating these patients are quite valid.[20,21] The reasons for preventing DVT/venous thromboembolism (VTE) and acute pulmonary embolism (PE) are obvious and critical to the provision of quality patient care.[21] In addition, vessel and graft patency are frequently dependent on adequate anticoagulation during both the intraoperative and postoperative periods. Finally, caution must be used to individually risk stratify each patient when considering the use of a neuraxial axis anesthetic in the presence of perioperative anticoagulation.

In this chapter we present a synopsis of the American Society for Regional Anesthesia (ASRA) Consensus Guidelines from 1998,[22,23] 2003,[24] and the proceedings of the 2007 Consensus Conference[25] for the use of spinal axis anesthesia techniques in patients who are receiving or will be receiving either unfractionated heparin (UH) or low-molecular-weight heparin (LMWH) in the perioperative period. We also present the current European thoughts and protocols regarding this issue and discuss how they differ from the North American guidelines.

THE CLINICAL RATIONALE FOR THROMBOPROPHYLAXIS AND THE RELATED HISTORICAL DATA

The rationale for thromboprophylaxis stems from the high prevalence of VTE among postsurgical patients; the incidence can run as high as 80% in patients undergoing total knee replacement (TKR) who are not receiving anticoagulation therapy.[26] The clinically silent presentation of the disease in most patients, and the morbidity and mortality frequently encountered when a VTE occurs, makes it imperative that all patients undergoing TKR, total hip replacement

(THR), hip fracture surgery (HFS), and certain abdominal and pelvic procedures receive DVT anticoagulation therapy.[26,27] Pulmonary embolism produces few specific symptoms and the presence of this devastating complication is often silent. Moreover, the clinical diagnosis of PE is very unreliable.[28-30] The first presentation of a VTE may be a catastrophic PE,[21,26] which requires that a preventive rather than a screening approach be taken to properly address the DVT/PE problem.[27] Routine screening of patients in the postoperative period for DVT and VTE has not been demonstrated to reduce the frequency of clinically significant outcomes such as VTE and PE,[27] and has been shown to be cost-prohibitive when compared with routine prophylactic regimens.[28,29,31-36]

Historical data derived from clinical trials and cohort studies provide practitioners with a base of information on the incidence of acute VTE associated with major orthopedic surgery on the lower extremities and other procedures, as well as relative information to help guide one's decisions on the implementation of thromboprophylaxis. The world standard test for the detection of postoperative DVT is contrast venography performed on the seventh to fourteenth postoperative day.[32] When one uses these methods on control patients, the prevalence of DVT at 7 to 14 days after TKR, THR, and HFS is about 50% to 60%.[26] In lower-extremity procedures it is usually the operative leg that is affected, but the nonoperative leg may be affected in about 20% of cases.[26] The standards for the detection of PE are either a ventilation-perfusion study, a spiral computed tomography (CT) scan, arteriography, or a postmortem examination.[37,38] The incidence of asymptomatic PE is less well defined. In studies routinely using ventilation-perfusion scans, 7% to 11% of THR and TKR patients had a high probability of PE as determined by scans performed on postoperative days 7 to 14.[26] Acute VTE and PE also occur after hospital discharge in a clinically significant number of patients. Venography studies show that in patients not receiving thromboprophylaxis, 10% to 20% will develop a DVT and 6% will develop an intermediate-to-high probability ventilation-perfusion scan, suggestive of subclinical PE at 4 to 5 weeks after discharge.[26]

The bottom line is that the risk of a patient developing an adverse event in the postoperative period such as myocardial infarction, DVT, or PE increases with age, and the elderly, particularly women over age 80, are at significant risk.[39] These data suggest that the risk of developing a VTE is substantial, be it a DVT or PE, without thromboprophylaxis. As previously mentioned, the potential severity of a VTE, and the difficulty and expense of screening for it postoperatively, warrants some type of thromboprophylaxis for all patients undergoing major lower-extremity orthopedic surgery.[26,38] Again, this chapter focuses on the relationships and benefits of spinal axis anesthesia in the patient requiring DVT prophylaxis. The areas of focus are limited to pharmacologic methods of thromboprophylaxis and there is no discussion of the available mechanical methods for reducing the incidence of VTE.

THE HEMOSTATIC PROCESSES

Understanding the mechanisms of the hemostatic cascades is important if one is to fully understand how anticoagulants work and the implications of their use in patients receiving spinal axis anesthetics. Because of space limitations, this chapter provides only a general overview of these intricate systems and focuses primarily on the intrinsic pathway; it is primarily this pathway that is altered by the heparins. The blood clotting system, or coagulation pathway, is a proteolytic cascade. Each enzyme of the pathway is present in the plasma as a zymogen, an inactive form, which on activation undergoes proteolytic cleavage to release the active factor from the precursor molecule. The pathway functions through both positive and negative feedback loops that control activation of this process. The ultimate goal of the pathway is to produce thrombin, which then converts soluble fibrinogen into fibrin, which in turn facilitates clot formation. The generation of thrombin can be divided into three phases: the intrinsic and extrinsic pathways that provide alternative routes for the generation of factor X, and the final common pathway that results in thrombin formation.[40]

The intrinsic pathway is activated when blood comes into contact with subendothelial connective tissue. Quantitatively the intrinsic pathway is the more important of the two pathways, but it cleaves fibrin more slowly than does the extrinsic pathway.[41] The Hageman factor (factor XII), factor XI, prekallikrein, and high-molecular-weight kininogen (HMWK) are involved in the activation of this pathway. The first step is the binding of factor XII to a subendothelial surface exposed by an injury. A complex of prekallikrein and HMWK interacts with the exposed surface in close proximity to the bound factor XII, which becomes activated. Activated factor XII in turn activates prekallikrein. The kallikrein produced by the aforementioned process can then cleave factor XII, and a further amplification mechanism is triggered. The activated factor XII activates factor XI, the next step in the intrinsic pathway, which to proceed efficiently requires calcium ions. Also involved at this stage is HMWK, which binds to factor XI and facilitates the activation process.[42] Eventually the intrinsic pathway activates factor X, a process that can also be brought about by the extrinsic pathway.[43] Factor X is the first molecule of the common pathway and is activated by a complex of molecules containing activated factor IX, factor VIII, calcium, and phospholipid, which is provided by the platelet surface where this reaction usually takes place. The precise role of factor VIII in this reaction is not clearly understood. However, its presence in the coagulation cascade is obviously essential, as evidenced by the serious consequences of factor VIII deficiency experienced by hemophiliacs. Factor VIII is modified by thrombin, a reaction that results in greatly enhanced factor VIII activity, which in turn promotes the activation of factor X.

The extrinsic pathway is an alternative route for the activation of the clotting cascade. It provides a very rapid response to tissue injury, generating activated factor X almost instantaneously; on the other hand, the intrinsic pathway requires seconds or even minutes to activate factor X. The main function of the extrinsic pathway is to augment the activity of the intrinsic pathway.[40] The intrinsic and extrinsic systems converge at factor X to form the final common pathway, which is ultimately responsible for the production of thrombin (factor IIa).[40] The end result, as mentioned earlier, is the production of thrombin for the conversion of fibrinogen to fibrin.

How Do the Heparins Interrupt the Coagulation Cascade?

Simply stated, the heparins all work primarily by inhibiting the intrinsic limb of the coagulation pathway. A large portion of the clinical effects of both UH and LMWH occurs through enhancement of the antithrombotic action of antithrombin III (ATIII), an important endogenous inhibitor of coagulation that acts primarily by inactivating factor IIa and factor Xa.[44] The fundamental biologic difference between UH and LMWH stems from the relative potency of the drug to accelerate the basal rate of ATIII-mediated IIa and Xa inactivation.[45] Unfractionated heparin enhances the inactivation of both IIa and Xa, whereas LMWH predominantly catalyzes factor Xa inactivation. The specific mechanism of action of both UH and LMWH will be discussed within the sections dedicated to them later in this chapter.

Monitoring of Anticoagulation in Patients Receiving Heparin Therapy

Monitoring of the level of therapeutic anticoagulation in patients receiving UH is achieved via the activated partial thromboplastin time (aPTT). In the aPTT test, a contact activator is used to stimulate the production of XIIa by providing a surface for the activation of HMWK, kallikrein, and factor XIIa. The contact activation is allowed to proceed at 37°C for a specified period of time. Calcium is then added to trigger further reactions, and the time (in seconds) required for clot formation is measured. Phospholipids are required to form complexes, which activate factor X and prothrombin. Normal values on the aPTT range from 24.3 to 35.0 seconds.[46]

The aPTT does not specifically measure anti-Xa activity, and there is little correlation between anti-Xa activity and aPTT levels.[47] Therefore aPTT is not generally used to monitor LMWH therapy. Because of the very predictable plasma levels obtained when one administers LMWH subcutaneously and the lack of correlation between LMWH plasma levels and aPTT and anti-Xa values, one should *not* attempt to monitor LMWH therapy with either of these laboratory studies. However, in cases of renal insufficiency and obesity monitoring may be justified.[48] Unfortunately, the anti-Xa level assay is only available at a few medical centers in North America.

What Is the Risk of Spinal/Epidural Hematoma Formation in the Anticoagulated Patient Undergoing Neuraxial Anesthesia?

Bleeding is a recognized complication associated with the placement of a regional anesthetic block in the anticoagulated patient.[49] However, the most significant risk is the development of a spinal axis hematoma.[50] The true incidence of neurologic complications caused from bleeding following spinal axis anesthesia is unknown; however,

the reported incidence is estimated to be less than 1 per 220,000 with spinal anesthesia and less than 1 per 150,000 with epidural anesthesia.[12]

A review of the 61 previously reported spinal hematoma formations in patients receiving neuraxial anesthesia between 1906 and 1994 was published in 1994 by Vandermeulen and colleagues.[14] In addition, the authors discussed the following possible risk factors[14]:

1. At the time of anesthetic administration, 42 of the 61 (68%) patients developing spinal hematoma had impaired coagulation. In 25 of 42 of the cases, some form of heparin therapy was present. An additional 5 of 42 patients had undergone a major vascular procedure in which heparin was likely used, but not reported. The remaining 12 of 42 patients had a variety of medical conditions that could have produced an impairment in their ability to form a quality clot. These conditions included thrombocytopenia, hepatic dysfunction, and renal insufficiency, or they had been treated with another anticoagulant/antiplatelet agent at the time the bleeding occurred.
2. The needle placement was reported as difficult in 15 of 61 patients (25%) and/or it was bloody in another 15 (25%) of the cases.
3. Multiple punctures were reported in 12 of 61 (20%) of the cases.
4. Pregnancy was noted in 5 of 61 (8%) of the cases.
5. Anatomic abnormalities, such as spina bifida occulta and vascularized tumor, were noted in 4 of 61 (6.5%) of the cases.
6. An epidural technique was used in 46 of 61 (75%) of the cases and an epidural catheter was placed in 32 of 46 (70%). In 15 of 32 (47%) of the epidural catheter cases the bleed occurred immediately on removal of the catheter.
7. A spinal technique was involved in 15 (25%) of the cases.

The extensive literature review conducted by Vandermeulen and colleagues[14] has served as the benchmark for all of us in ascertaining the risks of spinal/epidural hematoma formation in patients receiving a neuraxial block and who either have received or will receive medications that may/will alter their coagulation cascade. However, the Vandermeulen study[14] has two major shortcomings: it is a retrospective review of the literature and does not evaluate any primary data, and, more important, probably less than 1 in 10 adverse events that occur are reported in the literature. More recently, Moen and colleagues[51] conducted a retrospective review of all central neuraxial blocks placed in Sweden between 1990 and 1999. The study encompassed two phases. First, a postal survey letter was sent to the chairperson of all anesthesia departments in which they were asked to provide the number of spinal and epidural blocks placed in their department during 1998. In addition, they were asked to provide the number of block-related complications that occurred in their department during the decade 1990-1999. The specific complications that the study addressed were epidural hematoma, epidural abscess, meningitis, and cauda equina syndrome. No patient identification was sought or used during this study. The researchers then went to the National Board of Health and Welfare

(NBHW) and reviewed the quality assurance files associated with each complication. By Swedish law all serious complications must be reported to the NBHW. During the study period Moen and colleagues[51] ascertained that 1,260,000 spinal blocks were performed and 450,000 epidural blocks administered, including 200,000 labor epidural blocks. As a result of these blocks 127 serious complications occurred and 85 of 127 of these patients sustained permanent neurologic damage. There were 33 of 127 spinal axis hematomas. Other serious complications were cauda equina syndrome (32), meningitis (29), epidural abscess (13), and miscellaneous (20). The results of the Moen study[51] mirror those of Tryba[12] in that the incidence of complications after epidural blockade are much more frequent than after spinal blockade. In addition, more complications than expected were found by Moen and colleagues.[51] The incidence of epidural hematoma formation association with labor epidural block placement was quite low (1:200,000) while those placed in women undergoing knee arthroplasty were very high (1:3,600) and mirror the predictions made by Schroeder during the First ASRA Consensus Conference in 1998.[52] Perhaps the most alarming information reported by Moen and colleagues[51] is the fact that "one third of all spinal hematomas were seen in patients receiving thromboprophylaxis in association with a central neuraxial block (CNB) in accordance with the current guidelines and in the absence of any previously known risk factors. Consequently, adherence to the guidelines regarding LMWH and CNB may reduce but not completely abolish the risk of spinal hematoma after CNB." This latter fact is further reinforced by the case report by Sandhu and colleagues[53] in which they essentially followed the ASRA Guidelines and still had an epidural hematoma formation occur in their patient 1 day after the removal of her epidural catheter. However, this author must point out that the patient in the Sandhu case report had two risk factors. The patient was elderly, age 79 years, and a female. In brief, the Sandhu article[53] reports the placement of an epidural catheter on the third attempt, hours after the last dose of subcutaneous unfractionated heparin (UH) 5000 units. The catheter was removed on the third postoperative day, 6 hours after the last dose of UH 5000 units. This elderly female patient developed a symptomatic epidural hematoma the next day that required surgical evacuation. This patient's platelet count and aPTT were within normal limits at all times. Sandhu and colleagues[53] highlighted the need for all clinicians to be vigilant about the timing of epidural placement and removal, even in patients on standard-dose UH therapy, and they encouraged the monitoring of coagulation status.

The alarming information reported by Moen and colleagues[51] that more than one third of all epidural hematomas occur in patients in whom all guidelines were followed and that the incidence of this catastrophic event is still very likely underreported may be tempered by a recent meta-analysis by Kreppel and colleagues.[54] Kreppel and colleagues evaluated 613 case studies published between 1826 and 1996 and ascertained that in about one third of the cases (29.7%) no etiologic factor could be identified as the cause of the bleeding. This idiopathic group formed the largest group of patients who developed a spinal/epidural hematoma. Spinal and epidural anesthetics placed in conjunction with anticoagulation therapy were actually the fifth most common cause of spinal/epidural hematoma formations, and spinal and epidural anesthesia alone were the tenth most common etiologic factor. The second largest group was made up of cases in which the patients were undergoing anticoagulation therapy (17%). To this end, this author saw two cases in his pain clinic during the past decade in which spontaneous epidural hematoma formations occurred in anticoagulated patients. In both these cases the patients were referred for the emergent evaluation and treatment of their severe back pain of sudden onset without any other symptoms. In both cases grossly abnormal International Normalized Ratio (INR) values were noted as the result of warfarin therapy, and a magnetic resonance imaging (MRI) study showed the presence of an epidural hematoma. Neither of these patients had undergone any recent spinal manipulation or intervention. Unlike Moen and colleagues,[51] Kreppel and associates[54] found elderly men between 55 and 70 years of age to be at the greatest risk for the development of spinal hemorrhage. Sixty-four percent of the patients in the Kreppel series[54] were men; however, the etiologies of the spinal hemorrhages in the Kreppel study patients were from all causes and not just patients undergoing total joint replacement under spinal/epidural anesthesia in conjunction with perioperative anticoagulation, where elderly women are clearly at greatest risk.[51,52]

Spinal hematoma is a rare and catastrophic complication associated with both epidural and spinal anesthesia. It may occur with bleeding into either the epidural space or the subarachnoid space.[11,16,49] The prominent epidural venous plexus accounts for the majority of hematomas being formed in the epidural space. In addition, the radicular vessels along nerve roots can bleed either into the intrathecal or epidural space.[11]

Spinal hematoma is often occult, delaying both diagnosis and treatment.[16] The presenting symptom of spinal hematoma is not always radicular back pain. Vandermeulen and colleagues[14] found the presenting symptoms to be weakness (46%), radicular back pain (38%), and paresthesia (14%). The diagnosis is frequently complicated/delayed due to the residual paresthesia/anesthesia produced by the neuraxial block. Such delays can be averted by using a short-acting local anesthetic agent. The use of such agents facilitates immediate postoperative neurologic evaluation, and, if abnormal findings are uncovered, appropriate radiographic studies, if indicated, can then be obtained in a timely manner. There is certainly a temporal relationship between the onset of paraplegia, surgical evacuation of hematoma, and recovery (Table 51-1).[14,55] Full recovery of neurologic function is unlikely if surgery is postponed for more than 8 to 12 hours.[14] Like the patients in the Vandermeulen series,[14] patients in the Kreppel series[54] who underwent rapid diagnosis and surgical evacuation obtained the most ideal recovery of neurologic function. Thirty-one of 47 patients in the Kreppel study who received surgical treatment within 12 hours of the onset of their symptoms recovered completely (66%); more than half of the patients who did not obtain surgical decompression until 13 to 24 hours had elapsed did not recover any neurologic function.

Table 51-1	Neurologic Outcome* in Patients with Spinal Hematoma after Neuraxial Blockade		
Interval between Onset of Paraplegia and Surgery	**Good Recovery (*n* = 15)**	**Partial Recovery (*n* = 11)**	**Poor Recovery (*n* = 29)**
Less than 8 hr (*n* = 13)	6	4	3
Between 8-24 hr (*n* = 8)	2	2	4
Greater than 24 hr (*n* = 11)	1	0	10
No surgical intervention (*n* = 13)	4	1	8
Unknown (*n* = 10)	2	4	4

Modified from Vandermeulen EP, Van Aken H, Vermylen J: *Anesth Analg* 1994;79:1165-1177.

*Neurologic outcome was reported for 55 of 61 cases of spinal hematoma after neuraxial block.

CLINICALLY RELEVANT ASPECTS OF UNFRACTIONATED AND LOW-MOLECULAR-WEIGHT HEPARIN ADMINISTRATION

Unfractionated heparin was discovered by McLean in 1916 and has been used clinically as an antithrombotic agent for several decades.[56] It is an inexpensive and highly effective anticoagulant with which one can achieve graded anticoagulation in a partially dose-dependent fashion.[57] Unfractionated heparin is a highly negatively charged, water-soluble glycosamine composed of chains of alternating residues of D-glucosamine and a uronic acid. It is heterogeneous with respect to molecular weight, anticoagulant properties, and pharmacokinetics. The variable molecular weight of UH is attributed to the variable numbers of attached polysaccharide chains, with an average molecular weight of 15,000 daltons (range of 5000 to 30,000 daltons).[58] The major anticoagulant effect of UH is attributed to a unique pentasaccharide with a high-affinity binding to ATIII.[59] Binding of this pentasaccharide to ATIII accelerates its ability to inactivate thrombin (factor IIa), as well as factors IXa, Xa, XIa, and XIIa. Unfractionated heparin catalyzes the inactivation of IIa by ATIII/heparin complex formation, acting as a template to which both the enzyme and the inhibitor can bind to form a ternary complex.[59] This complex requires a chain length of at least 18 saccharide units and is the basis for the differences between LMWH and UH. Unlike UH, LMWH consists of primarily the pentasaccharide sequence and lacks the long polysaccharide unit required to bind to IIa and ATIII simultaneously. Thus LMWH has a Xa:IIa affinity ratio of approximately 3:1 and primarily inactivates Xa. The inactivation of Xa by ATIII/heparin does not require ternary complex formation and is achieved by binding of the enzyme to ATIII.[60] The anticoagulant effect of UH depends on both the number of heparin molecules with the pentasaccharide chain (Xa inhibition) and the size of the molecules containing the pentasaccharide sequence (IIa inhibition).[22]

Both UH and LMWH are derived from animal sources. This explains the uncommon, but serious, occurrence of heparin-induced thrombocytopenia and thrombosis (HITT). The HITT syndrome is an immunoglobulin G (IgG)–mediated decrease in platelets to below 150,000 that usually occurs 5 days after initiating heparin therapy[61] and may be complicated by pathologic thrombosis. In randomized clinical trials it has been shown to occur at a rate of about 3%.[61] Warkentin and colleagues[61] found that in a group of 665 patients randomized to receive either UH or LMWH, 9 of the 665 patients developed HITT. In this study 332 received UH and 333 received LMWH. None of the patients receiving LMWH developed HITT whereas nine of the patients receiving UH developed clinically significant HITT (2.7%). Eight of the nine (89%) who developed HITT also had significant thrombotic complications. Patients with a history of HITT syndrome should not receive LMWH because, as previously mentioned, it is also derived from animal sources and there is a high incidence of cross-reactivity. Clinical exposure to UH is clearly associated with a higher incidence of precipitating HITT syndrome than is LMWH.

Unfractionated Heparin Reversal

Serious bleeding associated with UH therapy may be controlled by the administration of protamine sulfate. Protamine is a strongly basic protein that binds to and neutralizes heparin.[62] Most of the anticoagulant effects of UH are reversed by equimolar doses of protamine. Protamine is a positively charged protein derived from salmon sperm. When administered intravenously (IV) in the presence of heparin, the positively charged protamine interacts with the negatively charged portion of the heparin molecule and forms a stable complex. The long polysaccharide chains of UH appear to increase attraction to protamine. The dose of protamine required to fully reverse heparin is 1 mg for each 100 units of circulating heparin. This dose is decreased if more than 15 minutes have elapsed since the last heparin administration.

Low-Dose Subcutaneous UH Therapy: How Effective Is It at Preventing DVT Formation?

The administration of 5000 units of UH subcutaneously every 8 to 12 hours has been used extensively and effectively for the prevention of DVT. In a review of 11 trials, Geerts and colleagues[26] found that the overall risk of DVT in patients undergoing THR was 30% with low-dose UH, compared with 54% in controls. The therapeutic basis for low-dose subcutaneous UH therapy is linked to the inhibition of activated factor X and the fact that the inhibition of small amounts of Xa prevents amplification of the coagulation cascade. Thus, only small doses of UH are required for prophylaxis whereas much larger doses are needed to treat thromboembolic disease. Maximum anticoagulation occurs 40 to 50 minutes after subcutaneous injection of UH and returns to baseline within 4 to 6 hours. The aPTT often remains in the normal range, but wide variances have occurred in individual patients.[63]

In their 1988 review of the results of randomized trials in urologic, orthopedic, and general surgery regarding fatal PE and venous thrombosis, Collins and colleagues[64] found that therapy with low-dose subcutaneous UH therapy, dosed at 5000 units 2 hours before surgery and every 8 to 12 hours postoperatively, reduced the risk of DVT by 70% and fatal PE by 50%. However, when comparing the efficacy of low-dose subcutaneous UH with LMWH, UH is slightly less effective in the prevention of DVT and PE. Significant protein binding creates variability in dose response to UH when compared with LMWH.[65]

Evidence Regarding the Safety of Neuraxial Anesthesia in Patients Who Are Receiving or Will Be Receiving UH

Multiple studies have demonstrated the relative safety of neuraxial anesthetic techniques in the presence of DVT prophylaxis with low-dose subcutaneous UH, and they have also demonstrated that there is little increased risk of spinal hematoma associated with this therapy.[8,9,13,66-68] There are nine published series involving more than 9000 patients who received this therapy without any complications.[9-11,67,69] Allemann and colleagues[68] and Lowson and Goodchild[13] similarly reported no cases of spinal hematoma in 204 epidural blocks and 119 spinal blocks on patients who had received 5000 units of UH subcutaneously 2 hours before needle placement. The large amount of data regarding both the safety and the efficacy of subcutaneous heparin for DVT prophylaxis in patients undergoing surgery with a neuraxial block suggests that UH is a reasonable alternative for DVT prophylaxis in patients undergoing lower-extremity orthopedic procedures, as well as general, urologic, and gynecologic operations.

There are very few data that would suggest that it is not safe to administer low-dose UH to patients who have received or will receive neuraxial anesthesia. There are currently only three case reports of spinal hematomas following neuraxial block in the presence of low-dose subcutaneous UH in the literature, two of which involved a continuous epidural anesthetic technique.[70-72] In one of these aforementioned case reports, an epidural catheter was placed despite elevation of the patient's aPTT. In another, blood was aspirated from the catheter during placement. In the last case, multiple attempts at spinal anesthesia were performed.

Deliberations on the Use of UH from the Third American Society of Regional Anesthesia (ASRA) Consensus Conference

The material presented at the Third American Society of Regional Anesthesia (ASRA) Consensus Conference (Vancouver, British Columbia, Canada, in April 2007) on the use of UH in conjunction with neuraxial anesthesia raised several questions but provided few new answers.[25] The last published guidelines, which were updated as a result of the Second ASRA Consensus Conference held in Chicago in spring 2002[24] with regard to the use of UH in conjunction with neuraxial anesthesia, remain in effect and were not superseded or altered in any way by the deliberations in Vancouver. The results of the Third Consensus Conference should be published in *Regional Anesthesia and Pain Medicine* in summer 2009.

In his update on the use of UH, Rowlingson pointed out that the surgeons at the University of Virginia are now using mini-dose heparin 5000 units administered three times a day (tid) rather than twice daily.[25] Rowlingson further indicated that there are no answers at this time to the following questions related to the use of tid UH: Can we safely leave an epidural catheter in place? Should we monitor platelet count while the catheter is in place? Should we obtain an aPTT before we remove the catheter and if so, what do the results mean clinically?

To this end a recent case report by Jooste and colleagues at the Children's Hospital of Pittsburgh[73] would suggest that it is safe to place and remove a thoracic epidural catheter in a pediatric patient who has been receiving long-term LMWH therapy by strictly adhering to the ASRA Guidelines. To comply with the 2002 ASRA Guidelines,[24] we[73] stopped the child's enoxaparin (1.5 mg/kg every 12 hours) 5 days before surgery and substituted low-dose tid UH (5000 units subcutaneously), and continued the tid UH into the postoperative period until the catheter was safely removed on postoperative day 7. The risk of spinal/epidural hematoma formation may be much less in children based on the data gleaned from the recent study by Kreppel and colleagues.[54] However, we did follow daily platelet counts and the child's aPTT, the results of which were always in the normal range, and removed his epidural catheter 6 hours after the last heparin dose. We performed a neurologic examination every 4 hours for the first 48 hours and then every 6 hours until 24 hours after the catheter was safely removed.[73]

ASRA 2002 Guidelines for Use of Neuraxial Techniques in Patients Receiving Low-Dose Subcutaneous UH[24]

During subcutaneous (mini-dose) prophylaxis, there is no contraindication to the use of neuraxial techniques. The risk of neuraxial bleeding may be reduced by delaying the heparin injection until 1 to 2 hours after the block, and it may be increased in debilitated patients or after prolonged therapy. Because heparin-induced thrombocytopenia may occur during heparin administration, patients receiving heparin for more than 4 days should have a platelet count assessed before neuraxial block.[24]

- Avoid neuraxial techniques in patients with other coagulopathies.
- Heparin administration should be delayed for 1 hour after needle placement.
- Remove the catheter 1 hour before any subsequent heparin administration or 2 to 4 hours after the last heparin dose.
- Monitor the patient postoperatively to provide early detection of motor blockade and consider use of minimal concentration of local anesthetics to enhance the early detection of a spinal hematoma.
- Although the occurrence of a bloody or difficult neuraxial needle placement may increase risk, there are no data to support mandatory cancellation of a case. Clinical

judgment is needed. If a decision is made to proceed, full discussion with the surgeon and careful postoperative monitoring are warranted.

The Safety of Neuraxial Anesthesia in the Patient Receiving Therapeutic and Full Anticoagulation with UH

These treatment/management modalities usually involve the injection of moderate amounts (5000 to 10,000 units) of IV UH intraoperatively. Injection is often done during vascular cases to prevent thrombus formation during arterial cross-clamping. Alternatively, one can inject 20,000 to 30,000 units of UH during a cardiac procedure to facilitate cardiac bypass. In both these situations, transient high levels of UH are present.

Several studies have demonstrated that spinal or epidural anesthesia followed by systemic heparinization with UH is relatively safe.[8,22,74,75] Perhaps the most significant study to evaluate the safety of therapeutic anticoagulation with UH in the presence of neuraxial anesthesia is by Rao and El-Etr.[8] These authors reported on the outcomes of 3146 patients receiving continuous epidural anesthesia and 847 patients receiving continuous spinal anesthesia for lower-extremity vascular procedures. Unfractionated heparin was administered 50 to 60 minutes after catheter placement to achieve an activated clotting time (ACT) of twice the normal value. The UH was given every 6 hours throughout the period of anticoagulation therapy, and the catheters were removed the next day, 1 hour before the administration of the next maintenance dose of UH. None of the patients developed spinal hematoma. This UH therapy was closely monitored, and catheters were removed when UH levels were relatively low.

In 1998 Liu and Mulroy[22] reported a total of greater than 1000 patients undergoing full intraoperative anticoagulation who also had received either a single-bolus spinal injection of opioids or an epidural opioid infusion without any incidence of spinal hematoma formation. The authors point out that communication with the surgeon regarding traumatic attempts and subsequent management of anticoagulation can be critical. Similarly, in 1998 Sanchez and Nygard[74] reported on 558 patients undergoing cardiac surgery who had epidural catheters placed following strict guidelines. These guidelines included placement of the epidural catheters the day before surgery; using a paramedian approach; obtaining an initial normal coagulation profile; carefully screening for preoperative drug use; and limiting catheter placement to two attempts. There was a zero incidence of spinal hematoma in this study.

Baron and colleagues[75] published a retrospective review in 1987 that evaluated 912 patients who had received continuous epidural analgesia while undergoing major vascular reconstruction of a lower extremity. The patients all received transient, full anticoagulation with UH at a dose of 75 IU/kg, in addition to a maintenance dose of 1000 IU/hr. None of these patients developed neurologic evidence of spinal hematoma. In this review 71% of the patients were male, the average age was 68.7 years, and the following hematologic studies were obtained preoperatively: hemoglobin level, platelet count, prothrombin time (PT), and aPTT. There was no reference to the timing of either catheter placement or removal in the Baron article.

The potential usefulness of thoracic epidural analgesia in patients undergoing cardiothoracic surgery has been shown in multiple studies. The benefits include improved pulmonary function[76] and postoperative hemodynamics in patients undergoing coronary artery bypass surgery.[77-79] Brodsky and colleagues[80] reported that the continuous lumbar epidural infusion of hydromorphone after thoracotomy provided excellent pain relief for patients.

In 2000 Ho and colleagues[81] published a statistical analysis suggesting that at most one spinal hematoma secondary to epidural catheter placement would occur for every 1520 patients undergoing coronary bypass surgery and receiving epidural analgesia. This analysis was based on the fact that a zero incidence of spinal hematoma formation had occurred in the more than 1500 reported uses of epidural analgesia in patients undergoing cardiac surgery. Thus, the aforementioned studies purporting the safety of epidural anesthesia in the fully anticoagulated patient may be tainted by small sample sizes and type II statistical error.

It is important to recognize that other members of the care team may institute an inappropriate therapeutic intervention with catastrophic results. Such an event recently happened to the author when a junior intensive care house officer administered an antithrombotic medication to one of our pediatric patients who had a functioning epidural catheter in place.[82] The patient had been up and ambulating before the administration of the alteplase. Almost immediately following the administration of the aforementioned drug, the child developed severe back pain and blood was noted in his epidural catheter. The house officer immediately removed the epidural catheter and within minutes our patient developed lower-extremity sensory and motor losses. Our anesthesia care team was promptly notified and a timely laminectomy and clot evacuation resulted in total recovery of neurologic function in this child 6 weeks later. This later case report reinforces the need for all members of the care teams involved in the management of complex cases to be familiar with the guidelines for the management of epidural or other indwelling catheters. Finally, this event occurred after the Rosen team had placed and managed slightly more than 1500 epidural catheters in infants and children undergoing total heparinization a cardiopulmonary bypass. I remind my readers of the Ho prediction[81] of one hematoma for each 1500 patients managed in this high-risk subgroup.

The studies in the previous section suggest that neuraxial anesthesia techniques in patients either therapeutically or fully anticoagulated with UH are relatively safe. However, Ruff and Dougherty[18] reported the occurrence of spinal hematomas in 7 of 347 patients who had initially presented with signs of cerebral ischemia. After a subarachnoid bleed had been ruled out, each patient immediately underwent a diagnostic lumbar puncture with a 20-gauge needle, followed by the institution of IV UH therapy. Unfortunately, the amount of UH administered to these patients was not reported in the Ruff and Dougherty[18] article. The article concludes that traumatic needle placement, initiation of IV UH within 1 hour of lumbar puncture, and concomitant aspirin therapy were all risk factors that led to the development of these seven spinal hematomas.

The risks and benefits of neuraxial anesthetic techniques in patients undergoing therapeutic and/or full anticoagulation with UH must be carefully considered. The complication of spinal hematoma formation, although rare, can be catastrophic. Risk factors contributing to spinal hematoma in these patients appear to be traumatic or difficult needle placement, preexisting coagulopathies, concomitant aspirin therapy, absence of monitoring of anticoagulation activity, and initiation of UH therapy within 1 hour of spinal or epidural needle placement.[8,18]

The therapeutic benefits of UH are limited by an increased risk of bleeding, which is at least a partially dose-dependent phenomenon.[83] To optimize the balance between efficacy and bleeding complications, physicians have adopted two dosing practices: (1) Frequent estimation of UH plasma concentrations using frequent serial evaluations of the aPTT, a relatively inexpensive laboratory test. However, with repeated serial testing, cost may become an issue. (2) Continuous IV administration of UH, in an attempt to allow multiple rapid dosage adjustments guided by aPTT values.[84]

As previously mentioned, the cost of the aPTT test is minimal; however, frequent testing does increase costs. Also, the requirement for repeated testing and need to maintain an IV infusion requires hospitalization for most patients,[85] which significantly increases the cost of therapy.[86] Therefore this increased cost and inconvenience associated with UH therapy must be considered when comparing it with the use of the more expensive drug, LMWH, which requires no laboratory monitoring or IV access. In addition, UH compared with LMWH has a higher incidence of bleeding complications when administered for therapeutic anticoagulation.

ASRA 2002 Guidelines for the Administration of Neuraxial Anesthesia in the Patient Fully Anticoagulated with UH[24]

Currently, insufficient data and experience are available to determine if the risk of neuraxial hematoma is increased when combining neuraxial techniques with the full anticoagulation of cardiac surgery. Postoperative monitoring of neurologic function and selection of neuraxial solutions that minimize sensory and motor block are recommended to facilitate detection of new or progressive neurodeficits.

Prolonged therapeutic anticoagulation appears to increase risk of spinal hematoma formation, especially if combined with other anticoagulants or thrombolytics. Therefore neuraxial blocks should be avoided in this clinical setting.

- If systemic anticoagulation therapy is begun with an epidural catheter in place, it is recommended to delay catheter removal for 2 to 4 hours after therapy discontinuation and evaluation of coagulation status. The concurrent use of medications that affect other components of the clotting mechanisms may increase the risk of bleeding complications for patients receiving standard heparin. These medications include antiplatelet medications, LMWH, and oral anticoagulants.

- The author believes that it is important to note that approximately one half of the spinal hematomas that have involved epidural catheters have occurred on the removal of the catheter. As previously mentioned, Vandermeulen and colleagues[14] found that between 1906 and 1994, 32 spinal hematomas occurred as the result of epidural catheter placements, and 15 of these 32 hematoma formations occurred immediately after catheter removal. Epidural catheter removal carries the same risk as catheter placement, and the same guidelines should be followed for both procedures.

THE EUROPEAN POSITION ON NEURAXIAL BLOCKADE IN PATIENTS WHO ARE RECEIVING OR WILL RECEIVE DVT PROPHYLAXIS WITH UH[87]

Since the early 1980s hospital patients in central continental Europe have primarily received either UH or LMWH as primary thromboprophylactic agents.[87] Tryba[87] found a low incidence of spinal hematoma formation in the large numbers of European patients who had received a spinal axis anesthetic and concurrent anticoagulation therapy. In Germany about 1.5 million patients per year receive this therapeutic and clinical management scheme. It is of note, however, that 70% to 75% of neuraxial blocks performed in Europe are single-shot spinal blocks.[87] Based on their experiences and available experimental data, Germany has promulgated guidelines regarding the dosing of the heparins in patients who had received or would receive a neuraxial anesthetic. The remainder of Europe has guidelines that differ little from those of Germany.[87] However, new updated European guidelines are in draft form at the time of this writing and should be published in summer 2009 (personal communication with ESRA President Giorgio Ivani). The evidence-based data used to draft the original European guidelines were derived primarily from papers/studies by Bergqvist,[88] Gogarten,[50,89] Heit,[21,90] Hirsh,[45,58,62,91,92] Horlocker,[24,93-95] Planes,[96] Tryba,[12,67,87,97] and Vandermeulen.[14,15]

Unfractionated Heparin in Low-Dose Regimen

- No increased risk of spinal hematoma has been observed with low-dose UH therapy, providing that a minimal interval between administration and puncture has been observed.[67,89,98]
- An interval of 4 hours between administration of UH and neuraxial block placement is recommended.[69,89]
- Unfractionated heparin should be administered 1 or more hours after neuraxial block placement.[89]
- No laboratory tests are suggested for the first 4 postoperative days; platelets should be checked on day 5 because of the risk of heparin-induced thrombocytopenia.[67,89]

Unfractionated Heparin in Full and Therapeutic Doses

- Compared with low-dose prophylaxis with UH, therapeutic doses of IV UH are associated with an increased risk of spinal bleeding. Thus, no neuraxial block or catheter removal should be performed in any patient receiving therapeutic anticoagulation.[14,87]

- If neuraxial block or catheter removal is required, UH administration must be stopped for at least 4 hours, and laboratory tests (ACT, aPTT, and platelets) evaluated before proceeding.[87]
- Because patients who receive intraoperative anticoagulation may benefit from a neuraxial block (e.g., patients undergoing vascular or cardiac surgery and patients with unstable angina),[2,99] IV UH (up to 5000 units) may not be considered an absolute contraindication, providing there is careful postoperative observation of the patient.[89]
- In the previous case, IV UH should be initiated no sooner than 1 hour after spinal puncture, the UH dose should be adjusted so that the aPTT does not exceed twice the normal value, and catheters should be removed no earlier than 2 to 4 hours after stopping the UH infusion.[87,89]
- If a bloody tap occurs during neuraxial puncture, surgery should be postponed for 12 hours. Alternatively, catheters may be inserted the night before the surgery.[87]
- Administration of low-dose IV UH (total dose 2000 units or less) has been shown to be effective in preventing thromboembolic complications during high-risk orthopedic surgery.[100] UH administration at this dosage does not result in a significant alteration of hemostasis and thus should not be considered as a contraindication to neuraxial blocks.[87]

EVIDENCE FOR PERFORMING NEURAXIAL BLOCKS IN THE PATIENT RECEIVING LOW-MOLECULAR-WEIGHT HEPARIN

Low-Molecular-Weight Heparin

Enoxaparin was the first commercially available LMWH. Low-molecular-weight heparins are produced by chemical or enzymatic depolymerization of UH, and they have a molecular weight of 4000 to 6500 daltons and contain polysaccharide chain lengths of 13 to 22 sugars.[90] The mechanism of action of LMWH is basically similar to that of UH in that both bind to ATIII and inhibit activation of coagulation factor Xa and to a lesser extent factor IIa. However, there is a difference in the relative potency of anti-Xa and anti-IIa when compared with UH; LMWH retains full anti-Xa activity with significantly less anti-IIa activity. The reason for this is that LMWH chain lengths that have a molecular weight of about 5000 daltons contain the pentasaccharide sequence, which preferentially inhibits factor Xa. It is not until the chain length is increased to about 15,000 to 30,000 daltons in weight that the chain is long enough to bind to factor IIa (thrombin). When compared with UH, LMWH does not usually prolong the aPTT to supranormal levels when prophylactic doses are used. A specific assay for anti-Xa activity may be used to monitor the biologic activity of LMWH; however, the monitoring of factor Xa levels is not recommended by ASRA.[24] This is because anti-Xa levels are not predictive of the development of hemorrhagic complications such as spinal hematoma formation. Finally,

the employment of ACT is not useful for assessing anticoagulation with LMWH.[101]

The reduction in molecular weight of LMWH creates pharmacologic advantages over UH because there is a marked reduction in the binding of LMWH to non-anticoagulant plasma proteins. This reduced binding reduces variations in plasma levels of the drug.[90] Low-molecular-weight heparin is dosed on a weight-adjusted scale, which results in very predictable and reproducible plasma levels. The bioavailability of LMWH is 90% when it is injected subcutaneously, compared with only 30% for UH. The plasma half-life of LMWH is 4.0 to 6.0 hours compared with 0.5 to 1.0 hours for UH. This longer half-life makes less frequent dosing possible. The peak anticoagulant effects of LMWH occur at approximately 3 to 4 hours following subcutaneous injection. Low-molecular-weight heparin is eliminated almost exclusively via renal excretion; consequently, significant accumulation occurs with renal insufficiency, and prophylactic therapy with LMWH should be avoided in patients with renal impairment.[90]

There is a difference in opinion between the United States (North America) and Europe with regard to DVT prophylaxis with LMWH when it is used in conjunction with a neuraxial anesthetic, and both views are presented in this chapter. A LMWH dose-response series by Planes and colleagues[96] is presented in some detail in the following paragraphs because it is the outcome of this trial that has been used to establish the current European dosing protocols. I leave it to my readers to decide which evidence-based protocol/guidelines (North American versus European) they wish to follow.

North American (United States) LMWH Dosing Regimens[102]

Abdominal Surgery

In patients undergoing abdominal surgery who are at risk for thromboembolic complications, the recommended dose of enoxaparin is 40 mg by subcutaneous injection, once daily. The initial administration is 2 hours before surgery.

Total Hip or Knee Arthroplasty

In patients undergoing THR or TKR, the recommended dose of enoxaparin is 30 mg injected subcutaneously every 12 hours. The initial administration should be 12 to 24 hours after surgery. Alternatively in patients undergoing THR, a dose of 40 mg injected subcutaneously once daily may be considered. The initial dose should be administered 12 ($\pm$3) hours before surgery. However, the usual dosing regimen for postsurgical DVT prophylaxis with enoxaparin in the United States is 30 mg injected subcutaneously every 12 hours, with the initial dose administered 12 to 24 hours postoperatively.

European LMWH Dosing Regimen

The European regimen is 40 mg injected subcutaneously once daily, with the initial dose usually administered 12 hours before surgery. The next dose is administered 24 hours after the initial dose.[97]

Safety and Efficacy of LMWH at Preventing DVT Formation

The results of three successive prospective clinical trials by Planes and colleagues,[103-105] attempting to define the once-daily dosing regimen protocol for enoxaparin in THR, suggest that 40 mg dosed once daily is the superior combination for THR.[96]

Planes and colleagues[103] randomized 228 patients to one of four groups. Group I ($n = 50$) received enoxaparin 60 mg once daily; group II ($n = 28$) received enoxaparin 30 mg twice daily; group III ($n = 50$) received enoxaparin 40 mg once daily; group IV ($n = 100$) received enoxaparin 20 mg twice daily. The groups were standardized to surgeon, operative approach, anesthesiologist, anesthetic, and postoperative physical prophylactic method. All therapies were initiated 12 hours before surgery. The number of red blood cell units transfused increased between doses of 40 and 60 mg ($p = 0.006$) and wound hematoma formation differed significantly between the groups. Group II (30 mg twice daily) had a wound hematoma occurrence rate of 22%; group I (60 mg once daily) had an occurrence of 12%; group III (40 mg once daily) had an occurrence of 6%; and group IV (20 mg twice daily) had an occurrence of 2%. In addition, the incidence of both distal and proximal DVT formation ranged from 6% to 8% in all of the groups. The proximal DVT rate in groups I, III, and IV ranged from 4% to 6%. However, no proximal DVT formations occurred in group II. It is this latter fact, no proximal DVT formations, coupled with a wound hematoma occurrence rate that prompted the U.S. Food and Drug Administration (FDA) to initially accept only the 30 mg twice-daily dosing regimen for enoxaparin. Finally, this author believes that the aforementioned data on the incidence of wound hematoma formation probably also apply to the relative risk that a patient will have the potential for the development of a spinal/epidural hematoma.

Planes and colleagues[104] studied two modes of administration enoxaparin 40 mg: group A, with two injections of 20 mg subcutaneously, and group B, with one injection of enoxaparin 40 mg, plus one injection of placebo, both administered subcutaneously. In all cases the first dose of enoxaparin was administered 12 hours before surgery. In group A, the patients received 20 mg in the evening of the first postoperative day (approximately 24 hours after initial dose) and every 12 hours thereafter. In group B, the patients received 40 mg at 8:00 PM on the day of surgery (approximately 24 hours after initial dose) and every evening thereafter. Patients with the following characteristics were excluded: age less than 45 years, weight less than 45 kg, past history of VTE, those receiving spinal anesthesia, those undergoing revision of THR, those with recent trauma, patients with thrombocytopenia, recent gastrointestinal (GI) bleeding, and ATIII deficiency, as well as those undergoing recent platelet therapy or anticoagulant therapy or having a preoperative aPTT 10 seconds longer than controls. The number of red blood cell units transfused did not differ significantly between groups. Wound hematoma formation occurred at the same frequency in both groups (5%). The incidence of total DVT was 1.7% in group A (20 mg twice daily) and 10.5% in group B

(40 mg once daily). The difference was found to be clinically insignificant ($p = 0.11$). No deaths or clinical signs and symptoms of PE were observed in either group.

Planes and colleagues[105] also performed a multicenter, double-blind, randomized, prospective study comparing enoxaparin with fixed doses of UH. Two hundred thirty-seven consecutive patients undergoing elective hip surgery received one of the following DVT prophylaxis regimens: (1) enoxaparin 40 mg, once daily, with initiation of therapy 12 hours before surgery ($n = 124$) and (2) UH 5000 IU, every 8 hours, initiated 2 hours before surgery ($n = 113$). The same exclusion and standardization criteria that were used in the enoxaparin trial (reference 97) were used in the present trial. Red blood cell transfusion requirements were higher in the UH group ($p = 0.035$). Wound hematoma formation was 6.4% in the enoxaparin group and 5% in the UH group, but three patients in the UH group required reoperation, whereas none of the patients in the enoxaparin group required surgical reintervention. There were no deaths in either group. Five patients developed PE, two in the enoxaparin group and three in the UH group. The incidence of total DVT in the enoxaparin group was 12.5%, compared with an incidence of 25% in the UH group ($p = 0.03$).

Data extrapolated from the Planes and colleagues series[96] demonstrate the relative safety and efficacy of enoxaparin 40 mg once daily, started the night before surgery. These data similarly show that the 40 mg daily regimen is superior to both the 60 mg daily and 30 mg twice-daily regimen in safety and that the efficacy of the higher doses is no better.

In a comprehensive review of the available literature, Geerts and colleagues[26] reported that LMWH is very effective for the prevention of DVT formation. Their review suggested that LMWH is more effective than UH for DVT prevention. The results of 21 trials involving 9364 patients[26] demonstrated a DVT risk reduction rate of 76% when LMWH therapy was employed and 68% reduction when low-dose UH was used, and these two therapeutic modalities were compared with control patients following general surgical procedures. In another series involving 30 trials and a total of 6216 patients,[26] a risk reduction of 78% was obtained with LMWH, 27% with low-dose UH, and 62% for adjusted-dose IV UH therapy when compared with controls after THR surgery.

In a double-blind randomized clinical trial, Turpie and colleagues[106] compared LMWH with placebo in patients undergoing elective hip surgery. Prophylactic treatment was begun postoperatively and continued for 14 days. In the placebo group ($n = 50$), 20 patients (51.3%) developed DVT. In the LMWH group ($n = 50$), four patients (10.8%) developed a DVT. The observed hemorrhagic rate was 4% in each group.

In a 1997 *New England Journal of Medicine* article, Weitz[107] reported that LMWH significantly reduced the risk of DVT formation in patients undergoing THR and TKR, as well as those sustaining multiple traumas. He also reported that LMWH was found to be more effective than low-dose subcutaneous UH,[108] and it was equal to[109] or superior to[110] adjusted-dose IV UH.

Evidence Regarding the Safety of Neuraxial Blockade in Patients Who Are Receiving or Will Be Receiving LMWH

A large number of patients have safely received neuraxial anesthesia in combination with prophylactic therapy with LMWH.[87,88,111] Tryba[87] reported that, in the European experience with LMWH, a dose of 40 mg or less once daily does not appear to increase the risk of spinal hematoma formation.

The administration of LMWH in patients undergoing neuraxial anesthesia was examined by Bergqvist and colleagues[88,111] in two reviews published in 1992 and 1993. In these reviews, they identified 19 articles involving 9013 patients who had safely received a combination of LMWH and neuraxial blockade.

Horlocker and Heit's 1997 review of the English language literature[7] identified 215 articles in which LMWH had been administered to surgical or obstetric patients. In 39 of the studies, representing 15,151 anesthetics, spinal or epidural anesthesia was used in combination with perioperative LMWH thromboprophylaxis. A single-dose spinal anesthetic was used in 7400 cases, a continuous spinal anesthetic in 20 cases, and an epidural anesthetic in 2957 cases. Low-molecular-weight heparin therapy was initiated preoperatively in almost 90% of the cases, typically using a regimen of 40 mg subcutaneously. There was a zero incidence of spinal hematoma formation in any of these patients.

Of the reports of spinal hematoma formation that have occurred in patients concurrently receiving DVT prophylaxis with LMWH and undergoing neuraxial blockade, the majority have occurred in patients receiving treatment in the United States. A large number of spinal hematomas have occurred since LMWH was introduced to the United States in 1993. Within 1 year of the introduction of enoxaparin into clinical practice in the United States there were two reported spinal hematomas.[112] The initial dosing regimen involved the utilization of 30 mg twice daily enoxaparin with the first dose administered as soon as possible after surgery. Unfortunately, more reports of epidural hematoma formations followed, and the manufacturer's prescribing information was changed in 1995 to recommend that the first dose be given 12 to 24 hours after surgery. By October 1995, 11 spinal hematomas had been reported to the MedWatch surveillance system. The drug label was again revised, expanding the Adverse Reactions and Warnings sections.[112] Between 1993 and 1997 more than 30 cases of spinal hematoma formations had been reported to the FDA's MedWatch surveillance system involving patients who had received LMWH therapy and a neuraxial block.[112] This prompted the FDA to issue a public health advisory in December 1997 asking physicians to carefully weigh the risks and benefits of neuraxial anesthesia in patients who had received or who would be receiving LMWH therapy in the postoperative period.[112] Within the FDA advisory it was noted that 75% of the spinal hematomas had occurred in elderly women undergoing orthopedic surgical procedures.

According to the MedWatch surveillance system, between 1993 and 2002 there were more than 80 reports of spinal or epidural hematoma formations in patients receiving neuraxial anesthesia with concurrent use of enoxaparin.[113] However, since 1998, the year in which the deliberations of the First ASRA Consensus Conference were published, there have only been 13 new cases of spinal hematomas following neuraxial blockade reported either through the MedWatch system or as a case report.[24] The majority of these patients had postoperative indwelling epidural catheters (10 of 13) or had received additional drugs affecting hemostasis, such as a nonsteroidal antiinflammatory drug (NSAID).[24,113]

The current FDA opinion is as follows:

1. When neuraxial anesthesia (epidural/spinal anesthesia) or spinal puncture is employed, patients anticoagulated or scheduled to be anticoagulated with LMWH or UH for prevention of thromboembolic complications are at risk for developing an epidural or spinal hematoma, which can result in long-term or permanent paralysis.
2. The risk of these events is increased by the use of indwelling epidural catheters for the provision of anesthesia/analgesia or by the concomitant use of drugs affecting hemostasis, such as NSAIDs, platelet inhibitors, and other anticoagulants.
3. Patients should be frequently monitored for signs and symptoms of neurologic impairment. If neurologic compromise is noted, urgent treatment is necessary.
4. Practitioners should carefully consider the potential benefit versus risk before performing a neuraxial intervention in patients anticoagulated or those who will be anticoagulated for thromboprophylaxis.

Guidelines for the Administration of Low-Molecular-Weight Heparin and the Concurrent Use of Neuraxial Anesthesia

The European Position on Neuraxial Blockade in Patients Who Are Receiving or Will Receive DVT Prophylaxis with LMWH[87,89]

The European experience surrounding the use of 40 mg or less of enoxaparin once daily clearly demonstrates that there is no increased risk of spinal hematoma formation, provided that a minimum interval of time between the administration of LMWH and neuraxial puncture is observed.[97] The current dosing regimen in Europe for enoxaparin (the most commonly used LMWH) is 40 mg subcutaneously once daily, with the initial dose administered 12 hours before surgery. However, several of my European colleagues have informed me that if they plan to place an epidural catheter for surgical anesthesia and postoperative analgesia, they administer the first dose of enoxaparin 12 or more hours after block placement. This usually translates into the morning following surgery. From the standpoint of epidural hematoma formation, this course of therapy is distinctly different from and has proven to be much safer than the regimen used in the United States (North America), in which 30 mg of enoxaparin is administered subcutaneously twice daily for TKR and THR, with the first administration 12 to 24 hours after surgery. However, the major distinction between the

European and North American protocols is the fact that spinal/epidural catheters can be left in place when one employs the European protocol/guidelines, whereas the North American (ASRA) guidelines call for their removal before the institution of anticoagulation therapy.[24] That said, 75% of the neuraxial blocks performed in Europe are single-shot spinal blocks.[87]

- An interval of at least 12 hours should elapse following the administration of LMWH and placement of neuraxial block.[87,89]
- The next dose of LMWH should be administered no sooner than 4 hours after puncture, resulting in an interval of approximately 8 hours until peak plasma concentrations occur.[87,89]
- In patients scheduled for neuraxial block, thromboembolism prophylaxis with LMWH should be initiated on the evening before surgery.[89] This dosage regimen results in a similar efficacy of thromboembolic prophylaxis, as with a dosage regimen starting on the morning of the surgery.[87,114,115]
- Catheter removal should occur at least 8 to 12 hours after the last LMWH administration or 1 to 2 hours before the next administration of LMWH. The next dose of LMWH should be delayed for 2 hours after catheter removal.[12,66]
- No laboratory tests are suggested for the first 4 postoperative days; however, a platelet count should be checked on day 5 because of the risk of heparin-induced thrombocytopenia.[89]

The ASRA 2002 Guidelines for the Safe Use of Neuraxial Anesthesia in the Patient Who Has Received Preoperative LMWH or Will Receive It in the Postoperative Period[24]

- The first subcutaneous dose of enoxaparin 30 mg is administered 12 to 24 hours following surgery (usually the morning following surgery), with the next 30 mg dose administered 12 hours later.
- It is imperative that all indwelling spinal/epidural catheters be removed at least 2 hours before the administration of the first dose of enoxaparin.
- Monitoring of the anti-Xa level is not recommended. The anti-Xa level is not predictive of the risk of bleeding and is therefore not helpful in the management of patients undergoing neuraxial blocks who have received LMWH.
- Antiplatelet or oral anticoagulant medications administered in combination with LMWH may increase the risks of spinal hematoma formation. Concomitant administration of medications affecting hemostasis, such as antiplatelet drugs, standard heparin, or dextran, represent an additional risk for the development of hemorrhagic complications during the perioperative period. This includes spinal/epidural hematoma formation. Education of the entire patient care team is necessary to avoid potentiation of the anticoagulant effects.
- The presence of blood during needle and catheter placement does not necessitate postponement of surgery. However, initiation of LMWH therapy in this setting should be delayed for 24 hours after surgery.

Traumatic needle or catheter placement may signify an increased risk of spinal hematoma, and it is recommended that this consideration be discussed with the surgeon.

Preoperative LMWH[24]

- Patients receiving preoperative LMWH can be assumed to have altered coagulation.
- A single-injection spinal anesthetic may be the safest neuraxial technique in patients receiving preoperative LMWH for thromboprophylaxis.
- In these patients needle placement should occur at least 10 to 12 hours after the last LMWH dose.
- Patients receiving higher doses of LMWH, such as enoxaparin 1 mg/kg q12h, enoxaparin 1.5 mg/kg daily, dalteparin 120 U/kg q12h, dalteparin 200 U/kg daily, or tinzaparin 175 U/kg daily will require delays of at least 24 hours before block placement.
- Neuraxial techniques should be avoided in patients who have received a dose of LMWH 2 hours before surgery (general surgery patients), because needle placement would occur during peak anticoagulant activity.

Postoperative LMWH[24]

- Patients with postoperative initiation of LMWH thromboprophylaxis may safely undergo single-injection and continuous catheter techniques. However, all catheters must be removed at least 2 hours before the administration of the first dose of LMWH. Management is based on total daily dose, timing of the first postoperative dose, and dosing schedule.

Twice-Daily Dosing[24]

- This dosage regimen approximates the United States' application (enoxaparin 30 mg q12h). This dosage may be associated with an increased risk of spinal hematoma.
- The first dose of LMWH should ideally be administered no earlier than 24 hours after surgery, regardless of anesthetic technique, and only in the presence of adequate hemostasis.
- Indwelling catheters should be removed before initiation of LMWH thromboprophylaxis. If a continuous technique is selected, the epidural catheter may be left indwelling overnight and removed the following day, with the first dose of LMWH administered 2 hours after catheter removal.

Once-daily Dosing[24]

- This dosing regimen approximates the European application (enoxaparin 40 mg/day).
- The first postoperative LMWH dose should be administered 6 to 8 hours after surgery.
- The second postoperative dose should occur no sooner than 24 hours after the first dose.
- Indwelling neuraxial catheters may be safely maintained. However, the catheter should be removed a

minimum of 10 to 12 hours after the last dose of LMWH. Subsequent LMWH dosing should occur at least 2 hours after catheter removal.

Deliberations on the Use of LMWH from the Third American Society of Regional Anesthesia (ASRA) Consensus Conference

The material presented at the Third American Society of Regional Anesthesia (ASRA) Consensus Conference (Vancouver, British Columbia, Canada, in April 2007) provided few new answers with respect to the use of LMWH in conjunction with neuraxial anesthesia.[25] The last published guidelines, which were updated as a result of the Second ASRA Consensus Conference held in Chicago in spring 2002,[24] remain in effect for the administration and management of LMWH and were not superceded or altered in any way by the deliberations in Vancouver. The author has been informed that the results of the Third Consensus Conference will be published in *Regional Anesthesia and Pain Medicine* in summer 2009.

At the Third Consensus Conference Horlocker and colleagues[25] indicated that the guidelines for antithrombotic therapy, including appropriate pharmacologic agent, degree of anticoagulation desired, and duration of therapy, continue to evolve. The American College of Chest Physicians (ACCP) updated its evidence-based guidelines in September 2004 based on the deliberations of the Seventh Conference on Antithrombotic and Thrombolytic Therapy.[116] The guidelines of the ACCP are derived from the presence or absence of asymptomatic thrombus formation, which are detected by ultrasonography or contrast venography and not clinical outcomes such as a reduction in the incidence of fatal PE or symptomatic DVT formation, and herein lies the problem. For an extensive discussion of this problem, see Chapter 50 of this text. In brief, many orthopedic surgeons do not believe that chest physicians, who do not perform surgery, should set the anticoagulation guidelines for surgeons.[25,117] The orthopedic surgeons point out that there has been no correlation between the reduction in the incidence of DVT formation and the incidence of fatal PE. The incidence of fatal PE remains 0.1% following joint surgery irrespective of the DVT rate.[117]

Horlocker summarized the new ACCP guidelines that apply to the use of LMWH as follows[25]:

1. There is a trend toward initiating thromboprophylaxis in close proximity to surgery. Early postoperative (and intraoperative) dosing of LMWH was associated with an increased risk of neuraxial bleeding.
2. The duration of prophylaxis has been extended to a minimum of 10 days following joint replacement or hip fracture surgery. The recommended duration for hip procedures is 28 to 35 days. It has been demonstrated that the risk of bleeding complications is increased with the duration of anticoagulation therapy. The interaction of prolonged thromboprophylaxis and previous neuraxial instrumentation, including difficult or traumatic needle insertion, is unknown.

AUTHOR'S RECOMMENDATIONS

There is very little question that patients undergoing surgical procedures that place them at a high risk for developing a postoperative thromboembolic complication will benefit from prophylactic anticoagulation. Choosing the best anticoagulant agent and dosing regimen for a particular patient undergoing a surgical procedure should be guided by the available literature and the individual patient. There are differences in the costs, convenience, safety, and efficacy of the available agents; however, patient safety has the highest priority when choosing an agent and dosing schedule. Nothing is as expensive as a bad outcome.

The practitioner must carefully consider each patient individually and weigh the risks of the procedure against the benefit of using a neuraxial technique. However, based on the current literature, it would appear that spinal anesthesia is associated with a lower risk of spinal/epidural hematoma formation,[12,14,70,72] and enoxaparin 40 mg once daily, with the first administration the evening before surgery, affords one the same efficacy of DVT prophylaxis as higher-dose regimens (30 mg twice daily), with less risk of surgical hematoma formation.[96] Although never prospectively studied, this reduced rate of surgical hematoma formation likely translates into a reduced risk of spinal/epidural hematoma formation as well. It is also important to consider the risks of spinal/epidural hematoma formation when removing an epidural catheter. Epidural catheter removal in the anticoagulated patient carries the same risk of hematoma formation as does catheter insertion.[14]

REFERENCES

1. Liu S, Carpenter RL, Neal JM: Epidural anesthesia and analgesia: Their role in postoperative outcome. *Anesthesiology* 1995;82: 1474-1506.
2. Christopherson R, Beattie C, Frank SM, et al: Perioperative morbidity in patients randomized to epidural or general anesthesia for lower extremity vascular surgery. Perioperative Ischemia Randomized Anesthesia Trial Study Group. *Anesthesiology* 1993;79:422-434.
3. Mathews ET, Abrams LD: Intrathecal morphine in open heart surgery. *Lancet* 1980;2:543.
4. Rosen DA, Rosen KR, Hammer GB: Pro: Regional anesthesia is an important component of the anesthetic technique for pediatric patients undergoing cardiac surgical procedures. *J Cardiothorac Vasc Anesth* 2002;16:374-378.
5. Keith I: Anaesthesia and blood loss in total hip replacement. *Anaesthesia* 1977;32:444-450.
6. Modig J, Borg T, Karlstrom G, et al: Thromboembolism after total hip replacement: Role of epidural and general anesthesia. *Anesth Analg* 1983;62:174-180.
7. Horlocker TT, Heit JA: Low molecular weight heparin: Biochemistry, pharmacology, perioperative prophylaxis regimens, and guidelines for regional anesthetic management. *Anesth Analg* 1997;85:874-885.
8. Rao TL, El-Etr AA: Anticoagulation following placement of epidural and subarachnoid catheters: An evaluation of neurologic sequelae. *Anesthesiology* 1981;55:618-620.
9. Horlocker TT, McGregor DG, Matsushige DK, et al: A retrospective review of 4767 consecutive spinal anesthetics: Central nervous system complications. Perioperative Outcomes Group. *Anesth Analg* 1997;84:578-584.
10. Horlocker TT, McGregor DG, Matsushige DK, et al: Neurologic complications of 603 consecutive continuous spinal anesthetics

using macrocatheter and microcatheter techniques. Perioperative Outcomes Group. *Anesth Analg* 1997;84:1063-1070.

11. Abel HT, Mesick JM, Strickland RA, Schroeder DR: Neurologic complications following placement of 4392 consecutive epidural catheters in anesthetized patients. *Reg Anesth Pain Med* 1998;23:3.

12. Tryba M: [Epidural regional anesthesia and low molecular heparin: Pro]. *Anasthesiol Intensivmed Notfallmed Schmerzther* 1993;28:179-181.

13. Lowson SM, Goodchild CS: Low-dose heparin therapy and spinal anaesthesia. *Anaesthesia* 1989;44:67-68.

14. Vandermeulen EP, Van Aken H, Vermylen J: Anticoagulants and spinal-epidural anesthesia. *Anesth Analg* 1994;79:1165-1177.

15. Vandermeulen E, Gogarten W, Van Aken H: [Risks and complications following peridural anesthesia]. *Anaesthesist* 1997;46(suppl)3:S179-S186.

16. Russell NA, Benoit BG: Spinal subdural hematoma. A review. *Surg Neurol* 1983;20:133-137.

17. Horlocker TT: Complications of spinal and epidural anesthesia. *Anesthesiol Clin North Am* 2000;18:461-485.

18. Ruff RL, Dougherty JH Jr: Complications of lumbar puncture followed by anticoagulation. *Stroke* 1981;12:879-881.

19. Horlocker TT: When to remove a spinal or epidural catheter in an anticoagulated patient. *Reg Anesth* 1993;18:264-265.

20. Hull RD, Pineo GF: Extended prophylaxis against venous thromboembolism following total hip and knee replacement. *Haemostasis* 1999;29(suppl)S1:23-31.

21. Heit JA: Venous thromboembolism epidemiology: Implications for prevention and management. *Semin Thromb Hemost* 2002;28(suppl)2:3-13.

22. Liu SS, Mulroy MF. Neuraxial anesthesia and analgesia in the presence of standard heparin. *Reg Anesth Pain Med* 1998;23:157-163.

23. Horlocker TT, Wedel DJ: Neuraxial block and low molecular weight heparin: Balancing perioperative analgesia thromboprophylaxis. *Reg Anesth Pain Med* 1998;23:164-177.

24. Horlocker TT, Wedel DJ, Benzon H, et al: Regional anesthesia in the anticoagulated patient: Defining the risks (the second ASRA Consensus Conference on Neuraxial Anesthesia and Anticoagulation). *Reg Anesth Pain Med* 2003;28:172-197.

25. Horlocker TT, Rowlingson JC, Wedel D, et al: Prevention of spinal hematoma—the Third ASRA Consensus Conference on Neuraxial Anesthesia and Anticoagulation, 32nd Annual Regional Anesthesia Meeting and Workshops Syllabus (Vancouver, BC, April 2007), pp 217-236.

26. Geerts WH, Heit JA, Clagett GP, et al: Prevention of venous thromboembolism. *Chest* 2001;119:132S-175S.

27. Hull RD, Pineo GF: Prophylaxis of deep venous thrombosis and pulmonary embolism. Current recommendations. *Med Clin North Am* 1998;82:477-493.

28. Hull RD, Feldstein W, Stein PD, Pineo GF: Cost-effectiveness of pulmonary embolism diagnosis. *Arch Intern Med* 1996;156:68-72.

29. Davidson BL, Elliott CG, Lensing AW: Low accuracy of color Doppler ultrasound in the detection of proximal leg vein thrombosis in asymptomatic high-risk patients. The RD Heparin Arthroplasty Group. *Ann Intern Med* 1992;117:735-738.

30. Kearon C, Ginsberg JS, Douketis J, et al: Management of suspected deep venous thrombosis in outpatients by using clinical assessment and D-dimer testing. *Ann Intern Med* 2001;135:108-111.

31. Hull R, Pineo G: A synthetic pentasaccharide for the prevention of deep-vein thrombosis. *N Engl J Med* 2001;345:291, author reply 292.

32. Hull RD, Feldstein W, Pineo GF, Raskob GE: Cost effectiveness of diagnosis of deep vein thrombosis in symptomatic patients. *Thromb Haemost* 1995;74:189-196.

33. Barnes RW, Nix ML, Barnes CL, et al: Perioperative asymptomatic venous thrombosis: Role of duplex scanning versus venography. *J Vasc Surg* 1989;9:251-260.

34. Comerota AJ, Katz ML, Greenwald LL, et al: Venous duplex imaging: Should it replace hemodynamic tests for deep venous thrombosis? *J Vasc Surg* 1990;11:53-59, discussion 59-61.

35. Agnelli G, Cosmi B, Ranucci V, et al: Impedance plethysmography in the diagnosis of asymptomatic deep vein thrombosis in hip surgery. A venography-controlled study. *Arch Intern Med* 1991;151:2167-2171.

36. Wells PS, Hirsh J, Anderson DR, et al: Accuracy of clinical assessment of deep-vein thrombosis. *Lancet* 1995;345:1326-1330.

37. Raskob GE, Hull RD: Diagnosis of pulmonary embolism. *Curr Opin Hematol* 1999;6:280-284.

38. Hull R, Hirsh J, Sackett DL, Stoddart G: Cost effectiveness of clinical diagnosis, venography, and noninvasive testing in patients with symptomatic deep-vein thrombosis. *N Engl J Med* 1981;304:1561-1567.

39. Mantilla CB, Horlocker TT, Schroeder DR, et al: Frequency of myocardial infarction, pulmonary embolism, deep venous thrombosis, and death following primary hip or knee arthroplasty. *Anesthesiology* 2002;96:1140-1146.

40. Brummel KE, Paradis SG, Butenas S, Mann KG: Thrombin functions during tissue factor-induced blood coagulation. *Blood* 2002;100:148-152.

41. Mann KG, Butenas S, Brummel K: The dynamics of thrombin formation. *Arterioscler Thromb Vasc Biol* 2003;23:17-25.

42. Meijers JC, Tekelenburg WL, Bouma BN, et al: High levels of coagulation factor XI as a risk factor for venous thrombosis. *N Engl J Med* 2000;342:696-701.

43. Bajaj SP, Joist JH: New insights into how blood clots: Implications for the use of APTT and PT as coagulation screening tests and in monitoring of anticoagulant therapy. *Semin Thromb Hemost* 1999;25:407-418.

44. Rosenberg RD, Damus PS: The purification and mechanism of action of human antithrombin-heparin cofactor. *J Biol Chem* 1973;248:6490-6505.

45. Hirsh J, Levine MN: Low molecular weight heparin. *Blood* 1992;79:1-17.

46. Van der Velde EA, Poller L: The APTT monitoring of heparin: The ISTH/ICSH collaborative study. *Thromb Haemost* 1995;73: 73-81.

47. Bratt G, Tornebohm E, Granqvist S, et al: A comparison between low molecular weight heparin (KABI 2165) and standard heparin in the intravenous treatment of deep venous thrombosis. *Thromb Haemost* 1985;54:813-817.

48. Rosenbloom DG Jr: Argument against monitoring levels of anti-factor Xa in conjunction with low molecular-weight heparin therapy. *Can J Hosp Pharm* 2002;15-19.

49. Evans RW: Complications of lumbar puncture. *Neurol Clin* 1998;16:83-105.

50. Gogarten W, Van Aken H, Wulf H, et al: [Para-spinal regional anesthesia and prevention of thromboembolism/anticoagulation. Recommendations of the German Society of Anesthesiology and Intensive Care Medicine, October 1997]. *Urologe A* 1998;37:347-351.

51. Moen V, Dahlgren N, Irestedt L: Severe neurological complications after central neuraxial blockades in Sweden 1990-1999. *Anesthesiology* 2004;101:950-959.

52. Schroeder DR: Statistics: Detecting a rare adverse drug reaction using spontaneous reports. *Reg Anesth Pain Med* 1998;23(suppl 2):183-189.

53. Sandhu H, Morley-Forster P, Spadafora S: Epidural hematoma following epidural analgesia in a patient receiving unfractionated heparin for thromboprophylaxis. *Reg Anesth Pain Med* 2000;25:72-75.

54. Kreppel D, Antoniadis G, Seeling W: Spinal hematoma: A literature survey with meta-analysis of 613 patients. *Neurosurg Rev* 2003;26:1-49.

55. Lawton MT, Porter RW, Heiserman JE, et al: Surgical management of spinal epidural hematoma: Relationship between surgical timing and neurological outcome. *J Neurosurg* 1995;83:1-7.

56. Crafoord CJB: Heparin as a prophylactic against thrombosis. *JAMA* 1941;2831.

57. Anand S, Ginsberg JS, Kearon C, et al: The relation between the activated partial thromboplastin time response and recurrence in patients with venous thrombosis treated with continuous intravenous heparin. *Arch Intern Med* 1996;156:1677-1681.

58. Hirsh J, Raschke R, Warkentin TE, et al: Heparin: Mechanism of action, pharmacokinetics, dosing considerations, monitoring, efficacy, and safety. *Chest* 1995;108:258S-75S.

59. Bjork I, Lindahl U: Mechanism of the anticoagulant action of heparin. *Mol Cell Biochem* 1982;48:161-182.

60. Ellis V, Scully MF, Kakkar VV: The relative molecular mass dependence of the anti-factor Xa properties of heparin. *Biochem J* 1986;238:329-333.

61. Warkentin TE, Levine MN, Hirsh J, et al: Heparin-induced thrombocytopenia in patients treated with low-molecular-weight heparin or unfractionated heparin. *N Engl J Med* 1995;332: 1330-1335.

62. Hirsh J, Warkentin TE, Raschke R, et al: Heparin and low-molecular-weight heparin: Mechanisms of action, pharmacokinetics, dosing considerations, monitoring, efficacy, and safety. *Chest* 1998;114:489S-510S.

63. Poller L, Taberner DA, Sandilands DG, Galasko CS: An evaluation of APTT monitoring of low-dose heparin dosage in hip surgery. *Thromb Haemost* 1982;47:50-53.

64. Collins R, Scrimgeour A, Yusuf S, Peto R: Reduction in fatal pulmonary embolism and venous thrombosis by perioperative administration of subcutaneous heparin. Overview of results of randomized trials in general, orthopedic, and urologic surgery. *N Engl J Med* 1988;318:1162-1173.

65. Young E, Cosmi B, Weitz J, Hirsh J: Comparison of the non-specific binding of unfractionated heparin and low molecular weight heparin (enoxaparin) to plasma proteins. *Thromb Haemost* 1993;70:625-630.

66. Schwander D, Bachmann F: [Heparin and spinal or epidural anesthesia: Decision analysis]. *Ann Fr Anesth Reanim* 1991;10: 284-296.

67. Tryba M: [Hemostatic requirements for the performance of regional anesthesia. Workshop on hemostatic problems in regional anesthesia]. *Reg Anesth* 1989;12:127-131.

68. Allemann BH, Gerber H, Gruber UF: [Perispinal anesthesia and subcutaneous administration of low-dose heparin-dihydergot for prevention of thromboembolism]. *Anaesthetist* 1983;32:80-83.

69. Gogarten W, Van Aken H: [Epidural administration of opioids in labor: pro]. *Anasthesiol Intensivmed Notfallmed Schmerzther* 1997;32: 253-255.

70. Darnat S, Guggiari M, Grob R, et al: [A case of spinal extradural hematoma during the insertion of an epidural catheter]. *Ann Fr Anesth Reanim* 1986;5:550-552.

71. Dupeyrat A, Dequire PM, Merouani A, et al: [Subarachnoid hematoma and spinal anesthesia]. *Ann Fr Anesth Reanim* 1990;9:560-562.

72. Metzger G, Singbartl G: Spinal epidural hematoma following epidural anesthesia versus spontaneous spinal subdural hematoma. Two case reports. *Acta Anaesthesiol Scand* 1991;35:105-107.

73. Jooste EH, Chalifoux T, Broadman LM: A perioperative strategy for the placement of a thoracic epidural catheter in a pediatric patient on high-dose enoxaparin. *Pediatr Anesth* 2007;17: 907-909.

74. Sanchez R, Nygard E: Epidural anesthesia in cardiac surgery: Is there an increased risk? *J Cardiothorac Vasc Anesth* 1998;12: 170-173.

75. Baron HC, LaRaja RD, Rossi G, Atkinson D: Continuous epidural analgesia in the heparinized vascular surgical patient: A retrospective review of 912 patients. *J Vasc Surg* 1987;6:144-146.

76. Stenseth R, Bjella L, Berg EM, et al: Effects of thoracic epidural analgesia on pulmonary function after coronary artery bypass surgery. *Eur J Cardiothorac Surg* 1996;10:859-865, discussion 866.

77. Liem TH, Booij LH, Hasenbos MA, Gielen MJ: Coronary artery bypass grafting using two different anesthetic techniques: Part I: Hemodynamic results. *J Cardiothorac Vasc Anesth* 1992;6: 148-155.

78. Liem TH, Hasenbos MA, Booij LH, Gielen MJ: Coronary artery bypass grafting using two different anesthetic techniques: Part 2: Postoperative outcome. *J Cardiothorac Vasc Anesth* 1992;6: 156-161.

79. Liem TH, Booij LH, Gielen MJ, et al: Coronary artery bypass grafting using two different anesthetic techniques: Part 3: Adrenergic responses. *J Cardiothorac Vasc Anesth* 1992;6:162-167.

80. Brodsky JB, Chaplan SR, Brose WG, Mark JB: Continuous epidural hydromorphone for postthoracotomy pain relief. *Ann Thorac Surg* 1990;50:888-893.

81. Ho AM, Chung DC, Joynt GM: Neuraxial blockade and hematoma in cardiac surgery: Estimating the risk of a rare adverse event that has not (yet) occurred. *Chest* 2000;117:551-555.

82. Rosen D, Hawkinberry D, Rosen K, et al: An epidural hematoma in an adolescent patient after cardiac surgery. *Anesth Analg* 2004; 98:966-969.

83. Wester JP, de Valk HW, Nieuwenhuis HK, et al: Risk factors for bleeding during treatment of acute venous thromboembolism. *Thromb Haemost* 1996;76:682-688.

84. Morris TA: Heparin and low molecular weight heparin: Background and pharmacology. *Clin Chest Med* 2003;24:39-47.

85. Hirsch DR, Lee TH, Morrison RB, et al: Shortened hospitalization by means of adjusted-dose subcutaneous heparin for deep venous thrombosis. *Am Heart J* 1996;131:276-280.

86. Gould MK, Dembitzer AD, Doyle RL, et al: Low-molecular-weight heparins compared with unfractionated heparin for treatment of acute deep venous thrombosis. A meta-analysis of randomized, controlled trials. *Ann Intern Med* 1999;130:800-809.

87. Tryba M: European practice guidelines: Thromboembolism prophylaxis and regional anesthesia. *Reg Anesth Pain Med* 1998; 23:178-182.

88. Bergqvist D, Lindblad B, Matzsch T: Low molecular weight heparin for thromboprophylaxis and epidural/spinal anaesthesia: Is there a risk? *Acta Anaesthesiol Scand* 1992;36:605-609.

89. Gogarten W, Van Aken H, Wulf H, Klose R, Vandermeulen E, Harenberg J: Regional anesthesia and thromboembolism prophylaxis/anticoagulation. *Anasthesiol Intensivmed Notfallmed Schmerzther* 1997;623-628.

90. Heit JA: Low-molecular-weight heparin: Biochemistry, pharmacology, and concurrent drug precautions. *Reg Anesth Pain Med* 1998;23:135-139.

91. Hirsh J, Levine MN: Low molecular weight heparin: Laboratory properties and clinical evaluation. A review. *Eur J Surg Suppl* 1994;9-22.

92. Hirsh J, Warkentin TE, Shaughnessy SG, et al: Heparin and low-molecular-weight heparin: Mechanisms of action, pharmacokinetics, dosing, monitoring, efficacy, and safety. *Chest* 2001;119:64S-94S.

93. Horlocker TT: Regional anesthesia and analgesia in the patient receiving thromboprophylaxis. *Reg Anesth* 1996;21:503-507.

94. Horlocker TT, Wedel DJ: Neurologic complications of spinal and epidural anesthesia. *Reg Anesth Pain Med* 2000;25:83-98.

95. Horlocker TT: Thromboprophylaxis and neuraxial anesthesia. *Orthopedics* 2003;26:S243-S249.

96. Planes A, Vochelle N, Fagola M, et al: Once-daily dosing of enoxaparin (a low molecular weight heparin) in prevention of deep vein thrombosis after total hip replacement. *Acta Chir Scand Suppl* 1990;556:108-115.

97. Tryba M, Wedel DJ: Central neuraxial block and low molecular weight heparin (enoxaparine): Lessons learned from different dosage regimes in two continents. *Acta Anaesthesiol Scand Suppl* 1997;111:100-104.

98. Prevention of postoperative venous thrombosis and pulmonary embolism. Consensus conference. *Rev Pneumol Clin* 1991;47 (6):265-269.

99. Christopherson R, Glavan NJ, Norris EJ, et al: Control of blood pressure and heart rate in patients randomized to epidural or general anesthesia for lower extremity vascular surgery. Perioperative Ischemia Randomized Anesthesia Trial (PIRAT) Study Group. *J Clin Anesth* 1996;8:578-584.

100. Huo MH, Salvati EA, Sharrock NE, et al: Intraoperative heparin thromboembolic prophylaxis in primary total hip arthroplasty. A prospective, randomized, controlled, clinical trial. *Clin Orthop* 1992;35-46.

101. Henry TD, Satran D, Knox LL, et al: Are activated clotting times helpful in the management of anticoagulation with subcutaneous low-molecular-weight heparin? *Am Heart J* 2001;142:590-593.

102. *Physicians' desk reference*. Montvale, NJ, Thompson Healthcare, 2003, p 57.

103. Planes A, Vochelle N, Ferru J, et al: Enoxaparine low molecular weight heparin: Its use in the prevention of deep venous thrombosis following total hip replacement. *Haemostasis* 1986;16: 152-158.

104. Planes A, Vochelle N, Mansat C: Prevention of deep venous thrombosis (DVT) after total hip replacement by enoxaparin (LOVENOX): One daily injection of 40 mg versus two daily injections of 20 mg. *Thromb Haemost* 1987;58:117.

105. Planes A, Vochelle N, Mazas F, et al: Prevention of postoperative venous thrombosis: A randomized trial comparing unfractionated heparin with low molecular weight heparin in

patients undergoing total hip replacement. *Thromb Haemost* 1988;60:407-410.

106. Turpie AG, Levine MN, Hirsh J, et al: A randomized controlled trial of a low-molecular-weight heparin (enoxaparin) to prevent deep-vein thrombosis in patients undergoing elective hip surgery. *N Engl J Med* 1986;315:925-929.

107. Weitz JI: Low-molecular-weight heparins. *N Engl J Med* 1997;337:688-698.

108. Nurmohamed MT, Rosendaal FR, Buller HR, et al: Low-molecular-weight heparin versus standard heparin in general and orthopaedic surgery: A meta-analysis. *Lancet* 1992;340:152-156.

109. TGHATG Group: Prevention of deep venous thrombosis with low molecular weight heparin in patients undergoing total hip replacement: A randomized trial. *Arch Orthop Trauma Surg* 1992;111:110-120.

110. Dechavanne M, Ville D, Berruyer M, et al: Randomized trial of a low-molecular-weight heparin (Kabi 2165) versus adjusted-dose subcutaneous standard heparin in the prophylaxis of deep-vein thrombosis after elective hip surgery. *Haemostasis* 1989;19:5-12.

111. Bergqvist D, Lindblad B, Matzsch T: Risk of combining low molecular weight heparin for thromboprophylaxis and epidural or spinal anesthesia. *Semin Thromb Hemost* 1993;19(suppl) 1:147-151.

112. Horlocker TT: Low molecular weight heparin and neuraxial anesthesia. *Thromb Res* 2001;101:V141-V154.

113. Food and Drug Administration: Available at www.fda.gov/medwatch, 2003.

114. Avikainen V, von Bonsdorff H, Partio E, et al: Low molecular weight heparin (enoxaparin) compared with unfractionated heparin in prophylaxis of deep venous thrombosis and pulmonary embolism in patients undergoing hip replacement. *Ann Chir Gynaecol* 1995;84:85-90.

115. Haas S, Flosbach CW: Prevention of postoperative thromboembolism with enoxaparin in general surgery: A German multicenter trial. *Semin Thromb Hemost* 1993;19(suppl)1:164-173.

116. Geerts WH, Pineo GF, Heit JA, et al: Prevention of venous thromboembolism: The Seventh ACCP Conference on Antithrombotic and Thrombolytic Therapy. *Chest* 2004;126(suppl): 338S-400S.

117. Callaghan JJ, Dorr LD, Engh GA, et al: Prophylaxis for thromboembolic disease: Recommendations from the American College of Chest Physicians—are they appropriate for Orthopaedic Surgeons? *J Arthroplasty* 2005;20:273-274.

52 Is Regional Anesthesia Appropriate for Outpatient Surgery?

Michael F. Mulroy, MD, and Wyndam Strodtbeck, MD

Outpatient surgery has increased dramatically in the last 25 years in the United States, both in volume and as a percentage of the total procedures done. It now constitutes over 60% of surgery performed in most medical centers, and it has initiated major revisions in the approach to anesthetic management and occasioned the development of new drugs and techniques. Outpatient anesthesia requires more rapid recovery and faster return to full mental function than standard inpatient procedures. It also requires minimum frequency of nausea, vomiting, and postoperative pain that might otherwise delay hospital discharge or precipitate unplanned overnight admission. The emphasis on home discharge has also elevated the patient's perception of "satisfactory" anesthesia, which now includes greater emphasis on alertness and a sense of well-being. Fortunately, new general anesthetic agents meet many of these requirements, especially rapid induction and emergence, which will theoretically improve the turnover in ambulatory surgery units.

Local anesthesia for the performance of surgery is ideal in that local anesthetics cause no loss of consciousness and provide excellent residual postoperative analgesia. This combination makes local anesthetic agents attractive options for outpatient surgery, where rapid discharge with minimal nausea and sedation is important to health care providers and patients.[1] Prospective comparisons of regional and general techniques confirm faster discharge with peripheral nerve blocks, as well as with local anesthesia.[2] Neuraxial techniques (spinal and epidural) have also been advocated because of their rapid onset of dense anesthesia. Neuraxial approaches, however, require resolution of the block before a patient can ambulate, and they obviously require some alternative method of postoperative analgesia.

Although there are several advantages to regional techniques, there are also questions raised about whether the performance of these blocks requires more time than the initiation of general anesthesia and thus may be deleterious to the overall efficiency of an outpatient unit. Similarly, there have been concerns that regional techniques, especially the peripheral nerve blocks, are not as reliable as the general anesthesia techniques and thus may further delay surgery. There is also the issue of possible complications associated with regional techniques, particularly the potential for postspinal headache and, more recently, transient neurologic symptoms (TNS) after spinal anesthesia.[3] Thus, it is legitimate to question whether regional anesthetic techniques are truly appropriate in the outpatient setting.

OPTIONS

Major options available in outpatient anesthesia are local, general, and regional techniques. For the sake of focus, this chapter will not include a discussion of local anesthesia techniques because these have universally been shown to be ideal techniques in outpatient anesthesia. This includes the use of local anesthesia for retrobulbar, peribulbar, or topical anesthesia for cataract surgery, which has been associated with a low risk of morbidity and with rapid discharge and high satisfaction in the elderly high-risk patient group undergoing this operation. Local techniques are also excellent for other superficial surgeries, such as hernia repair, breast biopsy, and perianal procedures.

General anesthesia has emerged as the most frequently used alternative because of the newer drugs available. The introduction of rapid-induction and fast-emergence general anesthetic agents (sevoflurane, desflurane, and propofol) in the last 20 years has produced dramatic improvement in the early emergence from general anesthesia. These advantages are balanced by side effects. The absence of analgesia in the postoperative period necessitates the addition of opioids and their attendant mental obtundation and nausea. The inhalation agents themselves continue to be associated with a 20% to 50% risk of postoperative nausea and vomiting,[4] although this can be minimized by generous use of prophylactic medication. Propofol appears to be associated with a significantly lower frequency of this complication but requires greater resources to administer and is no less expensive than the volatile drugs.

The regional techniques offer a third alternative, also with advantages and drawbacks. The two major categories are peripheral nerve blockade and neuraxial blockade, though one might include the use of continuous peripheral nerve catheters as an emerging third application.[5] There are multiple reports of peripheral nerve blockade, including intravenous regional anesthesia of the upper and lower extremities, as well as specific nerve blocks of the brachial and lumbar plexus (which have been summarized in a recent meta-analysis[6]). In general they require somewhat longer to perform and a longer time for initiation for adequate anesthesia than either general anesthesia or the neuraxial techniques. Neuraxial blockade includes the use of spinal as well as epidural and caudal injection. Caudal anesthesia is primarily limited to pediatric practice, where it is usually performed as an adjunct to a general anesthetic in this patient population. Spinal anesthesia should be the most effective example of regional techniques in the outpatient setting because of its simplicity of performance and rapidity of onset, but may be limited by prolonged discharge times.

EVIDENCE

There have been few prospective randomized comparative trials of regional techniques versus general anesthesia. Most of the reports are performed by enthusiastic supporters of regional anesthesia, who usually do not include a comparative general anesthesia group. All these reports are positive in their descriptions of analgesia, discharge times, and patient satisfaction. Although randomized blinded comparative studies are more desirable, it is impossible to perform a "blinded" study comparing the two because even the most naive of observers would be able to distinguish the presence of a local anesthetic block from a general anesthetic. It is also difficult for many procedures and many patient populations to successfully randomize patients to different techniques. Nevertheless, a literature search and meta-analysis has reviewed 15 studies comparing general anesthesia with neuraxial blockade (Table 52-1) and 7 comparing peripheral nerve blockade to general (Table 52-2).[6] These studies support the use of regional techniques when compared with general anesthesia in terms of superior analgesia, but raise concerns about the time involved and the impact on significant outcomes such as discharge time (Table 52-3).

The evidence regarding regional techniques compared with general anesthesia has been reviewed with respect to several outcomes. Seven studies of neuraxial block and six trials of peripheral nerve catheters that measured induction time showed an increase by 8 to 9 minutes in induction time associated with regional techniques. Two of the studies showed that blocks performed in an induction room outside the operating room during the room turnover process could allow for the total anesthesia time to be competitive with general anesthesia.[7,8] Two other studies looking at the utilization of block rooms showed actual reduction in induction time.[9,10] The use of rapid-acting drugs, such as 2-chloroprocaine, and the presence of experienced anesthesiologists also appear to reduce the additional time required for regional techniques.[11,12] Nevertheless, the overall data indicate that there is greater time required for the performance of blocks and the onset of satisfactory analgesia.

Ten studies of neuraxial blockade showed no decrease in postanesthesia care unit (PACU) time, or in the rate of PACU bypass, probably related to the persistent immobility associated with neuraxial anesthesia in the early

Table 52-1	Central Neuraxial Block versus General Anesthesia for Ambulatory Surgery			
Outcome	Number of Trials	Neuraxial (Mean)	General (Mean)	Odds Ratio or WMD (95% CI)
Induction time (min)	7	17.8	7.8	8.1 (4.1-12.1)[†]
PACU time (min)	10	56.1	51.9	0.42 (-7.1-7.9)
VAS in PACU	7	12.7	24.4	−9 (−15.5 to −2.6)*
Nausea	12	5%	14.7%0	0.40 (0.15-1.06)
Phase 1 bypass	4	30.8%	13.5%	5.4 (0.6-53.6)
Need for analgesia	11	31%	56%	0.32 (0.18-0.57)[†]
ASU discharge time (min)	14	190	153	34.6 (13-56.1)*
Patient satisfaction	11	81%	78%	1.5 (0.8-23.1)

Adapted from Liu SS, Strodtbeck WM, Richman JM, Wu CL: A comparison of regional versus general anesthesia for ambulatory anesthesia: A meta-analysis of randomized controlled trials. *Anesth Analg* 2005;101:1634-1642.
CI, confidence interval; WMD, weighted mean difference.
*p <0.01.
[†]p <0.001.

recovery phase. In contrast, peripheral nerve blockade allowed for earlier discharge from phase 1 PACU, as well as a higher percentage of eligibility to bypass phase 1 at the end of surgery.

Both neuraxial blockade and peripheral nerve block were associated with significantly lower visual analog scale (VAS) scores in the PACU, as well as a significantly reduced requirement for postoperative analgesics in the PACU. Despite better pain relief, as noted previously there was no difference in the PACU time with neuraxial blockade.

With neuraxial blockade, there was a 40% reduction in nausea associated with neuraxial blockade, but this was not statistically different from the general anesthesia group. Peripheral nerve blockade did provide a significant fivefold decrease in nausea.

Despite the significant advantages in pain, analgesic requirement, and nausea with peripheral nerve blockade, there was no difference in the total time for discharge from the ambulatory surgical unit (ASU). In contrast, neuraxial blockade actually required a longer discharge time than general anesthesia in the 14 trials that reported discharge times, with an average prolongation of 35 minutes. Although part of this prolonged discharge may have been related to the use of a longer-acting spinal anesthetic (bupivacaine was used in six trials, although in low doses), additional requirements frequently associated with neuraxial block in an ASU

Table 52-2	**Peripheral Nerve Block versus General Anesthesia for Ambulatory Surgery**			
Outcome	Number of Trials	Nerve Block (Mean)	General (Mean)	Odds Ratio or WMD (95% CI)
Induction time (min)	6	19.6	8.8	8.1 (2.6-13.7)*
PACU time (min)	6	45.2	72	−24.3 (−36.3 to −12)*
VAS in PACU	7	9.6	35.8	−24.5 (−35.7 to −13.3)*
Nausea	6	6.8%	30%	0.17 (0.08-0.33)*
Phase 1 bypass	6	81%	315	14.3 (7.5-27.4)*
Need for analgesia	6	6.2%	42.3%	0.11 (0.03 – 0.43)*
ASU discharge time (min)	6	133.3	159.1	−29.7 (−75.3 to 15.8)
Patient satisfaction	4	88%	72%	4.7 (1.8-12)*

*$p = <0.01$.
Adapted from Liu SS, Strodtbeck WM, Richman JM, Wu CL: A comparison of regional versus general anesthesia for ambulatory anesthesia: A meta-analysis of randomized controlled trials. *Anesth Analg* 2005;101:1634-1642.
CI, confidence interval; WMD, weighted mean difference.

Table 52-3	**Summary of Regional versus General Anesthesia for Outpatients**	
	Neuraxial Block	Peripheral Nerve Block
Induction time	Increased	Increased
PACU time	Same	Reduced
PACU VAS	Reduced	Reduced
Nausea	Same	Decreased
Phase 1 bypass	Same	Increased
Need for analgesics	Reduced	Reduced
ASU discharge time	Prolonged	Same
Patient satisfaction	Same	Greater

(for ambulation and voiding) may have contributed to the longer times. Only one study used procaine, and none employed 2-chloroprocaine, which has been reported to be associated with faster resolution and discharge times than lidocaine in three studies that did not include a general anesthesia comparison.[13-15]

General anesthesia is superior to regional techniques. In those studies that report results, success rates of 90% to 95% appear to be common, especially with peripheral nerve blocks. Spinal and epidural anesthesia have a high reliability, but none of the techniques equals the 100% efficacy of general anesthesia.

All the comparisons of pharmacoeconomics show that regional techniques are at least no more expensive than general anesthesia, and in most cases they are less expensive than general anesthetic techniques.[16,17]

Satisfaction with central neuraxial blockade was high (81%) but not significantly different from general anesthesia. With peripheral nerve blockade, there was a significant increase in patient satisfaction (88% versus 72%) compared with general anesthesia.

In the majority of the published series, the complications were equally proportioned between general and regional anesthesia. Minor complications of backache and postdural puncture headache were higher in the regional technique groups, whereas postoperative nausea and vomiting and sore throat were more frequent in the general anesthesia group. The incidence of overnight admission was higher following general anesthesia in the two series that reported this as an outcome after shoulder surgery. In both reports the admission rate was related to increased pain in the general anesthesia groups.

Peripheral Nerve Infusions

The latest development in the application of regional techniques in the outpatient setting has been the use of continuous local anesthetic infusions through peripheral nerve catheters in patients who are discharged home from an outpatient unit. The use of this technology does not fit into the same categories as the previously discussed comparison of regional techniques with general anesthesia for the performance of intraoperative anesthesia, but nevertheless represents a significant change and potential advantage for outpatient surgery. In a review of 11 published studies of the use of continuous catheters, Ilfeld and Enneking[5] found significant improvement in pain control after discharge in the patients who were treated with local anesthetic infusions compared with placebo in four trials. In all the published series, there is a decreased use of oral analgesic medications when peripheral nerve catheters are provided. This is associated with a reduction in several adverse side effects such as nausea and sleep disturbance. Others have found a faster return to normal activity[18] and greater patient satisfaction. None of these series have measured the extent of additional time that is required for the placement of the catheters, which would reasonably be expected to exceed the performance of a simple single-injection peripheral nerve block. Nevertheless, significant advantages have been demonstrated with these techniques, and serve as a further argument for the appropriate use of regional anesthesia in the outpatient setting.

AREAS OF UNCERTAINTY

The major discussion appears to be the perception of an increased time to perform regional techniques in the outpatient setting, and the lower level of reliability of regional anesthesia, which counterbalance the improved postoperative analgesia and a higher degree of alertness, superior analgesia, and the potential for more rapid discharge. Thus, the controversy is not necessarily whether regional anesthesia is appropriate in the outpatient setting, but whether it is a cost-effective, reasonable alternative in a specific clinical setting.

In addition to that global controversy, more specific controversies appear to be related to the use of spinal anesthesia in the outpatient setting. The issue of post-spinal headache remains a reality, although the use of new needles has appeared to reduce the incidence to less than 1% in adult outpatients. Another controversy associated with subarachnoid anesthesia is the phenomenon of TNS that has been associated most particularly with the use of lidocaine.[3] This is unfortunate because lidocaine historically is the drug associated with the most rapid resolution of blockade and readiness for discharge. Reduction of the dose or concentration does not appear to alleviate the frequency of the syndrome. Preliminary data suggest that the preservative-free 2-chloroprocaine may be a competitive alternative,[13-15] but further data are needed on the safety and reduced incidence with this drug. In the meantime, it appears that patients undergoing arthroscopy or lithotomy-position operations on an outpatient basis have a 15% to 40% risk of the TNS syndrome if lidocaine is used for spinal anesthesia. However, spinal anesthesia is the most reliable and rapid in onset of the regional anesthetic techniques, and it should be the ideal technique for other uses in the outpatient setting.

Another issue with spinal anesthesia is the concern about return of voiding function. Previous data had shown a high incidence of urinary retention with long-acting spinal blocks, but recent data suggest that urinary retention after a short-acting spinal anesthetic in low-risk patients (no history of retention, not hernia or urologic surgery) is not any more frequent than with general anesthesia.[19]

GUIDELINES

There are no formal guidelines on the use of regional anesthesia in the outpatient setting. There are some general guidelines based on the literature. Regional anesthesia is appropriate in the outpatient setting. Certain adjustments must be made to the techniques and the drugs to ensure an appropriate result.

1. Excessive sedation for the performance of blocks must be avoided if the advantage of a high degree of alertness and rapid discharge is to be maintained.
2. Rapid onset and highly reliable techniques will help resolve some of the issues of efficiency and cost-effectiveness. Spinal anesthesia and intravenous regional anesthesia are perhaps the most appropriate, given these considerations. Ultrasound guidance may prove useful in shortening performance time.
3. Peripheral nerve blocks appear to provide the greatest advantages in the outpatient setting in terms of discharge times, postoperative analgesia, PACU bypass, and reduction of nausea, but also are associated with slower onset than general anesthesia. The performance of these blocks in a *separate induction area* is therefore optimal.
4. Choice of drugs for peripheral nerve blocks has not been addressed by any of the comparative studies, but it remains an issue. Although long-acting amino-amides may provide 12 to 24 hours of postoperative analgesia, this benefit must be weighed against the risk of injury to a numb extremity after discharge, and thus appropriate guidelines should include clear written instructions for all patients regarding the protection of extremities that remain anesthetized after discharge.
5. The use of continuous peripheral nerve infusions adds significant improvement in postoperative analgesia, reduction of postdischarge complications, and patient satisfaction. The additional time required may well be offset by the advantages for the more painful outpatient procedures.
6. Spinal anesthesia is best performed with small-gauge, rounded bevel needles to reduce the incidence of post-spinal headache. Its use should be limited to patients who can return to the emergency department easily for evaluation and management of postdural puncture headache.
7. The problem of TNS has not yet been resolved. It appears to be lowest with the use of bupivacaine, although prolonged discharge may be associated with the use of this drug. Preliminary data suggest that 2-chloroprocaine may have a low incidence,[14] but further information regarding the safety of the preservative-free solution is needed.
8. Discharge times after spinal anesthesia also require careful selection of drug and dose. It appears that the addition of epinephrine to subarachnoid local anesthetics increases the potential for urinary retention and for prolonged discharge times. The use of fentanyl may be a better choice for intensifying local anesthetic effect without prolonging discharge due to urinary retention.
9. Urinary retention after a short-acting spinal anesthetic in low-risk patients is not any more frequent than with general anesthesia,[19] and these patients can be discharged without mandatory voiding.
10. The duration of spinal anesthesia is proportional to the total milligram dose of the local anesthetic involved, and thus high-dose techniques are generally best avoided. Preliminary data suggest that preservative-free 2-chloroprocaine may provide the shortest duration, potentially competitive with general anesthesia. Further data are needed on its safety and association with TNS.
11. Epidural anesthesia appears to be appropriate in the outpatient setting, although it should be limited to the use of short-acting drugs such as chloroprocaine and lidocaine. It does require a longer time for performance and onset than spinal anesthesia.

AUTHORS' RECOMMENDATIONS

Based on the data, we believe that regional anesthesia does have an appropriate role in the outpatient setting if appropriate techniques, drugs, and doses are selected.

- Local anesthesia is clearly ideal and should be used whenever possible as the sole anesthetic regimen, or at least included for postoperative analgesia after any technique.
- Peripheral nerve blockade is highly effective in providing postoperative analgesia and rapid discharge and should be used whenever possible for upper or lower extremity surgical procedures. It is also applicable for some of the truncal operations such as hernia repair. The use of continuous catheter techniques provides maximum benefit.
- Performance of a block in a separate induction room may reduce the additional time otherwise required for regional anesthesia.
- If neuraxial blockade is chosen, spinal anesthesia has the advantages of rapid onset and high reliability. Unfortunately, at the current time there appears to be a persistent risk of TNS with the drugs and doses that are available. A low dose of bupivacaine (less than 6 mg) will provide a low risk of TNS with the potential of a short discharge time, but with a high degree of variability and a limitation of adequate surgical anesthesia to the lower extremity and rectal area.
- Performance of an epidural anesthetic provides a more rapid discharge than with most of the current spinal techniques, and it provides the added advantage of flexibility in duration and extent of blockade if a catheter is placed.

REFERENCES

1. Carroll NV, Miederhoff P, Cox FM, Hirsch JD: Postoperative nausea and vomiting after discharge from outpatient surgery centers. *Anesth Analg* 1995;80:903-909.
2. Pavlin DJ, Rapp SE, Polissar NL, et al: Factors affecting discharge time in adult outpatients. *Anesth Analg* 1998;87:816-826.
3. Pollock JE: Transient neurologic symptoms: Etiology, risk factors, and management. *Reg Anesth Pain Med* 2002;27:581-586.
4. Apfel CC, Kranke P, Katz MH, et al: Volatile anaesthetics may be the main cause of early but not delayed postoperative vomiting: A randomized controlled trial of factorial design. *Br J Anaesth* 2002;88:659-668.
5. Ilfeld BM, Enneking FK: Continuous peripheral nerve blocks at home: A review. *Anesth Analg* 2005;100:1822-1833.
6. Liu SS, Strodtbeck WM, Richman JM, Wu CL: A comparison of regional versus general anesthesia for ambulatory anesthesia: A meta-analysis of randomized controlled trials. *Anesth Analg* 2005;101:1634-1642.
7. Brown AR, Weiss R, Greenberg C, et al: Interscalene block for shoulder arthroscopy: Comparison with general anesthesia. *Arthroscopy* 1993;9:295-300.
8. D'Alessio JG, Rosenblum M, Shea KP, Freitas DG: A retrospective comparison of interscalene block and general anesthesia for ambulatory surgery shoulder arthroscopy. *Reg Anesth* 1995;20:62-68.
9. Armstrong KP, Cherry RA: Brachial plexus anesthesia compared to general anesthesia when a block room is available. *Can J Anaesth* 2004;51:41-44.
10. Williams BA, Kentor ML, Williams JP, et al: Process analysis in outpatient knee surgery: Effects of regional and general anesthesia on anesthesia-controlled time. *Anesthesiology* 2000;93:529-538.
11. Hadzic A, Arliss J, Kerimoglu B, et al: A comparison of infraclavicular nerve block versus general anesthesia for hand and wrist day-case surgeries. *Anesthesiology* 2004;101:127-132.
12. Hadzic A, Karaca PE, Hobeika P, et al: Peripheral nerve blocks result in superior recovery profile compared with general anesthesia in outpatient knee arthroscopy. *Anesth Analg* 2005;100:976-981.
13. Casati A, Danelli G, Berti M, et al: Intrathecal 2-chloroprocaine for lower limb outpatient surgery: A prospective, randomized, double-blind, clinical evaluation. *Anesth Analg* 2006;103:234-238.
14. Casati A, Fanelli G, Danelli G, et al: Spinal anesthesia with lidocaine or preservative-free 2-chlorprocaine for outpatient knee arthroscopy: A prospective, randomized, double-blind comparison. *Anesth Analg* 2007;104:959-964.
15. Kouri ME, Kopacz DJ: Spinal 2-chloroprocaine: A comparison with lidocaine in volunteers. *Anesth Analg* 2004;98:75-80.
16. Chan VW, Peng PW, Kaszas Z, et al: A comparative study of general anesthesia, intravenous regional anesthesia, and axillary block for outpatient hand surgery: Clinical outcome and cost analysis. *Anesth Analg* 2001;93:1181-1184.
17. Li S, Coloma M, White PF, et al: Comparison of the costs and recovery profiles of three anesthetic techniques for ambulatory anorectal surgery. *Anesthesiology* 2000;93:1225-1230.
18. Capdevila X, Dadure C, Bringuier S, et al: Effect of patient-controlled perineural analgesia on rehabilitation and pain after ambulatory orthopedic surgery: A multicenter randomized trial. *Anesthesiology* 2006;105:566-573.
19. Mulroy MF, Salinas FV, Larkin KL, Polissar NL: Ambulatory surgery patients may be discharged before voiding after short-acting spinal and epidural anesthesia. *Anesthesiology* 2002;97:315-319.

53 Is Regional Anesthesia Superior to General Anesthesia for Hip Surgery?

Michael K. Urban, MD, PhD

Hip surgery is a common procedure, with approximately 300,000 total hip replacements and an equal number of surgical corrections of femoral neck fractures performed each year in the United States. Perioperative complications associated with this procedure include infection, bone-cement implantation syndrome, pulmonary embolism, myocardial infarction, and death. The mortality rate with total hip arthroplasty is about 0.15%. Factors associated with increased mortality rate are American Society of Anesthesiologists (ASA) level greater than 2, advanced age, history of cardiorespiratory disease, and a preoperative diagnosis of a femoral fracture.[1] There is at least some evidence to suggest that general anesthesia may also increase the risk of perioperative complications in these orthopedic procedures.[2]

OPTIONS

Anesthesia for hip surgery can be achieved by the following:

1. General anesthesia
2. Spinal anesthesia
3. Epidural anesthesia
4. Combined general anesthesia with spinal or epidural
5. Femoral nerve and sciatic nerve block

EVIDENCE

The controversy as to whether, when feasible, regional anesthesia has an advantage over general anesthesia has been debated at least since 1911, when George Crile reported improved outcome in high-risk surgical patients anesthetized with a regional anesthetic. Although regional anesthesia would simplistically appear to produce fewer physiologic perturbations than general anesthesia, the physiologic effects of both types of anesthesia are complex, and hence the *best* anesthetic choice for the procedure is not always inherently obvious. Furthermore, the question of which anesthetic type is best intraoperatively ignores the possibility that the benefits of regional anesthesia may depend on its use for postoperative analgesia.

There is, however, evidence to suggest that compared with general anesthesia, regional anesthesia reduces the incidence of perioperative complications (Table 53-1). Perka and colleagues,[2] in a prospective case-control study, showed general anesthesia to be a major risk for nonsurgical complications in knee arthroplasty. Rodgers and colleagues,[3] in a review of 141 trials of 9559 patients randomized to either regional or general anesthesia, reported that regional anesthesia reduced the risk of deep vein thrombosis (DVT), pulmonary embolism, blood loss, respiratory complications, and death. Regional anesthesia reduced the mortality rate by one third compared with general anesthesia.

Borghi and colleagues[4] studied 210 patients who were randomly selected to receive epidural, general, or combined anesthesia in hip arthroplasty. Intraoperative and postoperative blood loss was evaluated as either compensated or noncompensated blood loss by using Nadler's formula. The intraoperative and postoperative bleeding, referred to as compensated blood loss, was similar among groups. The circulating red blood cell (RBC) mass dropped on the first postoperative day to a similar extent among the groups, which recovered by the fifth day after surgery in patients who underwent epidural anesthesia, whereas no RBC recovery was observed in those who had received general anesthesia alone or combined with epidural anesthesia. The authors speculated that the presence of nitrous oxide in the anesthetic gas mixture might inhibit erythropoiesis by altering vitamin B_{12} functions.

Mauermann and colleagues[5] performed a meta-analysis of studies through August 2005 to determine whether anesthesia choice affected the outcome after elective total hip replacement. Ten independent trials, involving 330 patients under general anesthesia and 348 patients under neuraxial block, were identified and analyzed. Pooled results from five trials showed that neuraxial block significantly decreased the incidence of radiographically diagnosed DVT or pulmonary embolism. The odds ratio (OR) for DVT was 0.27 with 95% confidence interval (CI) 0.17 to 0.42. The OR for pulmonary embolism was 0.26 with 95% CI 0.12 to 0.56. Neuraxial block also decreased the operative time by 7.1 minutes per case (95% CI 2.3 to 11.9 minutes) and intraoperative blood loss by 275 mL per case (95% CI 180 to 371 mL). Data from three trials showed that patients under neuraxial block for total hip replacement were less likely to require blood transfusion than were patients under general anesthesia (21 of 177 = 12%

Table 53-1	Regional versus General Anesthesia for Hip Surgery		
	Regional	**General**	**Evidence***
Airway	Avoids manipulation of difficult airway and trauma to unstable cervical spine	It is safer to intubate difficult airway under controlled conditions before surgery.	NS
Respiratory	Reduced incidence of respiratory depression and failure	Embolization of bone marrow debris may result in respiratory complications independent of anesthetic.	BS
Cardiac	May diminish stress response. Postoperative epidural analgesia may be cardioprotective	A "cardiac" general anesthetic is just as safe as a regional anesthetic.	BS
DVT—pulmonary embolism	Significant reduction with regional anesthesia and analgesia		S
Blood loss	Reduced with regional anesthesia		S
Cognitive function	No advantage	No advantage	S

*Evidence: S, supported by well-controlled studies; BS, studies exist to support both regional and general anesthesia; NS, evidence does not exist to support either claim.

versus 62 of 188 = 33% of patients transfused, $p < 0.001$ by z-test). The OR for this comparison was 0.26 (95% CI 0.06 to 1.05).

The Case for Regional Anesthesia in Hip Surgery

Patients for elective arthroplasty often pose difficult airway management problems because of their generalized osteoarthritis or rheumatoid arthritis that also affects the cervical spine. In rheumatoid arthritis patients with atlantoaxial subluxation of the cervical spine, conventional endotracheal intubation with direct laryngoscopy can result in displacement of the odontoid with spinal cord or medullary compression. For general anesthesia, these patients require awake fiberoptic endotracheal intubation. Regional anesthesia avoids manipulation of the airway, and conscious patients can aid in positioning themselves in the safest and most comfortable positions.

General anesthesia has numerous effects on the respiratory system, leading to ventilation and perfusion inequalities and the development of atelectasis, shunts, and increased dead space. Neuraxial anesthesia does not interfere with the protective mechanisms of the airway, diaphragmatic function is maintained, and nonphysiologic ventilation/perfusion patterns are not established. Maximum breathing capacity and active exhalation can be reduced with the loss of abdominal and intercostal muscle strength with regional anesthesia, but usually not enough to produce hypoxemia. In the meta-analysis of Rodgers and colleagues,[3] regional anesthesia reduced the incidence of respiratory depression by 59% compared with general anesthesia. Several reports comparing regional with general anesthesia for vascular surgery have noted trends favoring reduced respiratory failure and pneumonia in the regional group. In 100 patients undergoing lower extremity vascular surgery randomly assigned to either regional or general anesthesia, the incidence of respiratory failure was reduced by more than 50% in the group randomized to regional anesthesia.[6] Pulmonary embolization of bone marrow debris and methylmethacrylate are common during hip arthroplasty. Some of these patients exhibit signs of the bone-cement implantation syndrome, which can progress to respiratory failure.[7] Because these events are probably independent of the anesthetic, it may be difficult to determine the role of anesthesia in respiratory complications.

Because regional anesthesia reduces the catecholamine stresses associated with myocardial ischemia (tachycardia and hypertension), cardiac outcome should be improved compared with general anesthesia. However, in several randomized trials only one was able to demonstrate an advantage of cardiac outcome with regional anesthesia.[4,8,9] In the meta-analysis of Rodgers and colleagues,[3] in 30 trials there were one third fewer myocardial infarctions in patients who received regional anesthesia, but the confidence intervals were compatible with no effect. At our institution, all patients for hip arthroplasty receive regional anesthesia and the incidence of postoperative cardiac events is about 3%, considerably below published levels (approximately 8%). However, these patients also receive epidural analgesia during the period of the highest incidence of adverse cardiac outcomes, postoperatively.

Surgery induces a hypercoagulable state that is attenuated with regional but not general anesthesia. Several randomized trials have demonstrated that regional anesthesia reduces the incidence of DVT after orthopedic surgery. In a meta-analysis of patients undergoing the repair of femoral neck fractures, the incidence of DVT was almost four times greater in the patients who received general versus regional anesthesia.[10] Pulmonary embolism is the leading cause of death after hip arthroplasty, and the current evidence suggests that this mortality rate is reduced with regional anesthesia.[11]

Significant blood loss can occur with hip surgery, particularly during hip arthroplasty in which 500 to 1800 mL of blood loss has been reported. Several studies have demonstrated a reduction in blood loss with regional anesthesia.[12] At our institution, employing hypotensive regional anesthesia with mean arterial pressures of 50 to 65 mm Hg, the intraoperative blood loss has been reduced to less than 300 mL.[13]

AREAS OF UNCERTAINTY

Because patients receiving regional anesthesia should theoretically be subjected to less systemic medications, their cognitive function should be preserved compared with those receiving general anesthesia. However, most trials have not been able to demonstrate an advantage of one type of anesthetic in maintaining postoperative cognitive function. Williams-Russo and colleagues[14] found no advantage in regional anesthesia and analgesia compared with general anesthesia and intravenous analgesia with regard to postoperative cognitive function in patients undergoing total knee arthroplasty.

GUIDELINES

There are no specific guidelines related to choice of anesthesia.

AUTHOR'S RECOMMENDATIONS

1. The preferred anesthetic for patients undergoing hip surgery is regional anesthesia. Patients with an abnormal coagulation profile, critical aortic stenosis, symptomatic idiopathic hypertrophic subaortic stenosis (IHSS), ankylosing spondylitis, and previous surgical spine fusions after excluded or combined femoral and sciatic nerve blocks with sedation may have to be excluded. We prefer a combined spinal-epidural anesthetic with plain 1.5% mepivacaine for operations of less than 2 hours and 0.5% bupivacaine for longer procedures.

2. Patients undergoing total hip arthroplasty should be monitored with an arterial catheter. Patients with significant medical comorbidities, repair of pathologic fractures, or revision arthroplasty should also have central venous access in the event of significant acute hemodynamic events. The insertion of a pulmonary artery catheter for patients with a significant risk for the bone-cement implantation syndrome is controversial.

3. Hypotensive anesthesia can be achieved by dosing with local anesthetic through the epidural catheter. To avoid bradycardia and severe hypotension, an epinephrine infusion is titrated to the desired mean arterial blood pressure (50 to 65 mm Hg).

4. The epidural catheter is infused postoperatively with a patient-controlled analgesia (PCA) pump using 0.06% bupivacaine and 10 µg/mL hydromorphone. This mixture usually controls pain and does not interfere with physical therapy and ambulation.

5. DVT prophylaxis is usually achieved with aspirin; however, for high-risk patients or procedures, warfarin (Coumadin) or low-molecular-weight heparin may be administered. The epidural catheter is removed 2 days after the initiation of warfarin (Coumadin) therapy and 2 hours before the initiation of low-molecular-weight heparin.

REFERENCES

1. Parvizi J, Johnson BG, Rowland C, Ereth MH, Lewallen DG: Thirty-day mortality after elective total hip arthroplasty. *J Bone Joint Surg Am* 2001;83:1524-1528.
2. Perka C, Arnold U, Buttgereit F: Influencing factors on perioperative morbidity in knee arthroplasty. *Clin Orthop* 2000;183:191/-196.
3. Rodgers A, Walker N, Schug S, McKee A, Kehlet H, Zundert AV, et al: Reduction of postoperative mortality and morbidity with epidural or spinal anesthesia: Results from overview of randomized trials. *BMJ* 2000;321:1-12.
4. Borghi B, Casati A, Iuorio S, Celleno D, Michael M, Serafini PL, et al: Effect of different anesthesia techniques on red blood cell endogenous recovery in hip arthroplasty. *J Clin Anesth* 2005;17(2):96-101.
5. Mauermann WJ, Shilling AM, Zuo Z: A comparison of neuraxial block versus general anesthesia for elective total hip replacement: A meta-analysis. *Anesth Analg* 2006;103(4):1018-1025.
6. Christopherson R, Beattie C, Frank SM, Norris EJ, Meinert CL, Gottlieb SO, et al: Perioperative morbidity in patients randomized to epidural or general anesthesia for lower extremity vascular surgery. *Anesthesiology* 1993;79:422-434.
7. Urban MK, Sheppard R, Gordon MA, Urquhart BL: Right ventricular function during revision total hip arthroplasty. *Anesth Analg* 1996;82:1225-1229.
8. Tuman KJ, McCarthy RJ, March RJ, Delaria GA, Patel RV, Ivankovich AD: Effects of epidural anesthesia and analgesia on coagulation and outcome after major vascular surgery. *Anesth Analg* 1991;73:696-704.
9. Bode RH, Lewis KP, Zarich SW, Pierce ET, Roberts M, Kowalchuk GJ, et al: Cardiac outcome after peripheral vascular surgery. *Anesthesiology* 1996;84:3-13.
10. Sorenson RM, Pace NL: Anesthetic technique during surgical repair of femoral neck fractures. *Anesthesiology* 1992;77:1095-1104.
11. Sharrock NE, Cazan MG, Hargett MJ, Williams-Russo P, Wilson PD: Changes in mortality after total hip and knee arthroplasty over a ten-year period. *Anesth Analg* 1995;80:242-248.
12. Twyman R, Kirwan T, Fennelly M: Blood loss reduced during hip arthroplasty by lumbar plexus block. *J Bone Joint Surg Am* 1990;72:1-8.
13. Sharrock NE, Mineo R, Urquhart B, Salvati EA: The effect of two levels of hypotension on intraoperative blood loss during total hip arthroplasty performed under epidural anesthesia. *Anesth Analg* 1993;76:580-584.
14. Williams-Russo P, Sharrock NE, Mattis S, Szatrowski TP: Cognitive effects after epidural vs general anesthesia in older adults. *JAMA* 1995;274:44-50.

54 Does Intraoperative Regional Anesthesia Decrease Perioperative Blood Loss?

Jeffrey M. Richman, MD; James F. Weller, MD; and Christopher L. Wu, MD

INTRODUCTION

Attempts to minimize exposure to allogeneic blood products remain a goal of perioperative care despite improvements in the safety of the blood supply. The risks of viral infection, bacterial contamination, hemolytic reactions, and transfusion-associated lung injury (TRALI) have been reviewed.[1] Evidence suggests that allogeneic blood transfusion may have immuno-suppressive effects leading to increased cancer recurrence, increased susceptibility to wound infections, and even increased mortality rate.[1] Thus, perioperative transfusion of blood products may be associated with an increase in perioperative morbidity and mortality rates.

Although there are many strategies to decrease intraoperative blood loss, use of regional anesthetic techniques has been suggested to diminish intraoperative blood loss and blood transfusions.[2] In addition to decreasing perioperative morbidity and mortality rates, neuraxial blockade has been shown to diminish the risk of postoperative deep venous thrombosis and pulmonary embolism.[3,4]

OPTIONS AND THERAPIES

Many strategies have been suggested to decrease perioperative exposure to allogeneic blood products. These can generally be divided into three categories: (1) pharmaceuticals (e.g., erythropoietin, epsilon-aminocaproic acid, aprotonin, blood substitutes); (2) techniques (e.g., minimally invasive and other surgical techniques, autologous donation, acute normovolemic hemodilution, deliberate hypotension); and (3) devices (e.g., intraoperative blood salvage). Many of these are discussed elsewhere. However, in comparison to these options, neuraxial regional techniques (e.g., spinal and epidural anesthesia) offer a particularly attractive alternative for reduction of perioperative hemorrhage, because they are inherent to the anesthetic itself; they require no modification of surgical technique or additional pharmacologic manipulation. The majority of randomized data supports the use of neuraxial regional anesthetic techniques in decreasing blood loss and need for blood transfusion; however, there is a lack of large-scale randomized data examining the effect of peripheral regional anesthesia on perioperative blood loss. Recently, two meta-analyses have been published

evaluating the effects of neuraxial techniques on surgical blood loss and blood transfusion requirements.[5,6] Data from these two studies confirm the benefits of neuraxial anesthesia in reducing blood loss and transfusion requirement,[5,6] although the combination of general anesthesia with epidural analgesia seems to negate the benefits of decreased blood loss.[5]

EVIDENCE

Since 1966, at least 76 studies comparing regional with general anesthesia have included either perioperative blood loss or transfusion requirement as an outcome measure. Of the two meta-analysis published in 2006, one identified 66 randomized controlled trials that compared neuraxial anesthesia to general anesthesia with a quantification of intraoperative blood loss,[5] and the other identified 24 trials.[6] The large difference in trials included by the two meta-analyses may be explained by a much broader search (667 articles reviewed for inclusion[5] versus 103 manuscripts[6]) or possibly by unpublished exclusion or inclusion criteria that differed between the two studies. A PubMed search through May 1, 2007, using the search criteria used by Richman and colleagues,[5] identified eight additional studies that would meet inclusion criteria if the analysis were repeated. A comparison of blood loss by location of surgery from the meta-analysis by Richman and colleagues[5] is shown in Table 54-1, and a comparison of blood loss from trials limited to direct comparisons of various techniques is shown in Table 54-2.

Some of the variability in the effect of regional anesthesia on blood loss may reflect differing mechanisms of hemorrhage during different surgical procedures. The largest body of literature on this subject has focused on surgery of the hip. Since 1966, at least 26 randomized controlled trials have measured differences in blood loss based on anesthetic technique with patients undergoing total hip arthroplasty or hip fracture repair. These studies have consistently reported significant decreases in blood loss with neuraxial versus general anesthesia. In 2000 Stevens and colleagues[7] published the first data associating peripheral nerve blockade with reduction in blood loss, although in this study the difference was eliminated when those patients with evidence of epidural spread of their

| Table 54-1 | Estimated Blood Loss: Comparison among Anesthetic Techniques and Type of Surgery |||||

Surgery	Anesthesia	Mean Difference*	95% CI	p-value
Abdominal		*Spinal vs.*		
	Epidural	−440	−698/−181	<0.001
	GA	−962	−1169/−756	<0.001
	EA-GA	−1344	−1561/−1128	<0.001
	Epidural vs.			
	GA	−523	−721/−324	<0.001
	EA-GA	−905	−1113/−696	<0.001
	General vs.			
	EA-GA	−382	−521/−243	<0.001
Pelvic		*Spinal vs.*		
	Epidural	−315	−375/−255	<0.001
	GA	−235	−280/−191	<0.001
	EA-GA	−150	−227/−72	<0.001
	Epidural vs.			
	GA	79	23/135	0.001
	EA-GA	165	81/249	<0.001
	General vs.			
	EA-GA	85	12/160	0.011
Lower Extremity		*Spinal vs.*		
	Epidural	−1	−62/61	1.0
	GA	−65	−111/−20	0.001
	EA-GA	−114	−194/−34	0.001
	Epidural vs.			
	GA	−65	−120/−9	0.014
	EA-GA	−114	−200/−27	0.003
	General vs.			
	EA-GA	−49	−125/27	0.529

From Richman JM, Rowlingson AJ, Maine DN, et al: Does neuraxial anesthesia reduce intraoperative blood loss? A meta-analysis. *J Clin Anesth* 2006;18(6):427-435.
*All data expressed in milliliters. A (-) mean difference favors the primary anesthetic. For instance, the first comparison (abdominal; spinal vs. epidural) would have favored the use of spinal anesthesia in decreasing blood loss by a mean of 440 mL.
CI, confidence interval; *EA*, epidural anesthesia; *EA-GA*, combined epidural-general anesthesia; *GA*, general anesthesia.

lumbar plexus blocks were eliminated from the analysis. The trial by Singelyn and colleagues[8] comparing general anesthesia, continuous femoral nerve block, and general anesthesia found no statistically significant difference in blood loss or transfusion in any of the three groups.[8] The association between regional anesthesia and reduced blood loss during hip fracture repair compared with total hip arthroplasty operation has been much weaker. A 1992 meta-analysis of 13 randomized controlled trials comparing regional versus general anesthesia for surgical repair of femoral neck fractures found no difference in estimated operative blood loss (use of general anesthesia was associated with a mean of +18 mL of blood loss; 95% CI: −99 to +116 mL).[9] Since

1992, at least one other investigation has revealed no difference in blood loss among patients operated on under continuous spinal, single-dose spinal, or general anesthesia with positive pressure ventilation.[10] This is supported in part by the meta-analysis by Guay,[6] in which a statistically significant difference in blood transfusion was seen for total hip replacement but not for fractured hip. Interestingly, blood loss was not decreased significantly for total hip arthroplasty, whereas it was for hip fracture.[6] Overall, total blood loss was much greater in total hip arthroplasty, possibly accounting for an increased need for transfusion.

Prostate surgery has also been evaluated extensively in outcomes research comparing regional and general

Table 54-2	Comparison of Estimated Blood Loss from Trials with Direct Comparison of GA versus SA, GA versus EA, or GA versus EA-GA				
	N (articles)	**Mean EBL**	**SD**	**95% CI**	**p-value**
EA	368 (17)	559	372	521-597	
GA	399 (17)	748	444	704-791	<0.001
	N (articles)	**Mean EBL**	**SD**	**95% CI**	**p-value**
SA	729 (14)	297	197	283-312	
GA	757 (14)	401	211	386-416	<0.001
	N (articles)	**Mean EBL**	**SD**	**95% CI**	**p-value**
EA-GA	399 (20)	1322	822	1241-1403	
GA	401 (20)	1244	811	1164-1323	0.175

From Richman JM, Rowlingson AJ, Maine DN, et al: Does neuraxial anesthesia reduce intraoperative blood loss? A meta-analysis. *J Clin Anesth* 2006;18(6):427-435.
CI, confidence interval; *EA*, epidural anesthesia; *EA-GA*, combined general anesthesia and epidural anesthesia; *EBL*, estimated blood loss (mean blood loss measured in milliliters); *GA*, general anesthesia; *N*, total number of patients in group; *SA*, spinal anesthesia; *SD*, standard deviation.

anesthesia. Numerous studies have been performed on patients undergoing transurethral resection of the prostate (TURP), with some investigators finding a decrease in blood loss attributable to neuraxial anesthesia,[11-13] whereas others have been unable to discern a statistically significant difference.[14-17] Because essentially all of the blood lost during TURP is aspirated into suction canisters by the resectoscope, this procedure allows for a relatively easy and extremely accurate estimate of hemorrhage. Several factors aside from anesthetic technique have been implicated as causes of increased blood loss during TURP, including infection and weight of prostate resected.[17] There are nine prospective studies evaluating blood loss in a randomized fashion for open prostatectomy with almost universal results of neuraxial techniques resulting in decreased blood loss.[18-26]

Fewer data are available on other general surgical patients. In a randomized study of the effects of epidural anesthesia on splanchnic blood flow during colorectal surgery, Mallinder and colleagues[27] noted a nonsignificant trend toward decreased blood loss among patients receiving epidural blockade in comparison with a total intravenous anesthetic control group. Bredtmann and colleagues[28] found similar results in a study of 116 colonic surgery patients randomized to receive general anesthesia followed by systemic opioids or combined general/epidural anesthesia followed by continuous epidural infusion of bupivicaine postoperatively. The authors found no significant difference in blood loss, despite a trend toward increased need for blood replacement among the regional anesthesia patients.[28] These findings are consistent with earlier retrospective reviews of patients undergoing gastrointestinal surgery, which failed to demonstrate a difference in blood loss between patients treated with regional versus general anesthesia.[29,30] Blood loss for many gastrointestinal procedures is relatively small when compared with hip arthroplasty or radical prostatectomy, which may account for inconsistency in individual clinical trials in demonstrating

reduced blood loss. One possible explanation for the lack of decreased blood loss noted for general surgical patients is the confounding factor of combined general-epidural anesthesia resulting in equivalent operative blood loss to general anesthesia alone. The meta-analysis by Richman and colleagues[5] demonstrates decreased blood loss for abdominal operations with spinal or epidural anesthesia compared with general anesthesia but no difference in blood loss with a combined technique. It is not clear why the combination of general anesthesia with epidural analgesia negates the benefits of decreased blood loss. The mechanism may be related to the use of spontaneous versus controlled ventilation (where controlled ventilation might result in slightly higher venous pressure and blood loss compared with spontaneous ventilation)[31] or other undetermined factors. In a study on radical prostatectomy, combined epidural-general anesthesia with spontaneous ventilation did result in a decrease in blood loss compared with general anesthesia alone.[26]

As in gastrointestinal surgery, the data for vascular surgery are limited and equivocal. Randomized trials of combined epidural/general anesthesia versus general anesthesia alone for patients undergoing repair of abdominal aortic aneurysms (AAAs) failed to discern a difference in blood loss or transfusion requirement.[32,33] A more recent retrospective review of endoluminal AAA repairs found similar results.[34] There is, however, at least one study demonstrating lower blood loss during vascular surgery with subarachnoid anesthesia. In 1986, Cook and colleagues[35] randomized 101 patients undergoing lower-extremity peripheral vascular surgery to receive either general or spinal anesthesia and found that blood loss was significantly lower in the spinal (560 ± 340 mL) than in the general anesthesia group (792 ± 440 mL). The spinal group also experienced significantly greater hypotension in this study.

A variety of other mechanisms have been proposed to explain the beneficial effects of regional anesthesia on perioperative hemorrhage. The most frequently cited explanation has been that neuraxial blockade predictably lowers arterial blood pressure, which, in turn, has been associated with decreased blood loss. However, in an elegant study of regional versus general anesthesia for total hip arthroplasty, Modig[36] demonstrated that the effects of regional anesthesia on peripheral venous pressure may be more relevant. Modig randomized 38 patients undergoing total hip arthroplasty to one of three anesthetics: (1) epidural anesthesia alone; (2) general anesthesia with spontaneous ventilation; or (3) general anesthesia with positive pressure mechanical ventilation. As expected, the epidural group experienced lower mean arterial blood pressure and less blood loss than either general anesthesia group. However, there was no significant correlation between arterial blood pressure and blood loss. Meanwhile, regression analysis revealed significant relationships between peripheral venous pressure (measured in the operative wound) and intraoperative blood loss for all three groups ($r = 0.92$ to 0.94).[36] Modig postulates that arterial bleeding contributes less to intraoperative hemorrhage than venous bleeding, because it is easier to control surgically.

AREAS OF UNCERTAINTY

Any legitimate study of the effects of anesthetic technique on surgical blood loss must a priori describe and utilize a validated, accurate technique of measuring the amount of blood actually lost. Unfortunately, much of the data available on anesthetic technique and blood loss is reported as a secondary outcome variable; however, subgroup analysis from a recent meta-analysis of intraoperative neuraxial regional versus general anesthesia trials demonstrated that use of neuraxial regional anesthesia decreased perioperative transfusion requirements by 50%.[3] Decreased blood loss and transfusion requirements have been confirmed by both the recent meta-analyses, although the analysis by Richman and colleagues[5] showed decreased transfusion only with spinal anesthesia and the decrease in transfusion noted in Guay's study[6] was negated if the effect of total hip arthroplasty is removed. Nevertheless, the methods used to calculate blood loss are often suspect. Other authors have chosen not to measure blood loss at all, but used transfusion requirement as a surrogate endpoint.[29] Although transfusion requirement may represent a clinically relevant marker for the efficacy of a technique to minimize blood loss, it is subject to individual variation in criteria for transfusion.

Several techniques for accurately measuring intraoperative and postoperative blood loss have been established, but none has gained uniform acceptance. The most commonly employed technique is the "gravimetric" method, which consists of adding the volume estimated from the weight of surgical sponges to that in suction canisters. More sophisticated photometric methods have been developed for transurethral surgery, during which essentially all the lost blood is conveniently collected through the suction port of the operative resectoscope.[37,38]

The most consistent methodologic problem in studies of regional versus general anesthesia and blood loss has been standardization of mean arterial pressure (MAP) and central venous pressure (CVP). Deliberate arterial hypotension has been shown to reduce blood loss in a variety of settings, including total hip arthroplasty.[39–41]

Meanwhile, deliberate central venous hypotension has been demonstrated to diminish blood loss during hepatic resection.[42] Another study, however, disputes the effects of profound hypotension (45 to 55 mm Hg) on blood loss, although this may have been the result of imprecision in the measurement technique (as in all studies) or a plateau in benefit of deliberate hypotension in decreasing blood loss.[43] Because major conduction blockade is well known for its ability to induce arterial and venous hypotension, any study of the effects of regional versus general anesthesia on blood loss should ideally include a description of hemodynamic responses to anesthesia.

The ability of regional anesthesia to decrease perioperative blood loss would not be predicted based on the known hematologic effects of local anesthetics. Studies attempting to elucidate the mechanisms behind the decreased risk of thromboembolic events following regional compared with general anesthesia have shown that local anesthetics exert numerous anticoagulant effects. These include (1) enhanced fibrinolytic activity produced via prevention of postoperative increases in plasminogen activator inhibitor 1 (PAI-1); (2) more rapid return of antithrombin III levels from increased to normal values; (3) attenuation of postoperative increases in platelet aggregation; and (4) epidurally administered local anesthetics reach plasma concentration sufficient to impair platelet aggregation and reduce blood viscosity directly.[44] Despite the suggestion that intraoperative regional anesthesia will decrease perioperative blood loss and blood transfusion requirements, the presence of methodologic issues in the randomized studies examining the effect of regional anesthesia on blood loss make it difficult to draw clear conclusions. The data from the recently published meta-analyses confirm the expected benefits of decreased blood loss and transfusion for neuraxial anesthesia when not combined with general anesthesia; however, the exact mechanism for this is still unclear. If reduced blood loss is primarily related to the effect of spontaneous rather than positive pressure ventilation, it may ultimately prove that there is no definitive link between decreased blood loss and neuraxial anesthesia.

GUIDELINES

No practice guidelines exist regarding the use of regional anesthesia in an attempt to decrease perioperative blood loss.

AUTHORS' RECOMMENDATIONS

- Based on the available evidence, neuraxial blockade induces both arterial and venous hypotension below the level of blockade. This relative hypotension appears to result in diminished blood loss during surgery and as long as the block is maintained postoperatively.
- The beneficial effects of neuraxial anesthesia on hemorrhage may be lost when positive pressure ventilation is employed. Therefore, if a combined regional/general anesthesia technique is employed, spontaneous ventilation should be maintained when possible and if there are no additional risks to the patient (with use of spontaneous ventilation) versus controlled ventilation.
- There is no current high-quality evidence to support an association between peripheral nerve blockade and reduction in blood loss.

REFERENCES

1. Goodnough LT, Brecher ME, Kanter MH, AuBuchon JP: Transfusion medicine: First of two parts: Blood transfusion. *N Engl J Med* 1999;340:438-447.
2. Salo M: Immunosuppressive effects of blood transfusion in anaesthesia and surgery. *Acta Anaesthesiol Scand Suppl* 1988;32: 26-34.
3. Rodgers A, Walker N, Schug S, et al: Reduction of postoperative mortality and morbidity with epidural or spinal anaesthesia: Results from overview of randomised trials. *BMJ* 2000;321: 1493-1496.
4. Modig J, Borg T, Karlstrom G, et al: Thromboembolism after total hip replacement: Role of epidural and general anesthesia. *Anesth Analg* 1983;62:174-180.
5. Richman JM, Rowlingson AJ, Maine DN, et al: Does neuraxial anesthesia reduce intraoperative blood loss? A meta-analysis. *J Clin Anesth* 2006;18:427-435.
6. Guay J: The effect of neuraxial blocks on surgical blood loss and blood transfusion requirements: A meta-analysis. *J Clin Anesth* 2006;18:124-128.
7. Stevens RD, Van Gessel E, Flory N, Fournier R, Gamulin Z: Lumbar plexus block reduces pain and blood loss associated with total hip arthroplasty. *Anesthesiology* 2000;93:115-121.
8. Singelyn FJ, Ferrant T, Malisse MF, Joris D: Effects of intravenous patient-controlled analgesia with morphine, continuous epidural analgesia and continuous femoral nerve sheath block on rehabilitation after unilateral total-hip arthroplasty. *Reg Anesth Pain Med* 2005;30(5):452-457.
9. Sorenson R, Pace N: Anesthetic techniques during surgical repair of femoral neck fractures. *Anesthesiology* 1992;77:1095-1104.
10. Juelsgaard P, Sand NP, Felsby S, et al: Perioperative myocardial ischaemia in patients undergoing surgery for fractured hip randomized to incremental spinal, single-dose spinal or general anaesthesia. *Eur J Anaesthesiol* 1998;15:656-663.
11. Mackenzie A: Influence of anaesthesia on blood loss in transurethral prostaectomy. *Scottish Med J* 1990;35:14-16.
12. Abrams PH, Shah PJ, Bryning K, et al: Blood loss during transurethral resection of the prostate. *Anaesthesia* 1982;37:71-73.
13. Madsen RE, Madsen PO: Influence of anesthesia form on blood loss in transurethral prostatectomy. *Anesth Analg* 1967;46:330-332.
14. Kirollos MM, Campbell N: Factors influencing blood loss in transurethral resection of the prostate (TURP): Auditing TURP. *Br J Urol* 1997;80:111-115.
15. Smyth R, Cheng D, Asokumar B, Chung F: Coagulopathies in patients after transurethral resection of the prostate: Spinal versus general anesthesia. *Anesth Analg* 1995;81:680-685.
16. Nielsen KK, Andersen K, Asbjorn J, Vork F, Ohrt-Nissen A: Blood loss in transurethral prostatectomy: Epidural versus general anaesthesia. *Int Urol Nephrol* 1987;19:287-292.
17. McGowan SW, Smith GF: Anaesthesia for transurethral prostatectomy. A comparison of spinal intradural analgesia with two methods of general anaesthesia. *Anaesthesia* 1980;35:847-853.
18. Salonia A, Suardi N, Crescenti A, et al: General versus spinal anesthesia with different forms of sedation in patients undergoing radical retropubic prostatectomy: Results of a prospective, randomized study. *Int J Urol* 2006;13(9):1185-1190.
19. O'Connor PJ, Hanson J, Finucane BT: Induced hypotension with epidural/general anesthesia reduces transfusion in radical prostate surgery. *Can J Anaesth* 2006;53(9):873-880.
20. Salonia A, Crescenti A, Suardi N, et al: General versus spinal anesthesia in patients undergoing radical retropubic prostatectomy: Results of a prospective, randomized study. *Urology* 2004;64(1):95-100.
21. Hendolin H, Mattila MA, Poikolainen E: The effect of lumbar epidural analgesia on the development of deep vein thrombosis of the legs after open prostatectomy. *Acta Chir Scand* 1981;147: 425-429.
22. Hendolin H, Alhava E: Effect of epidural versus general anaesthesia on peroperative blood loss during retropubic prostatectomy. *Int Urol Nephrol* 1982;14:399-405.
23. Hendolin H, Lansimies E: Skin and central temperatures during continuous epidural analgesia and general anaesthesia in patients subjected to open prostatectomy. *Ann Clin Res* 1982;14: 181-186.
24. Hendolin H, Penttila IM: Liver enzymes after retropubic prostatectomy in patients receiving continuous lumbar epidural analgesia or general anaesthesia. *Ann Clin Res* 1982;14:1-6.
25. Shir Y, Raja SN, Frank SM, Brendler CB: Intraoperative blood loss during radical retropubic prostatectomy: Epidural versus general anesthesia. *Urology* 1995;45:993-999.
26. Stevens RA, Mikat-Stevens M, Flanigan R, et al: Does the choice of anesthetic technique affect the recovery of bowel function after radical prostatectomy? *Urology* 1998;52:213-218.
27. Mallinder PA, Hall JE, Bergin FG, Royle P, Leaper DJ: A comparison of opiate- and epidural-induced alterations in splanchnic blood flow using intra-operative gastric tonometry. *Anaesthesia* 2000;55:659-665.
28. Bredtmann RD, Herden HN, Teichman W, et al: Epidural analgesia in colonic surgery: Results of a randomized prospective study. *Br J Surg* 1990;77:638-642.
29. Kanazi GE, Thompson JS, Boskovski NA: Effect of epidural analgesia on postoperative ileus after ileal pouch-anal anastamosis. *Am Surg* 1995;62:499-502.
30. Jensen M, Stokke D: Perioperative haemorrhage and epidural anaesthesia in major abdominal surgery. *Acta Anaesthesiol Scand* 1978;22:153-157.
31. Modig J: Beneficial effects on intraoperative and postoperative blood loss in total hip replacement when performed under lumbar epidural anesthesia. An explanatory study. *Acta Chir Scand Suppl* 1989;550:95-100.
32. Norris EJ, Beattie C, Perler BA, et al: Double-masked randomized trial comparing alternate combinations of intraoperative anesthesia and postoperative analgesia in abdominal aortic surgery. *Anesthesiology* 2001;95:1054-1067.
33. Davies MJ, Silbert BS, Mooney PJ, Dysart RH, Meads AC: Combined epidural and general anaesthesia versus general anaesthesia for abdominal aortic surgery: A prospective randomized trial. *Anaesth Intens Care* 1993;21:790-794.
34. Cao P, Zannetti S, Parlani G, et al: Epidural anesthesia reduces length of hospitalization after endoluminal abdominal aortic aneurysm repair. *J Vasc Surg* 1999;30:651-657.
35. Cook PT, Davies MJ, Cronin KD, Moran P: A prospective randomised trial comparing spinal anaesthesia using hyperbaric cinchocaine with general anaesthesia for lower limb vascular surgery. *Anaesth Intens Care* 1986;14:373-380.
36. Modig J: Regional anesthesia and blood loss. *Acta Anaesthesiol Scand Suppl* 1998;32:44-48.
37. Jansen H, Berseus O, Johansson JE: A simple photometric method for determination of blood loss during transurethral surgery. *Scand J Urol Nephrol* 1978;12:1-5.
38. Desmond J: A method of measuring blood loss during transurethral prostatic surgery. *J Urol* 1973;109:453-456.
39. Sharrock N, Mineo M, Urquhart B, Salvati E: The effect of two levels of hypotension on intraoperative blood loss during total hip arthroplasty performed under lumbar epidural anesthesia. *Anesth Analg* 1993;76:580-584.
40. Rosberg B, Fredin H, Gustafson C: Anesthetic techniques and surgical blood loss in total hip arthroplasty. *Acta Anaesthesiol Scand* 1982;26:189-193.
41. Niemi T, Pitkanen M, Rosenberg P: Comparison of hypotensive epidural anaesthesia and spinal anaesthesia on blood loss and coagulation during and after total hip arthroplasty. *Acta Anaesthesiol Scand* 2000;44:457-464.
42. Jones RM, Moulton CE, Hardy KJ: Central venous pressure and its effect on blood loss during liver resection. *Br J Surg* 1998;85:1058-1060.
43. Williams-Russo P, Sharrock N, Mattis S, et al: Randomized trial of hypotensive epidural anesthesia in older adults. *Anesthesiology* 1999;91:926-935.
44. Liu S, Carpenter R, Neal JM: Epidural anesthesia and analgesia: Their role in postoperative outcome. *Anesthesiology* 1995;82: 1474-1506.

55 What Is the Optimal Management of Post–Dural Puncture Headache?

David Wlody, MD

INTRODUCTION

Despite advances in equipment and regional anesthetic techniques, post–dural puncture headache (PDPH) remains a persistent problem. In many cases, the headache is mild in intensity and brief in duration, without significant sequelae. This is not always the case, however. PDPH is occasionally severe enough to leave patients bedridden, and often delays hospital discharge. PDPH can be prolonged, with reports of symptoms lasting months or even years.[1] Untreated PDPH can lead to the development of persistent cranial nerve palsies and even subdural hematoma.[2,3] Finally, despite the perception among physicians that PDPH is merely a nuisance, it is a surprisingly frequent, and a sometimes distressingly costly, source of litigation.[4]

A wide range of both conservative and invasive treatments for PDPH has been described in the literature, sometimes with scant scientific support. In this review, the rationale for the more common treatments of PDPH will be discussed, based on our current understanding of the pathophysiology of PDPH. The evidence supporting these techniques will be described, when such evidence exists. Because there are so few well-controlled studies of the treatment of PDPH, however, many of the treatment recommendations will be based on case reports, observational studies, and personal experience. A century after August Bier first described PDPH, the optimal management of PDPH is a question that remains unanswered.[5]

PATHOPHYSIOLOGY

Limitations of length require that this review deal primarily with the treatment of PDPH. It should not be forgotten, though, that our main goal should be the prevention of PDPH; as in many other areas of medicine, prevention is far preferable to treatment. There are numerous risk factors for PDPH that cannot be modified, but the two most important can be: needle shape and size. The use of small pencil-point needles for spinal anesthesia (25- or 27-gauge Whitacre, Sprotte, or Gertie Marx needles) will reduce the incidence of headache after dural puncture to 1% or less even in high-risk populations.[6] If a cutting needle (e.g., Quincke) is used, insertion of the needle with the bevel parallel to the longitudinal axis of the body will significantly decrease the risk of headache.[7] When performing epidural anesthesia, the option of using such small needles is not possible; we must instead rely on meticulous technique. The use of the combined spinal-epidural technique may reduce the risk of accidental dural puncture; the incidence of headache requiring autologous epidural blood patch has been reported to be no higher with this technique than with traditional epidural anesthesia.[8]

An understanding of the pathophysiology of PDPH is essential when considering its treatment. There are two competing yet somewhat complementary theories. The first is predicated on the belief that the continued leak of cerebrospinal fluid (CSF) from a dural puncture leads to a loss of fluid from the intracranial compartment. The loss of the cushioning effect of CSF allows the brain to sag within the skull, placing traction on the pain-sensitive meninges, an effect that becomes most apparent in the upright position. This suggests that the treatment of PDPH should be based on minimizing the leak of CSF, increasing CSF production, or translocating CSF from the spinal to the intracranial compartment.

The second theory postulates that the loss of CSF causes intracranial hypotension, which leads to compensatory cerebral vasodilation. This suggests that PDPH is similar to migraine headache, a theory supported by the similarly increased incidence of migraine and PDPH in women, and also by MRI studies that demonstrate enhanced cerebral blood flow in PDPH.[9] This theory suggests that PDPH will be relieved by restoration of intracranial CSF volume, but also that cerebral vasoconstrictors might provide symptomatic relief.

OPTIONS

The treatment of PDPH is traditionally divided into conservative and, for want of a better term, aggressive treatment. These will be described next.

Conservative Treatment

Bed rest
Hydration
Prone position
Abdominal binder

Caffeine, oral or parenteral
Triptans
Adrenocorticotropic hormone (ACTH)/corticosteroids

Aggressive Treatment

Intrathecal saline injection
Intrathecal catheter
Epidural saline
Epidural blood patch
Prophylactic epidural blood patch
Epidural dextran

EVIDENCE

Bed Rest

Bed rest will provide symptomatic relief of PDPH. However, a review of the literature demonstrated that bed rest after dural puncture did not reduce the risk of developing a headache; in fact, there was a trend toward increased headache in patients placed at rest.[10] There was no evidence that prolonging the duration of bed rest after dural puncture decreased the likelihood of headache. Early ambulation after dural puncture should be encouraged; patients with an established headache should ambulate as much as they are able to.

Hydration

Despite the widespread enthusiasm for aggressive hydration after dural puncture, there is only a single study of fluid supplementation after dural puncture; there was no evidence of any decrease in the incidence of PDPH.[11]

Prone Position

The prone position can relieve headache in some patients with PDPH, but there are no published studies supporting this common practice. Presumably, increased intraabdominal pressure translocates CSF from the lumbar spine to the intracranial compartment. The prone position may be worthwhile in patients whose surgical incision does not preclude this posture.

Abdominal Binder

A single study suggested that an abdominal binder prevents the development of spinal headache.[12] It may provide symptomatic relief by the same mechanism as prone positioning. Again, this may not be feasible in patients with an abdominal incision.

Caffeine, Oral or Parenteral

A study of 41 patients with headache unresponsive to conservative measures demonstrated that intravenous caffeine 500 mg led to permanent resolution of symptoms in 70% of subjects.[13] The small size of the study and the lack of a control group cast doubt on the routine use of this therapy. As intravenous caffeine is unavailable in many hospitals, the use of oral caffeine has been proposed as a substitute. Oral caffeine, 300 mg, produces a more significant decrease in headache intensity than placebo; the effect is short-lived, however, and there is no reduction in the percentage of patients requiring epidural blood patch.[14]

Sumatriptan

The serotonin agonist sumatriptan is a cerebral vasoconstrictor that is used to treat migraine. One study reported relief of PDPH in four of six patients treated with 6 mg subcutaneous sumatriptan.[15] A subsequent study did not replicate these results, and this treatment should be considered unproven.[16]

Corticosteroids/ACTH

A number of case reports have suggested a therapeutic role for corticosteroids or adrenocorticotropic hormone. A single randomized study demonstrated that high-dose hydrocortisone reduced the severity of spinal headache compared with placebo.[17] A randomized study could not demonstrate any benefit to the administration of ACTH.[18]

Intrathecal Saline

Injection of 10 mL of preservative-free saline via the Tuohy needle after accidental dural puncture decreased the incidence of headache from 62% to 32%. Injection of normal saline through an intrathecal catheter placed after accidental dural puncture also appeared to decrease headache, but the number of patients in this group was too small to achieve statistical significance.[19]

Intrathecal Catheter

After accidental dural puncture during attempted epidural placement, a catheter can be placed in the subarachnoid space to provide continuous spinal anesthesia. Some studies have suggested that this technique will reduce the incidence of subsequent spinal headache.[20] This result has not been consistently demonstrated, however, perhaps because of differing durations of subarachnoid catheterization in different studies.[21] In fact, one study did show improved results when the catheter remained in place for 24 hours after delivery.[22] If a spinal catheter is placed, it is critical to maintain the sterility of the catheter. It is also imperative that all anesthetic providers are aware of the subarachnoid location of the catheter, to prevent the injection of large (epidural) doses of local anesthetic.

Epidural Saline

Continuous epidural infusions of normal saline have been reported to prevent or relieve the symptoms of PDPH after accidental dural puncture during epidural placement.[23] Unfortunately, discontinuation of the infusion usually leads to recurrence of the headache. This technique may be useful in patients who refuse an epidural blood patch, providing symptomatic relief until the dural puncture spontaneously heals.

Epidural Blood Patch

The epidural blood patch (EBP) has been proposed as the gold standard for the treatment of PDPH, with early reports suggesting a success rate (permanent and complete relief of headache) of as high as 95%. Unfortunately, the great majority of these studies were not prospective, and a meta-analysis suggests that evidence for the efficacy of EBP is lacking.[24] Additionally, more recent reports suggest that the success rate of EBP may actually be as low as 65%.[25] EBP is least likely to be successful in patients with larger dural punctures, the very patients in whom headache is most likely to be severe and persistent. In those patients with recurrence of headache after EBP, a repeat procedure is usually successful. Failure of a second EBP should encourage a search for other possible causes of the headache.

There are technical aspects of a blood patch that increase the likelihood of its success. The spinal interspace chosen for the blood patch should be as close as possible to the initial puncture site, but if the volume of injected blood is sufficient, the spread of blood in the epidural space is usually extensive enough to reach the dural puncture site from any lumbar interspace. If significant back pain does not develop during injection, a volume of 15 to 20 mL of blood is optimal. The success rate of EBP is improved if the patient is allowed to remain supine for at least 1 hour, and possibly as long as 2 hours.[26] The patient should be advised to avoid heavy lifting or straining for at least 48 hours, because a forceful Valsalva maneuver may dislodge the patch, leading to recurrence of headache.

The decision to perform an EBP may be influenced by other considerations. The procedure is obviously contraindicated in patients thought to be bacteremic, but a low-grade fever is probably not a contraindication, especially if antibiotic therapy has been initiated. Despite early concerns that central nervous system involvement would be accelerated in human immunodeficiency virus (HIV)–infected patients receiving a blood patch, there is no evidence that this is the case, and EBP is not contraindicated in these patients.[27] Finally, for Jehovah's Witness patients who refuse EBP for religious reasons, the use of epidural dextran may be an effective alternative, although published experience with this technique is limited, and the patient should be fully informed about the speculative nature of this therapy.

Prophylactic EBP

EBP administered via an epidural catheter placed subsequent to accidental dural puncture has been reported to decrease the incidence of PDPH by as much as half, from 70% to 30%.[28] More recent work suggests that the usefulness of prophylactic EBP has been significantly overstated,[29] although there is evidence that while prophylactic EBP does not prevent headache, it may decrease its duration.[30] Because not all patients will develop PDPH after dural puncture, a substantial number of those who receive a prophylactic EBP will be treated for a complication that may never have developed even in the absence of the treatment. It is therefore essential that patients be fully informed of the potential complications of EBP, and that every effort is made to prevent those complications, particularly infection.

Epidural Dextran

In those patients who cannot receive EBP because of fever, or who refuse EBP because of religious reasons, epidural dextran has been used with some success.[31] This modality has never been studied in prospective fashion, and concerns about the potential for neurotoxicity and the risk of allergic reaction remain. Epidural dextran infusions must be considered nonstandard therapy at the present time.

AREAS OF UNCERTAINTY

Pharmacologic Management

In view of the mixed results of such interventions as caffeine, sumatriptan, and ACTH, yet acknowledging the benign nature of these treatments, is there any value to a trial of these agents, or should EBP be offered early in the course of PDPH?

Intrathecal Catheter Placement after Accidental Dural Puncture

Evidence as to the prophylactic value of this technique is sufficiently heterogeneous, and the potential risks of intrathecal catheterization (drug overdose, infection) are great enough that utilization of this technique or the placement of an epidural catheter at a different level can both be justified.

Neuroimaging

There is considerable overlap between the symptomatology of PDPH and intracranial venous thrombosis. In the setting of a failed initial EBP, it is not clear whether neuroimaging studies should be obtained before repeat EBP.[32]

GUIDELINES

The Therapeutics and Technology Assessment Subcommittee of the American Academy of Neurology has concluded that the use of an atraumatic spinal needle decreases the incidence of PDPH in adult patients, as does the use of smaller-sized needles.[33]

The American Society of Anesthesiologists Practice Guidelines for Obstetric Anesthesia recommends that pencil-point spinal needles should be used instead of cutting-bevel needles in order to decrease the risk of PDPH.[34]

AUTHOR'S RECOMMENDATIONS

It should be clear from the preceding discussion that PDPH can be debilitating, that it can cause serious morbidity, and that it may, in fact, result in significant litigation. In view of the multiple consequences of PDPH, the anesthesiologist should make every effort to minimize the risk of headache by optimizing those factors that can be controlled, namely needle size and shape. Despite our best efforts, though, these headaches will continue to occur, and we will continue to be called on to manage them.

Continued

AUTHOR'S RECOMMENDATIONS — Cont'd

Unfortunately, despite many years of research, it is still not clear what is the optimal treatment of PDPH. What follows, then, is one suggested management approach, based on the literature, but also on personal experience.

In patients who develop spinal headache, ambulation should not be restricted because bed rest has no demonstrated effect on the duration of spinal headache. The patient should therefore ambulate as much as he or she can tolerate. Although forced hydration is unlikely to augment CSF production to any significant degree, dehydration will worsen the headache, and intravenous fluids should be provided to patients who are unable to maintain adequate oral intake. Oral analgesics should be made available; in severe headache, narcotic analgesics may be required, and should be provided on a round-the-clock basis.

In patients who decline or who cannot receive an epidural blood patch, pharmacologic therapy should be considered. The only therapy that appears to be consistently effective is caffeine; if the intravenous preparation is available, one or two doses of caffeine benzoate 500 mg should be administered. Otherwise, 300 mg of oral caffeine can be administered every 6 hours. Until more supportive evidence is available, the routine use of sumatriptan cannot be recommended.

My practice is to wait at least 24 hours after the onset of symptoms before considering a blood patch because some headaches may resolve by that time, and I would prefer to avoid the possible complications of epidural blood patch in headaches that resolve that quickly. There are exceptions, however; in patients with a debilitating headache due to accidental dural puncture with a large epidural needle, the likelihood of rapid spontaneous resolution is small, and I will perform a blood patch soon after the development of symptoms. Bear in mind, however, that epidural blood patch performed within 24 hours of dural puncture has a lower success rate; whether this is because headaches treated within 24 hours are more severe, and thus more likely to lead to failed blood patch, or whether there is an intrinsic increased failure rate with early blood patch is unclear.

In the setting of a known accidental dural puncture during epidural placement, the likelihood of headache is so high that prophylactic measures should be considered. Because the evidence that placing an intrathecal catheter through a dural puncture decreases the incidence of headache is inconsistent, the decision to use a continuous spinal anesthetic should be made on the basis of other considerations, such as difficult airway or morbid obesity, in addition to the possible effect on the development of headache. If this is done, it is critically important for all caregivers to be notified of the intrathecal location of the catheter, to prevent the administration of what would be an appropriate epidural dose into the subarachnoid space. If a catheter is placed in the epidural space subsequent to a dural puncture, an infusion of epidural saline (20 to 30 mL/hr) will frequently prevent a headache from developing; however, a headache usually develops after the infusion is stopped. Finally, an immediate blood patch performed via an epidural catheter may prevent the development of a headache. Of course, as many as 50% of patients with a dural puncture from even a 17-gauge Touhy needle will not develop a headache, and these patients therefore would be treated unnecessarily; for this reason, I reserve immediate epidural blood patch for those patients in whom I suspect a repeated epidural procedure would be technically difficult. I also reserve immediate blood patch for those patients whose epidural catheters were treated in strict sterile fashion after the initial dural puncture, because the consequences of injecting blood through a contaminated catheter are potentially catastrophic.

REFERENCES

1. Gerritse BM, Gielen MJ: Seven months delay for epidural blood patch in post-dural puncture headache. *Eur J Anaesthesiol* 1999;16:650-651.
2. Bechard P, Perron G, et al: Case report: Epidural blood patch in the treatment of abducens palsy after a dural puncture. *Can J Anesth* 2007;54:146-150.
3. Zeiden A, Farhat O et al: Does postdural puncture headache left untreated lead to subdural hematoma? Case report and a review of the literature. *Int J Obstet Anesth* 2006;15:50-58.
4. Chadwick HS: An analysis of obstetric anesthesia cases from the American Society of Anesthesiologists closed claims project database. *Int J Obstet Anesth* 1996;5:258-263.
5. Bier A: Versucheüber cocainisirung des rückenmarkes. *Dtsch Zeitschr Chir* 1899;51:361-369.
6. Landau R, Ciliberto CF, et al: Complications with 25-gauge and 27-gauge Whitacre needles during combined spinal-epidural analgesia in labor. *Int J Obstet Anesth* 2001;10:168-171.
7. Richman JM, Joe EM, et al: Bevel direction and postdural puncture headache: A meta-analysis. *Neurologist* 2006;12:224-228.
8. Albright GA: The safety and efficacy of combined spinal and epidural analgesia/anesthesia (6002 blocks) in a community hospital. *Reg Anesth Pain Med* 1999;24:117-125.
9. Bakshi R, Mechtler LL, et al: MRI findings in lumbar puncture headache syndrome: Abnormal dural-meningeal and dural venous sinus enhancement. *Clin Imaging* 1999;23:73-76.
10. Sudlow C, Warlow C: Posture and fluids for preventing post-dural puncture headache. *Cochrane Database of Systematic Reviews* 2001, Issue 2. Art. no.: CD001790. DOI: 10.1002/14651858.CD001790.
11. Dieterich M, Brandt T: Incidence of post-lumbar puncture headache is independent of daily fluid intake. *Eur Arch Psychiatr Neurol Sci* 1988;237:194-196.
12. Mosavy SH, Shafei M: Prevention of headache consequent upon dural puncture in obstetric patient. *Anaesthesia* 1975;30:807-809.
13. Sechzer PH, Abel L: Post-spinal anesthesia headache treated with caffeine. Evaluation with demand method. Part I. *Curr Therap Res* 1978;24:307-312.
14. Camann WR, Murray RS, et al: Effects of oral caffeine on postdural puncture headache: A double-blind, placebo-controlled trial. *Anesth Analg* 1990;70:181-184.
15. Carp H, Singh PJ, et al: Effects of the serotonin-receptor agonist sumatriptan on postdural puncture headache: Report of six cases. *Anesth Analg* 1994;79:180-182.
16. Connelly NR, Parker RK, et al: Sumatriptan in patients with postdural puncture headache. *Headache* 2000;40:316-319.
17. Noyan Ashraf MA, Sadeghi A, et al: Hydrocortisone in postdural puncture headache. *Middle East J Anesthesiol* 2007;19:415-422.
18. Rucklidge MW, Yentis SM, Paech MJ: Synacthen depot for the treatment of postdural puncture headache. *Anaesthesia* 2004;59:138-141.
19. Charsly MM, Abram SE: The injection of intrathecal normal saline reduces the severity of postdural puncture headache. *Reg Anesth Pain Med* 2001;26:301-305.
20. Dennehy KC, Rosaeg OP: Intrathecal catheter insertion during labour reduces the risk of post-dural puncture headache. *Can J Anaesth* 1998;45:42-45.
21. Liu N, Montefiore A, et al: Prolonged placement of spinal catheters does not prevent postdural puncture headache. *Reg Anesth* 1993;18:110-113.
22. Ayad S, Demian Y, et al: Subarachnoid catheter placement after wet tap for analgesia in labor: Influence on the risk of headache in obstetric patients. *Reg Anesth Pain Med* 2003;28:512-515.
23. Shah JL: Epidural pressure during infusion of saline in the parturient. *Int J Obstet Anesth* 1993;2:190-192.
24. Sudlow C, Warlow C: Epidural blood patching for preventing and treating post-dural puncture headache. *Cochrane Database of Systematic Reviews* 2001, Issue 2. Art. no.: CD001791. DOI: 10.1002/14651858.CD001791.
25. Safa-Tisseront V, Thormann F, et al: Effectiveness of epidural blood patch in the management of post-dural puncture headache. *Anesthesiology* 2001;95:334-339.

26. Martin R, Jourdain S, et al: Duration of decubitus position after epidural blood patch. *Can J Anaesth* 1994;41:23-25.
27. Tom DJ, Gulevich SJ, et al: Epidural blood patch in the HIV-positive patient. Review of clinical experience. *Anesthesiology* 1992;76:943-947.
28. Cheek TG, Banner R, et al: Prophylactic extradural blood patch is effective. A preliminary communication. *Br J Anaesth* 1988;61:340-342.
29. Vasdev GM, Southern PA: Postdural puncture headache: The role of prophylactic epidural blood patch. *Curr Pain Headache Rep* 2001;5:281-283.
30. Scavone BM, Wong CA, et al: Efficacy of a prophylactic epidural blood patch in preventing post dural puncture headache in parturients after inadvertent dural puncture. *Anesthesiology* 2004;101:1422-1427.
31. Barrios-Alarcon J, Aldrete JA, Paragas-Tapia D: Relief of post-lumbar puncture headache with epidural dextran 40: A preliminary report. *Reg Anesth* 1989;14:78-80.
32. Lockhart EM, Baysinger CL: Intracranial venous thrombosis in the parturient. *Anesthesiology* 2007;107:652-658.
33. Armon C, Evans RW: Addendum to assessment: Prevention of post-lumbar puncture headaches. *Neurology* 2005;65:510-512.
34. American Society of Anesthesiologists Task Force on Obstetric Anesthesia: Practice guidelines for obstetric anesthesia. *Anesthesiology* 2007;106:843-863.

56 Should Ultrasound Guidance Be Used for Peripheral Nerve Blockade?

Michael Aziz, MD

INTRODUCTION

Ultrasound guidance for peripheral nerve blockade is gaining popularity among anesthesiologists for several reasons, including greater success rates and potentially fewer complications from nerve injury/paresthesia, local anesthetic toxicity, pneumothorax, painful muscle stimulation, and neuraxial anesthesia. Historically, peripheral nerve blocks were placed using a technique that elicited paresthesia on needle contact with a nerve. By adding nerve-stimulating devices, we have been able to more precisely locate peripheral nerves based on nerve twitch patterns. The improved resolution of modern ultrasound devices now allows us to visualize the peripheral nerves that we hope to anesthetize and/or their surrounding structures and to successfully guide our needle placement. Finally, in the growing number of outpatient procedures, ultrasound guidance techniques may improve control of postoperative pain.

Some basic knowledge of the physics of ultrasound technology may be useful here. An ultrasonographic image is produced by passing an electric voltage through a piezoelectric crystal, directing the pulse into tissue, and recording its reflection (echoes) off the tissue. Tissues are visualized as image structures, and their interfaces have differing acoustic impedance, so that the pulse is reflected, refracted, or scattered. A transducer that sends a high-frequency signal can gain higher resolution, but often for only very superficial structures because resolution decreases as penetration (depth) increases. Newer ultrasound machines, however, can produce higher resolution at deeper penetrations.

TECHNIQUE

Ultrasound-guided technique involves several steps. To begin, the probe orientation is critical to accurate identification of the structures; so, the anesthesiologist must know which end of the probe is orienting in which direction. To maintain proper orientation, some devices are equipped with a palpable dot on the side of the probe that corresponds to a dot on the screen. The appropriate probe is chosen based on patient size, the nerve to be blocked, and the resolution required. To visualize deep neural structures, we recommend using a curved array probe.

A preblock scan should be performed to identify the nerve and, perhaps more important, the surrounding structures such as bone, muscle, vascular structures, neuraxis, and pleura. To optimize the view, the anesthesiologist adjusts the transducer by sliding it along the skin, rotating it, and tilting it. After sterile prep, including a sterile sleeve around the ultrasound transducer, a needle is advanced close to the nerve without making direct contact. A needle kept in plane with the probe allows its entire course to be followed. Errors are described with this technique when the practitioner loses sight of the needle tip.[1] With the needle, nerve, and surrounding structures in view, a catheter can be placed for continuous perineural infusion or local anesthetic can be placed around the nerve. The local anesthetic should be seen completely surrounding the nerve[2]; however, if the nerve is directly injected, it will appear swollen.[3-5] For the brachial plexus, local anesthetic should be seen encircling all the relevant segments of the plexus.

EVIDENCE

Overall, data support the use of ultrasound guidance as a safe adjunct to nerve stimulation techniques or as a complete replacement for nerve stimulation. The most difficult question to answer is whether ultrasound guidance improves success rates and decreases complications. Studies have used various criteria to demonstrate higher success rates for ultrasound guidance compared with conventional techniques. However, because the rate of major complications from regional anesthesia is so low, only very large multicentered trials or meta-analyses could show that ultrasound guidance adds safety to regional anesthesia[6,7]; to date, no such studies exist. Although their outcome measures vary, randomized trials have demonstrated several benefits of ultrasound over nerve stimulation or other landmark techniques.

Procedure Attempts, Times, and Comfort

Findings indicate that less time and fewer attempts are needed to successfully perform a block using ultrasound guidance and that patient comfort is improved. Three randomized studies demonstrated quicker procedure times by measuring time intervals from first skin puncture to removal of the needle.[8-10] The elapsed time from probe placement through completion of injection was also shorter compared with nerve stimulation techniques.[11] Although these ultrasound techniques are approximately 2 to 6 minutes faster than landmark or nerve stimulation techniques, they do not account for prescanning and preparation of the ultrasound machine and probe, which could lengthen the procedural time. Fewer attempts have been reported for ultrasound-guided sciatic nerve blocks.[12] All these findings indicate that patient comfort is likely improved because the needle is in contact with the patient for a shorter period of time. In fact, children expressed lower pain scores during block performance with ultrasound compared with nerve stimulation.[13] There was also a lower incidence of paresthesia compared with landmark techniques.[14] In a patients with fractures of the extremity, painful muscle contractions that occur with nerve stimulation can be avoided with an ultrasound-guided nerve block.[15]

Block Onset Time

In several randomized trials, onset times were shorter for ultrasound-guided blocks than for blocks placed with conventional techniques. More specifically, shorter onset times have been documented for brachial plexus blocks in children and for femoral (three-in-one) blocks in adults.[13,16-18] Casati and colleagues[19] demonstrated a faster onset of sensory axillary brachial plexus block but found no difference in onset of motor block or in overall preparation time for surgery.[19] Similarly, sensory block onset was faster for supraclavicular brachial plexus blocks while the rate of motor block onset was unchanged.[20] Onset times were also faster for interscalene and axillary brachial plexus blocks under ultrasound compared with nerve stimulation,[17] although no difference in onset time was detected for sciatic nerve block.[12] The explanation for shorter onset times is not clear. However, with ultrasound guidance, we can see that the anesthetic is completely surrounding the nerve, which may not be occurring with nerve stimulation techniques.

Local Anesthetic Volume

Ultrasound may also provide the means to reduce the dose of local anesthetic necessary to achieve endpoints in a nerve block. For example, a lower volume of local anesthetic was required to encircle sciatic nerves (one-half volume) and femoral nerves (one-third volume) in children using ultrasound guidance compared with the set dose used for nerve stimulation. The ultrasound-guided group achieved successful blocks that also lasted longer than the nerve stimulation group.[21] For ilioinguinal/iliohypogastric nerve blocks, children needed less local anesthetic using ultrasound than using conventional "facial click" techniques (0.19 mL/kg versus 0.3 mL/kg). The ultrasound group of children also had better-quality blocks, based on a physical examination of sensory and motor block distribution.[22] An ultrasound-guided group that received 20 mL of local anesthetic for a femoral nerve block experienced a higher-quality block than a nerve

stimulation group that received 30 mL of local anesthetic.[16] Casati and colleagues[19] used the up-and-down staircase method to determine the amount of anesthetic required to achieve a sensory and a motor femoral nerve block. The minimum effective volume of ropivicaine 0.5% was 15 mL in the ultrasound-guided group and 26 mL in the nerve stimulation group.[23] Ultrasound guidance likely reduces local anesthetic dosing because reliable visualization of the local anesthetic spread around a nerve is possible to confirm the block. A lower total dose of local anesthetic may be a means to reduce the incidence of systemic local anesthetic toxicity.

Block Quality and Success

Success rates for nerve blocks can be difficult to assess, and criteria vary depending on the purpose of a block. For example, if a block is placed for postoperative pain relief, effectiveness may be measured by opiate consumption or distribution of sensory analgesia. If the purpose of the block is surgical anesthesia, measures of complete sensory and motor blocks, block supplementation, or the conversion rate to general anesthesia may be necessary to determine success. Lower intraoperative and postoperative analgesia was required in children receiving ilioinguinal/iliohypogastric nerve blocks with ultrasound placement compared with conventional "facial click" technique.[22]

Clinical studies favor ultrasound over conventional techniques for improved block quality as assessed by physical examination measurements. Several randomized studies have demonstrated reduced sensitivity to painful stimuli after ultrasound-guided femoral (3:1) blocks in adults and infraclavicular brachial plexus blocks in children.[13,16,18] Ultrasound-guided interscalene and axillary brachial plexus blocks also produced more complete sensory and motor blocks.[17] A higher incidence of complete sciatic nerve block and better tolerance of a tourniquet have been found with ultrasound compared with nerve stimulation.[12] Success rates are also higher in ultrasound-guided axillary brachial plexus blocks compared with the transarterial approach.[10] Half of the failures in the transarterial approach result from inability to locate the axillary artery, and the remainder are caused by inadequate intraoperative analgesia. In a quality study, Chan and colleagues[11] randomized three groups to receive axillary brachial plexus blocks using (1) ultrasound guidance, (2) nerve stimulation, or (3) both; success was defined as complete sensory block of the radial, median, and ulnar nerves. Ultrasound guidance with or without nerve stimulation was superior to nerve stimulation alone, and adding a nerve stimulator to the ultrasound technique did not provide any additional benefit. However, another study involving supraclavicular brachial plexus blocks did not report improved success or a reduced conversion rate to general anesthesia with ultrasound guidance and nerve stimulation techniques compared with nerve stimulation alone.[8]

Two studies have been published regarding the duration of analgesia and the benefits of ultrasound guidance compared with nerve stimulation. In one pediatric study, the time to first analgesic pain medicine was longer with ultrasound-guided sciatic and femoral nerve blocks.[21] This improved analgesic duration was also reported in children with ultrasound-guided infraclavicular brachial plexus blocks.[13]

Avoiding Intraneural Injection

Ultrasound may reduce the incidence of intraneural injection of local anesthetic. Most experts in regional anesthesia agree that intraneural injection is associated with postoperative neurologic dysfunction and should be avoided. Before ultrasound technology, the only indicators for intraneural needle placement were very painful

paresthesia, high injection pressures, or very low nerve stimulation current necessary to achieve a twitch. In an ultrasonographic study in pigs, Chan and colleagues[3] produced clear image differences between a perineural injection and a direct injection of a nerve in the axillary brachial plexus. According to these images, an intraneural injection is easily detected with ultrasound. The histologic examination of the nerves injected revealed infiltration of the injectate within the epineurium or perineurium. Interestingly, during axillary brachial plexus blocks, intraneural injection of low volumes of local anesthetic using ultrasound guidance may not cause neurologic dysfunction.[4] In this study, it appears that Bigeleisen[4] tried to achieve intraneural injection of anesthetics at low volumes

Table 56-1	Summary of Randomized Controlled Trials (RCTs) Comparing Ultrasound-guided with Nerve-stimulated Peripheral Nerve Blocks				
Study, Year	**Site (*n*)**	**Study Design**	**Intervention**	**Control**	**Outcomes**
Chan et al.,[11] 2007	Axillary brachial plexus (188)	Double-blinded RCT	Ultrasound alone or ultrasound and nerve stimulation	Nerve stimulation with multiple injection	Improved incidence of complete sensory block
Casati et al.,[23] 2007	Femoral (60)	Up-and-down staircase method for minimum effective volume	Ultrasound guided	Nerve stimulation	Reduces minimum effective anesthetic volume
Dingemans et al.,[9] 2007	Infraclavicular brachial plexus (73)	Prospective RCT	Ultrasound	Ultrasound and nerve stimulation	Faster onset
Casati et al.,[19] 2007	Axillary brachial plexus (60)	Prospective RCT	Ultrasound	Nerve stimulation with multiple injections	Faster onset
Domingo-Triado et al.,[12] 2007	Sciatic (61)	Prospective RCT	Ultrasound	Nerve stimulation	Improved quality of sensory block Improved tourniquet tolerance, reduced attempts
Oberndorfer et al.,[21] 2007	Pediatric femoral and sciatic (46)	Prospective RCT	Ultrasound	Nerve stimulation	Reduced volume of local anesthetic and longer duration of analgesia
Sites et al.,[10] 2006	Axillary brachial plexus (56)	Prospective RCT	Ultrasound	Perivascular technique	Reduced conversion to general anesthesia, reduced performance time
Willschke et al.,[22] 2005	Pediatric ilioinguinal/ iliohypogastric (100)	Prospective RCT	Ultrasound	Facial click	Lower local anesthetic volume, lower additional analgesic requirements
Marhofer et al.,[13] 2004	Infraclavicular brachial plexus (40)	Prospective RCT	Ultrasound	Nerve stimulation	Shorter onset time, lower pain scores during performance, longer sensory block, better sensory and motor block quality
Williams et al.,[8] 2003	Supraclavicular brachial plexus (80)	Prospective RCT	Ultrasound and nerve stimulation	Nerve stimulation alone	Shorter block performance time, better block distribution
Marhofer et al.,[16] 1998	3:1 femoral nerve block (60)	Prospective RCT	Ultrasound	Nerve stimulation at different volumes	Reduced onset time, improved quality of sensory block
Marhofer et al.,[18] 1997	3:1 femoral nerve block (40)	Prospective RCT	Ultrasound	Nerve stimulation	Reduced onset time, improved quality of sensory block

and show that ultrasound can help to guide such intra-neural injections. The relationship between neurologic dysfunction and intraneural injection is still unclear, but ultrasound imaging can show when a nerve is being injected and may help to avoid injecting high volumes of local anesthetic directly into a nerve (Table 56-1).

CONTROVERSIES

The referenced studies support a favorable argument for ultrasound guidance in regional anesthesia. These investi-gators have extensive experience with ultrasound guid-ance, and they acknowledge that ultrasonography takes quite some time to master. This should be taken into account when reviewing the data because it is not clear from the literature how an unsupervised novice would perform. For good performance of any regional anesthetic under ultrasound guidance, anatomy must be relearned, scanning must be practiced repeatedly, and images must be reviewed by experts. Therefore it seems unlikely that a novice would be able to quickly incorporate ultrasound guidance into his or her practice and achieve optimal benefits. Sites and colleagues[1] describe novice resident behaviors during the review of ultrasound images. Based on these observations, they created some target learning points for training and simulation.

Training in ultrasonography has become a contro-versial topic. Some experts believe that training and subsequent certification in this skill will improve the practice of regional anesthesia and avoid errors and com-plications. Others argue that training and certification pro-grams discourage the use of ultrasound and that even the novice can offer some benefits for our patients over nerve stimulation alone. Despite the clear benefits of ultra-sound, the lack of definitive data showing risk reduc-tion may discourage the considerable investment in the machine and training. Although machines are getting less expensive, few smaller anesthesiology groups can afford the expense, especially considering their low volume of regional anesthesia cases.

Although ultrasound guidance has become fairly com-mon in large academic centers and training institutions, many worry that graduating anesthesiology residents are no longer proficient in the conventional techniques of regional anesthesia, which they may well need if they take jobs in smaller community practices that do not have the benefit of ultrasound technology. I argue that ultrasound enhances a resident's knowledge of three-dimensional anatomy and thus improves the resident's performance of conventional techniques.

GUIDELINES

No guidelines have currently been issued by anesthesiol-ogy or pain medicine organizations for the use of ultra-sound during regional anesthesia. The data presented here are examples of recent findings regarding the benefit of incorporating ultrasound guidance into the practice of regional anesthesia. The safety of regional anesthesia before the use of ultrasound is well established.

AUTHOR'S RECOMMENDATIONS

- Compared with peripheral nerve stimulation, ultrasound-guided nerve blocks are faster to perform, less painful, and more successful. They also have a shorter onset time, result in a better-quality block, and last longer.
- It is presumed that ultrasound guidance may reduce complications by avoiding perineural structures such as vessels, pleura, and neuraxis, but no data confirm these presumptions.
- Data suggest that ultrasound guidance may also reduce complications by reducing the dose of local anesthetic, by diminishing painful paresthesia during performance, and by avoiding or limiting intraneural injection.
- Based on the data presented, it may be difficult to predict the successful performance of ultrasound-guided regional anesthesia by novices.
- For those interested in ultrasound-guided regional anesthesia, I recommend that they pursue training or mentorship to acquire this skill. Several training courses are now available, and a certification process may soon be offered.
- With ultrasound guidance techniques, anesthesiologists are gaining confidence in achieving successful nerve block placement. As this success rate improves, patients and surgeons will be encouraged, and the number of regional anesthesia cases will most likely increase.

REFERENCES

1. Sites BD, Spence BC, Gallagher JD, Wiley CW, Bertrand ML, Blike GT: Characterizing novice behavior associated with learning ultrasound-guided peripheral regional anesthesia. *Reg Anesth Pain Med* 2007;32:107-115.
2. Sandhu NS, Capal LM: Ultrasound-guided infraclavicular brachial plexus block. *Br J Anaesth* 2002;89:254-259.
3. Chan VWS, Brull R, McCartney CJL, XU D, Abbas S, Shannon P: An ultrasonographic and histological study of intraneuronal injection and electrical stimulation in pigs. *Anesth Analg* 2007; 104:1281-1284.
4. Bigeleisen PE: Nerve puncture and apparent intraneural injection during ultrasound-guided axillary block does not invariably result in neurologic injury. *Anesthesiology* 2006;105:779-783.
5. Chan VW: Ultrasound evidence of intraneural injection. *Anesth Analg* 2005;101:610-611.
6. Auroy Y, Benhamou D, Bargues L, Ecoffey C, Falissard B, Mercier F, et al: Major complications of regional anesthesia in France: The SOS Regional Anesthesia Hotline Service. *Anesthesiology* 2002;97:1274-1280.
7. Brull R, McCartney CJ, Chan VW, El Beheiry H: Neurological complications after regional anesthesia: Contemporary estimates of risk. *Anesth Analg* 2007;104:965-974.
8. Williams SR, Chouinard P, Arcand G, Harris P, Ruel M, Boudreault D, Girard F: Ultrasound guidance speeds execution and improves the quality of supraclavicular block. *Anesth Analg* 2003;97:1518-1523.
9. Dingemans E, Williams SR, Arcand G, Chouinard P, Harris P, Ruel M, Girard F: Neurostimulation in ultrasound-guided infra-clavicular block: A prospective randomized trial. *Anesth Analg* 2007;104:1275-1280.
10. Sites BD, Beach ML, Spence BC, Wiley CW, Shiffrin J, Hartman GS, Gallagher JD: Ultrasound guidance improves the success rate of a perivascular axillary plexus block. *Acta Anaesthesiol Scand* 2006;50:678-684.
11. Chan VW, Perlas A, McCartney CJ, Brull R, Xu D, Abbas S: Ultrasound guidance improves success rate of axillary brachial plexus block. *Can J Anesth* 2007;54:176-182.
12. Domingo-Triado V, Selfa S, Martinez F, Sanchez-Contreras D, Reche M, Teclas J, et al: Ultrasound guidance for lateral

midfemoral sciatic nerve block: A prospective, comparative, randomized study. *Anesth Analg* 2007;104:1270-1274.

13. Marhofer P, Sitzwohl C, Greher M, Kapral S: Ultrasound guidance for infraclavicular brachial plexus anaesthesia in children. *Anaesthesia* 2004;59:642-646.
14. Soeding PE, Sha S, Royse CE, Marks P, Hoy G, Royse AG: A randomized trial of ultrasound-guided brachial plexus anaesthesia in upper limb surgery. *Anaesth Intensive Care* 2005;33:719-725.
15. Plunkett AR, Brown DS, Rogers JM, Buckenmaier CC: Supraclavicular continuous peripheral nerve block in a wounded soldier: When ultrasound is the only option. *Br J Anaesth* 2006;97:715-717.
16. Marhofer P, Schrogendorfer K, Wallner T, Koinig H, Mayer N, Kapral S: Ultrasonographic guidance reduces the amount of local anesthetic for 3-in-1 blocks. *Reg Anesth Pain Med* 1998;23:584-588.
17. Soeding PE, Sha S, Royse CE, Marks P, Hoy G, Royse AG: A randomized trial of ultrasound-guided brachial plexus anaesthesia in upper limb surgery. *Anaesth Intensive Care* 2005;33:719-725.
18. Marhofer P, Schrögendorfer K, Koinig H, Kapral S, Weinstabl C, Mayer N: Ultrasonographic guidance improves sensory block and onset time of three-in-one blocks. *Anesth Analg* 1997;85:854-857.
19. Casati A, Danelli G, Baciarello M, Corradi M, Leone S, Di Canni S, Fanelli G: A prospective, randomized comparison between ultrasound and nerve stimulation guidance for multiple injection axillary brachial plexus block. *Anesthesiology* 2007;106:992-996.
20. Chan VW, Perlas A, Rawson R, Odukoya O: Ultrasound-guided supraclavicular brachial plexus block. *Anesth Analg* 2003;97:1514-1517.
21. Oberndorfer U, Marhofer P, Bosenberg A, Willschke H, Felfernig M, Weintraud M, et al: Ultrasonographic guidance for sciatic and femoral nerve blocks in children. *Br J Anaesth* 2007;98(6):797-801.
22. Willschke H, Marhofer P, Bosenberg A, Johnston S, Wanzel O, Cox SG, et al: Ultrasonography for ilioinguinal/iliohypogastric nerve blocks in children. *Br J Anaesth* 2005;95:226-230.
23. Casati A, Baciarello M, Cianni S, Danelli G, DeMarco G, Leone S, et al: Effects of ultrasound guidance on the minimum effective anaesthetic volume required to block the femoral nerve. *Br J Anaesth* 2007;98:823-827.

MONITORING

57 Does a Pulmonary Artery Catheter Influence Outcome in Noncardiac Surgery?

Glenn S. Murphy, MD, and Jeffery S. Vender, MD

The flow-directed pulmonary artery catheter (PAC) is a monitor used to guide the care of critically ill patients. It is estimated that approximately 25% of PACs are placed for the management of high-risk surgical and trauma patients.[1] The PAC provides the clinician with access to hemodynamic data that may not be obtained by routine clinical assessment.[2] Right heart catheterization (RHC) at the bedside allows for the immediate determination of intracardiac pressures, cardiac output, mixed venous oxygen saturation, and derived hemodynamic parameters (systemic and pulmonary vascular resistance).

Many clinicians believe that early detection and treatment of hemodynamic abnormalities in the critically ill patient will improve outcomes. Despite nearly 30 years of use in the operating room, there is still vigorous debate about the impact of pulmonary artery (PA) catheterization on morbidity and mortality rates in the perioperative setting. This debate has been intensified by the recent publication of several large-scale, randomized trials demonstrating no outcome benefit of PACs in patients with congestive heart failure, acute respiratory distress syndrome (ARDS), or shock, or in a heterogeneous intensive care unit (ICU) patient population.[3-6] Clinical trials in surgical patient populations have demonstrated that postoperative outcomes are improved, worsened, or unchanged with the use of PAC monitoring (Table 57-1). In response to a lack of clear evidence supporting a beneficial effect of PAC monitoring on outcomes, the use of PACs in medical and surgical patients has declined. A 63% decrease in PA catheterization use in all surgical admissions occurred between 1993 and 2004.[7] Despite the publication of randomized controlled trials, interpretation of most published studies remains limited by important flaws in study design. Uncertainty relating to optimal hemodynamic targets and therapies, appropriate patient populations to derive benefit from PAC use, and methods to control for user knowledge and experience complicates the design of appropriate outcome investigations.

OPTIONS

The PAC is simply a monitoring device. The central venous pressure (CVP) catheter can also measure central pressure, but not provide information on pulmonary artery pressure or cardiac output. In order for the PAC to influence outcome, the information provided by the catheter must modify treatment of the patient. The acquisition of hemodynamic data will not affect clinical outcomes unless the care of the surgical patient is significantly altered by this information. Several clinical trials have examined the clinical benefits and risks of PAC monitoring without defining how the therapeutic strategy was changed by the PAC data. In most studies, however, patient care was modified by the PAC to reach defined hemodynamic endpoints (goal-directed therapy). Goal-directed PAC trials use volume administration and vasoactive drugs to achieve "optimal" cardiac filling pressures, cardiac outputs, and/or oxygen delivery.

High-risk surgical patients may come to the operating room with significant physiologic abnormalities. Using invasive monitoring, Del Guercio and Cohn[8] determined that only 13.5% of elderly patients undergoing major surgery had normal hemodynamic and respiratory function. In several PAC outcome trials, goal-directed therapy has been used to normalize filling pressures and cardiac outputs in surgical patients with abnormal hemodynamics. In addition, investigators have observed that survivors of major operations had consistently higher postoperative cardiac outputs and oxygen delivery than nonsurvivors.[9,10] Goal-directed therapy, guided by the PAC, may also be used to achieve supranormal hemodynamic values in critically ill surgical patients. Although such therapy is controversial,[11] increasing the cardiac index and oxygen delivery to levels characteristic of survivors of high-risk surgery has been the goal of many investigations.

Other methods of measuring cardiac output and providing goal-directed therapy include transesophageal Doppler devices, transesophageal echocardiography, and transthoracic impedance.

EVIDENCE

Preoperative Monitoring

The role of the PAC in hemodynamic optimization before major noncardiac surgery remains controversial. Shoemaker and colleagues[12] randomized general surgical patients into three groups: a CVP group, a PAC control

Table 57-1 Effects of PAC Monitoring

Study	Number of Patients	Patient Population	Trial Design	Goal-directed Therapy	Outcomes
TRIALS DEMONSTRATING IMPROVED OUTCOME					
Whittemore et al[15] (1980)	110	Vascular surgical cohort	Prospective retrospective control preop optimization	Yes	Reduced mortality rate PAC group vs. historical control
Rao et al[20] (1983)	1097	Surgical patients cohort	Prospective retrospective control periop PAC	No	Reduced rate of reinfarction PAC group after MI
Hesdorffer et al[16] (1987)	61	Vascular surgical cohort	Prospective retrospective control preop optimization	Yes	Reduced renal dysfunction and mortality rates in PAC group vs. historical control
Shoemaker et al[12] (1988)	88	High-risk surgical	RCT periop PAC	Yes (supranormal)	Reduced morbidity/mortality rates in PAC protocol group vs. PAC control and CVP group
Berlauk et al[17] (1991)	89	Vascular surgical	RCT preop optimization	Yes	Reduced cardiac morbidity and graft thrombosis in PAC group vs. CVP group
Boyd et al[14] (1993)	107	High-risk surgical	RCT preop optimization	Yes (supranormal)	Reduced morbidity/mortality rates in PAC protocol group vs. PAC control group.
Wilson et al[13] (1999)	138	Major elective surgical	RCT preop optimization	Yes (supranormal)	Reduced mortality rate PAC protocol group vs. PAC control group
TRIALS DEMONSTRATING NO EFFECT ON OUTCOME					
Joyce et al[24] (1990)	40	Vascular surgical	RCT periop PAC	No	No differences in morbidity/mortality rates PAC group vs. CVP group
Isaacson et al[23] (1990)	102	Vascular surgical	RCT periop PAC	No	No differences in morbidity/mortality rates PAC group vs. CVP group
Yu et al[27] (1993)	67	ICU patients (subset surgical)	RCT postop PAC	Yes (supranormal)	No differences in morbidity/mortality rates PAC protocol group vs. PAC control group
Gattinoni et al[25] (1995)	762	ICU patients (subset surgical)	RCT postop PAC	Yes (supranormal)	No differences in morbidity/mortality rates PAC protocol vs. PAC control
Bender et al[19] (1997)	104	Vascular surgical	RCT preop optimization	Yes	No differences in morbidity/mortality rates PAC group vs. CVP group
Sandham et al[30] (2003)	1994	High-risk surgical	RCT	Yes (supranormal)	No differences in morbidity/mortality rates PAC group vs. standard therapy group
TRIALS DEMONSTRATING WORSENED OUTCOME					
Hayes et al[26] (1994)	109	ICU patients (subset surgical)	RCT postop PAC	Yes (supranormal)	Increased mortality rate PAC protocol group vs. PAC control group
Connors et al[29] (1996)	5735	ICU patients (subset surgical) cohort	Prospective postop PAC	No	Increased mortality rate in patients receiving PACs
Valentine et al[18] (1998)	120	Vascular surgical	RCT preop optimization	Yes	Increased intraop adverse events in PAC group vs. CVP group
Sandison et al[22] (1998)	145	Vascular surgical	Retrospective periop PAC	No	Increased mortality rate at hospital using more PACs
Polanczyk et al[21] (2001)	4059	Major noncardiac surgical cohort	Prospective periop PAC	No	Increased risk of major cardiac and noncardiac complications in patients receiving PACs

intraop, intraoperative; *MI*, myocardial infarction; *periop*, perioperative; *postop*, postoperative; *preop*, preoperative; *RCT*, randomized controlled trial.

group (normal hemodynamics), and a PAC protocol group (supranormal cardiac index and oxygen transport). Significant reductions in mortality rate, complications, and length of hospital stay were observed when fluids and inotropes were used to augment oxygen delivery preoperatively in the PAC protocol group. Two British studies in high-risk general surgical patients reported similar results.[13,14] Patients randomized to the protocol groups had oxygen delivery increased to greater than 600 mL/min/m^2 using PACs, fluids, and inotropes before surgery. When compared with the control groups receiving best standard perioperative care, a greater than 75% reduction in mortality rate was noted in the protocol groups.

Trials of preoperative optimization in vascular surgical patients have yielded conflicting results. Two studies reported that significant reductions in mortality rate[15,16] and renal dysfunction[16] occurred when hemodynamic values were normalized before surgery using PACs. However, both studies involved historical control groups. Three prospective randomized trials of preoperative optimization in vascular surgical patients have been published.[17-19] Patients in the PAC groups were administered fluids and vasoactive drugs until "optimal" values for wedge pressure, systemic vascular resistance, and cardiac index were obtained before surgery. Subjects in the control groups received CVP monitoring. No differences in mortality rate or hospital length of stay were observed between the PAC and control groups in any study. In the PAC group, morbidity was reported to be decreased (less cardiac morbidity and graft thrombosis),[17] increased (more adverse intraoperative events),[18] or unchanged.[19]

Intraoperative and Postoperative Monitoring

In a landmark study by Rao and colleagues,[20] the authors evaluated 733 patients with a history of myocardial infarction undergoing noncardiac surgery. Aggressive use of invasive monitoring and prompt correction of hemodynamic abnormalities was associated with a lower rate of myocardial reinfarction in these patients compared with a historical control group. Improvements in anesthetic techniques or ICU care that occurred over time may have accounted for the reduced cardiac morbidity in the prospective cohort group. Polanczyk and colleagues[21] examined the association between PAC use and postoperative cardiac complications in patients undergoing major noncardiac surgery. In this prospective observational cohort study, 4059 patients (221 had PACs and 3838 did not) were followed for major postoperative cardiac events. Patients monitored with PACs had a threefold increase in cardiac events. The investigators also performed a case-control analysis, using a propensity score to match patients who did and did not undergo PA catheterization. In this matched-pairs analysis, PAC use was associated with an increased risk of postoperative congestive heart failure and major noncardiac events.

Several clinical trials have compared outcomes in vascular surgical patients monitored with CVP versus PA catheters. Sandison and colleagues[22] examined morbidity and mortality rates in patients undergoing urgent or emergent abdominal aortic aneurysm (AAA) repair at two hospitals under the care of a single vascular surgeon. The authors observed that morbidity and mortality rates were significantly increased at the hospital that used PACs routinely. Two prospective randomized trials (PAC versus CVP) have been performed in low-risk AAA patients.[23,24] No significant differences in mortality rate, perioperative complications, or hospital length of stay were found between patients monitored with CVP or PA catheters.

Postoperative Monitoring

Oxygen consumption and delivery are increased in critically ill patients who survive major surgery. Four randomized clinical trials have evaluated the effect of using a PAC to achieve supranormal values of oxygen delivery in critically ill ICU patients. Fluids and inotropes were administered to reach defined treatment goals. High-risk postoperative patients made up a portion of each study population. In the largest trial, involving 762 patients in 56 ICUs, subjects were assigned to one of three treatments: a normal cardiac index, a cardiac index ≥ 4.5 L/min, or a mixed venous saturation $\geq 70\%$.[25] No differences in mortality rate, number of dysfunctional organs, or length of stay in the ICU were found among the three groups. Three additional studies randomized patients into a treatment group (oxygen delivery greater than 600 mL/min/m^2) or a control group ("normal" oxygen delivery or cardiac output).[26-28] In each trial, no improvement in in-hospital survival was observed in the treatment group.

Connors and colleagues[29] conducted a prospective cohort study involving 5735 critically ill adult patients at five medical centers. Postoperative patients meeting severity and other entry criteria were enrolled in the trial. The investigators evaluated the association between PAC monitoring and patient outcome using a propensity score. The propensity score was used to match patients managed with and without PACs for a variety of demographic and physiologic characteristics. Case-matching analysis revealed that patients managed with PACs had consistently higher mortality rates at 30, 60, and 180 days after study entry. Subgroup analysis revealed that the relative hazard of death with PAC monitoring was highest in patients receiving postoperative care.

In the largest randomized controlled trial enrolling surgical patients, Sandham and colleagues[30] compared outcomes in 1994 patients receiving goal-directed therapy guided by a PAC with standard care without the use of a PAC. The subjects were high-risk patients (ASA class III or IV with an age greater than 60) undergoing major operative procedures. Hemodynamic goals in the PAC group included an oxygen delivery index of 550 to 600 mL/min/m^2, a cardiac index of 3.5 to 4.5 L/min/m^2, and a wedge pressure of 18 mm Hg using fluids and vasoactive medications. In-hospital and one-year mortality rates were similar between groups. No differences in postoperative morbidity were observed between the groups, with the exception of a higher incidence of pulmonary embolism in the PAC group.

Summary

Studies examining the impact of PAC monitoring on clinical outcomes have yielded conflicting results. On the basis of currently available trials, it is difficult to draw meaningful conclusions about the safety and efficacy of PA catheterization in the perioperative setting. Presently there is insufficient evidence to determine if PACs improve or worsen outcomes in high-risk surgical patients.

There is a need for additional research to answer this important question. Significant design limitations are present in all the published studies. Unfortunately, nearly all randomized trials have been inadequately powered to detect meaningful clinical outcomes such as mortality rate. Combining data from smaller clinical trials by performing a meta-analysis may yield information on infrequent adverse effects related to PAC monitoring. A meta-analysis of the data from randomized controlled studies was published in 1997. No significant improvements in overall survival were observed.[31] However, a meta-analysis of morbidity data revealed significant reductions in major morbidity using PAC-guided strategies.[32] Most recently, a Cochrane Collaboration meta-analysis (amended in 2006) of randomized controlled trials revealed no effect of PAC monitoring on mortality rates in high-risk surgical patients (odds ratio of 0.98 [95% CI 0.73 to 1.33]).[33] Large-scale randomized controlled trials using carefully designed treatment interventions and clinically relevant outcome measures are needed to determine the benefits and harms associated with PA catheterization.

AREAS OF UNCERTAINTY/CONTROVERSY

The information provided by the PAC must be accurately interpreted in order to influence treatment strategies and outcomes. Misinterpretation of these data may alter decisions about patient therapy in a manner that can increase morbidity and mortality risks. Several studies have evaluated clinicians' knowledge of the PAC. Iberti and colleagues[34] administered a 31-question examination to 496 North American physicians to assess their understanding of PA catheterization. Significant deficiencies in clinicians' ability to interpret PAC data were identified; 47% of respondents were unable to determine pulmonary artery occlusion pressure (PAOP) from a clearly marked tracing. When a survey was provided to physician members of the Society of Critical Care Medicine in the United States, one third of respondents were unable to measure the PAOP on a clearly marked tracing or identify the major components of oxygen transport.[35] Nearly identical results were obtained when a similar multiple-choice examination was provided to European intensivists and American ICU nurses.[36,37] A cross-sectional survey of cardiovascular anesthesiologists demonstrated that most clinicians lack confidence in their ability to determine the PAOP from a sample pulmonary artery tracing.[38]

Outcomes will not be improved unless clinicians demonstrate competency in basic technical and cognitive aspects of PA catheterization. At the present time, no specific guidelines have been published relating to training, credentialing, or continuing medical education requirements for clinicians who use PACs. Some authors have suggested that PA catheterization should be restricted to individuals who have demonstrated expertise in catheter insertion and application of the data.[34,36] The American Society of Anesthesiologists (ASA) Task Force on Pulmonary Artery Catheterization recommends that all individuals who use PACs undergo supervised training and that quality improvement programs must be in place at centers where these catheters are used.[39,40] Variability in user competence may account for the lack of improvement in outcomes demonstrated in several PAC trials.

Randomized studies are needed to determine the clinical utility of PAC monitoring in surgical patients. However, there are ethical issues involved in randomizing the allocation of PACs in high-risk patients because many clinicians believe that PA catheterization improves outcomes. The Ontario Intensive Care Study Group abandoned a randomized PAC trial after 35% of the eligible subjects were excluded because the primary physician believed that PAC monitoring was ethically mandated.[41] Randomization in a clinical trial is ethically appropriate in settings where there is uncertainty about the benefits and harms of a particular therapy. Future randomized trials should examine patient populations in which expert opinion is divided about the clinical utility of PA catheterization (e.g., low-risk cardiac surgery).[1]

In some clinical trials, worsened outcomes have occurred in patients monitored with PACs. The information provided by the PAC often produces a more aggressive approach to patient care. Subjects randomized to PAC groups typically received more fluids and vasoactive drugs than control group patients. A more invasive and aggressive treatment strategy may benefit some patients by improving oxygen delivery. Other patients may be harmed using this approach because the risk of fluid overload, congestive heart failure, arrhythmias, and myocardial ischemia may be increased.

GUIDELINES

Several groups have published statements that address the clinical utility of PA catheterization in the perioperative setting. The National Heart, Lung, and Blood Institute and Food and Drug Administration Workshop Report on Pulmonary Artery Catheterization and Clinical Outcomes noted that there have been no randomized trials that clearly demonstrate that the use of PACs improves overall surgical outcomes.[1] The workshop recommended that methods to standardize and measure physician and nurse education be established and that further randomized trials in certain surgical populations be performed.

A report from the Pulmonary Artery Catheter Consensus Conference emphasized that there are limited data to support the use of PA catheterization in surgical patients and that the overall quality of published clinical trials was poor.[42] The conference participants recommended that clinicians should carefully weigh the risks and benefits of PAC monitoring in each patient.

In 1993 the ASA published guidelines on the role of the PAC in the perioperative setting.[39] These guidelines were updated in 2003.[40] The ASA Task Force acknowledged that there were significant deficiencies in the study designs of all of the published research examining the impact of PAC monitoring on outcomes. Therefore it was difficult to determine the safety and efficacy of PA catheterization based on scientific evidence. The expert opinion of the Task Force, however, was that access to PAC data, "coupled with accurate and appropriate treatment tailored to hemodynamic status, can reduce perioperative mortality and morbidity." Patients at increased risk for complications related to hemodynamic disturbances should be considered candidates for PA catheterization. Three interrelated variables should be assessed in determining the risks and benefits of PAC monitoring.

1. *Patient factors*: Patients should be evaluated for preexisting medical conditions that may increase the risk of hemodynamic instability (i.e., cardiovascular, pulmonary, or renal disease).
2. *Procedure factors*: Major surgical procedures may be associated with significant hemodynamic fluctuations, which may damage organ systems.
3. *Practice setting factors*: Complications from hemodynamic disturbances may be increased if the technical and cognitive skills of the physicians and nurses caring for the patient are poor.

Pulmonary artery catheterization is not required when the patient, procedure, and practice setting all pose a low risk for hemodynamic complications.

In 2007, the American College of Cardiology (ACC) and American Heart Association (AHA) jointly published the updated "ACC/AHA Guidelines on Perioperative Cardiovascular Evaluation and Care for Noncardiac Surgery."[43] After performing a formal literature review, evidence supporting the use of PACs in the setting of noncardiac surgery was weighed and graded. The reviewers concluded that "use of a PAC may be reasonable in patients at risk for major hemodynamic disturbances that are easily detected by a PAC; however, the decision must be based on 3 parameters: patient disease, surgical procedure and practice setting, because incorrect interpretation of the data from a PAC may cause harm (Class IIb [Benefit ≥ Risk; Procedure/Treatment may be considered], Level of Evidence: B [Recommendation's efficacy less well established; Conflicting evidence from single randomized trial or non-randomized studies])." Furthermore, the guidelines state that *routine* use of a PAC in the perioperative setting is not recommended, particularly in low-risk patients (Class III [Risk ≥ Benefit; Procedure should not be performed since it is not helpful], Level of Evidence: A [Sufficient evidence from multiple randomized trials or meta-analysis]).

AUTHORS' RECOMMENDATIONS

- At the present time the influence of PAC monitoring on perioperative outcomes remains uncertain because significant design flaws are present in all the published trials. Additional research is needed to clearly document the effectiveness or lack of effectiveness of PACs in surgical patients.
- Expert opinion suggests that PA catheterization may benefit patients who are at high risk for complications related to hemodynamic instability during the intraoperative and postoperative periods. Reductions in morbidity and mortality rates will not be observed if physicians and nurses using PACs lack competency in basic technical and cognitive skills.
- Clinician knowledge about the use of PACs in high-risk surgical patients should be improved and user knowledge benchmarks established.

REFERENCES

1. Bernard GR, Sopko G, Cerra F, et al: Pulmonary artery catheterization and clinical outcomes: National Heart, Lung, and Blood Institute and Food and Drug Administration Workshop Report. *JAMA* 2000;283(19):2568-2572.
2. Eisenberg PR, Jaffe AS, Schuster DP: Clinical evaluation compared to pulmonary artery catheterization in the hemodynamic assessment of critically-ill patients. *Crit Care Med* 1984;12:549-553.
3. Binanay C, Califf RM, Hasselblad V, et al: Evaluation study of congestive heart failure and pulmonary artery catheterization effectiveness: The ESCAPE trial. *JAMA* 2005;294:1625-1633.
4. Wheeler AP, Bernard GR, Thompson BT, et al: Pulmonary artery versus central venous catheter to guide treatment of acute lung injury. *N Engl J Med* 2006;354:2213-2224.
5. Richard C, Warszawski J, Anguel N, et al: Early use of the pulmonary artery catheter and outcomes in patients with shock and acute respiratory distress syndrome: A randomized controlled trial. *JAMA* 2003;290:2713-2720.
6. Harvey S, Harrison DA, Singer M, et al: Assessment of the clinical effectiveness of pulmonary artery catheters in management of patients in intensive care (PAC-Man): A randomized controlled trial. *Lancet* 2005;366:472-477.
7. Wiener RS, Welch HG: Trends in the use of the pulmonary artery catheter in the United States, 1993-2004. *JAMA* 2007;298:423-429.
8. Del Guercio LRM, Cohn JD: Monitoring operative risk in the elderly. *JAMA* 1980;243(13):1350-1355.
9. Shoemaker WC, Appel PL, Bland RD: Use of physiologic monitoring to predict outcomes and to assist in clinical decisions in critically ill postoperative patients. *Am J Surg* 1983;146:43-50.
10. Bland RD, Shoemaker WC: Common physiologic patterns in general surgical patients. *Surg Clin North Am* 1985;65:793-809.
11. Russell J: Adding fuel to the fire. The supranormal oxygen delivery trials controversy. *Crit Care Med* 1998;26(6):981-983.
12. Shoemaker WC, Appel PL, Kram HB, et al: Prospective trial of supranormal values of survivors as therapeutic goals in high-risk surgical patients. *Chest* 1988;94:1176-1186.
13. Wilson J, Woods I, Fawcett J, et al: Reducing the risk of major elective surgery: Randomized controlled trial of preoperative optimization of oxygen delivery. *BMJ* 1999;318(7191):1099-1103.
14. Boyd O, Grounds RM, Bennett ED: A randomized clinical trial of the effect of deliberate perioperative increase of oxygen delivery on mortality in high-risk surgical patients. *JAMA* 1993;270 (22):2699-2707.
15. Whittemore AD, Clowes AW, Hechtman HB, Mannick JA: Aortic aneurysm repair: Reduced operative mortality associated with maintenance of optimal cardiac performance. *Ann Surg* 1980;192 (3):414-421.
16. Hesdorffer CS, Milne JF, Meyers AM, et al: The value of Swan-Ganz catheterization and volume loading in preventing renal

failure in patients undergoing abdominal aneurysmectomy. *Clin Nephrol* 1987;28(6):272-276.

17. Berlauk JF, Abrams JH, Gilmour IJ, et al: Preoperative optimization of cardiovascular hemodynamics improves outcome in peripheral vascular surgery. A prospective, randomized clinical trial. *Ann Surg* 1991;214(3):289-299.

18. Valentine RJ, Duke ML, Inman MH, et al: Effectiveness of pulmonary artery catheters in aortic surgery: A randomized trial. *J Vasc Surg* 1998;27(2):203-212.

19. Bender JS, Smith-Meek MA, Jones CE: Routine pulmonary artery catheterization does not reduce morbidity and mortality of elective vascular surgery. Results of a prospective, randomized trial. *Ann Surg* 1997;226(3):229-237.

20. Rao TLK, Jacobs KH, El-Etr AA: Reinfarction following anesthesia in patients with myocardial infarction. *Anesthesiology* 1983;59:499-505.

21. Polanczyk CA, Rohde LE, Goldman L, et al: Right heart catheterization and cardiac complications in patients undergoing noncardiac surgery: An observational study. *JAMA* 2001;286(3):309-314.

22. Sandison AJ, Wyncoll DL, Edmondson RC, et al: ICU protocol may affect the outcome of non-elective abdominal aortic aneurysm repair. *Eur J Vasc Endovasc Surg* 1998;16:356-361.

23. Isaacson IJ, Lowdon JD, Berry AJ, et al: The value of pulmonary artery and central venous monitoring in patients undergoing abdominal aortic reconstructive surgery: A comparative study of two selected, randomized groups. *J Vasc Surg* 1990;12(6):754-760.

24. Joyce WP, Provan JL, Ameli FM, et al: The role of central hemodynamic monitoring in abdominal aortic surgery. A prospective randomized study. *Eur J Vasc Surg* 1990;4(6):633-636.

25. Gattinoni L, Brazzi L, Pelosi P, et al: A trial of goal-oriented hemodynamic therapy in critically ill patients. *N Engl J Med* 1995;333(16):1025-1032.

26. Hayes MA, Timmins AC, Yau EHS, et al: Elevation of systemic oxygen delivery in the treatment of critically ill patients. *N Engl J Med* 1994;330(24):1717-1722.

27. Yu M, Levy MM, Smith P, et al: Effect of maximizing oxygen delivery on morbidity and mortality rates in critically ill patients: A prospective, randomized, controlled study. *Crit Care Med* 1993;21(6):830-838.

28. Yu M, Takanishi D, Myers SA, et al: Frequency of mortality and myocardial infarction during maximizing oxygen delivery: A prospective, randomized trial. *Crit Care Med* 1995;23(6):1025-1032.

29. Connors AF, Speroff T, Dawson NV, et al: The effectiveness of right heart catheterization in the initial care of critically ill patients. *JAMA* 1996;276(11):889-897.

30. Sandham JD, Hull RD, Brant RF, et al: A randomized, controlled trial of the use of pulmonary-artery catheters in high-risk surgical patients. *N Engl J Med* 2003;348:5-14.

31. Ivanov R, Allen J, Sandham D, et al: Pulmonary artery catheterization: A narrative and systematic critique of randomized controlled trials and recommendations for the future. *New Horizons* 1997;5:268-276.

32. Ivanov R, Allen J, Calvin J: The incidence of major morbidity in critically ill patients managed with pulmonary artery catheters: A meta-analysis. *Crit Care Med* 2000;28(3):615-619.

33. Harvey S, Young D, Brampton W, et al: Pulmonary artery catheters for adult patients in intensive care. *Cochrane Database Syst Rev* 2006;(3):CD003408.

34. Iberti TJ, Fischer EP, Leibowitz, AB, et al: A multicenter study of physicians' knowledge of the pulmonary artery catheter. *JAMA* 1990;264(22):2928-2932.

35. Trottier SJ, Taylor RW: Physicians' attitudes toward and knowledge of the pulmonary artery catheter: Society of Critical Care Medicine membership survey. *New Horizons* 1997;5(3):201-206.

36. Gnaegi A, Feihl F, Perret C: Intensive care physicians' insufficient knowledge of right heart catheterization at the bedside: Time to act? *Crit Care Med* 1997;25(2):213-220.

37. Burns D, Burns D, Shively M: Critical care nurses' knowledge of pulmonary artery catheters. *Am J Crit Care* 1996;5:49-54.

38. Jacka MJ, Cohen MM, To T, et al: Pulmonary artery occlusion pressure estimation: How confident are anesthesiologists? *Crit Care Med* 2002;30(6):1197-1203.

39. Practice guidelines for pulmonary artery catheterization. A report by the American Society of Anesthesiologists Task Force on Pulmonary Artery Catheterization. *Anesthesiology* 1993;78:380-394.

40. Practice guidelines for pulmonary artery catheterization. An updated report by the American Society of Anesthesiologists Task Force on Pulmonary Artery Catheterization. *Anesthesiology* 2003;99:988-1014.

41. Guyatt G: A randomized controlled trial of right-heart catheterization in critically ill patients. Ontario Intensive Care Study Group. *J Intensive Care Med* 1991;6:91-95.

42. Pulmonary Artery Consensus Conference: Consensus statement. Pulmonary Artery Catheter Consensus Conference participants. *Crit Care Med* 1997;25(6):910-924.

43. Fleisher LA, Beckman JA, Brown KA, et al: ACC/AHA guidelines on perioperative cardiovascular evaluation and care for noncardiac surgery: Executive summary. A report of the ACC/AHA Task Force on Practice Guidelines. *Circulation* 2007;116:1971-1996.

58 What Is the Best Method of Diagnosing Perioperative Myocardial Infarction?

Martin J. London, MD

INTRODUCTION

Perioperative myocardial infarction (PMI) is a leading cause of postoperative morbidity and mortality in patients undergoing noncardiac surgery.[1] Although it appears that its incidence and associated mortality rate have declined substantially over the past 10 to 15 years, likely due to improvements in preoperative risk stratification, perioperative mangement, and prophylaxis (e.g., beta-blockers and other sympatholytic strategies), in aggregate it remains a costly and largely preventable complication. Prior reviews have estimated associated costs in the billions of dollars from resources consumed and adverse outcome.[2] However, these estimates are poorly supported by hard data and as of yet, no definitive large-scale prospective economic analyses have been reported.

Studies dating back to the 1950s have reported that PMIs tended to occur with a peak incidence several days after surgery (postoperative days 2 and 3); half were of the Q-wave variety, with the remainder non–Q-wave; they rarely caused classic chest pain (although other associated cardiac signs, such as pulmonary edema, reduction in cardiac output, new ventricular dysrhythmias, etc., are common); and the associated mortality rate was high, averaging 50%. Patients undergoing vascular surgery or those with prior myocardial infarction (MI) were at highest risk with incidences exceeding 5% and in some subgroups (e.g., high-risk vascular surgery) up to 20%. Patients sustaining PMI have been shown to have substantially elevated long-term cardiovascular mortality rate over the first 1 to 2 years after surgery.[3,4] More recent reports, in general, have reported lower rates of PMI with a temporal shift in the peak incidence earlier, closer to the first postoperative day, and, in some studies, the night of surgery.[5-7] A distinct predominance of non–Q-wave MIs are reported and the associated short-term mortality rate is appreciably lower, although long-term mortality and morbidity rates remain higher than in the non-MI population.[8]

In the mid to late 1990s a major shift occurred in the classic paradigms for diagnosing infarction.[9,10] The rise to prominence of the troponins, cardiac structural protein markers with high sensitivity and of particular interest

perioperatively, nearly 100% specificity, has radically changed cardiology practices and epidemiologic implications of this diagnosis. Much of this is based primarily on clinical studies in patients with acute coronary syndromes where the need for rapid decision making regarding thrombolysis and revascularization strategies is critical. Several large studies of ACS patients support the clinical efficacy of troponin over the previous "gold standard," the less specific cytoplasmic enzyme, creatine kinase (CK) (and its MB fraction). Older studies used CK-MB elevations (determined by a mass assay that supplanted older activity-based assays) usually exceeding 5% of the total as diagnostic of MI when accompanied by at least one of the two following signs or symptoms: associated chest pain or electrocardiogram (ECG) changes (Q-wave or ST-T changes) as defined by the World Health Organization (WHO).[11] These "WHO criteria" have been used in epidemiologic studies evaluating temporal patterns in coronary artery disease (CAD), and, as such, altering them has substantial implications.[12] Perioperatively, it has long been appreciated that the low specificity of total CK mass (due to muscle injury) and even the CK-MB fraction (due to gene expression in injured muscle), a lack of classic chest pain (attributed in part to analgesic use although not completely explained), and problems with ECG diagnosis (including sensitivity/specificity issues due to high resting sympathetic tone, changes in electrolyte and acid-base status, and patients with abnormal resting baseline ECGs) greatly complicated coding of MI using standard criteria.[13] Despite these difficulties, it is important to appreciate that nearly all the well-accepted studies of clinical risk stratification are based at least in part on diagnosis of PMI using adaptations of WHO critieria.[14]

In late fall 2007, shortly after the official release of the updated 2007 AHA/ACC perioperative guidelines, the Joint ESC/ACCF/AHA/WHF Task Force for the Redefinition of Myocardial Infarction released its extensive document providing a long-awaited "Universal Definition of Myocardial Infarction."[15] This task force essentially updated a widely cited and influential prior report that evaluated the changing diagnosis of MI given the rapidly expanding use of troponins in the late 1990s.[16]

Table 58-1	Universal Definition of Myocardial Infarction

CRITERIA FOR ACUTE MI (ONE OF THE FOLLOWING):

1. Rise and/or fall of cardiac biomarkers (troponin is preferred) with at least one value above the 99th percentile of the upper reference limit (URL) with at least one of the following:
   a. Ischemic symptoms
   b. Development of pathologic Q waves
   c. ECG changes indicative of ischemia (ST-T changes or new left bundle branch block [LBBB])
   d. Imaging evidence of loss of viable myocardium (includes echo regional wall motion change)
2. Sudden death or cardiac arrest with symptoms suggestive of ischemia accompanied by new ECG changes, evidence of thrombus at angiography or autopsy (in the situation when death occurred before blood sampling).
3. For PCI: biomarker elevation time times the 99th percentile URL.
4. For CABG: biomarker elevation five times the 99th percentile URL plus new Q waves or LBBB or angiographic evidence of graft or native vessel occlusion or imaging loss of viable myocardium.
5. Pathologic findings of acute MI.

CRITERIA FOR PRIOR MI (ONE OF THE FOLLOWING):

1. Development of new pathologic Q waves.
2. Imaging evidence of a region of loss of viable myocardium that is thinned and fails to contract.
3. Pathologic findings of a healed or healing myocardial infarction.

Adapted from the Joint ESC/ACCF/AHA/WHF Task Force for Redefinition of Myocardial infarction (2007).

The earlier report outlined recommendations for two specific categories: (1) acute, evolving, or recent MI and (2) established MI (Table 58-1), specifically incorporating use of either troponin I or T, criteria that have in some instances dramatically increased sensitivity in the diagnosis of MI in acute coronary syndrome (ACS) patients while appearing to maintain specificity. The recently updated "ACC/AHA Guidelines for the Management of Patients with Unstable Angina/Non-ST Elevation Myocardial Infarction" used these criteria, defining *necrosis* as elevation of troponin above the 99th percentile of normal and *infarction* as the latter along with a clinical finding such as ischemic ST- and T-wave changes, new left bundle branch block, new Q waves, percutaneous coronary intervention (PCI)-related marker elevation, or imaging showing a new loss of myocardium.[17] Although these guidelines state that CK-MB and myoglobin may be useful for diagnosis of early infarct extension or periprocedural MI, it is likely that introduction of more sensitive troponin I assays now commercially available will eventually supplant this recommendation.[18] A major change in the new ESC Universal Guidelines is adoption of a clinical classification system for different types of MI into five major types: type 1, spontaneous MI related to ischemia due to a primary coronary event; type 2, MI secondary to ischemia due to increased demand or decreased supply; type 3, sudden cardiac death; type 4a, MI associated with PCI; type 4b, MI associated with coronary stent thrombosis; and type 5, MI associated with coronary artery bypass graft (CABG).[15] The new definitions for diagnosis are presented in Table 58-1.

Despite the enthusiasm resulting from the widespread availability of troponin I, it was rapidly appreciated by clinicians and laboratory managers alike that there was substantial variability in the levels of detection (99th percentile) and variability of measurement (coefficient of variation) between different vendors. This has prompted substantial ongoing efforts toward standardization, although this area is as of yet unsettled.[19,20] Because troponin T is only available from one vendor, variability is not an issue.

Evidence is accumulating that other biochemical markers may further enhance sensitivity for MI or improve risk stratification in patients with ACS. In particular, both C-reactive protein (CRP) (a marker of inflammation that is increasingly appreciated as the primary acute physiologic process leading to plaque rupture and thrombosis) and N-terminal pro-brain natriuretic peptide (NT-proBNP), a sensitive but nonspecific response to left ventricular pressure or volume overload caused by severe ischemia or heart failure, are of intense interest in the ACS arena. Perioperatively, it is likely that CRP is of very limited value given its frequent elevation in surgical conditions. However, several recent publications have purported strong value for NT-proBNP in risk stratification for short- and long-term adverse outcomes in vascular and other major noncardiac surgery based on either isolated preoperative or postoperative measurements.[21-24]

OPTIONS/THERAPIES

A variety of diagnostic approaches are available to detect MI. The strengths and limitations of the most commonly used modalities are presented in Table 58-2. Older enzymes previously used to detect MI, including total CK (without MB fractionation), lactate dehydrogenase isoenzymes, and glutamic-oxaloacetic transaminase, are no longer recommended for clinical use because of their poor specificity. The specific criteria recommended by the ACC/ECS Joint Committee for MI are presented in Table 58-1.

EVIDENCE

Contemporary studies evaluating the efficacy of the troponins and CK-MB in detection of PMI are presented in Table 58-3.[5,8,9,25-32] In general, they note a higher specificity of the troponins over CK-MB (although conclusive demonstration of significant differences in sensitivity for MI are limited), apparent correlation of troponin leak with either short- or intermediate-term outcomes (although not conclusively in all studies). The low outcome rates of most of these single-center studies limits statistical power and thus the positive predictive values of most markers studied is very limited.

Table 58-2	**Strengths and Limitations of Modalities for Detecting PMI**		
	Strengths	**Limitations**	**Recommendations**
ECG	New Q waves, "tombstone" ST-segment elevation, horizontal or downsloping ST-segment depression, hyperacute T waves, deep symmetric T-wave inversion, involvement of multiple contiguous leads	Narrow septal or inferior Q waves, LVH, LBBB, repolarization-type ST-segment abnormalities, upsloping ST-segment depression, baseline ST-segment abnormalities, diffuse T-wave flattening, asymmetric T-wave inversion	At time of suspected event, for several days during clinical resolution, with suspected reinfarction.
Biochemical Markers			
CK-MB	Characteristic rise and fall, shorter time course than troponins, CK/CK-MB ratio > 5%, AUC time activity curve related to infarct size	Non–CAD-related cardiac and other noncardiac pathology, sustained elevation, gene expression in injured skeletal muscle, renal failure	Helpful to detect recurrent infarction with serial sampling
Troponin I	Later peak, more sustained duration, prognostic significance of low-level elevation	Non–CAD-related cardiac pathology, long duration of elevation, lack of a baseline measurement, multiple assays in use, variable detection limits	All patients with suspected PMI
Troponin T	Same as troponin I, only one assay in use, well-standardized detection limits	Release with nonischemic cardiac pathology, long duration of elevation, lack of a baseline measurement, low-level chronic elevation in ESRD	All patients with suspected PMI, troponin I preferable for patients with ESRD
Imaging Modalities			
TTE	New or worsening of baseline SWMA, akinesia, dyskinesia, reduction in ejection fraction, ischemic mitral regurgitation, change from prior TTE	Small Q-wave MI, non–Q-wave MI, prior MI with baseline SWMAs, reversible ischemia, stunning, hibernating myocardium	All patients with suspected PMI; document size of MI, impact on ventricular function
Perfusion imaging	Quantitative analysis, changes in flow	Prior MI, reversible ischemia, stunning, hibernating myocardium, technical/anatomic artifacts	Expensive, not recommended except possibly in patients with poor TTE imaging

ESRD, end-stage renal disease; *LBBB*, left bundle branch block; *LVH*, left ventricular hypertrophy; *SWMA*, segmental wall motion abnormality; *TTE*, transthoracic echocardiography.

AREAS OF UNCERTAINTY

Given continuing diagnostic advances (especially in biochemical markers), establishing a simple (e.g., binary) definition for PMI capable of rigorous categorization and standardization between centers remains problematic. This complicates uniform reporting of outcomes used for benchmarking of outcomes between hospitals. However, establishing an approximate quantitative index of damage using troponin elevation, ECG changes, NT-proBNP levels, and indices of ventricular function is a reasonable and necessary clinical goal. Comparison of perioperative studies has been difficult because of variable definitions of MI and different time periods for sampling and endpoint detection used. The recent contemporary studies are better designed, although they also suffer from variable or imprecise definitions and lack of a clear "gold standard" on which to assess predictive values of new markers. The value of perioperative surveillance looking for clinically asymptomatic troponin leakage, which may indicate patients at higher risk for intermediate-term morbidity or mortality, is controversial. It is likely that cost considerations in our increasingly resource-constrained health care systems and confidentiality issues related to insurance companies, with potential adverse patient-level economic impact, will limit such an approach despite its intellectual appeal.

GUIDELINES

The new ACC/AHA Perioperative Guidelines have extensively addressed the issue of PMI and presented recommendations for surveillance strategies in various risk groups (in contrast to the 2002 guidelines in which this was not addressed in detail)[13] (Table 58-4).

Table 58-3	**Contemporary Studies Evaluating Biochemical Markers of PMI**					
Reference	**Cohort**	**Variables**	**Gold Standard**	**Perioperative Findings**	**Mortality/Long-term**	**Comments**
Adams (1994)	108 patients, vascular or spine surgery	ECG, total CK, CK-MB, cTnI	New akinesia or dyskinesia on postop TTE	8 patients MI; sensitivity: cTn-I 100% vs. CK-MB 75%; specificity: cTn-I 99% vs. CK-MB 81%; CK-MB/total CK >2.5: sensitivity 63%	Three deaths, all with elevated cTn-I; periop FU only	First major study to evaluate periop use of cTnI
Lee (1996)	1175 NCS patients age >50	ECG; total CK, CK-MB, cTn-T	CK, CK-MB, and ECG changes	17 patients MI; cTnT (>0.1 ng/mL); sensitivity 87%, specificity 84%; ROC analysis for MI: no difference CK-MB vs. cTnT; ROC analysis for complications: cTnT superior	One sudden death with no elevation of either marker; periop FU only	cTnT very low PPV, 90% of patients with elevations without complications.
Lopez-Jimenez (1997)	772 NCS patients, age >50	Same as Lee (1996)	Same as Lee (1996); cTnT >0.1 ng/mL postop as risk factor for long-term outcome	12% of cohort had cTnT elevation postop; higher rates of postop CHF and new arrhythmias	2.5% had cardiac outcomes by 6 months, PPV 9%, RR 5.4; CK-MB not correlated with outcome	cTnT independent predictor of 6-month cardiac outcomes
Metzler (1997)	67 patients, known CAD or risk factors, vascular and other NCS	ECG, cTnT, CK-MB, cTnI for patients with elevated cTnT	CK-MB >12 IU/L and Q waves	13 patients elevated cTnT and cTnI; earlier rise in cTnI; CTnT >0.6 ng/mL PPV 87%, NPV 98%; CK-MB elevated 14 patients (7 patients discordant)	No perioperative deaths; periop FU only.	Favor cTnT with cutoff value of 0.6 ng/mL
Badner (1998)	323 NCS patients, age >50, known CAD	ECG, total CK, CK-MB, cTnT	Total CK >174 U/L and 2 of CK-MB >5%, new Q waves, cTnI >0.2 mcg/L, (+) pyrophosphate scan	18 patients with MI, 14 on POD 0-1, use of cTnT alone would double MIs	1-year FU: 2/15 MI patients death or unstable angina	cTnT not used in first 92 patients, lower rate of long-term complications than other studies
Neill (2000)	80 vascular or orthopedic patients;	Ambulatory ST monitoring, CK-MB, cTnI, cTnT	CK-MB >5 mcg/L and troponins >1 mcg/L, ECG changes	cTnT and I specificity for major complications 96/97%, sensitivity 29/43%	3-month FU: cTnT best correlated with complications	No correlation of serum markers with ST-segment ischemia
Godet (2000)	329 vascular patients	cTnI	ST depression >2 days or new Q wave or cTnI >1.5 ng/mL	13 patients with cardiac complications; peak cTnI POD 1; 27 patients cTnI >1.5 ng/mL; cTnI >0.54 ng/mL sensitivity 75%, specificity 89%	1-year FU; 9 patients (3%) with cardiac complications	1-year FU: no correlation with cTnI
Haggart (2001)	59 vascular patients; 24 emergent	cTnI	WHO criteria	Elective: 10/35 cTnI detected, no CK-MB >5%; emergent: 14/24 cTnI detected, 4 CK-MB >5%	Periop FU only: 0 deaths elective group; 8 deaths emergent group: 3 cTnI elevated	CK-MB low sensitivity
Jules-Elysee (2001)	85 patients CAD or risk factors, orthopedic surgery	CK-MB, cTnI	cTnI >3.1 ng/mL and CK-MB index >3.0	11 pts (+)CK-MB; 5/11 (+) cTnI; All others (-)cTnI; all (-)cTnI patients had uneventful course	No deaths; periop FU only	cTnI better specificity

(Continued)

Table 58-3 Contemporary Studies Evaluating Biochemical Markers of PMI—Cont'd

Reference	Cohort	Variables	Gold Standard	Perioperative Findings	Mortality/Long-term	Comments
Kim (2002)	229 patients vascular	cTnI	WHO criteria	Peak cTnI >1.5 ng/mL: 12% postop; 2/9 ESRD patients (+)cTnI	OR 5.9 cTnI >1.5 ng/mL for 6-month mortality; OR 27.1 for MI; dose-response relation	Diabetes only preop predictor of cTnI elevation
Le Manach (2005)	1316 patients vascular	cTnI	Abnormal cTnI >0.2-0.5 ng/mL; PMI cTnI >1.5 ng/mL	Abnormal cTnI (14%), PMI (5%)	Inhospital mortality: early MI 24% Delayed MI 21% Abnormal 7% Normal 3%	Early MI: increase in cTnI less than 24 hours, delayed MI >24-hour period of increased cTnI

cTnI, troponin I; *cTnT,* troponin T; *ESRD,* end-stage renal disease; *NCS,* noncardiac surgery; *OR,* odds ratio; *PACU,* postanesthesia care unit; *POD,* postoperative day; *PPV,* positive predictive value; *ROC,* receiver operator characteristic curve; *WHO,* World Health Organization.

Table 58-4 Recommendations of the ACC/AHA 2007 Guidelines on Perioperative Cardiovascular Evaluation for Noncardiac Surgery

Class I
Perioperative troponin measurement is recommended in patients with ECG changes or chest pain typical of acute coronary syndrome. (Level of Evidence: C)
Class IIb
The use of troponin measurement is not well established in patients who are clinically stable and have undergone vascular and intermediate-risk surgery. (Level of Evidence: C)
Class III
Postoperative troponin measurement is not recommended in asymptomatic stable patients who have undergone low-risk surgery. (Level of Evidence: C)
For patients with high or intermediate clinical risk undergoing high- or intermediate-risk surgical procedures obtaining an ECG at baseline, immediately after surgery, and daily for the first 2 days postoperatively appears to be the most cost-effective strategy.

Adapted from Fleisher LA, Beckman JA, Brown KA, Calkins H, Chaikof E, Fleischmann KE, et al: ACC/AHA 2007 guidelines on perioperative cardiovascular evaluation and care for noncardiac surgery. A report of the American College of Cardiology/American Heart Association Task Force on Practice Guidelines (Writing Committee to Revise the 2002 Guidelines on Perioperative Cardiovascular Evaluation for Noncardiac Surgery). *Circulation* 2007;116:e418-499.

AUTHOR'S RECOMMENDATIONS

1. The newly released "Universal Definition of Myocardial Infarction Guidelines" document and other cardiology-based guidelines of the ACC/AHA and National Academy of Clinical Biochemistry Laboratory Medicine provide a comprehensive framework for the diagnosis of MI. These

principles are applicable to the perioperative setting. At this point, troponin I is the most commonly used biomarker and will likely remain so for years to come. Wide variability in 99th percentile limits between manufacturers greatly complicate comparison of absolute values between centers.
2. Substantial evidence exists that even low levels of troponin elevation in otherwise clinically asymptomatic patients are associated with higher long-term (6 months to 1 year) cardiac morbidity and mortality rates. Whether this should change our current patterns of perioperative surveillance and the aggressiveness of postoperative cardiac risk stratification is uncertain.
3. Supplementing surveillance strategies with either preoperative or postoperative measurement of NT-proBNP in high-risk patients appears to be a promising approach, although its cost-effectiveness has not been validated.

REFERENCES

1. Devereaux PJ, Goldman L, Yusuf S, Gilbert K, Leslie K, Guyatt GH: Surveillance and prevention of major perioperative ischemic cardiac events in patients undergoing noncardiac surgery: A review. *CMAJ* 2005;173(7):779-788.
2. Mangano DT, Goldman L: Preoperative assessment of patients with known or suspected coronary disease. *N Engl J Med* 1995;333(26):1750-1756.
3. Mangano DT, Browner WS, Hollenberg M, Li J, Tateo IM: Long-term cardiac prognosis following noncardiac surgery. The Study of Perioperative Ischemia Research Group. *JAMA* 1992;268(2):233-239.
4. McFalls EO, Ward HB, Santilli S, Scheftel M, Chesler E, Doliszny KM: The influence of perioperative myocardial infarction on long-term prognosis following elective vascular surgery. *Chest* 1998;113(3):681-686.
5. Badner NH, Knill RL, Brown JE, Novick TV, Gelb AW: Myocardial infarction after noncardiac surgery. *Anesthesiology* 1998;88(3):572-578.
6. Landesberg G, Mosseri M, Zahger D, Wolf Y, Perouansky M, Anner H, et al: Myocardial infarction after vascular surgery:

The role of prolonged stress-induced, ST depression-type ischemia. *J Am Coll Cardiol* 2001;37(7):1839-1845.

7. Landesberg G: The pathophysiology of perioperative myocardial infarction: Facts and perspectives. *J Cardiothorac Vasc Anesth* 2003;17(1):90-100.

8. Kim LJ, Martinez EA, Faraday N, Dorman T, Fleisher LA, Perler BA, et al: Cardiac troponin I predicts short-term mortality in vascular surgery patients. *Circulation* 2002;106(18):2366-2371.

9. Adams JE, Sicard GA, Allen BT, Bridwell KH, Lenke LG, Dávila-Román VG, et al: Diagnosis of perioperative myocardial infarction with measurement of cardiac troponin I. *N Engl J Med* 1994;330(10):670-674.

10. Jaffe AS, Babuin L, Apple FS: Biomarkers in acute cardiac disease: The present and the future. *J Am Coll Cardiol* 2006;48(1):1-11.

11. Tunstall-Pedoe H, Kuulasmaa K, Amouyel P, Arveiler D, Rajakangas AM, Pajak A: Myocardial infarction and coronary deaths in the World Health Organization MONICA Project. Registration procedures, event rates, and case-fatality rates in 38 populations from 21 countries in four continents. *Circulation* 1994;90(1): 583-612.

12. Luepker RV, Apple FS, Christenson RH, Crow RS, Fortmann SP, Goff D, et al: Case definitions for acute coronary heart disease in epidemiology and clinical research studies: A statement from the AHA Council on Epidemiology and Prevention; AHA Statistics Committee; World Heart Federation Council on Epidemiology and Prevention; the European Society of Cardiology Working Group on Epidemiology and Prevention; Centers for Disease Control and Prevention; and the National Heart, Lung, and Blood Institute. *Circulation* 2003;108(20):2543-2549.

13. Fleisher LA, Beckman JA, Brown KA, Calkins H, Chaikof E, Fleischmann KE, et al: ACC/AHA 2007 guidelines on perioperative cardiovascular evaluation and care for noncardiac surgery. A report of the American College of Cardiology/American Heart Association Task Force on Practice Guidelines (Writing Committee to Revise the 2002 Guidelines on Perioperative Cardiovascular Evaluation for Noncardiac Surgery). *Circulation* 2007 Sep 27.

14. Devereaux PJ, Ghali WA, Gibson NE, Skjodt NM, Ford DC, Quan H, et al: Physician estimates of perioperative cardiac risk in patients undergoing noncardiac surgery. *Arch Intern Med* 1999;159(7):713-717.

15. Thygesen K, Alpert JS, White HD: Joint ESC/ACCF/AHA/WHF Task Force for the Redefinition of Myocardial Infarction. Universal definition of myocardial infarction. *Eur Heart J* 2007;28: 2525-2538.

16. Myocardial infarction redefined—a consensus document of the Joint European Society of Cardiology/American College of Cardiology Committee for the redefinition of myocardial infarction. *J Am Coll Cardiol* 2000;36(3):959-969.

17. Anderson JL, Adams CD, Antman EM, Bridges CR, Califf RM, Casey DE Jr, et al: ACC/AHA 2007 guidelines for the management of patients with unstable angina/non-ST-elevation myocardial infarction—Executive summary. A report of the American College of Cardiology/American Heart Association Task Force on Practice Guidelines (Writing Committee to Revise the 2002 Guidelines for the Management of Patients with Unstable Angina/Non-ST-Elevation Myocardial Infarction) developed in collaboration with the American College of Emergency Physicians, the Society for Cardiovascular Angiography and Interventions, and the Society of Thoracic Surgeons Endorsed by the American Association of Cardiovascular and Pulmonary Rehabilitation and the Society for Academic Emergency Medicine. *J Am Coll Cardiol* 2007;50(7):652-726.

18. Melanson SE, Morrow DA, Jarolim P: Earlier detection of myocardial injury in a preliminary evaluation using a new troponin I assay with improved sensitivity. *Am J Clin Pathol* 2007;128(2):282-286.

19. Christenson RH, Duh SH, Apple FS, Bodor GS, Bunk DM, Panteghini M, et al: Toward standardization of cardiac troponin I measurements part II: Assessing commutability of candidate reference materials and harmonization of cardiac troponin I assays. *Clin Chem* 2006;52(9):1685-1692.

20. Apple FS, Jesse RL, Newby LK, Wu AH, Christenson RH: National Academy of Clinical Biochemistry and IFCC Committee for Standardization of Markers of Cardiac Damage Laboratory Medicine Practice Guidelines: Analytical issues for biochemical markers of acute coronary syndromes. *Circulation* 2007;115(13): e352-e355.

21. Cuthbertson BH, Amiri AR, Croal BL, Rajagopalan S, Alozairi O, Brittenden J, et al: Utility of B-type natriuretic peptide in predicting perioperative cardiac events in patients undergoing major non-cardiac surgery. *Br J Anaesth* 2007;99(2):170-176.

22. Feringa HH, Bax JJ, Elhendy A, de Jonge R, Lindemans J, Schouten O, et al: Association of plasma N-terminal pro-B-type natriuretic peptide with postoperative cardiac events in patients undergoing surgery for abdominal aortic aneurysm or leg bypass. *Am J Cardiol* 2006;98(1):111-115.

23. Feringa HH, Schouten O, Dunkelgrun M, Bax JJ, Boersma E, Elhendy A, et al: Plasma N-terminal pro-B-type natriuretic peptide as long-term prognostic marker after major vascular surgery. *Heart* 2007;93(2):226-231.

24. Mahla E, Baumann A, Rehak P, Watzinger N, Vicenzi MN, Maier R, et al: N-terminal pro-brain natriuretic peptide identifies patients at high risk for adverse cardiac outcome after vascular surgery. *Anesthesiology* 2007;106(6):1088-1095.

25. Lee TH, Thomas EJ, Ludwig LE, Sacks DB, Johnson PA, Donaldson MC, et al: Troponin T as a marker for myocardial ischemia in patients undergoing major noncardiac surgery. *Am J Cardiol* 1996;77(12):1031-1036.

26. Lopez-Jimenez F, Goldman L, Sacks DB, Thomas EJ, Johnson PA, Cook EF, et al: Prognostic value of cardiac troponin T after noncardiac surgery: 6-month follow-up data. *J Am Coll Cardiol* 1997;29(6):1241-1245.

27. Metzler H, Gries M, Rehak P, Lang T, Fruhwald S, Toller W: Perioperative myocardial cell injury: The role of troponins. *Br J Anaesth* 1997;78(4):386-390.

28. Neill F, Sear JW, French G, Lam H, Kemp M, Hooper RJ, et al: Increases in serum concentrations of cardiac proteins and the prediction of early postoperative cardiovascular complications in noncardiac surgery patients. *Anaesthesia* 2000;55(7):641-647.

29. Godet G, Dumerat M, Baillard C, Ben Ayed S, Bernard MA, Bertrand M, et al: Cardiac troponin I is reliable with immediate but not medium-term cardiac complications after abdominal aortic repair. *Acta Anaesthesiol Scand* 2000;44(5):592-597.

30. Haggart PC, Adam DJ, Ludman PF, Bradbury AW: Comparison of cardiac troponin I and creatine kinase ratios in the detection of myocardial injury after aortic surgery. *Br J Surg* 2001;88(9):1196-1200.

31. Jules-Elysee K, Urban MK, Urquhart B, Milman S: Troponin I as a diagnostic marker of a perioperative myocardial infarction in the orthopedic population. *J Clin Anesth* 2001;13(8):556-560.

32. Le Manach Y, Perel A, Coriat P, Godet G, Bertrand M, Riou B: Early and delayed myocardial infarction after abdominal aortic surgery. *Anesthesiology* 2005;102(5):885-891.

59 Does Neurologic Electrophysiologic Monitoring Affect Outcome?

Michael L. McGarvey, MD, and Steven R. Messé, MD

INTRODUCTION

Neurologic injury from surgery results in substantial increased morbidity, mortality, and cost, and, most important, it is devastating to patients and their families. Thus, techniques to lessen, reverse, and even avoid neurologic injury are very valuable. Neurologic intraoperative electrophysiologic monitoring (NIOM) allows for the early identification of impending or ongoing intraoperative injury, thus allowing for interventions. Changes to a patient's neurologic electrophysiologic baselines during the procedure alert the operative team that a potential injury may be occurring. The goal of NIOM is to detect dysfunction caused by ischemia, mass effect, stretch, heat, and direct injury in real time before it causes permanent neurologic injury. Monitoring may also be useful in identifying and preserving neurologic structures during a procedure where they are at risk (mapping).

There are several challenges to establishing the efficacy of NIOM. The first is that there have been no blinded or randomized trials assessing the efficacy of NIOM in humans. Unfortunately, there will likely never be a substantial trial examining this issue.[1] The reason behind the lack of high-level evidence is that monitoring is well established and accepted in clinical practice. Moreover, it is generally extremely low risk to the patient. The general consensus in the surgical community is that monitoring is useful and there would be ethical and medicolegal dilemmas in withholding monitoring in patients who are at potential risk of injury. A second limitation in establishing outcomes for NIOM is that the goal of monitoring is to reverse a significant change if one is seen during a procedure. Thus, monitoring may detect an impending injury, which is reversed, but the benefit can never be confirmed because the patient wakes up with a normal examination. The utility of monitoring is based on animal studies and case series with comparisons to historical controls. The utility of NIOM may be supported by establishing that monitoring can in fact detect injury in cases where injury has occurred (true-positives), and limiting false-negative outcomes (injury occurred and was not detected) and persistent false-positive outcomes (injury was predicted by NIOM at the end of a procedure but did not occur). Multimodality monitoring is possible, so the ability of different NIOM techniques to predict injury can be compared in the same patient.

THERAPIES

Various portions of the nervous system can be monitored by using several NIOM techniques. The specific neurologic tissues at risk, as well as the type of potential injury, vary with different surgical procedures. Specific techniques include electroencephalograph (EEG) and evoked potentials, including somatotosensory evoked potentials (SSEPs), brainstem auditory evoked potentials (BAEPs), visual evoked potentials (VEPs), electromyography (EMG), nerve conduction studies (NCSs), and transcortical electrical motor evoked potentials (TcMEPs).

EEG is a measure of spontaneous electrical brain activity recorded from electrodes placed in standard patterns on a patient's scalp or directly on the cortex with sterile electrode strips or grids. The differences in activity between individual electrodes is amplified and then recorded as continuous wavelets that have different frequencies and amplitudes. These data can be displayed as a raw EEG on a display in a series of channels or broken down into the basic components of frequency and amplitude and displayed as a spectral analysis. A change in a patient's background EEG activity from baseline during a procedure may indicate ischemia of the cerebral cortex either focally or through a generalized loss of activity over the entire cortex. A 50% decrease in EEG amplitude is generally considered a significant change. EEG is routinely used intraoperatively during carotid endarterectomy (CEA), cerebral aneurysm, and arteriovenous malformation surgery or in other procedures that place the cortex at risk.[1-4]

Evoked potentials are measures of nervous system electrical activity resulting from a specific stimulus that is applied to the patient. Electrodes record responses to repetitive stimuli as averaged wavelets at different locations in the nervous system as this evoked activity propagates along its course.

SSEPs are produced by repetitive electrical stimulation of a peripheral nerve while recording averaged potentials as they travel through the afferent sensory system.

SSEP waveforms are recorded from peripheral nerve, spinal cord, brainstem, and primary somatosensory cortex. The recording of waveforms at sequential locations along the complete afferent sensory system allows for localization of dysfunction during procedures. This dysfunction could be caused by ischemia, mass effect, or local injury. SSEPs recorded from stimulation of the median nerve are used intraoperatively during carotid endarterectomy and intracranial surgery for anterior circulation vascular lesions.[5,6] SSEPs recorded from stimulation of the posterior tibial nerve in the leg are used during intracranial surgeries involving vascular lesions in the posterior cerebral circulation.[7] Monitoring both upper and lower extremity SSEPs during procedures that place the spinal cord at risk may be useful in procedures to treat scoliosis, spinal tumors, or descending aortic repairs. The accepted criterion for significant SSEP change, suggesting a potential injury, is a decrease of spinal or cortical amplitudes by 50% or an increase in latency by 10% from baseline.

BAEPs are wavelets generated by the auditory nerve and brainstem in response to repetitive clicks, delivered to the ear. Typically, five wavelets are recorded from electrodes place near the ear, with the first recorded wavelet representing the response from peripheral cochlear nerve, while the next four wavelets are generated from ascending structures in the brainstem. Changes in latency and amplitude of these five waves are used to assess the integrity of the auditory pathway during procedures that put them at risk.[8] BAEPs are commonly used in posterior fossa neurosurgical procedures such as acoustic neuroma resections, which place the eighth nerve at risk from either ischemia or stretch injury. BAEPs may also be useful in identifying and preventing injury in procedures such as tumor resections or arterio-venous malformation (AVM) repairs that place the brainstem itself at risk because of ischemia or mass effect.

VEPs are wavelets generated by the occipital cortex in response to visual stimuli (typically flashing lights delivered with light-emitting diode [LED] goggles in the operative setting). VEPs are recorded from electrodes overlying the occipital cortex and provide information about the integrity of the visual pathway during procedures. VEPs have been have been monitored during neurosurgical procedures involving mass and vascular lesions near the optic nerve and chiasm.

EMG and NCSs can be performed on both peripheral and cranial nerves to assess their integrity and to localize these nerves by recording compound motor action potentials (CMAPs) from the muscles they supply. Monitoring is performed by placing pins or electrodes in muscles and then identifying the nerve supplying the muscle by stimulating it during the procedure (mapping). NCSs can also be performed by determining whether a specific length of nerve will conduct electrical activity between a stimulating and recording electrode. If a nerve does not conduct the signal, this may indicate that it has been significantly injured along its course. Peripheral nerves are at risk of crush, stretch, ligation, ischemic, and hyperthermic injury during many surgical procedures due to malpositioning, electrocautery, or direct injury. Monitoring is also performed by observing spontaneous activity from the muscle, which may indicate that a nerve supplying it is suffering unexpected injury. Cranial motor nerves are often monitored in this fashion. Cranial nerve VII is often monitored during posterior fossa procedures where it is at high risk of injury and also during parotid gland procedures or other ear/nose/throat (ENT) procedures involving the face, ear, or sinuses. All peripheral nerves in the extremities and trunk can similarly be monitored. Monitoring of peripheral nerves can aid in localizing and protecting nervous tissue during nerve repairs or during tumor resections.

TcMEPs are performed by delivering electrical current to the motor cortex from electrodes on the scalp and recording either motor evoked potential (MEP) waveforms (D and I waves) from epidural electrodes near the spine itself or recording myogenic evoked potentials from muscles (CMAPs) in the upper and lower extremities. MEPs may also be recorded by direct electrical stimulation of the motor cortex following craniotomy (as a means of functional mapping of the motor cortex) or via transcortical magnetic stimulation. TcMEP provides a real-time assessment of the descending motor pathway from the cortex to muscle during procedures that place the corticospinal tracks at risk. TcMEP is becoming increasingly used in advanced neurosurgical, aortic, and orthopedic centers for monitoring motor pathways of the brain and spinal cord during procedures. MEPs appear to have a superior temporal resolution for detection of ischemia compared with SSEPs (less than 5 minutes versus 30 minutes). This is likely because TcMEP measures spinal gray matter, which is very sensitive to ischemia, in addition to spinal motor myelinated tracts. One downside is that there are no clear criteria in the literature to define a critical change warning that injury is occurring. Studies have used different losses in CMAP amplitude (25% versus 50% versus 80%) or threshold changes (that is, the amount of stimulation current it takes to obtain the CMAP) to signify a critical change.[9,10] The ability to perform TcMEP is also limited by its sensitivity to anesthetics, paralytic agents and temperature. The use of paralytic agents is discouraged and, if used at all, should be extremely limited and kept relatively constant (at less than 40% neuromuscular blockade). This also means that patients are at higher risk of injury due to spontaneous movements or stimulation during their procedures. Another limitation is the large concern that TcMEPs are often difficult to obtain from the leg. Whether this is because of technical limitations of the modality or preexisting injury in patients is unclear.[9-13] Complications are of greater concern than in other modalities because of the stimulus intensity required to induce the response and may include rare instances of seizures and tongue lacerations.[11,14,15] Finally, the establishment of efficacy for TcMEP has been limited by the lack of approved equipment and experience in performing the technique.

EVIDENCE

Evidence Supporting the Use of EEG in Carotid Endarterectomy

One of the most common uses of NIOM is EEG during CEA and other intracranial vascular procedures where the brain is at risk for ischemic injury from hypoperfusion.

Although commonly used to monitor CEAs, few data exist to support its use, including a lack of randomized trials. Intraoperative stroke is rare, occurring in approximately 2% to 3% of CEAs with a large proportion of these strokes due to embolism.[2-4] Despite this it is clear that a small proportion of these strokes are due to hypoperfusion, and it is known from both animal studies and human blood flow studies that loss of EEG activity reflects a reduction of blood flow in the brain.[16,17] In a large series of 1152 CEAs, a persistent significant change on intraoperative EEG (12 cases) had 100% predictive value for an intraoperative neurologic complication.[3] A critical point during CEA is clamping of the carotid artery in order to perform the endarterectomy. If ischemia is detected, elevating the blood pressure or placement of a carotid shunt may be used to alleviate the ischemia. Significant EEG changes can occur in up to 25% of cases during carotid clamping; however, strokes do not occur in a majority of these cases even without shunting.[3,17-19] In two separate series with a total of 469 patients undergoing CEA with EEG monitoring but without shunting, 44 patients suffered significant EEG changes and 6 of these suffered intraoperative strokes.[17-19] Although not all patient experiencing EEG changes during CEA in this cohort suffered a stroke, it is possible that the strokes may have been averted with use of selective shunting based on EEG. Use of selective shunting based on EEG is further supported by a series of 369 patients in which 73 patients were shunted based on significant EEG changes and no intraoperative strokes occurred and another study of 172 patients in which the use of EEG and selective shunting reduced neurologic complications from 2.3% to 1.1% in 93 patients.[2,21]

Evidence Supporting the Use of SSEPs to Detect Brain and Spinal Injury

Use of SSEPs to identify early spinal cord injury has become widespread. The risk of spinal injury varies with different surgeries but has reported to occur in 1% to 2% of scoliosis repairs. Significant changes in SSEPs have been predictive of injury in several small case series in complex cervical and thoracic spine procedures but false positives and false negatives do occur.[22-27] The risk for injury in cases involving intramedullary spinal lesions, such as tumors, has been reported to be up to 65.4%.[28,29] In a prospective and retrospective cohort study of 19 patients with adequate baseline SSEP signals undergoing intramedullary tumor resections, SSEPs successfully predicted a postoperative motor deficit in five patients with no false negatives.[30] In a large survey of 242 experienced surgical groups performing major spinal surgery, neurologic complications occurred twice as often in nonmonitored cases as in the monitored cases (51,263 total cases).[31] In the monitored cases, there were 184 neurologic complications of which 150 (81%) were predicted by SSEPs, although 34 were not identified, resulting in a false-negative rate of only 0.063%.[31] The authors concluded that SSEP monitoring detected greater than 90% of neurologic injuries with a sensitivity of 92% and a specificity of 98.9%. In a second large series by the same investigators, 33,000 SSEP-monitored spinal cases were retrospectively reviewed.[32] In this survey, a 0.75% false-positive, 0.48% true-positive, and 0.07% false-negative rate was reported for sensitivity of 86.5% and specificity of 99.2%. Specific data were collected for 77 patients who were injured in this group (30 injuries were severe): there were 17 false negatives and 60 true positives. Of the severe injuries, 5 were not detected by SSEP monitoring.

Permanent loss of SSEP signals in descending aortic repairs indicating spinal ischemia has accurately predicted paraplegia. Furthermore, good outcomes have been reported when a spinal SSEP change is reversed with maneuvers that improve spinal perfusion in small case series.[33-37] There is a direct correlation to the time of loss of SSEPs (40 to 60 minutes) and the incidence of paraplegia.[38] However, other data in a nonblinded prospective study of 198 patients undergoing thoracic aortic aneurysm (TAA) and thoracoabdominal aortic aneurysm (TAAA) repairs (99 patients underwent surgery with distal artery bypass and SSEP monitoring versus 99 patients without bypass and monitoring) demonstrated no significant differences in neurologic outcomes between the two groups (8% neurologic complication rate in the SSEP group versus 7% in the unmonitored group).[39] There was no statistical difference following logistic regression analysis between the two groups.

Upper-extremity SSEPs have been used for monitoring during CEA. A benefit of using SSEPs over EEG in CEA is that they allow for monitoring of subcortical structures, although EEG does provide neurophysiologic information for a much larger area of cortex. In a meta-analysis of seven large studies assessing the use of SSEPs during CEA in 3028 patients, significant central SSEP changes indicated ischemia in 170 patients (5.6%).[40] Although some of these 170 cases employed carotid shunting to reverse significant SSEP changes, 34 patients suffered an ischemic complication. Eight false negatives were reported in this analysis, but not every study included in the analysis reported false negatives. The authors concluded that SSEPs and EEG had similar sensitivities and specificities in detecting ischemia during CEA. Another meta-analysis of 15 studies of 3036 patients identified 10 false-negative patients. Of note, there was some overlap between this analysis and the previous review of seven large studies. This study also looked at the predictive value of significant SSEP change and concluded that it was poor in predicting outcome and in determining the need for carotid shunting. This was based on comparing similar outcomes in patients undergoing selective shunting with SSEP monitoring and 317 patients who had monitoring but were not shunted regardless of the changes seen on SSEP.[41]

The utility of SSEP monitoring during intracranial aneurysm repair has also been studied. In repairs of intracranial aneurysm, temporary occlusion of a proximal vessel such as the carotid may be necessary to increase the safety of aneurysm clip placement. During these periods, monitoring with SSEPs may enable longer periods of temporary ischemia, identification of inadequate collateral flow, or identification of malpositioning of aneurysm clips. In a series of 67 aneurysm clippings, 24 significant SSEP changes were noted during temporary clipping, yet only one patient awakened with deficit.[42] In a similar study involving 58 intracranial aneurysm repairs, 13 significant SSEP changes were demonstrated, only one of which was persistent and resulted in a neurologic deficit.[7] All the transient changes in this study resolved with intervention, including temporary clip removal, permanent clip adjustment, increase in systemic pressure, or retractor adjustment.[7]

Evidence Supporting the Use of BAEP in Posterior Fossa Neurosurgical Procedures

BAEP monitoring may be used to monitor surgical procedures involving the brainstem and posterior fossa that place the eighth cranial nerve and the auditory pathway at risk. In a series of 144 acoustic neuroma resections, the normal presence of wave V at the end of the resection, regardless of whether there was a transient change during the procedure, was consistent with preservation of useful hearing.[43] In a study of 46 posterior fossa procedures, 4 procedures had significant operative BAEP loss, each of which coincided with significant loss of hearing. The remaining patients without significant BAEP changes demonstrated normal hearing. A retrospective study of 70 patients undergoing microvascular decompression of the trigeminal nerve with BAEP monitoring was compared with 150 unmonitored patients. In the monitored group, none of the patients experienced hearing loss whereas 10 patients developed hearing loss in the unmonitored group.[44] In a retrospective study of 156 patients undergoing posterior fossa procedures, the permanent loss of wave V was significantly associated with hearing loss.[45] Finally, in a study of 90 acoustic neuroma resections with BAEP monitoring compared with 90 matched historical controls without monitoring, hearing loss was significantly less in those patients with tumors smaller than 1.1 cm who were monitored.[46]

Evidence Supporting the Use of EMG and Nerve Conduction Studies

Cranial nerve monitoring is employed in operations of the posterior fossa and brainstem. In a series of 104 acoustic neuroma resections in which only 29 underwent facial nerve monitoring with EMG, there were significantly better outcomes in monitored patients at 1 year.[47] In a study that compared 56 patients with facial nerve monitoring with EMG during parotidectomy with 61 patients who did not have monitoring, early facial weakness was significantly lower in the monitored group, 43.6% versus 62.3%, although the incidence of permanent facial weakness was not significantly different.[48] There are no large studies published evaluating the utility of monitoring other cranial and peripheral nerves.

Evidence Supporting the Use of VEP Monitoring

The evidence supporting VEP monitoring is sparse in part due to difficulty in obtaining signals in the operating room.[49,50] A group of 22 patients undergoing VEP monitoring during macroadenoma resection compared with 14 patients undergoing the procedure without monitoring demonstrated no significant difference in visual outcome.[51] Other small clinical case series have also reported no clear benefits of VEP monitoring.[52]

Evidence Supporting the Use of TcMEP in Spinal and Descending Aortic Surgery

The optimal approach to monitor the spinal cord during high-risk procedures is controversial, and it is unclear whether SSEP or TcMEP is superior. Procedures that may benefit from spinal cord monitoring include orthopedic procedures involving structural or vascular lesions, as well as repairs of the descending aorta, which put the spinal cord at risk of ischemia.[53,54] SSEP monitoring has been the traditional standard and it has been employed in routine clinical practice for spinal procedures since the 1980s.[1] However, SSEPs theoretically monitor only the sensory white matter tracts of the spinal cord, the posterior columns in particular. The question that arises is whether SSEPs are adequately sensitive for injury to the corticospinal tracts in the cord, which is of primary importance during these procedures. Multiple studies have reported improved outcomes with SSEP monitoring during aortic and spine surgery.[32,34,35,55] As noted previously, there are significant challenges associated with TcMEP use. Thus, the question is whether TcMEP provides greater sensitivity to injury of spinal cord structures that are most meaningful to outcome, thereby justifying its use over SSEP in procedures placing the spinal cord at risk.[11,14,56]

In a study of 142 patients undergoing complex spinal deformity repairs with TcMEP monitoring, 16 patients had significant changes indicating spinal cord motor tract dysfunction during their procedure.[10] In these 16 cases, 11 of the TcMEP changes were reversed during the procedure and no deficit occurred, whereas the 5 patients with persistent changes awoke with a motor deficit. In a cohort of 100 intramedullary spinal tumor resections, TcMEPs were detectable on all nonparaplegic patients. TcMEPs were 100% sensitive and 91% specific, and no patient with stable MEP signals throughout the case awoke with a deficit.[57] Similarly, a study of 50 patients monitored with TcMEP and SSEP during intramedullary tumor resection were compared with a group of 50 matched patients without monitoring from a historical cohort of 301 patients.[58] Neurologic outcomes were evaluated at discharge and at 3 months and demonstrated a strong trend at the time of discharge and significant improvement in outcomes at 3 months in the monitored group. Case series have shown a low rate of paraplegia in TAAA procedures when TcMEP are employed for monitoring. In a study of 75 TAAA repairs, all patients with normal TcMEP awoke without paraparesis, whereas 8 of 9 patients with significant changes consistent with spinal cord injury awoke with a deficit.[59] Twenty patients in this study had significant MEP changes that resolved intraoperatively and none of these patients awoke with a deficit. Other investigators have demonstrated that significant changes of intraoperative TcMEP during aortic surgery can be reversed with techniques that increase spinal perfusion, including reimplantation of intercostals and increasing systemic pressure.[60]

Several series have been performed in which TcMEPs and SSEPs were monitored during the same procedure (Table 59-1). This is a rare instance in which head-to-head comparisons have been performed between two monitoring techniques, although there are flaws in analyzing these data. In all cases, anesthesia was tailored to optimize TcMEP. Paralytic agents were not used, which increases the difficulty of optimally monitoring SSEPs because of motor artifacts generated from performing stimulation.

In a series of complex spine surgeries, 104 patients were monitored with both TcMEPs and SSEPs simultaneously.[13] Ninety patients had no significant changes and none of these patients awoke with a new deficit. In 7 of the remaining 14 cases changes were seen in both modalities: 5 patients had transient changes and awoke without a deficit whereas the remaining two patients had persistent SSEP or TcMEP changes that predicted one motor deficit and a sensory deficit. In the 7 remaining cases only TcMEP changes occurred: 4 patients had transient changes and aroused without a deficit. One patient had a permanent TcMEP change and awoke with a deficit and another had a transient TcMEP change and awoke with right leg weakness. One patient had a significant persistent TcMEP change without neurologic deficit. In a cohort of 427 patients undergoing anterior or posterior cervical spine repairs with both SSEPs and TcMEPs, the monitoring identified 12 patients who developed significant loss of signals indicating a spinal injury.[12] All 12 developed significant TcMEP changes with 4 also having significant SSEP changes. Seven of the patients with TcMEP-only changes and 3 of the patients with both TcMEP and SSEP changes were reversed with intraoperative adjustments. Of the remaining two patients with postoperative motor deficits, one had persistent TcMEP decrements and the other had both persistent TcMEP and SSEP changes, resulting in one patient in the cohort who had an intraoperative injury that was not identified by SSEPs. In a study of 118 patients undergoing TAAA repairs using both modalities, 42 patients had significant TcMEP changes whereas only 5 patients had significant SSEP changes.[61] Aggressive measures were taken to reverse the intraoperative monitoring changes, but despite these interventions, 18 patients had persistent TcMEP changes and 4 patients had persistent SSEP changes at the time of skin closure. Five patients awoke with paraplegia; four of these were predicted by TcMEPs and one by SSEPs. There are several smaller case series that appear to confirm the findings of these larger case studies except for an increase in false positives in both modalities.[9,58,62-65] TcMEPs appear to have increased sensitivity at predicting motor injury than SSEP.[9,12,13,61-63]

Controversies and Areas of Uncertainty

Although there is a legitimate concern regarding the unproven benefit of NIOM because of the lack of randomized trials, there are several situations in which monitoring appears to have an established utility. Specifically, the improved outcomes reported in large case series support the continued use of EEG in CEA, SSEP in spinal surgery, BAEP in posterior fossa procedures, and EMG in procedures placing the facial nerve at risk. There are several areas where the evidence has either not supported the use of monitoring or where further clinical research needs to be performed to demonstrate a clear benefit before recommending that these techniques become the standard of care in clinical practice. These techniques include VEP monitoring, SSEP and BAEP monitoring in procedures placing the brainstem at risk, EEG in neurosurgical vascular procedures, SSEP in CEA, and EMG in cases placing peripheral and cranial nerves at risk other than the seventh nerve.

There is early evidence supporting the use of TcMEP in complex cervical and thoracic spinal procedures and descending aortic procedures. It appears that TcMEP may be more sensitive than SSEP in detecting and predicting motor deficits in patients undergoing procedures that place their spinal cords at risk of motor deficits. This benefit must now be weighed against the potential risks of using TcMEP before it becomes the standard over SSEP for monitoring these procedures. The risks include potential skin injury, anesthetic restrictions, cost, oversensitivity, and the need for increased professional oversight. Further clinical research in the use of TcMEP is necessary to establish this promising technique. The exception at this time may be a clear benefit of the use of TcMEP in the treatment of intramedullary spinal cord tumors.

The difficulty of assessing the benefit of intraoperative monitoring techniques in isolation raises the question of whether using multiple electrophysiologic techniques or nonelectrical techniques during high-risk procedures adds any benefit. Adding multiple techniques during one procedure may aid in identifying injury but also may add confusion when the modalities do not correlate, as well as adding cost. Another benefit of dual monitoring is that if one modality fails for technical reasons the other modality is still available.

GUIDELINES

In 1990, the Therapeutics and Technology Subcommittee of the American Academy of Neurology (AAN) determined that the following techniques were useful and noninvestigational: EEG and SSEPs as adjuncts in CEA and brain surgeries where cerebral blood flow was compromised, SSEP monitoring performed in procedures involving ischemia or mechanical trauma to the spine, and BAEP and cranial nerve monitoring in surgeries performed in the region of the brainstem or ear are beneficial.[1] There have been no further recommendations from the AAN regarding NIOM.

Table 59-1 Motor Outcomes of Spinal and Aortic Procedures Using Both TcMEP and SSEP and a Comparison of Modalities

Study, Year (Type of Surgery: Cervical/Thoracic Spine,[1] TAAA[2])	Number of Patients	Number of Subjects with Significant Intraoperative SSEP/TCMEP Changes			Number of Subjects with Persistent Significant Changes Who Awoke with Motor Deficit (Additional False Negatives Bold, False Positives in Italics)				Sensitivity of Having a Significant Change and Having a Motor Deficit (%)		Specificity of Having a Significant Change and Having a Motor Deficit	
		Both SSEP/ TcMEP	TcMEP Alone	SSEP Alone	Total	Both SSEP/ TCMEP	TCMEP	SSEP	TcMEP	SSEP	TcMEP	SSEP
Pelosi, 2002[1]	104	7	7	0	3	1	2(1)(1)	1(2)	67	33	99	100
Hilibranbrand, 2004[1]	427	4	8	0	2	1	2	1(1)	100	50	100	100
Van Donegan, 2001[2]	118	5	37	0	5	1(4)	4(1)(14)	1(4)	80	20	88	100
Weinzierl, 2007[1]	69	6	12	2	10	2(1)(1)	8(2)(1)	2(8)(2)	80	20	98	97
Meylaerts, 1999[2]	38	5	13	11	0	0	0	0(15)	N/A	N/A	60	100
Costa, 2007[1]	38	3	0	1	1	1	1	1(1)	100	100	100	97
Total	794	30	77	14	21	6(1)(5)	17(4) (16)	6(16) (18)	81	27	98	98

AUTHORS' RECOMMENDATIONS

These recommendations serve as a guide only and are based on the authors' interpretation of the available data and should not replace clinical judgment. There should be judicial use of neurophysiologic monitoring. It should be reserved for surgical cases where the nervous system is at significant risk. When neurologic injury is expected, neurophysiologic monitoring becomes mandatory.

1. Although it is relatively rare, neurologic injury due to hypoperfusion may occur during carotid endarterectomy. EEG can identify this complication and appears to improve outcomes by indicating when carotid shunting is necessary. The available data support its use over other modalities at this time, although a randomized trial comparing modalities such as transcranial doppler ultrasound (TCD), SSEP, stump pressure, and nonselective shunting is needed. EEG's use in other procedures where the cerebral cortex is at risk may be beneficial but there is a lack of data to support it.

2. SSEPs are useful in identifying ischemia in the brain during complex neurosurgical vascular procedures, injury to the spinal cord in complex cervical and thoracic spinal procedures, and ischemia in descending aortic repairs. It is unclear whether SSEP or TcMEP is superior for detecting potential injury in the spinal cord given the current data available. This is deserving of further study. It is the current recommendation based on this review that SSEP be used during all complex cervical and thoracic spine and descending aortic procedures that place the spinal cord at any risk.

3. At this time, TcMEP should be considered as a useful adjunct in monitoring the spinal cord during procedures placing it at risk of injury, but more clinical data need to be collected before TcMEP should be considered the standard. SSEPs should also be monitored in all cases in which TcMEPs are attempted. A randomized controlled trial comparing TcMEP and SSEP spinal monitoring may be possible from an ethical standpoint and should be considered.

4. BAEPs are useful in identifying injury and improving outcomes during neurosurgical procedures involving the posterior fossa that place the eighth cranial nerve at risk and should be used. This is especially true in acoustic neuroma resections where the tumor is less than 2 cm in diameter. It is unclear whether BAEP and SSEP monitoring during procedures that put the brainstem at risk is useful, but given the potential benefit of monitoring during these procedures it should be continued while more outcome data are collected.

5. Seventh cranial nerve monitoring in surgeries performed in the region of the brainstem or ear using spontaneous EMG and mapping with direct simulation of seventh cranial nerves improves outcomes and should be used. Whether there is a benefit from monitoring of other cranial nerves or peripheral nerves during procedures that put them at risk is unclear, but a potential benefit does exist, so monitoring here should be continued while further outcome data are collected.

6. It is unclear whether VEP monitoring can adequately identify injury to the visual pathway and improve outcomes in surgical procedures placing it at risk, and its use should likely be limited to research protocols.

REFERENCES

1. Assessment: Intraoperative neurophysiology. Report of the Therapeutics and Technology Assessment Subcommittee of the American Academy of Neurology. *Neurology* 1990;40(11):1644-1646.

2. Sundt TM Jr, Sharbrough FW, Anderson RE, Michenfelder JD: Cerebral blood flow measurements and electroencephalograms during carotid endarterectomy. *J Neurosurg* 1974;41(3):310-320.

3. Sundt TM Jr, Sharbrough FW, Piepgras DG, Kearns TP, Messick JM Jr, O'Fallon WM: Correlation of cerebral blood flow and electroencephalographic changes during carotid endarterectomy: With results of surgery and hemodynamics of cerebral ischemia. *Mayo Clin Proc* 1981;56(9):533-543.

4. Sharbrough FW, Messick JM Jr, Sundt TM Jr: Correlation of continuous electroencephalograms with cerebral blood flow measurements during carotid endarterectomy. *Stroke* 1973;4(4):674-683.

5. Schramm J, Koht A, Schmidt G, Pechstein U, Taniguchi M, Fahlbusch R: Surgical and electrophysiological observations during clipping of 134 aneurysms with evoked potential monitoring. *Neurosurgery* 1990;26(1):61-70.

6. Buchthal A, Belopavlovic M: Somatosensory evoked potentials in cerebral aneurysm surgery. *Eur J Anaesthesiol* 1992;9(6):493-497.

7. Lopez JR, Chang SD, Steinberg GK: The use of electrophysiological monitoring in the intraoperative management of intracranial aneurysms. *J Neurol Neurosurg Psychiatry* 1999;66(2):189-196.

8. Manninen PH, Patterson S, Lam AM, Gelb AW, Nantau WE: Evoked potential monitoring during posterior fossa aneurysm surgery: A comparison of two modalities. *Can J Anaesth* 1994;41(2):92-97.

9. Weinzierl MR, Reinacher P, Gilsbach JM, Rohde V: Combined motor and somatosensory evoked potentials for intraoperative monitoring: Intra- and postoperative data in a series of 69 operations. *Neurosurg Rev* 2007;30(2):109-116, discussion 116.

10. Langeloo DD, Lelivelt A, Louis Journee H, Slappendel R, de Kleuver M: Transcranial electrical motor-evoked potential monitoring during surgery for spinal deformity: A study of 145 patients. *Spine* 2003;28(10):1043-1050.

11. Legatt AD: Current practice of motor evoked potential monitoring: Results of a survey. *J Clin Neurophysiol* 2002;19(5):454-460.

12. Hilibrand AS, Schwartz DM, Sethuraman V, Vaccaro AR, Albert TJ: Comparison of transcranial electric motor and somatosensory evoked potential monitoring during cervical spine surgery. *J Bone Joint Surg Am* 2004;86-A(6):1248-1253.

13. Pelosi L, Lamb J, Grevitt M, Mehdian SM, Webb JK, Blumhardt LD: Combined monitoring of motor and somatosensory evoked potentials in orthopaedic spinal surgery. *Clin Neurophysiol* 2002;113(7):1082-1091.

14. MacDonald DB: Safety of intraoperative transcranial electrical stimulation motor evoked potential monitoring. *J Clin Neurophysiol* 2002;19(5):416-429.

15. Macdonald DB: Intraoperative motor evoked potential monitoring: Overview and update. *J Clin Monit Comput* 2006;20(5):347-377.

16. Algotsson L, Messeter K, Rehncrona S, Skeidsvoll H, Ryding E: Cerebral hemodynamic changes and electroencephalography during carotid endarterectomy. *J Clin Anesth* 1990;2(3):143-151.

17. Zampella E, Morawetz RB, McDowell HA, et al: The importance of cerebral ischemia during carotid endarterectomy. *Neurosurgery* 1991;29(5):727-730, discussion 730–731.

18. Blume WT, Ferguson GG, McNeill DK: Significance of EEG changes at carotid endarterectomy. *Stroke* 1986;17(5):891-897.

19. Redekop G, Ferguson G: Correlation of contralateral stenosis and intraoperative electroencephalogram change with risk of stroke during carotid endarterectomy. *Neurosurgery* 1992;30(2):191-194.

20. Ballotta E, Dagiau G, Saladini M, et al: Results of electroencephalographic monitoring during 369 consecutive carotid artery revascularizations. *Eur Neurol* 1997;37(1):43-47.

21. Cho I, Smullens SN, Streletz LJ, Fariello RG: The value of intraoperative EEG monitoring during carotid endarterectomy. *Ann Neurol* 1986;20(4):508-512.

22. Luders H, Lesser RP, Hahn J, et al: Basal temporal language area demonstrated by electrical stimulation. *Neurology* 1986;36(4):505-510.

23. Minahan RE, Sepkuty JP, Lesser RP, Sponseller PD, Kostuik JP: Anterior spinal cord injury with preserved neurogenic "motor" evoked potentials. *Clin Neurophysiol* 2001;112(8):1442-1450.

24. More RC, Nuwer MR, Dawson EG: Cortical evoked potential monitoring during spinal surgery: Sensitivity, specificity, reliability, and criteria for alarm. *J Spinal Disord* 1988;1(1):75-80.

25. Mostegl A, Bauer R, Eichenauer M: Intraoperative somatosensory potential monitoring. A clinical analysis of 127 surgical procedures. *Spine* 1988;13(4):396-400.

26. Szalay EA, Carollo JJ, Roach JW: Sensitivity of spinal cord monitoring to intraoperative events. *J Pediatr Orthop* 1986;6(4):437-441.

27. Jones SJ, Edgar MA, Ransford AO, Thomas NP: A system for the electrophysiological monitoring of the spinal cord during operations for scoliosis. *J Bone Joint Surg Br* 1983;65(2):134-139.

28. Constantini S, Miller DC, Allen JC, Rorke LB, Freed D, Epstein FJ: Radical excision of intramedullary spinal cord tumors: Surgical morbidity and long-term follow-up evaluation in 164 children and young adults. *J Neurosurg* 2000;93(2 suppl):183-193.

29. Cristante L, Herrmann HD: Surgical management of intramedullary spinal cord tumors: Functional outcome and sources of morbidity. *Neurosurgery* 1994;35(1):69-74, discussion 76.

30. Kearse LA Jr, Lopez-Bresnahan M, McPeck K, Tambe V: Loss of somatosensory evoked potentials during intramedullary spinal cord surgery predicts postoperative neurologic deficits in motor function [corrected]. *J Clin Anesth* 1993;5(5):392-398.

31. Nuwer MR, Dawson EG, Carlson LG, Kanim LE, Sherman JE: Somatosensory evoked potential spinal cord monitoring reduces neurologic deficits after scoliosis surgery: Results of a large multicenter survey. *Electroencephalogr Clin Neurophysiol* 1995;96(1):6-11.

32. Dawson EG, Sherman JE, Kanim LE, Nuwer MR: Spinal cord monitoring. Results of the Scoliosis Research Society and the European Spinal Deformity Society survey. *Spine* 1991;16(8 suppl):S361-S364.

33. Galla JD, Ergin MA, Lansman SL, et al: Use of somatosensory evoked potentials for thoracic and thoracoabdominal aortic resections. *Ann Thorac Surg* 1999;67(6):1947-1952, discussion 1953-1958.

34. Grabitz K, Sandmann W, Stuhmeier K, et al: The risk of ischemic spinal cord injury in patients undergoing graft replacement for thoracoabdominal aortic aneurysms. *J Vasc Surg* 1996; 23(2):230-240.

35. Griepp RB, Ergin MA, Galla JD, et al: Looking for the artery of Adamkiewicz: A quest to minimize paraplegia after operations for aneurysms of the descending thoracic and thoracoabdominal aorta. *J Thorac Cardiovasc Surg* 1996;112(5):1202-1213, discussion 1213–1215.

36. Laschinger JC, Cunningham JN Jr, Nathan IM, Knopp EA, Cooper MM, Spencer FC: Experimental and clinical assessment of the adequacy of partial bypass in maintenance of spinal cord blood flow during operations on the thoracic aorta. *Ann Thorac Surg* 1983;36(4):417-426.

37. Robertazzi RR, Cunningham JN Jr: Monitoring of somatosensory evoked potentials: A primer on the intraoperative detection of spinal cord ischemia during aortic reconstructive surgery. *Semin Thorac Cardiovasc Surg* 1998;10(1):11-17.

38. Sloan TB, Jameson LC: Electrophysiologic monitoring during surgery to repair the thoraco-abdominal aorta. *J Clin Neurophysiol* 2007;24(4):316-327.

39. Crawford ES, Mizrahi EM, Hess KR, Coselli JS, Safi HJ, Patel VM: The impact of distal aortic perfusion and somatosensory evoked potential monitoring on prevention of paraplegia after aortic aneurysm operation. *J Thorac Cardiovasc Surg* 1988;95(3):357-367.

40. Fisher RS, Raudzens P, Nunemacher M: Efficacy of intraoperative neurophysiological monitoring. *J Clin Neurophysiol* 1995;12(1):97-109.

41. Wober C, Zeitlhofer J, Asenbaum S, et al: Monitoring of median nerve somatosensory evoked potentials in carotid surgery. *J Clin Neurophysiol* 1998;15(5):429-438.

42. Mizoi K, Yoshimoto T: Intraoperative monitoring of the somatosensory evoked potentials and cerebral blood flow during aneurysm surgery—safety evaluation for temporary vascular occlusion. *Neurol Med Chir (Tokyo)* 1991;31(6):318-325.

43. Nadol JB Jr, Chiong CM, Ojemann RG, et al: Preservation of hearing and facial nerve function in resection of acoustic neuroma. *Laryngoscope* 1992;102(10):1153-1158.

44. Radtke RA, Erwin CW, Wilkins RH: Intraoperative brainstem auditory evoked potentials: Significant decrease in postoperative morbidity. *Neurology* 1989;39(2 pt 1):187-191.

45. James ML, Husain AM: Brainstem auditory evoked potential monitoring: When is change in wave V significant? *Neurology* 2005;65(10):1551-1555.

46. Harper CM, Harner SG, Slavit DH, et al: Effect of BAEP monitoring on hearing preservation during acoustic neuroma resection. *Neurology* 1992;42(8):1551-1553.

47. Niparko JK, Kileny PR, Kemink JL, Lee HM, Graham MD: Neurophysiologic intraoperative monitoring: II. Facial nerve function. *Am J Otolaryngol* 1989;10(1):55-61.

48. Terrell JE, Kileny PR, Yian C, et al: Clinical outcome of continuous facial nerve monitoring during primary parotidectomy. *Arch Otolaryngol Head Neck Surg* 1997;123(10):1081-1087.

49. Cedzich C, Schramm J, Mengedoht CF, Fahlbusch R: Factors that limit the use of flash visual evoked potentials for surgical monitoring. *Electroencephalogr Clin Neurophysiol* 1988;71(2):142-145.

50. Sasaki T, Ichikawa T, Sakuma J, et al: [Intraoperative monitoring of visual evoked potentials]. *Masui* 2006;55(3):302-313.

51. Chacko AG, Babu KS, Chandy MJ: Value of visual evoked potential monitoring during trans-sphenoidal pituitary surgery. *Br J Neurosurg* 1996;10(3):275-278.

52. Herzon GD, Zealear DL: Intraoperative monitoring of the visual evoked potential during endoscopic sinus surgery. *Otolaryngol Head Neck Surg* 1994;111(5):575-579.

53. McGarvey ML, Cheung AT, Szeto W, Messe SR: Management of neurologic complications of thoracic aortic surgery. *J Clin Neurophysiol* 2007;24(4):336-343.

54. McGarvey ML, Mullen MT, Woo EY, et al: The treatment of spinal cord ischemia following thoracic endovascular aortic repair. *Neurocrit Care* 2007;6(1):35-39.

55. Schepens MA, Boezeman EH, Hamerlijnck RP, ter Beek H, Vermeulen FE: Somatosensory evoked potentials during exclusion and reperfusion of critical aortic segments in thoracoabdominal aortic aneurysm surgery. *J Card Surg* 1994;9(6):692-702.

56. Legatt AD, Ellen R: Grass lecture: Motor evoked potential monitoring. *Am J Electroneurodiagnostic Technol* 2004;44(4):223-243.

57. Kothbauer KF, Deletis V, Epstein FJ: Motor-evoked potential monitoring for intramedullary spinal cord tumor surgery: Correlation of clinical and neurophysiological data in a series of 100 consecutive procedures. *Neurosurg Focus* 1998;4(5):e1.

58. Sala F, Palandri G, Basso E, et al: Motor evoked potential monitoring improves outcome after surgery for intramedullary spinal cord tumors: A historical control study. *Neurosurgery.* 2006;58(6):1129-1143, discussion 1143.

59. Kawanishi Y, Munakata H, Matsumori M, et al: Usefulness of transcranial motor evoked potentials during thoracoabdominal aortic surgery. *Ann Thorac Surg* 2007;83(2):456-461.

60. Jacobs MJ, Elenbaas TW, Schurink GW, Mess WH, Mochtar B: Assessment of spinal cord integrity during thoracoabdominal aortic aneurysm repair. *Ann Thorac Surg* 2002;74(5):S1864-S1866, discussion S92-S98.

61. van Dongen EP, Schepens MA, Morshuis WJ, et al: Thoracic and thoracoabdominal aortic aneurysm repair: Use of evoked potential monitoring in 118 patients. *J Vasc Surg* 2001;34(6): 1035-1040.

62. Costa P, Bruno A, Bonzanino M, et al: Somatosensory- and motor-evoked potential monitoring during spine and spinal cord surgery. *Spinal Cord* 2007;45(1):86-91.

63. Meylaerts SA, Jacobs MJ, van Iterson V, De Haan P, Kalkman CJ: Comparison of transcranial motor evoked potentials and somatosensory evoked potentials during thoracoabdominal aortic aneurysm repair. *Ann Surg* 1999;230(6):742-749.

64. Dong CC, MacDonald DB, Janusz MT: Intraoperative spinal cord monitoring during descending thoracic and thoracoabdominal aneurysm surgery. *Ann Thorac Surg* 2002;74(5):S1873-S1876; discussion S92-S98.

65. DiCindio S, Theroux M, Shah S, et al: Multimodality monitoring of transcranial electric motor and somatosensory-evoked potentials during surgical correction of spinal deformity in patients with cerebral palsy and other neuromuscular disorders. *Spine* 2003;28(16):1851-1855, discussion 1855–1856.

CARDIOVASCULAR ANESTHESIA

Is Regional Superior to General Anesthesia for Infrainguinal Revascularization?

R. Yan McRae, MD, and Grace L. Chien, MD

INTRODUCTION

Infrainguinal revascularization includes bypass of the femoral artery or its branches. All patients having vascular surgery are at high risk for cardiac complications according to the American College of Cardiology Guidelines for Perioperative Evaluation for Noncardiac Surgery. Patients having lower-extremity vascular grafting are at high risk for perioperative complications including graft failure, myocardial infarction, respiratory failure, and death.[1] In a large cohort study, patients undergoing infrainguinal bypass had a 30-day mortality rate of 5.8% and a 1-year mortality rate of 16.3%.[2] About half of all perioperative deaths in this population are caused by cardiac complications.[3] Patients undergoing this type of surgery often have diabetes, histories of tobacco abuse, or hypertension, which are associated with peripheral and coronary artery disease. Risk factors for coronary artery disease have been associated with an increased risk of perioperative cardiac morbidity in numerous studies.[1]

Two types of benefit may come to such patients who receive neuraxial anesthesia. First, they may benefit with respect to outcomes related to their concomitant diseases, for example, reduction of myocardial infarction, respiratory complications, or infections. Second, they may benefit with respect to outcomes related directly to their surgery, for example, reduction of vascular graft failure that leads to a second procedure or even an amputation. Harm may also come to patients because of neuraxial anesthesia. The most obvious concern is for neurologic injury such as may occur with epidural or subdural hematoma. Evidence for and against these benefits and harms is given in this chapter.

THERAPEUTIC OPTIONS

Typical anesthetic options for patients having lower-extremity vascular grafting include general anesthesia (GA), epidural anesthesia, spinal anesthesia, and combinations thereof. It is important to consider that clinical practices in any hospital or study may differ in basic choices that in turn may influence outcomes to a similar or perhaps greater degree than the variable studied. When interpreting studies designed to address anesthetic choice

and infrainguinal revascularization outcomes, utilization of postoperative epidural infusion, invasive monitoring-guided hemodynamic optimization, and antithrombosis therapy are examples of "standardized" therapeutic choices that in fact vary between studies. The anesthesiologist must evaluate these choices in his or her own practice, as well as in the body of published evidence, in order to determine how best to serve his or her patients.

EVIDENCE

Benefits

Mortality and Morbidity in Mixed Surgical Populations

Rodgers and colleagues[4] performed a large meta-analysis of 141 randomized trials comparing neuraxial anesthesia with general anesthesia for all types of patients. Neuraxial anesthesia was associated with a significant (approximately 30%) reduction in postoperative mortality rate. When odds of dying were examined by type of surgery, neuraxial blockade appeared salutary for orthopedic surgery more than vascular, general, or urologic procedures. When odds of dying were examined by type of anesthesia, neuraxial blockade alone was superior to GA alone. Nonfatal operative morbidities including deep venous thrombosis, pulmonary embolism, perioperative transfusion, pneumonia, and respiratory depression were reduced for patients randomized to neuraxial blockade. Myocardial infarction was possibly reduced (odds ratio [OR] 0.67; 95% confidence interval [CI], 0.45 to 1.00) in patients receiving neuraxial blockade.

The Multicentre Australian Study of Epidural Anesthesia (the MASTER Anesthesia Trial) included 888 patients with high-risk comorbidities undergoing major abdominal surgery or esophagectomy, randomized between GA with epidural anesthesia/analgesia or GA with postoperative intravenous opioids.[5,6] Pain scores were lower at rest on the first postoperative day (POD) and with coughing on POD 1 to 3 in the epidural group. Respiratory failure was also reduced, but no significant differences in mortality rate or cardiovascular morbidity were demonstrated. The rate of death or at least one major complication was 57.1% in the epidural group and 60.7% in the GA group; to demonstrate a statistically significant 3.6% benefit of regional anesthesia/analgesia would require a study of roughly 6000 patients. Ultimately, it remains controversial whether or not a small but significant benefit of regional anesthesia exists in high-risk mixed surgical populations.

Bode and colleagues[7] tested the hypothesis that regional anesthesia reduces operative cardiovascular morbidity and mortality rate associated with infrainguinal revascularization. Four hundred twenty-three patients were randomly assigned to receive general (138), epidural (149), or spinal (136) anesthesia for femoral to distal artery bypass surgery. Epidural catheters were removed at the time of discharge from the postanesthesia care unit (PACU), but some patients received epidural morphine before catheter removal. All patients were monitored for at least 48 hours postoperatively with arterial lines and pulmonary artery catheters (but without standardized treatment protocol). Patients received subcutaneous heparin on POD 1 until ambulation, then aspirin 81 mg daily thereafter. There was no significant reduction of myocardial infarction, angina, or congestive heart failure, or all-cause mortality rate, between GA (16.7%), epidural (15.4%), or spinal anesthesia (21.3%). Because of study design, potential benefit of postoperative epidural infusion was not addressed. In sum, current evidence for significant reduction of mortality rate and *cardiac* risk by use of regional anesthesia during infrainguinal revascularization is limited. If favorable, the benefit of regional anesthesia is small.

Graft Failure in Lower-Extremity Revascularization

In two randomized studies, one (Christopherson and colleagues[8]) comparing epidural to GA for patients having lower-extremity grafts and the other (Tuman and colleagues[9]) comparing epidural-supplemented with unsupplemented GA for patients having either aortic or lower-extremity vascular surgery, vascular graft failure was reduced in patients with epidurals. Both these studies reported high rates of vascular graft failure, and both of them continued epidural analgesia into the postoperative period. In the study by Christopherson and colleagues,[8] preoperative aspirin was withheld and heparin was continued into the postoperative period only when there was suspicion of graft failure. Few patients in that study were monitored with pulmonary artery catheters.[8] In the study by Tuman and colleagues,[9] intraoperative heparin was reversed with protamine at the end of surgery. High rates of graft failure in these two studies might have been reduced had different antithrombosis strategies been used. However, high rates of adverse outcomes made it possible for these two studies to show significant reduction of graft failure in patients who received epidural anesthesia.

A focused retrospective chart review by Kashyap and colleagues[10] also showed possible benefit to regional anesthesia. This review examined graft survival after infrapopliteal revascularization with polytetrafluoroethylene (PTFE) graft material for critical ischemia. These criteria narrowed the results to 77 patients of 1500 lower-extremity revascularization surgeries over the period 1978–1998 and functionally selected for a study population with a high rate of graft failure, thus strengthening the ability to detect a small effect. GA accounted for 75%

of these cases and regional anesthesia, mostly spinal anesthetics, 25% of the cases. There were 11 incidents of acute graft thrombosis, all in the GA group. The regional group had prolonged primary graft patency at 36 months (35%) when compared with the GA group (15%). Specific breakdown of which patients had neuraxial analgesia continued into the postoperative period was not reported. Postoperative warfarin use was not statistically associated with an improvement in graft patency, but only some of the patients received warfarin in this retrospective, unrandomized study.

In contrast, a retrospective chart review by Schunn and colleagues[11] examined 294 primary femoral-popliteal-tibial bypass surgeries occurring between 1989–1994 and found no significant difference of early graft thrombosis rates between GA alone (9.4%) and epidural alone (14%). However, the article did not state if epidural analgesia was always continued into the postoperative period or continued selectively in certain cases and, as a chart review, there was no randomization between the two groups. In two prospective randomized trials, one (Cook and colleagues[12]) comparing spinal to GA and one (Pierce and colleagues[13]) in which patients were randomized to spinal, epidural, or GA, neuraxial analgesia was not continued into the postoperative period. There was no benefit associated with regional anesthesia. Rates of graft failure were lower overall, in fact so low in the study by Pierce and colleagues[13] that the study was underpowered to find a difference in rates of graft failure. In the study by Pierce and colleagues[13] no difference was found in the rate of postoperative amputation. All patients received aspirin and either subcutaneous heparin or oral Coumadin. Additionally, all patients were monitored with arterial lines and pulmonary artery catheters for 24 to 48 hours after surgery.[13] It has been shown that patients undergoing lower-extremity vascular surgery under GA had improved vascular graft survival if they were monitored and treated appropriately using pulmonary artery catheters.[14] Thus, use of neuraxial anesthesia may add no further benefit with respect to graft patency if antithrombosis therapy is used and hemodynamics are optimized. Furthermore, there appears to be little evidence supporting improved vascular graft patency after neuraxial anesthesia without continuation of neuraxial analgesia into the postoperative period.

Risks

Antithrombosis therapy is important in the maintenance of vascular graft patency. In some institutions aspirin is routinely given before surgery. Intravenous heparin is almost always given intraoperatively before clamping of the arteries to be grafted. Thus, a spinal or an epidural needle might be placed into a patient whose platelet function is impaired from aspirin, and subsequent to placing of an epidural catheter, an anticoagulant is almost always given. Furthermore, intravenous heparin may be continued into the postoperative period, or low-molecular-weight heparin may be given subcutaneously. Because of their concomitant diseases, vascular surgery patients may be on Coumadin or antiplatelet therapy.

The American Society of Regional Anesthesia and Pain Medicine (ASRA) has recently reviewed the evidence of risk of epidural hematoma for patients receiving neuraxial blockade while anticoagulated.[15] Pertinent recommendations related to heparin and antiplatelet agents are summarized below. For more details or for evidence-based management of neuraxial anesthesia for patients on other anticoagulants, the reader is referred to the ASRA consensus document, available at www.asra.com.

1. Unfractionated heparin: Patients undergoing vascular surgery, who will receive heparin intraoperatively, should not receive neuraxial anesthesia if they have other coagulopathies. If there is difficult or bloody needle placement, they may be at increased risk of neuraxial hematoma; there should be a discussion with the surgeon as to whether the case should proceed or be canceled. In general, heparin should not be given until at least 1 hour after needle placement. In the postoperative period, there should be careful monitoring of neurologic status, and concentrations of local anesthetics should be limited to those that allow assessment of motor strength. Epidural catheters should be removed at least 2 to 4 hours after a heparin dose. Patients on heparin for 4 days or longer are at risk for heparin-induced thrombocytopenia; therefore a platelet count should be obtained before neuraxial block is performed.

2. Low-molecular-weight heparin (LMWH): Patients receiving preoperative LMWH should be assumed to have impaired coagulation. The safest timing and type of anesthesia is likely a single-injection spinal anesthetic given at least 10 to 12 hours after the last thromboprophylaxis-dosed LMWH; patients receiving higher (treatment) doses of LMWH should not receive neuraxial anesthesia for at least 24 hours. If LMWH is to be started postoperatively, dosing and epidural catheter removal must be timed. Additional care and consideration of the risk and benefits of regional techniques should be considered when the patient is being treated with other drugs that may act synergistically with LMWH.

3. Antiplatelet medications: Nonsteroidal antiinflammatory drug therapy alone is not a contraindication to a regional technique. Before neuraxial regional anesthesia, an interval of 14 days is suggested for ticlopidine and 7 days for clopidogrel. The family of platelet glycoprotein (GP) IIb/IIIa inhibitors deserves special mention. Platelet aggregation is impaired for 24 to 48 hours following administration of abciximab, and for 4 to 8 hours following eptifibatide and tirofiban.

AREAS OF UNCERTAINTY

As far as we know, no studies have been published to date to determine whether spinal anesthesia affects graft survival, as epidural anesthesia does in some studies.

GUIDELINES

We recommend two guidelines published by national societies to address issues discussed in this chapter. Both can be found on websites, where they are updated from time to time as new information becomes available. With respect to perioperative cardiac morbidity and mortality rates, the reader is referred to the website of the American College of Cardiology (www.acc.org). With respect to management of neuraxial blockade for anticoagulated patients, the reader is referred to the website of the American Society of Regional Anesthesia and Pain Medicine (www.asra.com).

AUTHORS' RECOMMENDATIONS

Patients with peripheral vascular disease have a significant rate of perioperative mortality and cardiac morbidity. Therefore any reduction of risk would provide a relatively large decrease in the absolute number of operative complications. The literature reveals contradictory studies, which only hint that neuraxial techniques may show a small benefit to mortality and cardiac event rates in a mixed population of surgical patients. Specific to the current practice of regional anesthesia, in addition to the usual consideration of anatomy, risk of infection, and patient preference, increasing utilization of perioperative antithrombotic therapy adds complexity both to analysis of potential risks and benefits and to actual patient management.

Graft survival may be similar with general anesthesia as with neuraxial blockade, especially if patients receive optimized hemodynamic therapy and/or perioperative antithrombosis therapy. If epidural anesthesia is given, epidural therapy should be continued into the postoperative period because the only randomized studies that demonstrated reduction of graft failure were performed with continued postoperative epidural therapy.

In our hospital we have a very low rate of graft failure. Our patients receive aspirin before surgery. Arterial, central venous, and pulmonary artery catheters are used only for medical indications, and most patients do not receive these monitors. When deemed safe and feasible, regional anesthesia techniques are offered as options to patients undergoing infrainguinal revascularization, but with the acknowledgment that the most likely benefit is superior postoperative analgesia.

REFERENCES

1. Eagle et al: Perioperative cardiovascular evaluation for noncardiac surgery update. American College of Cardiology, 2002. Available at www.acc.org/clinical/guidelines/perio/update.htm.
2. Fleisher LA, Eagle KA, Shaffer T, Anderson GF: Perioperative and long-term mortality rates after major vascular surgery: The relationship to preoperative testing in the Medicare population. *Anesth Analg* 1999;89:849-855.
3. Hertzer NR: Basic data concerning associated coronary disease in peripheral vascular patients. *Ann Vasc Surg* 1987;1:616-620.
4. Rodgers A, Walker N, Schug S, McKee A, Kehlet H, van Zundert A, et al: Reduction of postoperative mortality and morbidity with epidural or spinal anaesthesia: Results from overview of randomised trials. *BMJ* 2000;321:1-12.
5. Peyton PJ, Myles PS, Silbert BS, Rigg JRA, Jamrozik K, Parsons R: Perioperative epidural analgesia and outcome after abdominal surgery in high-risk patients. *Anesth Analg* 2003;96:548-554.
6. Rigg JRA, Jamrozik K, Myles PS, Silbert BS, Peyton PJ, Parsons RW, Collins KS: Epidural anaesthesia and analgesia and outcome of major surgery: A randomized trial. *Lancet* 2002;359:1276-1282.
7. Bode RH, Lewis KP, Zarich SW, Pierce ET, Roberts M, Kowalchuck GJ, et al: Cardiac outcome after peripheral vascular surgery: Comparison of general and regional anesthesia. *Anesthesiology* 1996;84:3-13.

8. Christopherson R, Beattie C, Frank SM, Norris EJ, Meinert CL, Gottlieb SO, et al: Perioperative morbidity in patients randomized to epidural or general anesthesia for lower extremity vascular surgery. *Anesthesiology* 1993;79:422-434.

9. Tuman KJ, McCarthy RJ, March RJ, DeLaria GA, Patel RV, Ivankovich AD: Effects of epidural anesthesia and analgesia on coagulation and outcome after major vascular surgery. *Anesth Analg* 1991;73:696-704.

10. Kashyap MS, Ahn SS, Quinones-Baldrich WJ, Byung-Uk C, Dorey F, Reil TD, et al: Infrapopliteal-lower extremity revascularization with prosthetic conduit: A 20-year experience. *Vasc Endovascular Surg* 2002;36:255-262.

11. Schunn CD, Hertzer NR, O'Hara PJ, Krajewski LP, Sullivan TM, Beven EG: Epidural versus general anesthesia: Does anesthetic management influence early infrainguinal graft thrombosis? *Ann Vasc Surg* 1998;12:65-69.

12. Cook PT, Davies MJ, Cronin KD, Moran P: A prospective randomized trial comparing spinal anaesthesia using hyperbaric cinchocaine with general anesthesia for lower limb vascular surgery. *Anaesth Intensive Care* 1986;14:373-380.

13. Pierce ET, Pomposelli FB, Stanley GD, et al: Anesthesia type does not influence early graft patency or limb salvage rates of lower extremity arterial bypass. *J Vasc Surg* 1997;25:226-233.

14. Berlauk JF, Abrams JH, Gilmour IJ, O'Connor SR, Knighton DR, Cerra FB: Preoperative optimization of cardiovascular hemodynamics improves outcome in peripheral vascular surgery. *Ann Surg* 1991;289-297.

15. American Society of Regional Anesthesia and Pain Medicine: Regional anesthesia in the anticoagulated patient—defining the risks. 2002. Available at www.asra.com.

61 Evidence-Based Practice for Fast-Track Cardiac Anesthesia— Is It Safe?

Daniel Bainbridge MD, FRCPC, and Davy Cheng, MD, MSc, FRCPC, FCAHS

INTRODUCTION

Fast-track cardiac surgery was first proposed in 1977.[1] However, it was not until cost and resource utilization issues became increasingly important that the concept of fast-track anesthesia reemerged into prominence in the 1990s and has since become a widespread technique. Fast-track cardiac anesthesia (FTCA) can be considered a management protocol involving the perioperative care of patients with the goal of allowing rapid recovery following surgery.

The perioperative management of patients in a fast-track protocol encompasses several steps. Preoperative screening and optimization of patients is the first step to a successful fast-track program. In a study by Wong and colleagues,[2] preoperative risks for delayed tracheal extubation included age and female sex. Postoperative risk factors included bleeding, inotrope use, intra-aortic balloon pump (IABP) use, and atrial arrhythmias.[2] Intraoperatively, management consists of low narcotic dosages balanced with an inhaled agent and/or propofol to provide a more rapidly reversible state that facilitates early extubation. It also requires attention to patient temperature and associated management of coagulation and hemodynamic status to prevent complications, which will delay extubation. Postoperative care involves continued vigilance for and management of any complications (bleeding, arrhythmias, etc.) and nursing support to fast-track these patients. It is important to acknowledge that all patients are potential fast-track candidates and therefore, when clinically indicated, may be extubated within 4 hours of admission.

The potential benefits of such a protocol are clear. Early tracheal extubation in the intensive care unit (ICU) leads to early discharge to the floor. This in turn leads to early discharge from the hospital, which ultimately leads to cost savings, a reduction in resource utilization, or both.[3-6]

OPTIONS

Figure 61-1 outlines the post–cardiac surgery recovery models for the management of patients. The practice of higher-dose narcotics with a 16- to 24-hour ICU stay is the traditional approach to management of cardiac surgery patients. Recovery of fast-track protocol (FTP) patients can involve three cardiac recovery models that have been proposed to maximize the benefits of an FTP in cardiac surgery: one in which the cardiac recovery area (CRA) is separate from the ICU (free-standing model); one in which the CRA is adjacent to the ICU (parallel model); and the integrated model, in which the CRA and ICU are physically intertwined. What has been demonstrated from studies involving FTP for cardiac patients is that extubation itself reduces costs only marginally. Maximal costs savings are realized only with the adoption of different recovery structures. The greatest benefit of an FTP lies in its ability to reduce costs, and its ability to reduce costs requires a change in the structure of patient recovery. Therefore the change to an FTP approach should be accompanied by a change in patient recovery practice.

EVIDENCE

To change practice, three fundamental questions should be addressed. The first is safety; does this practice increase mortality or morbidity risks? For cardiac surgery, morbidity endpoints include stroke, cognitive decline, myocardial infarction, pneumonia, long-term ventilatory support, and renal failure. Second, how applicable is this practice to all cardiac patients, and in particular, does the evidence support the use of this technique in high-risk subgroups? Third, what is the benefit to using fast-track cardiac anesthesia?

The best available evidence for fast-track surgery is from a recent systematic review and meta-analysis of randomized trials comparing fast-track cardiac anesthesia with conventional anesthesia using high-dose narcotic regimens[7] (Figure 61-2). This review identified 10 trials involving over 1800 patients. The patients included in the review had mean ages ranging from 59 to 64 years, and the majority of patients were male. Many of the trials excluded elderly patients, those with respiratory disease, and those with poor left ventricle (LV) function. The majority of patients underwent elective coronary artery bypass graft (CABG) surgery. Addressing the issue of

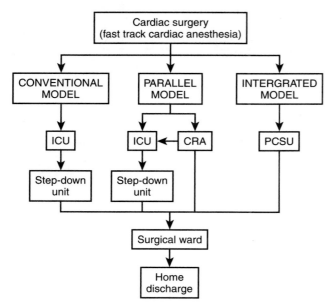

Figure 61-1. Post–cardiac surgical recovery models. ICU, intensive care unit; CRA, cardiac recovery area; PCSU, post–cardiac surgical unit. *(From Cheng DC: Fast track cardiac surgery pathways: Early extubation, process of care, and cost containment. Anesthesiology 1998;88:1429-1433.)*

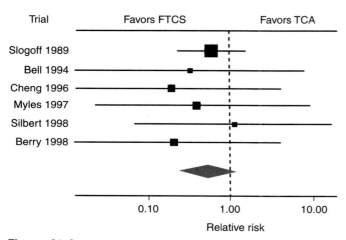

Figure 61-2. A systematic review of the safety and effectiveness of fast-track cardiac anesthesia. *(From Myles PS, Daly DJ, Djaiani G, et al: Anesthesiology 2003;99:982-987.)*

safety, the pooled analysis was unable to demonstrate a significant difference in outcomes with regard to mortality rate (relative risk [RR], 0.51 [95% confidence interval (CI): 0.23 to 1.13]), myocardial infarction (RR, 1.00 [95% CI 0.52 to 1.94]), stroke 0.74 (0.05 to 10.56), or acute renal failure 2.92 (0.32 to 27.1). This suggests that, in comparison with conventional anesthesia, fast-track cardiac anesthesia is safe. However, it is still possible that small differences exist because most adverse events were rare and thus the review lacked power to detect small differences. Only one patient in all the trials required reintubation. However, many patients in the early extubation groups failed to be extubated early, and this outcome was not reported in the meta-analysis. One other outcome of interest was not addressed in the meta-analysis, namely, awareness.

To address the issue of awareness, Dowd and colleagues[8] reported the results of their prospective observational study on 608 patients undergoing FTCA. All participants were interviewed 18 hours after surgery to determine if the patients had been aware during the surgical procedure. Only two patients (0.3%) reported awareness during surgery, which is consistent with reports for general surgical procedures.[9]

Ovrum and colleagues[10] published a prospective observational study on 5658 patients who underwent FTCA from 1989 until 1997. The mean age of patients was 63, and 16.9% were female. The average ejection fraction was 70%, with 70% reporting New York Heart Association (NYHA) class III or IV symptomatology. The median time to extubation was 1.5 hours, with 99.3% being extubated within 4 hours. A total of 1.09% of patients required reintubation in their cohort, with the reason for reintubation being bleeding in 0.62% and hemodynamic instability in 0.46%. The rate of reintubation is similar to other reports on reintubation rates during cardiac surgery (either conventional or FTCA), which range from 1% to 6%. The rates of myocardial infarction and in-hospital mortality were 2.53% and 0.41%, respectively. Although not a randomized trial, it included both high- and low-risk patient groups and included a sufficient sample size to accurately determine the absolute risk of adverse events associated with FTCA. This study suggests that the broad application of a fast-track protocol is safe and effective.

Myles and colleagues,[7] in addition to examining adverse events, also examined the potential benefits of an FTCA in reducing length of ventilation, length of ICU stay, and length of hospital stay. Of these, the duration of intubation was statistically different (weighted mean difference [WMD] 8.1 hours; 95% CI: 3.7 to 12.5; $p = 0.001$), as was the ICU length of stay (WMD 5.4 hours; 95% CI: 0.3 to 10.5; $p = 0.039$). Unfortunately, this did not result in an overall reduction in the length of hospital stay (WMD 0.61 days; 95% CI: 0.28 to 1.5; $p = 0.18$). One of the reasons why discharge times were reduced only moderately is likely because of the reluctance in most ICUs to discharge patients who meet discharge criteria in the evening or overnight.[9]

Taken collectively these papers all support the safety of fast-track protocols for elective CABG patients. Patients with poor left ventricular function, respiratory disease, and the elderly (age greater than 75 years) were not included in most of these studies; thus, care should be exercised in these subgroups when deciding on suitability for fast-track cardiac anesthesia.

CONTROVERSIES

The two most active areas of research currently are the type of intraoperative narcotic that best facilitates FTCA, and the method of pain control during the recovery period. There are several randomized trials examining the efficacy of remifentanyl, fentanyl, and sufentanyl for fast-track cardiac anesthesia. Fentanyl loads were from 7 to 15 mcg/kg with titration to control stimulation from surgery. Sufentanyl load was 1 to 4 mcg/kg again with titration to control stimulation from surgery. Remifentanil loading was from 0.5 to 1.0 mcg/kg with maintenance infusions of up to 1.0 mcg/kg/min. Times to extubation were no different in any of the studies.[3,11,12]

The use of regional anesthesia has also become an area of renewed interest both to aid in early extubation and to provide adequate pain control in the postoperative period. A systematic review with meta-analysis by Liu and colleagues[13] examined patients who had received either thoracic epidural analgesia (TEA) versus control or spinal narcotics versus control. For the TEA group a total of 15 trials enrolling 1178 patients was included. TEA reduced pulmonary complications (OR 0.41, 95% CI 0.27 to 0.60), dysrythmias (OR 0.52, 95% CI 0.29 to 0.93), time to tracheal extubation (WMD 4.5 hours, 95% CI -7 to -2), and visual analog scale (VAS) pain scores (WMD 7.8 mm, 95% CI -15 to -0.6). For intrathecal narcotic utilization a total of 17 trials enrolling 668 patients were included. No benefit was seen in time to tracheal extubation. VAS pain scores were improved and total narcotic consumption reduced. In a subset of trials, in those using intrathecal narcotic doses less than 7 mcg/kg morphine, a reduction in time to tracheal extubation was seen (WMD 1.2 hours, 95% CI -1.8 to -0.7). There still exists, however, concern over the use of regional techniques in cardiac patients, and the risk of epidural hematoma. The risk of epidural hematomas has been difficult to determine.[14]

Another meta-analysis reviewed the benefit of patient-controlled analgesic (PCA)–administered narcotics to nurse-administered narcotics in patients undergoing cardiac surgery.[15] The review covered 10 trials involving 666 patients. There was no difference in VAS pain scores at 24 hours (WMD 0.19, 95% CI -0.61 to 0.24). VAS pain scores at 48 hours were reduced by 25% (WMD 0.73, 95% CI -1.19 to -0.27). Narcotic consumption was increased by 7 mg at 24 hours postoperatively. This study suggests that there is little benefit to the use of PCA in patients undergoing cardiac surgery.

Nonsteroidal antiinflammatory drugs (NSAIDs) have commonly been used in noncardiac surgery as part of a multimodal anesthetic regimen to reduce pain following surgery. A recent meta-analysis reviewed 20 trials involving 1065 patients who underwent either thoracic or cardiac surgery and received NSAIDs or control.[16] The results demonstrated a reduction in VAS at 24 hours of 1 point and a reduction in morphine consumption of 5 mg in the first 24 hours in the cardiac surgical patients. Although the rates of renal dysfunction and renal failure were not different in these trials, most trials excluded patients with preoperative elevations of creatinine.

AUTHORS' RECOMMENDATIONS

The following recommendations are based on the aforementioned studies and the authors' personal experience and should be viewed as a guide to aid in the decision-making process. The entire cardiac care team must be involved when making the switch from conventional treatment of cardiac patients to a fast-track approach. Patients who are suitable for an FTC program must be identified preoperatively. The anesthetic must be tailored appropriately. In addition, close attention must be paid to the patients' coagulation profile, temperature, and hemodynamic profile in order to treat complications that will prevent early extubation. Finally, postoperative care must be tailored to the patients' needs. FTCA's primary benefits are cost reduction and improved resource utilization. These benefits are greatly enhanced by modifications in the basic recovery model. By adoption of cardiac recovery areas, maximum savings are realized.

- Identification of suitable candidates preoperatively. Patients under age 75 with good LV function (ejection fraction [EF] greater than 40%) are candidates for FTCA. However, patients over age 75 or with EF less than 40% should not necessarily be excluded from FTCA management; instead, it should be recognized that success is less likely and that a greater number of these patients will require prolonged postoperative ventilation.
- Except where the clinical situation does not allow, all patients should be treated with lower-dose narcotics (10 to 15 mcg/kg fentanyl, 2 to 6 mcg/kg sufentanil, 0.5 to 1.5 mcg/kg/min remifentanil) to allow for early extubation in the recovery area.
- Close attention must be paid to the patients' coagulation status, temperature, and hemodynamic stability. Bleeding, hypothermia, and cardiac instability will all prevent early extubation.
- Analgesia with nurse-administered or patient-administered narcotics with supplemental analgesia provided by NSAIDs (if no contraindications).
- Following surgery, the patient's status to fast-track must be communicated with the recovery care team.

REFERENCES

1. Prakash O, Jonson B, Meij S, Bos E, Hugenholtz PG, Nauta J, Hekman W: Criteria for early extubation after intracardiac surgery in adults. *Anesth Analg* 1977;56:703-708.
2. Wong DT, Cheng DC, Kustra R, Tibshirani R, Karski J, Carroll-Munro J, Sandler A: Risk factors of delayed extubation, prolonged length of stay in the intensive care unit, and mortality in patients undergoing coronary artery bypass graft with fast-track cardiac anesthesia: A new cardiac risk score. *Anesthesiology* 1999;91:936-944.
3. Cheng DC, Newman MF, Duke P, Wong DT, Finegan B, Howie M, et al: The efficacy and resource utilization of remifentanil and fentanyl in fast-track coronary artery bypass graft surgery: A prospective randomized, double-blinded controlled, multi-center trial. *Anesth Analg* 2001;92:1094-1102.
4. Cheng DC, Karski J, Peniston C, Raveendran G, Asokumar B, Carroll J, et al: Early tracheal extubation after coronary artery bypass graft surgery reduces costs and improves resource use. A prospective, randomized, controlled trial. *Anesthesiology* 1996;85:1300-1310.
5. Cheng DC: Fast track cardiac surgery pathways: Early extubation, process of care, and cost containment. *Anesthesiology* 1998;88:1429-1433.
6. Hadjinikolaou L, Cohen A, Glenville B, Stanbridge RD: The effect of a "fast-track" unit on the performance of a cardiothoracic department. *Ann R Coll Surg Engl* 2000;82:53-58.
7. Myles PS, Daly DJ, Djaiani G, Lee A, Cheng DC: A systematic review of the safety and effectiveness of fast-track cardiac anesthesia. *Anesthesiology* 2003;99:982-987.
8. Dowd NP, Cheng DC, Karski JM, Wong DT, Munro JA, Sandler AN: Intraoperative awareness in fast-track cardiac anesthesia. *Anesthesiology* 1998;89:1068-1073, discussion 9A.

9. Liu WH, Thorp TA, Graham SG, Aitkenhead AR: Incidence of awareness with recall during general anaesthesia. *Anaesthesia* 1991;46:435-437.

10. Ovrum E, Tangen G, Schiott C, Dragsund S: Rapid recovery protocol applied to 5,658 consecutive "on-pump" coronary bypass patients. *Ann Thorac Surg* 2000;70:2008-2012.

11. Engoren M, Luther G, Fenn-Buderer N: A comparison of fentanyl, sufentanil, and remifentanil for fast-track cardiac anesthesia. *Anesth Analg* 2001;93:859-864.

12. Mollhoff T, Herregods L, Moerman A, Blake D, MacAdams C, Demeyere R, et al: Comparative efficacy and safety of remifentanil and fentanyl in "fast track" coronary artery bypass graft surgery: A randomized, double-blind study. *Br J Anaesth* 2001; 87:718-726.

13. Liu SS, Block BM, Wu CL: Effects of perioperative central neuraxial analgesia on outcome after coronary artery bypass surgery: A meta-analysis. *Anesthesiology* 2004;101:153-161.

14. Ho AM, Chung DC, Joynt GM: Neuraxial blockade and hematoma in cardiac surgery: Estimating the risk of a rare adverse event that has not (yet) occurred. *Chest* 2000;117:551-555.

15. Bainbridge D, Martin JE, Cheng DC: Patient-controlled versus nurse-controlled analgesia after cardiac surgery—a meta-analysis. *Can J Anaesth* 2006;53:492-499.

16. Bainbridge D, Cheng DC, Martin JE, Novick R: NSAID-analgesia, pain control and morbidity in cardiothoracic surgery [L'analgesie avec des AINS, le controle de la douleur et la morbidite en chirurgie cardiothoracique]. *Can J Anaesth* 2006;53: 46-59.

62

Is There a Best Technique to Decrease Blood Loss and Transfusion after Coronary Artery Bypass Grafting?

John G. T. Augoustides, MD, FASE

INTRODUCTION

The importance of excessive blood loss after coronary artery bypass grafting (CABG) is related to its significant association with deleterious perioperative outcome, including all the risks of blood transfusion.[1-3] Blood transfusion after CABG significantly increases mortality risk, ischemic morbidity (stroke, myocardial infarction, and renal failure), infections (wound, pneumonia, and sepsis), hospital stay, and overall health costs.[3-5]

The techniques for reducing bleeding and transfusion should collectively be focused on all CABG patients, particularly the high-risk subgroups. The recent clinical practice guideline on blood transfusion and blood conservation in cardiac surgery by the Society of Thoracic Surgeons (STS) and Society of Cardiovascular Anesthesiologists (SCA) identified six important risk factors for increased bleeding and transfusion risk: advanced age, low preoperative red cell volume, preoperative antithrombotic or antiplatelet drugs, reoperative or combined procedures, emergency surgery, and noncardiac patient comorbidity.[4,5] These risk factors identify high-risk CABG subgroups that merit aggressive intervention to limit perioperative risk due to bleeding and transfusion.

Furthermore, it is essential to have guideline-driven transfusion of blood components in order to optimize the risk/benefit ratio of this intervention. The practice guidelines for blood component therapy by the American Society of Anesthesiologists (ASA) identified four considerations for transfusion of packed red blood cells in adults: (1) hemoglobin during cardiopulmonary bypass ≤ 6.0 g/dL; (2) hemoglobin ≤ 7.0 g/dL in patients older than 65 years or with chronic cardiac or respiratory disease; (3) acute blood loss greater than 1500 mL or 30% of blood volume; and (4) rapid uncontrolled blood loss.[6] This ASA guideline further suggests that in stable patients with hemoglobin between 7 and 10 g/dL, red blood cell transfusion may be considered, but the benefit of this approach is unclear.[6] It is important to note that these ASA guidelines are not specific to cardiac surgery and that they are not based on randomized controlled trials.

OPTIONS TO DECREASE BLOOD LOSS AND TRANSFUSION AFTER CABG

The perioperative options for limiting blood loss and transfusion after CABG are presented in Table 62-1. The evidence for each option will be reviewed to assess its quality and determine a recommendation, according to the schema of the American Heart Association, as outlined in Tables 62-2A (classes of recommendations) and 62-2B (levels of evidence). The recommendation classes and evidence levels are summarized for rapid review in Table 62-3 (class I recommendations), Tables 62-4A (class IIa recommendations) and 62-4B (class IIb recommendations), and Table 62-5 (class III recommendations). The discussion of the evidence will focus on selected representative references. A complete reference list of over 750 citations is available from the comprehensive STS/SCA guideline dedicated to this topic (available at www.scahq.org or www.sts.org, accessed February 24, 2008).[4]

EVIDENCE

1. Pharmacologic Hemostasis by Preoperative Recovery of Coagulation

Potent preoperative anticoagulants frequently increase bleeding and transfusion significantly after CABG. Therefore, when clinically feasible, they should be discontinued preoperatively to allow recovery of the coagulation system (class IIb recommendation; level C evidence). The timing of discontinuation depends on the half-life of the particular agent and the possibility of reversibility. The exception to this principle is unfractionated heparin, which may be discontinued shortly before CABG or not at all.

High-intensity platelet blockade with thienopyridines such as clopidogrel may be associated with life-threatening bleeding after CABG.[7] It is reasonable to discontinue this potent platelet blockade 5 to 7 days before surgery to limit blood loss and transfusion (class IIa recommendation;

Table 62-1 Perioperative Options to Minimize Blood Loss and Transfusion after CABG

Options	Examples
Preoperative intervention	Autologous donation
Erythropoietin	
Pharmacologic hemostasis	Antifibrinolytic agents
Desmopressin acetate	
Recombinant factor VIIa	
Discontinue preoperative anticoagulation	
Hemostasis with mechanical ventilation	Positive end-expiratory pressure
Avoidance of cardiopulmonary bypass	Off-pump coronary artery bypass grafting
Cardiopulmonary bypass	Oxygenator design
Pump type	
Heparin-coated circuits	
Minimized low-prime circuit	
Heparin management	
Protamine management	
Blood management	Acute normovolemic hemodilution
Intraoperative autotransfusion	
Red cell salvage	
Retrograde autologous priming	
Leukocyte filtration	
Platelet pheresis	
Plasmapheresis	
Hemofiltration	
Perioperative transfusion protocol	

Table 62-2A Definition of Classification Scheme for Clinical Recommendations

Clinical Recommendations	Definition of Recommendation Class
Class I	The procedure/treatment should be performed (benefit far outweighs the risk)
Class IIa	It is reasonable to perform the procedure/treatment (benefit still clearly outweighs risk)
Class IIb	It is not unreasonable to perform the procedure/treatment (benefit probably outweighs the risk)
Class III	The procedure/treatment should not be performed because it is not helpful and may be harmful (risk may outweigh benefit)

Taken from the American Heart Association/American Council of Cardiology Manual for Guideline Writing Committees at http://circ.ahajournals.org/manual/manual_IIstep6.shtml (accessed February 25, 2008).

Table 62-2B Definition of Classification Scheme for Supporting Evidence for Clinical Recommendations

Level of Evidence	Definition of Recommendation Class
Level A	Sufficient evidence from multiple randomized trials or meta-analyses
Level B	Limited evidence from a single randomized trial or multiple nonrandomized studies
Level C	Case studies and expert opinion

Taken from the American Heart Association/American Council of Cardiology Manual for Guideline Writing Committees at http://circ.ahajournals.org/manual/manual_IIstep6.shtml (accessed February 25, 2008).

Table 62-3 Class I Multimodal Recommendations to Minimize Bleeding and Transfusion after CABG

Recommendation	Class and Evidence
A multimodality evidence-based approach will limit bleeding and promote blood conservation after CABG. Multiple stakeholders, institutional support, transfusion algorithms, and point-of-care testing are important components.	I (level A)
Lysine analogs such as epsilon-aminocaproic acid and tranexamic acid reduce blood loss and transfusion.	I (level A)
Routine red-cell saving limits blood transfusion in CABG with cardiopulmonary bypass. This is not indicated in patients with infection or malignancy.	I (level A)

Adapted from the following guideline: Society of Thoracic Surgeons Blood Conservation Guideline Task Force, Ferraris VA, Ferraris SP, Saha SP, Hessel EA 2nd, Haan CK, Royston D, et al: Perioperative blood transfusion in cardiac surgery: The Society of Thoracic Surgeons and the Society of Cardiovascular Anesthesiologists clinical practice guideline. *Ann Thorac Surg* 2007;S27-S86.

level B evidence).[4] In the presence of coronary stents, whether bare-metal or drug-eluting stents, acute withdrawal of antiplatelet therapy can precipitate stent thrombosis.[8] The options to maintain stent patency must be considered, including preoperative hospitalization to substitute thienopyridine therapy with short-acting intravenous platelet blockade.[8-10]

It is reasonable to stop low-intensity antiplatelet therapy (e.g., aspirin) preoperatively in elective patients without acute coronary syndromes to reduce blood loss and transfusion after CABG (class IIa recommendation; level A evidence).[11] In the setting of emergent CABG, aspirin should be continued because the small bleeding

Table 62-4A Class IIa Multimodal Recommendations to Minimize Bleeding and Transfusion after CABG	
Recommendation	**Class and Evidence**
Off-pump CABG is reasonable for blood conservation, provided that emergent conversion to on-pump bypass is unlikely to be based on surgeon experience or patient characteristics.	IIa (level A)
Total quality management, including continuous assessment of existing and emerging blood conservation techniques, is reasonable for implementation of a complete blood conservation program.	IIa (level B)
A comprehensive multimodality blood conservation program in the intensive care unit is a reasonable means to limit bleeding and transfusion.	IIa (level B)
Patients with known qualitative platelet defects or severe thrombocytopenia ($<50,000/mm^2$) are at high risk for bleeding and should receive maximal multimodal blood conservation procedures.	IIa (level B)
It is reasonable to stop thienopyridine therapy (e.g., clopidogrel) 5-7 days before surgery to limit blood loss and transfusion. In the presence of drug-eluting coronary stents, care must be taken because acute withdrawal of antiplatelet therapy can precipitate stent thrombosis. The options to maintain stent patency must be considered, including preoperative hospitalization to convert substitute thienopyridine therapy with short-acting GP 2b/3a inhibitor therapy.	IIa (level B)
It is reasonable to stop low-intensity antiplatelet therapy (e.g., aspirin) preoperatively in elective patients without acute coronary syndromes to reduce blood loss and transfusion.	IIa (level A)
It is reasonable to transfuse hemostatic blood products based on clinical evidence of bleeding, preferably guided by timely and accurate point-of-care testing.	IIa (level C)
Preoperative autologous blood donation in selected patients is a reasonable step for blood conservation.	IIa (level A)
Recombinant erythropoietin is reasonable to boost red blood cell volume for patients undergoing preoperative autologous blood donation.	IIa (level A)
Recombinant erythropoietin is reasonable for anemic low-risk elective patients (hemoglobin <13 g/dL), provided that it is given with iron several days before surgery.	IIa (level A)

Adapted from the following guideline: Society of Thoracic Surgeons Blood Conservation Guideline Task Force, Ferraris VA, Ferraris SP, Saha SP, Hessel EA 2nd, Haan CK, Royston D, et al: Perioperative blood transfusion in cardiac surgery: The Society of Thoracic Surgeons and the Society of Cardiovascular Anesthesiologists clinical practice guideline. *Ann Thorac Surg* 2007;S27-S86.

risk is outweighed by its overall benefits (class IIa recommendation; level A evidence).[12]

2. Limiting Bleeding and Transfusion with Autologous Donation and Erythropoietin

Preoperative donation of at least 2 units of autologous blood is reasonable in elective CABG, especially when combined with appropriate erythropoietin and iron therapy (class IIa recommendation; level A evidence). This practice is associated with a significant reduction in allogeneic blood transfusion.[13-15] Erythropoietin in conjunction with iron therapy is also indicated to boost red blood cell mass in anemic patients (hemoglobin less than 13 g/dL) at least several days before elective CABG (class IIa recommendation; level B evidence).[14] This application of erythropoietin is especially useful in the perioperative management of Jehovah's Witnesses, patients in whom allogeneic blood transfusion must be avoided.[16] Preoperative augmentation of red blood cell mass will most likely be explored in detail by large randomized trials, given the recent high-quality evidence that preoperative anemia independently predicts for death, stroke, and renal failure after CABG.[17,18]

3. Pharmacologic Hemostasis with Antifibrinolytic Agents

The antifibrinolytic agent aprotinin has recently been withdrawn from the world market because of concerns about patient safety recently identified from interim outcome analysis from the BART trial (details available at www. trasylol.com, accessed February 19, 2008). BART is the acronym for a registered multicenter trial conducted across Canada: "Blood Conservation using Antifibrinolytics: A Randomized Trial in High-risk Cardiac Surgery Patients" (international standard randomized controlled trial number ISRCTN15166455; details available at the ISRCTN register at http://isrctn.org, accessed February 24, 2008). The BART study has been suspended until all trial data have been thoroughly analyzed for the apparent increase in mortality rate caused by aprotinin as compared with tranexamic acid and aminocaproic acid. Before this development, safety concerns related to anaphylaxis and renal dysfunction had already significantly limited the clinical application of aprotinin.[19] Two recent massive outcome analyses of aprotinin in CABG (cumulative $N = 88,474$) have also documented a significant increase in mortality rate in CABG patients exposed to perioperative aprotinin as compared with aminocaproic acid.[20,21] Further discussion of antifibrinolytics for CABG will now be limited to tranexamic acid and aminocaproic acid, the remaining two antifibrinolytics in clinical practice.

Recent high-quality meta-analyses of randomized trials consistently support the safety and efficacy of the lysine analogs, tranexamic acid and aminocaproic acid, for reduction of bleeding and transfusion after CABG.[22-24] These agents significantly reduce bleeding and blood component transfusion ($p < 0.05$) across multiple randomized trials. As a result, the application of these agents, particularly in high-risk CABG subgroups, has received a class I recommendation (level A evidence).

Table 62-4B Class IIb Multimodal Recommendations to Minimize Bleeding and Transfusion after CABG

Recommendation	Class and Evidence
Most high-intensity anticoagulants increase bleeding after CABG. It is not unreasonable to stop these agents preoperatively, taking into account the half-life and potential lack of reversibility. Unfractionated heparin is an exception because it may be discontinued very shortly before surgery or not at all.	IIb (level C)
In cardiopulmonary bypass, it is not unreasonable to maintain the hemoglobin ≥7 g/dL in patients at risk for critical end-organ injury.	IIb (level C)
In patients with critical noncardiac end-organ ischemia, it is not unreasonable to maintain the hemoglobin concentration ≥10 g/dL.	IIb (level C)
Desmopressin acetate therapy is not unreasonable to attenuate excessive bleeding in patients with platelet dysfunction secondary to uremia, cardiopulmonary bypass, and type I von Willebrand's disease.	IIb (level B)
Recombinant factor VIIa therapy is not unreasonable for the management of intractable nonsurgical bleeding that is unresponsive to routine hemostatic therapy.	IIb (level B)
A trial of therapeutic positive end-expiratory pressure to ameliorate excessive bleeding is not unreasonable.	IIb (level B)
Open venous reservoir membrane oxygenator systems during cardiopulmonary bypass are not unreasonable to reduce blood utilization.	IIb (level C)
All cardiopulmonary bypass pumps provide acceptable blood conservation. It is not unreasonable to prefer centrifugal pumps for their safety features.	IIb (level B)
It is not unreasonable to maintain higher heparin concentrations for CPB durations >2 hours to reduce hemostatic system activation, blood loss, and transfusion.	IIb (level B)
Protamine titration or empiric low-dose regimens (e.g., 50% of total heparin dose) to lower the total protamine dose at the end of CPB to reduce bleeding and transfusion.	IIb (level B)
Heparin-coated CPB circuits are not unreasonable to promote blood conservation.	IIb (level B)
Low-dose heparin therapy for CPB (ACT about 300 seconds) is not unreasonable to promote blood conservation, but all the safety concerns have not been well studied.	IIb (level B)
Minimized low-prime CPB circuits are not unreasonable as part of a multimodality blood conservation program.	IIb (level B)
Acute normovolemic hemodilution is not unreasonable for blood conservation in cardiac surgery.	IIb (level B)
Intraoperative autotransfusion directly from cardiotomy suction or recycled from a cell-saving device is not unreasonable to augment blood conservation.	IIb (level C)
After CPB, transfusion of pump blood is not unreasonable as a means of blood conservation.	IIb (level C)

Adapted from the following guideline: Society of Thoracic Surgeons Blood Conservation Guideline Task Force, Ferraris VA, Ferraris SP, Saha SP, Hessel EA 2nd, Haan CK, Royston D, et al: Perioperative blood transfusion in cardiac surgery: The Society of Thoracic Surgeons and the Society of Cardiovascular Anesthesiologists clinical practice guideline. *Ann Thorac Surg* 2007;S27-S86.

Table 62-5 Class III Multimodal Recommendations to Minimize Bleeding and Transfusion after CABG

Recommendation	Class and Evidence
Transfusion is not recommended for a hemoglobin concentration above 10 g/dL.	III (level C)
Routine prophylactic desmopressin acetate is not recommended to reduce bleeding and transfusion.	III (level A)
Prophylactic positive end-expiratory pressure does not reduce bleeding.	III (level B)
Routine intraoperative platelet or plasmapharesis is not recommended for blood conservation.	III (level A)
Leukocyte filtration during cardiopulmonary bypass is not indicated for perioperative blood conservation.	III (level B)
Direct infusion of shed mediastinal blood from postoperative chest tube drainage is not indicated for perioperative blood conservation.	III (level B)
Routine ultrafiltration in not recommended for blood conservation in adult CABG surgery.	III (level B)

Adapted from the following guideline: Society of Thoracic Surgeons Blood Conservation Guideline Task Force, Ferraris VA, Ferraris SP, Saha SP, Hessel EA 2nd, Haan CK, Royston D, et al: Perioperative blood transfusion in cardiac surgery: The Society of Thoracic Surgeons and the Society of Cardiovascular Anesthesiologists clinical practice guideline. *Ann Thorac Surg* 2007;S27-S86.

4. Pharmacologic Hemostasis with Desmopressin and Recombinant Factor VIIa

Routine prophylactic desmopressin acetate does not reduce bleeding and transfusion after CABG (class III recommendation; level A evidence).[25] Desmopressin acetate therapy is not unreasonable to attenuate excessive bleeding in patients with platelet dysfunction secondary to uremia, cardiopulmonary bypass, and type I von Willebrand's disease (Class IIb recommendation; level B evidence).[4] Furthermore, preoperative platelet dysfunction detectable by point-of-care testing can often be reversed by desmopressin therapy.[26,27] Thus, desmopressin is indicated perioperatively in selected cases with evidence of platelet dysfunction.

Recombinant factor VIIa therapy has demonstrated efficacy in the management of massive and refractory medical bleeding after CABG (class IIb recommendation; level of evidence B).[28] This efficacy is based on a consistent trend from multiple case series that recently have been systematically reviewed.[28] Randomized controlled trials are currently in progress to evaluate the safety and efficacy of this intervention in the reduction of bleeding and transfusion after CABG.

5. Mechanical Hemostasis with Positive End–Expiratory Pressure

Positive end-expiratory pressure (PEEP) exerts mechanical pressure on the heart and so may limit bleeding after CABG. Two clinical studies with no control group have documented control of excessive bleeding with escalating levels of PEEP up to a maximum of 20 cm H_2O.[29,30] A trial of therapeutic positive end-expiratory pressure to ameliorate excessive bleeding is not unreasonable (class IIb recommendation; level B evidence). Prophylactic PEEP does not reduce bleeding (class III recommendation; level B evidence).[31] When PEEP is effective, it is typically apparent within an hour. Further studies are required to assess the risks of cardiovascular compromise from high PEEP immediately after CABG.

6. Limiting Bleeding and Transfusion with Avoidance of Cardiopulmonary Bypass

CABG without cardiopulmonary bypass (CPB) is associated with decreased bleeding and transfusion (odds ratio 0.43; 95% CI 0.29 to 0.65) when compared by meta-analysis of randomized trials to CABG with CPB.[32] Off-pump CABG is reasonable for blood conservation, provided that emergent conversion to on-pump bypass is unlikely based on surgeon experience or patient characteristics (class IIa recommendation; level A evidence). Emergent conversion to CABG with CPB is associated with significantly greater bleeding and transfusion.[33]

7. Limiting Bleeding and Transfusion with Modified Cardiopulmonary Bypass

The conduct of cardiopulmonary bypass may significantly affect bleeding and transfusion after CABG. The design of the CPB circuit is the first major consideration. The hemostatic possibilities in CPB hardware design include oxygenator design (bubble or membrane), pump type (centrifugal or roller), and circuit type (heparin coating and/or minimized low-prime). The second major consideration is anticoagulation management for CPB with heparin and protamine. The evidence and recommendations for each of these considerations will now be reviewed.

A membrane oxygenator during cardiopulmonary bypass is not unreasonable to reduce blood utilization (class IIb recommendation; level C evidence).[4] Membrane oxygenators have largely replaced bubble oxygenators in contemporary clinical practice because they are associated with reductions in cerebral emboli and blood transfusion.[34,35] Cardiopulmonary bypass pump design, however, has less of a role in perioperative blood conservation after CABG. All pump designs, whether centrifugal or roller, provide acceptable hemostatic performance. The theoretic advantages of the centrifugal design over the roller design include reduced complement activation and preserved platelet function.[4,36] These advantages, however, have not translated into consistent clinical reductions in bleeding and transfusion after CABG in randomized trials.[37] It is not unreasonable, however, to prefer centrifugal pumps for their enhanced safety, including a lower risk of massive air embolism (class IIb recommendation; level B evidence).[4]

Heparin-coated CPB circuits are not unreasonable to promote blood conservation (class IIb recommendation; level B evidence).[38,39] Despite their increased cost, heparin-bonded circuits in a recent meta-analysis (41 randomized trials: total $N = 3434$) significantly improved perioperative outcome, including blood transfusion (odds ratio 0.8; 95% CI 0.6 to 0.9; $p = 0.004$) and mediastinal exploration for bleeding (odds ratio 0.6; 95% CI 0.4 to 0.8; $p = 0.002$).[39] These benefits, however, depend on the level of heparin therapy used for CPB (see discussion in next section).[40] Furthermore, the lack of a definitive cost/benefit analysis continues to result in debate about their routine application in CPB for CABG.[40,41]

Minimized low-prime CPB circuits are not unreasonable as part of a multimodality blood conservation program (class IIb recommendation; level B evidence). Recent clinical trials have documented significant reductions in bleeding and transfusion after CABG with the low-prime CPB circuit as compared with conventional CPB.[42,43] Furthermore, there is emerging high-quality evidence that these beneficial outcome effects are similar in magnitude to the hemostatic benefit from CABG without CPB.[44]

Anticoagulation for CABG with CPB is used to limit cellular and coagulation factor activation and to prevent circuit thrombosis. Unfractionated heparin is the anticoagulant of choice because it is effective, reversible with protamine, generally well tolerated, and inexpensive. The activated clotting time (ACT) is a standard point-of-care test to monitor heparin effect during CPB. An ACT time of greater than 400 seconds is the traditional standard for safe CPB, originally based on a 1978 primate study with bubble oxygenators.[45] There is no single ACT value that can be considered as the best or the standard, based on the literature to date. Low-dose heparin therapy to maintain an ACT of 300 seconds in conjunction with heparin-coated CPB circuits has been evaluated as a hemostatic intervention to limit bleeding and transfusion after CABG. This intervention was considered as not unreasonable to promote blood conservation, but safety concerns such as thrombosis have not been well studied (class IIb recommendation; level B evidence).[4] Although the results from multiple trials are not all in agreement, the trend of the evidence suggests that this intervention has net benefit for reduction of bleeding and promotion of blood conservation after CABG.[39]

In the setting of prolonged CPB, high-dose heparin therapy decreases thrombin generation, fibrinolytic activity, and platelet activation.[46,47] High-dose heparin therapy significantly preserves coagulation during CPB and may decrease bleeding and transfusion. There is, however, not complete agreement in the multiple clinical trials that have evaluated this rationale. An important randomized prospective trial demonstrated that intensive individualized high-dose heparin therapy monitored with point-of-care testing (heparin concentration and ACT) significantly decreased bleeding and hemoststatic blood component transfusion after CPB.[48] Considering all the evidence together, it is not unreasonable to use high-dose heparin therapy monitored with point-of-care testing to reduce hemostatic activation, blood loss, and transfusion in high-risk patients likely to require prolonged CPB for CABG (class IIb recommendation; level B evidence).

Heparin reversal with protamine can affect bleeding and transfusion after CABG with CPB because excess protamine is itself an anticoagulant. Protamine titration or empiric low-dose regimens not only lower the total protamine dose but also have been shown in clinical trials to reduce bleeding and transfusion, but not consistently.[49,50] The eight published trials that address this question are evenly divided: four show hemostatic benefit, and four do not. Although protamine titration or empiric low-dose protamine therapy is not unreasonable (class IIb recommendation; level B evidence), more consistent evidence of benefit is required before a higher class recommendation can be assigned.

8. Limiting Bleeding and Transfusion with Modified Blood Management

Conservation of the patient's red cell volume with a multimodal approach is the first principle of modified blood management for limitation of bleeding and transfusion after CABG. Routine red-cell saving limits blood transfusion in CABG with cardiopulmonary bypass (class I recommendation; level A evidence).[4] Because of safety concerns, this is not indicated in patients with infection (concern is septicemia) or malignancy (concern is metastasis). Intraoperative autotransfusion directly from cardiotomy suction or recycled from a cell-saving device is also not unreasonable to augment blood conservation (class IIb recommendation; level C evidence). Extensive cell-saving, however, leads to loss of coagulation factors and platelets, which may result in a bleeding diathesis.[51] This deleterious effect of extensive cell-saving can be offset after CPB by direct transfusion of pump blood, which is considered a not unreasonable means of blood conservation (class IIb recommendation; level C evidence). The heparin given with the anticoagulated pump blood must be reversed with adequate protamine.

Acute normovolemic hemodilution is not unreasonable for blood conservation in cardiac surgery (class IIb recommendation; level B evidence). The typical practice involves the removal of 1 to 2 units of autologous blood immediately before initiation of CPB. To maintain circulating blood volume, the volume of removed blood is replaced 1:1 with crystalloid or colloid. An advantage of this technique is that platelet function is preserved because autologous blood CPB is avoided. During CPB, transfusion is determined by the measured hematocrit. Relative contraindications to this technique include cardiogenic shock, preoperative anemia, and a low ejection fraction (less than 30%).[52]

Retrograde autologous priming is an intervention for blood conservation that, like acute normovolemic hemodilution, is instituted just before initiation of CPB. Typically, the arterial limb of the CPB circuit is cleared retrograde by back bleeding from the aortic cannula and the venous limb is cleared anterograde using the blood pump. Clinical trials have yielded conflicting results.[53,54] Despite this limitation, retrograde autologous priming is not unreasonable for blood conservation after CABG, especially when combined with a multimodal perioperative protocol (class IIb recommendation; level B evidence).

Routine intraoperative platelet pheresis before CPB is not recommended for blood conservation (class III recommendation; level A evidence).[55,56] Although there is the theoretic benefit of platelet preservation and protection through avoidance of CPB, meta-analysis of clinical trials failed to show meaningful perioperative reductions in bleeding and transfusion.[55,56] Plasmaphereis has also had a similar fate when clinically evaluated (class III recommendation; level A evidence).[4]

Because leukocyte activation during CPB is responsible for many harmful effects of CPB, leukocyte filtration during CPB may theoretically improve bleeding and transfusion after CABG. Clinical trials of this intervention have failed to show consistent hemostatic benefit after CABG.[57] Furthermore, there is evidence that leukocyte depletion during CPB may activate white cells.[58] Because of the lack of clinical benefit and possible harm, leukofiltration during CPB cannot be recommended for blood conservation in CABG (class III recommendation; level B evidence).

Ultrafiltration during CPB is able to remove the crystalloid priming volume of the CPB circuit, resulting in hemoconcentration and potential perioperative blood conservation. Clinical trials in cardiac surgery to date have not shown consistent hemostatic benefit of this intervention.[59,60] Consequently, routine ultrafiltration in not recommended for blood conservation in adult CABG (class III recommendation; level B evidence).

Although postoperative transfusion of shed mediastinal blood may limit blood transfusion, multiple clinical trials have failed to demonstrate consistent benefit. Furthermore, there is potential for harm, including sternal and systemic infection.[61,62] Given the lack of consistent clinical benefit and evidence of harm, direct infusion of shed mediastinal blood from postoperative chest tube drainage is not indicated for perioperative blood conservation after CABG (class III recommendation; level B evidence).

The second principle of modified blood management for limitation of bleeding and transfusion after CABG is a perioperative transfusion protocol to standardize institutional transfusion practice as far as possible. The following recommendations all relate to this principle: currently, they are all based on expert opinion and consensus.[4]

It is reasonable to transfuse hemostatic blood products based on clinical evidence of bleeding, preferably guided by point-of-care testing (class IIa recommendation; level C evidence). In cardiopulmonary bypass, it is not unreasonable to maintain the hemoglobin ≥ 7 g/dL in patients with risk for critical end-organ injury (class IIb recommendation; level C evidence). Transfusion is not recommended for a hemoglobin concentration above 10 g/dL (class III recommendation; level C evidence). In patients with critical noncardiac end-organ ischemia, it is not unreasonable to maintain the hemoglobin concentration ≥ 10 g/dL (class IIb recommendation; level C evidence).

AREAS OF UNCERTAINTY

The current controversy regarding the safety and efficacy of aprotinin awaits resolution with the publication of the prospective randomized data from the BART trial. The accumulating evidence to date supports the withdrawal of aprotinin from the world market until its safety is clarified. A second area of uncertainty is whether preoperative augmentation of red blood cell mass will improve outcome after CABG, given the recent high-quality evidence that preoperative anemia independently predicts for death, stroke, and renal failure after CABG.[17,18] This hypothesis should be tested with adequately powered randomized controlled clinical trials.

GUIDELINES AND AUTHOR'S RECOMMENDATIONS

The recent STS/SCA guideline on perioperative blood transfusion and blood conservation in cardiac surgery is comprehensive and current with respect to evidence-based reduction of bleeding and transfusion after CABG.[4] As per this guideline, this author endorses a multimodality approach to minimizing bleeding and transfusion after CABG (class I recommendation; level A evidence). This multimodality approach should involve all perioperative stakeholders in the operating room and the intensive care unit and should have full institutional support. All the aforementioned evidence-based interventions should be integrated appropriately and focused on the patient at high risk for bleeding and transfusion after CABG, as outlined in the introduction. There should be a perioperative transfusion protocol supplemented with point-of-care testing where indicated. Total quality management, including continuous assessment of existing and emerging blood conservation techniques, is strongly recommended for implementation of this complete blood conservation program (class IIa recommendation; level B evidence).

REFERENCES

1. Karthik S, Gravson AD, McCarron EE, Pullan DM, Desmond MJ: Reexploration for bleeding after coronary artery bypass surgery: Risk factors, outcomes, and effect of time delay. *Ann Thorac Surg* 2004;78:527-534.
2. Moulton MJ, Creswell LL, Mackey ME, Cox JL, Rosenbloom M: Reexploration for bleeding is a risk factor for adverse outcomes after cardiac operations. *J Thorac Cardiovasc Surg* 1996;111:1037-1046.
3. Murphy GJ, Reeves BC, Rogers CA, Rizvi SIA, Culliford L, Angelini GD: Increased mortality, postoperative morbidity, and cost after red blood cell transfusion in patients having cardiac surgery. *Circulation* 2007;116:2544-2552.
4. Society of Thoracic Surgeons Blood Conservation Guideline Task Force: Ferraris VA, Ferraris SP, Saha SP, et al; The Society of Cardiovascular Anesthesiologists Special Task Force on Blood Transfusion: Spiess BD, Shore-Lesserson L, Stafford-Smith M, et al: Perioperative blood transfusion and blood conservation in cardiac surgery: The Society of Thoracic Surgeons and the Society of Cardiovascular Anesthesiologists clinical practice guideline. *Ann Thorac Surg* 2007;S27-S86.
5. Ranucci M, Pazzaglia A, Bianchini C, Bozzetti G, Isgro G: Body size, gender, and transfusions as determinants of outcome after coronary operations. *Ann Thorac Surg* 2008;85:481-487.
6. American Society of Anesthesiologists: Practice guidelines for blood component therapy: A report by the American Society of Anesthesiologists's Task Force on Blood Component Therapy. *Anesthesiology* 1996;84:732-747.
7. Hongo RH, Lev J, Dick SE, Yee RR: The effect of clopidogrel in combination with aspirin when given before coronary artery bypass grafting. *J Am Coll Cardiol* 2002;40:231-237.
8. Grines Cl, Bonow RO, Casey DF Jr, et al: American Heart Association; American College of Cardiology; Society for Cardiovascular Angiography and Interventions; American College of Surgeons; American Dental Association; American College of Physicians. Prevention of premature discontinuation of dual antiplatelet therapy in patients with coronary artery stents: A science advisory from the American Heart Association, American College of Cardiology, Society for Cardiovascular Angiography and Interventions, American College of Surgeons, and American Dental Association, with representatives from the American College of Physicians. *Circulation* 2007;15:813-818.
9. Brilakis ES, Banerjee S, Berger PB. Perioperative management of patients with coronary stents. *J Am Coll Cardiol* 2007;49: 2145-2150.
10. Augoustides JG: Perioperative thrombotic risk of coronary stents: Possible role of intravenous platelet blockade. *Anesthesiology* 2007;107:516.
11. Ferraris VA, Ferraris SP, Joseph O, Wehner P, Mentzer RM Jr: Aspirin and postoperative bleeding after coronary artery bypass grafting. *Ann Surg* 2002;235:820-827.
12. Ferraris VA, Ferraris SP, Moliterno DJ, et al: The Society of Thoracic Surgeons practice guidelines series: Aspirin and other antiplatelet agents during operative coronary revascularization (executive summary). *Ann Thorac Surg* 2005;79:1454-1461.
13. Yoda M, Nonoyama M, Shimakura T: Autologous blood donation before elective off-pump coronary artery bypass grafting. *Surg Today* 2004;34:21-23.
14. Dietrich W, Thuermel K, Heyde S, Busley R, Berger K: Autologous blood donation in cardiac surgery: Reduction of allogeneic blood transfusion and cost-effectiveness. *J Cardiothorac Vasc Anesth* 2005;20:513-518.
15. Alghamdi AA, Albanna MJ, Guru V, Brister SJ: Does the use of erythropoietin reduce the risk of exposure to allogeneic blood transfusion in cardiac surgery? A systematic review and meta-analysis. *J Card Surg* 2006;21:320-326.
16. Sowade O, Warnke H, Scigalla P, et al: Avoidance of allogeneic blood transfusions by treatment with epoetin beta (recombinant human erythropoietin) in patients undergoing open-heart surgery. *Blood* 1997;89:411-418.
17. Kulier A, Levin J, Moser R, et al for the Investigators of the Multicenter Study of Perioperative Ischemia Research Group and the Ischemia Research and Education Foundation: Impact of preoperative anemia on outcome in patients undergoing coronary artery bypass graft surgery. *Circulation* 2007;116:471-479.
18. Karkouti K, Wijeysundera DN, Beattie WS for the Reducing bleeding in Cardiac Surgery Investigators: Risk associated with preoperative anemia in cardiac surgery: A multicenter cohort study. *Circulation* 2008;117:478-484.
19. Augoustides JG: Con: Aprotinin should not be used in cardiac surgery with cardiopulmonary bypass. *J Cardiothorac Vasc Anesth* 2007;21:302-304.

20. Schneeweiss S, Seeger JD, Landon J, Walker AM: Aprotinin during coronary artery bypass grafting and the risk of death. *N Engl J Med* 2008;158:771-783.

21. Shaw AD, Stafford-Smith M, White WD, et al: The effect of aprotinin on outcome after coronary artery bypass grafting. *N Engl J Med* 2008;158:784-793.

22. Henry DA, Carless PA, Moxey AJ, et al: Antifibrinolytic use for minimizing perioperative allogeneic blood transfusion. *Cochrane Database Syst Rev* 2007;17:CD001886.

23. Umscheid CA, Kohl BA, Williams K: Antifibrinolytic use in adult cardiac surgery. *Curr Opin Hematol* 2007;14:455-467.

24. Brown JR, Birkmeyer NJ, O'Connor GT: Meta-analysis comparing the effectiveness and adverse outcomes of antifibrinolytic agents in cardiac surgery. *Circulation* 2007;115:2801-2813.

25. Pleym H, Stenseth R, Wahba A, et al: Prophylactic treatment with desmopressin does not reduce postoperative bleeding after coronary surgery in patients treated with aspirin before surgery. *Anesth Analg* 2004;98:578-584.

26. Despotis GJ, Levine V, Saleem R, Spitznagel E, Joist JH: Use of point-of-care test in identification of patients who can benefit from desmopressin during cardiac surgery. *Lancet* 1999;354: 106-110.

27. Koscielny J, Ziemer S, Radtke H, et al: A practical concept for preoperative identification of patients with impaired primary hemostasis. *Clin Appl Thromb Hemost* 2004;10:195-204.

28. Warren O, Mandal K, Hadjianastassiou V, et al: Recombinant activated factor VII in cardiac surgery: A systematic review. *Ann Thorac Surg* 2007;83:707-714.

29. Ilabaca PA, Ochsner JL, Mills NL: Positive end-expiratory pressure in the management of a patient with a postoperative bleeding heart. *Ann Thorac Surg* 1980;30:281-284.

30. Hoffman WS, Tomasello DN, MacVaugh H: Control of post-cardiotomy bleeding with PEEP. *Ann Thorac Surg* 1982;34:71-73.

31. Collier B, Kolff J, Deviveni R, Gonzalez LS III: Prophylactic positive end-expiratory pressure and reduction of postoperative blood loss in open-heart surgery. *Ann Thorac Surg* 2002;74:1191-1194.

32. Cheng DC, Bainbridge D, Martin JE, Novick RJ for the Evidence-Based Perioperative Clinical Outcomes Research Group: Does off-pump coronary artery bypass reduce mortality, morbidity, and resource utilization when compared with conventional coronary artery bypass? A meta-analysis of randomized trials. *Anesthesiology* 2005;102:188-203.

33. Jin R, Hiratzka LF, Grunkemeier GL, Krause A, Page US: Aborted off-pump coronary artery bypass patients have much worse outcomes than on-pump or successful off-pump patients. *Circulation* 2005;112:I332-I337.

34. Lim MW: The history of extracorporeal oxygenators. *Anaesthesia* 2006;61:984-995.

35. Parker JL, Hackett JE, Clark D, Crane TN, Reed CC: Membrane versus bubble oxygenators: A clinical comparison of postoperative blood loss. *Cardiovasc Dis* 1979;6:78-84.

36. Salama A, Hugo F, Heinrich D, et al: Deposition of terminal C5b-9 complement complexes on erythrocytes and leukocytes during cardiopulmonary bypass. *N Engl J Med* 1988;318:408-414.

37. Scott DA, Silbert BS, Blyth C, O'Brien J, Santamaria J: Blood loss in elective coronary artery surgery: A comparison of centrifugal versus roller pump heads during cardiopulmonary bypass. *J Cardiothorac Vasc Anesth* 2001;15:322-325.

38. Kreisler KR, Vance RA, Cruzzavala J, Mahnken JD: Heparin-bonded cardiopulmonary bypass circuits reduce the rate of red blood cell transfusion during elective coronary artery bypass surgery. *J Cardiothorac Vasc Anesth* 2005;19:608-611.

39. Mangoush O, Purkayastha S, Haj-Yahia S, et al: Heparin-bonded circuits versus nonheparin-bonded circuits: An evaluation of their effect on clinical outcome. *Eur J Cardiothorac Surg* 2007;31: 1058-1069.

40. Jessen ME: Pro: Heparin-coated circuits should be used for cardiopulmonary bypass. *Anesth Analg* 2006;103:1365-1369.

41. Taneja R, Cheng DC. Con: Heparin-bonded cardiopulmonary bypass circuits should be routine for all cardiac surgical procedures. *Anesth Analg* 2006;103:1370-1372.

42. Remadi JP, Rakotoarivelo Z, Marticho P, Benamar A: Prospective randomized study comparing coronary artery bypass grafting with the new mini-extracorporeal circulation Jostra System or with a standard cardiopulmonary bypass. *Am Heart J* 2006;151: 198e1-198e7.

43. Immer FF, Ackermann A, Gygax E, et al: Minimal extracorporeal circulation is a promising technique for coronary artery bypass grafting. *Ann Thorac Surg* 2007;1515-1521.

44. Mazzel V, Nasso G, Salamone G, Castorino F, Tommasini A, Anselmi A: Prospective randomized comparison of coronary artery bypass grafting with minimal extracorporeal circulation system (MECC) versus off-pump coronary surgery. *Circulation* 2007;116:1761-1767.

45. Young JA, Kisker CT, Doty DB: Adequate anticoagulation during cardiopulmonary bypass determined by the activated clotting time and the appearance of fibrin monomer. *Ann Thorac Surg* 1978;26:231-240.

46. Gravlee GP, Haddon WS, Rothberger HK, et al: Heparin dosing and monitoring. A comparison of techniques with measurement of subclinical plasma coagulation. *J Thorac Cardiovasc Surg* 1990;99:518-527.

47. Okita Y, Takamoto S, Ando M, et al: Coagulation and fibrinolysis system in aortic surgery under deep hypothermic circulatory arrest with aprotinin: The importance of adequate heparinization. *Circulation* 1997;96(suppl 2):376-381.

48. Despotis GJ, Joist JH, Hogue CW Jr, et al: The impact of heparin concentration and activated clotting time monitoring on blood conservation. A prospective, randomized evaluation in patients undergoing cardiac operation. *J Thorac Cardiovasc Surg* 1995;110: 46-54.

49. Jobes DR, Aitken GL, Shaffer GW: Increased accuracy and precision of heparin and protamine dosing reduces blood loss and transfusion in patients undergoing primary cardiac operations. *J Thorac Cardiovasc Surg* 1995;110:36-45.

50. Shore-Lesserson L, Reich DL, DePerio M: Heparin and protamine titration do not improve haemostasis in cardiac surgical patients. *Can J Anaesth* 1998;45:10-18.

51. Despotis GJ, Filos KS, Zoya TN, Hogue CW Jr, Spitznagel E, Lappas DG: Factors associated with excessive postoperative blood loss and hemostatic transfusion requirements; a multivariate analysis in cardiac surgical patients. *Anesth Analg* 1996; 82:13-21.

52. Jamnicki M, Kocian R, van der Linden P, Zaugg M, Spahn DR: Acute normovolemic hemodilution: Physiology, limitations, and clinical uses. *J Cardiothorac Vasc Anesth* 2003;17:747-754.

53. Dalrymple-Hay MJ, Dawkins S, Pack L, et al: Autotransfusion decreases blood usage following cardiac surgery—a prospective randomized trial. *Cardiovasc Surg* 2001;9:184-187.

54. Murphy GS, Szokol JW, Nitsun M, et al: The failure of retrograde autologous priming of the cardiopulmonary bypass circuit to reduce blood use after cardiac surgical procedures. *Anesth Analg* 2004;98:1201-1207.

55. Rubens FD, Fergusson D, Wells PS, Huang M, McGowan JL, Laupacia A: Platelet-rich plasmapheresis in cardiac surgery: A meta-analysis of the effect on transfusion requirements. *J Thorac Cardiovasc Surg* 1998;116:641-647.

56. Carless PA, Rubens FD, Anthony DM, O'Connell D, Henry DA: Platelet-rich plasmapharesis for minimizing perioperative allogeneic blood transfusion. *Cochrane Database Syst Rev* 2003;2: CD004172.

57. Efstathiou A, Vlachveis M, Tsonis G, Asteri T, Psarakis A, Fessatidis IT: Does leukodepletion during elective cardiac surgery really influence the overall clinical outcome? *J Cardiovasc Surg (Torino)* 2003;44:197-204.

58. Ilmakunnas M, Pesonen EJ, Ahonen J, Ramo J, Siitonen S, Repo H: Activation of neutrophils and monocytes by a leukocyte-depleting filter used throughout cardiopulmonary bypass. *J Thorac Cardiovasc Surg* 2005;129:851-859.

59. Babka RM, Petress J, Briggs R, Helsal R, Mack J: Coventional haemofiltration during routine coronary bypass surgery. *Perfusion* 1997;12:187-192.

60. Grunenfelder J, Zund G, Schoeberlein A, et al: Modified ultra-filtration lowers adhesion molecules and cytokine levels after cardiopulmonary bypass without clinical relevance in adults. *Eur J Cardiothorac Surg* 2000;17:77-83.
61. Dial S, Nguyen D, Menzies D: Autotransfusion of shed mediastinal blood: A risk factor for mediastinitis after cardiac surgery? Results of a cluster investigation. *Chest* 2003;124:1847-1851.
62. Body SC, Birmingham J, Parks R, et al: Safety and efficacy of shed mediastinal blood transfusion after cardiac surgery: A multi-center observational study. Multicenter Study of Perioperative Ischemia Research Group. *J Cardiothorac Vasc Anesth* 1999;13:410-416.

63 Should Thoracic Epidural/Spinal Analgesia Be Used for CABG?

Mark A. Chaney, MD

INTRODUCTION

Adequate postoperative analgesia prevents unnecessary patient discomfort, may decrease morbidity, may decrease postoperative hospital length of stay, and may thus decrease cost. Achieving optimal pain relief after cardiac surgery may be difficult. Pain may be associated with many interventions, including sternotomy, thoracotomy, leg vein harvesting, pericardiotomy, or chest tube insertion, among others. Inadequate analgesia during the postoperative period may increase morbidity by causing adverse hemodynamic, metabolic, immunologic, and hemostatic alterations. Thus, aggressive control of postoperative pain may improve outcome in high-risk patients after noncardiac surgery,[1,2] as well as in cardiac surgery.[3,4] Postoperative analgesia may be attained via a wide variety of techniques (local anesthetic infiltration, nerve blocks, opioids, nonsteroidal antiinflammatory drugs, alpha-adrenergic drugs, etc.). Traditionally, analgesia after cardiac surgery has been obtained with intravenous opioids. However, intravenous opioid use is associated with definite detrimental side effects, and longer-acting opioids may delay tracheal extubation during the immediate postoperative period. In the current era of early extubation (fast-tracking) and minimally invasive surgical techniques (including off-pump surgery), cardiac anesthesiologists are exploring unique analgesic options other than traditional intravenous opioids for control of postoperative pain in patients following cardiac surgery. During the last decade, intrathecal and epidural techniques have been used more often in response to this changing surgical climate.[5] Intrathecal and epidural techniques clearly produce reliable analgesia in patients undergoing cardiac surgery. Additional potential benefits include stress response attenuation and thoracic cardiac sympathectomy. The quality of analgesia obtained with thoracic epidural techniques is sufficient to allow cardiac surgery to be performed in awake patients without general endotracheal anesthesia. However, applying regional anesthetic techniques to patients undergoing cardiac surgery is not without risk. Side effects of local anesthetics (hypotension) and opioids (pruritus, nausea/vomiting, urinary retention, respiratory depression), when used in this manner, may complicate perioperative management. Increased risk of hematoma formation in this scenario has generated much lively debate regarding the acceptable risk/benefit ratio of applying regional anesthetic techniques to patients undergoing cardiac surgery.

OPTIONS/THERAPIES

Inadequate analgesia (linked to an uninhibited stress response) during the postoperative period may lead to many adverse hemodynamic (tachycardia, hypertension, vasoconstriction), metabolic (increased catabolism), immunologic (impaired immune response), and hemostatic (platelet activation) alterations. In patients undergoing cardiac surgery, perioperative myocardial ischemia is most often observed during the immediate postoperative period and seems to be related to outcome. Intraoperatively, initiation of cardiopulmonary bypass causes substantial increases in stress response hormones (norepinephrine, epinephrine, etc.) that persist into the immediate postoperative period and may contribute (along with inadequate analgesia) to myocardial ischemia during this time. Furthermore, postoperative myocardial ischemia may be aggravated by cardiac sympathetic nerve activation, which disrupts the balance between coronary blood flow and myocardial oxygen demand. Thus, during the pivotal immediate postoperative period after cardiac surgery, adequate analgesia (coupled with stress response attenuation) may potentially decrease morbidity and enhance health-related quality of life.

It is clear that intrathecal and epidural techniques produce reliable postoperative analgesia in patients after cardiac surgery. Although numerous techniques have been successfully described (intrathecal opioids, intrathecal local anesthetics, epidural opioids, epidural local anesthetics, various combinations),[5] the most popular technique has become the use of epidural opioids/local anesthetics (perhaps because of flexibility in analgesic drug administration options). Additional potential advantages of using intrathecal and epidural techniques in this scenario include stress response attenuation and thoracic cardiac sympathectomy.

Intrathecal or epidural techniques may inhibit the stress response associated with surgical procedures.[6] Local anesthetics are more effective than opioids in stress response attenuation, perhaps because of their unique mechanism of action. Although still a matter of debate, perioperative stress response attenuation with epidural local anesthetics or opioids in high-risk patients after major noncardiac surgery may potentially improve outcome. In patients undergoing cardiac surgery, initiation of cardiopulmonary bypass causes significant increases in stress response hormones that persist into the immediate postoperative period. Attenuation of this component of the stress response with postoperative continuous intravenous infusion of opioids may also decrease morbidity and mortality rates in these patients. Intrathecal and epidural techniques (particularly with local anesthetics) are attractive alternatives to intravenous opioids in cardiac surgery patients for their potential to attenuate the perioperative stress response, yet still allow tracheal extubation to occur in the immediate postoperative period.

The myocardium and coronary vasculature are densely innervated by thoracic sympathetic nerve fibers that arise from T1 to T5 and profoundly influence total coronary blood flow and distribution. Cardiac sympathetic nerve activation initiates coronary artery vasoconstriction and paradoxic coronary vasoconstriction in response to intrinsic vasodilators. In patients with coronary artery disease, cardiac sympathetic nerve activation disrupts the normal matching of coronary blood flow and myocardial oxygen demand. Furthermore, myocardial ischemia initiates a cardio-cardiac reflex mediated by sympathetic nerve fibers, which augments the ischemic process. Cardiac sympathetic nerve activation likely plays a central role in initiating postoperative myocardial ischemia by decreasing myocardial oxygen supply via the mechanisms listed previously.[6] Thoracic epidural anesthesia with local anesthetics effectively blocks cardiac sympathetic nerve afferent and efferent fibers. Opioids, administered similarly, are unable to effectively block such cardiac sympathetic nerve activity. Patients with symptomatic coronary artery disease may benefit clinically from cardiac sympathectomy, and application of thoracic sympathetic blockade in the management of angina pectoris was described as early as 1965.[7] Thoracic epidural anesthesia with local anesthetics increases the diameter of stenotic epicardial coronary artery segments without causing dilation of coronary arterioles, decreases determinants of myocardial oxygen demand, improves left ventricular function, and decreases anginal symptoms. Furthermore, cardiac sympathectomy increases the endocardial-to-epicardial blood flow ratio, beneficially affects collateral blood flow during myocardial ischemia, decreases poststenotic coronary vasoconstriction, and attenuates the myocardial ischemia-induced cardio-cardiac reflex. In an animal model, thoracic epidural anesthesia with local anesthetics actually decreased myocardial infarct size after coronary artery occlusion. Thus, thoracic epidural techniques with local anesthetics may benefit patients undergoing cardiac surgery by effectively blocking cardiac sympathetic nerve activity and improving the myocardial oxygen supply-demand balance.

In summary, use of intrathecal/epidural techniques in patients undergoing cardiac surgery offers three potential clinical benefits: enhanced postoperative analgesia, stress response attenuation, and thoracic cardiac sympathectomy. The many clinical investigations involving intrathecal techniques indicate that administration of intrathecal

morphine produces reliable postoperative analgesia after cardiac surgery. Intrathecal techniques cannot reliably attenuate the perioperative stress response associated with cardiac surgery that persists during the immediate postoperative period. Although large amounts of intrathecal local anesthetics may induce thoracic cardiac sympathectomy, the hemodynamic changes (hypotension, bradycardia) associated with a "total spinal" make the technique unacceptable in patients with cardiac disease. The many clinical investigations involving epidural techniques indicate that administration of thoracic epidural opioids or local anesthetics produces reliable postoperative analgesia after cardiac surgery. Furthermore, administration of thoracic epidural local anesthetics can both reliably attenuate the perioperative stress response associated with cardiac surgery and induce thoracic cardiac sympathectomy. Thus, the technique chosen (intrathecal, epidural, opioids, local anesthetics) depends on specific clinical goals. If enhanced postoperative analgesia is the goal, this can be achieved via a wide variety of options: intrathecal morphine or epidural opioids and/or local anesthetics. The only way to reliably achieve stress response attenuation or thoracic cardiac sympathectomy is via epidural administration of local anesthetics.

EVIDENCE

Intrathecal Techniques

Most investigators have used intrathecal morphine (administered before induction of general anesthesia) in hopes of providing prolonged postoperative analgesia. Some investigators have used intrathecal fentanyl, sufentanil, or local anesthetics for intraoperative anesthesia (with stress response attenuation) or thoracic cardiac sympathectomy.

Two early randomized, blinded, placebo-controlled clinical studies reveal the ability of intrathecal morphine to induce significant postoperative analgesia after cardiac surgery.[8,9] Vanstrum and colleagues[8] prospectively randomized 30 patients to receive either intrathecal morphine (0.5 mg) or intrathecal placebo before induction of anesthesia. Patients who received intrathecal morphine required significantly less intravenous morphine than placebo controls during the initial 30 hours after intrathecal injection. Associated with this enhanced analgesia was a substantially decreased need for antihypertensive medications during the immediate postoperative period. However, time to tracheal extubation and postoperative arterial blood gas tensions were not significantly affected. Chaney and colleagues[9] prospectively randomized 60 patients to receive either intrathecal morphine (4.0 mg) or intrathecal placebo before induction of anesthesia. Tracheal extubation time was similar in all patients. Patients who received intrathecal morphine required significantly less intravenous morphine than placebo controls during the initial postoperative period. However, despite enhanced analgesia, there were no clinical differences between groups regarding postoperative morbidity rate, mortality rate, or duration of postoperative hospital stay.

The mid-1990s saw the emergence of fast-track cardiac surgery, with the goal being tracheal extubation in the immediate postoperative period. Chaney and colleagues[10,11] were the first to study the potential clinical benefits of intrathecal morphine when used in patients undergoing cardiac surgery and early tracheal extubation. In these two randomized, blinded, placebo-controlled clinical studies, the use of intrathecal morphine (10 mcg/kg) before induction of anesthesia was associated with significantly prolonged tracheal extubation times. Furthermore, patients receiving intrathecal morphine had similar intravenous morphine requirements during the immediate postoperative period when compared with placebo controls. There were no clinical differences between groups regarding postoperative morbidity rate, mortality rate, or duration of postoperative hospital stay. Since this time, however, other clinical investigators have revealed that certain combinations of intraoperative anesthetic technique (reduced amounts of intravenous anesthetics/analgesics) coupled with appropriate doses of intrathecal morphine will allow both tracheal extubation after cardiac surgery within the immediate postoperative period and enhanced analgesia.[5] However, no additional clinical benefits (reduced morbidity/mortality rate), beyond enhanced postoperative analgesia, have been revealed.

Numerous other nonrandomized clinical investigations (retrospective, observational, etc.) attest to the ability of intrathecal morphine to produce substantial postoperative analgesia in patients after cardiac surgery,[5] the quality of which depends not only on the intrathecal dose administered, but also on the type and amount of intravenous drugs used for the intraoperative baseline anesthetic. However, no additional clinical benefits, beyond analgesia, have been reliably obtained. The optimal dose of intrathecal morphine for achieving the maximum postoperative analgesia with minimum undesirable drug effects is uncertain. Naturally, when larger doses of intrathecal morphine are used, more intense and prolonged postoperative analgesia is produced at the expense of more undesirable drug effects.

Only a few clinical investigations have examined the ability of intrathecal morphine to potentially attenuate the intraoperative stress response associated with cardiopulmonary bypass.[5] The results of these few studies indicate that intrathecal morphine (even in relatively large doses) is unable to reliably attenuate the perioperative stress response (assessed via blood levels of certain mediators) associated with cardiac surgery and cardiopulmonary bypass.

Most clinical attempts at inducing thoracic cardiac sympathectomy in patients undergoing cardiac surgery have used thoracic epidural anesthesia with local anesthetics. However, some have attempted cardiac sympathectomy in this setting with an intrathecal injection of a large amount of local anesthetic. Typically, a large amount of hyperbaric local anesthetic is delivered intrathecally, and, in an attempt to produce a "total spinal" (thoracic cardiac sympathectomy), the Trendelenburg position is then maintained for a short time. Although stress response attenuation has been suggested, no real effect on clinical outcome variables has been observed. Hypotension or bradycardia (or both) is also commonly observed.

In summary, the many clinical investigations involving intrathecal techniques indicate that administration of intrathecal morphine before induction of general anesthesia produces reliable postoperative analgesia after cardiac surgery. However, it remains controversial whether such analgesia truly affects clinical outcome. Intrathecal techniques cannot reliably attenuate the perioperative stress response associated with cardiac surgery that persists during the immediate postoperative period. Although large amounts of intrathecal local anesthetics may induce thoracic cardiac sympathectomy, the hemodynamic changes associated with a "total spinal" makes the technique unacceptable in patients with cardiac disease.

Epidural Techniques

Most investigators have used thoracic epidural local anesthetics in hopes of providing analgesia, stress response attenuation, or thoracic cardiac sympathectomy. Some investigators have used thoracic epidural opioids to provide intraoperative and postoperative analgesia. Whereas some clinicians insert the epidural catheter immediately before induction of general anesthesia, most perform this maneuver the day before scheduled surgery (in hopes of decreasing the risk of hematoma formation).

Thoracic epidural techniques with local anesthetics or opioids produce significant postoperative analgesia in patients after cardiac surgery. Numerous clinical studies attest to this fact.[5] The quality of analgesia obtained with thoracic epidural techniques is sufficient to allow cardiac surgery to be performed in awake patients without general endotracheal anesthesia.[12] However, despite enhanced postoperative analgesia offered via thoracic epidural techniques, such analgesia does not decrease the incidence of persistent pain after cardiac surgery.

Many clinical investigations have proven that thoracic epidural techniques with local anesthetics significantly attenuate the stress response (assessed via blood levels of certain mediators) in patients undergoing cardiac surgery. Patients randomized to receive thoracic epidural local anesthetics during and after cardiac surgery have exhibited decreased blood levels of epinephrine, norepinephrine, and cortisol (as well as other mediators) when compared with patients managed similarly without thoracic epidural catheters. Other clinical studies suggest the ability of thoracic epidural techniques with local anesthetics to help promote hemodynamic stability (optimize heart rate, systemic vascular resistance) in patients undergoing cardiac surgery, which suggests stress response attenuation. However, it remains controversial whether or not such stress response attenuation truly affects clinical outcome.

Perioperative cardiac sympathectomy induced via thoracic epidural techniques with local anesthetics may clinically benefit patients undergoing cardiac surgery by increasing myocardial oxygen supply (via coronary vasodilation). Cardiac sympathectomy may also offer additional benefits to patients undergoing cardiac surgery. Clinical studies demonstrate that thoracic epidural techniques with local anesthetics significantly decrease heart rate and the need to administer beta-adrenergic blockers. Clinical studies also demonstrate that use of thoracic epidural techniques with local anesthetics significantly decreases systemic vascular resistance. Patients undergoing cardiac surgery who receive thoracic epidural local anesthetics may also exhibit decreases in postoperative electrocardiographic evidence of myocardial ischemia. However, it remains controversial whether such cardiac sympathectomy truly affects clinical outcome.

In 2001 a relatively large clinical investigation highlighted the potential clinical benefits of thoracic epidural techniques (along with difficulties determining clinical relevance of such studies) in cardiac surgical patients. Scott and colleagues[13] prospectively randomized (nonblinded) 420 patients undergoing cardiac surgery to receive either thoracic epidural bupivacaine/clonidine and general anesthesia or general anesthesia alone (control group). Epidural infusions were continued for 96 hours after surgery (titrated according to need). In control patients, postoperative analgesia was obtained with intravenous opioids. After surgery, striking clinical differences were observed between the two groups. Postoperative supraventricular arrhythmia, respiratory tract infection, renal failure, and acute confusion were all decreased in thoracic epidural patients when compared with control patients. However, data from this investigation must be viewed with caution. Somewhat surprisingly, the clinical protocol dictated that beta-adrenergic blockers could not be used during or after surgery for the 5 days of the study period. Because approximately 90% of this study's patients were taking beta-adrenergic blockers before surgery, this unique perioperative management (discontinuation of beta-adrenergic blockers) clouds interpretation of postoperative supraventricular arrhythmia data. Also, despite prospective randomization, substantially fewer patients receiving thoracic epidural catheters were active smokers before surgery when compared with controls, which clouds interpretation of postoperative respiratory tract infection data. These investigators also found that postoperative preextubation maximal expiratory lung volumes were increased in thoracic epidural patients and postoperative tracheal extubation was facilitated in these patients as well (yet thoracic epidural patients and control patients were managed somewhat differently during the immediate postoperative period). Postoperative analgesia was not definitively assessed in this clinical investigation. Although these results are intriguing, definitive conclusions regarding the use of thoracic epidural techniques in patients undergoing cardiac surgery cannot be drawn because of the study's substantial limitations.

Since the publication of the somewhat encouraging findings of Scott and colleagues[13] in 2001, three prospective, randomized, nonblinded investigations reveal that using thoracic epidural techniques in patients undergoing cardiac surgery may not offer substantial clinical benefits.[14-16] Priestley and colleagues[14] prospectively randomized 100 patients undergoing elective cardiac surgery to receive either thoracic epidural ropivacaine/fentanyl and general anesthesia or general anesthesia alone (control group). Thoracic epidural patients were tracheally extubated sooner than controls, yet this difference may have been secondary to differing amounts of intraoperative intravenous opioid administration. Postoperative pain scores were lower in epidural patients only on postoperative days 0 and 1 (equivalent on days 2 and 3). There were no differences between the two groups in

postoperative oxygen saturation on room air, chest radiograph changes, spirometry, postoperative mobilization goals, atrial fibrillation, or postoperative hospital discharge. In short, this investigation revealed that a thoracic epidural may provide enhanced postoperative analgesia (although brief) and enhance postoperative tracheal extubation, yet has no effect on important clinical variables. Royse and colleagues[15] prospectively randomized 80 patients undergoing cardiac surgery to receive either thoracic epidural ropivacaine/fentanyl and general anesthesia or general anesthesia alone (control group). Once again, thoracic epidural patients were tracheally extubated earlier than controls, yet this difference may have been secondary to differing amounts of intraoperative intravenous opioid administration. Postoperative pain scores at rest and with cough were significantly less in thoracic epidural patients on postoperative days 1 and 2 only (equivalent on postoperative day 3). Like the Priestley and colleagues[14] investigation, there were no substantial differences between the two groups regarding important postoperative clinical variables (respiratory function, renal function, atrial fibrillation, hospital length of stay). Last, a recently published (2006) clinical investigation by Hansdottir and colleagues[16] provides additional evidence that thoracic epidural techniques offer no real clinical benefits to patients undergoing cardiac surgery. This relatively large (113 patients) prospective trial randomized patients undergoing elective cardiac surgery to receive either patient-controlled thoracic epidural analgesia (catheter inserted the day before surgery, using bupivacaine, fentanyl, and adrenalin) or patient-controlled intravenous morphine analgesia during the immediate postoperative period. Perioperative care was standardized (all patients underwent general anesthesia and received a median sternotomy). When the two groups were compared, the only difference was a shorter time to postoperative tracheal extubation in patients receiving thoracic epidural analgesia. Absolutely no differences were observed regarding postoperative analgesia (at rest and during cough), degree of sedation, lung volumes (forced vital capacity, forced vital capacity at 1 second, peak expiratory flow), degree of ambulation, global quality of recovery score (including all five domains), cardiac morbidity, renal morbidity, neurologic outcome, intensive care unit stay, or hospital length of stay.

A recently published (2004) meta-analysis by Liu and colleagues[17] assessed effects of perioperative central neuraxial techniques on outcome after coronary artery bypass surgery. These authors, via MEDLINE and other databases, searched for randomized controlled trials of patients undergoing coronary artery bypass surgery with cardiopulmonary bypass. Fifteen trials enrolling 1178 patients were included for thoracic epidural analysis, and 17 trials enrolling 668 patients were included for intrathecal analysis. Thoracic epidural techniques did not affect incidences of mortality or myocardial infarction, yet seemed to reduce risk of dysrhythmias (atrial fibrillation and tachycardia), pulmonary complications (pneumonia and atelectasis), the time to tracheal extubation, and analog pain scores. Intrathecal techniques did not affect incidences of mortality, myocardial infarction, dysrhythmias, or time to tracheal extubation and seemed only to modestly decrease systemic morphine use and pain scores (while increasing incidence of puritus). These authors conclude that central neuraxial techniques do not affect mortality or myocardial infarction rates after revascularization, yet may be associated with improvements such as faster time to tracheal extubation, decreased pulmonary complications and cardiac dysrhythmias, and reduced pain scores. However, the authors also note that most potential clinical benefits offered by these techniques (earlier extubation, decreased dysrhythmias, enhanced analgesia) may be achieved in other (safer?) ways, such as using fact-track protocols, use of beta-adrenergic blockers or amiodarone, or use of alternative intravenous analgesics.

In summary, the many clinical investigations involving epidural techniques indicate that administration of thoracic epidural opioids or local anesthetics produces reliable postoperative analgesia after cardiac surgery. Administration of thoracic epidural local anesthetics can both reliably attenuate the perioperative stress response associated with cardiac surgery and induce thoracic cardiac sympathectomy. However, it remains controversial whether such analgesia, stress response attenuation, and thoracic cardiac sympathectomy truly affects clinical outcome.

CONTROVERSIES

Clinical problems associated with intrathecal/epidural local anesthetics (hypotension) and intrathecal/epidural opioids (pruritus, nausea and vomiting, urinary retention, respiratory depression) are well known. Furthermore, thoracic epidural analgesia may mask myocardial ischemia (angina) via analgesia or initiate myocardial ischemia via alterations in autonomic nervous system activity. Of the few patients who have received large amounts of intrathecal local anesthetics to produce a "total spinal" for cardiac surgery, most have required intravenous phenylephrine during surgery to increase arterial blood pressure, indicating that hypotension is a substantial problem with this technique. Hypotension also seems to be relatively common when thoracic epidural local anesthetics are used in this setting. Volume replacement, beta-adrenergic agonists, and alpha-adrenergic agonists are required in a fair proportion of patients, and coronary perfusion pressure may decrease in susceptible patients after cardiopulmonary bypass. The most important undesirable drug effect of intrathecal and epidural opioids is respiratory depression, which may delay tracheal extubation.

Thoracic epidural supplementation of general anesthesia in patients undergoing cardiac surgery may also produce temporary neurologic deficits in the immediate postoperative period that can complicate management. Chakravarthy and colleagues[18] describe two patients in whom high thoracic epidural local anesthetic supplementation of general anesthesia for cardiac surgery was used. In both patients, focal upper-extremity (unilateral) paresis was observed during the immediate postoperative period that resolved after epidural catheter repositioning. The deficits may have been caused by direct nerve irritation from the epidural catheter or unexpected spread of the local anesthetic to the brachial plexus. Whatever the cause, such focal neurologic deficits occurring in patients immediately after cardiac surgery require extra clinical effort to determine the origin.

Although most investigators agree that the risk of hematoma is increased when intrathecal or epidural instrumentation is performed in a patient before systemic heparinization required for cardiac surgery, the absolute degree of increased risk is somewhat controversial. An extensive mathematical analysis by Ho and colleagues[19] in patients subjected to systemic heparinization required for cardiopulmonary bypass (without a single episode of hematoma formation) reported in the literature as of the year 2000 estimated that the maximum risk may be as frequent as 1:2400. Similarly, for epidural instrumentation, maximum risk may be as frequent as 1:1000. Certain precautions, however, likely decrease risk. Most clinical studies use the technique only after demonstration of laboratory evidence of normal coagulation variables, delay surgery in the event of a traumatic tap, or require that the time from instrumentation to systemic heparinization exceeds 60 minutes. Whereas most studies investigating the use of epidural techniques insert catheters the day before scheduled surgery, recent investigators have performed instrumentation on the same day as surgery. These techniques should not be used in a patient with known coagulopathy from any cause. Additionally, systemic heparin effect and reversal should be tightly controlled (smallest amount of heparin used for the shortest duration compatible with therapeutic objectives), and patients should be closely monitored after surgery for signs and symptoms of hematoma formation.

As the use of thoracic epidural techniques in patients undergoing cardiac surgery has increased, reports of hematoma formation have surfaced. In 2004, the first report of hematoma formation associated with epidural instrumentation the day before scheduled cardiac surgery was published.[20] The first report of hematoma formation during the immediate postoperative period following cardiac surgery (catheter inserted immediately before surgery following induction of general anesthesia) occurred the same year.[21] Most recently, a letter to the editor in 2006 details permanent paraplegia in two patients undergoing cardiac surgery with thoracic epidural supplementation and hints at two additional patients who experienced hematoma formation associated with catheter insertion the day before scheduled cardiac surgery.[22] Furthermore, this author is aware of at least three additional cases of catastrophic (permanent paralysis) epidural hematoma formation in patients who had catheters inserted for elective cardiac surgery within the past few years in the United States alone (none published).

Whereas hematoma formation is always a concern, thromboembolic complications may also occur during the postoperative period when normalization of coagulation variables (in a patient requiring anticoagulation) are achieved to safely remove the epidural catheter. Chaney and Labovsky[23] detail such a case, where a patient had a thoracic epidural catheter inserted before elective cardiac surgery (intraoperative and immediate postoperative courses uneventful) and required postoperative anticoagulation for a mechanical aortic valve and atrial fibrillation. On the seventh postoperative day, coagulation parameters were normalized to safely remove the epidural catheter. On that same day, following normalization of coagulation parameters, the patient experienced a left temporal lobe stroke (verified by clinical examination and computed tomographic scan), which gradually resolved over the next 4 days.

AREAS OF UNCERTAINTY

Whether intrathecal and epidural techniques truly affect morbidity (cardiac function, pulmonary function, etc.) and mortality risks in patients undergoing cardiac surgery remains to be determined. All clinical reports involving the use of intrathecal and thoracic epidural techniques for cardiac surgery involve small numbers of patients, and few (if any) are well designed.[5] Only a handful of clinical studies involving intrathecal techniques are prospective, randomized, blinded, and placebo-controlled.[5] There are no blinded, placebo-controlled clinical studies involving thoracic epidural techniques in patients undergoing cardiac surgery.[5] Furthermore, none of these clinical studies uses clinical outcome as a primary endpoint (most focus entirely on postoperative analgesia). When critically reviewed, this body of literature suggests that these techniques reliably induce enhanced postoperative analgesia, yet (at the current time) have no clinically important effect on morbidity and mortality risks.

Cardiac surgery is unique, and because of this, involves unique risks not routinely associated with noncardiac surgery. Furthermore, as all clinicians know, for a wide variety of reasons, patients undergoing cardiac surgery continue to get older and "sicker" (more comorbidities: neurologic dysfunction, myocardial dysfunction, pulmonary dysfunction, renal dysfunction, etc.). Multiple factors interact in a complicated manner during the perioperative period that affect outcome and quality of life after cardiac surgery (Table 63-1). Although others may disagree, the factors listed in Table 63-1 are arranged in descending order of importance as viewed by this author. Obviously, depending on specific clinical situations, certain factors will be more important than others. It is extremely difficult (if not impossible) to determine exactly how important attaining adequate or "high-quality" postoperative analgesia truly is in relation to all these important clinical factors surrounding a patient undergoing cardiac surgery. For example, how important is it to obtain "high-quality" postoperative analgesia in an 80-year-old patient with preoperative myocardial dysfunction, renal dysfunction, and a heavily calcified aorta after double-valve replacement? It could be argued that factors other than quality of postoperative analgesia will determine clinical outcome in this patient. On the other hand, how important is it to obtain "high-quality" postoperative analgesia in an otherwise healthy 50-year-old patient after routine coronary artery bypass grafting? It is likely that this patient's clinical outcome will be satisfactory even if postoperative analgesia is suboptimal.

In summary, the use of spinal/epidural techniques in patients undergoing cardiac surgery remains extremely controversial.[24-29] When one thoughtfully and critically evaluates the published literature, it becomes clear that the only substantiated clinical benefit obtained is postoperative analgesia. However, such "enhanced postoperative analgesia" (attained via any method) has never been linked to improved patient outcome. On the other hand, there are clear disadvantages associated with these techniques, including labor intensivity, intrathecal/epidural local anesthetic problems, intrathecal/epidural opioid problems, potential complications of postoperative assessment, hematoma risk, thromboembolic risk, high failure rate (epidural techniques), and no proven clinically beneficial effects.

GUIDELINES

No formal practice guidelines have been published regarding the use of intrathecal or epidural techniques in patients undergoing cardiac surgery. The only substantiated clinical benefit obtained is enhanced postoperative analgesia (although this has never been linked to improved patient outcome). On the other hand, there are clear disadvantages and risks associated with these techniques in this patient population. It is up to the anesthesiologist to thoughtfully decide whether or not such benefit (analgesia) is worth the disadvantages and risks in each specific patient undergoing cardiac surgery.

AUTHOR'S RECOMMENDATIONS

The use of spinal/epidural techniques in patients undergoing cardiac surgery remains extremely controversial. It is this author's opinion that, at the current time, the disadvantages and risks associated with the use of intrathecal/epidural techniques in patients undergoing cardiac surgery far outweigh the lone substantiated clinical benefit (enhanced analgesia). Postoperative analgesia in these patients can be obtained via simpler and safer methods. Thus, it is this author's opinion that intrathecal/epidural techniques should not be used in patients undergoing cardiac surgery.

Table 63-1	Factors Affecting Outcome Following Cardiac Surgery

Type and quality of surgical intervention
Extent of postoperative neurologic dysfunction
Extent of postoperative myocardial dysfunction
Extent of postoperative pulmonary dysfunction
Extent of postoperative renal dysfunction
Extent of postoperative coagulation abnormalities
Extent of systemic inflammatory response
Quality of postoperative analgesia

REFERENCES

1. Tuman, KJ, McCarthy RJ, March RJ, et al: Effects of epidural anesthesia and analgesia on coagulation and outcome after major vascular surgery. *Anesth Analg* 1991;73:696-704.
2. Yeager MP, Glass DD, Neff RK, Brink-Johnsen T: Epidural anesthesia and analgesia in high-risk surgical patients. *Anesthesiology* 1987;66:729-736.
3. Mangano DT, Siliciano D, Hollenberg M, et al: Postoperative myocardial ischemia: Therapeutic trials using intensive analgesia following surgery. *Anesthesiology* 1992;76:342-353.
4. Anand KJS, Hickey PR: Halothane-morphine compared with high-dose sufentanil for anesthesia and postoperative analgesia in neonatal cardiac surgery. *N Engl J Med* 1992;326:1-9.

5. Chaney MA: Intrathecal and epidural anesthesia and analgesia for cardiac surgery (review article). *Anesth Analg* 2006;102:45-64.

6. Liu S, Carpenter RL, Neal MJ: Epidural anesthesia and analgesia: Their role in postoperative outcome (review article). *Anesthesiology* 1995;82:1474-1506.

7. Birkett DA, Apthorp GH, Chamberlain DA, et al: Bilateral upper thoracic sympathectomy in angina pectoris: Results in 52 cases. *BMJ* 1965;2:187-190.

8. Vanstrum GS, Bjornson KM, Ilko R: Postoperative effects of intrathecal morphine in coronary artery bypass surgery. *Anesth Analg* 1988;67:261-267.

9. Chaney MA, Smith KR, Barclay JC, Slogoff S: Large-dose intrathecal morphine for coronary artery bypass grafting. *Anesth Analg* 1996;83:215-222.

10. Chaney MA, Furry PA, Fluder EM, Slogoff S: Intrathecal morphine for coronary artery bypass grafting and early extubation. *Anesth Analg* 1997;84:241-248.

11. Chaney MA, Nikolov MP, Blakeman BP, Bakhos M: Intrathecal morphine for coronary artery bypass graft procedure and early extubation revisited. *J Cardiothorac Vasc Anesth* 1999;13:574-578.

12. Aybek T, Kessler P, Dogan S, et al: Awake coronary artery bypass grafting: Utopia or reality? *Ann Thorac Surg* 2003;75:1165-1170.

13. Scott NB, Turfrey DJ, Ray DAA, et al: A prospective randomized study of the potential benefits of thoracic epidural anesthesia and analgesia in patients undergoing coronary artery bypass grafting. *Anesth Analg* 2001;93:528-535.

14. Priestley MC, Cope L, Halliwell R, et al: Thoracic epidural anesthesia for cardiac surgery: The effects on tracheal intubation time and length of hospital stay. *Anesth Analg* 2002;94:275-282.

15. Royse C, Royse A, Soeding P, et al: Prospective randomized trial of high thoracic epidural analgesia for coronary artery bypass surgery. *Ann Thorac Surg* 2003;75:93-100.

16. Hansdottir V, Philip J, Olsen MF, et al: Thoracic epidural versus intravenous patient-controlled analgesia after cardiac surgery: A randomized controlled trial on length of hospital stay and patient-perceived quality of recovery. *Anesthesiology* 2006;104:142-151.

17. Liu SS, Block BM, Wu CL: Effects of perioperative central neuraxial analgesia on outcome after coronary artery bypass surgery: A meta-analysis. *Anesthesiology* 2004;101:153-161.

18. Chakravarthy M, Nadiminto S, Krishnamuthy J, et al: Temporary neurologic deficits in patients undergoing cardiac surgery with thoracic epidural supplementation. *J Cardiothorac Vasc Anesth* 2004;18:512-520.

19. Ho AMH, Chung DC, Joynt GM: Neuraxial blockade and hematoma in cardiac surgery: Estimating the risk of a rare adverse event that has not (yet) occurred. *Chest* 2000;117:551-555.

20. Sharma S, Kapoor MC, Sharma VK, et al: Epidural hematoma complicating high thoracic epidural catheter placement intended for cardiac surgery. *J Cardiothorac Vasc Anesth* 2004;18:759-762.

21. Rosen DA, Hawkinberry DW, Rosen KR, et al: An epidural hematoma in an adolescent patient after cardiac surgery. *Anesth Analg* 2004;98:966-969.

22. Ho AMH, Li PTY, Karmakar MK: Risk of hematoma after epidural anesthesia and analgesia for cardiac surgery. *Anesth Analg* 2006;103:1327-1328.

23. Chaney M, Labovsky J: Case report of thoracic epidural anesthesia and cardiac surgery: Balancing postoperative risks associated with hematoma formation and thromboembolic phenomenon. *J Cardiothorac Vasc Anesth* 2005;19:768-771.

24. O'Connor CJ, Tuman KJ: Editorial: Epidural anesthesia and analgesia for coronary artery bypass graft surgery: Still forbidden territory? *Anesth Analg* 2001;93:523-525.

25. Schwann NM, Chaney MA: Editorial: No pain, much gain? *J Thorac Cardiovasc Surg* 2003;126:1261-1264.

26. Mora Mangano CT: Editorial: Risky business. *J Thorac Cardiovasc Surg* 2003;125:1204-1207.

27. Castellano JM, Durbin CG: Editorial: Epidural analgesia and cardiac surgery: Worth the risk? *Chest* 2003;117:305-307.

28. Chaney MA. Editorial: Cardiac surgery and intrathecal/epidural techniques: At the crossroads? *Can J Anaesth* 2005;52:783-788.

29. Chaney MA. Editorial: How important is postoperative pain after cardiac surgery? *J Cardiothorac Vasc Anesth* 2005;19:705-707.

NEUROSURGICAL ANESTHESIA

64 Is There a Best Technique in the Patient with Increased Intracranial Pressure?

Kristin Engelhard, MD, PhD; Nicole Forster, MD; and Adrian W. Gelb, MBChB

The contents of the cranium can be divided into three compartments. The brain or tissue compartment accounts for greater than 85% of the total intracranial volume, cerebrospinal fluid (CSF) contributes approximately 10%, and the blood in the vasculature contributes approximately 2% to 5%. The majority of the cerebral blood volume (CBV) resides in the low-pressure venous system, whereas only 15% of the CBV is found in the arteries and 15% in the venous sinuses.

Intracranial pressure (ICP) is closely regulated, even in the presence of a space-occupying lesion, as long as compensatory mechanisms are operational and the pathologic process evolves slowly. Any increase in intracranial volume must be compensated by volume reduction of one of the other compartments to maintain normal ICP. The CSF system has the greatest buffering capacity through displacement of CSF from the cranium to the spinal subarachnoid space. Cerebral blood volume reduction occurs first by compression of the low-pressure venous system, followed by capillary collapse, and then arterial compression leading to cerebral ischemia. The impact of ICP on outcome lies in its role in determining cerebral perfusion pressure (CPP) (CPP = mean arterial pressure [MAP] − ICP). There is evidence, at least in head trauma, that a CPP less than 50 mm Hg is associated with poor outcome.[1] However, an improved outcome does not necessarily result from a higher CPP. For the calculation of CPP, the arterial pressure transducer should be at the level of the ear.

Increased ICP may be caused by changes in the volume of any one or a combination of the intracranial compartments, including hematomas caused by vascular rupture, increases in brain and interstitial volumes caused by tumors, and vasogenic and cytotoxic edema secondary to hypoxia and infection. Increased ICP can also result from obstruction of CSF pathways and alteration of CSF production or reabsorption.

OPTIONS

Management strategies include decisions about choice of (1) anesthetic drugs, (2) ventilation, (3) hyperosmolar therapy, (4) head and body position, and (5) decompressive craniectomy (Table 64-1). The effects are influenced by whether the ICP increase was acute or has developed slowly, which usually allows some compensation to take place.

EVIDENCE

What Are the Targets for ICP and CPP?

The intracranial pressure should be kept below 20 mm Hg, because higher values are associated with poorer neurologic outcome.[1] A CPP greater than 70 mm Hg should be avoided if it requires massive fluid infusion and high-dose catecholamines because hypervolemia and catecholamine therapy increase the incidence of acute respiratory distress syndome.[2] A spontaneous increase of CPP above 70 mm Hg can be accepted as long as cerebrovascular autoregulation is intact or the neurologic state seems to benefit clinically. When autoregulation is intact, an increase in CPP is associated with autoregulatory vasoconstriction and, thereby, a reduction of CBV and ICP. The critical lower threshold for CPP lies between 50 and 60 mm Hg. Therefore a CPP below 50 mm Hg should be avoided.[1]

What Are the Effects of Anesthetics on ICP?

The choice of anesthetic agents and adjunctive drugs is based on consideration of their effects on cerebral blood flow (CBF), CBV, cerebral metabolic rate of oxygen ($CMRO_2$), ICP, cerebrovascular autoregulation, and carbon dioxide (CO_2) reactivity. Most randomized trials have focused on these surrogate endpoints rather than on clinical or neurologic patient outcomes.

Volatile anesthetics depress cerebral metabolism in a dose-dependent fashion while directly inducing cerebral vasodilation, which results in increases in CBV and ICP. Sevoflurane causes less cerebral vasodilation compared with isoflurane or desflurane.[3] Cerebrovascular autoregulation and CO_2 response remain intact with sevoflurane up to 1 minimum alveolar concentration (MAC), and therefore it is suitable for neurosurgical patients as long as ICP is not markedly or acutely increased.

433

Table 64-1 Management of Acutely Increased Intracranial Pressure (ICP)

STANDARDS

No prophylactic hyperventilation

GUIDELINES

Monitoring of ICP
Barbiturate infusion for intractable increased ICP
Use of mannitol

OPTIONS

Cerebral perfusion pressure 50-70 mm Hg
Brief hyperventilation for acute neurologic deterioration
Propofol infusion
Positioning patient head up

Nitrous oxide is a potent cerebral vasodilator with resultant increase in ICP. Although there are no outcome studies to demonstrate a deleterious effect, nitrous oxide should not be used in patients with acutely elevated ICP.

Total intravenous anesthesia has received attention in neuroanesthesia as a means of avoiding the vasodilating effects of nitrous oxide and volatile anesthetics. Intravenous agents such as propofol and etomidate produce cerebral vasoconstriction and a reduction in CBF, CBV, and ICP secondary to a decrease in $CMRO_2$ while preserving autoregulation.[4] Propofol should be used intraoperatively in patients with markedly or acutely increased ICP. In the intensive care unit propofol can be used for up to 7 days with a maximal dosage of 4 mg/kg/hr. Propofol administered for longer or at higher concentrations might induce the "propofol infusion syndrome," which includes hyperkalemia, lipemia, metabolic acidosis, myocardial failure, rhabdomyolysis, and renal failure potentially resulting in death.[5]

Barbiturates similarly exert their ICP-lowering effects through vasoconstriction, with a reduction of CBF and CBV secondary to suppression of cerebral metabolism. Barbiturates can produce ICP control and improved CPP in patients with severe head trauma when other treatments have failed, but there is no evidence that prophylactic barbiturate therapy improves outcome.[6,7] Furthermore, high doses of barbiturates decrease immune function and can cause hypokalemia. The slow plasma clearance of barbiturates is another disadvantage because it causes a substantial delay in awakening. Barbiturate coma should be titrated to achieve an electroencephalogram (EEG) burst suppression ratio of 5% to 10% or ICP control.

Propofol and barbiturates reduce MAP, and intravenous (IV) fluids and vasopressors may be necessary. Etomidate causes less cardiovascular depression and may be the drug of choice in cardiovascular disease or hypovolemia, but its use should be confined to induction because it suppresses the adrenocortical response to stress.

There has been controversy about the effect of opioids on ICP. In one study transient increases in ICP without changes in middle cerebral artery blood flow velocity occurred concomitant with decreases in MAP, while in patients with stable blood pressure ICP was unchanged.[8] This suggests that increases in ICP seen with sufentanil and other opioids

may be due to autoregulatory vasodilation secondary to systemic hypotension. This is consistent with a more recent study of remifentanil in patients with head trauma.[9]

Nondepolarizing neuromuscular relaxants have no effect on CBF, $CMRO_2$, and ICP, whereas succinylcholine may transiently increase ICP. The increase in ICP occurred during periods of elevated CBF, which coincided with EEG evidence of cerebral arousal in dogs.[10] These effects were primarily related to succinylcholine-induced increases in muscle afferent activity and not the presence or absence of fasciculations.[10,11] The increases in ICP were much reduced in animals with brain injury. When rapid-sequence intubation is required, succinylcholine remains the drug of choice. However, rocuronium in high doses may be a suitable alternative.

What Is the Effect of Hyperventilation on ICP?

Arterial carbon dioxide tension is a potent modulator of cerebrovascular tone and CBF. Arterial hypercapnia dilates cerebral blood vessels, decreases cerebrovascular resistance, and increases CBF, CBV, and ICP, whereas hypocapnia has the opposite effect. Hyperventilation is often used in patients with increased ICP to reduce CBV. Because hyperventilation reduces ICP through vasoconstriction, this could critically affect the oxygen and glucose delivery to vulnerable brain areas.

Moderate hyperventilation lowers global hemispheric CBF, but does not alter $CMRO_2$. This mismatch between low CBF and normal or elevated $CMRO_2$ caused by hyperventilation after severe traumatic brain injury may lead to cerebral ischemia, which might further compromise neuronal outcome.[12]

There remains much controversy about the beneficial or detrimental effects of hyperventilation. Although hyperventilation may produce a rapid reduction in ICP and high ICP is one of the most common precursors of death or neurologic disability, there is little evidence to suggest that hyperventilation improves clinically relevant outcomes. In fact, a much-quoted study found a detrimental effect. Patients with severe traumatic brain injury were randomized to a hyperventilated group ($PaCO_2$ of 25 ± 2 mm Hg) or a normoventilated group ($PaCO_2$ of 35 ± 2 mm Hg) for 5 days.[13] Patients in the hyperventilation group had a significantly worse outcome at 3 months than did those in the normocapnic group.

In elective supratentorial craniotomy, aggressive hyperventilation ($PaCO_2$ 25 ± 2 mm Hg) has been found in a multicenter randomized trial to reduce ICP and improve operating conditions as assessed by surgeons blinded to treatment group.[14] This effect was independent of the use of propofol total intravenous anesthesia or less than 0.8 MAC isoflurane. The hyperventilation was not maintained for the duration of the surgery, and the study did not attempt to determine whether the hyperventilation altered neurologic outcomes. Therefore short periods of hyperventilation to manage acute increase in ICP can be recommended.

What Is the Effect of Mechanical Ventilation on ICP?

The effect of positive end-expiratory pressure (PEEP) on ICP has been reported by many investigators without a clear consensus. Mechanical ventilation and PEEP can increase intrathoracic pressure, may increase ICP by impeding venous drainage, or could reduce CPP by reducing blood pressure. Studies suggest that if CPP is maintained, PEEP (up to 15 cm H_2O) seems to have no significant adverse effect.[15] If an adverse effect of PEEP on ICP occurs, it can often be overcome by placing the patient in the head-up position.

Volume recruitment maneuvers with high-peak intrathoracic pressure reduce MAP, increase ICP, and decrease CPP. This technique affects cerebral hemodynamics and can only be recommended when severe lung injury is leading to hypoxia, which in turn can increase neuronal injury. Recruitment maneuvers should be performed carefully and under continuous control of ICP and CPP.

What Is the Effect of Hyperosmolar Therapy on ICP?

The administration of mannitol (0.25 to 1.0 g/kg) has become a cornerstone of ICP management. Because of side effects (e.g., tubular necrosis of the kidney) a dose of 4 g/kg/day should not be exceeded and the serum osmolarity has to be kept below 320 mOsm/L. Although there are many data regarding its mechanism of action, few studies exist that validate mannitol usage.[16]

Mannitol has an immediate plasma-expanding effect that reduces blood viscosity and thereby increases CBF, which in turn induces autoregulatory vasoconstriction. This rheologic effect might explain the early decrease of ICP. Osmotic agents withdraw more water from the brain tissue than from other organs because the blood-brain barrier (BBB) impedes penetration of the osmotic agent into the brain, thus maintaining an osmotic diffusion gradient. Osmotic diuretics may also reduce ICP by retarding CSF formation. Under normal circumstances, hypertonic agents slowly penetrate the BBB. When the BBB is disrupted, they may enter and raise brain osmolality, pulling water back into the brain. Interstitial accumulation of mannitol is most marked with continuous infusions, and therefore it is recommended that mannitol be administrated as repeated boluses rather than as a continuous infusion.[17]

Mannitol administration has become common practice in the management of head-injured patients with elevated ICP, but it has never been subjected to a controlled clinical trial against placebo. There are only three randomized controlled trials evaluating mannitol use in head injury.[16] One study in brain trauma patients compared mannitol with barbiturates for ICP control. Mannitol was superior to barbiturates at improving CPP, ICP, and outcome. A further study compared a bolus dose of mannitol given before hospital admission with the administration of a similar volume of saline. There was a slight reduction in mortality rate with mannitol. In 22 patients who received ventriculostomy drainage, mannitol or hyperventilation was used to control high ICP. Mannitol was found to be more effective than hyperventilation in reducing ICP.

Hypertonic saline also reduces the cerebral water content, and its effect on ICP seems to be equal or superior to mannitol.[18,19] Although the use of hypertonic saline is not yet included in management guidelines, it can be used in cases where mannitol is not effective.[20]

The evidence supporting mannitol is sufficiently strong to warrant guideline status. A bolus of mannitol is also recommended in patients with transtentorial herniation or progressive neurologic deterioration not attributable to extracranial causes.[1]

What Is the Effect of Patient's Position on ICP?

Flexion or torsion of the neck can obstruct cerebral venous outflow and increase brain bulk and ICP. A simple change in head position can immediately decrease ICP. Between 30° and 40° head-up or reverse Trendelenburg position is also effective in reducing ICP as long as MAP is maintained.[21]

What Is the Effect of Decompressive Craniectomy on ICP?

Decompressive craniectomy and opening of the dura mater may be a useful option when maximal medical treatment has failed to control ICP.[22] In children, decompressive craniectomy is recommended as a therapy to control ICP.[22] The prognosis after decompression depends on the clinical signs and symptoms at the time of admission, the patient's age, and the existence of major extracranial injuries.[23,24] One criticism of decompressive craniectomy is that more patients survive in a vegetative state. To avoid this, decompressive craniectomy should be restricted to patients younger than 50 years without multiple trauma and patients younger than 30 years in the presence of major extracranial injuries; it should *never* be used in patients with a primary brainstem lesion. Two major studies are currently ongoing to characterize the efficacy and the ideal time for the intervention (DECRAN and RescueICP).

AUTHORS' RECOMMENDATIONS

- In the patient with acutely elevated ICP, propofol provides the greatest margin of safety and ability to reduce ICP. Care must be taken not to compromise CPP through hypotension. High-dose barbiturate therapy may be considered in hemodynamically stable severe head injury patients with intracranial hypertension refractory to other ICP-lowering therapies.
- Mannitol is effective for the control of raised ICP after severe head injury. Limited data suggest that intermittent boluses are more effective than continuous infusion. The effective dose range is 0.25 to 1.0 g/kg. Serum osmolarity should be kept below 320 mOsm/L, and hypovolemia should be avoided.
- The use of prophylactic chronic hyperventilation ($PaCO_2$ less than 30 mm Hg) during the first 24 hours after severe traumatic brain injury should be avoided because it can compromise CBF. Hyperventilation may be used for short periods in acute neurologic deterioration or elective supratentorial craniotomy.

REFERENCES

1. Bullock M, Povlishock J: Guidelines for the management of severe traumatic brain injury. *J Neurotrauma* 2007;24(suppl 1):S1-S95.
2. Robertson GS, Valadka AB, Hannay HJ, Contant CF, Gopinath SP, Cormio M, et al: Prevention of secondary ischemic insults after severe head injury. *Crit Care Med* 1999;27:2086-2095.

3. Holmström A, Akeson J: Desflurane increases intracranial pressure more and sevoflurane less than isoflurane in pigs subjected to intracranial hypertension. *J Neurosurg Anesthesiol* 2004;16: 136-143.

4. Alkire MT, Haier RJ, Barker SJ, Shah NK, Wu JC, Kao YJ: Cerebral metabolism during propofol anesthesia in humans studied with positron emission tomography. *Anesthesiology* 1995;82: 393-403.

5. Cremer OL, Moons KG, Bouman EA, Kruijswijk JE, De Smet AM, Kalkman CJ: Long-term propofol infusion and cardiac failure in adult head-injured patients. *Lancet* 2001;357:117-118.

6. Roberts I: Barbiturates for acute traumatic brain injury (Cochrane Review). *Cochrane Library* 2002;2.

7. Cormino M, Gopinath S, Valadka AB, Robertson CS: Cerebral hemodynamic effects of pentobarbital coma in head-injured patients. *J Neurotrauma* 1999;16:927-936.

8. Werner C, Hoffman WE, Baughman VL, Albrecht RF, Schulte AM, Esch J: Effects of sufentanil on cerebral blood flow, cerebral blood flow velocity, and metabolism in dogs. *Anesth Analg* 1991;72:177-181.

9. Engelhard K, Reeker W, Kochs E, Werner C: Effect of remifentanil on intracranial pressure and cerebral blood flow velocity in patients with head trauma. *Acta Anaesthesiol Scand* 2004;48: 396-399.

10. Lanier W, Milde J, Michenfelder J: Cerebral stimulation following succinylcholine in dogs. *Anesthesiology* 1986;64:551-559.

11. Lanier W, Iaizzo P, Milde J: Cerebral function and muscle afferent activity following intravenous succinylcholine in dogs anesthetized with halothane: The effects of pretreatment with a defasciculating dose of pancuronium. *Anesthesiology* 1989;71: 87-95.

12. Coles JP, Fryer TD, Coleman MR, Smielewski P, Gupta AK, Minhas PS, et al: Hyperventilation following head injury: Effect on ischemic burden and cerebral oxidative metabolism. *Crit Care Med* 2007;35:568-578.

13. Muizelaar JP, Marmarou A, Ward JD: Adverse effects of prolonged hyperventilation in patients with severe head injury: A randomized clinical trial. *J Neurosurg* 1991;75:731-739.

14. Gelb AW, Craen R, Rao G, Reddy K, Megyesi J, Mohanty B, et al: Does hyperventilation improve operating condition during supratentorial craniotomy? A multicenter randomized crossover trial. *Anesth Analg* 2008;106:585-594.

15. McGuire G, Crossley D, Richards J, Wong D: Effects of varying levels of positive end-expiratory pressure on intracranial pressure and cerebral perfusion pressure. *Crit Care Med* 1997;25: 1059-1062.

16. Shierhout G, Roberts I: Mannitol for acute traumatic brain injury (Cochrane Review). *Cochrane Library* 2002.

17. Mendelow AD, Teasdale GM, Russell T, Flood J, Patterson J, Murray GD: Effect of mannitol on cerebral blood flow and cerebral perfusion pressure in human head injury. *J Neurosurg* 1985;63:43-48.

18. Vialet R, Albanèse J, Thomachot L, Antonini F, Bourgouin A, Alliez B, Martin C: Isovolume hypertonic solutes (sodium chloride or mannitol) in the treatment of refractory posttraumatic intracranial hypertension: 2 ml/kg 7.5% saline is more effective than 2 ml/kg 20% mannitol. *Crit Care Med* 2003;31:1683-1687.

19. Battison C, Andrews PJ, Graham C, Petty T: Randomized, controlled trial on the effect of a 20% mannitol solution and a 7.5% saline/6% dextran solution on increased intracranial pressure after brain injury. *Crit Care Med* 2005;33:196-202.

20. White H, Cook D, Venkatesh B: The use of hypertonic saline for treating intracranial hypertension after traumatic brain injury. *Anesth Analg* 2006;102:1836-1846.

21. Mavrocordatos P, Bissonette B, Ravussin P: Effects of neck position and head elevation on intracranial pressure in anaesthetized neurosurgical patients. *J Neurosurg Anesthesiol* 2000;12:10-14.

22. Sahuquillo J, Arikan F: Decompressive craniectomy for the treatment of refractory high intracranial pressure in traumatic brain injury. *Cochrane Database Syst Rev* 2006.

23. Meier U, Gräwe A: The importance of decompressive craniotomy for the management of severe head injuries. *Acta Neurochir* 2003;86(suppl):367-371.

24. Ruf B, Heckmann M, Schroth I, Hugens-Penzel M, Reiss I, Borkhardt A, et al: Early decompressive craniectomy and duraplasty for refractory intracranial hypertension in children: Results of a pilot study. *Crit Care* 2003;7:R133-138.

65 What Works for Brain Protection?

Izumi Harukuni, MD, and Stephen T. Robinson, MD

INTRODUCTION

Despite recent advances in anesthesia techniques and monitoring measures, intraoperative and postoperative neurologic events remain the most devastating complications and continue to concern anesthesia providers. Even without any significant intraoperative events, there is a considerable risk for cerebral ischemia in specific surgical populations, such as cardiac surgeries and vascular surgeries.

The neurologic sequelae range from frank stroke to cognitive dysfunction. The incidence of perioperative stroke is reported from 1.6% to 5.2% in coronary artery bypass grafting (CABG) and from 0.25% to 7% in carotid endarterectomy (CEA),[1] whereas the incidence of cognitive dysfunction ranges from 24% to 57% at 6 months after cardiac surgery.[2]

There is a substantial amount of interest in research to identify neuroprotective strategies; however, most of the clinical trials have resulted in disappointment, and there are no formal guidelines based on the strongest clinical evidence. This is thought to be because of the complexity of the mechanism in cerebral ischemia.

Most anesthesia providers strongly agree that maintaining adequate cerebral oxygenation and perfusion pressure is the most effective and important strategy in neuroprotection. There is also historical clinical evidence that advocates avoiding deleterious factors in the event of ongoing cerebral ischemia or in higher–risk populations.

OPTIONS

Neuroprotective strategies are classified into two concepts: passive, which refers to the avoidance of deleterious factors, and active, which refers to the application of beneficial interventions. Hans and Bonhomme[3] proposed categorizing the neuroprotecting measure into physiology, anesthetics, nonanesthetic pharmacologic agents, and preconditioning. Along with these strategies, the authors will discuss the role of monitoring in specific surgical populations.

1. *Physiology*: Avoidance of hyperthermia, hyperglycemia, cerebral hypoxia, and hypoperfusion.
2. *Anesthetics*: Use of certain anesthetics that are potentially neuroprotective because of reduction of energy requirement.
3. *Pharmacology*: Use of potentially neuroprotective agents, which can block the pathways of neuronal cell death.

This may include *N*-methyl-D-aspartate (NMDA) receptor antagonists, excitatory amino acid (EAA) receptor antagonists, and erythropoietin.
4. *Preconditioning*: The use of physiologic or pharmacologic alterations that could mimic preconditioning for high-risk populations.
5. *Monitoring*: Use of epiaortic echocardiography scanning to manage severe atherosclerotic disease and near-infrared reflectance spectroscopy (NIRS) for assessment of bifrontal regional cortical oxygen saturation (rSO_2) in cardiac surgery.

EVIDENCE (TABLE 65-1)

Physiology

To ensure adequate cerebral oxygenation and cerebral perfusion, measures that reduce cerebral metabolic rate (CMR) are known to be beneficial. Hypothermia has been proposed to offer neuroprotective effect for over several decades, but in a recent larger clinical trial in acute traumatic injury patients, hypothermia failed to improve neurologic outcome.[4,5] The effect of mild hypothermia (32°C to 35°C) on CMR is negligible, and only deep hypothermia (18°C to 22°C), which is employed in specific types of cardiac surgeries, is neuroprotective. However, two prospective randomized trials in comatose survivors of out-of-hospital cardiac arrest demonstrated better neurologic outcome in the patients treated with mild hypothermia.[6,7] It was also reported that intraischemic or delayed hyperthermia worsens outcome.[8] Grigore and colleagues[9] reported that the slower rewarming rate with lower peak cerebral temperatures results in significantly better cognitive performance after cardiac surgery with hypothermic cardiopulmonary bypass.

Tight glucose control is associated with reduced mortality and morbidity rates in critically ill patients and post-cardiac surgery patients.[10] Persistent hyperglycemia after stroke has been shown to increase the size of ischemic brain injury and worsen clinical outcome. There is a retrospective study that demonstrated decreased mortality rate by normalizing blood glucose level after acute ischemic stroke.[11] One should keep in mind that tight glucose control (80 to 110 mg/dL) is associated with a higher incidence of hypoglycemia.[12] Nonetheless, based on these clinical data, hyperglycemia should be avoided perioperatively.

The use of corticosteroids is not advocated in ischemic or traumatic brain injury because there is no strong

Table 65-1	Overview of Major Clinical Studies Evaluating Neuroprotective Strategies and Outcome					
Study (Year)	**Number of Subjects**	**Patient Population**	**Study Design**	**Intervention**	**Control**	**Outcomes**
PHYSIOLOGY						
Bernard (2002)	273	Comatose survivors of out-of-hospital cardiac arrest	Prospective randomized	Mild hypothermia	Normothermia	Favorable neurologic outcome
Kammersgaard (2002)	390	Acute stroke	Observational	Hypothermia ($\leq 37°C$)	Hyperthermia ($> 37°C$)	Low admission temperature is an independent predictor of good short-term outcome
Grigore (2001)	165	CABG with CPB	Prospective not randomized	Slower rate of rewarming	Conventional rewarming	Better cognitive performance at 6 weeks
Gentile (2006)	960	Acute ischemic stroke	Retrospective	Normlization of BG (<130 mg/dL) during first 48 hr	Hyperglycemia (BG $\geq$ 130 mg/dL)	Associated with a 4.6-fold decrease in mortality risk
Vicek (2003)	372	Acute ischemic stroke	Retrospective	Lowering DBP more than 25% from admission value	Maintained DBP	Associated with a 3.8-fold increased adjusted odds for poor neurologic outcome on day 5
Ahmed (2003)	201	Acute ischemic stroke	Retrospective	Lowering DBP with nimodipine	Maintained DBP	Worsened the neurologic outcome in nontotal anterior circulation infarct
Gold (1995)	251	CABG with CPB	Prospective randomized	High MABP (80-100 mm Hg) during CPB	MABP 50-60 mm Hg during CPB	Fewer myocardial and neurologic complications
ANESTHETICS						
Michenfelder (1987)	2223	Carotid endoarterectomy	Retrospective chart review	Isoflurane	Enflurane, halothane	Lower critical CBF (10 mL/100 g/min) vs. 15 in enflurane and 20 in halothane; lower incidence of EEG ischemic change (18% vs. 26% in enflurane and 25% in halothane)
Messick (1987)	6	Carotid endoarterectomy	Prospective single-arm	Isoflurane	Halothane	Lower critical CBF (less than 10 ml/100 g/min) vs 18-20 in halothane
Kanbak (2004)	20	CABG with CPB	Prospective randomized	Isoflurane	Propofol	Alleviated increase of S-100 beta protein
Hoffman (1998)	12	Middle cerebral artery occlusion	Prospective randomized	Desflurane	Etomidate	Increased brain tissue PO_2 and attenuated acidotic change
Mitchell (1999)	65	Left heart valve operation	Prospective randomized	Intravenous lidocaine	Placebo	Fewer incidences of decreased neuropsychologic performance
Wang (2002)	118	CABG with CPB	Prospective randomized	Intravenous lidocaine	Normal saline	Decreased the occurrence of early postoperative cognitive dysfunction

PHARMACOLOGY

Arrowsmith (1998)	171	CABG with CPB	Prospective randomized	Remacemide	Placebo	Overall postoperative change (reflecting learning ability in addition to reduced deficits) was favorable in treated group
Mathew (2004)	914	CABG with CPB	Prospective randomized	Pexelizumab	Placebo	Decreased visuospatial function impairment but not overall cognitive dysfunction
Ehrenreich (2002)	40	Acute ischemic stroke	Prospective randomized	Recombinant human erythropoietin	Saline	Improvement in clinical outcome at 1 month
MONITORING						
Royse (2000)	46	CABG with CPB	Prospective not randomized	Epiaortic echocardiography and exclusive Y graft	Digital palpation and aorta-coronary operations	Less incidence of late neuropsychologic dysfunction
Murkin (2007)	200	CABG with CPB	Prospective randomized	Cerebral regional oxygen saturation monitoring and treatment protocol	No intervention	Avoids profound cerebral desaturation and is associated with fewer incidences of major organ dysfunction

BG, blood glucose; *CABG,* coronary artery bypass grafting; *CPB,* cardiopulmonary bypass; *DBP,* diastolic blood pressure; *EEG,* electroencephalogram; *MABP,* mean arterial blood pressure.

evidence to support the benefit from treatment with corticosteroids.[13] There is a potential harm from hyperglycemia induced by its administration.[14]

Maintaining baseline blood pressure is an essential measure that ensures vital organ perfusion, including brain. Cerebral perfusion pressure is calculated by subtracting intracranial pressure from mean arterial blood pressure (MABP). Two clinical studies demonstrated that lowering diastolic blood pressure (DBP) in the acute phase of ischemic stroke worsened the neurologic outcome.[15,16]

Another retrospective study in patients who sustained sudden cardiac arrest demonstrated that good neurologic recovery was independently and directly related to MABP during the first 2 hours after return of spontaneous circulation.[17] Gold and colleagues[18] found fewer myocardial and neurologic complications after CABG surgery when targeted MABP during cardiopulmonary bypass (CPB) was between 80 and 100 mm Hg rather than 50 and 60 mm Hg. In this study, the incidence of cognitive dysfunction at 6 months after surgery was low and there was no relation between arterial pressure and cognitive outcome. However, maintaining "higher" MABP target strategy is considered to be acceptable, safe, and useful for patients at high risk for neurologic complications.[19]

Anesthetics

There is accumulating experimental evidence that confirms the neuroprotective effect of inhalational anesthetics in both focal and global ischemia. The mechanism involves inhibition of excitatory neurotransmission and potentiation of inhibitory receptors resulting in suppression of energy requirement. Preconditioning from inhalational agents is proposed as an additional mechanism of neuroprotection. The tolerance against ischemia is increased in the future event by activation of adenosine triphosphate (ATP)–dependent potassium channels and adenosine A_1 receptors.[1,20] In contrast to the multitude of experimental studies, clinical evidence on the neuroprotective effect of inhalational anesthetics has been scant. Hoffman and colleagues[21] reported that desflurane, in comparison with etomidate, increased brain tissue oxygen pressure and reduced acidosis in patients subjected to temporary middle cerebral artery occlusion. Another prospective study in patients undergoing CEA determined that the critical regional cerebral blood flow, which is the flow rate when electroencephalographic signs of ischemia are evident, during isoflurane anesthesia was much lower than during halothane or enflurane anesthesia.[22] In a retrospective study, the incidence of ischemic change was lower with isoflurane anesthesia when compared with halothane or enflurane anesthesia and there was no difference in neurologic outcome despite the fact that the isoflurane group had a higher risk of an adverse outcome.[23] Sufficiently powered, prospective randomized controlled studies evaluating the neurologic outcome using more appropriate endpoints such as long-term neurocognitive function are still needed. However, the use of volatile anesthetics can be considered as a part of an anesthetic plan when the risk of neuronal injury is anticipated.

Lidocaine was shown to have a neuroprotective effect in an in vivo study due to the reduction of energy consumption by delaying ischemia-induced membrane depolarization and also alleviation of apoptosis.[24-26] There is a small clinical trial in which a lidocaine infusion at the antiarrhythmic dose demonstrated improved long-term neuropsychologic performance in 65 patients with left heart valve procedures.[27] More recently, Wang and colleagues[28] reported that intraoperative administration of lidocaine decreased the occurrence of early postoperative cognitive dysfunction in patients who had undergone coronary artery bypass grafting surgery. Neither of these studies has enough power to conclude that lidocaine infusion should be used routinely as a neuroprotecting agent. Larger clinical trials with the optimal dosing regimen and long-term results are still needed.

There is a long history of postulating neuroprotective ability of barbiturates, which was considered to be from reduction of CMR and blocking glutamate receptors. However, there have been mixed results and its clinical perioperative efficacy remains controversial.[29,30] One of the problems with using barbiturates is their prolonged duration of action, thus causing delayed emergence. Since the volatile anesthetics have been shown to have similar effects as barbiturates, except shorter emergence time, the popularity of barbiturates has declined.

Propofol and ketamine have also been postulated as neuroprotecting agents; however, both drugs failed to improve long-term neurocognitive performance.[31-33]

Pharmacology

A few clinical trials with encouraging results deserve mention. Remacemide, the NMDA receptor antagonist, has been shown to improve some measures of postoperative psychometric performance in cardiac surgery patients.[34]

Mathew and colleagues[35] reported that pexelizumab, a humanized monoclonal antibody against the C5 complement component, led to less visuospatial impairment up to 1 month after CABG surgery, but failed to decrease the overall incidence of cognitive dysfunction.

Erythropoietin (EPO) has been used for the treatment of anemia and is known to be safe. It blocks apoptosis, blocks inflammation, and induces vasculogenesis and neurotrophic factors. In a clinical trial, high-dose intravenous EPO was shown to improve clinical outcome at 1 month in acute ischemic stroke patients.[36]

Numerous pharmacologic agents have been investigated for their potential ability to limit neuronal injury. Despite promising data from laboratory work, all had disappointing clinical results. This is mainly due to the complexity of the mechanisms of neuronal injury and the difficulty in controlling physiologic factors. The combination of multiple strategies, including the use of compounds targeting different pathways and the control of physiologic variables, may afford the most meaningful results in perioperative neuroprotection.

Preconditioning

Preconditioning is a novel concept of neuroprotection in which a prior exposure to minor insults will induce an increased tolerance to more serious injury.[1] The mechanism of preconditioning is activation of ATP-dependent potassium channels and adenosine A_1 receptors.[1] Other than history of transient ischemic attack before acute stroke promoting ischemic tolerance in human brain, many factors and various drugs can mimic preconditioning, such as hyperoxia, hypothermia, electroconvulsive shock, volatile anesthetics, and the potassium channel opener diazoxide, and erythromycin.[3]

Monitoring

In some specific surgical procedures, the use of specific monitoring measures may have impact on neurologic outcome. The change of surgical approach led by intraoperative epiaortic echocardiography has been shown to lower the incidence of late neurologic dysfunction in a large observational study[37] and also in a smaller case-control study.[38] This strategy is rated as class IIb (acceptable, safe, and useful) for patients undergoing CABG surgery at high risk for neurologic injury in an evidence-based rating by Hogue and colleagues.[19]

The use of near-infrared reflectance spectroscopy (NIRS) for assessment of bifrontal regional cortical oxygen saturation (rSO_2) has demonstrated correlation between CAB patients having low rSO_2 values and cognitive dysfunction, prolonged hospital length of stay, and cerebrovascular accident. A recent randomized control study by Murkin and colleagues[39] demonstrated that the treatment of declining rSO_2 prevented prolonged desaturations and was associated with a shorter intensive care unit (ICU) length of stay and a significantly reduced incidence of perioperative major organ morbidity and mortality. This result may have been the reflection of the good clinical practice to optimize organ perfusion instead of the direct effect of rSO_2 monitoring. However, the monitoring would allow early detection and rapid improvement of end-organ compromise.

AREAS OF UNCERTAINTY

An important cause of the mixed results in clinical trials to evaluate perioperative neurologic outcomes is the complexity of the mechanism of neuronal injury. Many layers of pathways and various transmitters and their receptors are involved. The mechanism of global ischemia differs from focal ischemia. For instance, the avoidance of hypoxia and hypoperfusion is essential to the perioperative brain protection, and rapid restoration of oxygen supply is critical after the ischemic insults; however, hyperoxia and excessive hypertension should be avoided because there is increased concern regarding worsening outcome with hyperoxia after global ischemia.[14]

The problem in interpreting the results from most of the clinical studies is that the endpoints of these trials are not uniform. Because the mechanism of early neuronal injury is more likely necrosis and that of delayed injury is apoptosis, the clinical manifestation would be different. Caution must be taken in terms of appropriate timing of treatment and neurobehavioral testing when evaluating the results from these studies.

GUIDELINES

There are no formal practice guidelines regarding perioperative neuroprotection. The clinical evidence of most of the neuroprotective strategies is weak because of lack of large, prospective, randomized controlled trials. The Internal Liaison Committee on Resuscitation published an advisory statement in 2003 regarding therapeutic hypothermia after cardiac arrest based on two prospective randomized trials that demonstrated promising results with improved neurologic outcome in the hypothermia group. In addition to ventricular fibrillation of out-of-hospital cardiac arrest, it states that cooling to 32°C to 34°C for 12 to 24 hours after the insult may also be beneficial for other rhythms or an in-hospital cardiac arrest.[40]

AUTHORS' RECOMMENDATIONS

Presently, there are no definitive neuroprotective strategies supported by strong clinical evidence. The available data do not support a definite benefit even for some of the strategies that have been historically used to provide neuroprotection. One example is the use of thiopental and steroids in cardiac surgery with deep hypothermic circulatory arrest. Furthermore, some strategies have been revealed as harmful. Based on very limited aforementioned clinical evidence, the following recommendations can be made when anticipating ischemic insult in patients at high risk or managing patients after the occurrence of a significant insult. These recommendations mainly consist of avoidance of deleterious interventions rather than beneficial measures.

- Hyperthermia, hyperglycemia, hypoxemia, and hypoperfusion should be avoided at all times. Mild induced hypothermia (32°C to 34°C) may be beneficial after recovery from out-of-hospital cardiac arrest or in-hospital cardiac arrest. Insulin therapy should be used to maintain normoglycemia. Hyperoxemia should be avoided in cases of global ischemia. After restoration of spontaneous circulation, oxygen saturation should be maintained within the range of 94% to 96%.
- Volatile anesthetics can be used during the intraoperative period to obtain the benefit of reduced energy requirement and potential preconditioning.
- The use of corticosteroids should be avoided in global ischemia.
- In the management of CPB in patients at high risk for neurologic injury (e.g., advanced age, prior stroke, atherosclerosis of the ascending aorta), higher mean arterial blood pressure should be maintained.
- In CABG surgery, the use of epiaortic echocardiography scanning and the change of surgical approach may be warranted to prevent macroembolism from manipulation of atherosclerosis in the aorta.

REFERENCES

1. Kitano H, Kirsch JR, Hurn, PD, Murphy SJ: Inhalational anesthetics as neuroprotectants or chemical preconditioning agents in ischemic brain. *J Cereb Blood Flow Metab* 2007;27:1108-1128.
2. Sanders RD, Ma D, Maze M: Anaesthesia induced neuroprotection. *Best Practice and Research Clinical Anaesthesiology* 2005;19:461-474.
3. Hans P, Bonhomme V: The rationale for perioperative brain protection. *Eur J Anesth* 2004;21:1-5.
4. Clifton GC, Miller ER, Choi SC, Levin HS, McCauley GC, Smith KR, et al: Lack of effect of induction of hypothermia after acute brain injury. *N Engl J Med* 2001;344:556-563.
5. Peterson K, Carson S, Carney N: Hypothermia treatment for traumatic brain injury: A systematic review and meta-analysis. *J Neurotrauma* 2008;25:62-71.
6. Hypothermia after Cardiac Arrest Study Group: Mild therapeutic hypothermia to improve the neurologic outcome after cardiac arrest. *N Engl J Med* 2002;346:549-556.
7. Bernard SA, Gray TW, Buist MD, Jones, BM, Silvester W, Gutteridge G, Smith K: Treatment of comatose survivors of out-of-hospital cardiac arrest with induced hypothermia. *N Engl J Med* 2002;346:557-563.
8. Kammersgaard LP, Jørgensen HS, Rungby JA, Reith J, Nakayama H, Weber UJ, et al: Admission body temperature predicts long-term mortality after acute stroke. *Stroke* 2002;33:1759-1762.
9. Grigore AM, Grocott HP, Mathew JP, Phillips-Bute B, Stanley TO, Butler A, et al, and the Neurologic Outcome Research Group of the Duke Heart Center: The rewarming rate and increased peak temperature alter neurocognitive outcome after cardiac surgery. *Anesth Analg* 2002;94:4-10.
10. Van den Berghe G, Wouters P, Weekers F, Verwaest C, Bruyninckx F, Schetz M, et al: Intensive insulin therapy in critically ill patients. *N Engl J Med* 2001;345:1359-1367.
11. Gentile NT, Seftchick MW, Huynh T, Kruus LK, Gaughan J: Decreased mortality by normalizing blood glucose after acute ischemic stroke. *Acad Emerg Med* 2006;13:174-180.
12. Preiser JC, Devos P: Clinical experience with tight glucose control by intensive insulin therapy. *Crit Care Med* 2007;35:S503-S507.
13. CRASH Trial Collaborators: Final results of MRC CRASH, a randomized placebo-controlled trial of intravenous corticosteroid in adults with head injury—outcomes at 6 months. *Lancet* 2005;365:1957-1959.
14. Fukuda S, Warner DS: Cerebral protection. *Br J Anesth* 2007;99:10-17.
15. Vicek M, Schillinger M, Lang W, Lalouschek W, Bur A, Hirchl MM: Association between course of blood pressure within the first 24 hours and functional recovery after acute ischemic stroke. *Ann Emerg Med* 2003;42:619-626.
16. Ahmed N, Wahlgren NG: Effect of blood pressure lowering in the acute phase of total anterior circulation infarcts and other stroke subtypes. *Cerebrovasc Dis* 2003;15:235-243.
17. Müllner M, Sterz F, Binder M, Hellwagner K, Meron G, Herkner H, Laggner A: Arterial blood pressure after human cardiac arrest and neurological recovery. *Stroke* 1996;27:59-62.
18. Gold JP, Charlson ME, Williams-Russo P, Szatrowski TP, Peterson JC, Pirraglia PA, et al: Improvement of outcomes after coronary artery bypass. A randomized trial comparing intraoperative high versus low mean arterial pressure. *J Thorac Cardiovasc Surg* 1995;110:1302-1314.
19. Hogue CW, Palin CA, Arrowsmith JE: Cardipulmonary bypass management and neurologic outcome: An evidence-based appraisal of current practices. *Anesth Analg* 2006;103:21-37.
20. Koerner IP, Brambrink AM: Brain protection by anesthetic agents. *Curr Opin Anesthesiol* 2006;19:481-486.
21. Hoffman WE, Charbel FT, Edelman G, Mukesh M, Ausman JI: Comparison of the effect of etomidate and desflurane on brain tissue gasses and pH during prolonged middle cerebral artery occlusion. *Anesthesiology* 1998;88:1188-1194.
22. Messick JM, Casement B, Sharbrough FW, Milde LN, Michenfekder JD, Sundt TM: Correlation of regional cerebral blood flow (rCBF) with EEG changes during isoflurane anesthesia for carotid endarterectomy: Critical rCBF. *Anesthesiology* 1987;66:344-349.
23. Michenfelder JD, Sundt TM, Fode N, Sharbrough FW: Isoflurane when compared to enflurane and halothane decreases the frequency of cerebral ischemia during carotid endarterectomy. *Anesthesiology* 1987;67:336-340.
24. Lei B, Cottrell JE, Kass IS: Neuroprotective effect of low-dose lidocaine in rat model of transient focal verebral ischemia. *Anesthesiology* 2001;95:445-451.

25. Lei B, Popp S, Capuano-Waters C, Cottrell JE, Kass IS: Lidocaine attenuates apoptosis in the ischemic penumbra and reduces infarct size after transient focal cerebral ischemia in rats. *Neuroscience* 2004;125:691-701.

26. Seyfried FJ, Adachi N, Arai T: Suppression of energy requirement by lidocaine in the ischemic mouse brain. *J Neurosurg Anesthesiol* 2005;17:75-81.

27. Mitchell S, Pellet O, Gorman DF: Cerebral protection by lidocaine during cardiac operations. *Ann Thorac Surg* 1999;67:1117-1124.

28. Wang D, Wu X, Ki J, Xiao F, Liu X, Meng M: The effect of lidocaine on early postoperative cognitive dysfunction after coronary artery bypass surgery. *Anesth Analg* 2002;95:1134-1141.

29. Nussmeier NA, Arlund C, Slogoff S: Neuropsychiatric complications after cardiopulmonary bypass: Cerebral protection by a barbiturate. *Anesthesiology* 1986;64:165-170.

30. Zaidan JR, Klochany A, Martin WM, Ziegler JS, Harless DM, Andrews RB: Effect of thiopental on neurologic outcome following coronary artery bypass grafting. *Anesthesiology* 1991;74: 406-411.

31. Roach GW, Newman MF, Murkin JM, Martzke J, Ruskin A, Li J, et al: Ineffectiveness of burst suppression therapy in mitigating perioperative cerebrovascular dysfunction. Multicenter Study of Perioperative Ischemia (McSPI) Research Group. *Anesthesiology* 1999;90:1255-1264.

32. Kanbak M, Saricaoglu F, Avci A, Ocal T, Koray Z, Aypar U: Propofol offers no advantage over isuflurane anesthesia for cerebral protection during cardiopulmonary bypass: A preliminary study of S-100 protein levels. *Can J Anesth* 2004;51:712-717.

33. Nagles W, Demeyere R, Van Hemelrijck J, Vandenbussche E, Gijbels K, Vandermeersch E: Evaluation of neuroprotective effects of S(+)-ketamine during open-heart surgery. *Anesth Analg* 2004;98:1595-1603.

34. Arrowsmith JE, Harrison MJG, Newman SP, Stygall J, Timberlake N, Pugsley WB: Neuroprotection of brain during cardiopulmonary bypass. A randomized trial of remacemide during coronary artery bypass in 171 patients. *Stroke* 1998;29:2357-2362.

35. Mathew JP, Sherman SK, White WD, Fitch JCK, Chen JC, Bell L, Newman MF: Preliminary report of the effects of complement suppression with pexelizumab on neurocognitive decline after coronary artery bypass graft surgery. *Stroke* 2004;35:2335-2339.

36. Ehrenreich H, Hasselblatt M, Dembowski C, Cepek L, Lewczuk P, Stiefel M, et al: Erythropoietin therapy for acute stroke is both safe and beneficial. *Molec Med* 2002;8:495-505.

37. Wareing TH, Dávila-Román VG, Barzilia B, Murphy SF, Kouchoukos NT: Management of the severely atherosclerotic ascending aorta during cardiac operations. A strategy for detection and treatment. *J Thorac Cardiovasc Surg* 1992;103:453-462.

38. Royse AG, Royse CF, Ajani AE, Symes E, Maruff P, Karagiannis S, et al: Reduced neuropsychological dysfunction using epiaortic echocardiography and the exclusive Y graft. *Ann Thorac Surg* 2000;69:1431-1438.

39. Murkin JM, Adams SJ, Novick RJ, Quantz M, Bainbridge D, Iglesias I, et al: Monitoring brain oxygen saturation during coronary bypass surgery: A randomized, prospective study. *Anesth Analg* 2007;104:51-58.

40. International Liaison Committee on Resuscitation: Therapeutic hypothermia after cardiac arrest. An advisory statement by the Advanced Life Support Task Force of the International Liaison Committee on Resuscitation. *Circulation* 2003;108:118-121.

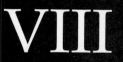

OBSTETRIC ANESTHESIA

66 Anesthesia for Cesarean Delivery—Regional or General?

Yaakov Beilin, MD

INTRODUCTION

The cesarean delivery rate has been steadily increasing and in 2005 climbed above 30%.[1] The most common indications for cesarean delivery include prior cesarean delivery, dystocia, breech, multiple gestation, and fetal distress. The cesarean section rate is likely to increase further as women are requesting an elective cesarean delivery even for their first delivery, also known as "cesarean on demand." Although controversial, the American College of Obstetricians and Gynecologists (ACOG) has opined that it is ethical for an obstetrician to perform an elective cesarean delivery if the physician believes that the cesarean delivery promotes the health of the mother and fetus more than a vaginal delivery.[2] The selection of regional or general anesthesia for cesarean delivery depends on the experience of the anesthesiologist, past medical history of the patient, and the indication for and urgency of the cesarean delivery. The anesthetic considerations will be discussed separately for the elective case, where there is little controversy that regional anesthesia is the preferred technique, and the emergent case, where controversy exists.

OPTIONS/THERAPIES

When choosing regional or general anesthesia for cesarean delivery, one must consider both maternal and neonatal outcome. Maternal outcome studies have primarily focused on maternal mortality, and neonatal outcome studies have focused on umbilical cord pH, Apgar score, the need for ventilatory assistance at birth, and neurobehavior scores.

EVIDENCE

Elective Cesarean Delivery

Maternal outcome is better with regional anesthesia than with general anesthesia. Hawkins and colleagues[3] found that the case fatality rate for cesarean delivery was 32 per million when general anesthesia was used but only 2 per million when regional anesthesia was used. The reason for this difference is primarily related to the respiratory system of the parturient. Difficult tracheal intubation is 10 times more difficult in the parturient than in the general population,[4]

hypoxemia develops quickly during periods of apnea, and the parturient is at increased risk for pulmonary aspiration. Furthermore, airway management experience is decreasing among U.S.-trained physicians. In a recent survey of anesthesiology residents training in the United States, 13% had never intubated the trachea of a parturient during their residency training and 65% performed fewer than three tracheal intubations.[5] Hawthorne and colleagues[6] reviewed the incidence of failed intubation on their maternity unit. They found that the incidence of failed tracheal intubation, defined as the inability to successfully intubate the trachea with one dose of succinylcholine thus necessitating initiation of the failed intubation protocol, increased from 1 in 250 in 1984 to 1 in 300 in 1994. In a recent review of maternal mortality causes, Mhyre and colleagues[7] found that "airway problems" is still a leading cause of maternal mortality, but that the problems occurred during emergence or tracheal extubation and not during tracheal intubation.

Neonatal outcome is also better when regional anesthesia is used. A number of retrospective studies have evaluated the effect of anesthetic technique on neonatal outcome, and essentially all have found the same results.[88-12] In one of the larger studies, Roberts and colleagues[10] reviewed the medical records of women who underwent an elective cesarean delivery. There were 1601 women in their database of which 371 had a general anesthetic, 286 had an epidural anesthetic, 231 had a spinal anesthetic, and 659 had a combined spinal-epidural anesthetic. They found that umbilical artery pH was greater in the neonate delivered with general anesthesia, but clinical parameters (e.g., Apgar score and the need for assisted ventilation) were better when regional anesthesia was used. The acidemia found in the regional anesthesia groups was greatest in the spinal group and lowest in the epidural group. However, it should be noted that the acidemia was almost always (80%) respiratory in nature, which is not associated with an increase in neonatal complications. For these reasons, most elective cesarean deliveries in the United States are now performed under regional anesthesia.[13] A flaw with this study and most of the other retrospective ones was that the amount of prehydration before the regional anesthetic,[14] the duration of the hypotension,[15] and the duration from uterine incision until delivery,[16] all important variables with regard to the development of fetal acidemia, were not controlled.

This author is aware of four prospective, randomized studies evaluating anesthetic technique on neonatal outcome.[17-20] In only one of these studies was the fetal pH lower in the regional versus the general anesthesia group, but even in that study there were no infants with fetal acidemia as defined by a pH less than 7.20.[20] In the other three studies, acid-base status was either better in the spinal anesthesia group[17,18] or unchanged.[19] All the investigators either found no difference in Apgar scores or greater Apgar scores in the regional anesthesia group (Table 66-1).

Spinal anesthesia is commonly used rather than epidural anesthesia for elective cesarean delivery because with spinal anesthesia the speed of onset is quicker and the failure rate is lower. Riley and colleagues[21] found that spinal anesthesia leads to a more efficient utilization of operating room time than epidural anesthesia because time from entering the operating room until skin incision is faster with spinal anesthesia. The most common complication from spinal anesthesia is hypotension, which may explain the decreased umbilical artery pH as compared with both epidural and general anesthesia.[15]

Numerous techniques have been attempted to prevent hypotension following spinal anesthesia, with varying success. The most important preventive measure is to ensure left uterine displacement so as to avoid the supine hypotensive syndrome.[22] Prehydration is not necessarily an effective measure to prevent hypotension. Rout and colleagues[23] randomized women to receive no prehydration or 20 mL/kg of a crystalloid before cesarean delivery. They found a smaller incidence of hypotension in the prehydrated group (55%) as compared with the control group (71%), but the total amount of fluid, the total amount of ephedrine, and the severity of the hypotension did not differ between groups. Also, there was still a fair amount of hypotension in the prehydrated group. Park and

Table 66-1   Results of Studies Comparing Anesthetic Techniques for Elective Cesarean Delivery

Author	Design	Average UA Ph Spin/Epid/GA	UA Ph < 7.20 Spin/Epid/GA %	Avg 1 min Apgar Spin/Epid/GA	Avg 5 min Apgar Spin/Epid/GA	Apgar 1 min <7 Spinal/Epid/GA %	Apgar 5 min <7 Spinal/Epidl/GA %	Comment
Evans[8] (1989)	Retro	NA/7.28/7.28	NA/4.8/3.9	NA/NA/NA	NA/NA/NA	NA/4.0/22	NA/0/6	
Ratcliffe[9] (1993)	Retro	7.25/7.29/7.3	NA/NA/NA	NA/NA/NA	NA/NA/NA	7/4/25	0/0/9	
Roberts[10] (1995)	Retro	NA/NA/NA	34/10/4	8/8/9‡	9/9/9‡	0/0/1†	0/0/0†	Assisted ventilation at birth required more often with GA
Mueller[11] (1997)	Retro	NA/NA/NA	13.9/14.0/7.8	NA/NA/NA	NA/NA/NA	NA/NA/NA	2.2/2.9/4.5*	Assisted ventilation at birth required more often with GA
Sendag[12] (1999)	Retro	NA/7.32/7.35	NA/5/0	NA/8.9/8.4	NA/9.9/9.8	NA/0/0†	NA/0/0	
Dick[17] (1992)	Prosp	NA/7.30/7.27	NA/NA/NA	NA/NA/NA	NA/NA/NA	NA/38/13	NA/8/0	Assisted ventilation at birth required more often with GA
Kolatat[18] (1999)	Prosp	7.30/7.31/7.29	NA/NA/NA	8.2/8.3/6.7	9.8/9.7/9.2	NA/NA/NA	NA/NA/NA	1 and 5 min Apgar similar but numbers not reported
Kavak[19] (2001)	Prosp	7.24/NA/7.25	7.2/NA/7.2	8.9/NA/8.7	9.9/NA/9.9	NA/NA/NA	0/NA/0	
Petropoulos[20] (2003)	Prosp	7.26/7.28/7.29	0/0/0	NA/NA/NA	NA/NA/NA	5/4/6	3/3/4	

*Apgar <8.
†Apgar <4.
‡Median.
Epid, epidural; *GA*, general anesthesia; *min*, minute; *NA*, not applicable; *Prosp*, prospective; *Retro*, retrospective; *Spin*, spinal; *UA*, umbilical artery.

colleagues[24] randomized women to receive 10, 20, or 30 mL/kg of crystalloid before cesarean delivery. They found less hypotension as the amount of prehydration increased (67% versus 56% versus 47% in the 10, 20, and 30 mL/kg groups, respectively) that did not reach statistical significance. But even in those who received 30 mL/kg of crystalloid prehydration there was almost a 50% incidence of hypotension. Prehydration is still recommended because neonatal outcome, Apgar score, and the percentage of neonates with a normal acid-base balance is improved when the mother is prehydrated.[14] Colloid prehydration may be more promising and deserves further study. Ueyama and colleagues[25] randomized women undergoing cesarean delivery to receive either 1500 mL of lactated Ringer's or 500 mL or 1000 mL of a colloid solution (hydroxyethylstarch). The incidence of hypotension was 75% in those who received lactated Ringer's, 58% in those who received 500 mL of hydroxyethylstarch, and only 17% in those who received 1000 mL of hydroxyethylstarch. Prophylactic intravenous ephedrine[26] or phenylephrine[27] before spinal anesthetic placement has been studied to prevent hypotension, and is generally not recommended because of the risk of reactive hypertension.[28]

Emergency Cesarean Delivery

Maternal outcome is also improved when regional anesthesia is used for an emergent cesarean delivery as compared with an elective cesarean delivery because of the difficulty with tracheal intubation. Indeed, airway concerns during an emergency cesarean delivery are even greater than in the elective scenario. Endler and colleagues[29] reviewed maternal deaths in the state of Michigan from 1972 through 1984. They found that the emergent situation was a risk factor for difficult tracheal intubation and that in 11 of 15 patients the inability to successfully intubate the trachea was the principal cause of death.

Neonatal outcome for the emergent cesarean delivery is also better with regional anesthesia than with general anesthesia. The author is aware of four studies, three retrospective studies[30-32] and one prospective study,[33] that addressed anesthetic technique during urgent cesarean delivery. The authors of the three retrospective studies all found the incidence of low Apgar scores at 1 and 5 minutes and the incidence of neonates requiring assisted ventilation greater in those who received general anesthesia. Bowring and colleagues[32] also found that umbilical cord pH was the same (pH = 7.22) in those who received regional and general anesthesia. In the only prospective and partially randomized study, Marx and colleagues[33] evaluated neonatal outcome in women who underwent a cesarean delivery for fetal distress. The choice of anesthetic, general, spinal, or extension of an existing epidural catheter, was made by the mother immediately before administration of the anesthetic. There were 126 women in the study of whom 71 chose general anesthesia, 33 chose spinal anesthesia, and 22 chose extension of their epidural anesthetic. The time from decision to perform a stat cesarean delivery until skin incision was less than 20 minutes in all patients. However, the time from decision to perform the cesarean delivery until skin incision was greater in the regional anesthesia groups as compared with the general anesthesia group. Despite this difference in starting time, they were unable to detect a significant difference in 5-minute Apgar scores or umbilical arterial or venous pH among the three groups, but the 1-minute Apgar score was greater in the regional anesthesia groups than in the general anesthesia group (Table 66-2).

A potential flaw with the Marx study is that many of the cases that were classified as "stat" were not true emergencies and therefore the results should not be extrapolated to the true emergency. Indeed, the findings of Marx and colleagues[33] are controversial and many contend that general anesthesia is the preferred technique for a true emergency cesarean delivery. The concern is

Table 66-2 Results of Studies Comparing Anesthetic Techniques for Emergent Cesarean Delivery

Author	Design	n	Average UA PH	Apgar 1 min <8	Apgar 5 min <8	Comment
		Spinal/Epid/GA	*Spinal/Epid/GA %*	*Spinal/Epid/GA %*	*Spinal/Epidl/GA %*	
Gale[30] (1982)	Retro	NA/NA/NA	NA/NA/NA	NA/NA/NA	NA/NA/NA	Assisted ventilation at birth required more often with GA
Ong[31] (1989) Bowring[32] (2006)	Retro Retro	Total = 390 With few spinal Regional = 57 General = 17	NA/NA/NA Regional = 7.22 General = 7.22	NA/18/43* NA	NA/3/8* Regional = 12% General = 5%	Tracheal intubation at birth and neonatal death more often with GA; ICU admission greater in the GA group
Marx[33] (1984)	Prosp	33/22/71	Regional = 7.22 General = 7.22	21/23/49	3/0/15	Only partia lly randomized study

*Apgar <5.
Epid, epidural; *GA*, general anesthesia; *ICU*, intensive care unit; *Prosp*, prospective; *Retro*, retrospective; *UA*, umbilical artery.

related to the greater time it may take to administer a regional anesthetic as compared with a general anesthetic in a case where time is of the essence.

AREAS OF UNCERTAINTY

Most clinicians agree that for elective cesarean delivery, regional anesthesia is safer than general anesthesia for both the mother and the baby and is therefore the preferred technique. The area of uncertainty is in regard to emergent cesarean delivery. There are two concerns when administering a spinal anesthetic for emergent cesarean delivery. One is that the placement of a spinal anesthetic may take "too long," and the second is that hypotension from a spinal anesthetic may further worsen uteroplacental blood flow and neonatal outcome. However, choosing a general anesthetic should not be taken lightly, because the leading cause of maternal morbidity and mortality remains failed endotracheal intubation and aspiration pneumonia.

Obstetricians tend to use the terminology "emergent cesarean delivery" to describe many different scenarios where there is concern about the fetus. A more useful classification may be to further classify the emergency as either "urgent" or "stat." An urgent cesarean delivery is one where there is some concern about the fetus and the baby should be delivered before there is further deterioration, such as the case where there are variable fetal heart rate decelerations with prompt recovery. A "stat" cesarean delivery is one where time is of the essence such as a cord prolapse with a slow fetal heart rate or maternal hemorrhage. The anesthetic choice will differ based on whether the indication for the emergent cesarean delivery is urgent or stat.

GUIDELINES

There are two guidelines published by the American College of Obstetricians and Gynecologists (ACOG), one in conjunction with the American Academy of Pediatrics (AAP), that address the issue of emergent cesarean deliveries.[34,35] The first guideline[34] states that hospitals should have the capability of initiating a cesarean delivery within 30 minutes. The second guideline[35] asserts in part that (1) failed intubation and pulmonary aspiration is the leading cause of morbidity and mortality for the mother; (2) the obstetrician should be able to identify those factors that place the patient at greater risk for general anesthesia and should request an antepartum anesthesia consultation; (3) strategies to reduce the need for emergency induction of general anesthesia should be developed, including the early placement of an epidural anesthetic; (4) the term *fetal distress* is imprecise, and a better term is *nonreassuring fetal heart rate pattern*; and (5) a cesarean delivery for a nonreassuring fetal heart rate pattern does not preclude the use of regional anesthesia. The American Society of Anesthe-

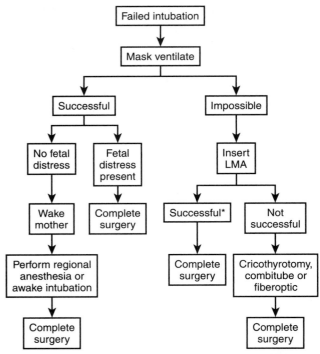

Figure 66-1. Management of the Unanticipated Difficult Airway. LMA, laryngeal mask airway. *Consider endotracheal intubation through the LMA.

siologists has developed "Practice Guidelines for Management of the Difficult Airway."[36] These parameters are an excellent guide to the management of the unanticipated difficult endotracheal intubation, and a plan based on these guidelines is summarized in Figure 66-1.

AUTHOR'S RECOMMENDATIONS

ELECTIVE CESAREAN DELIVERY (TABLE 66-3)

Spinal anesthesia can be used for the majority of elective cesarean deliveries. Hyperbaric bupivacaine 0.75%, 1.5 mL, will reliably give a T-4 level of anesthesia. De Simone and colleagues[37] compared the duration, highest dermatomal level achieved, and success rate of 1.5 mL of bupivacaine 0.75% versus 2 mL of the same drug. They found that the quality of analgesia was satisfactory in all patients, but the duration of anesthesia was longer in those who received 2 mL as compared with those who received 1.5 mL (162 versus 140 min). The highest dermatomal level achieved was on average 2.2 spinal segments higher in those who received the 2 mL dose, with 7 of 12 in that same group achieving a cervical level of anesthesia. Cervical levels of anesthesia are not needed for a cesarean delivery and may be uncomfortable for the patient, which is why this author uses 1.5 mL of hyperbaric bupivacaine.

Continued

Some opt to use the combined spinal epidural technique for cesarean delivery in case the procedure is prolonged. This decision should be made on an individual basis taking into account the speed of the surgeon and specific patient factors, for example, repeat cesarean delivery or previous abdominal procedures.

Epidural anesthesia is generally reserved for the parturient who has an epidural in situ, or where there may be a benefit to slow titration of local anesthetic such as a woman with severe hypertension or valvular heart disease. Lidocaine 2% with epinephrine is a commonly used epidural anesthetic regimen. General anesthesia is never used unless the patient refuses a regional anesthetic technique.

EMERGENCY CESAREAN DELIVERY

When the indication is urgent (not stat), this author uses a spinal anesthetic or an epidural in situ. When administering a spinal anesthetic for urgent cesarean delivery, the fetal tracing should be continuously monitored in the operating room. Do not wait for complete prehydration before placing the spinal anesthetic. Bupivacaine 0.75% (1.5 mL) will confer adequate and quick analgesia for the cesarean delivery. This author encourages early placement of an epidural anesthetic in a woman likely to require a cesarean delivery or in a woman in whom general anesthesia may be deleterious (history of a difficult airway). Lidocaine 2% with 1:200,000 epinephrine or 2-chloroprocaine 3% can be used to provide safe and rapid anesthesia for the cesarean delivery.

When confronted with a stat cesarean delivery (time is of the essence), the anesthesiologist must accomplish the anesthetic quickly and efficiently and must take into account both the mother and the fetus. Maternal concerns include any preexisting medical condition and a full evaluation of the airway. A nonparticulate antacid should be administered. Airway evaluation should start with an external examination of the head and neck. A receding mandible (micrognathia) and other external anomalies should be noted. Difficulty in neck extension and flexion may predict suboptimal alignment of the oral, pharyngeal, and laryngeal axes. The relation of the size of the tongue to the oral cavity can be estimated using the Mallampati classification. Combining all this information will help the clinician decide if a difficult tracheal intubation is anticipated. Clinical experience is the key to making this decision. If the mother has a known or suspected difficult airway, either an awake intubation should be performed or a spinal anesthetic should be used. However, under *no* circumstance should the patient receive a general anesthetic before the airway is secured. If the mother does not have a suspected difficult airway, this author would proceed with a general anesthetic.

General endotracheal anesthesia must be accomplished in a rapid-sequence manner (Table 66-4). After preoxygenation and application of cricoid pressure, general anesthesia proceeds with an induction agent and succinylcholine for paralysis. Although subtle differences exist among induction agents in regard to maternal and neonatal outcome, they are essentially all safe. This author commonly uses either thiopental or etomidate. Anesthesia is maintained with 50% N_2O in O_2 and 0.3% to 0.5% of a potent inhaled anesthetic agent to ensure amnesia.

Table 66-3 A Suggested Technique for Performing Regional Anesthesia for Elective Cesarean Delivery

1. Check the anesthesia machine. Prepare resuscitative equipment and drugs.
2. Administer a nonparticulate antacid by mouth.
3. Transport to the operating room with left uterine displacement.
4. Prehydrate with 1000-1500 mL crystalloid solution intravenously.
5. Place routine monitors including blood pressure cuff, electrocardiogram (ECG), and pulse oximeter.
6. Administer oxygen via face mask.
7. **For spinal anesthesia**: Use small-gauge (25-27) pencil-point needle. Administer 1.5 mL of 0.75% hyperbaric bupivacaine with 0.1-0.5 mL of preservative-free morphine sulfate.
8. **For epidural anesthesia**: After placing epidural catheter, administer 3 mL of 2% lidocaine with epinephrine 1:200,000 as a test dose. Wait 5 minutes, observing for signs of either intravascular or subarachnoid injection. After confirming catheter position, inject same medication in 5-mL increments, no more frequently than every 5 minutes, until Thoracic-4 level of anesthesia is achieved.
9. Monitor vital signs every 2 minutes for the first 20 minutes and then every 5 minutes thereafter, if stable.
10. If hypotension occurs, administer 250-500 mL boluses of additional crystalloid, ephedrine in 5-mg increments, or phenylephrine in 50-mcg doses until blood pressure returns to normal.

Table 66-4 A Suggested Method of Performing a General Anesthetic for Stat Cesarean Delivery

1. Check the anesthesia machine. Prepare resuscitative equipment and drugs.
2. Administer a nonparticulate antacid by mouth
3. Rapidly prehydrate with 1000-1500 mL crystalloid.
4. Transport to the operating room with left uterine displacement.
5. Place routine monitors including blood pressure cuff, ECG, and pulse oximeter.
6. Administer oxygen via face mask.
7. After denitrogenation induce anesthesia with thiamylal 4 mg/kg followed by succinylcholine, 100 mg, with cricoid pressure. Do not administer a defasciculating dose of a nondepolarizing agent.
8. Maintain anesthesia with 50% N_2O, O_2, and 0.3%-0.5% isoflurane or 0.5%-0.7% enflurane until the baby is delivered. After delivery of the baby, administer fentanyl 100 mcg and increase N_2O concentration to 70%. Keep concentration of halogenated agent below 0.5 MAC to avoid uterine relaxation.
9. Administer neostigmine 0.04-0.07 mg/kg and glycopyrrolate 0.01-0.15 mg/kg to antagonize residual neuromuscular blockade.
10. Tracheally extubate patient when fully awake.

REFERENCES

1. Ecker JL, Frigoletto FD Jr: Cesarean delivery and the risk-benefit calculus. *N Engl J Med* 2007;356:885-888.
2. American College of Obstetricians and Gynecologists: Surgery and patient choice. In *Ethics in obstetrics and gynecology*, ed 2. Washington, DC, American College of Obstetricians and Gynecologists, 2004, pp 21-25.
3. Hawkins JL, Koonin LM, Palmer SK, Gibbs CP: Anesthesia-related deaths during obstetric delivery in the United States, 1979-1990. *Anesthesiology* 1997;86:277-284.
4. Samsoon GL, Young JR: Difficult tracheal intubation: A retrospective study. *Anaesthesia* 1987;42:487-490.
5. Bhavani-Shankar K, Camann W: General anesthesia for cesarean delivery. The status of current resident training and experience. *Anesthesiology* 2001;94:A31.
6. Hawthorne L, Wilson R, Lyons G, Dresner M: Failed intubation revisited: 17-yr experience in a teaching maternity unit. *Br J Anaesth* 1996;76:680-684.
7. Mhyre JM, Riesner MN, Polley LS, Naughton NN: A series of anesthesia-related maternal deaths in Michigan, 1985-2003. *Anesthesiology* 2007;106:1082-1084.
8. Evans CM, Murphy JF, Gray OP, Rosen M: Epidural versus general anaesthesia for elective caesarean section. Effect on Apgar score and acid-base status of the newborn. *Anaesthesia* 1989;44:778-782.
9. Ratcliffe FM, Evans JM: Neonatal well being after elective caesarean delivery with general, spinal, and epidural anaesthesia. *Eur J Anaesthesiol* 1993;10:175-181.
10. Roberts SW, Leveno KJ, Sidawi JE, et al: Fetal acidemia associated with regional anesthesia for elective cesarean delivery. *Obstet Gynecol* 1995;85:79-83.
11. Mueller MD, Bruhwiler H, Schupfer GK, Luscher KP: Higher rate of fetal acidemia after regional anesthesia for elective cesarean delivery. *Obstet Gynecol* 1997;90:131-134.
12. Sendag F, Terek C, Oztekin K, Sagol S, Asena U: Comparison of epidural and general anaesthesia for elective caesarean delivery according to the effects of Apgar scores and acid-base status. *Aust N Z J Obstet Gynaecol* 1999;39:464-468.
13. Hawkins JL, Gibbs CP, Orleans M, et al: Obstetric anesthesia work force survey, 1981 versus 1992. *Anesthesiology* 1997;87:135-143.
14. Caritis SN, Abouleish E, Edelstone DI, Mueller-Heubach E: Fetal acid-base state following spinal or epidural anesthesia for cesarean section. *Obstet Gynecol* 1980;56:610-615.
15. Corke BC, Datta S, Ostheimer GW, Weiss JB, Alper MH: Spinal anaesthesia for caesarean section. The influence of hypotension on neonatal outcome. *Anaesthesia* 1982;37:658-662.
16. Datta S, Brown WU Jr, Ostheimer GW, Weiss JB, Alper MH: Epidural anesthesia for cesarean section in diabetic parturients: Maternal and neonatal acid-base status and bupivacaine concentration. *Anesth Analg* 1981;60:574-578.
17. Dick W, Traub E, Kraus H, Tollner U, Burghard R, Muck J: General anaesthesia versus epidural anaesthesia for primary caesarean section—a comparative study. *Eur J Anaesthesiol* 1992; 9:15-21.
18. Kolatat T, Somboonnanonda A, Lertakyamanee J, Chinachot T, Tritrakarn T, Muangkasem J: Effects of general and regional anesthesia on the neonate (a prospective, randomized trial). *J Med Assoc Thai* 1999;82:40-45.
19. Kavak ZN, Basgul A, Ceyhan N: Short-term outcome of newborn infants: Spinal versus general anesthesia for elective cesarean section. A prospective randomized study. *Eur J Obstet Gynecol Reprod Biol* 2001;100:50-54.
20. Petropoulos G, Siristatidis C, Salamalekis E, Creatsas G: Spinal and epidural versus general anesthesia for elective cesarean section at term: Effect on the acid-base status of the mother and newborn. *J Matern Fetal Neonatal Med* 2003;13:260-266.
21. Riley ET, Cohen SE, Macario A, et al: Spinal versus epidural anesthesia for cesarean section: A comparison of time efficiency, costs, charges, and complications. *Anesth Analg* 1995;80:709-712.
22. Scott DB: Inferior vena caval occlusion in late pregnancy and its importance in anaesthesia. *Br J Anaesth* 1968;40:120-128.
23. Rout CC, Rocke DA, Levin J, et al: A reevaluation of the role of crystalloid preload in the prevention of hypotension associated with spinal anesthesia for elective cesarean section. *Anesthesiology* 1993;79:262-269.
24. Park GE, Hauch MA, Curlin F, et al: The effects of varying volumes of crystalloid administration before cesarean delivery on maternal hemodynamics and colloid osmotic pressure. *Anesth Analg* 1996;83:299-303.
25. Ueyama H, He YL, Tanigami H, et al: Effects of crystalloid and colloid preload on blood volume in the parturient undergoing spinal anesthesia for elective cesarean section. *Anesthesiology* 1999;91:1571-1576.
26. Kee WD, Khaw KS, Lee BB, et al: A dose-response study of prophylactic intravenous ephedrine for the prevention of hypotension during spinal anesthesia for cesarean delivery. *Anesth Analg* 2000;90:1390-1395.
27. Kee WD, Khaw KS, Ng FF: Prevention of hypotension during spinal anesthesia for cesarean delivery: An effective technique using combination phenylephrine infusion and crystalloid cohydration. *Anesthesiology* 2005;103:744-750.
28. Beilin Y: The treatment should not be worse than the disease. *Anesthesiology* 2006;104:1348-1349.
29. Endler GC, Mariona FG, Sokol RJ, Stevenson LB: Anesthesia-related maternal mortality in Michigan, 1972 to 1984. *Am J Obstet Gynecol* 1988;159:187-193.
30. Gale R, Zalkinder-Luboshitz I, Slater PE: Increased neonatal risk from the use of general anesthesia in emergency cesarean section. A retrospective analysis of 374 cases. *J Reprod Med* 1982;27:715-719.
31. Ong BY, Cohen MM, Palahniuk RJ: Anesthesia for cesarean section—effects on neonates. *Anesth Analg* 1989;68:270-275.
32. Bowring J, Fraser N, Vause S, Heazell AE: Is regional anaesthesia better than general anaesthesia for caesarean section? *J Obstet Gynaecol* 2006;26:433-434.
33. Marx GF, Luykx WM, Cohen S: Fetal-neonatal status following caesarean section for fetal distress. *Br J Anaesth* 1984;56:1009-1013.
34. Hauth JC, Merenstein GB, editors: *Guidelines for perinatal care*, ed 4. Elk Grove Village, IL: American Academy of Pediatrics and American College of Obstetricians and Gynecologists, 1997, p 112.
35. American College of Obstetricians and Gynecologists Committee on Obstetrics: Maternal and fetal medicine. Anesthesia for emergency deliveries. ACOG Committee Opinion no. 104. Washington, DC, 1992. (This opinion was reaffirmed in 1998.)
36. Task Force Members: Practice guidelines for management of the difficult airway. A report by the American Society of Anesthesiologists Task Force on Management of the Difficult Airway. *Anesthesiology* 1993;78:597-602.
37. De Simone CA, Leighton BL, Norris MC: Spinal anesthesia for cesarean delivery. A comparison of two doses of hyperbaric bupivacaine. *Reg Anesth* 1995;20:90-94.

67 When Should a Combined Spinal-Epidural (CSE) Be Used?

Rolf A. Schlichter, MD, and Valerie A. Arkoosh, MD

INTRODUCTION

The combined spinal-epidural (CSE) technique produces the reliable and rapid onset of spinal anesthesia combined with the flexibility to extend the height and duration of a block provided by continuous epidural anesthesia. CSE has become a popular technique in both obstetrics and orthopedic surgery. CSE was originally described in 1979 by Curelaru,[1] and in 1981 by Brownridge,[2] as a double-segment technique with the epidural and spinal procedures performed at different interspaces of the lumbar spine. Advances in needle design led to the more popular and practical single-segment technique (SST) in use today. In 1982 clinicians described the use of the SST for lower limb surgery and in 1984 for cesarean section.[3,4]

The SST involves locating the epidural space with either a standard or a specialized epidural needle using the loss of resistance technique. Once the epidural space has been identified, a small-gauge spinal needle is introduced via the epidural needle into the cerebrospinal fluid. A spinal dose of opioid or local anesthetic (or both) is given through the spinal needle, and then the spinal needle is removed. An epidural catheter is then inserted through the epidural needle to the appropriate depth. A specialized epidural needle with a back hole is available that enables the spinal needle to exit the epidural needle in the horizontal plane perpendicular to the dura, rather than through the curved tip of a standard epidural needle. The technique can be performed in the sitting or lateral position.

OPTIONS/THERAPIES

The CSE technique is widely used for labor analgesia, anesthesia for cesarean section, lower-extremity orthopedic surgery, and urologic procedures. Once popular, the role of CSE in lower-extremity vascular procedures has declined secondary to the use of antithrombotic and antiplatelet therapies for the treatment of vascular disease.

CSE produces rapid onset of analgesia for the woman in advanced labor while simultaneously maintaining maternal ability to push during the second stage.[5] In early labor, an initial dose of intrathecal opioid alone maintains maternal mobility and may increase the speed of cervical dilation.[6,7] Concurrent placement of the epidural catheter enables additional doses of local anesthetic with or without opioid to produce prolonged labor analgesia or cesarean section anesthesia.

CSE for cesarean section provides the benefit of a quick onset of neuraxial blockade with the ability to use the epidural if the spinal block recedes or the surgery is unexpectedly prolonged. Secondarily, the epidural can be used to provide postoperative analgesia with both low-dose local anesthetics and epidural opioids.

In orthopedic procedures, the CSE technique is used in lower-extremity surgeries, such as total hip and total knee arthroplasties. The technique can be as efficient as a general anesthetic,[8] may reduce the incidence of postoperative deep vein thrombosis,[9] and can be used for postoperative analgesia in the absence of antithrombotic therapy.

The low-dose sequential CSE technique is a modification of the original technique that uses a deliberately subanesthetic intrathecal dose with the expectation of extending the block height by the subsequent epidural injection of either local anesthetic or saline. This technique has been shown to enhance cardiovascular stability in high-risk cases, including pregnant women with severe preeclampsia.[10,11]

CONTRAINDICATIONS

Patients receiving a CSE must be appropriate candidates for a neuraxial technique. Contraindications include patient refusal, coagulopathy, and some infections. American Society of Regional Anesthesia (ASRA) guidelines recommend that a patient have normal coagulation before undergoing instrumentation of the neuraxis.[12] Aspirin or nonsteroidal antiinflammatory agent therapy is not a contraindication; however, other antiplatelet therapies such as clopidogrel require cessation 7 days before undergoing the procedure. Patients taking Coumadin should undergo 5 days without therapy or have a current normal prothrombin time (PT) and international normalized ratio (INR). Patients receiving prophylactic doses of low-molecular-weight heparin (LMWH), such as enoxaparin 30 to 40 IU or dalteparin 5000 IU every 24 hours, must wait 12 hours after the last dose before undergoing neuraxial blockade. Patients receiving therapeutic doses of LMWH, such as enoxaparin 1 mg/kg every 12 hours, enoxaparin 1.5 mg/kg daily, dalteparin 120 U/kg every 12 hours, dalteparin 200 U/kg daily, or tinzaparin 175 U/kg daily, must wait 24 hours from the last dose before receiving a neuraxial block. Subcutaneous heparin is not a contraindication to regional anesthesia.[12]

Evaluating the coagulation status of the obstetric patient can present a special challenge. Pregnancy may be complicated by conditions that lower the platelet count or inhibit platelet function such as preeclampsia, eclampsia, or the syndrome of hemolysis, elevated liver enzymes, and low platelets (HELLP syndrome). Given the hypercoaguable condition of pregnancy, the absolute platelet count is less concerning than the trend in platelet numbers. There is no evidence for a specific platelet count below which neuraxial techniques are contraindicated in the obstetric patient. Thus it would seem, as a practical matter, that a risk/benefit assessment should be undertaken on any pregnant woman with a platelet count of less than $75,000/mm^3$ or with a sudden, substantial drop from her baseline, and an individualized decision reached regarding the safety of a neuraxial technique. Patients with a platelet count less than $75,000/mm^3$ should be examined for stigmata of coagulopathy (easy bruising, petechiae, bleeding from the intravenous site or Foley catheter) before instrumentation. A PT, a partial thrombin time, and a platelet count should be reviewed before proceeding. If any of the aforementioned tests are abnormal, a fibrinogen level and a d-dimer level are useful to assess the patient for the presence of disseminated intravascular coagulation.

Obstetric patients may be receiving anticoagulation therapy for a variety of obstetric or nonobstetric indications. Ideally, women on long-acting anticoagulants (e.g., for deep vein thrombosis prophylaxis or prosthetic heart valves) should be converted from their long-acting therapies (e.g., LMWH) to subcutaneous heparin at 36 weeks of gestational age. A patient on therapeutic LMWH who is in labor must wait a minimum of 24 hours from the last dose before undergoing CSE analgesia or anesthesia.

Patients with infection at the needle insertion site, suspected meningitis (bacterial or viral), or sepsis should not undergo neuraxial blockade. Patients with suspected chorioamnionitis can receive regional anesthesia following the administration of appropriate intravenous antibiotics.[13,14] Parturients with a primary herpes simplex outbreak are at increased risk for herpetic meningitis with neuraxial techniques. Human immunodeficiency virus/acquired immunodeficiency syndrome (HIV/AIDS) is not a contraindication to CSE.[12]

EVIDENCE FAVORING THE USE OF CSE

CSE for Labor Analgesia

The benefits of CSE for labor analgesia have been described in comparison to either traditional epidural or modern low-dose epidural analgesia. These benefits include faster onset of analgesia, better pain relief in advanced labor, improved maternal mobility, and less chance of an instrumented vaginal delivery. Because there is no standard drug regimen for either CSE, traditional, or low-dose epidural analgesia, it is difficult to compare and contrast studies. Nonetheless, a Cochrane Systematic Review, which included data from 19 randomized trials (2658 laboring women), has attempted to assess the evidence behind some of the stated benefits of CSE.[15] This analysis found that analgesic onset is faster with CSE compared with low-dose epidural analgesia, with the likelihood of patient comfort at 10 minutes to be nearly twice as high in patients receiving CSE. This finding is important to the laboring woman rapidly approaching the second stage of labor, for whom both comfort and maintenance of adequate motor strength to push are important therapeutic goals.

Two studies have suggested that the CSE technique has no negative influence on obstetric outcome when administered in very early labor. The first, a randomized study of the combination of intrathecal sufentanil and bupivacaine compared with epidural bupivacaine for early (cervical dilation less than 5 cm) analgesia, demonstrated a faster rate of cervical dilation in parturients receiving CSE analgesia (2.1 cm/hr versus 1 cm/hr; $p = 0.0008$).[5] The parturients receiving CSE analgesia also had a quicker analgesic onset and superior pain scores for 110 minutes compared with the women with epidural analgesia. There was no difference in the rate of cesarean section or instrumental delivery between the two groups.[5] A randomized trial of intrathecal fentanyl (25 mcg) compared with systemic hydromorphone (1 mg intravenously [IV] and 1 mg intramuscularly [IM]) for early (median cervical dilation 2 cm) labor analgesia followed by epidural analgesia in both groups demonstrated that the CSE group experienced superior analgesia, shorter analgesic onset, and a shorter interval to complete cervical dilation (295 versus 385 minutes; $p = 0.001$), and gave birth to infants with higher Apgar scores ($p < 0.01$). There was no difference in rate of cesarean section or instrumental delivery between the two groups.[6] The Cochrane analysis compared the likelihood of an instrumental vaginal delivery in patients receiving CSE, traditional epidural analgesia, and low-dose epidural analgesia. There was no difference between CSE and low-dose epidurals, but the relative risk of 0.82 (95% confidence interval [CI] 0.67 to 1.00) was at the border of favoring CSE over traditional epidurals.[15]

CSE for Cesarean Section

The CSE technique has been associated with positive outcomes and low failure rates when used as the anesthetic technique for cesarean delivery. A controlled study of intrathecal bupivacaine compared with epidural bupivacaine demonstrated that 100% of the women receiving a CSE anesthetic had adequate anesthesia compared with 74% of women receiving epidural anesthesia.[16] The total dose of bupivacaine used was three times higher in women with epidural anesthesia (125 mg) compared with those using the CSE technique (40 mg). Maternal and fetal blood concentrations of bupivacaine were higher in the women with epidural anesthesia (604 mg and 186 mg, respectively) compared with the women with intrathecal anesthesia (205 mg and 45 mg, respectively). There was no difference in Apgar scores, umbilical cord blood gases, or the neonatal neurobehavioral examination between the two groups.[16]

A randomized, prospective study of 120 women comparing CSE with epidural anesthesia assessed both objective outcomes and subjective maternal experience.[17] The women receiving intrathecal bupivacaine and fentanyl had quicker onset of a T4 level of anesthesia (10 versus 16 minutes), a shorter time to surgical incision (29 versus 36 minutes), and more reliable motor blockade (54% versus 11%) than the women receiving epidural lidocaine with epinephrine and fentanyl. Significantly more women in the CSE group reported no pain, lower anxiety, and greater satisfaction than the epidural group. There were no significant differences in incidence of hypotension, nausea, pruritus, post–dural puncture headache (PDPH), or neonatal outcomes between the two groups.[17]

Hypotension can be an important side effect of spinal anesthesia for cesarean section. The CSE technique enables the successful use of small doses of spinal medication coupled with epidural supplementation, if needed.[10,11] A recent study compared the spinal administration of 6.5 mg of hyperbaric bupivacaine combined with sufentanil 2.5 mcg versus 9.5 mg of hyperbaric bupivacaine with sufentanil 2.5 mcg for CSE anesthesia for cesarean delivery. Patients in the high-dose group experienced significantly more hypotension than the low-dose group (68% versus 16%, $p < 0.05$), and significantly more patients required treatment. The anesthetic duration was shorter in the low-dose group, pointing out the necessity of having an epidural catheter in place.[18]

CSE for Orthopedic Surgery

Patients undergoing orthopedic procedures may also benefit from the CSE technique. A retrospective chart review of 62 total hip arthroplasties found that patients undergoing either the CSE technique, single-injection spinal anesthesia, or general anesthesia had the same time interval from anesthesia start to surgical incision (59 minutes) whereas those receiving epidural anesthesia had a longer interval (73 minutes).[8] A randomized controlled study of patients undergoing hip arthroplasty compared time to adequate block and adequacy of muscle relaxation in patients receiving either intrathecal bupivacaine as a single injection, as part of the CSE technique, or through an epidural.[19] Time to adequate block was significantly shorter in the two intrathecal groups, 11 minutes for single-injection spinal and 14 minutes for the CSE technique, compared with 36 minutes for the epidural group. Similarly, muscle relaxation was adequate in 100% of those receiving intrathecal bupivacaine compared with 12% of those receiving epidural bupivacaine. Four of the 25 patients receiving epidural bupivacaine were converted to general anesthesia because of inadequate anesthesia whereas none of the patients receiving intrathecal bupivacaine were. Four of the 25 patients receiving the CSE technique received supplemental bupivacaine via the epidural catheter. There were no differences demonstrated in terms of hemodynamic changes ($p > 0.005$) among the three groups.[19]

CONTROVERSIES

Controversy with the CSE technique has largely centered on the incidence and significance of side effects. For instance, patients who receive a lipid-soluble opioid as part of a CSE technique experience more pruritus than patients who receive a local anesthetic alone or the same opioid by the epidural route.[20] This mu receptor–mediated side effect is not dangerous but can be annoying

to the individual patient. The incidence of pruritus can be reduced with lower doses of intrathecal opioid.[21]

Of greater concern is the observation by some authors of an increased incidence of fetal bradycardia following the CSE technique for labor analgesia. A 2002 meta-analysis of studies conducted in the 1990s, administering higher doses of intrathecal opioids than are generally in use today, found an odds ratio of 1.8 for occurrence of fetal bradycardia within the first 60 minutes of intrathecal opioid administration versus neuraxial analgesia without intrathecal opioids. However, these episodes did not result in an increase in the rate of cesarean deliveries.[21] Also reassuring are the results from the 2007 Cochrane Systematic Review, which found no difference in neonatal outcomes, as measured by neonatal Apgar scores or need for neonatal intensive care unit admission, between CSE and epidural techniques.[15] Dose of intrathecal medication appears to have an impact on the incidence of fetal bradycardia. A randomized controlled (low-dose epidural group) study of 7.5 mcg intrathecal sufentanil alone compared with 1.5 mcg intrathecal sufentanil combined with 2.5 mg bupivacaine found that the lower-dose combination of sufentanil and bupivacaine was associated with a 12% incidence of fetal bradycardia, the low-dose epidural group with an 11% incidence, and the higher-dose sufentanil group with a 24% incidence. There were no differences in maternal pain scores or mobility between the two groups.[21]

Failed epidural is another theoretic concern with the CSE technique. The data from four randomized controlled studies in which epidural failure rate was measured demonstrated an equal or lower failure rate of an epidural when inserted as part of the CSE technique (0.7% to 1.49%) compared with epidural insertion alone (0.7% to 3.18%).[22-24]

Meningitis, including viral, bacterial, and aseptic, has been reported following instrumentation of the epidural and intrathecal space. With proper sterile technique, the incidence has been shown to be 0% to 0.04%.[25,26] There are no data that demonstrate an increased rate of meningitis following the CSE technique compared with other neuraxial techniques.[14]

Since the CSE technique requires dural puncture, PDPH is a possible side effect of this technique. The use of a small-gauge pencil-point needle, however, reduces this risk. In two controlled studies the rate of PDPH after the CSE technique was found to be 0.44% to 1.7%. There was a 0.65% to 1.6% incidence of dural puncture using a 17-gauge epidural needle; however, that dural puncture was associated with a 38% incidence of PDPH.[27,28] It appears that puncture with the larger epidural needle is associated with an increased risk of PDPH versus the smaller pencil-point needle used for the actual spinal.

GUIDELINES

There are currently no formal guidelines published by national societies that specifically address the indications for CSE. However, broader guidelines from two organizations include information about CSE and many of the issues raised in this chapter. The American Society of

Anesthesiologists' "Practice Guidelines for Obstetric Anesthesia" is an excellent resource for best practices in the care of the obstetric patient and supports the use of CSE for both labor analgesia and cesarean delivery.[29] In 2002, the American Society of Regional Anesthesia and Pain Medicine published the results of a consensus conference, "Regional Anesthesia in the Anticoagulated Patient—Defining the Risks."[12] This document is in the process of being updated from the results of the consensus conference held in 2007. Finally, the American Society of Regional Anesthesia and Pain Medicine recently published a series of articles based on the 2004 "Conference on Infectious Complications of Neuraxial Blockade."[30]

AUTHORS' RECOMMENDATIONS

CSE can play a role in any procedure in which rapid onset of analgesia or anesthesia is desirable and the duration of the expected procedure is likely to outlast a single dose of spinal medication, or in which postoperative pain management with an epidural catheter is warranted. The best evidence supporting the use of CSE is derived from the meta-analysis of numerous, relatively small, randomized studies carried out at single institutions. This evidence supports the use of CSE for the following indications. It must be kept in mind, however, that there are inadequate data to demonstrate the difference, if any, between CSE and epidural analgesia for extremely rare events, such as meningitis.

- Labor analgesia—CSE has been shown to be advantageous both very early in labor and in advanced labor. Early in labor, small doses of spinal opioids, with or without local anesthetic, have been associated with excellent maternal pain relief and favorable obstetric outcomes. In advanced labor, CSE reliably produces maternal analgesia while simultaneously maintaining maternal ability to participate in the second stage of labor.
- Cesarean section—CSE is advantageous in any setting where the cesarean section may outlast the duration of a single injection of spinal medication. Low-dose CSE should also be considered for patients in whom hemodynamic stability is a particular concern.
- Orthopedic surgery—CSE can be considered for long procedures, as well as for those patients who would benefit from postoperative epidural analgesia.
- CSE may be associated with an increased risk of fetal bradycardia in the laboring patient. Thus, in the situation where a laboring mother has a fetus already having episodes of fetal bradycardia, an epidural alone may be preferable.

REFERENCES

1. Curelaru I: Long duration of subarachnoid anesthesia with continuous epidural blocks. 1979.
2. Brownridge P: Epidural and subarachnoidal analgesia for elective cesearean section. *Anaesthesia* 1981;36.
3. Coates MB: Combined subarachnoid and epidural techniques. *Anaesthesia* 1982;89-90.
4. Mumtaz MH: Another single space technique for orthopedic surgery. *Anaesthesia* 1982;90.
5. Abouleish A, Abouleish E, Camann W: Combined spinal-epidural analgesia in advanced labour. *Can J Anaesth* 1994;41:575-578.
6. Tsen L et al: Is combined spinal-epidural analgesia associated with more rapid cervical dilatation in nulliparous patients when compared to conventional epidural analgesia? *Anesthesiology* 1999;91:920-925.
7. Wong C et al: The risk of cesarean delivery with neuraxial analgesia given early versus late in labor. *N Engl J Med* 2005;352 (7):655-665.
8. Rosenblatt MA, Czuchlewski D, Hossain S: Combined spinal-epidural anesthesia is an efficient technique for conserving operating room time during total joint replacement. ASA abstract.
9. McNaught, AF, Stocks GM: Epidural volume extension and low-dose sequential combined spinal-epidural blockade: Two ways to reduce spinal dose requirement for caesarean section. *Int J Obstet Anesth* 2007;16:346-353.
10. Rodgers et al: Reduction of postoperative mortality and morbidity with epidural or spinal anaesthesia: Results from overview of randomized trials. *BMJ* 2000;321:1-9.
11. Van de Veld et al: Combined spinal-epidural anesthesia for cesarean delivery: Dose-dependent effects of hyperbaric bupivacaine on maternal hemodynamics. *Anesth Analg* 2006;100:187-190.
12. American Society of Regional Anesthesia and Pain Medicine Consensus Conference: Regional anesthesia in the anticoagulated patient—Defining the risks. American Society of Regional Anesthesia and Pain Medicine, 2002. Available at www.asra.com/consensus-statements/2.html.
13. Carp H, Bailey S: The association between meningitis and dural puncture in bacteremic rats. *Anesthesiology* 1992;76:739-742.
14. Loo CC, Dahlgren G, Irestedt L: Neurological complications in obstetric regional anaesthesia. *Int J Obstet Anesth* 2000;9:99-124.
15. Simmons SW, Cyna AM, Dennis AT, Hughes D: Combined spinal-epidural versus epidural analgesia in labour. *Cochrane Database of Systematic Reviews* 2007, issue 3. Art. no.: CD003401. DOI: 10.1002/14651858.CD003401.pub2.
16. Narinder R et al: Epidural versus combined spinal epidural for cesarean section. *Acta Anaesthesiol Scand* 1988:32:61-66.
17. Davies S et al: Maternal experience during epidural or combined spinal-epidural anesthesia for cesarean section: A prospective, randomized trial. *Anesth Analg* 1997;85:607-613.
18. Van De Velde M et al: Intrathecal sufentanil and fetal heart rate abnormalities: A double blind, double placebo-controlled trial comparing two forms of combined spinal epidural analgesia with epidural analgesia in labor. *Anesth Analg* 2004;98:1153-1159.
19. Holmstrom B: Combined spinal epidural versus spinal and epidural block for orthopaedic surgery. *Can J Anesth* 1993;40:601-606.
20. Norris M et al: Complications of labor analgesia: Epidural versus combined spinal epidural techniques. *Anesth Analg* 1994;79:529-537.
21. Mardirosoff C, Dumont L, Boulvain M, Tramer MR: Fetal bradycardia due to intrathecal opioids for labour analgesia: A systematic review. *Br J Obstet Gynaecol* 2002;109:274-281.
22. Eappen S, Blinn A, Segal S: Incidence of epidural catheter replacement in parturients, a retrospective chart review. *Int J Obstet Aneth* 1998;7:220-225.
23. D'Angelo R et al: Intrathecal sufentanil compared to epidural bupivicaine for labor analgesia. *Anesthesiology* 1994;80:1209-1215.
24. Correl DJ, Visicusi ER, Witkowski TA, et al: Success of epidural catheters placed for postoperative analgesia: Comparison of a combined spinal-epidural vs. a standard epidural technique. *Anesthesiology* 1998;89:A1095.
25. Bouhemad B et al: Bacterial meningitis following combined spinal-epidural analgesia for labour. *Anaesthesia* 1998;53:290-295.
26. Harding SA et al: Meningitis after combined spinal-extradural anaesthesia in obstetrics. *Br J Anaesth* 1994;73:545-547.
27. Van De Velde M et al: Post dural puncture headache following combined spinal epidural or epidural anaesthesia in obstetric patients. *Anaesth Intensive Care* 2001;29:595-599.
28. Felsby S et al: Combined spinal and epidural anesthesia. *Anesth Analg* 1995;80:821-826.
29. Practice guidelines for obstetric anesthesia: An updated report by the American Society of Anesthesiologists Task Force on Obstetric Anesthesia. *Anesthesiology* 2007;106:843-863.
30. American Society of Regional Anesthesia and Pain Medicine: Conference on infectious complications of neuraxial blockade, 2004. Available at www.asra.com/consensus-statements/3.html.

68 Does Labor Analgesia Affect Labor Outcome?

B. Scott Segal, MD

INTRODUCTION

In 1847, only months after the first demonstration of anesthesia, James Simpson, an obstetrician, administered ether to a woman in labor for childbirth. He was quite impressed with the analgesia the new drug induced, as was his patient. However, his journal notes on the case indicated his concern over the possible adverse effects of anesthesia on labor and delivery[1]:

> It will be necessary to ascertain anesthesia's precise effect, both upon the action of the uterus and on the assistant abdominal muscles; its influence, if any, upon the child; whether it has a tendency to hemorrhage or other complications.

Thus began, more than a century and a half ago, perhaps the longest-lived controversy in the history of obstetric anesthesia, one that continues to this day in both academic and lay circles.

OPTIONS

The modern debate has centered on several main issues:

1. Does regional analgesia for labor affect the length of labor or the rate of cervical dilation? In particular, does the timing of initiation of epidural analgesia play a role?
2. Does regional labor analgesia increase the risk of instrumental vaginal delivery?
3. Does regional labor analgesia increase the risk of cesarean section?

No definitive study has adequately addressed any of these questions, and methodologic problems have plagued all available evidence. The principal difficulty is that risk factors for dysfunctional labor also predispose a woman to request an epidural. This chapter will review the available literature, focusing on randomized controlled trials (RCTs) but considering other forms of evidence, and will emphasize the different conclusions reached by observational and prospective randomized designs.

EVIDENCE

Evidence Regarding Rate of Cervical Dilation and Timing of Initiation

Conventional wisdom holds that if started too early in labor (during the latent phase), epidural analgesia may markedly slow or even arrest the progress of labor.

Amazingly, this widely accepted clinical dogma has never been proved in carefully performed studies. Its origin can be traced to early case series of caudal or epidural anesthesia for labor, which probably resulted in dense sacral as well as lumbar blocks. In these uncontrolled reports, although some women in whom blocks were initiated very early may not have progressed through labor, it is unclear whether they would have progressed more quickly without the block.[2]

Some nonrandomized studies have found an association between earlier epidural placement and dystocia. Thorp and colleagues[3] compared various groups of nulliparous women defined by their early cervical dilation rate, their cervical dilation at the time of initiation of analgesia, and the choice of epidural or alternative analgesia. Among women with dilation less than 5 cm and dilation rate less than 1 cm/hr, epidural analgesia was associated with a sixfold increase in cesarean section for dystocia. Other comparisons demonstrated smaller relative risks or no difference. In a secondary analysis of the same group's randomized trial,[4] the increased risk of cesarean section was greatest in women requesting analgesia earlier, though women were not randomly assigned to dilation at time of initiation of analgesia. Using a case-control methodology, Malone and colleagues[5] identified epidural initiation at less than 2 cm dilation as a significant risk factor for prolonged nulliparous labor (odds ratio [OR] 42.7). In a sophisticated observational study using a variant of multivariate regression (propensity score analysis) to control for multiple simultaneous confounders, Lieberman and colleagues[6] identified both cervical dilation less than 5 cm and station less than 0 at the time of epidural initiation as strong risk factors for cesarean delivery.

Evidence from RCTs has failed to confirm this finding (Table 68-1). Chestnut and colleagues[7] randomized women requesting epidural analgesia to early or late groups (approximately 4 and 5 cm dilation). No differences in labor outcome were seen in either spontaneous labors[7] or induced labors.[8] However, the early and late groups in these studies were not markedly different in their cervical dilation at the time of epidural placement. Three more recent trials randomized women to early epidural placement or opioids until later in labor[9,10] or to intrathecal opioids followed by later epidural initiation.[11] In each case progress through the first stage of labor was either equivalent or faster in the early group than in the

Table 68-1   Randomized Trials Comparing Early versus Later Epidural Initiation

Author, Year	Outcome	CERVICAL DILATION IN CM (N)		RESULTS		
		Early	Late	Early	Late	p
Chestnut, 1994[7]*	First stage (min)	4 (172)	5 (162)	329	359	NS
	Second stage (min)			85	88	NS
	CS (%)			10	8	NS
	IVD (%)			37	43	NS
Chestnut, 1994[8]†	First stage (min)	3.5 (74)	5 (75)	318	273	NS
	Second stage (min)			91	77	NS
	CS (%)			18	49	NS
	IVD (%)			43	19	NS
Luxman, 1998[9]	First stage (min)	2.5 (30)	4.5 (30)	342	317	NS
	Second stage (min)			41	38	NS
	CS (%)			7	10	NS
	IVD (%)			13	17	NS
Ohel, 2006[10]	First stage (min)	2.4 (221)	4.6(228)	354	396	.04
	Second stage (min)			95	105	.12
	CS (%)			13	11	.77
	IVD (%)			17	19	.63
Wong, 2005[11]‡	First stage (min)	<4 (366)	>4 (362)	295	385	<.001
	Second stage (min)			71	82	.67
	CS (%)			18	21	.31
	IVD (%)			20	16	.13

*Spontaneous labor; cervical dilation given as median.
†Oxytocin-receiving subjects; cervical dilation given as median.
‡Subjects randomized at <4 cm to intrathecal fentanyl 25 mcg or IM + IV hydromorphone; all subjects received epidural analgesia at second request for analgesia
    (systemic group) or >4 cm or at third request for analgesia (intrathecal group).
CS, Cesarean section; IVD, instrumental vaginal delivery.

later group. No differences in second-stage duration or mode of delivery were found in any of the trials. The difference between the RCTs and the retrospective studies may be due to selection bias, in that women requesting analgesia earlier in labor may be experiencing pain due to anatomic or physiologic factors predisposing them to dystocia.

The effect of epidural analgesia on cervical dilation in established labor is probably minimal. Some earlier retrospective studies finding slower cervical dilation were probably hampered by selection bias. Meta-analyses of randomized trials of epidural analgesia versus opioid analgesia have concluded that the first stage of labor is not prolonged by epidural analgesia.[12-14]

Evidence Concerning Risk of Instrumental Vaginal Delivery

The incidence of instrumental vaginal delivery may be increased by epidural analgesia, though this practice varies tremendously between obstetricians and hospitals. Table 68-2 shows the results of 15 randomized trials, published in English as full papers, comparing epidural analgesia to systemic opioids. Seven of the trials found a significant difference in rates. However, the overall use of forceps varied from 0% to 55% in the opioid groups and from 2% to 80% in the epidural groups, indicating substantial variation in practice style. Indeed, meta-analysis of randomized trials has found the total instrumental delivery rate to be 1.38 to 2.19 times more likely

in patients receiving epidural analgesia, but with a very broad confidence interval indicative of the variation between studies.[12-16] Moreover, there is strong evidence that many instrumental deliveries in epidural patients are done for reasons other than dystocia, perhaps for teaching purposes.[17] Most recently, Sharma and colleagues[18] demonstrated in one of the best randomized trials performed to date that the rate of instrumental delivery was increased from 3% in a group receiving intravenous opioids to 12% in the epidural group among 459 nulliparous women. Careful written guidelines for the use of forceps were established before the study.

Evidence Concerning Risk of Cesarean Section

Evidence regarding cesarean section represents the most important aspect of the issue of the effect of epidural analgesia on labor. Both randomized clinical trials and an important type of observational study have been reported. Data from 15 randomized trials reported in final form in which epidural analgesia was compared with systemic opioids are given in Table 68-2. Only one trial, when analyzed on an intent-to-treat basis, has found a difference in the risk of cesarean section.[4] One other, by Ramin and colleagues,[19] was originally reported on a protocol-compliant basis, after excluding from the analysis approximately one third of the randomized patients. In this form, a significant difference in cesarean section rates was observed. Unfortunately, the reasons for noncompliance were not

Table 68-2	Randomized Trials Comparing Mode of Delivery with Epidural or Opioid Analgesia							
		RATE OF FORCEPS DELIVERY[a]				RATE OF CESAREAN SECTION FOR DYSTOCIA[b]		
Author, Year	**Parity**	**Epidural Group**	**Opioid Group**	**p**		**Epidural Group**	**Opioid Group**	**p**
Robinson, 1980[54]	Nulliparas	17/28 (51%)	8/30 (27%)	<.02		0	0	—
	Mulitparas	5/17 (30%)	1/18 (6%)	NS				
Philipsen, 1989[55]	Nulliparas	1/57 (2%)	0/54 (0%)	NS		10/57 (17%)	6/54 (11%)	NS
Thorp, 1993[4]	Nulliparas	4/48 (8.3%)	3/45 (6.7%)	NS		8/48 (16.7%)	1/45 (2.2%)	<.05
Ramin, 1995[19c]	Mixed	41/432 (10%)	13/437 (3%)	<.0001		43/664 (6%)	37/666 (6%)	NS
Bofill, 1997[17]	Nulliparas	39/49 (80%)	28/51 (55%)	.004		4/49 (4%)	3/51 (3%)	NS
Sharma, 1997[56]	Mixed	26/358 (7%)	15/357 (4%)	NS		13/358 (4%)	16/357 (5%)	NS
Clark, 1998[57]	Nulliparas	24/156 (15%)	20/162 (12%)	NS		15/156 (9.6%)	22/162 (14%)	NS
Gambling, 1998[58d]	Mixed	51/616 (8%)	34/607 (6%)	.08 NS		39/616 (6%)	34/607 (6%)	NS
	Nulliparas	37/336 (13%)	32/314 (13%)			30/336 (10%)	25/314 (9%)	NS
Loughnan, 2000[59]	Nulliparas	88/304 (29%)	81/310 (26%)	NS		36/304 (12%)	40/310 (13%)	NS
Howell, 2001[60]	Nulliparas	55/184 (30%)	36/185 (19%)	.03		13/184 (7%)	17/185 (9%)	NS
Lucas, 2001[61e]	Mixed	51/372 (14%)	27/366 (7%)	.005		46/372 (12%)	54/366 (15%)	NS
Dickinson, 2002[62f]	Nulliparas	169/493 (34%)	148/499 (30%)	NS		85/493 (17%)	71/499 (14%)	NS
Sharma, 2002[18]	Nulliparas	26/226 (12%)	7/233 (3%)	<.001		13/226 (6%)	17/233 (7%)	NS
Head, 2002[65e]	Mixed	3/56 (5%)	3/60 (5%)	NS		7/53 (13%)	6/52 (12%)	NS
Jain, 2003[63]	Nulliparas	12/43 (28%)	8/83 (10%)	<.01		9/45 (20%)	12/83 (14%)	NS
Long, 2003[64]	Mixed					1/30 (3%)	6/50 (12%)	NS

[a]Total forceps rate (outlet + "low") when separately reported.
[b]Cesarean section rate for dystocia if separately analyzed, otherwise total cesarean section rate.
[c]Ramin et al. was originally reported in 1995 only as a protocol compliant analysis, which is inappropriate in primary analysis of randomized trials. The data given in the table are taken from the authors' 2000 published reanalysis by intention-to-treat, the correct method, for cesarean section.[9] Only protocol-compliant analysis has been reported for forceps.
[d]Combined spinal-epidural vs. opioid.
[e]Patients with pregnancy-induced hypertension.
[f]Control group received continuous midwifery care and a variety of nonepidural analgesics; crossover to epidural group was 61.3%.

given. It is likely that some excluded patients in the epidural group were low-risk patients who delivered quickly without the need for analgesia. Conversely, some opioid patients probably demanded epidural analgesia because of inadequate analgesia during a protracted, painful labor (i.e., high risk). Therefore the protocol-compliant analysis probably overemphasized the difference between groups. Indeed, the authors published a revised analysis on an intent-to-treat basis that found no difference in cesarean section, and is given in Table 68-2.[20]

Several meta-analyses of various groups of these RCTs and sometimes including some reported only as abstracts or in languages other than English are shown in Table 68-3. Despite inclusion of different studies, these analyses have consistently shown no difference in the total rate of cesarean delivery or the rate of cesarean for dystocia.[12-16]

Another body of evidence concerns studies in which the availability of epidural analgesia in an institution has suddenly changed.[21-31] The results of 11 such studies are given in Table 68-4. None has found an association between higher utilization of epidural analgesia and a higher rate of cesarean section. Not surprisingly, meta-analysis showed no association between greater availability of epidural analgesia and cesarean section.[32] Though nonrandomized, these "sentinel event" or "natural

experiment" studies offer some unique insights. The investigations span two decades and studied widely varying practice settings. All patients in the hospital are included, so external validity is not a problem as it may be with the RCTs. An assumption of these studies is that the patient population and obstetric practice styles are likely to change little, or at least slowly, when compared with the sudden availability of epidural analgesia. This assumption has generally proven valid but not all sentinel event studies have addressed it directly, and some documented subtle changes in the patient population.[28-31]

Obstetric Practice Style

As evidence has accumulated discounting the direct effect of epidural analgesia on labor, greater emphasis has been placed on the role of the obstetric caregiver as the primary determinant of the risk of cesarean section. One early study demonstrated that after nulliparity, the greatest risk factor for cesarean section among a cohort of women was the identity of the individual obstetrician.[33] Other investigators have reported variation in cesarean section rates between indigent patients and those with private health insurance, despite similar rates of epidural analgesia use.[34,35] Three studies have reported 50% decreases in

Table 68-3		Meta-analysis of RCTs Comparing Epidural with Nonepidural Analgesia				
Author, Year	**Number of Trials**	**Outcome**	**Number of Subjects (Epidural/ Nonepidural)**	**Epidural**	**Nonepidural**	**OR, RR, or WMD (95% CI) Epidural vs. Nonepidural**
Halpern, 1998[12]	10	First stage (min)	524/555	8.2	5.6	+42 min (17-68)
	5	Second stage (min)	581/609	15.5	8.9	+14 min (5-23)
	6	CS (%)	1183/1186	12.2	17.1	1.50 (0.81-2.76)
	7	IVD (%)	1155/1164			2.19 (1.32-7.78)*
	9	IVD dystocia (%)	106/105			0.68 (0.31-1.49)
	2					
Zhang, 1999[16]*	4	First stage (min)	397/409			1.19 (1.01-1.39)*
		Second stage (min)				1.37 (1.07-1.76)*
		CS (%)				1.66 (0.59-4.68)
		IVD (%)				1.57 (0.92-2.68)
Liu, 2004[15]	7	Second stage (min)	1473/1489	64.5	49.3	+15 min (2.1-28.2)*
	4	CS (%)	1473/1489	12.1	11.3	1.18 (0.71-1.48)
	7	IVD (%)	1276/1300	27.8	22.2	1.63 (1.12-2.37)*
	6	IVD nonelective (%)	1071/1087	27.3	22.2	1.56 (0.99-2.46)
	4					
Leighton, 2002[13]	14	First stage (min)	2161/2136	7.7	8.0	+26 min (-8-60)
	7	Second stage (min)	1012/1050	19.0	12.3	+15 min (9-22)*
	8	CS (%)	1068/1103	7.2	4.2	1.0 (0.77-1.28)
	14	IVD (%)	2161/2136			2.08 (1.48-2.93)*
	12	IVD dystocia (%)	1813/1840			1.53 (0.29-8.08)
	3		538/542			
Anim-Somuah, 2005[14]	21	First stage (min)	1165/1163	11.0	10.2	+24 min (-19-67)
	9	Second stage (min)	1796/1784	6.3	7.0	+16 min (7.5-24)*
	11	CS (%)	3326/3308	19.3	14.2	1.07 (0.93-1.23)
	20	CS dystocia (%)	2311/2295			0.90 (0.73-1.12)
	11	IVD (%)	3044/3118			1.38 (1.24-1.53)*
	17					

*Also analyzed observational studies and comparisons of epidurals continued or discontinued during second stage. Only trials comparing epidural with nonepidural analgesia are included in the table. Pooled estimates of various parameters were not reported.
CS, Cesarean section; *IVD,* instrumental vaginal delivery.

Table 68-4	Sentinel Event Studies Comparing Cesarean Section Rate before and after a Rapid Change in Epidural Availability		
	RATE OF CESAREAN SECTION (EPIDURAL RATE)		
Author, Year	**Low Epidural Use Period**	**High Epidural Use Period**	**p**
Bailey, 1983[21]	7.1% (0%)	9.3% (27%)	NS
Gribble, 1991[22]	9.0% (0%)	8.2% (47%)	NS
Larson, 1992[23]	27.5% (0%)	22.9% (32%)	NS
Mancuso, 1993[24]	14.9% (19%)	12.3% (67%)	NS
Johnson, 1995[25]	18.4% (21%)	17.2% (71%)	NS
Lyon, 1997[26]	11.8% (13%)	10.0% (59%)	NS
Fogel, 1998[27]	9.1% (1%)	9.7% (29%)	NS
Yancey, 1999[29]	19.4% (1%)	19.0% (59%)	NS
Impey, 2000[28]	3.8% (10%)	4.0% (57%)	NS
Zhang, 2001[30]*	14.4% (1%)	12.1% (84%)	NS
Vahratian, 2004[31]*	18% (2%)	18% (92%)	NS

*Zhang and Vahratian studied the same institution at slightly different time periods, and Vahratian confined the analysis to nulliparas admitted in spontaneous labor and who received epidural analgesia at ≤4 cm dilation.

hospital-wide cesarean rates by peer review, physician education, and publishing individual obstetricians' rates of operation, while simultaneously doubling the rate of epidural analgesia usage.[36-38] Another found no correlation between 110 individual obstetricians' rates of cesarean section and the rates of epidural analgesia utilization among their patients.[39] Two others have documented no relationship between epidural rates and cesarean rates across hospitals in Belgium and Sweden.[40,41]

However, indirect effects of the presence of a regional analgesic block may affect obstetric decision making on the mode of delivery. For example, it is well known that patients with epidural blocks will experience a gradual rise in temperature during the course of labor.[42] Maternal fever or its consequences (e.g., fetal tachycardia) may be one of the factors leading an obstetrician to decide to perform a cesarean section.[43] Similarly, most anesthesiologists request that patients remain in bed after an epidural block is initiated. Some obstetric caregivers believe that ambulation speeds the progress of labor and therefore that the presence of an epidural block could indirectly slow the rate of cervical dilation. However, controlled trials have failed to confirm a beneficial effect of walking in labor, both in patients with and without regional analgesia.[44,45] Finally, it has also been suggested that a patient who desires epidural analgesia may be one who is more amenable to a more interventional management of her labor, including assisted vaginal or cesarean modes of delivery.

CONTROVERSIES

General Methodologic Difficulties

It is generally agreed that the ideal clinical study is prospective, randomized, double-blind, and placebo-controlled. No study of epidural analgesia's effect on labor and delivery has met this standard, and none probably ever will. By far the majority of studies meet none of these criteria, but are instead retrospective comparisons of women who self-selected epidural analgesia with those who did not. Such comparisons introduce selection bias. Bias is introduced by comparing two groups of patients who do not share equivalent risk of the outcome being studied. In this case, the outcomes of interest may include the duration of labor, the need for oxytocin, or the risk of cesarean section. Similar problems arise when looking retrospectively at outcomes such as perineal trauma, maternal fever, or neonatal sepsis evaluations.

Indeed, investigators have identified many characteristics of patients requesting epidural analgesia that independently predict longer labor and nonspontaneous delivery. They are more frequently nulliparous, tend to come to the hospital earlier in labor and with higher fetal station, have slower cervical dilation before analgesia, more frequently are already receiving oxytocin for induction or augmentation of labor, deliver larger babies, and may have received epidural analgesia because of other perceived risk factors for operative delivery such as poor fetal status or maternal systemic disease.[3,46-48] Floberg and colleagues[49] used radiographic pelvimetry to demonstrate that women requesting epidural analgesia have smaller pelvic outlets, an obvious risk factor for operative delivery.

Another important and often overlooked difference is the pain of labor itself. Pain in early labor is associated with slower labor and forceps or cesarean delivery.[50] Of course, more pain in labor is associated with a higher likelihood of selecting epidural analgesia. Investigators have also related the ongoing analgesic requirements of patients who are already receiving epidural analgesia to dysfunctional labor. These studies suggest that women who require denser blocks or more "top-up" doses of local anesthetic have slower labors and are at increased risk of operative vaginal or cesarean delivery.[51] Panni and Segal[52] further extended this observation by demonstrating a greater local anesthetic requirement in nulliparous women in early labor who later go on to require cesarean section for dystocia than in those who deliver vaginally. Others have demonstrated similar findings in women receiving patient-controlled intravenous meperidine for labor analgesia.[53]

Several randomized, prospective trials comparing epidural analgesia with an alternative (usually parenteral opioids) have appeared.[4,17-19,54-65] Although these studies represent a far better approach than retrospective comparisons, there are still potential problems with them. First, in none was a placebo control employed. Performing randomized prospective trials with placebo controls may raise ethical concerns, or at least it may be very difficult to get patients to give their consent and minimize cross-over between groups. Because parenteral opioids may themselves affect the course of labor,[66] these trials cannot specifically define the influence of epidural analgesia relative to natural childbirth. Nonetheless, the analgesia is consistently better with epidural than systemic opioid analgesia. Consequently, a second, essentially insurmountable problem is posed by the practical impossibility of blinding patients and obstetricians, nurses, and anesthesiologists to the presence or absence of a functional epidural block. Since the decision to proceed with operative delivery is ultimately a subjective clinical one made by the obstetrician, the absence of blinding may be very important. Obstetricians and midwives may not treat their patients with epidural analgesia the same way they treat those without it. For example, forceps-assisted delivery may be more common among patients with epidural analgesia partly because obstetricians know their patients will be comfortable and have relaxed pelvic musculature for the procedure.[17]

Third, several of the randomized trials have been severely underpowered. Detecting a moderate difference in typical cesarean section rates of 10% to 20% requires several hundred patients per group. Many of the trials that have concluded that epidural analgesia does not affect the rate of cesarean section have studied only a small fraction of this number. Hence their conclusions could at least theoretically be due to the small sample sizes involved.

Fourth, protocol noncompliance has been a persistent problem. Approximately one third of patients in most randomized trials do not ultimately receive the randomly assigned treatment. Analysis of only protocol-compliant patients introduces bias, because patients excluded from an epidural group may be low-risk patients progressing easily through labor with minimal pain, whereas those excluded from an opioid group may be high-risk patients experiencing slow, painful labor. Analysis by intent-to-treat, though correct, is complicated when such large numbers of patients fail to receive their assigned analgesic, and at least further reduces the statistical power of the study. One recent trial was both sufficiently powered and achieved low crossover (8%).[18]

Finally, it may not be easy to extrapolate the findings of even well-conducted randomized trials to the general labor and delivery population (i.e., external validity). Most parturients have strong opinions about their desire for labor analgesia. Patients who do consent to randomized trials (in which they have a 50% chance of being assigned to not receive epidural analgesia) may make up a subset of patients who are ambivalent about labor analgesia, and thus not representative of the general labor and delivery population.

GUIDELINES

The American College of Obstetricians and Gynecologists (ACOG) has recently revised its guidelines for obstetric anesthesia services. Previously, ACOG had suggested that epidural analgesia be delayed until a cervical dilation of 4 to 5 cm is reached. Anesthesiologists were not well represented in the formation of these guidelines and the evidence cited in support of them was incomplete.[67] Recently, ACOG updated this statement, no longer endorsing a delay and explicitly disavowing consideration of fear of increasing the risk of cesarean delivery.[68] ACOG and the American Society of Anesthesiologists have also jointly endorsed a statement that "maternal request is a sufficient medical indication for pain relief during labor" and that epidural analgesia is usually the preferred method.[69]

AUTHOR'S RECOMMENDATIONS

- Methodologic problems are likely to continue to make definitive answers to the controversies of the effects of epidural analgesia on labor elusive.
- Earlier administration of epidural analgesia does not cause longer labor or an increase in operative delivery. In the absence of a contraindication, women should be offered an epidural whenever labor pain is intensive enough to elicit a request for analgesia.
- Epidural analgesia minimally affects the progress of established labor. Second stage is prolonged approximately 15 minutes; first stage may not be prolonged at all, or at most less than 30 minutes.
- Instrumental vaginal delivery is probably increased by effective epidural analgesia. Variation in obstetric practice style, however, makes it difficult to assess the magnitude of this risk for any given patient.
- The risk of cesarean section is not increased by epidural analgesia.
- Appreciation of indirect effects of the presence of an epidural on the practice style of obstetricians or the decision-making process of patients may further our understanding of the possible effects of epidural analgesia on labor outcome.

REFERENCES

1. Simpson J: In Simpson W, editor: *The works of Sir J. Y. Simpson.* Edinburgh, Adam & Charles Black, 1871.
2. Siever JM, Mousel LH: Continuous caudal anesthesia in three hundred unselected obstetric cases. *JAMA* 1943;122:424-426.
3. Thorp JA, Eckert LO, Ang MS, Johnston DA, Peaceman AM, Parisi VM: Epidural analgesia and cesarean section for dystocia: Risk factors in nulliparas. *Am J Perinatol* 1991;8:402-410.
4. Thorp JA, Hu DH, Albin RM, McNitt J, Meyer BA, Cohen GR, Yeast JD: The effect of intrapartum epidural analgesia on nulliparous labor: A randomized, controlled, prospective trial. *Am J Obstet Gynecol* 1993;169:851-858.
5. Malone FD, Geary M, Chelmow D, Stronge J, Boylan P, D'Alton ME: Prolonged labor in nulliparas: Lessons from the active management of labor. *Obstet Gynecol* 1996;88:211-215.
6. Lieberman E, Lang JM, Cohen A, D'Agostino R Jr, Datta S, Frigoletto FD Jr: Association of epidural analgesia with cesarean delivery in nulliparas. *Obstet Gynecol* 1996;88:993-1000.
7. Chestnut DH, McGrath JM, Vincent RD Jr, Penning DH, Choi WW, Bates JN, McFarlane C: Does early administration of epidural analgesia affect obstetric outcome in nulliparous women who are in spontaneous labor? *Anesthesiology* 1994;80:1201-1208.
8. Chestnut DH, Vincent RD Jr, McGrath JM, Choi WW, Bates JN: Does early administration of epidural analgesia affect obstetric outcome in nulliparous women who are receiving intravenous oxytocin? *Anesthesiology* 1994;80:1193-1200.
9. Luxman D, Wolman I, Groutz A, Cohen JR, Lottan M, Pauzner D, David MP: The effect of early epidural block administration on the progression and outcome of labor. *Int J Obstet Anesth* 1998;7:161-164.
10. Ohel G, Gonen R, Vaida S, Barak S, Gaitini L: Early versus late initiation of epidural analgesia in labor: Does it increase the risk of cesarean section? A randomized trial. *Am J Obstet Gynecol* 2006;194:600-605.
11. Wong CA, Scavone BM, Peaceman AM, McCarthy RJ, Sullivan JT, Diaz NT, et al: The risk of cesarean delivery with neuraxial analgesia given early versus late in labor. *N Engl J Med* 2005; 352:655-665.
12. Halpern SH, Leighton BL, Ohlsson A, Barrett JF, Rice A: Effect of epidural vs parenteral opioid analgesia on the progress of labor: A meta-analysis. *JAMA* 1998;280:2105-2110.
13. Leighton BL, Halpern SH: Epidural analgesia: Effects on labor progress and maternal and neonatal outcome. *Semin Perinatol* 2002;26:122-135.
14. Anim-Somuah M, Smyth R, Howell C: Epidural versus non-epidural or no analgesia in labour. *Cochrane Database Syst Rev* 2005: CD000331.
15. Liu EH, Sia AT: Rates of caesarean section and instrumental vaginal delivery in nulliparous women after low concentration epidural infusions or opioid analgesia: Systematic review. *BMJ* 2004;328:1410.
16. Zhang J, Klebanoff MA, DerSimonian R: Epidural analgesia in association with duration of labor and mode of delivery: A quantitative review. *Am J Obstet Gynecol* 1999;180:970-977.
17. Bofill JA, Vincent RD, Ross EL, Martin RW, Norman PF, Werhan CF, Morrison JC: Nulliparous active labor, epidural analgesia, and cesarean delivery for dystocia. *Am J Obstet Gynecol* 1997; 177:1465-1470.
18. Sharma SK, Alexander JM, Messick G, Bloom SL, McIntire DD, Wiley J, Leveno KJ: Cesarean delivery: A randomized trial of epidural analgesia versus intravenous meperidine analgesia during labor in nulliparous women. *Anesthesiology* 2002;96:546-551.
19. Ramin SM, Gambling DR, Lucas MJ, Sharma SK, Sidawi JE, Leveno KJ: Randomized trial of epidural versus intravenous analgesia during labor. *Obstet Gynecol* 1995;86:783-789.
20. Sharma SK, Leveno KJ: Update: Epidural analgesia during labor does not increase cesarean births. *Curr Anesth Rep* 2000;2:18-24.
21. Bailey PW, Howard FA: Forum. Epidural analgesia and forceps delivery: Laying a bogey. *Anaesthesia* 1983;38:282-285.
22. Gribble RK, Meier PR: Effect of epidural analgesia on the primary cesarean rate. *Obstet Gynecol* 1991;78:231-234.
23. Larson DD: The effect of initiating an obstetric anesthesiology service on rate of cesarean section and rate of forceps delivery.

Abstracts of the 24th Annual meeting of the Society for Obstetric Anesthesia and Perinatology 1992;13.

24. Mancuso JJ: Epidural analgesia in an army medical center: Impact on cesarean and instrumental vaginal deliveries. *Abstracts of the 25th Annual meeting of the Society for Obstetric Anesthesia and Perinatology* 1993;13.

25. Johnson S, Rosenfeld JA: The effect of epidural anesthesia on the length of labor. *J Fam Pract* 1995;40:244-247.

26. Lyon DS, Knuckles G, Whitaker E, Salgado S: The effect of instituting an elective labor epidural program on the operative delivery rate. *Obstet Gynecol* 1997;90:135-141.

27. Fogel ST, Shyken JM, Leighton BL, Mormol JS, Smeltzer JS: Epidural labor analgesia and the incidence of cesarean delivery for dystocia. *Anesth Analg* 1998;87:119-123.

28. Impey L, MacQuillan K, Robson M: Epidural analgesia need not increase operative delivery rates. *Am J Obstet Gynecol* 2000;182:358-363.

29. Yancey MK, Pierce B, Schweitzer D, Daniels D: Observations on labor epidural analgesia and operative delivery rates. *Am J Obstet Gynecol* 1999;180:353-359.

30. Zhang J, Yancey MK, Klebanoff MA, Schwarz J, Schweitzer D: Does epidural analgesia prolong labor and increase risk of cesarean delivery? A natural experiment. *Am J Obstet Gynecol* 2001;185:128-134.

31. Vahratian A, Zhang J, Hasling J, Troendle JF, Klebanoff MA, Thorp JM Jr: The effect of early epidural versus early intravenous analgesia use on labor progression: A natural experiment. *Am J Obstet Gynecol* 2004;191:259-265.

32. Segal S, Su M, Gilbert P: The effect of a rapid change in availability of epidural analgesia on the cesarean delivery rate: A meta-analysis. *Am J Obstet Gynecol* 2000;183:974-978.

33. Goyert GL, Bottoms SF, Treadwell MC, Nehra PC: The physician factor in cesarean birth rates. *N Engl J Med* 1989;320:706-709.

34. Neuhoff D, Burke MS, Porreco RP: Cesarean birth for failed progress in labor. *Obstet Gynecol* 1989;73:915-920.

35. Cary AJ: Intervention rates in spontaneous term labour in low risk nulliparous women. *Aust N Z J Obstet Gynaecol* 1990;30:46-51.

36. Iglesias S, Burn R, Saunders LD: Reducing the cesarean section rate in a rural community hospital. *Can Med Assoc J* 1991;145:1459-1464.

37. Socol ML, Garcia PM, Peaceman AM, Dooley SL: Reducing cesarean births at a primarily private university hospital. *Am J Obstet Gynecol* 1993;168:1748-1754, discussion 1754-1758.

38. Lagrew DC Jr, Morgan MA: Decreasing the cesarean section rate in a private hospital: Success without mandated clinical changes. *Am J Obstet Gynecol* 1996;174:184-191.

39. Segal S, Blatman R, Doble M, Datta S: The influence of the obstetrician in the relationship between epidural analgesia and cesarean section for dystocia. *Anesthesiology* 1999;91:90-96.

40. Cammu H, Martens G, Van Maele G: Epidural analgesia for low risk labour determines the rate of instrumental deliveries but not that of caesarean sections. *J Obstet Gynaecol* 1998;18:25-29.

41. Eriksson SL, Olausson PO, Olofsson C: Use of epidural analgesia and its relation to caesarean and instrumental deliveries—a population-based study of 94,217 primiparae. *Eur J Obstet Gynecol Reprod Biol* 2006;128:270-275.

42. Camann WR, Hortvet LA, Hughes N, Bader AM, Datta S: Maternal temperature regulation during extradural analgesia for labour. *Br J Anaesth* 1991;67:565-568.

43. Lieberman E, Cohen A, Lang J, Frigoletto F, Goetzl L: Maternal intrapartum temperature elevation as a risk factor for cesarean delivery and assisted vaginal delivery. *Am J Public Health* 1999;89:506-510.

44. Nageotte MP, Larson D, Rumney PJ, Sidhu M, Hollenbach K: Epidural analgesia compared with combined spinal-epidural analgesia during labor in nulliparous women. *N Engl J Med* 1997;337:1715-1719.

45. Bloom SL, McIntire DD, Kelly MA, Beimer HL, Burpo RH, Garcia MA, Leveno KJ: Lack of effect of walking on labor and delivery. *N Engl J Med* 1998;339:76-79.

46. Studd JW, Crawford JS, Duignan NM, Rowbotham CJ, Hughes AO: The effect of lumbar epidural analgesia on the rate of cervical dilatation and the outcome of labour of spontaneous onset. *Br J Obstet Gynaecol* 1980;87:1015-1021.

47. Willdeck-Lund G, Lindmark G, Nilsson BA: Effect of segmental epidural analgesia upon the uterine activity with special reference to the use of different local anaesthetic agents. *Acta Anaesthesiol Scand* 1979;23:519-528.

48. Moore J, Murnaghan GA, Lewis MA: A clinical evaluation of the maternal effects of lumbar extradural analgesia for labour. *Anaesthesia* 1974;29:537-544.

49. Floberg J, Belfrage P, Ohlsen H: Influence of the pelvic outlet capacity on fetal head presentation at delivery. *Acta Obstet Gynecol Scand* 1987;66:127-130.

50. Wuitchik M, Bakal D, Lipshitz J: The clinical significance of pain and cognitive activity in latent labor. *Obstet Gynecol* 1989;73:35-42.

51. Hess PE, Pratt SD, Soni AK, Sarna MC, Oriol NE: An association between severe labor pain and cesarean delivery. *Anesth Analg* 2000;90:881-886.

52. Panni MK, Segal S: Local anesthetic requirements are greater in dystocia than in normal labor. *Anesthesiology* 2003;98:957-963.

53. Alexander JM, Sharma SK, McIntire DD, Wiley J, Leveno KJ: Intensity of labor pain and cesarean delivery. *Anesth Analg* 2001;92:1524-1528.

54. Robinson JO, Rosen M, Evans JM, Revill SI, David H, Rees GA: Maternal opinion about analgesia for labour. A controlled trial between epidural block and intramuscular pethidine combined with inhalation. *Anaesthesia* 1980;35:1173-1181.

55. Philipsen T, Jensen NH: Epidural block or parenteral pethidine as analgesic in labour; a randomized study concerning progress in labour and instrumental deliveries. *Eur J Obstet Gynecol Reprod Biol* 1989;30:27-33.

56. Sharma SK, Sidawi JE, Ramin SM, Lucas MJ, Leveno KJ, Cunningham FG: Cesarean delivery: A randomized trial of epidural versus patient-controlled meperidine analgesia during labor. *Anesthesiology* 1997;87:487-494.

57. Clark A, Carr D, Loyd G, Cook V, Spinnato J: The influence of epidural analgesia on cesarean delivery rates: A randomized, prospective clinical trial. *Am J Obstet Gynecol* 1998;179:1527-1533.

58. Gambling DR, Sharma SK, Ramin SM, Lucas MJ, Leveno KJ, Wiley J, Sidawi JE: A randomized study of combined spinal-epidural analgesia versus intravenous meperidine during labor: Impact on cesarean delivery rate. *Anesthesiology* 1998;89:1336-1344.

59. Loughnan BA, Carli F, Romney M, Dore CJ, Gordon H: Randomized controlled comparison of epidural bupivacaine versus pethidine for analgesia in labour. *Br J Anaesth* 2000;84:715-719.

60. Howell CJ, Kidd C, Roberts W, Upton P, Lucking L, Jones PW, Johanson RB: A randomised controlled trial of epidural compared with non-epidural analgesia in labour. *Br J Obstet Gynecol* 2001;108:27-33.

61. Lucas MJ, Sharma SK, McIntire DD, Wiley J, Sidawi JE, Ramin SM, et al: A randomized trial of labor analgesia in women with pregnancy-induced hypertension. *Am J Obstet Gynecol* 2001;185:970-975.

62. Dickinson JE, Paech MJ, McDonald SJ, Evans SF: The impact of intrapartum analgesia on labour and delivery outcomes in nulliparous women. *Aust N Z J Obstet Gynaecol* 2002;42:59-66.

63. Jain S, Arya VK, Gopalan S, Jain V: Analgesic efficacy of intramuscular opioids versus epidural analgesia in labor. *Int J Gynaecol Obstet* 2003;83:19-27.

64. Long J, Yue Y: Patient controlled intravenous analgesia with tramadol for labor pain relief. *Chin Med J (Engl)* 2003;116:1752-1755.

65. Head BB, Owen J, Vincent RD Jr, Shih G, Chestnut DH, Hauth JC: A randomized trial of intrapartum analgesia in women with severe preeclampsia. *Obstet Gynecol* 2002;99:452-457.

66. Kowalski WB, Parsons MT, Pak SC, Wilson L Jr: Morphine inhibits nocturnal oxytocin secretion and uterine contractions in the pregnant baboon. *Biol Reprod* 1998;58:971-976.

67. American College of Obstetricians and Gynecologists, Committee on Obstetrical Practice: *Evaluation of cesarean delivery*. Washington, DC, American College of Obstetricians and Gynecologists, 2000.

68. American College of Obstetricians and Gynecologists, Committee on Obstetrical Practice: ACOG committee opinion. No. 339: Analgesia and cesarean delivery rates. *Obstet Gynecol* 2006;107:1487-1488.

69. American College of Obstetricians and Gynecologists, Committee on Obstetrical Practice. *ACOG committee opinion No. 231: Pain relief in labor*. Washington, DC, American College of Obstetricians and Gynecologists, 2000.

69 Does Anesthesia Increase the Risk to the Parturient Undergoing Nonobstetric Surgery?

Donald H. Penning, MD, MS, FRCP

Anesthesia during pregnancy is a fairly common event. It is estimated that up to 2% of pregnant women will undergo surgery during pregnancy, but that figure is probably low because underreporting is common, or the patient may not know she is pregnant at the time of surgery.[1] One study of adolescent patients documented an overall 1.2% pregnancy rate, which increased to 2.4% in patients greater than 15 years old.[2] Appendectomy and cholecystectomy are the most common surgical procedures performed.[3,4] The anesthetic considerations include maternal safety, fetal toxicity including teratology, fetal asphyxia, and preterm labor.[5] The independent, detrimental effects from anesthesia alone are poorly understood. This is understandable because maternal anesthesia rarely if ever occurs without surgery (and vice versa). The stress of surgery; the duration, location, and nature of the surgical event; and the underlying pathophysiology of the surgical condition, in addition to anesthetic effects, all play a role in the overall risk to the mother. Though not a risk to the parturient per se, some new information on the fetal toxicity of anesthesia is included in this edition.

The anesthetic implications of nonobstetric surgery is a well-reviewed topic, and many of the standard texts deal with it well.[6,7] This chapter explores areas where there is confusing or recent literature and where controversy still exists. Specific topics include how, when, and why to monitor the fetus during and after surgery; the risk to the fetus from exposure to anesthetic agents, including maternal occupational exposure to trace gases; and a discussion of the effect of mode of abdominal surgery (i.e., laparoscopic versus open laparotomy) on fetal outcome.

EVIDENCE

Monitoring the Fetus during Surgery

Fetal heart rate (FHR) and uterine contraction monitoring are frequent dilemmas in nonobstetric surgery. The usual problems are logistic and medical. The proposed site of surgery may interfere with monitoring. Vaginal ultrasound probes have been used when the abdominal wall cannot be used. The issue of who will perform and evaluate the fetal tracing is also a common problem. Most anesthesiologists are either uncomfortable in this role or do not wish to have their attention diverted from the mother. In most hospitals, a labor and delivery room nurse stays with the patient to interpret the FHR and uterine contraction tracing in the operating room (OR) and into the recovery period. Commonly, these skilled personnel are in scarce supply so there can be considerable production pressure to reduce, or in some cases omit, the monitoring altogether.

The principal goals of monitoring are to identify fetal compromise and preterm labor. Both these goals are problematic. Electronic FHR monitoring has been used by obstetricians for many years to assess fetal well-being in labor. The use of electronic FHR monitoring has not been shown to be superior to intermittent auscultation in fetal assessment.[8,9] Nevertheless, FHR monitoring combined with the current medicolegal climate is the major reason for the increase in cesarean delivery rate in the United States and other countries. It is estimated that the false-positive rate for performing a cesarean section to prevent a case of cerebral palsy using electronic FHR monitoring is 99.8%.[10] With this in mind, is it reasonable to ignore FHR monitoring for nonobstetric surgery? Not necessarily. It is often incorrectly argued that FHR monitoring is unnecessary or cumbersome in a given patient because "we wouldn't do a cesarean section anyway" if an FHR abnormality was detected either because the surgery was impractical or because the fetus was previable. However, although immediate cesarean section may not be useful or practical, there are many possible therapeutic options short of cesarean delivery that can be employed. Changes in patient position, maternal cardiovascular manipulations to improve placental blood flow, and increasing fetal oxygenation via increasing maternal oxygenation (via manipulating ventilation or hemoglobin concentration) may have a salutary effect on the fetus. The detection of uterine contractions could lead the anesthesiologist to deepening anesthetic depth, thus decreasing uterine tone and improving the uteroplacental circulation for the fetus. Alternatively, FHR monitoring may be useful in defining the limits of manipulations that can be safely employed. For example, permissive hypoventilation, hemodilution, or hypotension might be required, and the FHR serves as a rough guide for threshold values that are permissible. No absolute agreed-on values exist in these circumstances. Rather than expressing "threshold values" in terms of fetal health, most clinicians prefer terms such as "lack of nonreassuring FHR abnormalities." Such carefully worded phrases reflect the reality of the poor predictive value of FHR analysis and the medicolegal environment in the United States and elsewhere.

The reliability of FHR monitoring is gestational age–dependent. It is often possible as early as 18 weeks of gestation but generally only reliable after 22 weeks.[11,12] The kinds of surgery amenable to monitoring are generally nonabdominal cases, but, as mentioned, vaginal ultrasound has been used even in these situations. The interpretation of the FHR trace requires knowledge of the effects of anesthetic agents. Except under situations of very light sedation, most narcotics and general anesthetics decrease or obliterate long- and short-term FHR variability,[11] hence one is left interpreting changes in baseline FHR. Thus, tachycardia (greater than 160 beats/min), bradycardia (less than 100 beats/min), or decelerations in conjunction with uterine contractions are the main diagnostic criteria remaining under general anesthetics. The question as to how long one should measure FHR following surgery is also controversial. The most common monitoring period is 12 to 24 hours, but again data are lacking.

Anesthetic Toxicity to the Fetus, Including Teratology

The majority of anesthetic agents cross the placenta and enter the fetal circulation. The major exception is the muscle relaxants, which are highly charged and generally do not cross to the fetus in clinically important amounts. Halogenated general anesthetics, such as isoflurane or halothane, rapidly cross the placenta, but fetal levels remain lower than maternal for a significant period of time.[5] At least in sheep, the values for minimum alveolar concentration (MAC) appear to be lower in the fetus than in the mother.[13] Excessive levels of inhalation anesthetics may depress cardiac output in the fetus, possibly leading to progressive fetal acidosis. The exact level at which this may occur has been studied in fetal lambs but is much less well understood in humans. In sheep, maternal administration of 1.5% halothane reduced fetal blood pressure but was without significant effect on fetal cardiac output, acid-base balance, or brain blood flow.[14,15] With 2% isoflurane there was no significant decline in fetal cardiac index or any progressive fetal acidosis.[16] This should be contrasted with an older fetal lamb study that showed 1.5% halothane or 2% isoflurane reduced fetal blood pressure and led to progressive fetal acidosis.[17] If this were not confusing enough, what about exposure to anesthetic agents in the already compromised fetus? Again there are conflicting data. In one experiment there were no detrimental effects,[18] but in another there was aggravation of fetal acidosis.[19] These fetal experiments are not easy to perform, and they exhibit a large degree of variability. The individual variations in experimental methodology explain much of the conflicting results without actually

clarifying which is "right." Factors such as gestational age, adjunct anesthetic agents, and other uncontrolled reasons for fetal compromise make the prediction of anesthetic effects and their extrapolation to human subjects difficult. However, it seems likely that long exposure to 1 MAC or less of an inhalation agent is probably safe.

In order for a drug to have a teratogenic effect it must be given to a susceptible species, at a critical dose, and at a critical period of development.[20] Animal studies can be very useful in establishing potential risk in humans, but results can be misleading. For instance, benzodiazepines in high doses can be associated with oral clefts in animals but not in humans at clinically relevant dosages.[21,22]

The actual effect of anesthetic agents themselves on fetal development, particularly in earlier gestation, is an area of great concern but also great controversy. New drugs themselves are almost never tested for detrimental fetal effects in humans before release. They usually carry general admonitions on the label such as "use in pregnancy is not recommended unless the potential benefits justify the risks to the fetus."[21] At the very earliest stage of gestation there is some incomplete information on the effects of anesthetic agents. For instance, data exist in humans that assisted reproductive techniques such as in vitro fertilization (IVF) are more successful in narcotic MAC cases than some general anesthetics.[23,24] However, comprehensive, evidence-based information on anesthesia and IVF technology is largely incomplete.

The fetal consequences resulting from environmental or workplace exposure to anesthetic agents is an important but hard-to-study topic. Vecchio and colleagues[25] have recently summarized a great deal of work in this area. There have been numerous epidemiologic studies performed in health care workers. For example, OR personnel exposed to trace nitrous oxide and isoflurane levels had increased chromosomal and lymphocyte abnormalities compared with nonexposed personnel.[26] The authors ranked the genetic risk equal to that of smoking 11 to 20 cigarettes daily. The same group studied in vitro tests of occupational exposure. Genotoxicity was assessed by the formation of micronucleated lymphocytes in 25 anesthetists and anesthetic nurses, compared with a group of nonexposed personnel of the same hospital. There was an increased fraction of micronucleated lymphocytes per 1000 binucleated cells in the high-level exposure group (median 14.0, range 9.0 to 26.7 versus median 11.3, range 3.2 to 19.4; $p < 0.05$) but not in the low-level exposure group (median 9.8, range 4.2 to 20.0 versus median 10.5, range 5.0 to 20.5). They concluded that a high-level exposure to inhaled anesthetics is associated with an increase in chromosome damage. Further, a high level of occupational exposure to inhaled anesthetics was associated with genotoxicity (as defined by formation of micronucleated lymphocytes), whereas a low-level exposure (within National Institute of Occupational Safety and Health [NIOSH] limits) was not.[27]

A number of large epidemiologic studies have reviewed this issue. In one large retrospective study (by questionnaire), 8032 personnel exposed to anesthetic gases in ORs and recovery rooms in Ontario (Canada) hospitals were compared with 2525 nonexposed hospital staff.

The response was 78.8% for the exposed and 87.2% for the unexposed personnel during the study period (1981–1985). Logistic regression analysis, with age and smoking standardized, showed that women in the exposed group had significantly increased frequencies of spontaneous abortions, and their children had significantly more congenital abnormalities ($p < 0.05$). No chronic disease was significantly associated with the exposed group. The authors concluded that it is prudent to minimize exposure to waste anesthetic gases.[28] A large study was performed by Boivin[29] to determine the association between maternal occupational exposure to anesthetic gases and risk of spontaneous abortion. He performed a meta-analysis of published epidemiologic studies identified from literature reviews, unsystematic perusal of reference lists of relevant publications, and two Medline searches (1984–1992, keywords: anaesthetic gases; anaesthetics; anaesthetics, local; operating rooms; operating room nursing; pregnancy; abortion; 1985–1992, keywords: anaesthetics; adverse effects; occupational exposure; anaesthesia, inhalation; operating room nursing; pregnancy; abortion). All peer-reviewed studies were retained. Student theses were excluded, as were conference abstracts, unpublished material, and two studies in which data on paternal and maternal occupational exposures were pooled. Overall, 24 comparisons between exposed and unexposed women were obtained from 19 reports. From these, the relative risk of spontaneous abortion was estimated. The overall relative risk was 1.48 (95% confidence interval [CI], 1.4 to 1.58). To test whether this result was influenced by the quality of the studies, the validity of the reviewed papers was rated on the basis of three criteria: appropriateness of the unexposed comparison group, control for nonoccupational confounding variables, and response rate. The estimate of risk increased to 1.9 (95% CI, 1.72 to 2.09) when analysis was restricted to the six comparisons that were rated the most rigorous. In summary, the author found that epidemiologic studies based on data obtained in the pre-scavenging era indicate an increased risk of spontaneous abortion. Despite the limitations of meta-analysis, the results of this large study indicate that the OR may be a dangerous environment. Some of the previous studies indicate that attention to scavenging to NIOSH standards may help reduce the risk to exposed personnel and their offspring. The overall contribution of risk factors apart from anesthetic agents is harder to control for. Personnel in the OR are commonly subjected to a stressful environment, surrounded by pathogens, and working long hours where a premium is placed on endurance. It remains to be seen if subsequent studies will identify risks in the OR beyond or in conjunction with anesthetic agents. At this time it seems prudent to comply or do better than comply with published NIOSH standards.

Of recent concern are the effects of many anesthetics on fetal and neonatal brain development. One prominent neuroscientist has recently suggested that anesthetic agents cause developing neurons to commit suicide.[30] Most general anesthetics studied can, under experimental conditions in neonatal or fetal laboratory animals, either kill brain cells or increase apoptotic processes. This includes drugs such as isoflurane, benzodiazapines, nitrous oxide, ethanol, phencyclidine, propofol, ketamine, and even barbiturates.[31] Ketamine and propofol have received much of the attention as a neurotoxic agents. The ketamine controversy was the subject of a review and the conclusion was that ketamine remains a valuable drug that should not be abandoned.[32] The U.S. Food and Drug Administration (FDA) produced a review of the available literature to assess risk in pediatric patients requiring anesthesia.[33] The authors state, "The FDA views this communication as opening a dialog with the anesthesia community to address this issue." The review highlights the lack of human data corroborating the laboratory findings but finds the laboratory data compelling enough to warrent concern and further research. A volume of a recent major anesthetic journal was largely devoted to the issue. McGowan and Davis[34] summarized the issues in an accompanying editorial. This will clearly be a hot subject area for research in the coming years.

Laparoscopic Abdominal Surgery in Pregnancy

The use of laparoscopic surgery in pregnancy has increased with overall experience and the evolution of improvements in laparoscopic technique and equipment. What is unclear is whether this approach confers any benefit or risk to the mother or fetus. The topic of safety and risks of laparoscopy in pregnancy has been recently reviewed.[35] Well-documented advantages of laparoscopic surgery include decreased blood loss, decreased postoperative analgesia requirements, shorter hospital stays, and an earlier return to normal activities.[36] Because many acute surgical problems (e.g., appendicitis) are more difficult to diagnose during pregnancy, laparoscopic diagnostic procedures may make it possible to rule out a problem at decreased maternal and fetal morbidity. Earlier mobilization after laparoscopic procedures may decrease thromboembolic events, to which pregnant women are more prone.[37]

Possible disadvantages include direct uterine or fetal injury from trocar insertion, alterations in maternal and fetal blood gases through direct absorption of CO_2, and hypoventilation secondary to interference with diaphragmatic excursion. Additionally, excessive abdominal pressure may lead to decreased uterine blood flow by reducing venous return and decreasing cardiac output or by restricting uterine venous drainage, thus decreasing the gradient to uterine flow unless there is a concomitant increase in mean uterine arterial pressure.

The laparoscopic approach has been used successfully during pregnancy in many common abdominal procedures, including some in the first trimester.[38] Less common, yet successful, applications during pregnancy include a laparoscopic splenectomy in a morbidly obese woman[39] and several patients undergoing transabdominal cervical cerclage procedures.[36] Although these successful cases demonstrate the potential value of laparoscopy, no large series exist that demonstrate its clear superiority, for mother or fetus, over open procedures. A case series describes seven patients undergoing either appendectomy or cholecystectomy between 12 and 33 weeks of gestational age.[40] All the patients had general anesthesia and CO_2 insufflation to 12 mm Hg. The surgery was successful in all cases, and each pregnancy ended in full-term, healthy babies. No long-term follow-up was provided. Rizzo[40] has published the 1- to 8-year follow-up of 11 laparoscopic cases in pregnancy. All cases were performed between the sixteenth and twenty-eighth weeks of pregnancy. CO_2 insufflation pressure was maintained at 10 mm Hg, and the case duration ranged from 25 to 90 minutes. Surgery was performed for appendectomy (3 patients), cholecystectomy (5 patients), or diagnostic laparotomy with intraoperative diagnosis of small bowel obstruction (2 patients). Another patient was converted to open laparotomy because the adhesion could not be approached because of excessive uterine size. All surgeries were successful, and all patients undergoing laparoscopic surgery were discharged in under 48 hours. The one open laparotomy patient spent 5 days in the hospital. All patients, even those previable at surgery, were monitored for 24 hours postoperatively. All pregnancies reached term, and all babies were healthy at birth. Chart review and telephone follow-up for 1 to 6 years has revealed no medical problems or failure to thrive in the offspring. No details are provided regarding the quality or extent of the follow-up. The opinion of the authors was that "laparoscopic surgery in pregnancy is now proving to be safe and efficacious." As more experience is obtained, laparoscopy may become the standard of care.

Several attempts have been made to explore the maternal-fetal physiology of laparoscopy in pregnancy. One such study explored the fetal response to CO_2 pneumoperitoneum using the instrumented fetal sheep. The study was performed in 110-day gestation fetal sheep, which is considered midgestation (term is 147 days). This is important because the results may not apply later when the uterus is larger and abdominal compliance is reduced. Laparoscopy was performed under general anesthesia under controlled ventilation. The abdomen was insufflated to 20.7 mm Hg. Maternal and fetal blood gases and organ blood flows (using radioactive microspheres) were determined at set intervals. It was calculated that maternal perfusion pressure decreased 22%, inferior vena cava pressure rose 53%, and maternal placental blood flow decreased 61% from control measures after 1 hour of insufflation. All these findings were statistically significant. Despite these findings, fetal placental blood flow, perfusion pressure, and blood gases were unchanged, as were maternal blood gases. No mention of fetal brain blood flow was made. These results prompted the authors to conclude that the sheep fetus has enough reserves to tolerate 1 hour of insufflation to 20 mm Hg. This should not be extrapolated to human fetuses or later gestational ages or fetuses that may be chronically stressed or with decreased reserves. Two studies by a different surgical group addressed the fetal cerebral effects of laparoscopy in pregnancy. Both these studies were performed in preterm pregnant guinea pigs. The first study measured fetal brain histology 3 to 5 days after an in utero exposure to 40-minute laparoscopic CO_2 insufflation.[41] Animals were divided in three groups: anesthesia only, CO_2 pneumoperitoneum (5 mm Hg), or laparotomy. The fetal brains were harvested 3 to 5 days later and fixed for histologic examination. A separate animal underwent laparotomy and 20 minutes of total uterine artery occlusion as a positive control. There were two main findings: there was no increase in maternal/fetal morbidity in any of the groups, and CO_2 pneumoperitoneum at 5 mm Hg for 40 minutes did not produce any detectable fetal brain injury. This same group did a further study to examine for early postnatal behavioral deficits that may exist but not manifest in histologic evidence of brain injury.[42] The experiments were similar except the pneumoperitoneum was 7 mm Hg for 45 minutes. The experimental group exhibited hyperactivity significantly more than the control group at postnatal days 10 and 20. What this means for humans is uncertain but does raise potential concerns. The use of laparoscopic surgery in pregnancy is on the rise and offers many potential advantages. However, more physiologic research is necessary to properly evaluate the potential risks.

GUIDELINES

There are no authoritative guidelines for anesthesia for nonobstetric surgery. One must rely on the comprehensive chapters in the major texts cited earlier and take into account the normal physiologic changes of pregnancy to determine the risk of anesthesia for the parturient undergoing nonosbstetric surgery. In general, one should avoid aorta-caval compression after 20 weeks, limit drugs to those with a demonstrated track record of safety in pregnancy, and regard each pregnant woman as a potential aspiration risk. Fetal monitoring should be employed if staffing and surgical site allow. The duration of monitoring into the recovery period and use of tocolytic agents is unclear. Operating and recovery room facilities should be periodically monitored for waste gas scavenging and appropriate NIOSH standards observed. As far as laparoscopic surgery during pregnancy is concerned, the benefits probably outweigh the risks, but care must be taken to avoid trocar injury and the lowest possible insufflation pressures should be used.

AUTHOR'S RECOMMENDATIONS

- Remember to check pregnancy tests where available before anesthesia and surgery.
- Long exposures to 1 MAC or less of inhalation agents are probably safe for mother and fetus.
- Pregnant women should avoid unnecessary exposures to anesthetic agents in the workplace, but if that is unavoidable, NIOSH standards are probably safe and the risk, if any, is very small.
- Laparoscopic surgery during pregnancy is likely a useful modality that will continue to find a place in the surgical approach to some conditions. Scrupulous care should be taken to avoid excessive abdominal distending pressures (greater than 20 mm Hg is suggested, although definitive data are lacking). If surgery is anticipated to be long or difficult, early consideration of open laparotomy seems reasonable.
- FHR and uterine contraction monitoring can be useful and should not be reserved for viable pregnancies only. If monitoring is practical, it is possible for the surgical and anesthetic team to tailor their actions, taking fetal responses into account.
- Anesthetics render FHR beat-to-beat variability unreliable, and only changes in baseline FHR should be considered. FHR monitoring is generally not reliable before 18 weeks of gestation and is most useful at or beyond 22 weeks of gestation.

REFERENCES

1. Cohen SE: Nonobstetric surgery during pregnancy. In Chestnut DH, editor: *Obstetric anesthesia: Principles and practice*, ed 2. St Louis, 1999, Mosby.

2. Azzam FJ, Padda GS, DeBoard JW, Krock JL, Kolterman SM: Preoperative pregnancy testing in adolescents. *Anesth Analg* 1996;82(1):4-7.

3. Barnard JM, Chaffin D, Droste S, Tierney A, Phernetton T: Fetal response to carbon dioxide pneumoperitoneum in the pregnant ewe. *Obstet Gynecol* 1995;85(5 pt 1):669-674.

4. Allen JR, Helling TS, Langenfeld M: Intraabdominal surgery during pregnancy. *Am J Surg* 1989;158(6):567-569.

5. Rosen MA: Anesthesia for fetal procedures and surgery. *Yonsei Med J* 2001;42(6):669-680.

6. Chestnut DH: *Obstetric anesthesia: Principles and practice*, ed 2. St Louis, 1999, Mosby.

7. Hughes SC, Levinson G, Rosen MA, editors: *Shnider and Levinson's anesthesia for obstetrics*, ed 4. Philadelphia, 2002, Lippincott Williams & Wilkins.

8. Friedman EA: The obstetrician's dilemma: How much fetal monitoring and cesarean section is enough? *N Engl J Med* 1986; 315(10):641-643.

9. Leveno KJ, Cunningham FG, Nelson S, et al: A prospective comparison of selective and universal electronic fetal monitoring in 34,995 pregnancies. *N Engl J Med* 1986;315(10):615-619.

10. Hankins GD, Erickson K, Zinberg S, Schulkin J: Neonatal encephalopathy and cerebral palsy: A knowledge survey of Fellows of the American College of Obstetricians and Gynecologists. *Obstet Gynecol* 2003;101(1):11-17.

11. Liu PL, Warren TM, Ostheimer GW, Weiss JB, Liu LM: Foetal monitoring in parturients undergoing surgery unrelated to pregnancy. *Can Anaesth Soc J* 1985;32(5):525-532.

12. Biehl DR: Foetal monitoring during surgery unrelated to pregnancy. *Can Anaesth Soc J* 1985;32(5):455-459.

13. Gregory GA, Wade JG, Beihl DR, Ong BY, Sitar DS: Fetal anesthetic requirement (MAC) for halothane. *Anesth Analg* 1983;62(1):9-14.

14. Biehl DR, Cote J, Wade JG, Gregory GA, Sitar D: Uptake of halothane by the foetal lamb in utero. *Can Anaesth Soc J* 1983;30(1):24-27.

15. Biehl DR, Tweed WA, Cote J, Wade JG, Sitar D: Effect of halothane on cardiac output and regional flow in the fetal lamb in utero. *Anesth Analg* 1983;62(5):489-492.

16. Biehl DR, Yarnell R, Wade JG, Sitar D: The uptake of isoflurane by the foetal lamb in utero: Effect on regional blood flow. *Can Anaesth Soc J* 1983;30(6):581-586.

17. Palahniuk RJ, Shnider SM: Maternal and fetal cardiovascular and acid-base changes during halothane and isoflurane anesthesia in the pregnant ewe. *Anesthesiology* 1974;41(5):462-472.

18. Yarnell R, Biehl DR, Tweed WA, Gregory GA, Sitar D: The effect of halothane anaesthesia on the asphyxiated foetal lamb in utero. *Can Anaesth Soc J* 1983;30(5):474-479.

19. Palahniuk RJ, Doig GA, Johnson GN, Pash MP: Maternal halothane anesthesia reduces cerebral blood flow in the acidotic sheep fetus. *Anesth Analg* 1980;59(1):35-39.

20. Levinson G: Anesthesia for surgery during pregnancy. In Hughes SC, Levinson G, Rosen MA, editors: *Shnider and Levinson's anesthesia for obstetrics*, ed 4. Philadelphia, 2001, Lippincott Williams & Wilkins.

21. Koren G, Pastuszak A, Ito S: Drugs in pregnancy. *N Engl J Med* 1998;338(16):1128-1137.

22. Rosenberg L, Mitchell AA, Parsells JL, Pashayan H, Louik C, Shapiro S: Lack of relation of oral clefts to diazepam use during pregnancy. *N Engl J Med* 1983;309(21):1282-1285.

23. Wilhelm W, Hammadeh ME, White PF, Georg T, Fleser R, Biedler A: General anesthesia versus monitored anesthesia care with remifentanil for assisted reproductive technologies: Effect on pregnancy rate. *J Clin Anesth* 2002;14(1):1-5.

24. Vincent RD Jr, Syrop CH, Van Voorhis BJ, et al: An evaluation of the effect of anesthetic technique on reproductive success after laparoscopic pronuclear stage transfer. Propofol/nitrous oxide versus isoflurane/nitrous oxide. *Anesthesiology* 1995;82(2):352-358.

25. Vecchio D, Sasco AJ, Cann CI. Occupational risk in healthcare and research. *Am J Ind Med* 2003;43:364–369.

26. Hoerauf KH, Wiesner G, Schroegendorfer KF, et al: Waste anaesthetic gases induce sister chromatid exchanges in lymphocytes of operating room personnel. *Br J Anaesth* 1999;82(5): 764–766.

27. Wiesner G, Hoerauf K, Schroegendorfer K, Sobczynski P, Harth M, Ruediger HW: High-level, but not low-level, occupational exposure to inhaled anesthetics is associated with genotoxicity in the micronucleus assay. *Anesth Analg* 2001;92(1):118-122.

28. Guirguis SS, Pelmear PL, Roy ML, Wong L: Health effects associated with exposure to anaesthetic gases in Ontario hospital personnel. *Br J Ind Med* 1990;47(7):490-497.

29. Boivin JF: Risk of spontaneous abortion in women occupationally exposed to anaesthetic gases: A meta-analysis. *Occup Environ Med* 1997;54(8):541-548.

30. Olney JW, Young C, Wozniak DF, Jevtovic-Todorovic V, Ikonomidou C: Do pediatric drugs cause developing neurons to commit suicide? *Trends Phamacol Sci* 2004;25(3):135-139.

31. Soriano SG, Anand KJS, Rovnaghi CR, Hickey PR: Of mice and men: Should we extrapolate rodent experimental data to the care of human neonates? *Anesthesiology* 2005;102:866-868.

32. Bhutta AT, Venkatesan AK, Rovnaghi CR, Anand KJS: Anesthetic neurotoxicity in rodents: Is the ketamine controversy real? *Foundation/Acta Paediatrica* 2007;96:1554-1556.

33. Mellon RD, Simone AF, Rappaport BA: Use of anesthetic agents in neonates and young children. *Anesth Analg* 2007;104(3):509–520.

34. McGowan FX, Davis PJ: Anesthetic-related neurotoxicity in the developing infant: Of mice, rats, monkeys and, possibly, humans. *Anesth Analg* 2008;106:1599-1602.

35. Al-Fozan H, Tulandi T: Safety and risks of laparoscopy in pregnancy. *Curr Opin Obstet Gynecol* 2002;14(4):375-379.

36. Lemaire BM, van Erp WF: Laparoscopic surgery during pregnancy. *Surg Endosc* 1997;11(1):15-18.

37. Schwartzberg BS, Conyers JA, Moore JA: First trimester of pregnancy laparoscopic procedures. *Surg Endosc* 1997;11(12):1216-1217.

38. Allran CF Jr, Weiss CA 3rd, Park AE: Urgent laparoscopic splenectomy in a morbidly obese pregnant woman: Case report and literature review. *J Laparoendosc Adv Surg Tech A* 2002;12(6):445-447.

39. Gallot D, Savary D, Laurichesse H, Bournazeau JA, Amblard J, Lemery D: Experience with three cases of laparoscopic transabdominal cervico-isthmic cerclage and two subsequent pregnancies. *Br J Obstet Gynecol* 2003;110(7):696-700.

40. Rizzo AG: Laparoscopic surgery in pregnancy: Long-term follow-up. *J Laparoendosc Adv Surg Tech A* 2003;13(1):11-15.

41. Garcia-Oria M, Ali A, Reynolds JD, et al: Histologic evaluation of fetal brains following maternal pneumoperitoneum. *Surg Endosc* 2001;15(11):1294-1298.

42. Fuente SG, Pinheiro J, Gupta M, Eubanks WS, Reynolds JD: Early postnatal behavior deficits after maternal carbon dioxide pneumoperitoneum during pregnancy. *Surg Endosc* [E-pub June 17] 2003.

PEDIATRIC ANESTHESIA

70 How Young Is the Youngest Infant for Outpatient Surgery?

Lucinda L. Everett, MD

INTRODUCTION/BACKGROUND

Outpatient surgery accounts for a significant percentage of anesthetics delivered annually in the United States. Many pediatric procedures, including myringotomy and tubes, endoscopy, circumcision, and hernia repair, are performed in infants and may occur on an outpatient basis.

Apnea is the most common serious adverse event after general anesthesia in an infant. Premature and former premature infants are at higher risk of apnea than healthy term babies; there is little evidence regarding apnea risk in term patients. In addition, infants (younger than 1 year) are at higher risk of intraoperative anesthetic cardiac arrest and other complications,[1] and require careful anesthetic management by practitioners with training and ongoing experience in this population.

PATHOPHYSIOLOGY

Apnea of prematurity is found in 50% of premature infants, and is almost universal in infants who are 1000 g at birth. Clinically significant apnea in infants is defined as breathing pauses of 20 seconds, or 10 seconds with bradycardia or oxygen desaturation. However, there is no consensus as to what is pathologic in terms of the duration of apnea, degree of change in oxygen saturation, and severity of bradycardia, and the relationship with conditions such as gastroesophageal reflux is unclear.[2]

In the perioperative setting, 1982 brought Steward's publication of a small series of infants having herniorrhaphy, which showed that preterm infants were more prone to apnea and other airway complications.[3] A larger prospective study of infants having general anesthesia for a variety of procedures found that a much higher proportion of premature infants required postoperative ventilation.[4] The authors postulated that "anesthetics may unmask a defect in ventilatory control of prematurely born infants younger than 41–46 weeks conceptual age with preanesthetic history of idiopathic apnea." Apnea of prematurity and postoperative apnea are primarily central in nature, although a minority of children have an obstructive or mixed pattern.

EVIDENCE

Overall Risk in Pediatric Anesthesia

Few studies specifically address risk in infants for outpatient surgery. Patel and Hannallah[5] assessed anesthetic complications in a large series of pediatric outpatients and did not note any specific issues in approximately 350 patients under 6 months of age.

Further evaluation of overall risk requires extrapolation from studies of particular patient populations or from adverse outcomes in infants who are not necessarily outpatients. Several studies have demonstrated an increased incidence of complications in infants (younger than 1 year of age) compared with other pediatric age-groups. A prospective survey of 40,240 anesthetics in infants and children from 1978 to 1982 found an overall complication rate of 4.3% in infants compared with 0.5% in children 1 to 14 years of age; the cardiac arrest rate was 1.9% in infants compared with 0.2% in the older patients.[6] Risk increased with increasing ASA status and in emergency procedures; the majority of "accidents" in the infant group occurred during the maintenance of anesthesia and were initiated by respiratory events. Analysis of anesthetics conducted in more than 29,000 children from 1982 to 1987 found a high incidence of adverse events in very small infants (younger than 1 month), but patients were more likely to have a higher ASA status and/or be undergoing major cardiac or intraabdominal surgery.[7] A large prospective French audit reflecting currently available drugs and monitoring techniques showed that respiratory events accounted for 53% of all intraoperative events, and that there remains a higher risk of adverse events in infants compared with older children.[8]

Analysis of closed claims information as published in 1993 showed that pediatric claims were more often related to respiratory events, and the mortality rate was greater than in adults.[9] The complications in pediatric cases were more frequently thought to have been preventable with better monitoring. Analysis of pediatric closed claims from 1990 to 2000 showed a decrease in the proportion of respiratory claims, particularly those for inadequate oxygenation and ventilation, compared with pediatric claims from the earlier period.[10]

The initial observations from the closed claims data led to the creation of the Pediatric Perioperative Cardiac Arrest (POCA) Registry.[1] Basic demographic information from participating institutions was submitted along with case reports of cardiac arrest. Although overall denominator data are available, more specific information such as breakdown of anesthetic agents in all cases or qualifications of the anesthesia caregivers is not. The incidence of cardiac arrest for the institutions studied for the first report (1994 to 1997) was 1.4 per 10,000 anesthetics, with a mortality rate of 26%. Cardiac arrest occurred most often in patients less than 1 year of age and in patients with severe underlying disease. Patients with concurrent diseases and those having emergency surgery were most likely to have a fatal outcome. In patients who were ASA status 1 or 2, 64% of the cardiac arrests were medication related; two thirds of the medication-related arrests were due to cardiovascular depression from halothane alone or in combination with other drugs. Cases from the POCA registry for the years 1998 to 2004 demonstrated a declining proportion of cardiac arrest related to medications, in parallel with the transition from halothane to sevoflurane in clinical practice.[11]

Apnea Risk

Term Infants

There is relatively little specific evidence about apnea risk following anesthesia in term infants. Some evidence exists for individual procedures, which is not generalizable, but may help in setting limits for outpatient surgery. Infants with pyloric stenosis require admission because of the need for preoperative fluid resuscitation and the risk of postoperative apnea (related to metabolic abnormalities). Data from 60 full-term neonates and infants undergoing pyloromyotomy showed a significant incidence of apnea (27% preoperatively and 16% postoperatively), some in patients with normal preoperative pneumograms.[12] Although currently not considered appropriate for outpatient surgery because of airway concerns, Stephens and colleagues[13] report a retrospective analysis of 50 neonates (3 to 56 days; 11 former prematures of less than 45 weeks postconceptual age) having cleft lip repair who had minimal respiratory complications.[13] Ongoing reassessment of practice and refinement of techniques, however, continue to lead to additional procedures being done in a short-stay or day-surgery setting in selected patients: 23-hour admission has been described for otherwise healthy, nonsyndromic patients having primary cleft palate surgery at ages from 6 to 20 months.[14] Large population studies are needed to truly evaluate risk.

Premature Infants

The bulk of evidence regarding apnea risk after anesthesia relates to former premature infants rather than term babies. A number of small case series tried to more accurately define risk; the data from several of these were pooled into a "combined analysis" in 1995 by Coté and colleagues.[15] The combined series contains data from 255 former preterm infants having general anesthesia for inguinal hernia repairs; infants receiving caffeine were excluded. Using a standardized definition of apnea (greater than 15 seconds without bradycardia, or less than 15 seconds when accompanied by bradycardia), they looked for associated risk factors to better define the population at risk. There was considerable variation between institutions in the reported incidence, which was thought to be related to differences in monitoring techniques. The combined analysis showed that apnea was strongly and inversely related to both gestational age and postconceptual age, and that continuing apnea at home and anemia were also risk factors. No association was found with a number of other historical factors or anesthetic variables, but this may have been due to the relatively small numbers.

The Coté combined analysis does not define a strict cutoff age for all patients, but rather defines confidence intervals for the risk of apnea at various combinations of gestational and postconceptual age. For nonanemic infants free of recovery room apnea, the probability of apnea was not less than 1% until postconceptual age 56 weeks with gestational age 32 weeks, or postconceptual age 54 weeks with gestational age 35 weeks. The authors note that individual clinicians must decide on acceptable risk in a given practice setting.

Some question the clinical relevance of apnea detected only by sophisticated monitoring techniques, and one group has published a series of 124 former preterm infants, including 67 patients below 46 weeks of postconceptual age, where those having uncomplicated anesthetics were discharged after an average recovery room stay of 94 minutes with no apparent adverse consequences.[16] One episode of apnea, responsive to stimulation, was noted in an infant on an apnea monitor at home. A retrospective review of respiratory complications in 57 former premature infants having hernia repair noted that all instances of postoperative apnea/bradycardia and laryngospasm occurred within the first four hours postoperatively.[17] Caution is urged in generalizing these findings without larger studies to demonstrate the safety of outpatient care in this patient population.

Methylxanthines. A prospective randomized trial of caffeine versus placebo for apnea of prematurity in 2006 infants with birth weights of 500 to 1250 g showed that fewer caffeine-treated infants required supplemental oxygen (36% versus 47%) and treated infants had positive airway pressure discontinued on average 1 week earlier.[18] The follow-up phase of the same study showed a modest improvement in survival, and a modest decrease in the incidence of cerebral palsy and cognitive dysfunction, in caffeine-treated very low birth weight infants.[19]

Caffeine has been shown to decrease the risk of apnea in former premature infants undergoing general anesthesia, but studies are relatively small. Welborn and colleagues[20] randomized 32 former preterm infants (37 to 44 weeks postconceptual age) to receive either caffeine 10 mg/kg or placebo in conjunction with general anesthesia for inguinal hernia repair. No patients in the caffeine group had postoperative bradycardia, prolonged apnea, periodic breathing, or postoperative oxygen saturation less than 90%; 81% of patients in the control group had prolonged apnea at 4 to 6 hours postoperatively.[20] Systematic review of the available studies concluded that evidence supports that caffeine reduces apnea risk, but that because of small numbers and questionable clinical significance of apneic

Table 70-1	**Summary of Meta-analysis on Prophylactic Caffeine to Prevent Postoperative Apnea following General Anesthesia in Former Preterm Infants**				
Study, Year	**Number of Trials**	**Number of Subjects**	**Intervention**	**Control**	**Outcomes**
Ref. 21, 2001	3	78	Caffeine (10 mg/kg in two studies, 5 mg/kg in one)	Placebo	Apnea/bradycardia occurred in fewer treated infants. In two studies, oxygen desaturation was evaluated; fewer episodes occurred in the treatment group.

episodes in clinical trials to date, caution should be used in applying these results to routine clinical practice[21] (Table 70-1).

Anesthetic Technique and Apnea Risk. In a prospective comparison by Welborn and colleagues,[22] spinal anesthesia alone had a lower incidence of postoperative apnea and bradycardia in former preterm infants when compared with spinal plus sedation, or general anesthesia. Other studies have confirmed a lower incidence of oxygen desaturation and bradycardia,[23] although Krane and colleagues[24] did not find a difference in the incidence of central apnea, suggesting that airway obstruction may also play a role in postoperative clinical events. The incidence of apnea after unsupplemented spinal anesthesia in former premature infants is low[25]; however, cardiopulmonary events occur frequently enough in this population[26] to warrant postoperative observation as for general anesthesia. A Cochrane review analyzed four small trials comparing spinal with general anesthesia in the repair of inguinal hernia in former preterm infants[27] (Table 70-2). The authors found no significant difference in the proportion of infants having postoperative apnea/bradycardia or oxygen desaturation. Meta-analysis supported a reduction in postoperative apnea in infants having spinal anesthesia without sedation, as well as a borderline significant decrease in the use of postoperative assisted ventilation.

The majority of studies of spinal anesthesia in former preterm infants used comparison with older volatile agents, primarily halothane; however, a comparison with sevoflurane still showed a lower incidence of postoperative cardiorespiratory complications with spinal anesthesia.[28] Because both groups received supplemental caudal analgesia, this study actually examined whether a "light" general anesthetic with caudal block would lower the risk to the same level as with unsupplemented spinal, and found that it did not.

Clonidine has good safety and efficacy in children for caudal block, but several case reports have suggested that it is associated with postoperative apnea.[29,30] A prospective series of term and preterm infants having spinal anesthesia with bupivacaine and clonidine found a significant increase in apneic episodes postoperatively but no change in the incidence of desaturation[31]; there was not a study group without clonidine.

Regarding general anesthetic agents, one study comparing halothane with remifentanil for infants undergoing pyloromyotomy found that none of the 38 patients receiving remifentanil developed new pneumogram abnormalities after anesthesia, whereas 3 of 22 infants receiving halothane did.[32] Coté and colleagues[15] did not find a specific influence of opioids on postoperative apnea, but note that very few of the infants in their study received opioids. In a comparison of general anesthetic techniques in term and former preterm infants less than 60 weeks of postconceptual age having hernia repairs, patients having thiopental or halothane induction with desflurane maintenance had significantly shorter times to extubation than those having the entire anesthetic with either halothane or sevoflurane. None of the 40 infants in this study had significant postoperative apnea.[33] A prospective comparison of sevoflurane and desflurane in former premature infants having hernia repair found no difference in the incidence of respiratory events, and no difference between the preoperative and postoperative incidence of apnea in either group.[34]

Expertise of Anesthesia Providers

Although not extensively studied, some evidence suggests fewer adverse outcomes in the hands of anesthesiologists with frequent ongoing experience in anesthetizing children. Keenan and colleagues[35] found a lower incidence of bradycardia in infants when a pediatric

Table 70-2	**Summary of Meta-analysis on Regional versus General Anesthesia in Preterm Infants**				
Study, Year	**Number of Trials**	**Number of Subjects**	**Intervention**	**Control**	**Outcomes**
Ref. 27, 2003	4	108	Spinal anesthesia (local anesthetic only)	General Volatile plus muscle relaxant	Significant reduction in postoperative apnea for unsupplemented spinal anesthesia

anesthesiologist was present. Mamie and colleagues[36] showed a lower incidence of respiratory complications in the hands of pediatric anesthesiologists. The exact definition of a pediatric anesthesiologist, and how to best balance adequate ongoing practice with broad availability, remains controversial.[37] The American Academy of Pediatrics Section on Anesthesiology[38] has stated that anesthesiologists "providing or directly supervising the anesthesia care of patients in categories designated by the facility's Department of Anesthesia as being at increased anesthesia risk should be graduates of an ACGME pediatric anesthesiology fellowship training program or its equivalent or have documented demonstrated historical and continuous competence in the care of such patients." (See below, under Guidelines.)

CONTROVERSIES

Current evidence does not define an exact "safe" age for former premature infants to be discharged after general anesthesia, nor does it completely delineate the appropriate length of postoperative monitoring for general anesthesia with or without caffeine, or for spinal anesthesia. There is a lack of consensus on what constitutes a "significant" postoperative apnea event, and different studies report apnea in different ways (i.e., absolute number of episodes, versus change from preoperative). Although evidence supports an advantage to the use of spinal anesthesia in former premature infants, the optimal anesthetic/analgesic regimen for all infants is not known.

In addition, the overall postoperative risk in healthy term infants having outpatient surgery is not well delineated although apnea risk after minor procedures appears to be low.

GUIDELINES

There are no formal practice guidelines from major anesthesia or pediatric organizations regarding outpatient surgery in infants. However, many individual hospitals have developed such guidelines, particularly for ex-premature infants. These frequently establish a cutoff age of 50 to 56 weeks of postconceptual age in infants born before 37 weeks, and may also consider factors such as anemia, prior apnea, and coexisting disease. Postoperative monitoring recommendations range from 12- to 24-hour admission for cardiorespiratory monitoring to include oxygen saturation, heart rate, and impedance pneumography. Some facilities also restrict the lower age for day surgery procedures to above 44 to 46 weeks of postconceptual age in term infants, or require a longer observation period (e.g., 4 hours) in phase II recovery.

A practice guideline from the American Academy of Pediatrics Section on Anesthesiology does have implications for facilities providing anesthesia care for infants.

The document "Guidelines for the Pediatric Perioperative Anesthesia Environment" makes recommendations for facilities, equipment, and provider considerations in caring for various classes of pediatric patients, and recommends that patients considered by the facility to be at "high risk," including small infants, be cared for by anesthesiologists with fellowship training or expertise based on ongoing experience.[38] The American Society of Anesthesiologists has made similar recommendations.

AUTHOR'S RECOMMENDATIONS

KEY FINDINGS BASED ON DATA

- Postoperative apnea in former premature infants is inversely proportional to both gestational age and postconceptual age.
- Caffeine decreases the risk of postoperative apnea in former premature infants.
- Spinal anesthesia without sedation has a lower incidence of postoperative apnea in premature infants than general anesthesia or spinal with sedation.
- No specific general anesthetic agent or regimen has been shown to be superior in minimizing complications in former premature infants.
- Anesthesia for healthy term infants having simple surgical procedures appears to be safe on an outpatient basis, although there are few data.

SPECIFIC CLINICAL RECOMMENDATIONS

- Appropriate short-acting anesthetic agents may facilitate emergence and discharge.
- Where possible, regional anesthetic techniques and nonopioid analgesics should be used instead of opioids.
- A loading dose of caffeine citrate 20 mg/kg may decrease postoperative apnea in former premature infants.
- If the surgical procedure is suitable, consider spinal anesthesia without sedation in former premature infants; however, postoperative monitoring is still recommended in the at-risk age range.
- Former premature infants should be admitted for observation unless they are over 54 to 56 weeks of postconceptual age (depending on degree of prematurity) and are without anemia, ongoing apnea, or other significant medical problems. Infants meeting these criteria need also to have had an uneventful anesthetic and recovery room course to allow consideration of discharge. More refined recommendations regarding exact postconceptual age and gestational age can be made on an individual patient basis using data from Coté's combined analysis.[15]
- Term infants are acceptable for outpatient procedures providing they are otherwise healthy, the procedure is not likely to result in significant physiologic changes or postoperative pain requiring opioid medications, and the anesthetic proceeds uneventfully. It may be prudent to monitor these patients in the recovery area for several hours postoperatively (Figure 70-1).
- All infants should be cared for in a facility with adequate and appropriately sized equipment, and medical and nursing staff with appropriate expertise and adequate ongoing experience in caring for this age-group.

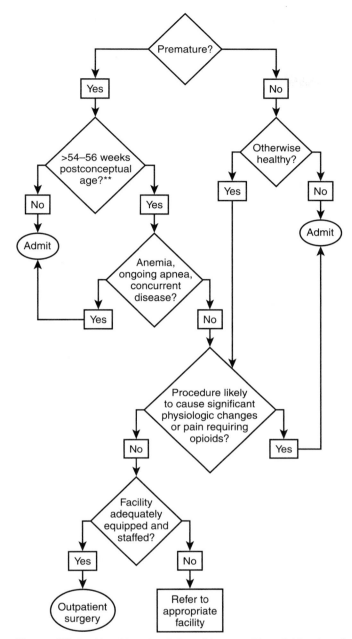

Figure 70-1. Algorithm for Infants Younger Than 6 Months of Age Having Outpatient Surgery

REFERENCES

1. Morray JP, Geiduschek J, Ramamoorthy C, et al: Anesthesia-related cardiac arrest in children: Initial findings of the Pediatric Perioperative Cardiac Arrest (POCA) Registry. *Anesthesiology* 2000;93:6-14.
2. Finer NN, Higgins R, Kattwinkel J, et al: Summary proceedings from the Apnea of Prematurity Group. *Pediatrics* 2006;117: S47-S51.
3. Steward DJ: Preterm infants are more prone to complications following minor surgery than are term infants. *Anesthesiology* 1982;56:304-306.
4. Liu LMP, Coté CJ, Goudsouzian NG, et al: Life-threatening apnea in infants recovering from anesthesia. *Anesthesiology* 1983;59: 506-510.
5. Patel RI, Hannallah RS:, Anesthetic complications following pediatric ambulatory surgery: A 3-yr study. *Anesthesiology* 1988;69:1009-1012.
6. Tiret L, Nivoche Y, Hatton F, et al: Complications related to anaesthesia in infants and children. *Br J Anaesth* 1988;61: 263-269.
7. Cohen MM, Cameron CB Duncan PG, Pediatric anesthesia morbidity and mortality in the perioperative period. *Anesth Analg* 1990;70:160-167.
8. Murat I, Constant I, Maud'huy H, et al: Perioperative anaesthetic morbidity in children: A database of 24 165 anaesthetics over a 30-month period. *Pediatr Anesth* 2004;14:158-166.
9. Morray JP, Geiduschek JM, Caplan RA, et al: A comparison of pediatric and adult anesthesia closed malpractice claims. *Anesthesiology* 1993;78:461-467.
10. Jimenez N, Posner KL, Cheney FW, et al: An update on pediatric anesthesia liability: A closed claims analysis. *Anesth Analg* 2007; 104:147-153.
11. Bhananker SM, Ramamoorthy C, Geiduschek JM, et al: Anesthesia-related cardiac arrest in children: Update from the pediatric Perioperative Cardiac Arrest Registry. *Anesth Analg* 2007;105: 344-350.
12. Galinkin JL, Davis PJ, McGowan FX, et al: A randomized multi-center study of remifentanil compared with halothane in neonates and infants undergoing pyloromyotomy. II. Perioperative breathing patterns in neonates and infants with pyloric stenosis. *Anesth Analg* 2001;93:1387-1392.
13. Stephens P, Saunders P, Bingham R: Neonatal cleft lip repair: A retrospective review of anaesthetic complications. *Paediatr Anaesth* 1997;7:33-36.
14. Cronin ED, Williams JL, Shayani P, et al: Short stay after cleft palate surgery. *Plast Reconstr Surg* 2001;108:838-840.
15. Coté CJ, Zaslavsky A, Downes JJ, et al: Postoperative apnea in former preterm infants after inguinal herniorrhaphy. *Anesthesiology* 1995;82:809-821.
16. Melone JH, Schwartz MZ, Tyson RT, et al: Outpatient inguinal herniorrhapy in premature infants: Is it safe? *J Pediatr Surg* 1992;27:203-208.
17. Allen GS, Cox CS, White N: Postoperative respiratory complications in ex-premature infants after inguinal hemiorrhaphy. *J Pediatr Surg* 1998;39:1095-1099.
18. Schmidt B, Roberts RS Davis P, et al: Caffeine therapy for apnea of prematurity. *N Engl J Med* 2006;354:2112-2121.
19. Schmidt B, Roberts RS Davis P, et al: Long-term effects of caffeine therapy for apnea of prematurity. *N Engl J Med* 2007; 357:1893-1902.
20. Welborn LG, Hannallah RS, Fink R, et al: High-dose caffeine suppresses postoperative apnea in former preterm infants. *Anesthesiology* 1989;71:347-349.
21. Henderson-Smart DJ, Steer P: Prophylactic caffeine to prevent postoperative apnea following general anesthesia in preterm infants. *Cochrane Database of Systematic Reviews* 2001;4: CD000048.
22. Welborn LG, Rice LJ, Hannallah RS, et al: Postoperative apnea in former preterm infants: Prospective comparison of spinal and general anesthesia. *Anesthesiology* 1990;72:838-842.
23. Somri M, Gaitin L, Vaida S, et al: Postoperative outcome in high-risk infants undergoing herniorrhaphy: Comparison between spinal and general anaesthesia. *Anaesthesia* 1998;53:762-766.
24. Krane EJ, Haberkern CM, Jacobson LE: Postoperative apnea, bradycardia, and oxygen desaturation in formerly premature infants: Prospective comparison of spinal and general anesthesia. *Anesth Analg* 1995;80:7-13.
25. Frumiento C, Abajian JC, Vane DW: Spinal anesthesia for preterm infants undergoing inguinal hernia repair. *Arch Surg* 2000;135: 445-451.
26. Shenkman Z, Hopperstein D, Litmanowitz I, et al: Spinal anesthesia in 62 premature, former-premature or young infants—technical aspects and pitfalls. *Can J Anesth* 2002;49:262-269.
27. Craven PD, Badawi N, Henderson-Smart DJ, et al: Regional (spinal, epidural, caudal) versus general anaesthesia in preterm infants undergoing inguinal herniorrhaphy in early infancy. *Cochrane Database of Systematic Reviews* 2003;6:CD003669.
28. Williams JM, Stoddart PA, Williams SAR, et al: Post-operative recovery after inguinal herniotomy in ex-premature infants: Comparison between sevoflurane and spinal anaesthesia. *Br J Anaesth* 2001;86:366-371.

29. Breschan C, Krumpholz R, Likar R, et al: Can a dose of 2μg/kg caudal clonidine cause respiratory depression in neonates? *Paediatr Anaesth* 1999;9:81-83.

30. Fellmann C, Gerber AC, Weiss M: Apnoea in a former preterm infant after caudal bupivacaine with clonidine for inguinal herniorrhaphy. *Paediatr Anaesth* 2002;12:637-640.

31. Rochette A, Troncin R, Raux O, et al: Clonidine added to bupivacaine in neonatal spinal anesthesia: A prospective comparison in 124 preterm and term infants. *Paediatr Anaesth* 2005;15:1072-1077.

32. Davis PJ, Galinkin J, McGowan FX, et al: A randomized multicenter study of remifentanil compared with halothane in neonates and infants undergoing pyloromyotomy. I. Emergence and recovery profiles. *Anesth Analg* 2001;93:1380-1386.

33. O'Brien K, Robinson DN, Morton NS: Induction and emergence in infants less than 60 weeks post-conceptual age: Comparison of thiopental, halothane, sevoflurane and desflurane. *Br J Anaesth* 1998;80:456-459.

34. Sale SM, Read JA, Stoddart PA, et al: Prospective comparison of sevoflurane and desflurane in formerly premature infants undergoing inguinal herniotomy. *Br J Anaesth* 2006;96:774-778.

35. Keenan RL, Shapiro JH, Kane FR, Simpson PM: Bradycardia during anesthesia in infants. An epidemiologic study. *Anesthesiology* 1994;80:976-982.

36. Mamie C, Habre W, Delhumeau C, et al: Incidence and risk factors of perioperative respiratory adverse events in children undergoing elective surgery. *Paediatr Anaesth* 2004;14:218-224.

37. McNicol R: Paediatric anaesthesia—who should do it? The view from the specialist hospital. *Anaesthesia* 1997;52:513-516.

38. American Academy of Pediatrics: Guidelines for the pediatric perioperative anesthesia environment. *Pediatrics* 1999;103:512-515.

71 Should a Child with a Respiratory Tract Infection Undergo Elective Surgery?

Christopher T. McKee, DO; Lynne G. Maxwell, MD; and
R. Blaine Easley, MD

INTRODUCTION

Acute respiratory infections are one of the leading medical causes for surgery cancellation in children.[1] Anesthesiologists are often confronted with patients demonstrating symptoms of upper respiratory tract infections (URIs; runny nose, congestion, cough, etc.) and lower respiratory tract infections (LRIs; crackles, rales, wheezing, sputum production) on the day of surgery. Additional pressures to proceed with anesthesia and surgery despite respiratory symptoms often involve nonmedical issues, which may be social, emotional, and even financial in nature, and these pressures can come from the patient's family, the surgeon, and the hospital.[1]

What is the evidence regarding risk of proceeding with anesthesia and surgery in the face of acute URI/LRI symptoms? Many large retrospective studies have shown an increased risk for adverse intraoperative and perioperative events such as croup, laryngospasm, and bronchospasm.[2,3] Physiologic experiments in animals and humans have shown increased small airway reactivity during and after viral respiratory tract infections.[4-7] Although the exact mechanisms are unknown, it appears that the airways are affected for up to 6 weeks following a viral respiratory infection.

Another confounding issue in dealing with respiratory tract infections in children is the frequency with which they occur. The average child less than 5 years of age is reported to suffer from five to six URIs per year with a duration of 7 to 10 days of active symptoms and residual pulmonary effects of 2 to 6 weeks.[8] This creates a practical problem of children becoming reinfected as often as every 2 weeks, especially during the winter months. Adverse respiratory events such as bronchospasm and laryngospasm have been shown to occur more frequently in all pediatric patients even in the absence of respiratory infections, especially in children under 1 year of age. Pediatric patients have an incidence of laryngospasm of 17.4 per 1000 in ages 0 to 9 years, which increases in patients with reactive airway disease to 63.9 per 1000. The ratio rises to 95.8 per 1000 when children have a history of respiratory tract infections.[3] Children with underlying chronic pulmonary diseases (e.g., reactive airway disease, asthma, cystic fibrosis, and lung disease of prematurity) have been shown

to have an increased risk for perioperative events such as prolonged intubation, reintubation, hypoxemia, bronchospasm, and laryngospasm.[9-13] There is some evidence that risk of airway events is also increased in children who are exposed to secondhand smoke even in the absence of a history of reactive airway disease or infection.[14]

OPTIONS

Although there is a great deal of anecdotal information in the literature concerning adverse events in children with respiratory infections,[15,16] the clinical dilemma of managing those patients who are demonstrating symptoms of URI or LRI persists for many practitioners. Numerous studies have attempted to elucidate the risks of anesthesia in children with respiratory infections. The following studies and their results are reviewed to better understand the current state of anesthetic care for infants and children with respiratory tract infections, as they relate to the following issues:

1. Appropriately identifying children with acute or recent respiratory tract infections
2. Evidence to proceed with a general anesthetic in children with and without endotracheal intubation
3. Evidence to support delaying nonemergent surgery for 2 weeks or up to 6 weeks

EVIDENCE FOR PERIOPERATIVE RISK OF CHILDREN WITH RESPIRATORY INFECTIONS

No randomized prospective studies have evaluated the different management options and the relationship to perioperative respiratory complications in acutely symptomatic children or in those who are recovering from a respiratory tract infection. The studies that have been done have been limited to patients having brief outpatient procedures. There are no studies to evaluate children with URI who undergo prolonged or invasive procedures to address the possibility of benefit from delaying versus proceeding with nonurgent surgery. Therefore one must rely on cohort studies for determining the clinical evidence that exists for management of children with symptomatic and resolving respiratory tract infections (Table 71-1).

Table 71-1 Overview of Study Design and Findings of Major Studies Involving Risk of General Anesthesia in Children with URI

Study	Design	Number of Patients Studied	Number of Children with URI	Number of Children with Recent URI	Intubation	LMA	Facemask	Adverse Events	Conclusions
Tait (1987)[17]	Retrospective	3585	122	133	Yes	Yes		L, B, S, A	No increased risk if URI, no difference between ETT versus facemask, if recent URI had a 3 times higher rate of bronchospasm
Tait (1987)[19]	Prospective	489	78	84	No	Yes		L, Dy, A	No increased rate of complications in groups with acute or recent URI
DeSoto (1988)[21]	Prospective	50	25	—	Yes	Yes		D	If URI present, increased risk for desaturation
Cohen (1991)[25]	Prospective	22159	1283	—	Yes	Yes	Yes	L, B, S, A	If URI then 2 to 3 times more likely to have event, 11 times more likely if URI and ETT
Rolf (1992)[23]	Prospective	402	30	—	Yes	Yes	Yes	L, B, D	If URI then increase in minor desaturation, if URI and ETT then higher frequency of bronchospasm
Kinouchi (1992)[22]	Prospective	61	20	—	No	Yes		D, A	Desaturation occurs more frequently in young children and is of longer duration
Levy (1992)[20]	Prospective	130	22	28	No	Yes		D	If acute or recent URI then an increased risk for desaturation
Schreiner (1996)[24]	Case control	15183	30	17	Yes	Yes	Yes	L	Laryngospasm was more likely to occur in patients with URI, younger children, no correlation between mask versus ETT versus LMA
Skolnick (1998)[14]	Prospective	602	?	?	Yes	Yes		L, B, S, A	Increased risk for adverse events if URI, smoking exposure increase
Tait (1998)[26]	Prospective	82	82	?	Yes	Yes	Yes	C, A, L, B, D	LMA suitable alternative to ETT
Homer (2007)[27]	Prospective	335	?	?	Yes	Yes	Yes	D, C	
Tait (2001)[43]	Prospective	1078	407	335	Yes	Yes	Yes	B, L, A, C, D	Child with active or recent URI at increased risk for adverse events, but most can be safely anesthetized

A, apnea/breath holding; B, bronchospasm; C, coughing; D, desaturation; Dy, dysrhythmia; ETT, endotracheal tube; L, laryngospasm; LMA, laryngeal mask airsay; S, stridor; URI, upper respiratory tract infection.

Appropriately Identifying Children with Respiratory Tract Infections

The diagnosis of a respiratory tract infection is made based on symptoms. There are no laboratory tests or radiographic findings that make the diagnosis more or less accurate. As mentioned earlier, symptoms can involve the upper respiratory tract, the lower respiratory tract, or both (Table 71-2). Unfortunately, other chronic conditions such as nasal foreign body or allergic rhinitis can occur acutely with similar symptoms as a respiratory tract infection. There are no published guidelines on diagnosing a child with a respiratory tract infection. Studies have used varying definitions ranging from rigid criteria to simply asking parents, "Does your child have an upper respiratory tract infection?" An early study by Tait and Knight[17] used two symptoms of the following list for the diagnosis of URI. These were sore or scratchy throat, sneezing, rhinorrhea, congestion, malaise, cough, fever (greater than 38.3°C), or laryngitis. The most prevalent and statistically significant symptoms for URI were sneezing (24.4%, $n = 78$), congestion (53.8%, $n = 78$), and nonproductive cough (76.9%, $n = 78$), more common when compared with asymptomatic controls. In a later study, Tait and colleagues[18] surveyed 212 pediatric anesthesiologists and found the following symptoms being used by anesthesiologists in diagnosing respiratory tract infection. The single symptoms used as contraindications to surgery were fever (64%, $n = 125$), productive cough (62.4%, $n = 121$), wheezing (80.3%, $n = 163$), and rales and/or rhonchi (78.2%, $n = 151$). Further, the most frequently cited combination of symptoms resulting in cancellation of the case were fever and productive cough (45.4%) or fever and yellow/green rhinorrhea (40.5%). Of note, the average temperature cutoff for cancellation of surgery was 100.8°F (38.3°C). After deciding if a patient is acutely symptomatic, one must also consider how to manage a "recently" symptomatic child. The following studies often use a 1- to 2-week period after resolution of acute symptoms as having a "recent" or "resolving" URI. This is one of the confounding elements in dealing with these studies.

Evidence to Proceed with General Anesthesia in Children Not Requiring Endotracheal Intubation with Symptoms of Acute and Resolving Respiratory Tract Infection

A prospective cohort study by Tait and Knight[19] of 489 patients investigated the prevalence of respiratory complications in children with URI, or recent URI, undergoing general anesthesia by facemask. No increased rate of complications (laryngospasm, dysrhythmia, or apnea) was found in the URI children ($n = 243$) when compared with the control group.[19]

Tait and Knight[17] also retrospectively evaluated the prevalence of adverse perianesthetic respiratory events (stridor, laryngospasm, and bronchospasm) in 3585 children; 122 had an active URI, and 133 had recent URI symptoms. No increased rate of respiratory complications during and after anesthesia was noted in the symptomatic group when compared with historical controls, but a threefold increase in bronchospasm and laryngospasm was demonstrated in the patients with a history of recent URI regardless of intubation requirement.[17]

Levy and colleagues[20] prospectively studied 130 children undergoing general anesthesia by facemask with either acute or recently resolved URI symptoms. They demonstrated an increased incidence of hypoxemia (despite oxygen administration) during transport to the postanesthesia care unit (PACU) in both the acutely infected and recently infected groups when compared with children without URI. Increased rates of desaturation persisted in the acutely infected group during their stay in the PACU.

Though some respiratory events still occur in children with a URI undergoing general anesthesia by facemask, the risk for laryngospasm and bronchospasm does not appear to be significantly increased, though the incidence of desaturation intraoperatively and postoperatively may be higher. It would seem that the decision to proceed with elective surgery can be made with caution, but there is less risk for adverse respiratory events if endotracheal intubation of children with URI symptoms is avoided.

Table 71-2	Signs and Symptoms of Respiratory Tract Infections in Children with URI and LRI			
	Mild URI	**Severe URI**	**LRI**	**Allergic Rhinitis**
History	No fever Minimal cough Clear runny nose Sneezing	Malaise Fever Purulent coryza Sneezing Cough	Severe cough Sputum production Wheezing +/− fever	Atopy Seasonal history Sneezing
General examination	Nontoxic appearance Clear runny nose	Toxic appearance Malaise Fever	+/− toxic appearance Tachypneic +/− irritability	No fever Allergic shiners
Pulmonary examination	Clear lungs +/− upper airway congestion	Maybe clear lungs Upper airway congestion	Rales Rhonchi	

LRI, lower respiratory tract infection; *URI*, upper respiratory tract infection; +/−, may be present or absent.

Evidence to Proceed with General Anesthesia in Children Requiring Endotracheal Intubation with Symptoms of Acute and Resolving Respiratory Tract Infection

Endotracheal intubation in patients with acute or recent URI symptoms has been shown in a variety of studies to be associated with a higher incidence of adverse respiratory events such as perioperative hypoxia, bronchospasm, and laryngospasm. An increased incidence of intraoperative and postoperative hypoxemia in children with an acute URI has been well studied and demonstrated in children.

DeSoto and colleagues[21] prospectively studied 50 children (25 with URI) ages 1 to 4 years who underwent general anesthesia and found that 20% ($n = 5$) of the URI group had postoperative hypoxemia (defined as SpO_2 <95%) (p <0.03). Of note, no supplemental oxygen was being administered in the recovery period unless desaturation was noted. Another study of hypoxemia in children with URI by Kinouchi and colleagues[22] found that the time period for desaturation to SpO_2 95% in preoxygenated children was 30% shorter during induction in those with an acute respiratory infection.

Rolf and Cote[23] conducted a prospective study of 402 children who were either asymptomatic ($n = 372$) or symptomatic with nonpurulent coryza URI ($n = 30$) undergoing general anesthesia. They compared perioperative events such as desaturation, laryngospasm, and bronchospasm between the two groups and found a higher frequency of minor desaturations (SpO_2 <95% for 60 seconds or more) and a higher frequency of bronchospasm in patients with URI who had endotracheal tubes placed for surgery.[23] Schreiner and colleagues[24] performed a case-control study to examine whether children who experienced laryngospasm were more likely to have a URI on day of surgery. URI symptoms were evaluated by questionnaire in 15,183 children. Laryngospasm was found to occur more often in children with active URI, in children of young age (less than 1 year of age), and in children whose anesthetics were supervised by less experienced attending anesthesiologists.[24]

Cohen and Cameron[25] conducted a large prospective study involving 22,159 children. URI symptoms were present in 1283 of these children with a two to seven times higher incidence of respiratory events intraoperatively and postoperatively when compared with asymptomatic children. They also found that the use of an endotracheal tube in a child with URI symptoms increased the risk for adverse respiratory events by elevenfold.[25]

Based on these studies and the strong correlation demonstrated between adverse events and URI symptoms in the setting of endotracheal intubation, the decision to delay elective surgery that requires general anesthesia with endotracheal intubation seems prudent until the adverse effects of the infection have resolved.

Evidence to Proceed with General Anesthesia in Children Using a Laryngeal Mask Airway with Symptoms of Acute and Resolving Respiratory Tract Infection

Some surgical procedures that require endotracheal intubation may be amenable to airway management using a laryngeal mask airway (LMA). In a series of 82 patients, Tait and colleagues[26] in an observational study demonstrated that use of LMA ($n = 41$) in place of endotracheal intubation ($n = 41$) had a significantly lower incidence of mild bronchospasm (12.2% versus 0%, p <0.05). There was no significant difference in larygnospasm, coughing, breath holding, or oxygen desaturation.[26] The coughing observed on emergence following LMA usage was subjectively thought to be less severe than with endotracheal tube (ETT) usage in this study. Further, the authors demonstrated no difference in the incidence of complications with endotracheal extubation under deep anesthesia versus awake, although the incidence of complications was higher for the ETT groups compared with LMA (adverse events 40.5% ETT versus 24.2% LMA, p <0.05). There are no randomized controlled trials comparing the effects of deep versus awake endotracheal extubation in patients with URI.

Homer and colleagues[27] using data collected from several prospective studies, showed that airway management had an impact on postanesthetic respiratory complications, such as laryngospasm, desaturation, and coughing ($p = 0.003$). When compared with LMA removed at a deep level of anesthesia, deep endotracheal extubation had a higher incidence of adverse respiratory events (odds ratio [OR] = 2.39). The protective effect of LMA was minimized when the airway device was removed with the patient awake. This same study showed that use of facemask alone decreased such events (OR = 0.15).[27]

Based on the available evidence, there may be a role for the use of LMA anesthesia in children with URI symptoms. In patients in whom mask anesthesia would be cumbersome, LMA may be a suitable alternative. Although it does carry more risk for laryngospasm, bronchospasm, and desaturation when compared with facemask, it appears to have a lower incidence in comparison with endotracheal intubation regardless of circumstance (whether removed awake or during deep anesthesia).

Evidence for Delaying Surgery 2 to 6 Weeks following an Acute Respiratory Infection

The majority of anesthesiologists who choose to delay an elective surgery will establish a period of time that must pass before they believe the child will be "safe" or at a "lower risk" to undergo anesthesia. The exact duration of time is unknown. Physiologic studies performed in animals studying respiratory infections and anesthesia demonstrate alterations in arterial oxygen tension, distribution of ventilation and perfusion, shunt, and functional residual capacity before and after viral infection. The exact mechanism is unknown. Perhaps it is a convergence of multiple processes such as changes in airway secretions,[28] smooth muscle responsiveness to tachykinins,[29] and altered muscarinic receptors.[30] Studies in adults evaluating pulmonary function tests before and following a respiratory tract infection have shown changes in small airway hyperreactivity that persist for up to 7 weeks[31] and general respiratory muscle weakness for up to 12 days.[32] Similar pulmonary function test changes have been demonstrated in children ages 6 and older with upper respiratory infections.[6]

Skolnick and colleagues[14] prospectively studied 499 children, of whom 26.8% had some history of passive smoke exposure, who received general anesthesia. Adverse respiratory events or complications were identified as severe coughing on induction/emergence, desaturation to SpO_2 less than 95% in the operating room, breath holding, severe coughing in the recovery room, and laryngospasm. The incidence of respiratory complications was 44% in smoke-exposed children compared with 25.5% in non–smoke-exposed children. However, children with an active URI were not found to have an increased risk of events whereas patients with a recent URI and passive smoke exposure had a higher incidence of events. Presence of a URI in this study was determined only by parental survey. As mentioned earlier, Tait and Knight[17] found that a threefold increase in bronchospasm and laryngospasm was demonstrated in patients with a recent history of URI regardless of intubation requirement. These findings would suggest that waiting would eliminate the higher risk of these adverse events. Unfortunately, no study has determined a correlation between duration of surgical delay, severity of respiratory tract symptoms, and a decreased incidence of respiratory complications.

In summary, these studies fail to generate a consensus.[33-39] They do suggest a higher risk of developing laryngospasm, bronchospasm, and desaturation events with endotracheal tube placement in acute and recently infected children. Also, both physiologic and patient-based studies provide evidence that supports the decision to delay surgery for 2 to 6 weeks following a respiratory tract infection in children, especially in the presence of high risk factors (e.g., reactive airway disease and presence of increased nasal congestion/sputum).

CONTROVERSIES

One area of difficulty raised by these studies is defining and differentiating symptoms for acute and recent respiratory tract infections. Attempting to define the condition is easy; however, the particular symptoms used to make the diagnosis and assigning severity to those symptoms is difficult within a single study. Importantly, the definition of "respiratory tract infection" and "resolving respiratory tract infection" differed greatly between studies and makes comparison difficult.

A criticism that exists for all the aforementioned studies is their failure to identify alternative causes of "runny nose" and "cough." Children can have other underlying diseases that mimic the symptoms of an "acute URI." For instance, both allergic rhinitis or foreign body can cause a runny nose and should be sought as possible etiologies and not incorrectly diagnosed as URI.

Although many texts and articles cite an increased incidence of pulmonary complications in children with underlying concomitant chronic medical disease and URI, there are no data in the literature to support this notion. Children with conditions such as congenital heart disease, asthma, and cystic fibrosis are commonly identified as being at increased risk for anesthetic complications. Whether the presence of an acute or recent respiratory tract infection further increases anesthetic risk has not been well studied. One

study in children with asthma and URI symptoms undergoing anesthesia with and without endotracheal tube placement demonstrated no increased incidence of adverse events.[10] Another study on children with congenital heart disease undergoing cardiac surgery who had URI symptoms evaluated the incidence of adverse respiratory events compared with asymptomatic children undergoing similar procedures and found no increased incidence, and actually an improvement in symptoms.[39] Further studies need to be performed to better understand if anesthetic risk is increased in children with chronic diseases such as asthma, cystic fibrosis, and congenital heart disease who experience URI. However, current biases and perceptions in anesthetic practice may make such studies difficult.

GUIDELINES

There are no formal practice guidelines regarding management of patients with respiratory tract infections from any major pediatric or anesthesia society. The difficulty of providing a consensus statement or practice guideline is perhaps accented by a survey by Tait and colleagues,[18] sent 400 questionnaires to members of the Society for Pediatric Anesthesia (SPA). Of the 212 respondents, 35% reported seldom canceling cases secondary to URI symptoms versus 20% indicating they usually canceled in the event of a URI. Factors considered to be of major importance were urgency of surgery, underlying asthma, procedure requiring intubation, fear of perioperative complications, and past experience anesthetizing patients with URI. Delay of surgery was up to 4 weeks for URI symptoms and greater than 4 weeks for LRI symptoms. The single symptoms identified as contraindications to surgery were fever, productive cough, wheezing, and rales and/or rhonchi. Currently, the only published "guidelines" are for general pediatric practitioners when evaluating children immediately before surgery, but these "guidelines," for reasons stated earlier, are not evidence based.[40]

AUTHORS' RECOMMENDATIONS

The following suggestions have been derived from the aforementioned studies. These recommendations are neither clinical guidelines nor a consensus statement and should not replace clinical judgment, but they should serve as a guide to help anesthesiologists make a rational decision with parents, surgeons, and patients. As with all children, the perioperative evaluation can serve as an important time to screen children for risk factors for anesthetic complications and begin educating parents about the anesthetic and operative process.[41-43] However, the absence of a visit for preoperative evaluation does not eliminate the need for an exchange of information between families and the center, which should occur before the day of surgery. Efforts should be made to make parents aware of the problems with respiratory tract infections and anesthesia, and parents should be encouraged to call before the day of surgery to discuss the symptoms and possible need for delay with the anesthesiologist and surgeon. There may be a role for pediatricians and other primary care practitioners to play in the process of perioperative evaluation and education.

Continued

AUTHORS' RECOMMENDATIONS—Cont'd

First, an emergency case mandates judicious airway management and logically must proceed regardless of the presence or absence of respiratory symptoms. In patients undergoing elective (nonurgent) surgery, initial consideration should be with respect to the severity of respiratory tract symptoms (Figure 71-1). Acute symptoms, such as runny nose and cough, must be differentiated from chronic symptoms related to underlying diseases such as allergic rhinitis (clear runny nose) and asthma (cough). Often, careful questioning of parents can differentiate acute from chronic symptoms. Patients with severe symptoms such as fever greater than 38.4°C, malaise, productive cough, wheezing, or rhonchi should be considered for delay of elective surgery. A reasonable period of delay would be 4 to 6 weeks. If mild symptoms are present, such as nonproductive cough, sneezing, or mild nasal congestion, surgery could proceed for those having regional or general anesthesia without endotracheal tube placement. The intraoperative plan should include early use pulse oximetry, decision of facemask or LMA use, and careful suctioning of the nasal and oropharynx under deep anesthesia before emergence. Additional management considerations for patients with URI or LRI undergoing anesthesia include hydration status, use of airway humidification, and the potential benefit of pharmacologic agents to help with airway secretions and airway hyperreactivity (e.g., anticholinergics and beta-agonists). However, for those patients who require ETT placement for anesthesia, especially children less than 1 year of age, it is important to identify risk factors such as passive smoke exposure and underlying conditions (asthma, chronic lung disease, etc.) because these children may benefit from a slight delay of 2 to 4 weeks. Finally, those patients with resolving respiratory tract infections with severe symptoms or mild symptoms should have the same relative waiting periods fulfilled to minimize risks of proceeding with surgery (i.e., 2 to 4 weeks after resolution of minor URI and 4 to 6 weeks after resolution of severe URI or LRI).

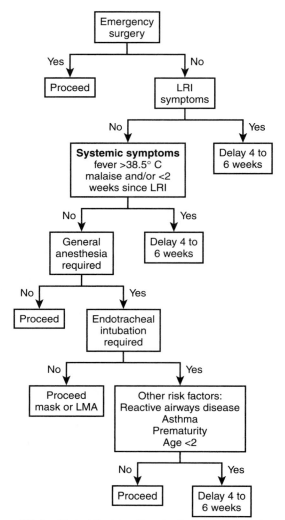

Figure 71-1. Clinical Decision Tree for Proceeding with Surgery in Children with Respiratory Tract Infections.

REFERENCES

1. Tait AR, Voepel-Lewis T, Munro HM, et al: Cancellation of pediatric outpatient surgery: Economic and emotional implications for patients and their families. *J Clin Anesthesiol* 1997;9:213-219.
2. Olsson GL: Bronchospasm during anaesthesia. A computer-aided incident study in 136,929 patients. *Acta Anesthesiol Scand* 1987;31:244-252.
3. Olsson GL, Hallen B: Laryngospasm during anaesthesia. A computer-aided incident study in 136,929 patients. *Acta Anesthesiol Scand* 1984;28:567-575.
4. Campbell NN: Respiratory tract infection and anaesthesia. *Anaesthesia* 1990;45:561.
5. Fridy WW Jr, Ingram RH Jr, Hierholzer JC, et al: Airway function during mild viral respiratory illnesses. *Ann Intern Med* 1974;80:150.
6. Collier AM, Pimmel RL, Hasselblad V, et al: Spirometric changes in normal children with upper respiratory infections. *Ann Rev Respir Dis* 1978;117:47-53.
7. Hirshman CA: Airway reactivity in humans: Anesthetic implications. *Anesthesiology* 1983;58:170-177.
8. Monto AS, Ullman BM: Acute respiratory illness in an American community. The Tecumseh study. *JAMA* 1974;227:164-169.
9. Morray JP, Geiduschek JM, Caplan RA, et al: A comparison of pediatric and adult anesthesia closed malpractice claims. *Anesthesiology* 1993;461-467.
10. Pradal M, Vialet R, Soula F, Dejode JM, Lagier P: The risk of anesthesia in the asthmatic child. *Pediatr Pulmonol* 1995;11(suppl):51-52.
11. Harnik EV, Hoy GR, Potolicchio S, et al: Spinal anesthesia in premature infants recovering from respiratory distress syndrome. *Anesthesiology* 1986;64:95-99.
12. Warner DO, Warner WA, Barnes RD, Offord KP, Schroeder DR, Gray DT, Yunginger JW: Peri-operative respiratory complications in patients with asthma. *Anesthesiology* 1996;85:460-467.
13. Stringer DA, Spragg A, Joudis E, et al: The association of cystic fibrosis, gastroesophageal reflux, and reduced pulmonary function. *Can Assoc Radiol J* 1988;39:100.
14. Skolnick ET, Vomvolakis MA, Buck KA, Mannino SF, Sun LS: Exposure to environmental tobacco smoke and the risk of adverse events in children receiving general anesthesia. *Anesthesiology* 1998;88:1144-1153.
15. Konarzewski WH, Ravindran N, Findlow D, Timmis PK: Anaesthetic death of a child with a cold. *Anaesthesia* 1992;47:624.
16. Williams OA, Hills R, Goddard JM: Pulmonary collapse during anaesthesia in children with respiratory tract symptoms. *Anaesthesia* 1992;47:411.
17. Tait AR, Knight PR: Intraoperative respiratory complications in patients with upper respiratory tract infections. *Can J Anaesth* 1987;34:300-303.
18. Tait AR, Reynolds PI, Gutstein HB: Factors that influence an anesthesiologist's decision to cancel elective surgery for the

child with an upper respiratory tract infection. *J Clin Anesth* 1995;7:491-499.

19. Tait AR, Knight PR: The effect of general anesthesia on upper respiratory tract infections in children. *Anesthesiology* 1987;67:930-935.
20. Levy L, Pandit UA, Randel GI, Lewis IH, Tait AR: Upper respiratory infections and general anaesthesia in children. Peri-operative complications and oxygen saturation. *Anaesthesia* 1992;47:678-682.
21. DeSoto H, Patel RI, Soliman IE, Hannallah RS: Changes in oxygen saturation following general anesthesia in children with upper respiratory infection signs and symptoms undergoing otolaryngological procedures. *Anesthesiology* 1988;68:276-279.
22. Kinouchi K, Tanigami H, Tashiro C, et al: Duration of apnea in anesthetized infants and children required for desaturation of hemoglobin to 95%: The influence of respiratory infection. *Anesthesiology* 1992;77:1105-1107.
23. Rolf N, Cote CJ: Frequency and severity of desaturation events during general anesthesia in children with and without upper respiratory infections. *J Clin Anesth* 1992;200-203.
24. Schreiner MS, O'Hara I, Markakis DA, Politis GD: Do children who experience laryngospasm have an increased risk of upper respiratory tract infection? *Anesthesiology* 1996;3:475-480.
25. Cohen MM, Cameron CB: Should you cancel the operation when a child has an upper respiratory tract infection? *Anesth Analg* 1991;72:282-288.
26. Tait AR, Pandit UA, Voepel-Lewis T, et al: Use of laryngeal mask airway in children with upper respiratory tract infections: A comparison with endotracheal intubation. *Anesth Analg* 1998;86:706-711.
27. Homer JR, Elwood T, Peterson D, Rampersad S: Risk factors for adverse events in children with colds emerging from anesthesia: A logistic regression. *Pediatr Anesth* 2007;17:154-161.
28. Dueck R, Prutow R, Richman D: Effect of parainfluenza infection on gas exchange and FRC response to anesthesia in sheep. *Anesthesiology* 1991;74:1044-1051.
29. Dusser DJ, Jakoby DB, Djokic TD, Rubenstein I, et al: Virus induces airway hyperresponsiveness to tachykinins: Role of neutral endopeptidase. *J Appl Physiol* 1989;67:1504-1511.
30. Fryer AD, Jacoby DB: Parainfluenza virus infection damages inhibitory M2 muscarinic receptors on pulmonary parasympathetic nerves in the guinea pig. *Br J Pharmacol* 1991;102:267-271.
31. Empey DW, Laitinen LA, Jacobs L, et al: Mechanisms of bronchial hyperreactivity in normal subjects following upper respiratory tract infection. *Am Rev Respir Dis* 1976;113:131-139.
32. Mier-Jedrzejowicz A, Brophy C, Green M. Respiratory muscle weakness during upper respiratory tract infections. *Am Rev Respir Dis* 1988;138:5.
33. Martin LD: Anesthetic implications of an upper respiratory infection in children. *Pediatr Clin North Am* 1994;41:121-130.
34. Rice LJ: Common problems in pediatric ambulatory surgery: Upper respiratory infection, heart murmur, or sickle-cell disease. *J Clin Anesth* 1993;5(suppl 1):34S-38S.
35. Fennelly ME, Hall GM. Anaesthesia and upper respiratory tract infections—a nonexistent hazard? *Br J Anaesth* 1990;64:535-536.
36. Jacoby DB, Hirshman CA: General anesthesia in patients with viral respiratory infections: An unusual sleep? *Anesthesiology* 1991;74:969-972.
37. Goresky GV: Respiratory complications in patients with upper respiratory tract infections. *Can J Anesth* 1987;34:655
38. Hinkle AJ: What wisdom is there in administering elective general anesthesia to children with active upper respiratory tract infections? *Anesth Analg* 1989;68:413.
39. Malviya S, Voepel-Lewis T, Siewert M, et al: A prospective evaluation of the risks of upper respiratory infections in children undergoing open heart surgery. *Anesthesiology* 1997;87:A1073.
40. Means LJ, Ferrari LR, Fisher QA, Kingston HGG, Schreirner MS: Evaluation and preparation of pediatric patients undergoing anesthesia. *Pediatrics* 1996;98:502-508.
41. Maxwell LG, Yaster M: Peri-operative management issues in pediatric patients. *Anesthesiol Clin North Am* 2000;18(3):601-632.
42. Tait AR, Malviya S: Anesthesia for the child with an upper respiratory tract infection: Still a dilemma? *Anesth Analg* 2005;100:59-65.
43. Tait AR, Malviya S, Voepel-Lewis T, et al: Risk factors for perioperative adverse respiratory events in children with upper respiratory tract infections. *Anesthesiology* 2001;95:283-285.

PAIN MANAGEMENT

72 Optimal Postoperative Analgesia

Michael A. Ashburn, MD, MPH, and Jane C. Ballantyne, MD, FRCA

INTRODUCTION

For several decades before the 1980s, postoperative pain management in the United States was fairly standardized. Mild-to-moderate pain was treated with acetaminophen or a nonsteroidal antiinflammatory drug (NSAID), and moderate-to-severe pain was treated with intermittent, intramuscular opioids as needed. In the 1980s, the options for managing postoperative pain expanded. When endogenous opioids and their receptors were identified in the late 1970s, the value of neuraxially administered opioids was realized, and epidural analgesia became popular. During the 1980s and 1990s, infusion pump technology improved dramatically; microprocessors became increasingly miniaturized, and infusion pumps became portable. As a result, patient-controlled analgesia (PCA) became practical and started to enjoy widespread use.

Brian Ready and his colleagues introduced the concept of a formalized acute pain service to provide coordinated, interdisciplinary acute pain care.[1] This prompted investigation into the process of patient care and its impact on pain outcomes.[2] Interest was also generated on the use of multimodal analgesia, rather than reliance on one single treatment modality. This opened the door to further investigations into the use of nonopioid analgesics, including NSAIDs, acetaminophen, and gabapentin, in the perioperative period.[3] The goal of therapy was not necessarily to replace opioids with these medications, but rather to improve acute pain control and lower the incidence and severity of chronic pain following selected surgical procedures.

We have seen a renewed interest in the perioperative use of regional anesthesia for acute pain control, made possible by the development of ultrasound guidance techniques that appear to improve the efficacy and safety of these blocks.[4] The trend in postoperative pain management appears to be away from systemic opioids and toward multimodal analgesic techniques.

When the era of evidence-based medicine dawned at the end of the twentieth century, most existing trials of postoperative pain management compared newer approaches (epidural analgesia, PCA, and adjunctive use of NSAIDs) with conventional analgesia, often defined as systemic opioids. Therefore early attempts at formulating an evidence-based approach to postoperative pain management focused on assessing whether these new approaches offered superior analgesia, or a better effect on surgical outcome, compared with conventional analgesia. As a result, our first attempts at providing evidence-based recommendations focused on assessing the outcomes associated with the use of a single approach to postoperative pain management.[5]

There are many factors, some of which are not obvious, that can affect the results observed in clinical trials. The decisions made by health care providers throughout the surgical period can affect outcomes in a number of ways, from patient selection for the surgical procedure, to the conduct of anesthesia and surgery, to the care provided in the immediate postoperative period. Therefore variability exists within and outside the context of pain care, and this variability can have an impact on the outcomes of pain-related clinical trials. This variability may also make it difficult to document the outcomes related only to the pain therapy of interest.

Many experts advocate the use of perioperative rehabilitation, often defined as the use of an integrated, interdisciplinary process of care for patients undergoing the same kind of surgical procedure.[6] With perioperative rehabilitation, a team approach is advocated. Pain management is integrated into this care, and is often multimodal, no longer relying only on one pain therapy technique. Therefore the way pain therapy is applied may well be another treatment variable that has to be considered when evaluating the outcomes associated with pain therapy.

TREATMENT OPTIONS

It is hard to imagine that 20 years ago patients undergoing major surgery would stay in the hospital for up to 2 weeks (sometimes longer); would stay immobile in bed for days on end, unable to move because of severe pain; and would not be given water or food until the bowels started moving. Not surprisingly, the incidence of thrombosis, embolus, infarction, and infection was much higher than it is today. Improvements in pain care have played an important role in efforts to improve perioperative outcomes.

The thrust of postoperative care has changed from one of passively waiting for recovery to one of actively encouraging a rapid return to normal function. Although pain control is critical to rapid recovery, the clinician must balance the risk of harm with the potential for benefit. Although uncontrolled pain will delay a return to normal function by making patients afraid to move, breathe deeply, or cough, systemic opioids may delay recovery by slowing the bowels, causing sedation, and (rarely) causing clinically important compromise of ventilation.

An important role of postoperative pain management is to maximize pain relief while minimizing side effects. Treatment options are evaluated not only according to their ability to provide satisfactory analgesia, but also by their ability to promote recovery and rehabilitation. In this chapter, we consider the evidence supporting the use of intravenous patient-controlled analgesia, epidural analgesia, and NSAIDs.

Outcomes associated with a pain treatment modality will vary based on the specific characteristics of the patient, as well as the procedure the patient is going to undergo. The discussion in this chapter focuses on the evidence supporting the use of individual analgesic techniques specified previously. However, guidelines have been recently published regarding the evidence for the use of multimodal analgesic techniques in specific surgical procedures,[7] and more guidelines are under development.[8]

EVIDENCE

Epidural Analgesia

Epidural analgesia can be accomplished by infusing a variety of drugs (typically low-dose local anesthetics and opioids) into the epidural space. Epidural *analgesia* must be distinguished from epidural *anesthesia*, which implies dense epidural local anesthetic blockade and is generally reserved for intraoperative use. Conceptually, the provision of epidural analgesia is an attractive means of minimizing opioid requirement while providing excellent analgesia, thereby promoting recovery after surgery. Epidural opioid doses are much smaller than those required systemically (in the order of one tenth), and low-dose epidural local anesthetics, apart from producing analgesia without overt sensory/motor blockade or opioid-associated adverse effects, can have additional beneficial effects on bowel mobility. Does the evidence support the superior analgesic efficacy of epidural analgesia and its ability to promote recovery after surgery?

It is important to separate the potential benefits of intraoperative epidurals from the benefits of postoperative epidural analgesia. There are significant differences in the way epidurals are used during surgery: sometimes complete epidural anesthesia is provided, sometimes only epidural analgesia, sometimes the epidural is not used at all intraoperatively, and of course there is a range of practice in between. Some benefits are likely to pertain chiefly to the use of profound blockade during surgery (e.g., lower incidence of thromboembolic events, lower incidence of graft failure in the case of major vascular surgery, lower blood loss, lowering of the metabolic stress response, lower incidence of chronic pain). This chapter concentrates on the benefits likely to pertain specifically to postoperative epidural analgesia.

Many of the early trials of epidural analgesia (during the 1970s and early 1980s) were small, randomized studies that attempted to confirm the clinically apparent superior analgesia of postoperative epidurals compared with conventional analgesia, some also assessing aspects of postoperative recovery. These early trials (and meta-analyses) overwhelmingly supported the superior analgesic efficacy

of epidural analgesia compared with conventional analgesia.[9] Assessments of postoperative recovery focused on differences in minor morbidities, including pulmonary function, bowel function, and mobility.[10-12]

A goal of epidural analgesia is to restore normal physiologic function as rapidly as possible to avoid adverse outcomes associated with prolonged immobilization and hospital stay. As evidenced by small randomized controlled trials (RCTs) and subsequent meta-analysis (and in some cases, confirmed by the large RCTs), epidural analgesia fulfills this goal extremely well. Epidural analgesia has been shown to promote early mobilization and reduce rehabilitation time, particularly after joint surgery.[13-15] In addition, it has been shown to reduce pulmonary morbidity,[11,16-19] reduce time to extubation of the trachea after major thoracic and vascular procedures,[16-18,20-22] reduce cardiac ischemia and dysrhythmia in high-risk patients,[20,23] and reduce postoperative ileus,[24] thereby reducing length of hospital stay.[25-28] A meta-analysis by Beattie and colleagues[23] found a reduction in the incidence of myocardial infarction associated with the use of postoperative epidural anesthesia (odds ratio [OR] 0.56; confidence interval [CI] 0.30 to 1.03).

Several clinical trials have been conducted to evaluate the impact of epidural analgesia on mortality rate and major morbidity (including major cardiac morbidity, pulmonary embolus, and stroke). Early results suggested that combined epidural and general anesthesia (GA) followed by postoperative epidural analgesia had a favorable effect on major morbidity, and possibly also on mortality rate.[29,30] The findings of Yeager and colleagues[30] were particularly striking because they showed remarkable decreases in surgical morbidity and mortality rates attributable to epidural analgesia in high-risk patients undergoing major surgical procedures. Interestingly, this study was stopped after the completion of 53 patients by the monitoring committee because the early results favored the epidural treatment so strongly that the committee believed it would be unethical to continue the trial. This study certainly contributed to the belief that epidural analgesia improves surgical outcome, particularly in sick patients.

However, the validity of the results of the Yeager study has been questioned,[31] and this skepticism led investigators to set about assessing the possible effects of epidural analgesia on major morbidity in high-risk patients. Two large RCTs were later published. Unfortunately, neither confirmed the earlier findings that epidural analgesia has a favorable effect on major morbidity.[16,17]

Well-designed, large randomized trials such as those by Park and colleagues[16] and Rigg and colleagues[17] constitute strong evidence about the efficacy of epidural analgesia. (Meta-analysis is considered stronger evidence, but it must be carefully conducted and must select only well-designed and relatively homogeneous studies.) In terms of analgesic efficacy, these studies lend further support to the findings of earlier smaller trials and meta-analyses that confirmed the superior analgesic efficacy of epidural analgesia. However, these two large studies were designed specifically to assess the value of epidural analgesia in terms of its ability to reduce major morbidity and mortality rates in high-risk patients. In these respects, the results were disappointing for those who believed, on the basis of earlier small trials,[29,30] that the treatment has a major impact on major morbidity and mortality rates.

Epidural analgesia may play an important role following abdominal surgery. In this setting, epidural analgesia has been reported to lower the incidence of myocardial infarction, stroke, and death in patients undergoing abdominal aortic surgery.[16] A recent meta-analysis evaluated the impact of epidural analgesia versus systemic opioids following abdominal aortic surgery.[32] This analysis included 13 studies involving 1224 patients. The epidural analgesia group showed significantly improved pain control on movement up to the third postoperative day. In addition, postoperative duration of tracheal intubation and mechanical ventilation was significantly shorter by about 20%. The overall incidence of cardiovascular complications, myocardial infarction, acute respiratory failure, gastrointestinal complications, and renal insufficiency were all significantly lower in the epidural analgesia group, especially in trials that used thoracic epidural analgesia. The incidence of mortality, however, was not reduced.

Another study provided indirect evidence that epidural analgesia may lower mortality rate following major surgery.[33] This study examined a cohort of 3501 patients who underwent lung resection. These patients represented a 5% random sample of patients who underwent lung resection procedures between 1997 and 2001, and who were listed in the Medicare claims database. Multivariate regression analysis showed that the presence of epidural analgesia was associated with a significantly lower odds of death at 7 days (OR 0.39; 95% CI 0.19 to 0.80; $p = 0.001$) and 30 days (OR 0.53; 95% CI 0.35 to 0.78; $p = 0.002$). Interestingly, this study reported no difference in major morbidity.

It is easy to forget that the evolution of epidural analgesia has occurred alongside the evolution of postoperative management in general, and that differences in serious morbidity and mortality rates that might be expected to emanate from the benefits outlined earlier may not be obvious because of improvements in postoperative care in general. A policy of early oral fluid administration, early nasogastric tube removal, and forced early mobilization, in combination with optimized pain management, has resulted in earlier hospital discharge and a decrease in postoperative mortality rate when compared with that 20 years ago. It may be impossible to show the benefit of postoperative epidural analgesia in isolation, whereas studies of this mode of analgesia used with regard to its specific effects on certain outcomes (e.g., postoperative ileus); with attention to appropriate level of catheter placement, drug choice, and drug dose in order to achieve the desired outcome; and its combination with other aspects of postoperative care are needed before we can discount the value of epidural analgesia in terms of major morbidity and mortality rates.[34] At the same time, major morbidity and mortality rates have become so low that even larger trials or patient numbers in meta-analyses may be required to show a difference.[17]

In summary, the superior analgesic efficacy of epidural analgesia compared with conventional analgesia seems absolutely clear, and benefits in terms of morbidity and length of hospital stay (by contributing to an accelerated return to normal physiologic function) have been demonstrated. The evidence is even stronger for thoracic epidural catheters. It remains unclear whether epidural analgesia has a role in reducing mortality.

Patient-Controlled Analgesia

The use of microcomputer-controlled infusion pumps to enable patients to self-deliver doses of analgesic drugs (patient-controlled analgesia [PCA]) was popularized in the 1980s when microprocessors became small enough to be incorporated into portable pumps. Patients and nurses seemed to like PCA—patients because of the greater control they achieved over their analgesic dosing, and nurses because of the convenience of this mode of analgesia. PCA is now available in most large hospitals in the United States, as well as many small hospitals,[35] and it has become an important tool to aid hospitals' compliance with mandated pain assessment and treatment standards. Although there are many clinical indications for PCA, its most common application is for postoperative pain management, usually opioids delivered intravenously.

Intravenous PCA differs from conventional analgesia in two important ways: (1) provided patients dose appropriately, peaks and troughs in serum analgesic level are less extreme, and analgesic level is better matched to analgesic need, and (2) patients' anxiety over obtaining analgesia is obviated. The question we must ask is, do these factors result in better analgesia, lower opioid requirements, superior patient satisfaction with treatment, fewer side effects, and better surgical outcome? In this chapter, we compare intravenous PCA with conventional analgesia. The use of patient-controlled epidural analgesia (PCEA) in the management of postoperative pain is also increasing in popularity,[36] but this treatment will not be addressed here.

Three meta-analyses of PCA versus conventional analgesia have been published, one in 1993,[37] the second in 2001,[38] and the third in 2006.[39] Apart from updating the first analysis, the second incorporated trials in which control group opioids are given by the subcutaneous and intravenous as well as the intramuscular route. Fifteen trials (787 patients) were included in the first analysis, 32 (2072 patients) in the second, and 55 (3861 patients) in the third. All but one trial (which used meperidine) in the first analysis used morphine in both experimental and control group patients (699 patients). In the second and third analyses, morphine was used in the majority of studies, but various opioids were also used, including hydromorphone, meperidine, piritramide, nalbuphine, and tramadol.

The first meta-analysis demonstrated that patients prefer PCA to conventional analgesia and that PCA has slightly better analgesic efficacy. The mean difference in satisfaction is 42% ($p = 0.02$), whereas the mean difference in pain score on a scale of 0 to 100 is 5.6 ($p = 0.006$). However, there was no difference in opioid usage, side effects, or length of hospital stay.

Despite the passing of almost 10 years and the addition of 12 trials (1000 patients) to the first meta-analysis, the results of the second analysis differ very little from those of the first. Patients' preference for PCA is confirmed, as was slightly better analgesic efficacy. In three morphine trials and one meperidine trial, PCA is preferred (relative risk [RR] 1.41; CI 1.1 to 1.80). Combined data on pain intensity and relief from one piritramide, one nalbuphine, and eight morphine trials also demonstrated a preference for PCA (RR 1.22; CI 1.00 to 1.50). There was no difference in opioid usage or side effects, and no convincing evidence of a difference in surgical outcome, although the limited data (152 patients) available on pulmonary function did suggest an improvement.

The third meta-analysis included yet more studies (55) and patients (2023 receiving PCA and 1838 receiving conventional analgesia).[39] Even with an increase in the number of trials and patients, the results were similar, in that PCA was demonstrated to provide better pain control and patient satisfaction than conventional analgesia. However, patients using PCA consumed higher amounts of opioids than the control, had a higher incidence of pruritus, but had a similar incidence of other adverse effects. There was no difference in the length of hospital stay.

Another meta-analysis evaluated PCA compared with conventional analgesia following cardiac surgery.[40] This study used patient-reported pain intensity as the primary outcome, and cumulative opioid use, intensive care unit (ICU) and hospital length of stay, postoperative nausea and vomiting, sedation, respiratory depression, and all-cause mortality rate as secondary outcome measures. The authors identified 10 RCTs involving 666 patients. Compared with conventional analgesia, PCA significantly reduces the Visual Analog Scale (VAS) at 48 hours, but not at 24 hours following surgery. PCA *increased* cumulative 24- and 48-hour opioid consumption. Ventilation times, length of ICU stay, length of hospital stay, patient satisfaction scores, sedation scores, and incidence of postoperative nausea and vomiting, respiratory depression, and death were not significantly different.

Do these meta-analyses represent the best evidence we have about the utility of intravenous PCA compared with conventional analgesia? Certainly the meta-analyses help by providing a quantitative summary of existing data. However, because many of the trials contributing to these meta-analyses were small, treatment effects may have been distorted because of deficiencies inherent in small trials, including Type I error, distortions that can possibly be compounded in meta-analyses.[41-45] Another problem encountered here (and, indeed, in many epidural trials) is that neither patients nor assessors were blinded to treatment; thus, there is a high likelihood of assessor bias, which might be expected to exaggerate treatment effects.[38,46] One should also be concerned with the degree of differences observed in the analysis. Some meta-analyses have demonstrated a small improvement in analgesic efficacy, and possibly pulmonary function, with PCA use. However, we not only need to question the clinical significance of these findings because of the small effect size, but also because of the weakness in the design of the contributing studies as a result of blinding.

It is also worth noting that in real life there are wide variations in factors such as patient education and nursing workload that have a profound effect on the doses of analgesic actually received, and thus on the efficacy of either

method.[47] In addition, there may be significant differences in outcomes in patients participating in clinical trials evaluating pain outcomes when compared with patients receiving routine postoperative care outside the context of an analgesic trial. Thus, the efficacy of PCA compared with conventional analgesia is likely to differ between trials and real life, individual patients, and institutions.

Patients' preference for PCA seems to be an important reason that PCA has been established as the standard of care for routine management of moderate-to-severe postoperative pain. In view of the lack of evidence of any other real advantage to PCA, other than a slight improvement in analgesic efficacy, it seems that the reason that patients prefer PCA is that it provides them with a sense of autonomy and control over their own analgesic management.[48,49] In today's health care climate, patient preference is an important and valid reason for a treatment choice.

Given the lack of evidence of other benefits, one has to ask whether the cost of PCA is justified. Preliminary cost-benefit analyses suggest that postoperative analgesia using PCA is more expensive than conventional analgesia,[50-52] despite the hope that nursing involvement would be reduced, and reduced nursing costs would offset the increase in equipment costs. However, the results of cost-effectiveness studies are often based on cost data specific to one institution at a specific time, and therefore may not be valid at other institutions or at different times.

Nonsteroidal Antiinflammatory Drugs

NSAIDs have been demonstrated to be effective analgesics for the treatment of pain after surgery. This has been proven in single-dose studies in mild-to-moderate pain,[53] as well as in multiple-dose studies in moderate-to-severe pain.[54] NSAIDs have been demonstrated to have an opioid-sparing effect.[55,56]

When considering the use of NSAIDs in the postoperative period, there are several key issues to consider. First, does the addition of an NSAID improve pain control and/or lower the incidence of opioid-induced adverse side effects? Second, does the addition of an NSAID present new risk of harm to the patient? Third, are there any benefits to the use of COX-2 selective agent in this setting?

Following major surgery, NSAIDs alone cannot provide effective pain relief. Therefore they are added to other pain therapy, such as systemic opioids. When given in combination with other opioids after surgery, NSAIDs result in better pain relief and lower opioid consumption.[57,58] A recent meta-analysis evaluated the administration of NSAIDs on morphine PCA.[59] This analysis included 33 trials with 1644 patients. In the trials evaluating multiple-dose regimens of NSAIDs, there was an average reduction in 24-hour morphine consumption of 19.7 mg, which was equal to a 40% opioid-sparing effect. In addition, the use of an NSAID lowered pain intensity from approximately 3 to 2 on the 10 cm VAS when compared with morphine PCA alone.

The addition of an NSAID with the resultant reduction in opioid consumption may not lower the overall incidence of adverse events.[55] It seems clear that the incidence and degree of respiratory depression is reduced,[58,60,61] but improvements in pulmonary function (less opioid-induced hypercapnic responses) have not been convincingly demonstrated.[57] The adjunctive use of NSAIDs reduces the incidence of nausea in several studies, although an equal number of studies do not show any benefit.[57] The literature is equivocal about whether or not opioid sparing by NSAIDs promotes rapid recovery. A limited number of studies demonstrate accelerated recovery in association with less nausea and sedation, improved mobility and earlier return of bowel function,[62,63] but others fail to show any benefit in terms of recovery.[58,64,65]

A recent meta-analysis evaluated the effect of NSAID administration on PCA morphine side effects.[66] This study included 22 randomized, double-blind clinical trials published between 1991 and 2003, with 1316 patients receiving NSAIDs and 991 patients receiving PCA morphine only. This study demonstrated that NSAIDs significantly decreased the incidence of postoperative nausea and vomiting by 30%, and the incidence of sedation by 29%. Pruritus, urinary retention, and respiratory depression were not significantly decreased by NSAIDs.

NSAID use may be associated with a number of potential adverse events, including inhibition of platelet function, alteration in renal function, peptic ulceration, and alterations in bone healing.[67-71] However, it appears that short-term use of NSAIDs around the time of surgery may not be associated with a compromise of bone healing.[72] The risk of NSAID-induced adverse events is higher with higher doses and longer durations of therapy. In addition, the risk of harm is higher in the elderly.

A recent meta-analysis evaluated the effects of NSAIDs on postoperative renal function in adults with normal renal function.[73] This analysis included 23 trials with 1459 patients. Perioperative administration of NSAIDs reduced creatinine clearance by 16 mL/min (95% CI 5 to 28) and potassium output by 38 mmol/day (95% CI 19 to 56) on the first day after surgery compared with placebo. However, there was no significant difference in serum creatinine on the first day (0 µmol/L, 95% CI 3 to 4). No significant reduction in urine volume during the early postoperative period was found, and there were no cases of postoperative renal failure requiring dialysis. Other studies have demonstrated that the risk of adverse renal effects is increased in patients with preexisting compromise of renal function, hypovolemia, hypotension, or the concomitant use of other nephrotoxic drugs.[74]

Concern has developed over the last several years about the cardiovascular consequences of NSAID administration.[75] This concern was triggered by evidence that the COX-2 inhibitors may lack the thrombotic-protective and cardioprotective effects of aspirin and other standard NSAIDs, but now extends to the demonstrated deleterious effects of NSAIDs in general on cardiac function and blood pressure, especially in susceptible patients. A recent meta-analysis that included 55 trials with 99,087 patients evaluated the impact of COX-2 selective agents on risk for MI.[76] The overall pooled OR for myocardial infarction (MI) risk for any coxib compared with placebo was 1.46 (95% CI 1.02 to 2.09). This study concluded that celecoxib, rofecoxib, etoricoxib, valdecoxib, and lumiracoxib were all associated with higher MI risk compared with placebo. The pooled OR for any coxib compared with other NSAIDs was 1.45 (95% CI 1.09 to 1.93). Another meta-analysis reported that all NSAIDs increase the risk of MI and cerebrovascular accidents, and COX-2 selective agents confer the highest risk.[77]

In summary, perioperative NSAID administration is associated with significant opioid-sparing effects and a resultant reduction in several opioid-induced side effects. Other than the differences in the effect on platelet function, there appears to be little advantage to the use of COX-2 selective agents, and the use of these agents may be associated with an increased risk of cardiovascular adverse events.

AREAS OF UNCERTAINTY

The focus of postoperative pain trials has been on assessing new modes of analgesia with particular regard both to their analgesic efficacy and to their ability to improve surgical outcome. In this chapter, trials assessing epidural analgesia, PCA, and NSAIDs used as adjuncts were reviewed. The studies leave no doubt that these modes of analgesia provide effective analgesia, and in the case of epidurals and adjunctive NSAIDs, the analgesia is better than conventional analgesia.

The opioid-sparing effects of epidural analgesia and adjunctive NSAIDs (not PCA) is confirmed. The incidence of some opioid-induced adverse side effects is lower. It is not clear, however, whether opioid sparing per se actually improves recovery, and the evidence from the literature is equivocal.

Epidural analgesia offers a number of distinct benefits and appears to hasten recovery (largely because of its favorable effects on the bowel). However, although improvements in morbidity have been demonstrated, analysis of current trials suggests that epidural analgesia offers no benefit in terms of major morbidity and mortality.

Despite the apparent certainty of these stated findings, many questions remain unanswered. We do not know whether the marked improvements in surgical morbidity and mortality rates that have occurred over the last few decades, due to improvements in postoperative care in general, mask the benefits of improved postoperative pain control. Trials have tended to segregate treatments and have not assessed pain treatments as part of a multimodal approach, or in terms of their integration into accelerated recovery programs. Issues such as choice of drug, dosage, and site of administration, and their relationship to specific benefits, have largely been ignored, particularly in epidural and PCA trials. Hopefully, future studies will examine the role of analgesia in rehabilitation after surgery. Uncertainty about the benefits of various modes of analgesia will remain until we can be clearer about the importance of pain control to the overall goal of restoring normal physiologic function as rapidly as possible.

GUIDELINES

Guidelines on acute and postoperative pain management abound. One of the first comprehensive evidence-based guidelines was published by the Agency for Health Care

Policy and Research (AHCPR) in 1992. Anesthesia and pain societies around the world have published their own guidelines on acute pain management.[2,25,78-80] The message has been consistent. They emphasize the importance of optimizing pain management. They reinforce the value of alternatives to conventional analgesia, particularly epidurals, PCA, and NSAIDs, in terms of their ability to improve analgesia, reduce opioid doses, and improve surgical outcome. They also recommend nonmedical approaches such as transcutaneous electrical nerve stimulation (TENS) and relaxation, which are not normally the province of anesthesiologists and are not discussed in this chapter.

AUTHORS' RECOMMENDATIONS

Current evidence demonstrates convincingly that epidurals, PCA, and adjunctive NSAIDs improve postoperative analgesia. Epidural analgesia, but not PCA, has the additional benefit of sometimes promoting rapid recovery after surgery, although an effect on major morbidity or mortality has not been demonstrated. In the case of PCA, improvements in pain relief are slight, but patients clearly prefer PCA. The material costs of epidural analgesia and PCA are substantial, and the labor costs of epidural management even greater. Epidurals and PCA are recommended for their demonstrated ability to provide good analgesia, improve patient satisfaction, and, in the case of epidurals, hasten recovery.

The use of NSAIDs to supplement systemic and neuraxial opioid therapy also has demonstrated benefit in terms of improved analgesia, opioid sparing, and a moderate reduction in some opioid-induced adverse effects. However, NSAID opioid sparing has not been demonstrated to improve overall surgical outcome, and care must be taken to balance the benefits of NSAID administration with the risk for harm. Having said that, it appears that many patients can benefit from perioperative NSAID administration.

One of the best clinical practice guidelines available to guide acute pain practice is the guideline prepared by the Australian and New Zealand College of Anaesthesia and Faculty of Pain Medicine.[81] These guidelines are evidence-based and provide clear, detailed information regarding acute pain treatment options.

Individual institutions must be prepared to devote the necessary resources before offering advanced analgesic technologies. Because it has not yet been possible to demonstrate improvements in major morbidity and mortality in association with epidurals (or PCA), the question of whether to offer these advanced pain treatments often turns on cost and feasibility. Institutional differences in drug and equipment costs, staffing levels (particularly anesthesia staffing levels), and patients (and their expectations) may determine whether or not an institution chooses to offer epidural analgesia or PCA.

REFERENCES

1. Ready LB, Oden R, Chadwick HS, Benedetti C, Rooke GA, Caplan R, Wild LM: Development of an anesthesiology-based postoperative pain management service. *Anesthesiology* 1988;68:100-106.
2. Practice guidelines for acute pain management in the perioperative setting: An updated report by the American Society of Anesthesiologists Task Force on Acute Pain Management. *Anesthesiology* 2004;100:1573-1581.
3. Tiippana EM, Hamunen K, Kontinen VK, Kalso E: Do surgical patients benefit from perioperative gabapentin/pregabalin? A systematic review of efficacy and safety. *Anesth Analg* 2007;104:1545-1556, table of contents.
4. Marhofer P, Chan VW: Ultrasound-guided regional anesthesia: Current concepts and future trends. *Anesth Analg* 2007;104:1265-1269, table of contents.
5. Acute pain management: Operative or medical procedures and trauma, Part 1. Agency for Health Care Policy and Research. *Clin Pharm* 1992;11:309-331.
6. Kehlet H, Buchler MW, Beart RW Jr, Billingham RP, Williamson R: Care after colonic operation—is it evidence-based? Results from a multinational survey in Europe and the United States. *J Am Coll Surg* 2006;202:45-54.
7. Fischer HB, Simanski CJ: A procedure-specific systematic review and consensus recommendations for analgesia after total hip replacement. *Anaesthesia* 2005;60:1189-1202.
8. Kehlet H, Wilkinson RC, Fischer HB, Camu F: PROSPECT: Evidence-based, procedure-specific postoperative pain management. *Best Pract Res Clin Anaesthesiol* 2007;21:149-159.
9. Ballantyne J: *Acute pain management: AHCPR guideline technical report.* Rockville, MD, Department of Health and Human Services, Agency for Health Care Policy and Research, 1995.
10. Atanassoff PG: Effects of regional anesthesia on perioperative outcome. *J Clin Anesth* 1996;8:446-455.
11. Ballantyne JC, Carr DB, deFerranti S, Suarez T, Lau J, Chalmers TC, et al: The comparative effects of postoperative analgesic therapies on pulmonary outcome: Cumulative meta-analyses of randomized, controlled trials. *Anesth Analg* 1998;86:598-612.
12. de Leon-Casasola OA, Lema MJ: Postoperative epidural opioid analgesia: What are the choices? *Anesth Analg* 1996;83:867-875.
13. Gottschalk A, Smith DS, Jobes DR, Kennedy SK, Lally SE, Noble VE, et al: Preemptive epidural analgesia and recovery from radical prostatectomy: A randomized controlled trial. *JAMA* 1998;279:1076-1082.
14. Singelyn FJ, Deyaert M, Joris D, Pendeville E, Gouverneur JM: Effects of intravenous patient-controlled analgesia with morphine, continuous epidural analgesia, and continuous three-in-one block on postoperative pain and knee rehabilitation after unilateral total knee arthroplasty. *Anesth Analg* 1998;87:88-92.
15. Williams-Russo P, Sharrock NE, Haas SB, Insall J, Windsor RE, Laskin RS, et al: Randomized trial of epidural versus general anesthesia: Outcomes after primary total knee replacement. *Clin Orthop Relat Res* 1996:199-208.
16. Park WY, Thompson JS, Lee KK: Effect of epidural anesthesia and analgesia on perioperative outcome: A randomized, controlled Veterans Affairs cooperative study. *Ann Surg* 2001;234:560-569, discussion 569-571.
17. Rigg JR, Jamrozik K, Myles PS, Silbert BS, Peyton PJ, Parsons RW, Collins KS: Epidural anaesthesia and analgesia and outcome of major surgery: A randomised trial. *Lancet* 2002;359:1276-1282.
18. Scott NB, Turfrey DJ, Ray DA, Nzewi O, Sutcliffe NP, Lal AB, et al: A prospective randomized study of the potential benefits of thoracic epidural anesthesia and analgesia in patients undergoing coronary artery bypass grafting. *Anesth Analg* 2001;93:528-535.
19. Gupta A, Fant F, Axelsson K, Sandblom D, Rykowski J, Johansson JE, Andersson SO: Postoperative analgesia after radical retropubic prostatectomy: A double-blind comparison between low thoracic epidural and patient-controlled intravenous analgesia. *Anesthesiology* 2006;105:784-793.
20. Boylan JF, Katz J, Kavanagh BP, Klinck JR, Cheng DC, DeMajo WC, et al: Epidural bupivacaine-morphine analgesia versus patient-controlled analgesia following abdominal aortic surgery: Analgesic, respiratory, and myocardial effects. *Anesthesiology* 1998;89:585-593.
21. Norris EJ, Beattie C, Perler BA, Martinez EA, Meinert CL, Anderson GF, et al: Double-masked randomized trial comparing alternate combinations of intraoperative anesthesia and postoperative analgesia in abdominal aortic surgery. *Anesthesiology* 2001;95:1054-1067.
22. Priestley MC, Cope L, Halliwell R, Gibson P, Chard RB, Skinner M, Klineberg PL: Thoracic epidural anesthesia for cardiac surgery: The effects on tracheal intubation time and length of hospital stay. *Anesth Analg* 2002;94:275-282, table of contents.

23. Beattie WS, Badner NH, Choi P: Epidural analgesia reduces postoperative myocardial infarction: a meta-analysis. *Anesth Analg* 2001;93:853-858.
24. Taqi A, Hong X, Mistraletti G, Stein B, Charlebois P, Carli F: Thoracic epidural analgesia facilitates the restoration of bowel function and dietary intake in patients undergoing laparoscopic colon resection using a traditional, nonaccelerated, perioperative care program. *Surg Endosc* 2007;21:247-252.
25. Practice guidelines for acute pain management in the perioperative setting. A report by the American Society of Anesthesiologists Task Force on Pain Management, Acute Pain Section. *Anesthesiology* 1995;82:1071-1081.
26. Carli F, Trudel JL, Belliveau P: The effect of intraoperative thoracic epidural anesthesia and postoperative analgesia on bowel function after colorectal surgery:A prospective, randomized trial. *Dis Colon Rectum* 2001;44:1083-1089.
27. Steinbrook RA: Epidural anesthesia and gastrointestinal motility. *Anesth Analg* 1998;86:837-844.
28. Stevens RA, Mikat-Stevens M, Flanigan R, Waters WB, Furry P, Sheikh T, et al: Does the choice of anesthetic technique affect the recovery of bowel function after radical prostatectomy? *Urology* 1998;52:213-218.
29. Tuman KJ, McCarthy RJ, March RJ, DeLaria GA, Patel RV, Ivankovich AD: Effects of epidural anesthesia and analgesia on coagulation and outcome after major vascular surgery. *Anesth Analg* 1991;73:696-704.
30. Yeager MP, Glass DD, Neff RK, Brinck-Johnsen T: Epidural anesthesia and analgesia in high-risk surgical patients. *Anesthesiology* 1987;66:729-736.
31. McPeek B: Inference, generalizability, and a major change in anesthetic practice. *Anesthesiology* 1987;66:723-724.
32. Nishimori M, Ballantyne JC, Low JH: Epidural pain relief versus systemic opioid-based pain relief for abdominal aortic surgery. *Cochrane Database Syst Rev* 2006;3:CD005059.
33. Wu CL, Sapirstein A, Herbert R, Rowlingson AJ, Michaels RK, Petrovic MA, Fleisher LA: Effect of postoperative epidural analgesia on morbidity and mortality after lung resection in Medicare patients. *J Clin Anesth* 2006;18:515-520.
34. Basse L, Madsen JL, Kehlet H: Normal gastrointestinal transit after colonic resection using epidural analgesia, enforced oral nutrition and laxative. *Br J Surg* 2001;88:1498-1500.
35. Stamer UM, Mpasios N, Stuber F, Maier C: A survey of acute pain services in Germany and a discussion of international survey data. *Reg Anesth Pain Med* 2002;27:125-131.
36. Vercauteren MP: PCA by epidural route (PCEA). *Acta Anaesthesiol Belg* 1992;43:33-39.
37. Ballantyne JC, Carr DB, Chalmers TC, Dear KB, Angelillo IF, Mosteller F: Postoperative patient-controlled analgesia: Meta-analyses of initial randomized control trials. *J Clin Anesth* 1993;5:182-193.
38. Walder B, Schafer M, Henzi I, Tramer MR: Efficacy and safety of patient-controlled opioid analgesia for acute postoperative pain. A quantitative systematic review. *Acta Anaesthesiol Scand* 2001;45:795-804.
39. Hudcova J, McNicol E, Quah C, Lau J, Carr DB: Patient-controlled opioid analgesia versus conventional opioid analgesia for postoperative pain. *Cochrane Database Syst Rev* 2006;CD003348.
40. Bainbridge D, Martin JE, Cheng DC: Patient-controlled versus nurse-controlled analgesia after cardiac surgery—a meta-analysis. *Can J Anaesth* 2006;53:492-499.
41. Jadad AR, McQuay HJ: Meta-analyses to evaluate analgesic interventions: A systematic qualitative review of their methodology. *J Clin Epidemiol* 1996;49:235-243.
42. Moore RA, Gavaghan D, Tramer MR, Collins SL, McQuay HJ: Size is everything—large amounts of information are needed to overcome random effects in estimating direction and magnitude of treatment effects. *Pain* 1998;78:209-216.
43. Moore RA, Tramer MR, Carroll D, Wiffen PJ, McQuay HJ: Quantitative systematic review of topically applied non-steroidal anti-inflammatory drugs. *BMJ* 1998;316:333-338.
44. Pogue J, Yusuf S: Overcoming the limitations of current meta-analysis of randomised controlled trials. *Lancet* 1998;351:47-52.
45. Souter MJ, Signorini DF: Meta-analysis:Greater than the sum of its parts? *Br J Anaesth* 1997;79:420-421.

46. Schulz KF, Chalmers I, Hayes RJ, Altman DG: Empirical evidence of bias. Dimensions of methodological quality associated with estimates of treatment effects in controlled trials. *JAMA* 1995;273:408-412.
47. Wilder-Smith CH, Schuler L: Postoperative analgesia: Pain by choice: The influence of patient attitudes and patient education. *Pain* 1992;50:257-262.
48. Cooper DW, Turner G: Patient-controlled extradural analgesia to compare bupivacaine, fentanyl and bupivacaine with fentanyl in the treatment of postoperative pain. *Br J Anaesth* 1993;70:503-507.
49. Gil KM, Ginsberg B, Muir M, Sykes D, Williams DA: Patient-controlled analgesia in postoperative pain: The relation of psychological factors to pain and analgesic use. *Clin J Pain* 1990;6:137-142.
50. Chan VW, Chung F, McQuestion M, Gomez M: Impact of patient-controlled analgesia on required nursing time and duration of postoperative recovery. *Reg Anesth* 1995;20:506-514.
51. Choiniere M, Rittenhouse BE, Perreault S, Chartrand D, Rousseau P, Smith B, Pepler C: Efficacy and costs of patient-controlled analgesia versus regularly administered intramuscular opioid therapy. *Anesthesiology* 1998;89:1377-1388.
52. Vercauteren M, Vereecken K, La Malfa M, Coppejans H, Adriaensen H: Cost-effectiveness of analgesia after caesarean section. A comparison of intrathecal morphine and epidural PCA. *Acta Anaesthesiol Scand* 2002;46:85-89.
53. Edwards JE, Loke YK, Moore RA, McQuay HJ: Single dose piroxicam for acute postoperative pain. *Cochrane Database Syst Rev* 2000;CD002762.
54. Reuben SS, Connelly NR: Postoperative analgesic effects of celecoxib or rofecoxib after spinal fusion surgery. *Anesth Analg* 2000;91:1221-1225.
55. Bainbridge D, Cheng DC, Martin JE, Novick R: NSAID-analgesia, pain control and morbidity in cardiothoracic surgery. *Can J Anaesth* 2006;53:46-59.
56. Camu F, Beecher T, Recker DP, Verburg KM: Valdecoxib, a COX-2-specific inhibitor, is an efficacious, opioid-sparing analgesic in patients undergoing hip arthroplasty. *Am J Ther* 2002;9:43-51.
57. Kehlet H, Rung GW, Callesen T: Postoperative opioid analgesia: Time for a reconsideration? *J Clin Anesth* 1996;8:441-445.
58. Moote C: Efficacy of nonsteroidal anti-inflammatory drugs in the management of postoperative pain. *Drugs* 1992;44(suppl 5):14-29, discussion 29-30.
59. Elia N, Lysakowski C, Tramer MR: Does multimodal analgesia with acetaminophen, nonsteroidal antiinflammatory drugs, or selective cyclooxygenase-2 inhibitors and patient-controlled analgesia morphine offer advantages over morphine alone? Meta-analyses of randomized trials. *Anesthesiology* 2005;103:1296-1304.
60. Gillies GW, Kenny GN, Bullingham RE, McArdle CS: The morphine sparing effect of ketorolac tromethamine. A study of a new, parenteral non-steroidal anti-inflammatory agent after abdominal surgery. *Anaesthesia* 1987;42:727-731.
61. Hodsman NB, Burns J, Blyth A, Kenny GN, McArdle CS, Rotman H: The morphine sparing effects of diclofenac sodium following abdominal surgery. *Anaesthesia* 1987;42:1005-1008.
62. Grass JA, Sakima NT, Valley M, Fischer K, Jackson C, Walsh P, Bourke DL: Assessment of ketorolac as an adjuvant to fentanyl patient-controlled epidural analgesia after radical retropubic prostatectomy. *Anesthesiology* 1993;78:642-648, discussion 21A.
63. Reasbeck PG, Rice ML, Reasbeck JC: Double-blind controlled trial of indomethacin as an adjunct to narcotic analgesia after major abdominal surgery. *Lancet* 1982;2:115-118.
64. Higgins MS, Givogre JL, Marco AP, Blumenthal PD, Furman WR: Recovery from outpatient laparoscopic tubal ligation is not improved by preoperative administration of ketorolac or ibuprofen. *Anesth Analg* 1994;79:274-280.
65. Thind P, Sigsgaard T: The analgesic effect of indomethacin in the early post-operative period following abdominal surgery. A double-blind controlled study. *Acta Chir Scand* 1988;154:9-12.
66. Marret E, Kurdi O, Zufferey P, Bonnet F: Effects of nonsteroidal antiinflammatory drugs on patient-controlled analgesia morphine side effects: Meta-analysis of randomized controlled trials. *Anesthesiology* 2005;102:1249-1260.

67. Goodman S, Ma T, Trindade M, Ikenoue T, Matsuura I, Wong N, et al: COX-2 selective NSAID decreases bone ingrowth in vivo. *J Orthop Res* 2002;20:1164-1169.
68. Goodman SB, Ma T, Genovese M, Lane Smith R: COX-2 selective inhibitors and bone. *Int J Immunopathol Pharmacol* 2003;16:201-205.
69. Goodman SB, Ma T, Mitsunaga L, Miyanishi K, Genovese MC, Smith RL: Temporal effects of a COX-2-selective NSAID on bone ingrowth. *J Biomed Mater Res A* 2005;72:279-287.
70. Long J, Lewis S, Kuklo T, Zhu Y, Riew KD: The effect of cyclooxygenase-2 inhibitors on spinal fusion. *J Bone Joint Surg Am* 2002; 84-A:1763-1768.
71. McGlew IC, Angliss DB, Gee GJ, Rutherford A, Wood AT: A comparison of rectal indomethacin with placebo for pain relief following spinal surgery. *Anaesth Intensive Care* 1991;19:40-45.
72. Reuben SS, Ablett D, Kaye R: High-dose nonsteroidal anti-inflammatory drugs compromise spinal fusion. *Can J Anaesth* 2005;52:506-512.
73. Lee A, Cooper MG, Craig JC, Knight JF, Keneally JP: Effects of nonsteroidal anti-inflammatory drugs on postoperative renal function in adults with normal renal function. *Cochrane Database Syst Rev* 2007;CD002765.
74. Tannenbaum H, Bombardier C, Davis P, Russell AS: An evidence-based approach to prescribing nonsteroidal antiinflammatory drugs. Third Canadian Consensus Conference. *J Rheumatol* 2006;33:140-157.
75. Hillis WS: Areas of emerging interest in analgesia: Cardiovascular complications. *Am J Ther* 2002;9:259-269.
76. Chen LC, Ashcroft DM: Risk of myocardial infarction associated with selective COX-2 inhibitors: Meta-analysis of randomised controlled trials. *Pharmacoepidemiol Drug Saf* 2007;16:762-772.
77. Abraham NS, El-Serag HB, Hartman C, Richardson P, Deswal A: Cyclooxygenase-2 selectivity of non-steroidal anti-inflammatory drugs and the risk of myocardial infarction and cerebrovascular accident. *Aliment Pharmacol Ther* 2007;25:913-924.
78. Walker SM, Macintyre PE, Visser E, Scott D: Acute pain management: Current best evidence provides guide for improved practice. *Pain Med* 2006;7:3-5.
79. Windsor AM, Glynn CJ, Mason DG: National provision of acute pain services. *Anaesthesia* 1996;51:228-231.
80. Laubenthal H, Becker M, Neugebauer E: [Guideline: Treatment of acute perioperative and posttraumatic pain. Updating from the S2- to the S3-level: A preliminary report]. *Anasthesiol Intensivmed Notfallmed Schmerzther* 2006;41:470-472.

81. Australian and New Zealand College of Anaesthetists: *Acute pain management: Scientific evidence.* Australian and New Zealand College of Anaesthetists, http://nhmrc.gov.au/publications/synopses/cp104syn.htm, May 22, 2008.
82. Carli F, Mayo N, Klubien K, Schricker T, Trudel J, Belliveau P: Epidural analgesia enhances functional exercise capacity and health-related quality of life after colonic surgery: Results of a randomized trial. *Anesthesiology* 2002;97:540-549.
83. de Leon-Casasola OA, Karabella D, Lema MJ: Bowel function recovery after radical hysterectomies: Thoracic epidural bupivacaine-morphine versus intravenous patient-controlled analgesia with morphine: A pilot study. *J Clin Anesth* 1996;8:87-92.
84. Jorgensen H, Wetterslev J, Moiniche S, Dahl JB: Epidural local anaesthetics versus opioid-based analgesic regimens on postoperative gastrointestinal paralysis, PONV and pain after abdominal surgery. *Cochrane Database Syst Rev* 2000;CD001893.
85. Williams BA, DeRiso BM, Figallo CM, Anders JW, Engel LB, Sproul KA, et al: Benchmarking the perioperative process: III. Effects of regional anesthesia clinical pathway techniques on process efficiency and recovery profiles in ambulatory orthopedic surgery. *J Clin Anesth* 1998;10:570-578.
86. Davies MJ, Silbert BS, Mooney PJ, Dysart RH, Meads AC: Combined epidural and general anaesthesia versus general anaesthesia for abdominal aortic surgery: A prospective randomised trial. *Anaesth Intensive Care* 1993;21:790-794.
87. Garnett RL, MacIntyre A, Lindsay P, Barber GG, Cole CW, Hajjar G, et al: Perioperative ischaemia in aortic surgery: Combined epidural/general anaesthesia and epidural analgesia vs general anaesthesia and I.V. analgesia. *Can J Anaesth* 1996;43:769-777.
88. Rodgers A, Walker N, Schug S, McKee A, Kehlet H, van Zundert A, et al: Reduction of postoperative mortality and morbidity with epidural or spinal anaesthesia: Results from overview of randomised trials. *BMJ* 2000;321:1493.
89. Capdevila X, Barthelet Y, Biboulet P, Ryckwaert Y, Rubenovitch J, d'Athis F: Effects of perioperative analgesic technique on the surgical outcome and duration of rehabilitation after major knee surgery. *Anesthesiology* 1999;91:8-15.
90. Moiniche S, Hjortso NC, Hansen BL, Dahl JB, Rosenberg J, Gebuhr P, Kehlet H: The effect of balanced analgesia on early convalescence after major orthopaedic surgery. *Acta Anaesthesiol Scand* 1994;38:328-335.

73 Is Preemptive Analgesia Clinically Effective?

Allan Gottschalk, MD, PhD, and E. Andrew Ochroch, MD

INTRODUCTION

The concept of preemptive analgesia originated at a time of growing appreciation for the dynamic characteristics of the pain pathway. Experimental studies made it clear that noxious stimuli could sensitize both the peripheral and central components of the nociceptive pathway. This insight guided the interpretation of several clinical studies,[1-3] which appeared to demonstrate that subjects who underwent surgery having first received opioids or regional blockade experienced less postoperative pain, and raised "the possibility that preemptive preoperative analgesia has prolonged effects which outlast the presence of drugs."[4] Since then, a considerable number of laboratory and clinical studies of preemptive analgesia have been performed.

Interpretation of this growing body of data is encumbered by evolving concepts as to what constitutes preemptive analgesia.[5] Preemptive analgesia in the widest sense recognizes that noxious stimuli at any point throughout the entire perioperative period can sensitize the nervous system. More recently, the term *preventive* analgesia has been applied to clinical and laboratory studies that seek to demonstrate a beneficial effect of an analgesic intervention that outlasts the pharmacologic presence of the intervention. Such studies typically determine whether some long-term benefit is observed in those who received the analgesic intervention compared with those who did not. In contrast, preemptive analgesia in the narrow sense addresses only a small portion of the perioperative period such as the time of incision or the time of surgery. Clinical and laboratory studies of preemptive analgesia defined in this manner typically administer identical analgesic interventions at different times to the test and control groups, where typical times would be preincision and postincision or preoperatively and postoperatively. Subjects in such trials could receive considerable benefit from the intervention provided to the control group. Of late, trials such as this are considered tests of *preemptive* analgesia as opposed to *preventive* analgesia. Meta-analyses of clinical trials with a *preemptive* structure[6,7] have been conflicting, with the most recent being supportive of preemptive epidural analgesia, local anesthetic infiltration, and nonsteroidal antiinflammatory drug (NSAID) administration (Figure 73-1). Another meta-analysis demonstrated that studies with a *preventive* design as opposed to a *preemptive* design were more likely to lead to measurable benefits, particularly for use of N-methyl-D-aspartate (NMDA) antagonists.[8] In interpreting data from any one of these study designs, the timing and duration of the analgesic intervention may mean little if the intervention is not capable of preventing sensitization of the nociceptive pathways.[9]

The motivation for use of preemptive analgesic strategies is twofold. First, one seeks to minimize perioperative pain as well as pain during the typical recovery period for a given surgical procedure. Apart from the relief offered to patients, there is the expectation of reaping any functional benefits that may be associated with effective analgesic therapy. Second, preemptive analgesic approaches recognize that acute painful events can lead to long-term painful consequences, where pain persists even when tissue healing appears to be complete. Although the best-known long-term painful syndromes are associated with limb amputation, where about 70% of patients report pain 1 year following surgery,[10] long-term painful sequelae are reported for many other types of surgery.[11] In general, prior painful experience is predictive of increased pain and analgesic use following subsequent surgery.[12,13] Even relatively limited surgery can lead to long-term alterations in the response to noxious stimuli. For example, pain-related behavior is increased during vaccination for boys who previously underwent circumcision compared with those who did not.[14] Pain is reported 1 year following surgery in at least half of patients undergoing major thoracotomy[15-17] or breast surgery.[18] About half of patients undergoing lower abdominal surgery will still report some degree of residual pain several months following the surgical procedure.[19,20] Inguinal herniorrhaphy is associated with residual pain in 25% of patients 1 year following surgery.[21] Even low levels of residual pain are associated with decreases in activity and perception of health.[20,22] Thus, long-term alterations in pain perception occur frequently following a broad range of surgical procedures, and these alterations may affect quality of life. These long-term changes in pain perception motivate the use of preemptive analgesia. The underlying hypothesis is that such changes can be prevented by initiating an effective analgesic regimen before the onset of the procedure and maintaining it for a sufficient duration.

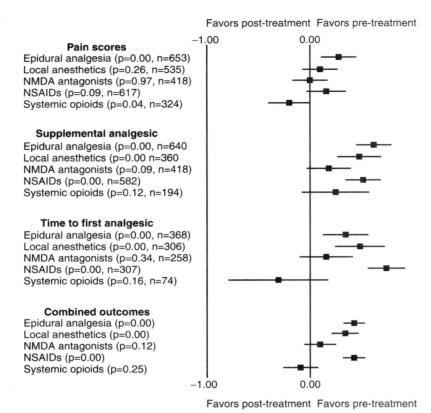

Figure 73-1. Summary of Results from a Recent Meta-analysis of Preemptive Analgesia.[7] The plot indicates the effect size (standardized mean difference) for preemptive treatment compared with control and the 95% confidence interval. For each intervention and outcome measure, the total number of subjects included in the meta-analysis and the significance of the result is indicated. Results when all three outcomes are combined are given at the bottom. NMDA, N-methyl-D-aspartate; NSAID, nonsteroidal antiinflammatory drug. (*Adapted from Figs. 1-4 of Ong CK, Lirk P, Seymour RA, Jenkins BJ: The efficacy of preemptive analgesia for acute postoperative pain management: A meta-analysis. Anesth Analg 2005;100:757-773, with permission.*)

OPTIONS

Therapeutic options for preemptive analgesia can include virtually all analgesic modalities and pharmacologic classes, individually and in combination. Analgesics can be administered systemically, at the site of surgery, along a peripheral nerve, or neuraxially. Analgesics include opioids, alpha$_2$ agonists, NMDA antagonists, muscarinic stimulation by administration of an anticholinesterase, NSAIDs, anticonvulsants, and local anesthetics.

Timing of the initiation of the analgesic regimen is central to the use of preemptive analgesia. Because most practitioners recognize the need for postoperative analgesia, most studies of preemptive analgesia have emphasized interventions initiated before the start of surgery and lasting for some portion of the surgical procedure. However, the quality of postoperative analgesia may be an important factor. Periods of intense pain on emergence or during recovery may lead to sensitization of the nociceptive pathway, overwhelming the benefits of preventing intraoperative sensitization. Conversely, highly effective postoperative analgesic regimens could mask the benefits of intraoperative efforts to prevent sensitization, and even limit sensitization in control groups. For procedures characterized by a long and painful postoperative course, preventing sensitization in the postoperative period may

be just as important as doing so intraoperatively. For analgesics that can take some time to exert their full effect (e.g., NSAIDs, see later discussion), initiation of the analgesic regimen well in advance of the start of surgery is required for preemption to occur. Along with the decision of when in the perioperative period to initiate analgesic therapy, the necessary dose and duration of analgesic therapy to prevent sensitization during each phase of the perioperative period requires elucidation, and may vary with the type of surgery.

EVIDENCE

Laboratory evidence of preemptive analgesia

Laboratory studies suggested the clinical applicability of preemptive analgesia by identifying the underlying mechanisms and the factors that may play important clinical roles. Painful stimuli can sensitize both the peripheral and central components of the nervous system.[23] In the periphery, repeated applications of noxious stimuli increase the magnitude of the response to subsequent applications of the same stimulus.[24] There is a complex interaction between peripheral nociceptors and inflammatory mediators released in response to tissue injury, which can enhance the response of peripheral nociceptors.[25]

This enhanced response can be attenuated with local anesthetics, opioids, and NSAIDs as described later in this chapter.

Neurons in the dorsal horn of the spinal cord exhibit a biphasic response to formalin injection of the skin.[26] Intrathecal opioids are effective at preventing both phases of this response.[27] However, the second phase is still prevented even after administration of an opioid antagonist after the initial response, indicating that alteration of neural behavior by a noxious stimulus can be prevented. Substance P and excitatory amino acid transmitters acting at NMDA receptors play a crucial role in sensitizing neurons in the dorsal horn.[28-31] Local anesthetic infiltration before formalin injection can limit longer-term pain-related behavior.[32] When noxious inflammatory stimuli of longer duration are used, longer-term reductions in pain-related behavior are seen only with local anesthetics whose duration of action matches that of the noxious stimulus.[33,34] Administration of local anesthetic before nerve section can decrease pain-related behavior for a considerable period of time.[35] In a laboratory model of incisional pain, rats receiving intrathecal opioid or local anesthetic before an incision in their hindpaw exhibited decreased wound hyperalgesia on the day of surgery, but not longer, when compared with those who received the same analgesics immediately after incision.[36]

Although laboratory studies of nociception suggested the clinical potential of preemptive approaches, many explicit laboratory tests of preemptive analgesia have been negative.[37-39] However, the quality and duration of the preemptively administered analgesic relative to the intensity of the experimental stimulus may play an important role in whether preemptive analgesic administration is beneficial.[40] Moreover, the extent that laboratory models of surgical pain replicate the nociceptive processing that takes place during major surgical procedures has not been fully determined. However, a new rat model of thoracotomy has been more successful in demonstrating the capacity of systemic and intrathecal analgesics to decrease long-term pain.[41]

Laboratory studies may also help to delineate the contribution of the general anesthetics to preemptive analgesic effects. Clinically effective concentrations of volatile anesthetics do not prevent central sensitization.[42] but they can potentiate the effects of neuraxial opioids.[43] Nitrous oxide has been shown to have a preemptive analgesic effect that is not observed when a volatile anesthetic is also present.[44]

Clinical evidence of preemptive analgesia

There are hundreds of studies evaluating the clinical use of preemptive analgesia. These vary considerably with respect to timing, intensity, and duration of the intervention, the analgesic used in the control group, and the type of surgery. In this section, we consider systemic interventions with opioids, NMDA antagonists, and NSAIDs, and regional administration of local anesthetics and opioids.

Systemic fentanyl administered as a bolus before incision and maintained with an infusion reduced wound hyperalgesia 24 and 48 hours after surgery when compared

with controls, all of whom received identical postoperative opioid analgesia.[45] Consequently, it is surprising that multiple studies of preemptive opioid administration for hysterectomy have, collectively, been somewhat disappointing, with multiple meta-analyses revealing no benefit of preincisional opioid administration (see Figure 73-1), and even a paradoxic effect in favor of analgesics administered postoperatively.[6,7] However, in all these studies, the same bolus dose of opioid was administered either before incision or at the conclusion of surgery. Consequently, especially since many of the studies employed relatively short-acting opioids, it is conceivable that intraoperative opioid levels were inadequate for preventing sensitization in the intervention group. Furthermore, the group receiving an opioid bolus at the conclusion of surgery would have been relatively comfortable during the often painful period immediately following surgery when sensitization is still possible. When intraoperative opioid levels were maintained with an infusion, reduced pain and analgesic consumption were seen for the 48 hours following surgery.[46] An additional potentially confounding factor is that acute opioid tolerance could have developed in the group receiving opioids before incision, rendering analgesics administered in the immediate postoperative period less effective.[47-49]

NMDA antagonists have the potential to limit central sensitization[30,31] and, through an additional consequence of their action at the NMDA receptor, decrease the acute tolerance that develops with opioid administration.[50,51] Systemic ketamine administered before surgery can decrease wound hyperalgesia measured 48 hours after surgery, although this was not associated with decreases in pain.[45] Other studies with lower doses of ketamine conflict as to whether preemptive ketamine administration by itself can lead to reductions in postoperative pain.[52,53] Systemic ketamine used in combination with epidural analgesics led to persistent reductions in postoperative pain.[54,55] Preoperative systemic dextromethorphan decreased pain and analgesic consumption in a dose-dependent manner,[56-59] and augmented the efficacy of performing surgery under epidural blockade with a combination of lidocaine and morphine.[60] A meta-analysis of eight trials comparing preincisional administration of ketamine or dextromethorphan with postincisional administration found no consistent benefit of preincisional ketamine administration, but did observe a benefit for the two trials of dextromethorphan that were included in the meta-analysis.[6] This negative result for NMDA antagonists was echoed (see Figure 73-1) by a more recent meta-analysis.[7] However, studies of NMDA antagonists that were more *preventive* in their design were associated with beneficial effects.[8] Importantly, NMDA antagonists can also enhance the benefits of epidural analgesia.[61-63]

Peripheral inflammation in response to tissue injury is painful and can enhance the sensitivity of the peripheral nociceptors, which are themselves a source of proinflammatory mediators.[25,64] The analgesic effects of NSAIDs are due to both their ability to reduce peripheral nociceptor output by modulating the peripheral inflammatory response and to their more central effects.[65] Therefore it is reasonable to hypothesize that NSAIDs may complement the use of other analgesics in the control of perioperative pain by limiting the nociceptor barrage that may contribute to central sensitization, by limiting peripheral sensitization induced by the inflammatory response, and through central mechanisms that are either additive or synergistic. A considerable number of studies demonstrate the ability of NSAIDs to reduce perioperative pain and limit the need for other analgesics.[66] Although the mechanism of action of NSAIDs suggests that administering them before the onset of surgery should be beneficial, the available studies indicate that expectations and strategies for the use of these drugs in a preemptive manner need revision.

In an initial meta-analysis of 19 trials of preincisional versus postincisional administration of NSAIDs, only 4 studies demonstrated any reduction in pain, decreased analgesic consumption, or delay until first analgesic request with preincisional NSAIDs.[6] However, a more recent meta-analysis of 17 studies (see Figure 73-1) was more supportive of a preemptive analgesic effect.[7] One favorable study not included in the first meta-analysis compared the effects of intravenous NSAID administration 30 minutes before induction with its administration at the conclusion of surgery. Preemptive administration resulted in improvement in pain scores, increased time until first analgesic request, and decreased analgesic consumption for the 4-hour period of study.[67] A follow-up study demonstrated similar results when the same NSAID was administered either 30 minutes before induction in the intervention group or at the time of induction, as opposed to the conclusion of surgery, in the control group,[68] emphasizing the importance of timing to observe a preemptive effect.[69] Even assuming that NSAIDs are administered preemptively at the optimal time, studies emphasizing only the intraoperative and immediate postoperative periods will miss any longer-term benefits of decreasing postoperative inflammation.

The anticonvulsant gabapentin appears to contribute to perioperative pain relief in studies where it was used in a preventive fashion. Decreased pain and opiate sparing have been demonstrated for lumbar spine surgery,[70] breast surgery,[71] and laparoscopic surgery.[72] Preventive use of gabapentin in combination with local anesthetics has demonstrated a reduction in acute pain, as well as chronic pain, six months after breast surgery.[73]

Local anesthetic infiltration is a relatively safe and simple analgesic modality that can decrease peripheral sensitization and reduce or prevent the nociceptor barrage at the spinal cord. Local anesthetic administered before a surgical procedure can have benefits that outlast the duration of action of the local anesthetic. Pain-related behavior by boys during vaccination is reduced in those who previously underwent circumcision after application of a local anesthetic cream compared with those who did not receive a local anesthetic for the procedure.[74] Local anesthetic infiltration with bupivacaine before surgery for inguinal herniorrhaphy reduced wound hyperalgesia compared with general anesthesia alone. This difference was seen 10 days following surgery, and was superior to spinal anesthesia.[75] Patients undergoing inguinal herniorrhaphy under general anesthesia who received preincisional infiltration of the incision site with lidocaine waited longer until their first analgesic request and were less likely to request analgesics than those who received

lidocaine infiltration at the time of closure.[76] When inguinal herniorrhaphy is performed under spinal anesthesia, subjects who had an ilioinguinal-iliohypogastric nerve block experienced less pain and had decreased analgesic consumption during the first 2 postoperative days.[77] Preemptive incisional[78] or peritoneal[79] use of local anesthetic for laparoscopic surgery may also have benefits.

Collectively, these studies of preemptive local anesthetic use imply that the pain pathways can be sensitized during both the intraoperative and postoperative phases of the perioperative period, and that interruption of this sensitization can lead to effects that outlast the duration of action of the drug used in the intervention. A systematic review of studies using local infiltration that contrasted interventions performed before incision with those performed before the conclusion of the procedure was generally not supportive of preincisional interventions with local anesthetics except during herniorrhaphy.[80] A subsequent meta-analysis was generally not supportive of preincisional local anesthetic infiltration compared with postincisional infiltration (weighted mean difference [±95% confidence interval (CI)] with respect to a 100-mm visual analog pain scale: 0 [−3,4]).[6] Another review stressed the importance of using a local anesthetic block of adequate strength and duration.[40] A more recent meta-analysis (see Figure 73-1) was more supportive of local anesthetic infiltration of the wound.[7]

Neuraxial blockade with a single dose of local anesthetic placed in the subarachnoid space produces profound, but not complete,[81] blockade for the duration of surgery and the immediate postoperative period. The use of spinal anesthesia may confer some longer-term benefits,[2,75,82] but when administration of a spinal anesthetic either before the start of surgery or after its conclusion was compared, only small differences in analgesic use were sometimes seen.[83,84]

Use of epidural catheters for the neuraxial administration of local anesthetics, opioids, and other drugs continues to be an important technique for perioperative pain control for major surgery. Because epidural catheters are often placed to provide postoperative pain relief and have been shown to do this effectively,[85] studies involving preemptive epidural analgesia often focus on the somewhat narrower question of whether or not there is a benefit to intraoperative use of the epidural catheter. This debate is made complex by variation in the procedures studied, the quality of intraoperative blockade achieved in the various studies, and the quality of the postoperative analgesia. Epidural anesthesia by itself may confer an analgesic benefit that outlasts the duration of the blockade.[1,3,86] Neuraxial fentanyl administered immediately before incision reduced pain in the immediate postoperative period compared with the same intervention given shortly after incision.[87] A single preoperative dose of epidural morphine appears to have analgesic benefits that outlast the drug's duration of action for certain types of procedures.[88,89] When local anesthetic alone or in combination with opioids is administered through epidural catheters during surgery, the impact on postoperative analgesia is often, but not always, beneficial,[19,90-102] as reflected by meta-analyses (see Figure 73-1) with different conclusions regarding the benefits of preemptive epidural analgesia.[6,7] However, with the exception of studies addressing long-term pain following amputation or major thoracotomy (see below), studies addressing pain or functionality after discharge are rare, but often favorable.[19,103]

Given the aforementioned ability of preemptively administered local anesthetic to limit long-term pain-related behavior following nerve section in the laboratory,[35] it might be anticipated that a preemptive analgesic approach might be particularly effective in preventing the long-term pain syndromes that are associated with thoracotomy and limb amputation. Initiation of epidural blockade before the onset of surgery as compared with after surgery, and then maintained for 48 hours in both groups, has had a positive long-term impact on the rate of postthoracotomy pain after the procedure.[99,101] In contrast, a study that initiated epidural analgesia before incision or at the start of closure, and then maintained the block until thoracostomy tube removal, demonstrated only short-term analgesic sparing effects when comparing the two groups.[104] However, this study reported substantially lower rates of postthoracotomy pain than the prior studies. Several early studies of long-term pain following amputation[3,86] demonstrated a benefit of preemptive approaches that was not observed in a larger study with a somewhat weaker intervention.[105] The editorial that accompanied this last study reviews the related literature in detail and concludes that the likelihood of benefits when epidural analgesia is used to prevent long-term pain following limb amputation varies with the quality and duration of the blockade.[106] Effective regimens used significant local anesthetic blockade for up to a day before surgery, during the surgical procedure, and for several days afterward.

AREAS OF UNCERTAINTY

As emphasized earlier, preemptive analgesia is a controversial area with a large and growing clinical and experimental literature that can be selectively mobilized to support multiple points of view. Whether preemptive anesthesia is defined in the wide (preventive analgesia) or narrow sense, there is a relative lack of studies that address long-term outcomes, particularly other than pain and analgesic use. However, even for rather narrow definitions of preemptive analgesia, long-term benefits have been demonstrated for major abdominal surgery[19,103] and thoracic surgery.[99,101] Apart from the timing of the intervention, there is considerable debate about the magnitude of the intervention. This applies to both the initial drug doses and to whether this level of intervention is maintained throughout surgery and into the postoperative period. Interventions must be capable of preventing sensitization of the pain pathways.[9] Studies defining and testing preemptive analgesia in the narrow sense generally use interventions and study designs that permit patients in both the control and intervention groups a comfortable transition to the postoperative period. Consequently, even the control groups often receive an analgesic regimen that might be expected to limit peripheral or central sensitization.[9] When considering outcomes other than pain, it remains uncertain how much any benefit of the intervention is due to reductions in pain and how much is a consequence of other effects of the intervention. For example, intraarticular local anesthetic infiltration reduces postoperative pain, and this pain reduction is associated with improved tissue oxygenation.[107] In contrast, epidural analgesia modulates a number of physiologic variables[108] that may contribute to favorable outcomes.[109-113] Last, few economic data are available to guide the choice of interventions and to assess the cost of inadequately treated pain.[114]

GUIDELINES

The studies that present a less than overwhelming case for preemptive analgesia generally define preemptive analgesia narrowly, using relatively limited interventions for a brief portion of the perioperative period. These studies should not obscure the importance of providing continuous outstanding pain relief throughout the entire perioperative period. There are enough studies demonstrating residual pain remaining once tissue healing appears to be complete and analgesic benefits that outlast the duration of action of the intervention to motivate aggressive perioperative pain control. At the very least, this involves the use of sufficient systemic analgesics, local infiltration, nerve blocks, and neuraxial analgesic administration to permit patients to emerge comfortably from surgery and remain comfortable throughout the postoperative period while achieving milestones for rehabilitation. One thing remains clear: modest interventions by themselves are unlikely to be beneficial, regardless of the timing of their administration.

AUTHORS' RECOMMENDATIONS

Given the current state of research, we continue to recommend regional anesthetics alone or in combination with systemic adjuncts and/or general anesthesia to smooth out the course of surgery and optimize perioperative pain control. Systemic adjuncts may be particularly useful in patients with preexisting pain. Epidural analgesia is frequently an option for major surgery. When possible, use combinations of opioids and local anesthetic administered epidurally well in advance of incision, and maintain the block with infusions or frequent bolus doses of the same medications throughout the procedure. Analgesia should be maintained with patient-controlled epidural infusions of opioid and local anesthetic initiated before the end of surgery. Nonfunctioning epidural catheters should be identified before the conclusion of surgery and either replaced or supplanted with intravenous analgesics. Although many anesthesiologists are concerned about the loss of sympathetic tone that accompanies the use of intraoperative local anesthetics,[115] there should be little concern about the use of intraoperative opioids, and it should be recognized that the sympathectomy that accompanies epidural blockade may actually be protective.[116,117]

When epidural catheter placement is not appropriate for the given surgical procedure, there are clear contraindications to epidural catheter placement, or epidural catheter placement is not technically feasible, we combine presurgical administration of systemic opiates and NSAIDs, and local infiltration of the incision site or nerve block with a long-acting local anesthetic. For procedures longer than 90 to 120 minutes, we recommend reinfiltration of the wound with a long-acting local anesthetic at the conclusion of surgery.

ACKNOWLEDGMENTS

Supported in part by National Institutes of Health grants 1-R01-NH-40545 and 1-K23-HD/NS-40914.

REFERENCES

1. Smith CM, Guralnick MS, Gelfand MM, Jeans ME: The effects of transcutaneous electrical nerve stimulation on post-cesarean pain. *Pain* 1986;27:181-193.
2. McQuay HJ, Carroll D, Moore RA: Postoperative orthopaedic pain—the effect of opiate premedication and local anaesthetic blocks. *Pain* 1988;33:291-295.
3. Bach S, Noreng MF, Tjellden NU: Phantom limb pain in amputees during the first 12 months following limb amputation, after preoperative lumbar epidural blockade. *Pain* 1988;33:297-301.
4. Wall PD: The prevention of postoperative pain. *Pain* 1988;33:289-290.
5. Kissin I: Preemptive analgesia: Terminology and clinical relevance. *Anesth Analg* 1994;79:809-810.
6. Moiniche S, Kehlet H, Dahl JB: A qualitative and quantitative systematic review of preemptive analgesia for postoperative pain relief: The role of timing of analgesia. *Anesthesiology* 2002;96:725-741.
7. Ong CK, Lirk P, Seymour RA, Jenkins BJ: The efficacy of preemptive analgesia for acute postoperative pain management: A meta-analysis. *Anesth Analg* 2005;100:757-773.
8. Katz J, McCartney CJ: Current status of preemptive analgesia. *Curr Opin Anaesthesiol* 2002;15:435-441.
9. Kissin I: Preemptive analgesia. Why its effect is not always obvious. *Anesthesiology* 1996;84:1015-1019.
10. Sherman RA, Devor M, Jones D, et al: *Phantom pain*. New York, Plenum, 1997.
11. Perkins FM, Kehlet H: Chronic pain as an outcome of surgery. A review of predictive factors. *Anesthesiology* 2000;93:1123-1133.
12. Taenzer P, Melzack R, Jeans ME: Influence of psychological factors on postoperative pain, mood and analgesic requirements. *Pain* 1986;24:331-342.
13. Bachiocco V, Scesi M, Morselli AM, Carli G: Individual pain history and familial pain tolerance models: Relationships to post-surgical pain. *Clin J Pain* 1993;9:266-271.
14. Taddio A, Goldbach M, Ipp M, et al: Effect of neonatal circumcision on pain responses during vaccination in boys. *Lancet* 1995; 345:291-292.
15. Dajczman E, Gordon A, Kreisman H, Wolkove N: Long-term postthoracotomy pain. *Chest* 1991;99:270-274.
16. Katz J, Jackson M, Kavanagh BP, Sandler AN: Acute pain after thoracic surgery predicts long-term post-thoracotomy pain. *Clin J Pain* 1996;12:50-55.
17. Gottschalk A, Cohen SP, Yang S, Ochroch EA: Preventing and treating pain after thoracic surgery. *Anesthesiology* 2006;104:594-600.
18. Wallace MS, Wallace AM, Lee J, Dobke MK: Pain after breast surgery: A survey of 282 women. *Pain* 1996;66:195-205.
19. Gottschalk A, Smith DS, Jobes DR, et al: Preemptive epidural analgesia and recovery from radical prostatectomy: A randomized controlled trial. *JAMA* 1998;279:1076-1082.
20. Haythornthwaite JA, Raja SN, Fisher B, et al: Pain and quality of life following radical retropubic prostatectomy. *J Urol* 1998;160:1761-1764.
21. Callesen T, Kehlet H: Postherniorrhaphy pain. *Anesthesiology* 1997;87:1219-1230.
22. Bay-Nielsen M, Perkins FM, Kehlet H: Pain and functional impairment 1 year after inguinal herniorrhaphy: A nationwide questionnaire study. *Ann Surg* 2001;233:1-7.
23. Fields HL: *Pain*. New York, McGraw-Hill, 1987.
24. Meyer RA, Campbell JN: Myelinated nociceptive afferents account for the hyperalgesia that follows a burn to the hand. *Science* 1981;213:1527-1529.
25. Kelly DJ, Ahmad M, Brull SJ: Preemptive analgesia I: Physiological pathways and pharmacological modalities. *Can J Anaesth* 2001;48:1000-1010.
26. Woolf CJ, King AE: Dynamic alterations in the cutaneous mechanoreceptive fields of dorsal horn neurons in the rat spinal cord. *J Neurosci* 1990;10:2717-2726.
27. Dickenson AH, Sullivan AF: Subcutaneous formalin-induced activity of dorsal horn neurones in the rat: Differential response to an intrathecal opiate administered pre or post formalin. *Pain* 1987;30:349-360.
28. Mantyh PW, Rogers SD, Honore P, et al: Inhibition of hyperalgesia by ablation of lamina I spinal neurons expressing the substance P receptor. *Science* 1997;278:275-279.
29. Malmberg AB, Chen C, Tonegawa S, Basbaum AI: Preserved acute pain and reduced neuropathic pain in mice lacking PKCγ. *Science* 1997;278:279-283.
30. Liu H, Mantyh PW, Basbaum AI: NMDA-receptor regulation of substance P release from primary afferent nociceptors. *Nature* 1997;386:721-724.
31. Woolf CJ, Thompson SW: The induction and maintenance of central sensitization is dependent on N-methyl-D-aspartic acid receptor activation; implications for the treatment of post-injury pain hypersensitivity states. *Pain* 1991;44:293-299.
32. Coderre TJ, Vaccarino AL, Melzack R: Central nervous system plasticity in the tonic pain response to subcutaneous formalin injection. *Brain Res* 1990;535:155-158.
33. Fletcher D, Kayser V, Guilbaud G: Influence of timing of administration on the analgesic effect of bupivacaine infiltration in carrageenin-injected rats. *Anesthesiology* 1996;84:1129-1137.
34. Kissin I, Lee SS, Bradley EL Jr: Effect of prolonged nerve block on inflammatory hyperalgesia in rats: Prevention of late hyperalgesia. *Anesthesiology* 1998;88:224-232.
35. Gonzalez-Darder JM, Barbera J, Abellan MJ: Effects of prior anaesthesia on autotomy following sciatic transection in rats. *Pain* 1986;24:87-91.
36. Zahn PK, Brennan TJ: Incision-induced changes in receptive field properties of rat dorsal horn neurons. *Anesthesiology* 1999;91: 772-785.
37. Pogatzki EM, Zahn PK, Brennan TJ: Effect of pretreatment with intrathecal excitatory amino acid receptor antagonists on the development of pain behavior caused by plantar incision. *Anesthesiology* 2000;93:489-496.
38. Brennan TJ, Umali EF, Zahn PK: Comparison of pre- versus post-incision administration of intrathecal bupivacaine and intrathecal morphine in a rat model of postoperative pain. *Anesthesiology* 1997;87:1517-1528.
39. Zahn PK, Brennan TJ: Lack of effect of intrathecally administered N-methyl-D-aspartate receptor antagonists in a rat model for postoperative pain. *Anesthesiology* 1998;88:143-156.
40. Pasqualucci A: Experimental and clinical studies about the preemptive analgesia with local anesthetics. Possible reasons of the failure. *Minerva Anestesiol* 1998;64:445-457.
41. Buvanendran A, Kroin JS, Kerns JM, et al: Characterization of a new animal model for evaluation of persistent postthoracotomy pain. *Anesth Analg* 2004;99:1453-1460.
42. Abram SE, Yaksh TL: Morphine, but not inhalation anesthesia, blocks post-injury facilitation. The role of preemptive suppression of afferent transmission. *Anesthesiology* 1993;78:713-721.
43. O'Connor TC, Abram SE: Halothane enhances suppression of spinal sensitization by intrathecal morphine in the rat formalin test. *Anesthesiology* 1994;81:1277-1283.
44. Goto T, Marota JJ, Crosby G: Nitrous oxide induces preemptive analgesia in the rat that is antagonized by halothane. *Anesthesiology* 1994;80:409-416.
45. Tverskoy M, Oz Y, Isakson A, et al: Preemptive effect of fentanyl and ketamine on postoperative pain and wound hyperalgesia. *Anesth Analg* 1994;78:205-209.
46. Katz J, Clairoux M, Redahan C, et al: High-dose alfentanil preempts pain after abdominal hysterectomy. *Pain* 1996;68:109-118.
47. Guignard B, Bossard AE, Coste C, et al: Acute opioid tolerance: Intraoperative remifentanil increases postoperative pain and morphine requirement. *Anesthesiology* 2000;93:409-417.
48. Celerier E, Rivat C, Jun Y, et al: Long-lasting hyperalgesia induced by fentanyl in rats: Preventive effect of ketamine. *Anesthesiology* 2000;92:465-472.
49. Eisenach JC: Preemptive hyperalgesia, not analgesia? *Anesthesiology* 2000;92:308-309.

50. Mao J, Price DD, Mayer DJ: Mechanisms of hyperalgesia and morphine tolerance: A current view of their possible interactions. *Pain* 1995;62:259-274.
51. Price DD, Mayer DJ, Mao J, Caruso FS: NMDA-receptor antagonists and opioid receptor interactions as related to analgesia and tolerance. *J Pain Symptom Manage* 2000;19:S7-S11.
52. Dahl V, Ernoe PE, Steen T, et al: Does ketamine have preemptive effects in women undergoing abdominal hysterectomy procedures? *Anesth Analg* 2000;90:1419-1422.
53. Roytblat L, Korotkoruchko A, Katz J, et al: Postoperative pain: The effect of low-dose ketamine in addition to general anesthesia. *Anesth Analg* 1993;77:1161-1165.
54. Aida S, Yamakura T, Baba H, et al: Preemptive analgesia by intravenous low-dose ketamine and epidural morphine in gastrectomy: A randomized double-blind study. *Anesthesiology* 2000;92:1624-1630.
55. De Kock M, Lavand'homme P, Waterloos H: "Balanced analgesia" in the perioperative period: Is there a place for ketamine? *Pain* 2001;92:373-380.
56. Grace RF, Power I, Umedaly H, et al: Preoperative dextromethorphan reduces intraoperative but not postoperative morphine requirements after laparotomy. *Anesth Analg* 1998;87:1135-1138.
57. Helmy SA, Bali A: The effect of the preemptive use of the NMDA receptor antagonist dextromethorphan on postoperative analgesic requirements. *Anesth Analg* 2001;92:739-744.
58. Wu CT, Yu JC, Yeh CC, et al: Preincisional dextromethorphan treatment decreases postoperative pain and opioid requirement after laparoscopic cholecystectomy. *Anesth Analg* 1999;88:1331-1334.
59. Wu CT, Yu JC, Liu ST, et al: Preincisional dextromethorphan treatment for postoperative pain management after upper abdominal surgery. *World J Surg* 2000;24:512-517.
60. Weinbroum AA, Lalayev G, Yashar T, et al: Combined preincisional oral dextromethorphan and epidural lidocaine for postoperative pain reduction and morphine sparing: A randomised double-blind study on day-surgery patients. *Anaesthesia* 2001;56:616-622.
61. Kararmaz A, Kaya S, Karaman H, et al: Intraoperative intravenous ketamine in combination with epidural analgesia: Postoperative analgesia after renal surgery. *Anesth Analg* 2003;97:1092-1096.
62. Yeh CC, Jao SW, Huh BK, et al: Preincisional dextromethorphan combined with thoracic epidural anesthesia and analgesia improves postoperative pain and bowel function in patients undergoing colonic surgery. *Anesth Analg* 2005;100:1384-1389.
63. Suzuki M, Haraguti S, Sugimoto K, et al: Low-dose intravenous ketamine potentiates epidural analgesia after thoracotomy. *Anesthesiology* 2006;105:111-119.
64. Stein C: The control of pain in peripheral tissue by opioids. *N Engl J Med* 1995;332:1685-1690.
65. Yaksh TL, Dirig DM, Malmberg AB: Mechanism of action of nonsteroidal anti-inflammatory drugs. *Cancer Invest* 1998;16:509-527.
66. Jin F, Chung F: Multimodal analgesia for postoperative pain control. *J Clin Anesth* 2001;13:524-539.
67. Colbert ST, O'Hanlon DM, McDonnell C, et al: Analgesia in day case breast biopsy—the value of pre-emptive tenoxicam. *Can J Anaesth* 1998;45:217-222.
68. O'Hanlon DM, Thambipillai T, Colbert ST, et al: Timing of pre-emptive tenoxicam is important for postoperative analgesia. *Can J Anaesth* 2001;48:162-166.
69. Katz J: Pre-emptive analgesia: Importance of timing. *Can J Anaesth* 2001;48:105-114.
70. Turan A, Karamanlioglu B, Memis D, et al: Analgesic effects of gabapentin after spinal surgery. *Anesthesiology* 2004;100:935-938.
71. Dirks J, Fredensborg BB, Christensen D, et al: A randomized study of the effects of single-dose gabapentin versus placebo on postoperative pain and morphine consumption after mastectomy. *Anesthesiology* 2002;97:560-564.
72. Pandey CK, Priye S, Singh S, et al: Preemptive use of gabapentin significantly decreases postoperative pain and rescue analgesic requirements in laparoscopic cholecystectomy. *Can J Anaesth* 2004;51:358-363.
73. Fassoulaki A, Triga A, Melemeni A, Sarantopoulos C: Multimodal analgesia with gabapentin and local anesthetics prevents acute and chronic pain after breast surgery for cancer. *Anesth Analg* 2005;101:1427-1432.
74. Taddio A, Katz J, Ilersich AL, Koren G: Effect of neonatal circumcision on pain response during subsequent routine vaccination. *Lancet* 1997;349:599-603.
75. Tverskoy M, Cozacov C, Ayache M, et al: Postoperative pain after inguinal herniorrhaphy with different types of anesthesia. *Anesth Analg* 1990;70:29-35.
76. Ejlersen E, Andersen HB, Eliasen K, Mogensen T: A comparison between preincisional and postincisional lidocaine infiltration and postoperative pain. *Anesth Analg* 1992;74:495-498.
77. Bugedo GJ, Cárcamo CR, Mertens RA, et al: Preoperative percutaneous ilioinguinal and iliohypogastric nerve block with 0.5% bupivacaine for post-herniorrhaphy pain management in adults. *Reg Anesth* 1990;15:130-133.
78. Ke RW, Portera SG, Bagous W, Lincoln SR: A randomized, double-blinded trial of preemptive analgesia in laparoscopy. *Obstet Gynecol* 1998;92:972-975.
79. Pasqualucci A, de Angelis V, Contardo R, et al: Preemptive analgesia: Intraperitoneal local anesthetic in laparoscopic cholecystectomy. A randomized, double-blind, placebo-controlled study. *Anesthesiology* 1996;85:11-20.
80. Moiniche S, Mikkelsen S, Wetterslev J, Dahl JB: A qualitative systematic review of incisional local anaesthesia for postoperative pain relief after abdominal operations. *Br J Anaesth* 1998;81: 377-383.
81. Lang E, Erdmann K, Gerbershagen HU: High spinal anesthesia does not depress central nervous system function as measured by central conduction time and somatosensory evoked potentials. *Anesth Analg* 1990;71:176-180.
82. Wang JJ, Ho ST, Liu HS, et al: The effect of spinal versus general anesthesia on postoperative pain and analgesic requirements in patients undergoing lower abdominal surgery. *Reg Anesth* 1996;21:281-286.
83. Dakin MJ, Osinubi OY, Carli F: Preoperative spinal bupivacaine does not reduce postoperative morphine requirement in women undergoing total abdominal hysterectomy. *Reg Anesth* 1996;21:99-102.
84. Vaida SJ, Ben David B, Somri M, et al: The influence of preemptive spinal anesthesia on postoperative pain. *J Clin Anesth* 2000;12:374-377.
85. Carr DB, Cousins MJ: Spinal route of analgesia: Opioids and future options. In Cousins MJ, Bridenbaugh PO, editors: *Neural blockade in clinical anesthesia and management of pain.* New York, Lippincott-Raven, 1998, pp 915-983.
86. Jahangiri M, Jayatunga AP, Bradley JW, Dark CH: Prevention of phantom pain after major lower limb amputation by epidural infusion of diamorphine, clonidine and bupivacaine. *Ann R Coll Surg Engl* 1994;76:324-326.
87. Katz J, Kavanagh BP, Sandler AN, et al: Preemptive analgesia. Clinical evidence of neuroplasticity contributing to postoperative pain. *Anesthesiology* 1992;77:439-446.
88. Nègre I, Guéneron JP, Jamali SJ, et al: Preoperative analgesia with epidural morphine. *Anesth Analg* 1994;79:298-302.
89. Aida S, Baba H, Yamakura T, et al: The effectiveness of preemptive analgesia varies according to the type of surgery: A randomized, double-blind study. *Anesth Analg* 1999;89:711-716.
90. Dahl JB, Hansen BL, Hjortso NC, et al: Influence of timing on the effect of continuous extradural analgesia with bupivacaine and morphine after major abdominal surgery. *Br J Anaesth* 1992; 69:4-8.
91. Espinet A, Henderson DJ, Faccenda KA, Morrison LM: Does pre-incisional thoracic extradural block combined with diclofenac reduce postoperative pain after abdominal hysterectomy? *Br J Anaesth* 1996;76:209-213.
92. Katz J, Clairoux M, Kavanagh BP, et al: Pre-emptive lumbar epidural anaesthesia reduces postoperative pain and patient-controlled morphine consumption after lower abdominal surgery. *Pain* 1994;59:395-403.
93. Nakamura T, Yokoo H, Hamakawa T, Takasaki M: [Preemptive analgesia produced with epidural analgesia administered prior to surgery]. *Masui* 1994;43:1024-1028.

94. Norris EJ, Beattie C, Perler BA, et al: Double-masked randomized trial comparing alternate combinations of intraoperative anesthesia and postoperative analgesia in abdominal aortic surgery. *Anesthesiology* 2001;95:1054-1067.

95. Pryle BJ, Vanner RG, Enriquez N, Reynolds F: Can pre-emptive lumbar epidural blockade reduce postoperative pain following lower abdominal surgery? *Anaesthesia* 1993;48:120-123.

96. Richards JT, Read JR, Chambers WA: Epidural anaesthesia as a method of pre-emptive analgesia for abdominal hysterectomy. *Anaesthesia* 1998;53:296-298.

97. Rockemann MG, Seeling W, Pressler S, et al: Reduced postoperative analgesic demand after inhaled anesthesia in comparison to combined epidural-inhaled anesthesia in patients undergoing abdominal surgery. *Anesth Analg* 1997;84:600-605.

98. Rockemann MG, Seeling W, Bischof C, et al: Prophylactic use of epidural mepivacaine/morphine, systemic diclofenac, and metamizole reduces postoperative morphine consumption after major abdominal surgery. *Anesthesiology* 1996;84:1027-1034.

99. Sentürk M, Özcan PE, Talu GK, et al: The effects of three different analgesia techniques on long-term postthoracotomy pain. *Anesth Analg* 2002;94:11-15.

100. Shir Y, Raja SN, Frank SM: The effect of epidural versus general anesthesia on postoperative pain and analgesic requirements in patients undergoing radical prostatectomy. *Anesthesiology* 1994;80:49-56.

101. Obata H, Saito S, Fujita N, et al: Epidural block with mepivacaine before surgery reduces long-term post-thoracotomy pain. *Can J Anaesth* 1999;46:1127-1132.

102. Katz J, Cohen L, Schmid R, et al: Postoperative morphine use and hyperalgesia are reduced by preoperative but not intraoperative epidural analgesia: Implications for preemptive analgesia and the prevention of central sensitization. *Anesthesiology* 2003;98:1449-1460.

103. Katz J, Cohen L: Preventive analgesia is associated with reduced pain disability 3 weeks but not 6 months after major gynecologic surgery by laparotomy. *Anesthesiology* 2004;101:169-174.

104. Ochroch EA, Gottschalk A, Augostides J, et al: Long-term pain and activity during recovery from major thoracotomy using thoracic epidural analgesia. *Anesthesiology* 2002;97:1234-1244.

105. Nikolajsen L, Ilkjaer S, Christensen JH, et al: Randomised trial of epidural bupivacaine and morphine in prevention of stump and phantom pain in lower-limb amputation. *Lancet* 1997;350:1353-1357.

106. Katz J: Prevention of phantom limb pain by regional anaesthesia. *Lancet* 1997;349:519-520.

107. Akca O, Melischek M, Scheck T, et al: Postoperative pain and subcutaneous oxygen tension. *Lancet* 1999;354:41-42.

108. Kehlet H: Modification of responses to surgery by neural blockade: Clinical implications. In Cousins MJ, Bridenbaugh PO, editors: *Clinical anesthesia and management of pain.* New York, Lippincott-Raven, 1998, pp 129-175.

109. Yeager MP, Glass DD, Neff RK, Brinck-Johnsen T: Epidural anesthesia and analgesia in high-risk surgical patients. *Anesthesiology* 1987;66:729-736.

110. Liu S, Carpenter RL, Neal JM: Epidural anesthesia and analgesia. Their role in postoperative outcome. *Anesthesiology* 1995;82:1474-1506.

111. Williams-Russo P, Sharrock NE, Haas SB, et al: Randomized trial of epidural versus general anesthesia: Outcomes after primary total knee replacement. *Clin Orthop* 1996;199-208.

112. Rodgers A, Walker N, Schug S, et al: Reduction of postoperative mortality and morbidity with epidural or spinal anaesthesia: Results from overview of randomised trials. *BMJ* 2000;321:1493.

113. Carli F, Mayo N, Klubien K, et al: Epidural analgesia enhances functional exercise capacity and health-related quality of life after colonic surgery: Results of a randomized trial. *Anesthesiology* 2002;97:540-549.

114. Carr DB: Preempting the memory of pain. *JAMA* 1998;279:1114-1115.

115. Cousins MJ, Veering B: Epidural neural blockade. In Cousins MJ, Bridenbaugh PO, editors: *Neural blockade in clinical anesthesia and management of pain.* New York, Lippincott-Raven, 1998, pp 243-322.

116. Shibata K, Yamamoto Y, Murakami S: Effects of epidural anesthesia on cardiovascular response and survival in experimental hemorrhagic shock in dogs. *Anesthesiology* 1989;71:953-959.

117. Shibata K, Yamamoto Y, Kobayashi T, Murakami S: Beneficial effect of upper thoracic epidural anesthesia in experimental hemorrhagic shock in dogs: Influence of circulating catecholamines. *Anesthesiology* 1991;74:303-308.

Index

Note: Page numbers followed by '*f*' indicate figures, '*t*' indicate tables, and '*b*' indicate boxes.